NURSING

DIAGNOSIS &

INTERVENTION

Planning for Patient Care

NURSING
DIAGNOSIS &
INTERVENTION

Planning for Patient Care

Third Edition

Gertrude K. McFarland, DNSc, RN, FAAN

Health Scientist Administrator
Nursing Research Study Section
Division of research grants
National Institutes of Health
Bethesda, Maryland

Elizabeth A. McFarlane, DNSc, RN, FAAN

Associate Professor
School of Nursing
The Catholic University of America
Washington, D.C.

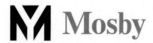 Mosby

St. Louis Baltimore Boston Carlsbad Chicago Naples
New York Philadelphia Portland London Madrid
Mexico City Singapore Sydney Tokyo Toronto Wiesbaden

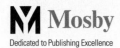

Mosby

Dedicated to Publishing Excellence

A Times Mirror Company

Vice President and Publisher: Nancy L. Coon
Editor: Loren S. Wilson
Developmental Editor: Brian Dennison
Project Manager: Carol Sullivan Weis
Production Editor: Florence Achenbach
Manuscript Editor: Hal Lockwood
Layout Artist: Myrna Vladic
Designer: Renée Duenow
Manufacturing Manager: Bill Winneberger
Cover Art: Jen Marmarinos

Third edition
Copyright © 1997 by Mosby–Year Book, Inc.

Previous editions copyrighted 1993, 1989

Printed in the United States of America

Composition by Penmarin Books
Printing/binding by R.R. Donnelley & Sons, Crawfordsville

Mosby–Year Book, Inc.
11830 Westline Industrial Drive
St. Louis, Missouri 63146

ISBN: 0-8151-7026-2

96 97 98 99 00 / 9 8 7 6 5 4 3 2 1

Contributors

NOLA M. BECKET, MS, RN

Nursing Quality Assurance Coordinator
University Hospital
Oregon Health Sciences University
Portland, Oregon

SISTER MARY ROSITA BRENNAN, CSSF, DNSc, RN

Chair, Department of Associate Nursing Program
Felician College
Lodi, New Jersey

HOWARD K. BUTCHER, PhD, RN, CS

Assistant Professor
School of Nursing
Pacific Lutheran University
Tacoma, Washington

SUSAN L. CARLSON, MSN, RN, CS

Director of Education
Baptist Medical Center
San Antonio, Texas

CLAIRE SHEINMAN COWAN, MSN, RN

Clinical Assistant Professor
Faculty of Nursing
University of Toronto
Toronto, Ontario
Canada

DOROTHY M. CRAIG, MScN, RN

Professor
Faculty of Nursing
University of Toronto
Toronto, Ontario
Canada

CAROLYN RUPPEL d'AVIS, MSN, RN

Director, Baccalaureate Program
School of Nursing
The Catholic University of America
Washington, D.C.

JACQUELINE DIENEMANN, PhD, RN, CNAA, FAAN

Associate Professor
School of Nursing
Johns Hopkins University
Baltimore, Maryland

JULIEANN DuBEAU, MSN, RN°

Regulatory Health Project Manager
Food and Drug Administration
Rockville, Maryland

CHRISTINE D. EHLERS, MSN, RN°

Commander, Navy Nurse Corps
Division Head
Ambulatory Procedures Department and
    Postanesthesia Care Unit
Portsmouth Naval Hospital
Portsmouth, Virginia

° The opinions expressed in chapters written by the contributors designated by an asterisk are those of the authors and do not necessarily reflect those of the National Institutes of Health or Food and Drug Administration, USPHS, U.S. Department of Health and Human Services; the Veterans Administration; or the Army, Navy or Department of Defense.

PHYLLIS A. ENFANTO, MS, RN

Nurse Coordinator
Pediatric and Adolescent Specialties
Beth Israel Hospital and Children's Hospital Medical
    Care Center
Lexington, Massachusetts

MARGARET I. FITCH, PhD, RN

Oncology Nurse Researcher and Head
Oncology Nursing
Toronto-Sunnybrook Regional Cancer Center
North York, Ontario
Canada
Assistant Professor
Faculty of Nursing
University of Toronto
Toronto, Ontario
Canada

CHERYL FORCHUK, PhD, RN

Nurse Scientist
Victoria Hospital
London, Ontario
Associate Professor
University of Western Ontario
London, Ontario
Canada

MARGIE L. FRENCH, MS, RN°

Clinical Manager, Comprehensive Rehabilitation Unit
Clinical Specialist, Gerontological Nursing
Veterans Administration Medical Center/Vancouver
    Division
Portland, Oregon

CHRISTINE M. GALANTE, PhD, RN°

Colonel, Army Nurse Corps
Deputy Chief of Staff for Regulatory Compliance
    and Quality
U.S. Army Medical Research and Materiel Command
Fort Detrick, Maryland

PATRICIA M. GARVER, DNSc, RN, CS

Assistant Professor
School of Nursing
University of San Diego
San Diego, California

LAUREL S. GARZON, DNSc, RN

Associate Professor
Old Dominion University
Norfolk, Virginia

ELIZABETH KELCHNER GERETY, MS, RN, CS, FAAN°

Clinical Nurse Specialist, Psychiatry
Psychiatry Consultation Service
Portland Veterans Affairs Medical Center
Portland, Oregon

LINDA D. GERSON, PhD, RN, CS-P

Nurse Psychotherapist
Ellicott City, Maryland

PAULINE McKINNEY GREEN, PhD, RN

Associate Professor
College of Nursing
Howard University
Washington, D.C.

JANICE C. HALLAL, DNSc, RN

Associate Professor
School of Nursing
The Catholic University of America
Washington, D.C.

KATHRYN VAN DYKE HAYES, DNSc, RN, C

Assistant Professor
Holy Family College
Philadelphia, Pennsylvania

JOAN HEATHER, MS, RN, CNA

Consultant
DBJ Enterprises
Portland, Oregon

LINDA K. HEITMAN, MSN, RN, CS

Clinical Nurse Specialist
Regional Heart Center Coordinator
Southeast Missouri Hospital
Cape Girardeau, Missouri

KAYE A. HERTH, PhD, RN, FAAN

Chair and Professor
Department of Nursing
Georgia Southern University
Statesboro, Georgia

KAREN E. INABA, MS, RN, CS

Psychiatric Mental Health Nurse Practitioner
Corrections Health
Multnomah County Health Department
Portland, Oregon

MAUREEN A. KNIPPEN, DNSc, RN*

Consumer Safety Officer
Food and Drug Administration
Center for Biologics Evaluation and Research
Rockville, Maryland

CANDICE S. KORB, MS, RN

Staff Nurse
Cross Country Health Care
Boca Raton, Florida

CAROL E. KUPPERBERG, MSN, RN

Nurse Coordinator
Montgomery County Infants and Toddlers Program
Rockville, Maryland

LORNA A. LARSON, DNSc, RN

Mental Health Home-Visiting Nurse
Adventist Home Health Services, Inc.
Southern Maryland Office
Waldorf, Maryland

PRISCILLA LeMONE, DSN, RN

Assistant Professor
Sinclair School of Nursing
University of Missouri-Columbia
Columbia, Missouri

MARGARET LUNNEY, PhD, RN, CS

Professor
Hunter-Bellevue School of Nursing
Hunter College of the City University of New York
New York, New York

SISTER JUDITH MARONI, CSJ, DNSc, RN, CS

Associate Professor
Carlow College
Pittsburgh, Pennsylvania

ANGELA M. MARTINELLI, DNSc, RN, CNOR

Postdoctoral Fellow
School of Nursing
University of Michigan
Ann Arbor, Michigan

GERTRUDE K. McFARLAND, DNSc, RN, FAAN*

Health Scientist Administrator
Nursing Research Study Section
Division of Research Grants
National Institutes of Health
Bethesda, Maryland

ELIZABETH A. McFARLANE, DNSc, RN, FAAN

Associate Professor
School of Nursing
The Catholic University of America
Washington, D.C.

MARGARET J. McGOVERN, MScN, RN

Assistant Professor
Faculty of Nursing
University of Toronto
Toronto, Ontario
Canada

KAREN A. McWHORTER, MN, RN, CS*

Clinical Nurse Specialist
Adult Day Health Care
Veterans Administration Medical Center/Vancouver
    Division
Portland, Oregon

VICTORIA L. MOCK, DNSc, RN

Director of Oncology Nursing Research
Johns Hopkins Oncology Center
Johns Hopkins Hospital
Baltimore, Maryland

MARTHA M. MORRIS, EdD, RN

Associate Professor
School of Nursing
St. Louis University
St. Louis, Missouri

GLORIA J. MORRISON, MSN Candidate, ARNP

Pacific Lutheran University
Tacoma, Washington
Nurse Practitioner
Providence General Sexual Assault Center
Everett, Washington

M. ELETTA MORSE, MSN, RN, GNPC

Geriatric Nurse Practitioner
Washington Hospital Center
Washington, D.C.

TYE R.-B. MULLIKIN, MSN, RN, CETN°

Clinical Nurse IV, Oncology
Clinical Center
National Institutes of Health
Bethesda, Maryland

CHARLOTTE E. NASCHINSKI, MS, RN°

Deputy Director
Continuing Education for Health Professionals
Uniformed Services University of the Health Sciences
Bethesda, Maryland

JOYCE NEUMANN, MS, RN, OCN

Clinical Nurse Specialist
Bone Marrow Transplant Unit
University of Texas
MD Anderson Cancer Center
Houston, Texas

COLLEEN K. NORTON, MSN, RN, CCRN

Doctoral Candidate
School of Nursing
The Catholic University of America
Washington, D.C.
Clinical Assistant Professor
School of Nursing
Georgetown University
Washington, D.C.

LINDA O'BRIEN-PALLAS, PhD, RN

Associate Professor and Career Scientist
Director, Quality of Worklife Research Unit
Faculty of Nursing
University of Toronto
Toronto, Ontario
Canada

ANNETTE M. O'CONNOR, PhD, RN

Associate Professor
School of Nursing
University of Ottawa
Ottawa, Ontario
Canada

SALLY PICKETT, MS, RN, CCRN, CS

Principal
Cynosure International
Ipswich, Massachusetts

BARBARA E. POKORNY, MSN, RN, CS

Family Nurse Practitioner
Community Health Center
New London, Connecticut

M. GAIE RUBENFELD, MS, RN

Associate Professor
Department of Nursing Education
Eastern Michigan University
Ypsilanti, Michigan

ANDREA BOURQUIN RYAN, MSN, RN, CRRN

Clinical Nurse Specialist
National Rehabilitation Hospital at Washington
   Hospital Center
Washington, D.C.

SISTER MARIA SALERNO, OSF, DNSc, RNCS, NP

Associate Professor
School of Nursing
The Catholic University of America
Washington, D.C.

ROSEMARIE F. DiMAURO SATYSHUR, DNSc, RN

Assistant Professor
School of Nursing
The Catholic University of America
Washington, D.C.

MARY ANN KADOW SCHROEDER, DNSc, RN, CS

Associate Professor
School of Nursing
The Catholic University of America
Washington, D.C.

CAROLE A. SHEA, PhD, RN, CS

Director, Graduate School of Nursing
Northeastern University
Boston, Massachusetts

SISTER MAURITA SOUKUP, RSM, DNSc, RN, CCRN

Director
The Center for Advanced Nursing Practice
Bryan Memorial Hospital
Lincoln, Nebraska

KAREN A. STEVENS, PhD, RN, FNP

Graduate Coordinator
Department of Nursing
Bowie State University
Bowie, Maryland

SYLVIA RAE STEVENS, MS, RN, CS

Adjunct Assistant Professor
School of Nursing
The Catholic University of America
Washington, D.C.
Private Practice, Psychotherapy
Washington, D.C.

BARBARA L. STRUNK, BSN, AB, CETN

Wound Care Clinical Nurse Specialist
Kaiser Permanente
Portland, Oregon

JANICE M. THAPE, MSN, RNC

Neonatal Clinical Specialist
Columbia Hospital for Women
Washington, D.C.

SISTER LINDA THIEL, OP, MS, RN, CFNP

Doctoral Candidate
School of Nursing
The Catholic University of America
Washington, D.C.

ANNA MAE TICHY, EdD, RN

Director of Nursing
Associate Degree Nursing Program
Mt. Hood Community College
Gresham, Oregon

JEAN O. TROTTER, MS, RN, C

Instructor
School of Nursing
Johns Hopkins University
Baltimore, Maryland

JOAN C. VELOS, MSN, CRNP

Doctoral Candidate and Lecturer
School of Nursing
University of Pennsylvania
Philadelphia, Pennsylvania

KAREN WADE, MScN, RN

Clinical Nurse Specialist
North York Public Health Department
North York, Ontario
Canada

ELEANOR A. WALKER, PhD, RNC

Chair, Department of Nursing
Bowie State University
Bowie, Maryland

THOMAS WALSH, MN, ARNP

Program Manager
Behavioral Health Services
Valley Medical Center
Renton, Washington

BENITA WALTON-MOSS, DNS, RNCS, FNP

Assistant Professor
School of Nursing
The Catholic University of America
Washington, D.C.

EVELYN L. WASLI, DNSc, RN

Chief Nurse
Emergency Psychiatric Response Division
D.C. Community Mental Health Service
Washington, D.C.

JUDITH H. WATT-WATSON, MScN, RN

Clinical Associate Professor
Faculty of Nursing
University of Toronto
Toronto, Ontario
Canada

JANET R. WEBER, EdD, MSN, RN

Associate Professor
Department of Nursing
Southeast Missouri State University
Cape Girardeau, Missouri

LINDA K. WEINBERG, MSN, RN, CRRN, CNA

Director
Home Health, Hospice, and Life Care
Anne Arundel Medical Center
Annapolis, Maryland

TO

**ALL PROFESSIONAL NURSES AND
NURSING STUDENTS**

who use and test
nursing diagnoses in practice

Preface

Nurses engaged in contemporary practice use the nursing process in their delivery of care. The nursing process is a problem-solving process that includes the following phases: (1) assessing; (2) diagnosing; (3) identifying expected patient outcomes; (4) planning; (5) implementing; and (6) evaluating. The work of the North American Nursing Diagnosis Association (NANDA) has done much to stimulate developments in nursing diagnosis, particularly as it relates to assessment, outcome identification, and selection of appropriate interventions.

This book provides comprehensive information that will enhance the understanding of all currently accepted NANDA diagnoses. Chapter 1 presents an overview of evolving issues and trends that have implications for the delivery of nursing care to communities, groups, families, and individuals, and consequently for nursing diagnosis. The development of NANDA'S diagnostic taxonomy is discussed, and competing taxonomic structures linking diagnoses to interventions and outcomes are presented.

Nursing diagnosis as an essential phase of the nursing process and a critical element of the Functional Health Patterns is described in Chapter 2. The 11 Functional Health Patterns serve as an organizing framework for categorizing all NANDA diagnoses that are presented in this book. The 11 patterns include Health-Perception—Health-Management Pattern, Nutritional-Metabolic Pattern, Elimination Pattern, Activity-Exercise Pattern, Sleep-Rest Pattern, Cognitive-Perceptual Pattern, Self-Perception—Self-Concept Pattern, Role-Relationship Pattern, Sexuality-Reproductive Pat-

tern, Coping—Stress-Tolerance Pattern, and Value-Belief Pattern. The relative ease with which nurses can understand this framework and apply it in a variety of settings has prompted its use in classifying the nursing diagnoses.

Comprehensive content is presented on each nursing diagnosis and cluster of diagnoses, including:

1. A definition that incorporates the accepted NANDA definition
2. An overview that integrates theory and research findings and that includes developmental, family, community, and cultural considerations
3. An assessment section that includes assessment strategies and guidelines relevant to the identification of defining characteristics and related factors for actual diagnoses and risk factors for risk diagnoses
4. A diagnosis section that differentiates the diagnosis being addressed from other nursing diagnoses and that addresses medical and psychiatric diagnoses that are commonly related to the nursing diagnosis
5. A description of outcome identification, planning, and implementation focusing on the interventions that must be planned to achieve specified patient outcomes
6. Nursing Care Guidelines that provide a generic plan of care for each diagnosis being addressed, including expected patient outcomes, interventions to achieve each outcome, and rationales for the interventions.
7. An evaluation section that addresses achievement of the expected patient outcomes

8. A case study with a plan of care that provides an example for individualizing care for patients with a particular nursing diagnosis
9. Critical thinking exercises that can assist the reader in analyzing and synthesizing content presented for each diagnosis or cluster of diagnoses

This book will assist nurses and nursing students in (1) conducting a comprehensive assessment, (2) formulating a nursing diagnosis, (3) identifying realistic patient outcomes, (4) implementing an outcome-directed plan of care, and (5) evaluating the effectiveness of the nursing care. It is hoped that the book will encourage nurses to contribute to the ongoing development and classification of nursing diagnoses.

NEW TO THIS EDITION

To present the most recent information on the development and application of nursing diagnoses, the following additions and revisions have been made to this edition:

- All new and revised nursing diagnoses approved by NANDA are included to provide the most up-to-date information.
- Nursing Interventions Classification (NIC) and Nursing-Sensitive Outcomes Classification (NOC) are discussed in relation to NANDA diagnoses, and pertinent NIC and NOC materials are presented in the appendixes.
- A section for each diagnosis or cluster of diagnoses on differential nursing diagnosis helps the reader discriminate between closely related diagnoses.
- Outcome identification is emphasized in the out-

come identification, planning, and implementation sections and in the Nursing Care Guidelines to demonstrate how the plan of care is derived from the nursing diagnosis.
- Collaborative interventions are distinguished from nursing interventions in the Nursing Care Guidelines (generic care plans) to indicate those interventions performed by nurses in conjunction with other health care providers.
- Rationales for nursing interventions are included in the Nursing Care Guidelines where appropriate to explain the basis of nursing actions.
- Critical thinking exercises for each diagnosis or cluster of diagnoses related to the case study with plan of care help the reader comprehend how nursing diagnoses apply to specific situations.

ACKNOWLEDGMENTS

We are grateful to our many nurse colleagues and nursing students who continue to stimulate our thinking about the development and application of nursing science, particularly nursing diagnosis. Sincere appreciation is extended to our many contributors, who are experts in using nursing diagnoses in practice. To our husbands, Al McFarland and Tom McFarlane, we are thankful for their continuing support, tolerance, and patience during this project. Finally our gratitude is extended to the Mosby staff, including Loren Wilson, Editor, and Brian Dennison, Developmental Editor, for their encouragement, support, and skills.

GERTRUDE K. MCFARLAND
ELIZABETH A. MCFARLANE

Contents

NURSING
DIAGNOSIS &
INTERVENTION

Planning for Patient Care

Nursing Diagnosis: Evolving Issues and Trends

During the first half of the 1990s, the focus of health care in the United States changed from an illness-oriented model to a wellness model. Terms such as *health promotion, disease prevention, managed care,* and *continuous quality improvement* have become commonplace in the health care literature. The health care delivery system has shifted from a system in which escalating costs were viewed as necessary to combat disease and illness to a system in which costs are to be reduced while quality and access are to be improved.

PARADIGM SHIFT

Health care consumers and providers alike have struggled to grasp the nature of the rapidly changing and evolving health care delivery system. Efforts to identify consequences that the evolving system has for the recipients and the providers of care have been frustrated by fear that the changes will not meet the personal or professional needs of either group. Although the frustrations may continue, a concerted effort is being made to reform a once fragmented system of health care into a system that will meet the health care needs of all people in the United States.

Healthy People 2000

The publication of *Healthy People 2000: National Health Promotion and Disease Prevention Objectives*[33] in 1990 provided a landmark document that offered support to those who had identified the need for health care reform. Because the federal government facilitated its development, the document is seen as having far-reaching implications. It is of interest to note that the document builds on two previous federal publications: *Healthy People: The Surgeon General's Report on Health Promotion and Disease Prevention,* published in 1979, and *Promoting Health/Preventing Disease: Objec-*

tives for the Nation, published in 1980. The latter document initiated and established the nation's health promotion and disease prevention objectives to be achieved by 1990.

Healthy People 2000 specifically addresses three broad public health goals for the 1990s: (1) increasing the span of healthy life for Americans; (2) reducing health disparities among Americans; and (3) achieving access to preventive services for all Americans. The health promotion and disease prevention objectives (measurable targets) have been organized into 22 priority areas; 21 of these areas are grouped into three categories: health promotion, health protection, and preventive services. The priority areas incorporate objectives that address the health care needs of children, adolescents and young adults, adults, and older adults. A fourth category addressing the last priority area, surveillance and data systems, was established to monitor progress toward stated targets and to assure the integrity of data collection efforts at every level.

After reviewing *Healthy People 2000,* it becomes apparent that health care reform has been stimulated by the report. Attention is being directed to providing accessible care of high quality to improve the health of population groups that are at the highest risk for premature death, disease, or disability.[33] These groups include people with low income, people who are members of racial or ethnic minorities, and people with disabilities. The focus of federal funding for health-related demonstration and research projects also has been influenced by the report. It is expected that such projects will include priority areas and address high-risk groups.

The issues of cost containment and the need to assure quality care and access to health care services focusing on health promotion and disease prevention have changed the environment of health care. The settings in which health care is provided have shifted. Hospital-based care is on the decline, and community-based care settings are rapidly increasing. This shift can be seen in the growing number of community-based clinics and care centers. Urgent care and primary care clinics are appearing in most cities and suburban areas, often in local shopping centers, which makes them more accessible. Home health care agencies are increasing, and many hospitals, to compensate for the decrease in bed utilization, have joined the home care business.

Nursing's Social Policy Statement

Nursing, like other health care professions, is evolving to meet the demands of the changing health care environment. *Nursing: A Social Policy Statement,* published in 1980 by the American Nurses' Association (ANA), presented a definition of *nursing:* "Nursing is the diagnosis and treatment of human responses to actual or potential health problems."[3] The definition reflects four defining characteristics of nursing: (1) *phenomena* of which nurses should be aware (i.e., human responses to actual or potential health problems); (2) *theory,* which is used to enhance an understanding of the phenomena of concern to nurses; (3) *actions,* which are taken to ameliorate, improve, or correct conditions or to prevent illness and promote health; and (4) *effects* that occur because of nursing actions and relate to the identifiable human responses.

In 1995 the ANA published a revision of the work done 15 years earlier entitled *Nursing's Social Policy Statement.*[4] Rather than offering a single definition of nursing, this document includes the 1980 definition along with the definitions of Florence Nightingale and Virginia Henderson. These definitions are provided as an attempt to "illustrate the consistent orientation of nurses to the provision of care that promotes well-being in the people being served."[4]

The importance of theory and research to the knowledge base for nursing practice, which is highlighted in this latest version of *Nursing's Social Policy Statement,* becomes apparent when examining the interrelationship of the phases of the nursing process. Analysis of objective and subjective data related to the phenomena of concern (*assessment*) leads to clinical judgments (*diagnoses* and *outcome identification*); theoretical, practical, and scientific knowledge about the relationships between potential interventions and desired outcomes provide the basis for planning *interventions;* and examination of the effectiveness of the interventions in terms of outcome attainment is the basis for *evaluation.*

The importance of the role of the nursing process in the provision of professional nursing care has received further support from the ANA through the development and publication of standards that provide direction for professional nursing practice. The outcome of the ANA's most recent efforts was published in December 1991 as *Standards of Clinical Nursing Practice.*[2] The publication presents two sets of standards: (1) standards of care that describe "a competent level of nursing care as demonstrated by the nursing process, involving assessment, diagnosis, outcome identification, planning, implementation, and evaluation" and (2) standards of professional performance that describe "a competent level of behavior in the professional role, including activities related to quality of care, performance appraisal, education, collegiality, ethics, collaboration, research, and resource utilization." Both sets of standards include criteria by which each identified standard is measured.

The relationship among the characteristics of nursing, the nursing process, and the Standards of Care is shown in Figure 1. Diagnosis culminates the assessment phase of the process, and provides the impetus for outcome identification. Outcome identification in turn is the pivotal link between the diagnosis phase and planning, implementing, and evaluating interventions.

Interdisciplinary Collaboration

It is nursing's phenomenon of concern that provides the nursing perspective when implementing the phases of the "process." Other health care providers approach the patient from different per-

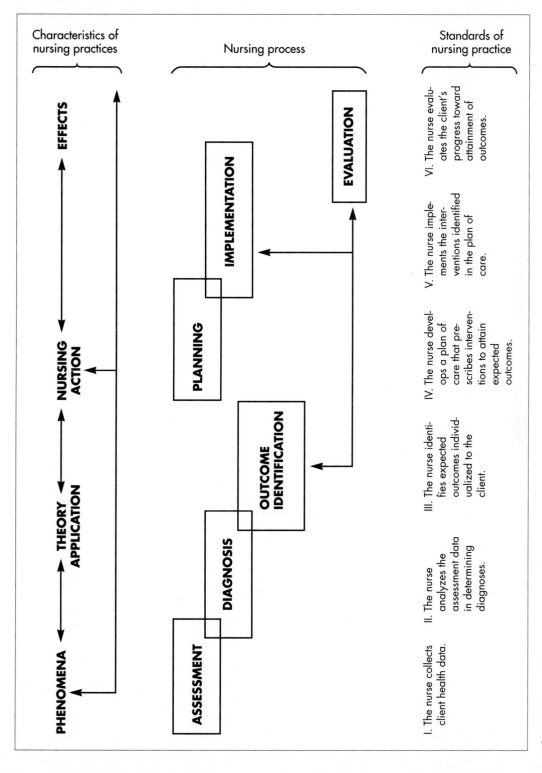

Figure 1 Relationship among defining characteristics of nursing practice, the nursing process, and the standards of clinical practice. Adapted from *Nursing: a social policy statement*, Kansas City, Missouri, 1980, and *American Nurses' Association and Standards of Clinical Practice*, Kansas City, Missouri, 1991, American Nurses' Association.

spectives; yet their approaches are also centered around assessment, diagnosis, outcome identification, planning, intervention, and evaluation. The variation in perspective of different health care providers makes collaborative care essential in terms of the patient's holistic nature. To assure appropriate collaboration, educational programs must socialize future health care providers into roles that support and are supported by interdisciplinary collaboration.[20]

A collaborative approach provides assurance that one's discipline perspective will not be emphasized more than another's. For example, a patient with the nursing diagnosis Risk for Activity Intolerance may also have a medical diagnosis of coronary artery disease. The two diagnoses require a team approach in managing the patient's care. A nurse, a physician, a physical therapist, a dietitian, and a clinical pharmacist could comprise the team. Each member would identify the patient's strengths and limitations (diagnosis) based on an assessment, and recommend outcomes and interventions. Such an approach is most supportive of health promotion and illness prevention for patients at any point on the wellness-illness continuum.

Scope of Nursing Practice

Traditionally the differentiation among the roles a nurse could assume was relatively simple. Roles were categorized into four major groups: practitioner, a general role indicating that the nurse provided patient care; nurse manager, usually referring to a middle management role; nurse educator, indicating a primary role of teaching students in a school of nursing or other nurses in an employment setting; and nurse researcher, referring to the nurse's active involvement in research projects.

The changing nature of health care delivery has shifted and expanded the traditional nursing roles. The ANA describes the scope of nursing practice in terms of educational preparation, experience, roles, and the nature of the patient population served.[4] Such a description supports the concept of collaborative practice, which involves shared functions among health care providers with a focus

on a common goal. A further distinction in nursing practice is made based on preparation, namely, for basic nursing practice or advanced nursing practice. This includes registered nurses educated for the basic or entry level of practice. Experience and continuing education may provide opportunities to "specialize" in a particular area of practice.

Advanced nursing practice requires education at an advanced level (a master's degree), experience, and certification in an area of specialization. The term is used to refer to clinical nurse specialists, nurse practitioners, nurse midwives, and nurse anesthetists. These advanced practice nursing roles have clouded the distinction between the traditional responsibilities of the nurse and the physician. Although nurse educators, administrators, and researchers may hold master's or doctoral degrees, they are not considered to be advanced practice registered nurses unless they are prepared and certified in an advanced clinical practice area.

Further changes in nursing roles may occur as a result of the report of the Pew Health Professions Commission, *Critical Challenges: Revitalizing the Health Professions for the Twenty-First Century*.[29] The commission addresses the effect that emerging systems of integrated care will have on the nation's 10 million health care workers.

Recommendations include preparing the next generation of professionals to practice in settings that will be more intensely managed and integrated, forming partnerships between professional schools and managed care, and incorporating interdisciplinary content in curricula. Recommendations specific to nursing include expanding the number of nurse practitioner programs at the master's degree level and distinguishing between practice responsibilities of nurses with different levels of basic nursing education. Many nursing schools are attempting to incorporate the recommendations of the Pew Commission and to restructure curricula to prepare nurses for practice in the future.[12,24,34]

Professional nursing must be proactive in developing models for practice and work force strategies that complement the changing nature of health care.[1,8,35] Regardless of the level or area of practice, nurses will be working closely with other health care professionals in the new arena of health care services. Therefore nursing must direct its attention to defining terms, standardizing terminology, and developing classification systems in ways that support collaborative care.

IMPLICATIONS FOR NURSING DIAGNOSIS

The term *nursing diagnosis* provides nurses with an accurate description of a critical nursing activity. The North American Nursing Diagnosis Association (NANDA) defines *nursing diagnosis* as a "clinical judgment about individual, family, or community responses to actual or potential health problems/life processes. Nursing diagnoses provide the basis for selection of nursing intervention to achieve outcomes for which the nurse is accountable."[6] The ANA offers an explicit definition of nursing diagnosis in *Standards of Clinical Practice: Nursing diagnosis* is "a clinical judgment about the client's response to actual or potential health conditions or needs."[2] The term is also the focus of Standard II, which is entitled "Diagnosis" and which states that "the nurse analyzes the assessment data in determining diagnoses." The importance of nursing diagnosis is further emphasized in Standard III, which focuses on outcome identification and includes a measurement criterion stating that "outcomes are derived from the diagnoses."

Classification System for Nursing Diagnosis

Although a definition of nursing diagnosis was not offered by NANDA until 1990 at the Ninth Conference for the Classification of Nursing Diagnoses, work on labeling and classifying diagnoses actually began in 1973.[10] Nurses recognized the need for a taxonomic system that would provide a frame of reference for nursing diagnoses, and efforts to create such a classification system were initiated. One hundred interested nurses participated in the First National Conference on Classification of Nursing Diagnoses.[10] The purpose of the conference was "to initiate the process of

preparing an organized, logical, comprehensive system for classifying those health problems or health states diagnosed by nurses and treated by means of nursing intervention." In essence, work had begun to make communication among health care professionals supportive of what is now known as collaborative practice. Although several classification systems had been discussed at the first conference, none was selected for use. At the conclusion of the conference, the participants realized that the development of a system for classifying nursing diagnoses and the process for identifying diagnostic labels was just beginning. One hundred nursing diagnoses were proposed and described at the conference, but no attempt was made to categorize these. However, participants agreed that such efforts would continue at subsequent conferences.

Significant progress occurred in the 17 months between the First and Second Conferences. The Clearinghouse–National Group for Classification of Nursing Diagnoses was established at St. Louis University School of Nursing, and plans to publish a newsletter were made. The Clearinghouse assumed responsibility for coordinating data collection for a project that would "accumulate data on nursing diagnoses identified on a wide range of patients in many nursing care organizations across the country."[9] These data were analyzed and used to evaluate the diagnoses identified at the First National Conference and to identify more diagnoses.

In March 1975, 119 nurses who represented nursing practice, education, and research convened for the Second National Conference on Classification of Nursing Diagnoses in St. Louis, Missouri. Three conference objectives were established:[9]

1. To consider further issues relevant to the development of nomenclature and taxonomy of those health conditions diagnosed by nurses.
2. To revise or evaluate those diagnoses identified at the First National Conference on Classification of Nursing Diagnoses.
3. To identify and describe additional diagnoses.

Although information was shared about the process of taxonomic development, many issues related to the introduction of a taxonomic system remained unsolved.

Those attending the Second Conference did make progress in the areas of evaluation of the diagnoses identified at the First Conference and identification of new diagnoses. Thirty-seven diagnostic labels or categories were accepted at the Second Conference. It should be noted that acceptance was relative to particular diagnostic concepts. Nurses were cautioned that the approved labels with their defining characteristics were neither exhaustive nor mutually exclusive. In essence, specific diagnostic labels with defining characteristics were accepted with the recognition that further data were needed to substantiate and support the validity of the diagnostic labels or categories. The participants at the conference identified an additional 19 labels that were recommended for consideration at future conferences.

Considerable progress toward the development of a system of classification of nursing diagnoses occurred at the Third and Fourth National Conferences,[19] which were held in 1978 and 1980. At the Third Conference, 14 nurse theorists met for the purpose of reaching consensus on a framework to place diagnostic terms into a taxonomy. After the theorists' initial efforts, three clinical specialists worked with the theorists at the Fourth Conference, and conscientious efforts were made to integrate the views of practitioners into the nurse theorists' framework. Participants at the Third and Fourth Conferences witnessed the maturing of the nursing diagnosis movement. The conference agenda included the presentation of papers that reflected theoretical and practical perspectives on the classification and use of nursing diagnoses. Five research papers on the development and use of nursing diagnoses were presented at each of the two conferences.

Concurrent with the contributions that resulted from the conferences, the nursing literature of the 1970s reflected the growing acceptance of the term *nursing diagnosis* and the increased application of nursing diagnosis in clinical practice and education. Journal articles increased in frequency, and books addressing a theoretical and practical knowledge base were published. This growing acceptance and interest indicated that support existed for a professional organization committed to the development of a diagnostic taxonomy.

Ongoing Efforts in Taxonomy Development

The formal organization of the North American Nursing Diagnosis Association (NANDA) was presented to the participants at the Fifth National Conference on Classification of Nursing Diagnoses in April 1982, and the bylaws were accepted by the members later that year. The purpose of the association, as described in the bylaws, is "to develop, refine, and promote a taxonomy of nursing diagnostic terminology of general use to professional nurses."[17]

The Fifth Conference also provided a forum for the presentation of the outcome of work done by the nurse theorists since the previous conference. A diagnostic framework that identified the health of unitary man/human as the phenomenon of concern to nursing was presented to the participants. Nine interactional patterns were proposed as concepts inherent to the diagnostic framework. These patterns, described at the Sixth Conference as patterns of unitary persons, were renamed the nine central human response patterns at the Seventh Conference.

The Sixth and Seventh Conferences convened in 1984 and 1986, respectively. The proceedings from the two conferences[13, 23] documented the ongoing development of a taxonomy and presented research studies on the identification and validation of nursing diagnoses. The foundational work for the emerging taxonomy was presented at the Sixth Conference, and Taxonomy I was presented at the Seventh Conference with subsequent approval by NANDA members. The effect of nursing diagnosis on clinical practice and education can be seen in the breadth of issues related to nursing diagnosis that were addressed at the conferences: diagnosis-related groups (DRGs), cost reimbursement, quality assurance, clinical competence, and computerization. Although no new diagnoses were presented at the Sixth Conference, 22 diagnoses were presented at the Seventh Conference. The members of NANDA accepted 21 of these, which were added to the list of diagnostic categories that had been developed and refined through the previous conferences.

The list of diagnoses was expanded further in 1988. Fifteen new diagnoses and two recommendations for revisions of diagnoses accepted at earlier conferences were presented at the Eighth Conference on Classification of Nursing Diagnoses.[5] All but one of the proposed new diagnoses were accepted by the members of NANDA. The need to continue work on Taxonomy I was evident at the Eighth Conference, and minor revisions were made, resulting in Taxonomy I, Revised.

The Ninth Conference on Classification of Nursing Diagnoses convened in 1990.[6] Two new nursing diagnoses were presented at the conference; both were accepted by NANDA members after the conference, bringing the total of diagnostic labels that have been approved for clinical use and testing to 100. Of special interest to those in attendance were two major topics: (1) the work of the Diagnosis Review Committee and the NANDA board of directors on developing a working definition of nursing diagnosis, clarification of terms used in relation to nursing diagnoses, and refinement of the nursing diagnosis submission guidelines and diagnostic review process; and (2) the work of the Taxonomy Committee on the development of Taxonomy II and the submission to the International Classification of Diseases, Tenth Edition (ICD-10) of "Conditions that Necessitate Nursing Care."

Work done during and between the Tenth and Eleventh Conferences focused on attempts to resolve several issues affecting the further development and refinement of the taxonomic system. Ten new diagnoses were approved at the Tenth Conference on Classification of Nursing Diagnoses[17] convened in 1992 in San Diego. Although the presentation of Taxonomy II was anticipated, no substantial progress was made beyond that which was presented at the ninth conference. A revision of Taxonomy I, Revised, 1992, incorporated the newly approved diagnoses and was published in the proceedings of the conference.[7]

The Eleventh Conference on Classification of Nursing Diagnoses, held in Nashville in 1994, focused on advancing professional practice with nursing diagnosis.[30] Participants struggled with taxonomic issues that seemed both frustrating and exciting. Jean Jenny's presentation on "Advancing the Science of Nursing" drew attention and support as she suggested that a new organizing structure be explored.[16] No new diagnoses were approved at the Eleventh Conference, but a new process for the submission and staging of diagnoses in the taxonomy was announced.[25]

Later in 1994, NANDA's board of directors incorporated 19 new diagnoses into the taxonomy,[26] resulting in a total of 129 diagnostic labels approved for clinical use and testing. NANDA's publication, *Nursing Diagnoses: Definitions and Classification, 1995–1996*,[28] presents the taxonomy with the new diagnoses incorporated (see Appendix A) as well as the definitions, defining characteristics, risk factors, and related factors for the approved diagnoses.

A frequent criticism of the NANDA taxonomy is that it lacks a conceptual link to practice. Whether or not the taxonomy will remain an independent entity remains to be seen. Late in 1994 NANDA initiated collaborative efforts with the Nursing Diagnosis Extension and Classification (NDEC) research team. The NDEC team has set as its goals to "(1) validate existing NANDA diagnoses, labels, etiologies, and defining characteristics that have not been validated; (2) identify and develop additional diagnoses from a broad database of diagnoses and problems in the literature, care plans, and nursing information system databases; and (3) work collaboratively with NANDA to develop a taxonomy inductively.[26]

Many nurses have expressed concern over NANDA diagnostic terminology, feeling it is cumbersome and not consistent with terminology used by other nurses and care providers. NANDA was represented on the ANA Steering Committee on Databases to Support Clinical Nursing Practice

(ANASCD), which reviewed nursing concepts to be included in the 1995 version of the Unified Medical Language System (UMLS).[27] This work, along with collaboration with NDEC, should prompt revisions and standardization of language that result in clearer communication of concepts among nurses and other health care providers.

Nursing diagnosis as the keystone to the development of a unified nursing language was the focus of the Twelfth Conference on the Classification of Nursing Diagnoses, held in Pittsburgh in April 1996. The conference provided a forum for identifying and discussing the role of nursing diagnosis as the nursing profession works toward a unified language. Although no new nursing diagnoses were presented, NANDA's Diagnosis Review Committee (DRC) reported that work had begun on (1) staging the 129 diagnoses currently approved for clinical use and testing, (2) revision of the staging criteria, and (3) revision of the process for submission and revision of diagnoses. During the summer of 1996 a diagnosis was approved by the DRC, bringing the number of approved diagnoses to 130. NANDA's continued collaboration with NDEC and ANASCD should support development of a nursing diagnosis taxonomy that is conceptually linked to practice and that reflects user-friendly terminology.

Linking Diagnoses with Interventions

Attempts at developing a diagnostic classification system have not been limited to the work done through the Conferences on the Classification of Nursing Diagnoses. Several proponents of nursing diagnosis have identified the need to develop taxonomic structures that link diagnoses with interventions, therefore making them more meaningful to practicing nurses.

One of the most notable of these systems for the categorization of nursing diagnoses is the Functional Health Patterns proposed by Marjory Gordon.[11] These 11 patterns provide a structure for assessment, that is, the initial and continued health status evaluation of a person, family, or community. In addition to supporting a deliberative and systematic assessment, the Functional

Health Patterns have been described as having the following advantages:

1. Not having to be continually relearned (application is expanded as clinical knowledge accumulates)
2. Leading directly to nursing diagnosis
3. Encompassing a holistic approach to human functional assessment in any setting and with any age group at any point in the health-illness continuum.[11]

The relative ease with which the nurse can understand this framework and apply it in a variety of settings has promoted its acceptance as a valuable guide for assessment and for planning care. Appendix B presents the categories of NANDA-accepted nursing diagnoses according to Gordon's Functional Health Patterns.

A second organizing framework, which is particularly useful to nurses practicing in community health settings, is the classification scheme developed and used by the Visiting Nurse Association of Omaha.[21] This classification scheme focuses on nursing problems (or nursing diagnoses) and has three basic components: a problem classification scheme, a problem rating scale for outcomes, and an intervention scheme. The problems are divided into the four domains representative of community health nursing practice: environmental, psychosocial, physiological, and health behaviors. Use of the classification scheme has positively influenced the agency's orientation plan, clinical records, computerized management information system, and quality assurance program.

Saba's Home Health Care Classification (HHCC)[31, 32] and Coding Scheme includes nursing diagnoses and interventions. The HHCC grew out of an effort to develop a classification of home health Medicare patients that would assist in predicting the need for nursing and other home health care services. Saba surveyed 646 home health care agencies; the agencies collected data on the entire episode of home health care of 8961 study patients. Twenty Home Health Care Components were developed that served as a framework for the classification and coding of nursing diagnoses, patient problems, and 4 nursing interventions. The resulting nursing diagnosis classification scheme consists of 145 nursing diagnoses, 3 nursing diagnosis modifiers, 160 unique nursing interventions, and 4 nursing intervention modifiers. Saba's Home Health Care Classification (HHCC) and Coding Scheme is presented in Appendix C.

Efforts to develop classification systems of patient outcomes and nursing interventions are also under way. Worthy of note are two major research projects, both funded through the National Institute of Nursing Research (NINR): the Nursing-Sensitive Outcomes Classification (NOC) project and the Nursing Interventions Classification (NIC) project. Both projects have implications in terms of language and classification and the use of nursing diagnoses.

The identification of expected patient outcomes creates the critical link between a nursing diagnosis and the selection of appropriate nursing interventions. Outcomes should be identified that, if achieved, eliminate or contribute to the elimination of the etiology of the diagnosis. The purpose of the Nursing-Sensitive Outcomes Classification project is to "(1) identify, label, validate, and classify nursing-sensitive patient outcomes and indicators, (2) evaluate the validity and usefulness of the classification in clinical field testing, and (3) define and test measurement procedures for the outcomes and indicators."[17] It is anticipated that the NOC project will provide a standardized language and measurement for patient outcomes, thus allowing "nurses to compare outcomes for large numbers of patients across settings, diagnoses, age groups, and other aggregates of interest."[17] Outcomes have been approved for clinical testing or are under development (see Appendix D).

The seminal work of the Iowa Intervention Project Research Team for Nursing Intervention Classification (NIC) supports the development of a standardized language for nursing interventions.[14,15,22] A total of 433 interventions are located in a validated and coded taxonomic structure (see Appendix E). The interventions are linked, when appropriate, to the diagnostic labels approved by

NANDA. The project responds to the need to standardize nomenclature about nursing treatment. Specifically the classification was developed to (1) address the links among diagnoses, treatment, and outcomes; (2) facilitate the development of information systems; (3) facilitate the teaching of decision making skills; (4) assist in determining the costs of nursing services; (5) assist in planning for resources; (6) provide a language to communicate the unique functions of nursing; and (7) articulate with classification systems of other health care providers.

Although some may view the energy invested in developing different classification systems as detracting from the development of a unified diagnostic taxonomy, such efforts have opened the lines of communication. The need for systems that support and guide diagnosis and intervention in a variety of settings cannot be disputed. The major contribution of these efforts has been the development of "competing" diagnostic and intervention classification systems. Through the collaborative efforts of NANDA, the ANA, and research teams, these classification systems will be refined and revised. This activity must draw from the collective wealth of nursing knowledge and understanding that resides in the membership of the ANA, NANDA, and other professional organizations. It will be through such collaborations that the seeds of nursing diagnosis, which were planted in 1973, will continue to germinate and take root. The use and ongoing evaluation of nursing diagnosis will enrich the fields of nursing education, practice, and research.

REFERENCES

1. Aiken LH: Transformation of the nursing workforce, *Nurs Outlook* 43:201–209, 1995.
2. American Nurses' Association: *Standards of clinical nursing practice,* Kansas City, Missouri, 1991, The Association.
3. American Nurses' Association: *Nursing: a social policy statement,* Kansas City, Missouri, 1980, The Association.
4. American Nurses' Association: *Nursing's social policy statement,* Washington, D.C., 1995, The Association.
5. Carroll-Johnson RM: *Classification of nursing diagnoses: proceedings of the Eighth Conference,* Philadelphia, 1989, JB Lippincott Co.

6. Carroll-Johnson RM and Paquette M: *Classification of nursing diagnoses: proceedings of the Ninth Conference,* Philadelphia, 1991, JB Lippincott Co.

7. Carroll-Johnson RM: *Classification of nursing diagnoses: proceedings of the Tenth Conference,* Philadelphia, 1994, JB Lippincott Co.

8. Chamberlain P and others: Innovative culture shock prescribed for health care, *Nurs Outlook* 43:232–234, 1995.

9. Gebbie KM: *Summary of the Second National Conference: classification of nursing diagnoses,* St. Louis, 1976, Clearinghouse–National Group for Classification of Nursing Diagnoses.

10. Gebbie KM and Lavin MA: *Classification of nursing diagnoses: proceedings of the First National Conference,* St. Louis, 1975, The CV Mosby Co.

11. Gordon M: *Nursing diagnosis: process and application,* St. Louis, 1994, Mosby–Year Book.

12. Hegge M: Restructuring registered nurse curricula, *Nurs Educator* 20(6):39–44, 1995.

13. Horley ME: *Classification of nursing diagnoses: proceedings of the Sixth Conference,* St. Louis, 1986, The CV Mosby Co.

14. Iowa Intervention Project: The NIC taxonomy structure, *Image* 25:187–192, 1993.

15. Iowa Intervention Project: Validation and coding of the NIC taxonomy structure, *Image* 27:43–49, 1995.

16. Jenny J: Advancing the science of nursing. In Rantz MJ and LeMone P: *Classification of nursing diagnoses: proceedings of the Eleventh Conference,* Glendale, California, 1995, CINAHL Information Systems.

17. Johnson M and Maas M: Nursing-sensitive outcomes classification: an overview. In speaker handouts, Twelfth National Conference on the Classification of Nursing Diagnoses, pp. 23–28, 1996.

18. Kim MJ, McFarland GK, and McLane AM: *Classification of nursing diagnoses: proceedings of the Tenth Conference,* St. Louis, 1984, The CV Mosby Co.

19. Kim MJ and Moritz DA: *Classification of nursing diagnosis: proceedings of the Third and Fourth National Conferences,* New York, 1982, McGraw-Hill.

20. Larson EL: New rules for the game: interdisciplinary education for health professionals, *Nurs Outlook* 43(4):180–185, 1995.

21. Martin KS and Scheet NJ: The Omaha system: applications for community health nursing, Philadelphia, 1992, WB Saunders Co.

22. McCloskey JC and Bulechek GM: *Nursing interventions classification (NIC),* ed 2, St. Louis, 1996, Mosby–Year Book.

23. McLane AM: *Classification of nursing diagnoses: proceedings of the Seventh Conference,* St. Louis, 1987, The CV Mosby Co.

24. Mueller A, Johnston M, and Bopp A: Changing associate degree nursing curricula to meet evolving health care delivery system needs, *Nurs Educator* 20(6):23–28, 1995.

25. NANDA News, *Nurs Diagnosis* 5:96–101, 1994.

26. NANDA News, *Nurs Diagnosis* 6:5–8, 1995.

27. NANDA News, *Nurs Diagnosis* 6:53–56, 1995.

28. North American Nursing Diagnosis Association: *NANDA nursing diagnoses: definitions and classification, 1995–1996,* Philadelphia, 1994, The Association.

29. Pew Health Professions Commission: *Critical challenges: revitalizing the health professions for the twenty-first century,* San Francisco, 1995, The Commission.

30. Rantz MJ and LeMone P: *Classification of nursing diagnoses: proceedings of the Eleventh Conference,* Glendale, California, 1995, CINHAL.

31. Saba VK: A new nursing vision: the information highway, *Nurs Leadership Forum* 1(2):44–50, 1995.

32. Saba VK: Diagnoses and interventions: the classification of home health care nursing, *Caring* 11(3):50–57, 1992.

33. U.S. Department of Health and Human Services: *Healthy people 2000: national health promotion and disease prevention objectives* (DHHS Pub No (PHS)91-50213), Washington, D.C., 1990, U.S. Government Printing Office.

34. Worrell JD and others: The RN-BSN student: developing a model of empowerment, *J Nurs Educ* 35:127–130, 1996.

35. Wolf GA, Boland S, and Aukerman M: A transformational model for the practice of professional nursing, *JONA* 24(4):51–57, 1994.

Nursing Diagnosis: The Critical Link in the Nursing Process

PROFESSIONAL TRENDS

A number of professional trends have led to acceptance of the nursing diagnosis as a component of the nursing process. As described in Chapter 1, the National Conferences on the Classification of Nursing Diagnoses focused on the need to specify more clearly what nurses contribute to resolve specific patient problems and the need to store such information by means of automated record keeping. Each national conference* had built on previous work in the identification and development of nursing diagnoses and has served to institutionalize further the acceptance of nursing diagnosis as a critical link in the nursing process. Ongoing research on the identification and development of nursing diagnoses also is now published in *Nursing Diagnosis,* the official Journal of the North American Nursing Diagnosis Association (NANDA).

The American Nurses' Association (ANA) through its published standards for generic and specialty nursing, lent considerable support to the acceptance of the nursing diagnosis as a part of the nursing process,[3] as did the 1980 ANA publication *Nursing: A Social Policy Statement* and the 1995 ANA publication *Nursing's Social Policy Statement.*[1,2]

Other professional trends have increased the use of nursing diagnoses as part of the nursing process in clinical practice. Among them are state nurse practice acts that hold the nurse accountable for nursing diagnosis in clinical practice, as well as professional standards. For example, the Joint Commission on Accreditation of Healthcare Organizations 1992 Standard NC.1.3.5 states, "Nursing care data related to patient assessments, the nursing diagnoses and/or patient needs, nursing inter-

---

*References 4–6, 8, 11, 12, 14, 15, 17, 21.

ventions and patient outcomes are permanently integrated into the clinical information system (for example, the medical record)"[20] (p. 6).

Pressure for adopting and using nursing diagnoses also comes from current endeavors, such as computerized nursing care records, reimbursement models based on nursing diagnoses, patient classification based on nursing diagnoses, and standardized methods of reporting nursing information, as in the Minimum Nursing Data Set.

NURSING PROCESS— A PROBLEM-SOLVING PROCESS

The nursing process is a problem-solving process that nurses use in interacting with patients, their families, or significant others in providing nursing care.

The commonly accepted components of the nursing process are (1) assessment (data collection), (2) nursing diagnosis (problem identification), (3) planning (goal setting), (4) implementation (nursing intervention and treatment), and (5) evaluation. Figure 1 in Chapter 1 clearly shows the relationship between components of the nursing process and the standards of nursing practice previously discussed. The diagram shows that nursing diagnosis provides a clear focus for care planning; that is, for goal setting and the selection of nursing interventions, based on the concept that symptoms of conditions diagnosed can be alleviated or modified by nursing actions. Therefore nursing diagnosis is a critical link in the nursing process.

DEFINITIONS OF NURSING DIAGNOSIS

An officially accepted definition of the concept of nursing diagnosis was approved by the Ninth Conference on NANDA.[4] This definition states,

"Nursing Diagnosis is a clinical judgment about individual, family, or community responses to actual or potential health problems/life processes. Nursing diagnoses provide the basis for selection of nursing interventions to achieve outcomes for which the nurse is accountable"[18] (p. 7).

This definition serves as the definition for understanding the use of nursing diagnosis in this text. An example of nursing diagnosis is Dysfunctional Grieving, or, if the related factor has been identified, Dysfunctional Grieving related to inadequate social supports. Of course, more than one related factor could be involved, in which case the nursing diagnosis could be Dysfunctional Grieving related to inadequate social supports and inability to attend to grieving because of other tasks. An alternate way of addressing multiple related factors is to state each as a separate nursing diagnosis, such as (1) Dysfunctional Grieving related to inadequate social supports and (2) Dysfunctional Grieving related to inability to attend to grieving because of other tasks.

The Nursing Diagnosis Category

To understand the concept of nursing diagnosis more fully, it is essential to explore its three basic components, known as PES.[9]

Health Problems

P refers to the health problems or health state of an individual, family, or community expressed in a short, clear, and precise word, words, or phrase. Examples of such health states or problems, as exemplified by nursing diagnoses categories, are Risk for Injury, Anxiety, and Knowledge Deficit (Specify). Note that Risk for Injury refers to a "risk for" rather than an actual problem. The majority of nursing diagnosis labels could, in fact, be considered simultaneously a risk for or an actual problem, for instance, Risk for Sleep Pattern Disturbance or Sleep Pattern Disturbance.

Related Factors

E, the second component, stands for related factors. Related factors are any internal or external elements that have an effect on the person, family, or community and that contribute to the existence, or maintenance of the person's health problem. Such factors are associated with or related to the patient's health problem.[9] Related factors, where applicable and when they can be identified, should be written as concisely as possible and included in the nursing diagnostic statement.

Because additional research is needed on the related factors for any one of the NANDA nursing diagnoses, the identification of the related factors is somewhat tentative. Linking the health problem or nursing diagnosis category with only one related factor may imply a single cause, which can inhibit the implementation of holistic nursing care. Thus at times the use of the nursing diagnosis category itself (such as Diversional Activity Deficit) may be sufficient as a working nursing diagnosis for a patient and can provide direction for planning care without narrowing the focus to only one aspect of a larger, more complex health problem. Multiple specific nursing diagnostic statements that include very specific related factors can also be formulated to encapsulate the complex needs of a specific patient.

In the plans of care for the case studies in this text, usually one specific nursing diagnosis is the focus of planning. This is to help the reader understand the particular nursing diagnosis category under discussion: it does not imply that additional nursing diagnoses should not also be identified and used to develop the plan of care.

This logic can be taken a step further. It may at times be important to use a diagnostic category at a higher level of abstraction in the NANDA taxonomy to capture the essence of complexities and interrelatedness of a patient's health state, thereby providing direction for holistic nursing intervention. An example of such a nursing diagnosis is Altered Self-Concept: Body Image Disturbance, Personal Identity Disturbance, Self-Esteem Disturbance: Chronic Low, and Self-Esteem Disturbance: Situational have all been identified as components of the self-concept and have been incorporated into nursing diagnoses in previous NANDA work, thereby clarifying the abstract diagnosis Altered Self-Concept. At present, Body Image Disturbance, Personal Identity Disturbance, Self-Esteem Disturbance: Chronic Low, and Self-Esteem Disturbance: Situational are listed under Altered Self-Concept in the NANDA taxonomy.

An even higher level of abstraction may be very useful in some clinical situations. Much is being written in the literature about Functional Health Patterns, one of which is the Self-Perception-Self-Concept pattern. In one text,[9] 12 nursing diagnostic labels are identified as part of this pattern, among them being Self-Esteem Disturbance, Body Image Disturbance, and Personal Identity Disturbance. If carried out in time, clinical observation and testing lend credence to this classification scheme; then the functional pattern—that is, the Self-Perception—Self-Concept Pattern—may itself be a useful nursing diagnosis in the clinical arena, especially in those clinical conditions where a very abstract nursing diagnosis would be useful to capture holistically very complex and interrelated elements. In this text, the Functional Health Patterns serve as an organizing framework for the NANDA nursing diagnoses that are addressed later in the chapter.

In the Nursing Care Guidelines in this text the level of abstraction addressed is at the nursing diagnosis category level; that is, nursing interventions are identified for nursing diagnoses, such as Personal Identity Disturbance or Impaired Verbal Communication. Thus a nurse or student nurse can select nursing interventions from these guidelines to develop a plan of care for a patient; for example, with a nursing diagnosis of Personal Identity Disturbance.

Whether a "related to" phrase is added to the nursing diagnosis category along with a related factor for a given patient must be determined by a practicing nurse who has clinical judgment and experience. The related factor determined from the assessment data by the nurse further directs the selection of the nursing interventions made from the Nursing Care Guidelines; that is, the practicing nurse tailors the nursing interventions to the specific nursing diagnosis and needs of an individual patient. Examples of this are provided in the Case Study with Plan of Care in each chapter.

■ Defining Characteristics

S, the third component, stands for defining characteristics. This is the cluster of subjective and objective signs and symptoms indicating the presence of a condition that corresponds to a given nursing diagnosis. Research has been conducted with the purpose of validating nursing diagnoses so that eventually the cluster of defining characteristics identified for a given nursing diagnosis category will be supported.[10,13]

Some of the defining characteristics are, however, still based on clinical observation. The clinician must use clinical reasoning to formulate the most appropriate nursing diagnosis or diagnoses for a given patient. To review, the usual way of stating a nursing diagnosis is not to include the signs and symptoms in the diagnoses but to state the nursing diagnosis category plus the related factor or factors, if known.

Critical Versus Supporting Defining Characteristics. Some authors differentiate defining characteristics that are critical for formulating a given nursing diagnosis from those defining characteristics that are supporting but not critical. For example, Gordon[9] (p. 26) states that "critical defining characteristics are the criteria for making a diagnosis. They are fewer in number than the supporting characteristics . . . They are almost always observed when the diagnosis is present and are usually absent when the diagnosis is absent. Thus the critical characteristics of each category permit diagnosticians to discriminate among diagnoses." In addition, the NANDA taxonomy differentiates between major and minor defining characteristics for some nursing diagnoses. Caution is warranted in such an approach, however. Differentiating critical defining characteristics from supporting characteristics at this stage of the art and science of nursing diagnosis should be considered developmental because there is little research on which to base such differentiation.

NURSING PROCESS AND PLANNING FOR PATIENT CARE

Assessment

The first phase of the nursing process is assessment. The purpose of this phase is to collect data about a patient, family, community, environment, or culture to (1) assess the wellness state and the patient's desire for additional lifestyle improvements to benefit health, (2) assess for risk factors to identify potential nursing diagnoses, (3) assess for any alterations in the wellness state, (4) assess for response to any alterations in wellness and the effect of any nurse or medical therapy already implemented in order to determine the patient's, family's, or community's actual nursing diagnoses, (5) assess strengths and potential strengths, along with a history of coping strategies used, and (6) assess the patient's family, health care, other relevant resources available, and other relevant environmental or cultural factors.

There are a number of variables to keep in mind while assessing a patient, family, or community. (1) The patient, family, or community must always be viewed holistically, while at the same time considering their uniqueness during the assessment process. It is thus important to collect data on the physiological, sociocultural, spiritual, psychological, developmental, and environmental aspects of functioning, as relevant in assessing wellness and strengths, patterns, alterations, and risk factors. (2) The nurse must be aware of self so he or she can be as objective as possible and understand the patient, family, or community from the patient's, family's, or community's own perspective. Yura and Walsh[22] (p. 111) describe this well: "The nurse maintains a clear distinction between meaning that originates in him- or herself and that which originates in the patient. The nurse attempts to understand these meanings at a particular moment with the idea that this understanding is subject to correction and change as new data become available." This will enable the nurse to collect objective data and differentiate between the cues actually manifested by the patient, family, or community and the nursing judgments or inferences made about these cues. (3) The interview and data collection process, including any guides or tools developed and used, must be adapted to the patient's or family's setting; that is, home versus hospital. (4) The setting in which the interview is conducted must be conductive to the collection of the nursing data—there should be minimal interruptions and noise, a pleasant decor, comfortable seats, and a comfortable temperature. (5) A number of data collection strategies should be used, such as the nursing interview and history; observation; physical examination; medical records, including previous nursing notes and care plans; interviews of family members and significant others; observation of the environment; interviews to collect information about the patient's culture; and collaboration with nurse colleagues and other health members on a one-to-one basis or in patient care planning conferences. Communicating effectively and observing systematically are, of course, very important throughout the entire assessment process.

The Initial Interview. The assessment phase includes a general initial interview and a focused assessment. The initial data-based interview focuses on the patient, family, and/or community and allows the nurse to collect data for the second phase of the nursing process—nursing diagnosis. Because of their apparent relevance to clinical practice, the Functional Health Patterns are useful in categorizing the NANDA nursing diagnoses[9] and providing some conceptual direction for the initial assessment of a patient. There are 11 functional health patterns,[9] each of which is defined below with the purpose of assessing the pattern. An assessment guide based on the Functional Health Patterns is presented in Appendix F.

Functional Health Patterns. The *Health-Perception—Health-Management Pattern* refers to the patient's perceptions of his or her own health state and how his or her health goals and beliefs shape personal health care practices. The purpose of the assessment is to determine past and current health-seeking behaviors, compliance with recommendations for nursing and medical treatment, resources available for health maintenance, injury prevention practices, and whether and how the patient is seeking a higher level of well-being.

The *Nutritional-Metabolic Pattern* refers to the biopsychosocial states linked to food and water supply and the patient's nutrient and fluid intake. The purpose of assessment is to determine the patient's functional or dysfunctional fluid and food patterns along with possible reasons, condition of the skin as a reflection of nutrition, and metabolic problems in temperature regulation. Weight, temperature, diet, fluid intake, and skin integrity are all assessed.

The *Elimination Pattern* describes a patient's urinary and bowel elimination patterns. The purpose of the assessment is to determine the adequacy of these patterns by assessing urinary and bowel routines, habits, and practices.

The *Activity-Exercise Pattern* refers to a patient's motivation and capability to engage in energy-consuming activities and conditions that affect these activities. The purpose of the assessment is to determine the patient's desire, choice, and actual involvement in leisure, work, self-care, and exercise. Also assessed are nursing diagnoses that can influence the activity pattern, such as tissue perfusion, cardiac output, breathing pattern, and gas exchange.

The *Sleep-Rest Pattern* refers to the patient's rest and sleep perceptions and practices. The purpose of the assessment is to determine the quality of the sleep and rest, as well as the patient's methods for promoting rest and sleep.

The *Cognitive-Perceptual Pattern* refers to the ability of the patient to perceive, understand, remember, and make decisions about information from the internal and external environments. The purpose of the assessment is to determine the status of the five senses and the use of any aids (e.g., a hearing aid), the degree of discomfort or pain, any perceptual alterations, and the patient's ability to understand, make decisions, and use good judgment. Also assessed is the patient's understanding of health care self-management practices and knowledge.

The *Self-Perception—Self-Concept Pattern* includes the patient's patterns of perception, attitudes, and self-competency. The purpose of the assessment is to determine the patient's attitudes and beliefs about personal abilities, identity, self-

worth, and body image. Emotions and feelings such as grieving, anxiety, hopelessness, and powerlessness, are also assessed

The *Role-Relationship Pattern* involves the patient's needs and actual interactions with others at work, in the family, or in the community. The purpose of the assessment is to determine the patient's role and responsibility at work, in the family life, or in social life, including his or her communication skills and patterns. Areas in which the patient is adequate or experiences difficulty are both assessed. Also assessed are risk factors for self-harm and potential for inflicting physical harm on others.

The *Sexuality-Reproductive Pattern* refers to the patient's actual and perceived satisfaction or dysfunction in sexuality or reproduction. The purpose of the assessment is to determine the patient's degree of satisfaction or dissatisfaction in fulfilling sexual and reproductive needs. Assessed are the patient's reproductive and associated problems and concerns.

The *Coping—Stress-Tolerance Pattern* refers to the patient's or family's adaptive or maladaptive response to stress and challenging life events. The purpose of the assessment is to determine the nature and degree of stressors, stress response, and coping pattern. Assessed are the patient's perceptions of the stress and of his or her coping strategies and the resources available to the patient and the family.

The *Value-Belief Pattern* includes the beliefs and values that guide a person's choices and lifestyle. The purpose of the assessment is to determine these life beliefs and values, including spiritual, religious, and philosophical beliefs.

The Focused Assessment. The general initial interview can often determine the need for a focused assessment involving the collection of very specific data about alterations in a particular functional pattern and, more specifically, in a given diagnostic category. This focused assessment rules out or validates the alterations or potential alterations in health or the desire for additional health-seeking opportunities as suggested by the data gathered during the initial interview. Each of the following nursing diagnosis sections in the text contains an assessment section useful in developing a good, focused assessment, along with clearly identified defining characteristics and related factors for each diagnostic category. A focused assessment can be completed as part of the initial interview if the data already collected suggest the need. Another focused assessment should be conducted after the initial one as additional data indicate a change in the patient's condition. The patient's verbalizations or information from other sources, such as the family or other health care team members, can all indicate a need for this second, focused assessment.

Formulating Nursing Diagnoses

To formulate accurate nursing diagnoses with a given patient, family, or community, the nurse must consider a number of important factors. Knowledge of nursing science and other related biopsychosocial and anthropological sciences is important for the practicing nurse to move from the assessment phase of the nursing process to formulating accurate nursing diagnoses. Clinical practice guided by experienced faculty, clinical nurse specialists, and experienced clinicians facilitate growth and assurance of the nurse's diagnostic reasoning skills. The opportunity to practice in a protected setting, such as the classroom or the continuing education workshop, likewise facilitates growth in the nurse's ability to formulate accurate nursing diagnoses. Equally essential is the need for the practicing nurse to consult quality nursing practice reference texts and manuals, which should be found in the library of every health care setting, and to consult with nurse peers, nurse consultants and specialists, and other health team members, either individually or in nursing staff or team conferences. It is likewise important to understand that the nursing diagnosis or diagnoses that the nurse formulates when beginning to care for a patient are working diagnoses subject to change and ongoing revision. The nurse may identify alternative explanations and confirm or rule these out, based on the data initially available; the nurse may obtain more data about the patient over time; or the patient's condition may change. Indeed, unless openness to alternative explanations is maintained, one alternative may be over-

valued, and the resulting narrow focus may not allow for all data to be considered, thus causing an inaccurate nursing diagnosis. Finally, the nurse's ability to understand the clinical reasoning process is an asset when the nurse actually assumes responsibility for formulating accurate nursing diagnoses in the clinical setting.

Diagnosis as a Process. One of the most commonly accepted models of diagnosis as a process contains four activities—collecting information, interpreting the information, clustering the information, and naming the cluster—occurring as an ongoing cyclical process that involves cognitive and perceptual activities.[9] Data collected by means of the strategies discussed above and in subsequent sections need to be interpreted to have meaning. Gordon elucidates that interpreting means assigning meaning or determining what is significant. Interpretation involves the ability to (1) pay attention to and recognize diagnostic cues, (2) clarify or search for a clearer understanding of the cues, (3) verify or double-check the cues, (4) recognize the direct or concealed meaning of the cues, and (5) evaluate the cues so that the initial cues are put together to have meaning.

In evaluating cues, the observed baseline data are compared with population norms or standards. The baseline data are also very useful in ongoing monitoring of the patient's progress. Through inferential reasoning, the nurse determines whether the cues fall within the expected norms or indicate some type of health problem. Interpretation must also take into account the whole patient situation, environment, and culture. Diagnostic hypotheses (the possible meanings of a cue or cue cluster) are then formed, providing further structure to the diagnostic tasks. Checkpoints for hypothesis generation and testing include the following:[9]

1. Has the collected data been clarified and verified?
2. Has attention been given to diagnostic cues in the data that have been collected?
3. Have the cues been interpreted for meaning and compared against norms?
4. Have the cues been adequately analyzed for the possibility of alternative explanations?

5. Have the defining characteristics for the hypotheses being tested been addressed?
6. Objectively, are sufficient cues or defining characteristics present to formulate tentative nursing diagnoses?

The diagnostic process involves ongoing information clustering; that is, relating and clustering the collected cues. The generated diagnostic hypothesis facilitates this activity. The collected cues may not lead directly and easily to the formulation of a nursing diagnosis. Inconsistencies among cues may be the result of (1) conflicting reports from health care team members, the patient, or the family, (2) measurement errors resulting from miscommunication or faulty instruments, (3) faulty expectations resulting from a nurse's lack of experience or knowledge, or (4) unreliable information.[9] Besides resolving such inconsistencies the clinician must weigh cues so he or she can arrive at the best working hypothesis and eventually formulate the actual nursing diagnostic statement that is the very best statement possible until an even more precise one can be formulated.

As previously described, the nursing diagnostic statement includes the health problem along with the related factor or factors when known. The health problem can be selected from the list of NANDA nursing diagnosis categories (each is discussed in depth in the following sections) if the cluster of signs and symptoms collected during assessment corresponds, at least in part, to the defining characteristics for a given nursing diagnosis category. Not all of the defining characteristics for a specific nursing diagnosis need be observed in or reported by a patient to use the diagnosis, but this determination requires clinical expertise and knowledge. Based on the collected data, the related factor or factors can also be identified. Common related factors for each of the nursing diagnoses in the following chapters are listed and can be used in formulating a specific nursing diagnosis if supported by the collected data.

In addition to naming the actual specific nursing diagnosis (e.g., Dysfunctional Grieving related to multiple unresolved previous losses), other assessment conclusions can be reached at the naming stage of the diagnostic process. First, the assessment conclusion often results in more than one nursing diagnosis, and they must be prioritized to identify those requiring immediate intervention. The assessment may also determine that the patient does not have an actual or evident health problem. The patient's history, current lifestyle, and other data sources may present evidence of risk factors, and the assessment conclusion may indicate a high-risk nursing diagnosis such as Risk for Violence: Self-Directed or Directed at Others related to a lengthy history of violent behavior. Depending on the patient's identified risk factors, any of the nursing diagnoses can be high-risk, such as Risk for Social Isolation. Such diagnoses address the preventive aspect of nursing care. A health promotion diagnosis may also result from the assessment (e.g., Health-Seeking Behaviors [Specify]).

Planning

The third phase of the nursing process is planning. "Planning is the determination of a plan of action to assist the client toward the goal of optimal wellness based on the highest level of fulfillment [in relation to the Functional Health Patterns] and to resolve the nursing diagnosis [or diagnoses]"[22] (p. 138). The formulated nursing diagnosis or diagnoses provide direction to the planning process and in selecting nursing interventions to achieve the desired outcomes. In other words, patient goals—referred to as *expected patient outcomes* in many contemporary practice settings and in this text—are developed for each of the nursing diagnoses formulated for a given patient. For each nursing diagnosis, one or more expected patient outcomes may be identified. The expected patient outcomes are desirable and measurable patient health states, including biological, physiological, psychological, sociocultural, and spiritual aspects, and the knowledge or skills related to these health states. The expected patient outcomes denote progress toward the resolution or modification of the condition that corresponds to an actual nursing diagnosis or the prevention of a condition that corresponds to a high risk for nursing diagnosis; or progress toward a higher level of optimal wellness in a patient who is healthy but desires to engage in further health-seeking behaviors. In a deteriorating health state or terminal illness, the expected patient outcome may be directed toward achieving satisfactory adaptation or coping.

The development of expected patient outcomes is guided by a number of factors:

(1) They should be stated in patient behavioral terms, with measurable verbs, and should be specific in content; for example, "The patient will [expected patient outcome]." or "The patient will be able to [expected patient outcome]." Examples of expected patient outcomes for a patient with the nursing diagnosis of Post-Trauma Response are the following: Patient will resolve the physiological changes suffered in the trauma; patient will express feelings about the effect of the trauma on personal lifestyle; patient will experience increasingly longer periods free of impaired concentration; patient will maintain old interpersonal relationships and develop new ones; patient will abstain from drugs and alcohol; and patient will integrate traumatic experience into his or her lifestyle and perception of self. For a patient with a nursing diagnosis of Impaired Verbal Communication, the expected patient outcomes could include: patient will attend to, perceive, and process relevant stimuli; patient will send precise, understandable messages, using congruent verbal and nonverbal communications; and patient will send and receive feedback.

(2) The development of any expected patient outcome is guided by the formulated nursing diagnosis, including the related factor, if identified and stated. This is evident because the desired overall outcome is to modify or resolve the condition that corresponds to an actual nursing diagnosis or, in the case of a potential nursing diagnosis, to prevent the occurrence of the actual condition in a patient with known risk factors.

(3) The overall database collected during the initial interview and focused assessment is also critically important because the expected patient outcomes must be realistic and attainable for a given patient and must take into account his or her strengths and potential, lifestyle, family, living arrangements, the community in which the patient resides, and the culture or subculture to which the patient belongs.

(4) Expected patient outcomes can be developed as both short-term and long-term outcomes and must be reviewed or modified as the patient progresses. This is especially important when the nursing diagnosis itself is modified or resolved.

(5) A time frame can be specified wherein the expected patient outcome or outcomes should be achieved for a particular patient.

(6) If the focus is the family or the community, expected outcomes refer to achievable behaviors for the family or the community. That is, the phrase for the family would be "The family will [expected family outcome]" or "The family will be able to [expected family outcome]." For example, for the nursing diagnosis Ineffective Family Coping: Compromised, expected family outcomes could be the following: The family will promote health to maintain integrity, or the family will use additional resources to preserve family supportive capacity.

In each of the sections of this text, sample expected patient outcomes are identified. Based on the data collected on a given patient and the actual nursing diagnosis formulated, these expected patient outcomes can be selected and used in developing a patient care plan. Major expected patient outcomes are identified for each nursing diagnosis in the Nursing Care Guidelines and are further discussed in the Outcome Identification, Planning, and Implementation section of each subsequent chapter in this text.

As described in Chapter 1, efforts are under way to classify nursing-sensitive outcomes.[12] The planning process also involves selecting nursing interventions (the action the nurse must take or assist the patient, family, or community in taking) to achieve the specified expected patient, family, or community outcome or outcomes. Nursing interventions are categorized by the level of assistance that the nurse offers the patient; these categories range from interventions that the nurse totally performs for a patient who is unable to assist to those that offer support and encouragement for a patient who actively participates in his or her own care. Nursing interventions involve ongoing assessment and monitoring, coordination of resources and health care services, emotional support or therapy, guidance or counseling, teaching, acting for or doing for the patient, collaborating with the patient, referring the patient to other health team members, monitoring the environment, and supporting and teaching the family. Similar to the expected patient outcomes, nursing diagnoses and related factors guide the selection of nursing interventions. The intended result of the implementation of the nursing interventions is to meet the expected patient outcomes.

In each of the nursing diagnosis sections of this book, sample nursing interventions are clearly identified in the Nursing Care Guidelines and discussed in detail, including the rationale for their use in the Outcome Identification, Planning, and Implementation sections. These nursing interventions are useful in developing a patient's plan of care and must be selected based on a particular patient's specific nursing diagnostic statement and expected outcomes, along with such collected data as the patient's particular strengths, coping skills, and resources available.

Approaches to writing actual nursing orders differ. Nursing orders can be stated more generally, as in the multiple sample interventions described in the following sections, or these nursing interventions can be specified further in terms of behaviors tailored to a particular patient. For example, one expected patient outcome for the nursing diagnosis Altered Nutrition: Less Than Body Requirements listed in this text is that the patient will improve and maintain food intake to meet metabolic demands. Among the nursing interventions identified for this expected patient outcome is encouraging verbalization by the patient and his or her family of their preferences regarding mealtimes, meal locations, and food likes and dislikes. Developed into a more specific nursing order, this nursing intervention could be "Meet with Mrs. Karen J. and her husband on Wednesday afternoon during visiting hours to discuss preferred mealtimes, meal locations, and

food likes and dislikes." Or "Schedule procedures so they do not conflict with mealtimes" can be developed into a more specific nursing order, such as "Schedule Mrs. Karen J. for a chest X-ray examination at 10 A.M. on Friday." Nursing orders can include the date, an action or directive verb, the action and when it should occur, how frequently and how long the action should occur, where the action is to take place, and the nurse's signature. The nursing interventions in the following sections can serve as useful guidelines if such specific nursing orders are desired. As mentioned in Chapter 1, efforts are under way to classify nursing interventions.[16]

Based on the collected data, a number of nursing diagnoses may be formulated for a particular patient. In the planning phase, attention must be given to assigning priority to these concomitant nursing diagnoses because it may be unreasonable to develop and implement expected patient outcomes and a corresponding plan of action for each of them. Therefore the nurse, in collaboration with the patient, may need to determine which nursing diagnoses should be addressed first in the care plan.

Implementing

Implementing is the fourth phase of the nursing process and "is the initiation and completion of actions necessary to accomplish the defined goal of optimal wellness for the client"[22] (p. 154). Depending on the nature of the patient's problem and his or her condition, ability, and resources, as well as the nature of the action planned, the nursing care plan may be implemented primarily by the nurse or by the nurse in collaboration with the patient, the patient's family, community resources, or other health care team members to whom selected aspects of care are delegated. Yura and Walsh[22] (p. 154) further note that "the implementation phase for the nursing process draws heavily on the intellectual, interpersonal, and technical skills of the nurse. Decision making, observation, and communication are significant skills enhancing the success of actions." The nursing care plan serves as a blueprint for action, and the nurse must monitor the patient's progress and achievement of the specified expected outcomes.

For each nursing diagnosis in the following sections, a sample Case Study with Plan of Care follows the description of the case study. The sample care plan is designed to help the reader understand the nursing diagnosis discussed in that section and is not intended to address other nursing diagnoses that could also be formulated for the specific patient in the case study.

The following quotation provides an excellent conclusion to the implementation section of the nursing process:

The success or failure of the nursing care plan depends on the nurse's intellectual, interpersonal, and technical abilities. This includes the ability to judge the value of new data that becomes available to the nurse during implementation and the nurse's innovative and creative ability in making adaptations to compensate for unique characteristics—physical, emotional, cultural, and spiritual—that become known during interaction with the patient. The nurse must have the ability to react to verbal and nonverbal cues, validating inferences based on observation. Paramount during the interaction is the nurse's acceptance of him- or herself as a person and the confidence in his or her ability to perform the independent nursing functions inherent in the planned action, recognizing those that are interdependent. . . . The nurse must have a realistic understanding of self, recognizing and accepting strengths and limitations; be convinced of his or her own personal worth and find meaning in his or her life; meet his or her own human needs reasonably well. . . . The more wholesome the nurse's view of him- or herself as a person and the stronger the philosophy of life, the less likely the client will experience depersonalizing encounters with the nurse[22] (p. 154).

Evaluation

The fifth phase of the nursing process is evaluating, which follows the implementation phase. In the implementation phase, the patient is monitored and data are collected to determine whether progress toward the achievement of the expected patient outcomes is being made and, in turn, whether the patient's condition has improved. The improvement can relate to actual nursing diagnoses being modified or resolved; actual nursing diagnoses being prevented, in the case of potential nursing diagnoses: or health-seeking behaviors being enhanced, in the case of the patient with the nursing diagnosis Health-Seeking Behaviors. Specific outcome criteria can be delineated to indicate whether the stated expected patient outcomes are being achieved.

Each of the following sections contains a description of relevant criteria that must be monitored to evaluate a patient's progress. Evaluation is very important in the nursing process because it is on the results of evaluation that nursing diagnoses are reexamined and perhaps restated, expected patient outcomes are altered, and different nursing interventions are implemented.

The work of the North American Nursing Diagnosis Association (NANDA) in identifying and developing nursing diagnoses and a taxonomy is an evolving, ever-changing process. Although the past 20 years of effort have resulted in a clinically useful list of nursing diagnoses and a beginning taxonomy, ongoing clinical observation and research will result in deletions, modifications, and additions to this system.

Nurse researchers are encouraged to continue the progress in research on nursing diagnosis, as reflected in the review of nursing diagnosis research by Gordon[10] and Kim[13] in the *Annual Review of Nursing Research.*

The practicing nurse is encouraged to use the nursing diagnoses recently developed and to test them in clinical practice, providing feedback to the professional organization when changes are needed in the system.

The work of specialty organizations—for example, the ANA Psychiatric Mental Health Nursing Groups, which has been working since 1984 to develop a "comprehensive working list on the phenomena of concern for psychiatric mental health (PMH) nurses"[19]—is encouraged, and they have submitted their work to NANDA for inclusion in the NANDA Taxonomy. Currently these diagnostic labels are listed in Appendix G, NANDA Diagnoses Received for Review and Developmental Staging.[18]

Finally, the nurse should keep in mind that the processes of clinical decision making and diagnostic reasoning are very complex and that more nursing research is needed to understand these complex processes. As the NANDA Taxonomy of nursing knowledge evolves in practice, nursing will continue to evolve as a true profession.[18]

REFERENCES

1. American Nurses' Association: *Nursing: a social policy statement,* Kansas City, Missouri, 1980, The Association.
2. American Nurses' Association: *Nursing's social policy statement,* Washington, D.C., 1995, The Association.
3. American Nurses' Association: *Standards of clinical nursing practice,* Kansas City, Missouri, 1991, The Association.
4. Carroll-Johnson RM, editor: *Classification of nursing diagnoses: proceedings of the Ninth Conference,* Philadelphia, 1991, JB Lippincott Co.
5. Carroll-Johnson RM: *Classification of nursing diagnoses: proceedings of the Eighth Conference,* Philadelphia, 1989, JB Lippincott Co.
6. Carroll-Johnson RM and Paquette M: *Classification of nursing diagnoses: proceedings of the Tenth Conference,* Philadelphia, 1994, JB Lippincott Co.
7. Gebbie KM: *Summary of the Second National Conference,* St. Louis, 1976, The Clearinghouse–National Group for Classification of Nursing Diagnoses.
8. Gebbie K and Lavin M: *Classification of nursing diagnoses: proceedings of the First National Conference,* St. Louis, 1975, The CV Mosby Co.
9. Gordon M: *Nursing diagnoses: process and application,* ed 3, St. Louis, 1994, Mosby–Year Book.
10. Gordon M: Nursing diagnosis, *Ann Rev Nurs Res* 3:127–146, 1985.
11. Hurley ME, editor: *Classification of nursing diagnoses: proceedings of the Sixth Conference,* St. Louis, 1986, The CV Mosby Co.
12. Johnson M and Maas M: *Nursing-sensitive outcomes classification. An overview,* Speaker Handout. Twelfth National Conference on the Classification of Nursing Diagnoses, Pittsburgh, Pennsylvania, April 11–14, 1996.
13. Kim MJ: *Nursing diagnosis, Ann Rev Nurs Res* 7:117–142, 1989.
14. Kim MJ, McFarland GK, and McLane AM, editors: *Classification of nursing diagnosis: proceedings of the Fifth National Conference,* St. Louis, 1984, The CV Mosby Co.
15. Kim MJ and Moritz DA, editors: *Classification of nursing diagnosis: proceedings of the Third and Fourth Conferences,* New York, 1982, McGraw-Hill.
16. McCloskey JC and Bulechek GM: *Nursing interventions classification (NIC),* ed 2, St. Louis, 1996, Mosby–Year Book.
17. McLane AM, editor: *Classification of nursing diagnoses: proceedings of the Seventh Conference,* St. Louis, 1988, Mosby–Year Book.
18. North American Nursing Diagnosis Association: *NANDA nursing diagnoses: definitions and classification, 1995–1996,* Philadelphia, 1994, The Association.
19. O'Toole AW and Loomis ME: Revision of the phenomena of concern for psychiatric mental health nursing, *Arch Psychiatr Nurs* III (5):288–299, 1989.
20. Parsek JD: Did JCAHO abolish care plans? *Am Nurs* 23(8):6, 1991.
21. Rantz MJ and LeMone P: *Classification of nursing diagnoses: proceedings of the Eleventh Conference,* Glendale, California, 1995, CINHAL Information Systems.
22. Yura H and Walsh M: *The nursing process: assessing, planning, implementing, evaluating,* Norwalk, Connecticut, 1988, Appleton & Lange.

HEALTH-PERCEPTION— HEALTH-MANAGEMENT PATTERN

Energy Field Disturbance

▶

Energy Field Disturbance *is a condition in which a disturbance of the human energy field manifests a disharmony in the human-environmental energy field mutual process.*

OVERVIEW

The postulate that the universe is a dynamic web of energy is not new. Perhaps what is new is that modern physics lends significant support to what many ancient civilizations had known. Ancient Indian tradition speaks of a universal energy as the source of all life, calling it *prana*, or the "basic breath of life." The Chinese in 3000 B.C. posited the existence of vital energy called *ch'i* or *qi*. Today the human energy system, *ch'i*, guides the practice of acupuncture. Kabbalah, the Jewish mystical philosophy that arose in the sixth century B.C., refers to the vital principle *nefish* and teaches that an iridescence or "astral light" surrounds the human body. Throughout the last two millennia, artists have depicted halos around Christian saints to signify their expanded energy and enlightenment.[28] Many cultures, past and present, have described human energy fields. In their book *Future Science*, White and Kripper[62] list 97 different cultures that refer to a human energy field with 97 different names. For example, the Hawaiians call this energy *mana*, and the Japanese call it *ki*. The human energy field is the basis of such practices as yoga, acupuncture, acupressure, shiatzu, Tai Chi, Reiki, Healing Touch, and many others.

Many scientists who believed that Eastern mysticism was vague, mysterious, and highly unscientific have found that mystical thought provides a consistent and relevant philosophical background to theories advanced in contemporary science.[14] Capra,[13] a theoretical physicist, found profound and striking parallels between modern physics and the great Eastern mystical traditions. An understanding of modern physics is essential to understanding that energy fields are the fundamental nature of reality. Contrary to Newton, who viewed matter as always "similar and immutable,"[15] Einstein[20] determined that all matter is composed of a "universal energy." The universe, including the human being, is not really composed of matter. The basic component is energy, as expressed in Einstein's famous equation, $E = mc^2$ (energy [E] equals mass [m] multiplied by the speed of light [c] squared). Thus mass and energy are interchangeable; two manifestations of the same reality, differing in degree and function but not in kind.[20] When viewed at the microcosmic level, all mass is a dynamic pattern of energy. Matter is merely "momentary manifestations of interacting fields."[65] Therefore the basic stuff of the universe is not matter but energy.[20,25]

Quantum theory also describes the basic oneness of the universe as characterized by patterns of energy rather than bounded substance. Furthermore, quantum theory has replaced the classic view of the world as a collection of distinct yet interacting parts, divisible into particles, with a new view of the universe as an "undivided wholeness."[7,27] Energy fields cannot be explained in terms of matter; rather, matter is explained in terms of energy within fields. Matter and everything experienced by the human senses are manifestations of the energy field. Because energy fields are unbounded, all is connected to everything else. An energy field has a continuous, holistic quality and cannot be separated into parts.[7,13,18,27,58] Therefore what appears to our senses as isolated entities, patterns, or events are actually manifestations of the whole field. All energy is dynamic and in continuous motion. Thus the universe is best described as a dynamic web of inseparable energy patterns.[14,65]

There is a mass of scientific literature supporting the existence of energy fields. Harold Saxon Burr,[8] in his life's work at Yale University, used very sensitive voltmeters to measure bioenergy fields, which he called "Life-fields" or "L-fields," emanating from and/or surrounding the body. Through studies of healthy and ill persons, Burr found changes in the voltage gradient. For example, studies of menstrual cycles demonstrated a sharp rise in the voltage gradient associated with ovulation. Ravitz[52] found that the human energy field fluctuates with a person's mood. Kirlian[33] studied the same energy fields using electrophotography. Kirlian photography provides a direct image of the human energy field on sensitive film, evidence that the human energy field extends outward from the body. Moss, Hubacher, and Saba[46] studied the differences in the intensity and quality of human energy fields using Kirlian photography of human finger pads. Persons experiencing tension demonstrate a narrow and constricted "corona" or energy field emanating around a finger pad, whereas relaxed persons have a large, bright, and vivid corona.

Robert Becker,[6] an orthopedic surgeon, demonstrated that pattern shapes and strengths of the body's energy field change in correlation with psychological and physiological changes. Another method of measuring human energy is thermography. *Thermography* is a technique for detecting and measuring variations in the heat emitted by various regions of the body and transforming them into visible signals that are recorded photographically. Several studies have demonstrated the validity and sensitivity of thermography in the assessment of thermal field changes associated with pain.[59,60,61] Motoyama,[47] a Japanese physicist, developed several electrode devices that measured a bioelectrical field at various distances from the surface of the body and found a strong correlation between meridians that were out of balance and the presence of underlying disease. Hunt et al.[29] used silver/silver chloride electrodes placed on the skin to record the frequency of low-voltage signals emanating from a person's body while being massaged. The recorded wave patterns were analyzed using Fourier analysis and a sonogram frequency analysis, which yielded band frequencies that were translated into colors. At the same time, a person able to see auras described changes in the energy field that correlated with the Fourier and sonogram frequency analyses.

Within the discipline of nursing, Rogers' Science of Unitary Human Beings[53,54,55] presents a view of humans and the environment consistent with the findings of progressive contemporary science. The science of Unitary Human Beings provides a theoretical foundation for the concept of Energy Field Disturbance. Rogers describes humans and the environment as open systems of energy. "The human field extends beyond the discernible mass which we perceive as man. The human field and the environmental field . . . are coextensive with the universe."[53] Rogers asserts that human beings do not have energy fields but *are* energy fields.[55] The physical body is a manifestation of the energy field. However, Rogers' conceptualization of the energy field transcends the narrow view of physical fields. According to Rogers, the human energy field is more than a physical field. The human energy and environmental fields are not biological fields, physical fields, social fields, psychological fields, or their summation.[55] Thus, as opposed to the concept of an energy field is defined in physics, Rogers is not referring to electromagnetic fields, biofields, or gravitational fields. For Rogers a field is a unifying concept, and energy signifies the dynamic nature of the field. Fields are finite, irreducible, indivisible, and in continuous motion. Rogers' term *unitary* refers to the indivisible and irreducible nature of energy fields. Energy fields are the fundamental unit of the living and the nonliving. Rogers[55] identifies two energy fields, the human energy field and the environmental energy field, and states that the two fields are integral with one another. *Integral* means that the human and the environmental fields are without boundaries and thus are inseparable. Both are continuously open to each other and in mutual process with one another. *Mutual process* signifies the dynamic, integral, and simultaneous process of change in both the human and the environmental fields. They co-evolve together.

Although Rogers' definition of an energy field may differ somewhat from contemporary physics, the idea that everything is energy patterning is consistent. Each person is a unique pattern within the larger fabric of the universe. One cannot see an energy field but one can perceive manifestations of a pattern emerging from the human-environmental field mutual process. Numerous colloquialisms suggest corollaries between energy fields and the observed world.[53] Disturbances in the human-environmental energy field emerge as manifestations of patterning. Behaviors, movements, thoughts, feelings, emotions, experiences, expressions, and perceptions are all examples of energetic manifestations of patterning emerging from the human-environmental field mutual process. Patients often use such terms as *charged, energized, low or high spirits, drained,* or *depleted.* Such expressions are not simply metaphors but, within an energy field perspective, are reflections of the nature of the human energy field. Kunz and Peper[37] also describe in detail how every thought, emotion, and action are energetic manifestations of the energy field. For example, Butcher[10] conceptualized the experience of dispiritedness within an energy field perspective, which he described as the experience of "dissipating energy" and "dissonant rhythmicity."

Rogers' Science of Unitary Human Beings reflects a radically new way of viewing humans and their universe. A practice model derived from Rogers' energy field perspective must be consistent with the concepts and principles of Rogerian Science. Rogers has repeatedly stated that the nursing process is inconsistent with a view of humans as irreducible energy fields in a pandimensional universe.[2,17] Instead, the Rogerian practice methodology consists of two phases: Pattern Manifestation Appraisal and Deliberative Mutual Patterning. *Pattern Manifestation Appraisal* is the continuous process of identifying manifestations of the human and environmental fields that relate to current health events.[2] *Deliberate Mutual Patterning* is the second phase of the Rogerian practice methodology and is defined as the continuous process whereby the nurse and the patient pattern the human-environmental field to promote harmony related to health events.[2]

ASSESSMENT

Pattern Manifestation Appraisal

The process of Pattern Manifestation Appraisal is used to identify energy field disturbances. There are several strategies for appraising the rhythm, quality, form, and intensity of the human energy field. Nurses engaging in Pattern Manifestation Appraisal need to focus completely on the well-being of the patient with unconditional love, compassion, and empathy.[9] Nurses also approach patient situations with intentionality. A nurse's intentionality is expressed by approaching patients with the intention of helping and healing guided by a scientific base for practice, a commitment to serve the well-being of the patient, and a willingness to confront oneself.[35]

To enhance the nurse's awareness and ability to sense and "tune into" the subtle manifestations and rhythms of energy field disturbances, the nurse initially centers him- or herself. In a centered condition, the outflow of one's energies becomes conscious and focused and heightens one's openness and awareness. Centering is a process of self-relatedness that can be thought of as a place of inner being, a place of calmness within oneself where one can feel integrated, united, and focused.[35] In addition, the centered nurse is better able to draw consciously on the universal energy in the environment to replenish both the patient and the nurse.

Krieger[36] described in detail the process of centering in the following manner. Centering is accomplished by first sitting in a comfortable position and taking quiet, full breaths. Your eyes can be open or closed. Then explore your own being and notice feelings that edge into your consciousness. Follow the thoughts that cross your mind without getting too involved with them. Distinguish which thoughts belong to you and which belong to other people. Concentrate on your attributes. Gradually become more sensitive to your own subtle energies. Become aware of your breathing; notice how your breath fills your lungs. Sense how your breath permeates the tissue of your body. Then identify in your mind through your mood or feelings with the facet of your consciousness that senses energies and creates visualizations or emotions. As you become more aware of these deeper levels of being, notice the increasing stillness and sense of timelessness. At this moment of quietude, you will feel a sense of well-being and relaxation, and you will be in control of yourself.

The two main avenues for appraising for energy field disturbances are therapeutic touch and dialogue. Therapeutic touch is a learned technique taught in more than 80 major colleges in the United States and in more than 60 other countries through presentations and classes.[36] Therapeutic touch is a knowledgeable and deliberate patterning of the patient-environmental energy field process in which the nurse assumes a meditative awareness and uses the hands as a focus for patterning of the mutual patient-environmental energy field process.[45]

After the nurse achieves a meditative awareness through the process of centering, the nurse uses the hands to assess the patient's energy field. The energy field, which flows through and extends beyond the patient's physical body, is felt easily when the hands are held about 3 to 5 inches from the surface of the skin.[42] Moving the hands through the entire field, head to toe, the nurse assesses for sensations or cues of pattern and rhythmicity of the field. Through the natural sensitivity of the hands, the nurse perceives the condition of the energy flow as differences in subtle sensations. The sensations are usually perceived as feelings of congestion, pressure, coolness, or tin-

gling. The nurse senses how far the field extends, its symmetry, vibration, texture, and fullness or depletion. Theoretically a disturbance in the energy field that occurs over specific regions of the body represents a block in the energy flow. Although these perceptions are highly subjective, Lionberger[39] found that nurses also perceive information about the patient through intuitive and somatic cues. Macrae,[42] a very experienced practitioner of therapeutic touch, notes that it is difficult to express the cues verbally. Often a skilled person performing therapeutic touch implicitly knows there is an energy disturbance and how to care for that disturbance.

Although therapeutic touch is a direct method for appraising the human-environmental energy field, engaging in a dialogue focusing on health-related events and experiences is also a means of appraising for energy pattern disturbances emerging from the human-environmental process. After centering, the nurse enters into a rhythmic dialogue and communion with the patient. The nurse relies on multiple modes of awareness in apprehending manifestations of the human-environmental field mutual process. Intuition and tacit knowing are multiple modes of awareness that enable the nurse to see the whole of the health situation and uncover hidden patterns and meanings. Data are not divided into categories such as spiritual, physical, emotional, mental, cultural, or biological. Rather, all data or information are conceived as energetic manifestations of the human-environmental energy field.[16,17]

The nurse asks the patient to describe his or her current health situation. Specifically the nurse focuses on apprehending the patient's perceptions, experiences, and expressions associated with the health situation. *Experience* refers to the patient's raw encounter of living loaded with sensation. *Perception* is the apprehending of experience, or the ability to reflect while experiencing. *Expression* is the manifestation of experience and perception and is reflective of the human field pattern.[17] Pattern manifestation appraisal for energy field disturbances should also include particular emphasis on the appraisal of the patient's thoughts, feelings, and emotions associated with the health event. Communication patterns, sleep-wake cycles, sense of time, activity and mobility patterns, sense of comfort-discomfort, sense of awareness, sense of connectedness to the environment, sense of power or control of the situation, degree of participation in the situation, and the patient's hopes and dreams are additional areas of focus when appraising manifestations of energy field patterning. All these data assist in providing unitary information about the patient's underlying energy field pattern. The nurse's openness and sensitivity to the subtlest of cues is critical in apprehending the patient's energy field pattern.

In addition, several tools have been developed that nurses can use in pattern manifestation appraisal. Each tool was developed to be consistent with Rogers' Science of Unitary Human Beings and identifies manifestations of pattern emerging from human-environmental energy field mutual process. Wright[64] developed the Energy Field Assessment Form as a means of recording the location of the field disturbance, the strength of the field, and the intensity of the field disturbance when appraising a patient's energy field using therapeutic touch. Ference[21] developed the Human Field Motion Tool as a measure of the wave frequency pattern of the human energy field. Higher human field motion has been found to correlate with relaxation,[23,41] a sense of timelessness,[12] experiencing higher frequencies manifest in blue light,[40] and risk-taking behaviors.[38]

Barrett[4,5] developed the Power as Knowing Participation in Change Tool as a way of appraising a patient's energy field pattern in relation to his or her capacity to participate knowingly in the continuous patterning of human and environmental fields as manifest in frequencies of awareness, choice-making ability, sense of freedom to act intentionally, and degree of involvement in creating change. Barrett[2] found a significant relationship between power and human field motion and concluded that as human field motion increases, the ability to participate knowingly in change also increases. Hastings-Tolsma's Diversity of Human Field Pattern Scale[24] may be used as a means for appraising patients' perceptions of the diversity

of their energy field patterns, and Johnson's Human Image Metaphor Scale[30] can be used as a way to appraise patients' perceptions of the wholeness of their energy fields. Disturbances in energy field patterning may manifest as a low score in power, human field motion, diversity, or human field image. The nurse shares and discusses with patients the pattern manifested from the appraisal tools to facilitate their own pattern recognition, to assist their knowing participation in change, and as a means for them to identify deliberate mutual patterning strategies. A holistic assessment such as the one developed by Dossey, Keegan, Guzzetta, and Kolkmeier[19] may also be used as a means of appraising disturbances of the energy field pattern. As the Science of Unitary Human Beings evolves, additional tools will be developed as indices of the human energy field pattern.

■ Defining Characteristics

The presence of the following disharmonic energetic manifestations from a direct assessment of the energy field using therapeutic touch indicates that the patient may be experiencing Energy Field Disturbance:

Disturbances in energy field *flow*
- Congestion of energy field patterns
- Slow or rapid field patterns
- Strong or weak energy field patterns
- Pulsating to pounding frequency patterns
- Tumultuous field patterns

Disturbances in the *rhythm* of energy field patterns
- Dissonant rhythms
- Random and irregular patterns
- Arrhythmic field patterns

Imbalances of energy flow
- Temperature differentials of heat or cold
- Attraction or magnetic pull to an area
- Energy deficit or hyperactivity
- Congestion or blockage of energy flow
- Tingling or slight electrical shocks
- Pulsations or unsynchronized rhythms

The presence of the following experiences, perceptions, and expressions may reflect an underlying Energy Field Disturbance:

- Discomfort
- Anxiety
- Fear
- Anger
- Agitation
- Grief
- Dispiritedness
- Depression
- Loneliness
- Loss
- Powerlessness
- Low energy
- Disruption in sleep-awake patterns
- Disruption in time perception
- Low-frequency power as measured by the Power as Knowing Participation in Change Tool
- Low-frequency human field motion as measured by the Human Field Motion Tool
- Low-frequency diversity as measured by the Diversity of Human Field Pattern Scale
- Low-frequency human field image as measured by the Human Field Image Tool

■ **Related Factors**

The following related factors are associated with Energy Field Disturbance:

- Changes in the environmental field (specify)
- A situational crisis (specify)
- An illness or injury (specify)
- Treatment for an illness or injury (specify)
- Immobility
- Pain

DIAGNOSIS

■ **Differential Nursing Diagnosis**

The diagnosis of Energy Field Disturbance is unique. It is the first diagnosis directly linked to a specific nursing conceptual framework, the Science of Unitary Human Beings, and is the first diagnosis with a specific assessment strategy, therapeutic touch. Thus the use of this diagnosis is differentiated from other nursing diagnoses by the nurse's theoretical perspective and/or use of ther-

apeutic touch as a method of pattern appraisal and strategy for deliberative mutual patterning. Nurses basing their practice on other theoretical perspectives may use such diagnoses as Anxiety, Fear, Sleep-Pattern Disturbance, Grieving, Altered Comfort, Ineffective Breathing Patterns, Fatigue, Acute or Chronic Pain, and Powerlessness; but within an energy field perspective, these diagnoses and others are viewed and assessed as disturbances in the nature of the human-environmental energy field. Nurses practice from many different theoretical perspectives. Although the diagnosis of Energy Field Disturbance may be unconventional and controversial to some, many nurses in the United States and around the world practice therapeutic touch and/or use Rogerian Science as the framework of their practice. In addition, advances in contemporary science and philosophy provide substantial support for this emerging world view. Furthermore, numerous controlled research studies support the effectiveness of therapeutic touch.

■ **Medical and Psychiatric Diagnoses**

Energy Field Disturbance may be associated with any major or minor illness. Therapeutic touch has demonstrated effectiveness in accelerating wound healing, decreasing pain, decreasing diastolic blood pressure, and reducing hospital stress. Clinical practice has shown that therapeutic touch is particularly useful for upper respiratory tract infections, allergies, and headaches, and in the treatment of musculoskeletal conditions. Therapeutic touch has also been used in the treatment of PMS, AIDS, elevated temperatures, nausea and vomiting, chronic fatigue syndrome, seasonal affective disorders, and during labor and delivery. Many potential DSM-IV diagnoses may be associated with Energy Field Disturbance. In particular, therapeutic touch has been used in the treatment of mood disorders such as major depression and anxiety disorders, including panic disorders.[28,36,57] It is important to note that therapeutic touch is not being advocated as a substitute for more conventional assessment and treatment measures. Rather, therapeutic touch is an adjunct to other assessment and treatment measures.

I

OUTCOME IDENTIFICATION, PLANNING, AND IMPLEMENTATION (DELIBERATIVE MUTUAL PLANNING)

Patient Potentials

The Rogerian nursing practice model has been described in several articles and books concerning the use of the Science of Unitary Human Beings in nursing practice.[*] Within Rogers' Science of Unitary Human Beings, outcomes are referred to as Patient Potentials. Expected outcomes infer predictability. Rogers' principle of *helicy* states that the nature of change in the human-environmental field process is unpredictable. Rather, in an energy field perspective, nurses assist patients in actualizing their field potentials by enhancing their ability to participate knowingly in the process of change. In addition, the Rogerian practice methodology does not use the term intervention. *Intervention* means "to come, appear, or lie between two things."[1] Within an energy field perspective, the nurse and the patient are energy fields and are integral to one another. Energy fields, by definition, are infinite, continuously open, and in mutual process. Thus there is no "coming between" if the nurse and the patient are integral. In Rogerian Science, the concept of Deliberative Mutual Patterning Strategy replaces the concept of nursing intervention. Deliberative Mutual Patterning Strategy more appropriately reflects the integral and mutual relationship of the patient and the nurse. Patterning is a key word because energy fields are identified by pattern, and the term *deliberative* connotes the intentionality of the nurse's engagement with the patient.

After Pattern Manifestation Appraisal, the nurse and the patient mutually explore strategies to facilitate the actualization of the patient's desired goals.[18] There are several innovative energy-patterning strategies the nurse can use. In relation to therapeutic touch, Deliberative Mutual Patterning consists of "unruffling" the field by gently

making sweeping motions with the hands 1 to 6 inches above the body. Unruffling is done over the entire body, with concentration over areas of disturbance. Patients commonly report a sensation of relaxation during unruffling. In situations where the patient is experiencing discomfort or pain of a physical or emotional nature, unruffling may noticeably diminish these symptoms.[31] Krieger[35] believes unruffling allows patients to mobilize their own resources so that self-healing can occur.

Deliberative Mutual Patterning also includes the next phase of therapeutic touch, referred to as modulation. *Modulation* is the direct laying on of hands for 3 to 5 minutes over the identified area of energy field disturbance. During this phase, the nurse relies on imagery to conceptualize areas of imbalance and to direct the flow of energy. For example, images of flowing light or water may be directed toward an area of congestion with the intent of dissipating the congestion or smoothing the energy flow.[31] The goal is to bring balance and harmony to the areas of the field that are blocked or congested. The cues of energy change are subtle: an area that was blocked and cool becomes warm and flowing; a hot area cools down; a pulsing area may stop throbbing; and pain may quietly subside. The last phase of therapeutic touch, closure, includes reappraisal of the energy field to assure that the disturbances are no longer present. The entire process usually lasts between 15 and 20 minutes. The patient may then rest quietly for about 20 minutes.

There are many controlled research studies documenting the effectiveness of therapeutic touch. Therapeutic touch has been found to increase human hemoglobin levels,[34] induce physiological relaxation,[34] decrease anxiety,[22,26,48,49] decrease diastolic blood pressure,[50] decrease pain,[32] enhance immunologic functioning,[51] decrease the use of pain medication,[45] and accelerate wound healing.[63] The National Institutes of Health (NIH) and the recently established NIH Office of Alternative Medicine have funded several studies on therapeutic touch. Therapeutic touch is taught at beginning, intermediate, and advanced levels in continuing education programs, graduate nursing programs, and summer intensive workshops.

[*]References 3, 5, 9, 11, 16, 17, 43.

◢ NURSING CARE GUIDELINES
Nursing Diagnosis: Energy Field Disturbance

Expected Outcome (Patient Potential): The patient will report relief of experiences, perceptions, and expressions that reflect an Energy Field Disturbance.

- Prepare by centering yourself before engaging with the patient. *Centering creates a calmness and establishes a basis for a continuum of awareness throughout the nurse-patient mutual process.*
- Develop a harmonious nurse-patient mutual process by approaching the patient with openness, unconditional love, compassion, and empathy with the intention of enhancing well-being and human betterment. *A harmonious nurse-patient mutual process maximizes the patient's potential to achieve desired goals.*
- Initiate the Pattern Manifestation Appraisal by engaging in a dialogue with the patient, focusing on uncovering the patient's experiences, perceptions, and expressions concerning health-related events. *Apprehending the patient's experiences, perceptions, and expressions provides clues to the nature of Energy Field Disturbances.*
- Consider using additional Pattern Manifestation Appraisal tools such as the Human Field Motion Tool, the Power as Knowing Participation in Change Tool, the Diversity in Human Field Pattern Scale, and the Human Image Metaphor Scale. *These tools were developed as indicators of the human-environmental field mutual process and provide useful information concerning the patient's energy field patterning in relation to human field motion, knowing participation in change, diversity of the energy field, and human image.*
- Consider using therapeutic touch as a means to assess for Energy Field Disturbance. Explain the procedures and purpose of therapeutic touch and obtain verbal permission before initiating therapeutic touch. *Knowledge and choice making enhances knowing participation in change.*
- Appraise the client's energy field with your hands held 3 to 5 inches from the surface of the skin from head to toe, using smooth, light movements. *Energy fields are fundamental units of the living and the nonliving. Human beings are energy fields. Energy fields are infinite and extend beyond what is seen as the visible body.*
- Sense for cues reflecting Energy Field Disturbances such as congestion, dissonant rhythms, and temperature differentials. *Disturbances in the flow, rhythm, and balance of the energy field reflect disturbances in the human-environmental field mutual process.*
- Initiate Deliberative Mutual Patterning by unruffling and modulating the energy field. *Unruffling and modulation of the energy field pattern strengthens the coherence and the integrity of the human-environmental field by patterning areas of disturbances toward harmony.*
- Provide an opportunity for the patient to rest. *Opportunities for rest promote relaxation and peacefulness.*
- Construct a Pattern Profile of the patient's energy field pattern by writing a narrative statement describing the essence of the patient's experiences, perceptions, and expressions concerning the health situation. Share the Pattern Profile with the patient. *A Pattern Profile is an image of the patient's underlying field pattern as reflected in the patient's experiences, perceptions, and expressions revealed during the Pattern Manifestation Appraisal process. Sharing the profile with the patient provides an opportunity to verify the profile with the patient, facilitate the patient's pattern recognition, and enhance knowing participation in change.*
- Explore with the patient additional Deliberative Mutual Patterning Strategies such as music, guided imagery, meditation, exercise, dance, color, light, and fragrance. *Each of the listed Deliberative Mutual Patterning Strategies are noninvasive techniques identified within the Science of Unitary Human Beings as having potential for patterning the human-environmental energy field toward the realization of optimum well-being and human betterment.*
- Enhance the patient's involvement in creating desired changes by teaching Deliberative Mutual Patterning Strategies so the patient can use these strategies whenever desired. *Integrating wellness strategies on a continuous basis facilitates the enhancement of harmony, well-being, and human betterment.*

■ = nursing intervention (Deliberative Mutual Patterning Strategy); ▲ = collaborative intervention (Deliberative Mutual Patterning Strategy).

In addition to therapeutic touch, Rogers advocates the use of noninvasive techniques to facilitate the actualization of well-being and human betterment. Guided imagery has been used within the Rogerian system as a means to facilitate increased human field motion.[12] Ludomirski-Kalmonson[40] in a study of blue and red light demonstrated that persons experiencing the higher wave frequency pattern manifested in blue light experienced higher human field motion than persons experiencing the lower frequency red light. McDonald[44] found that women with arthritis pain experienced a greater reduction in pain when exposed to blue light than women exposed to light of other wave lengths. Interestingly, light therapy has also been very successful in the treatment of seasonal depression.[56] Other holistic modalities such as diet, exercise, meditation, and music are all energy field–patterning strategies that can be explored with patients as methods to heal energy field disturbances.[11,19,54] Rather than focusing on physiological or psychological parts, each of these strategies is a treatment modality that affects the whole person. For this reason, they are consistent with a view of persons and the environment as irreducible wholes.

EVALUATION

Evaluation is continuous. While performing therapeutic touch, the nurse is continuously evaluating for changes in the human-environmental field. Changes are new patterns emerging from the human-environmental field mutual process. Changes are revealed in the form of relief of experiences, perceptions, and expressions that were indicators of a disturbance of the energy field. When using therapeutic touch, indices of harmony include a sense of balance where there was imbalance, warmth where there was coolness or heat, synchronous rhythms where there were dissonant rhythms, and smoothness and flow of the field where there were congested or tumultuous field patterns. Expressions of relaxation, well-being, increased energy, and pain relief are indicators that may reflect a harmonious human-environmental mutual field process. In addition, the Human Field Motion Tool, the Power as Knowing Participation in Change Tool, the Diversity of Human Field Pattern Scale, and the Human Field Metaphor Scale can be administered periodically as a means of evaluating changes in the human-environmental field mutual process.

■ CASE STUDY WITH PLAN OF CARE

Ms. Martha R. has been living in the Pacific Northwest for 2 years, and this year she noticed that during the winter months she experienced much lower energy. There is a wellness clinic at the health club that M.R. usually attends and although she has not attended the health club for 2 months, she decided to make an appointment to meet with the nurse in the wellness clinic. When meeting with the nurse, the nurse and M.R. engaged in the Pattern Manifestation Appraisal process as a means to reveal M.R.'s experiences, perceptions, and expressions concerning her decreased energy. The nurse then wrote and shared with M.R. the following Pattern Profile:

"I dislike these long cloudy, rainy, and foggy Northwest days. I lived in Arizona up until 2 years ago. There was always lots of sun. I noticed last winter, and now at the beginning of this fall, that my energy level has dropped. In the summer I have lots of energy and spend time out-

doors. But now I feel dispirited. I have little energy or enthusiasm. I lose interest when it's rainy and dark. I feel tired most of the time and make excuses not to spend time with friends or go to the health club. Even my work productivity goes down. I dread getting out of bed in the dark mornings and feel like I'm dragging myself to work. In the evenings, I spend most of my time snoozing in front of the television. I've also noticed that I have more appetite and have cravings for food high in sugar. I gained back the weight I lost this past summer. I can't wait until the spring, but I'm dreading the rest of this winter."

M.R. was administered the Human Field Motion Tool and the Power as Knowing Participation in Change Tool, and her scores revealed low-frequency human field motion and low-frequency power. M.R. agreed to a session of therapeutic touch, which revealed that her energy field was generally contracted, slow, cool, blocked, and congested.

▰ PLAN OF CARE FOR MS. MARTHA R.
Nursing Diagnosis:* Energy Field Disturbance Related to Seasonal Changes

Expected Outcome (Patient Potential): M.R. will actualize her desired potentials by experiencing inspiritedness as manifested by increased energy and enthusiasm, increased productivity at work, increased physical activity, the loss of 5 pounds, and reconnection with friends.
- Encourage M.R. to reestablish her pattern of attending the health club and exercising for 30 minutes three to four times a week.
- Teach M.R. how to use visualization exercises daily that involve images of bright, sunny summer days.
- ▲ Arrange for M.R. to experience 30 minutes of 10,000 lux of light on awaking.
- Encourage M.R. to reconnect with her close friends by spending time with them on weekends and at least two evenings a week.
- Provide dietary information and teaching concerning the importance of eating regular meals that are rich in fresh vegetables and fruit and of reducing the intake of foods high in carbohydrates.
- Experience 30 minutes of therapeutic touch at least three times a week.
- Administer the Human Field Motion Tool and Power as Knowing Participation in Change Tool weekly to monitor progress toward higher wave frequency patterning of the human-environmental fields.

■ = nursing intervention (Deliberative Mutual Patterning Strategy); ▲ = collaborative intervention (Deliberative Mutual Patterning Strategy).
*Author's note: Nurses using the Science of Unitary Human Beings as a practice methodology would not make a NANDA nursing diagnosis. Rather, the Pattern Profile would serve as a guide for planning care only.

▰ CRITICAL THINKING EXERCISES

1. What are the manifestations of patterning emerging from the human-environmental mutual field process?
2. Why would light therapy, guided imagery, diet changes, exercise, and therapeutic touch be appropriate as mutual patterning strategies within Rogers' Science of Unitary Human Beings?
3. In Rogers' Science, there is no cause and effect. There is only mutual process. So how can you explain the relationship between the seasonal changes and M.R.'s mood change?

REFERENCES

1. American River Dictionary, ed 3, New York, 1992, Houghton Mifflin Co.
2. Barrett EAM: Investigation of the principle of helicy: the relationship of human field motion and power. In Malinski VM, editor: *Explorations on Martha Rogers' science of unitary human beings*, Norwalk, Connecticut, 1986, Appleton-Century-Crofts.
3. Barrett EAM: Using Rogers' science of unitary human beings in nursing practice, *Nurs Sci Quart* 1:50–51, 1988.
4. Barrett EAM: A nursing theory of power for nursing practice: derivation from Rogers' paradigm. In Riehl-Sisca J, editor: *Conceptual models for nursing practice*, ed 3, Norwalk, Connecticut, 1989, Appleton-Century-Crofts.
5. Barrett EAM: Health patterning with clients in a private practice environment. In Barrett EAM, editor: *Visions of Rogers' science-based practice*, New York, 1990, National League for Nursing.
6. Becker RO and Selden G: *The body electric: electromagnetism and the foundation of life*, New York, 1985, Quill/William Morrow & Co.
7. Bohm D: *Wholeness and the implicate order*, London, 1980, Routledge and Kegan Paul.
8. Burr HS: *The fields of life: our links with the universe*, New York, 1972, Ballantine Books.
9. Butcher HK: Kaleidoscoping in life's turbulence: from Seurat's art to Rogers' nursing science. In Parker ME, editor: *Patterns of nursing theories in practice*, New York, 1993, National League for Nursing.
10. Butcher HK: A unitary field pattern portrait of dispiritedness in later life, doctoral dissertation, Columbia, South Carolina, 1994, University of South Carolina.
11. Butcher HK and McFarland GK: Conceptual frameworks for psychiatric mental health nursing practice. In McFarland GK and Thomas MD, editors: *Psychiatric mental health nursing: application of the nursing process*, Philadelphia, 1991, JB Lippincott Co.
12. Butcher HK and Parker NI: Guided imagery within Rogers' science of unitary human beings: an experimental study, *Nurs Sci Quart* 1:103–110, 1988.

13. Capra F: *The tau of physics,* New York, 1977, Bantam Books.

14. Capra F: *The turning point: science, society, and the rising culture,* New York, 1982, Bantam Books.

15. Caprk M: *The philosophical impact of contemporary physics,* Princeton, 1961, D Van Nostrand.

16. Cowling WR III: A template for unitary pattern-based nursing practice. In Barrett EAM, editor: *Visions of Rogers' science-based nursing,* New York, 1990, National League for Nursing.

17. Cowling WR III: Unitary knowing in nursing practice, *Nurs Sci Quart* 2:201–207, 1993.

18. Cowling WR III: Unitary practice: revisionary assumptions. In Parker ME, editor: *Patterns of nursing theories in practice,* New York, 1993, National League for Nursing.

19. Dossey B, Keegan L, Guzzetta C, and Kolkmeier, L: *Holistic nursing: a handbook for practice,* ed 2, Gaithersburg, Maryland, 1995, Aspen Publishers, Inc.

20. Einstein A: *The principle of relativity,* New York, 1923, Dorer.

21. Ference HF: The relationship of time experience, creativity traits, differentiation, and human field motion: an empirical investigation of Rogers' correlates of synergistic human development, doctoral dissertation, New York, 1979, New York University.

22. Gagne D and Toyne RC: The effects of therapeutic touch and relaxation therapy in reducing anxiety, *Arch Psych Nurs* 3(3):184–189, 1994.

23. Gueldner SH: The relationship between imposed motion and human field motion in elderly individuals living in nursing homes. In Malinski V, editor: *Explorations on Martha Rogers' science of unitary human beings,* Norwalk, Connecticut, 1986, Appleton-Century-Crofts.

24. Hastings-Tolsma M: The relationship of diversity of human field pattern to risk-taking and time experience, doctoral dissertation, New York, 1993, New York University.

25. Hawking SJ: *A brief history of time,* New York, 1988, Bantam Books.

26. Heidt P: Effect of therapeutic touch on anxiety level of hospitalized patients, *Nurs Research* 30(1):32–37, 1981.

27. Herbert N: *Quantum reality: beyond the new physics: an excursion into the metaphysics and the meaning of reality,* New York, 1985, Anchor Books.

28. Hover-Kramer D: *Healing touch: a resource for health care professionals,* San Francisco, 1996, Delmar Publishers.

29. Hunt V, Massey W, Weinberg R, Bruyere R, and Hahn P: *Project report, a study of structural integration from neuromuscular, energy field, and emotional approaches,* UCLA, 1977.

30. Johnson LW: The development of the human field image metaphor scale, *Dissertation Abstracts International* 54(5):1890-B, 1993.

31. Jurgens A, Meehan TC, and Wilson HL: Therapeutic touch as a nursing intervention, *Holistic Nurs Prac* 2(1):1–13, 1987.

32. Keller E and Bzdek VM: Effects of therapeutic touch on tension headache pain, *Nurs Research* 35(2):101–105, 1986.

33. Kirlian S and Kirlian V: Photographic and visual observation by means of high frequency currents, *J Sci App Photography* 6:397–403, 1961.

34. Krieger D: The response of in vivo human hemoglobin to an active healing therapy by laying on hands, *Human Dimensions* 1:12–15, 1972.

35. Krieger D: *The therapeutic touch: how to use your hands to help or heal,* Englewood Cliffs, New Jersey, 1979, Prentice-Hall.

36. Krieger D: *Accepting your power to heal: the personal practice of therapeutic touch,* Santa Fe, New Mexico, 1993, Bear & Company Publishing.

37. Kunz D and Peper E: Fields and their implications. In Kunz D: *Spiritual aspects of the healing arts,* Wheaton, Illinois, 1985, Theosophical Publishing House.

38. Lindley PA: An empirical study of the relationship of sensation seeking to the human energy field motion within Rogers' science of unitary human beings, master's thesis, Rochester, New York, 1981, University of Rochester.

39. Lionberger H: An interpretive study of nurses' practice of therapeutic touch. *Dissertation Abstracts International* 46:2624-b, 1985.

40. Ludomirski-Kalmonson B: The relationship between the environmental energy wave frequency pattern manifest in red light and blue light and human field motion in adult individuals with visual sensory perception and those with total blindness, doctoral dissertation, New York, 1983, New York University.

41. Macrae J: A comparison between meditating subjects and non-meditating subjects on time experience and human field motion, doctoral dissertation, New York, 1983, New York University.

42. Macrae J: *Therapeutic touch: a practical guide,* New York, 1987, Alfred A Knopf.

43. Madrid M and Barrett EAM, editors: *Rogers' scientific art of nursing practice,* New York, 1994, National League for Nursing.

44. McDonald S: The relationship between visible lightwaves and the experience of pain. In Malinski V, editor: *Explorations on Martha Rogers' science of unitary human beings,* Norwalk, Connecticut, 1986, Appleton-Century-Crofts.

45. Meehan TC: The science of unitary human beings and theory-based practice: therapeutic touch. In Barrett EAM, editor: *Visions of Rogers' science-based nursing,* New York, 1990, National League for Nursing.

46. Moss T, Hubacher J, and Saba F: Kirlian photography: visual evidence of bioenergetic interactions between people? In Dean SR, editor: *Psychiatry & Mysticism,* Chicago, 1975, Nelson-Hall Publishers.

47. Motoyama H: A biophysical elucidation of the meridian and ki-energy, *Int Assoc Religion Parapsych* 7(1):1981.

48. Olson M and Sneed N: Anxiety and therapeutic touch, *Iss Mental Health Nurs* 16: 97–108, 1995.

49. Quinn JF: Therapeutic touch as energy exchange: testing the theory, *Adv Nurs Sci* 6(2):42–49, 1984.

50. Quinn JF: Therapeutic touch as energy exchange: replication and extension, *Nurs Sci Quart* 2:79–87, 1989.

51. Quinn JF and Stelkauskas A: Psychoimmunologic effects of therapeutic touch on practitioners and recently bereaved recipients: a pilot study, *Adv Nurs Sci* 15(4):13–26, 1993.

52. Ravitz LJ: Bioelectric correlates of emotional states, *Conn State Med J* 16:499–505, 1952.

53. Rogers ME: *An introduction to the theoretical basis for nursing,* Philadelphia, 1970, FA Davis Co.

54. Rogers ME: Nursing science and art: a prospective, *Nurs Sci Quart* 1:99–102, 1988.

55. Rogers ME: Nursing science in the space age, *Nurs Sci Quart* 5:27–37, 1992.

56. Rosenthal N and Blehar MC: *Seasonal affective disorders and phototherapy,* New York, 1989, Gilford Press.

57. Sayre-Adams J and Wright S: *The theory and practice of therapeutic touch,* Edinburgh, 1995, Churchill Livingstone.

58. Sheldrake R: *The presence of the past: morphic resonance and the habits of nature,* New York, 1988, Times Books.

59. Sherman RA, Barja RH, and Bruno GM: Thermographic correlates of chronic pain: an analysis of 125 patients incorporating evaluations by a blind panel, *Arch Phys Med Rehab* 68:273–279, 1987.

60. Uricchio J: Thermography: the clinical use of thermography in orthopedic practice, *Postgrad Med* March:62–64, 1986.

61. Weinstein SA and Weinstein G: A clinical comparison of cervical thermography with EMG, CT scanning, myelography and surgical procedures in 500 patients, *Postgrad Med* March:40–44, 1986.

62. White J and Kripper S: *Future science,* New York, 1977, Anchor Books.

63. Wirth D: The effects of non-contract therapeutic touch on the healing rate of full thickness dermal wounds, *Subtle energies* 1(1):1–20, 1990.

64. Wright SM: Validity of the human energy field assessment form, *Western J Nurs Research* 13:635–647, 1991.

65. Zukav G: *The dancing wu-li masters,* New York, 1979, Bantam Books.

Altered Health Maintenance

Altered Health Maintenance *is the inability to identify, manage, and/or seek out help to maintain health.*[6]

OVERVIEW

There is an established pattern of behaviors that do not support health maintenance. The person may be unable to identify factors that contribute to Altered Health Maintenance because of knowledge deficits, cognitive limitations, or mental impairments. Altered Health Maintenance may also occur when the person has the knowledge but not the resources or opportunity to manage or seek out help because of socioeconomic barriers such as poverty. Altered Health Maintenance is not the result of an individual's lack of motivation.

Few diagnostic categories fall so clearly within the scope of nursing practice as does Altered Health Maintenance. Tripp and Stachowiak[11] contrast health maintenance with health promotion. Health maintenance is primarily a static state, one that defends or protects against disease and is not oriented toward wellness or health promotion. The goal of health maintenance is neutral health or health protection—traditionally a major focus in nursing practice. However, a shift toward health promotion and wellness is nursing's future.

Donley[3] projects that the new health care environment will include more persons being covered by health insurance—primarily mothers and children, many of whom are minorities, immigrants, and children living in single-parent families. This primary and preventive care initiative may provide services to underserved persons with health problems such as infectious diseases, inadequate immunizations, and poor prenatal care. More favorable U.S. health statistics for prenatal care have already been reported. "In 1992, 78 percent of mothers received prenatal care in the first trimester of pregnancy, the highest level ever recorded."[12] However, racial and ethnic disparities continue to exist, with the lowest percentage of prenatal care provided to American Indian, Mexican-American, and black women.[12]

By the year 2000, people over age 65 will represent an estimated 13% of the population of the United States, in contrast to 8% in 1950.[13] This trend is predicted to continue as a result of an increase in life expectancy at birth. In 1992 the average life expectancy at birth for males was 75.8 years, a record high, with a life expectancy at birth for females of 79.1 years.[12] As the aged population grows, so does the demand for nurses who are educated in and informed of the needs of the elderly.

The nursing diagnosis of Altered Health Maintenance is not limited to the elderly. In 1993 health care accounted for 13.9% of the gross domestic product (GDP) in the United States (up from 9.3% in 1980), compared to 10.3% in Canada, 8.7% in Germany, and 6.9% in Japan.[12] Despite significantly higher health expenditures, positive health outcomes lag behind those in many other developed countries. For instance, "in 1991 the infant mortality rate in Japan was one half that of the United States."[12]

According to *Health United States 1994*,[12] "The percent of Americans who have no health insurance has been increasing. The age-adjusted percent of persons under the age of 65 who were not covered by health insurance increased from 12.5% in 1980 to 17.3% in 1993." The age group most likely to be uninsured were those 15 to 44 years of age. Data from the 1992 National Health Interview Survey (NHIS)[5] indicate that "people who have a specific source of ongoing primary care show a slight decline from the 1986 baseline as a whole and for blacks, Hispanics, and people with low incomes." Clearly the overall state of health and health care practices in the United States is not favorable. Significant to nurses is that these trends indicate that vulnerable populations with inadequate access to basic primary care and preventive services will continue to experience Altered Health Maintenance. Individuals will likely turn to the self-care mode of health care treatment.

The increased personal responsibility for one's own health can render positive outcomes relative to wellness, given adequate resources such as education and support to maintain an acceptable level of health. In reality, vulnerable populations in lower socioeconomic groups, minorities, women and children, and the elderly may not have access to information and services to assist them. Nurses are often the most appropriate persons to manage individuals and populations who experience Altered Health Maintenance.

A relatively new model for care delivery is that of population-based managed care (PBMC),[8] which focuses on improving care for groups of patients or subpopulations with common health care needs. One criterion for the use of PBMC is that the clinical condition responds to preventive measures. Altered Health Maintenance may in the future become a community diagnosis. Interventions for group or population-based health alterations may be determined through participatory action research (PAR)[7]—"a combination of community participation, research, and action that supports local insights and abilities regarding the resolution of community issues." Issues commonly identified are alcohol and tobacco use, exercise, mental health, and dietary choices—each strongly associated with Altered Health Maintenance. The goal is to enhance self-care measures, to strengthen existing skills, and to develop new self-care competencies.

Responsibility for health maintenance falls primarily on adults because they usually care for themselves and are legally bound to care for dependent children. However, Altered Health Maintenance is an appropriate diagnosis for minors who exhibit defining characteristics such as lack of adequate immunizations, frequent infections, or inadequate accident prevention practices such as using bike helmets and seat belts. After diagnosing Altered Health Maintenance, the nurse intervenes by counseling and teaching the responsible adult or minor.

Altered Health Maintenance was accepted by NANDA as a diagnosis suitable for study and testing in 1982,[6] yet little research has been done on assessment, interventions, or evaluation of interventions. Swehla[10] conducted a descriptive study to identify nursing diagnoses of 100 gynecologic ambulatory-care patients. The most frequent diagnosis was practicing preventative health care and maintenance (17%). This label was derived from several defining characteristics, some of them similar to those from Altered Health Maintenance as described by NANDA. The focus on positive rather than negative health behaviors has applications for nursing in the future as nursing diagnoses become more oriented toward wellness. Boynton[2] describes the use of Altered Health Maintenance as a nursing diagnosis of the elderly in community settings. She emphasizes that the idea behind the diagnosis "is not to solve the problems of clients but to help them solve their own . . . and intervention by the nurse seeks a balance between the extremes of interference and neglect."

Although often considered a nursing diagnosis most appropriate for the community setting, Altered Health Maintenance is not frequently found in documentation of retrospective chart reviews. One study conducted by Zink[14] examined the relationship between nursing diagnosis documentation in home care and select patient and visit variables. Out of a sample of 199 records and 269 initial nursing diagnoses, Altered Health Maintenance was not identified among the 10 most frequently cited diagnoses. Perhaps one reason may be the broad scope of the diagnosis. Nurses favor specificity. Third-party reimbursement of services requires specificity. Any documentation that could be interpreted as vague and nondescript may be rejected as a billable visit—something nurses are keenly aware of in today's health care reimbursement environment.

ASSESSMENT

Assessment in the Health-Perception—Health-Management Pattern begins with determining how an individual perceives his or her health. Health must also be viewed within the context of family and community values. Presumptions made about a patient's culture may lead to a misdiagnosis of an actual problem or the identification of a "problem" that is simply an ethnic variant. An individual's behavior and beliefs must be assessed within the context of their culture and value system.

Care must also be taken to avoid misinterpreting subjective and objective data as defining characteristics of this nursing diagnosis. For example, if a patient arrives in the hospital for a PTCA and states, "They say I've got a little heart trouble, but you know, a guy can't live forever and you got to die from something," several questions need to be answered to make an accurate nursing diagnosis. Without further clarification, it may first appear that the patient is denying his illness, lacks knowledge regarding his illness, or believes that he has little control of his health. To conclude a diagnosis of Denial or Knowledge Deficit would be premature. A more focused assessment relative to his statement must be done. Additional interviewing may validate his casual attitude as a coping mechanism that compensates for his overwhelming fear of being hospitalized for a potentially life-threatening condition. Isolated cues or responses may initially be misleading and result in an incorrect nursing diagnosis.

▪ Defining Characteristics

The presence of the following characteristics indicates that the patient may be experiencing Altered Health Maintenance:

- Frequent infections, anorexia, obesity, headaches, or malaise

- Poor diet
- Lack of adequate immunizations
- Needs for alcohol, drugs, or tobacco
- Emotional fragility or behavior disorders
- Verbalization of inaccurate information
- Inability to take responsibility for basic health practices
- Impairment of adaptive behavior
- Inadequate accident prevention practices
- Lack of knowledge regarding health
- Failure to manage stress
- Lack of equipment, finances, and/or other resources
- Lack of adequate housing
- Illiteracy

▪ Related Factors

The following related factors are associated with Altered Health Maintenance:

- Lack of gross and/or fine motor skills
- Unachieved developmental skills
- Inability to make judgments
- Inadequate information
- Failure to practice age-related preventive practices
- Lack of perceived threat to health
- Perceptual or cognitive impairment
- Poor learning skills
- Ineffective coping (individual or family)
- Emotional difficulties
- Failure to assume responsibility for primary prevention
- Alteration in communication skills
- Loss of independence
- Inadequate resources
- Changing support systems
- Lack of access to health care services
- Disabling spiritual distress
- Dysfunctional grieving

DIAGNOSIS

▪ Differential Nursing Diagnosis

Defining characteristics appropriate to more than one nursing diagnosis will raise questions regarding which diagnostic label is the most accurate in describing the condition or situation the patient is experiencing. Differentiating among diagnoses requires examination of all of the defining characteristics. The nurse may have to ask, "Which defining characteristics are the most predominant and relevant to the individual's experience?" For example, Knowledge Deficit is the absence or deficiency of cognitive information.[6] This is frequently present in Altered Health Maintenance, so the question arises as to which nursing diagnosis is "best." Consider why Altered Health Maintenance is listed under Pattern 6: Moving of the NANDA classification. If it were listed under Pattern 8: Knowing, the scope of the problem of Altered Health Maintenance would be limited only to Knowledge Deficit. Human behaviors related to health maintenance are far more complex and must be evaluated from a holistic viewpoint. An individual may not have sufficient information related to a specific topic such as the required childhood immunizations; however, other significant social, economic, cultural, and emotional factors may be present that would rule out the nursing diagnosis of Knowledge Deficit.

Another nursing diagnosis often associated with Altered Health Maintenance is Ineffective Individual Coping. The definition is "impairment of adaptive behaviors and problem-solving abilities of a person in meeting life's demands and roles."[6] Impaired coping, as a defining characteristic of Altered Health Maintenance, pertains more specifically to health maintenance issues rather than difficulty in meeting life's responsibilities in general. Both diagnoses, however, predispose the person to illness and accidents, and a more focused assessment of the person's ability to solve problems will help the nurse differentiate between the two. The person's ability to solve problems is more severely impaired or absent in Ineffective Individual Coping.

Ineffective Management of Therapeutic Regimen (Individuals) was added to the NANDA list in 1992. It is a "pattern of regulating and integrating into daily living a program for treatment of illness and the sequelae of illness that are unsatisfactory for meeting specific health goals."[6] Similar to Altered Health Maintenance, it includes a pattern of behaviors that do not support the attainment of health goals. However, one difference is that Altered Health Maintenance does not generally apply to persons who are following a specified therapeutic regimen or prevention program. The major defining characteristic of Ineffective Management of Therapeutic Regimen (Individuals) is that the person makes choices in daily living that are ineffective for meeting treatment goals.[6] Intent to choose an unhealthy behavior is not always present in Altered Health Maintenance.

■ Medical and Psychiatric Diagnoses

Altered Health Maintenance may be associated with several medical and psychiatric diagnoses. Acute trauma may result from unnecessary risk-taking behavior such as driving under the influence of alcohol or drugs. *Alcohol dependence*, according to the DSM-IV,[1] is a physiological dependence on alcohol resulting in tolerance to increasing amounts of alcohol or symptoms of withdrawal when abstaining from alcohol. Because symptoms of alcohol withdrawal are so unpleasant, the individual may continue to drink to relieve the symptoms, thus being at an even higher risk for falls and serious accidents. Cognitive symptoms of dementia such as disorientation, apathy, poor concentration, and memory loss are associated with Altered Health Maintenance because the individual may not be aware of even the most basic needs for fluid and nutrition. Major depressive disorder,[1] both single episode and recurrent, is characterized by many of the behaviors associated with dementia and may also inhibit an individual's ability to manage personal health needs. Dementia of the Alzheimer's type[1] has a gradual onset with a continuing cognitive decline. Because of its gradual progression, Altered Health Maintenance should be anticipated so that support and services are provided when appropriate. Anorexia nervosa[1] is suspected if the individual fails to make expected weight gains and has a misperception of body shape and size. Anorexia nervosa may result in anemia, impaired renal function, cardiovascular problems, dental problems, and osteoporosis. Most of the related medical and psychiatric diagnoses are complex, chronic conditions that may never be completely resolved even with the most aggressive treatment. Ongoing collaboration among the multidisciplinary health teams, both during hospitalization and after discharge, is critical for affecting favorable patient outcomes.

OUTCOME IDENTIFICATION, PLANNING, AND IMPLEMENTATION

In planning care for the individual with Altered Health Maintenance, the nurse and the patient and family should begin by discussing the long-term goal relative to the patient's perception of what constitutes an acceptable level of health. An understanding of the patient's cultural traditions and values can profoundly affect the nurse-patient relationship. For example, if the nurse identifies the need for the patient to be referred to an adult day care center for socialization purposes, but the patient prefers to remain at home during the day, a conflict will result. Leininger[4] stresses that nurses must look beyond the physiological needs of patients and focus on the aspects of their lifeways, living conditions, stresses, and concerns that are transculturally based. Placed in the context of what the patient and family believe to be reasonable and expected, the nurse, the patient, and the family should discuss options for discharge referrals. Open dialogue about the services available to them will help the patient and family define expectations and prevent misunderstandings. Social Services may need to be consulted to discuss the details of the patient's community, social, and financial resources.

An expected patient outcome is the verbalization of the need for appropriate referrals. The nursing strategy to achieve this outcome includes further assessment of the patient's home situation.

Data to be collected include the patient's ability to care for personal needs; the patient's functional status, current medications, and treatments; follow-up appointments; and the availability of caregivers to assist the patient. The physical layout of the home should be discussed; the presence and number of steps and the location of rooms relative to the patient's needs and abilities should be noted. A prompt referral to Social Services after the diagnosis of Altered Health Maintenance is suspected assists in the planning process. Asking questions related to the concerns or worries the patient may have helps to individualize the plan of care based on what the patient identifies as a priority. Sometimes unrealistic patient expectations are identified, and the nurse may need to address the realities as they relate to health maintenance. For instance, if a patient living alone is not able to drive, the nurse should inquire as to how the patient will get to scheduled appointments or therapies.

The second expected outcome in the Nursing Care Guidelines is that the patient will actively participate in the decision-making process regarding determination of appropriate support services. Possible exceptions to using this outcome would be situations where a patient may be reluctant because of cultural norms or values to assume responsibility for decision making. Negotiation may be necessary to reach agreement on a mutually acceptable level of patient participation relative to discharge planning. It is important to realize that the "team approach" is not a universally accepted concept among all people. After the level of patient involvement is determined, specific information about the services to be provided must be given to the patient and family in writing to assure legal and professional accountability. The patient's record must show evidence that the appropriate interventions and patient education materials were provided. Regulatory agencies may also require that documentation reflects collaboration and coordination of planning efforts among members of the multidisciplinary health care team.

◢ NURSING CARE GUIDELINES
Nursing Diagnosis: Altered Health Maintenance Related to Lack of Adequate Resources/ Materials Necessary for Discharge Home

Expected Outcome: The patient will verbalize the need for assistance in obtaining appropriate referrals —if hospitalized, within 2 days of hospital discharge and, if at home, by the second home visit.

▲ Address specific issues related to health maintenance: the patient's ability to care for personal needs, ambulatory status, medication therapy, follow-up treatment, and the availability of friends or family to assist the patient. *This engages the patient in assessment of his or her needs and establishes collaboration between the patient and the multidisciplinary team.*

■ Discuss the physical layout of the home, noting the presence and the number of steps and the location of rooms in relation to the patient's present needs and functional ability. *This further assists the patient in the problem identification phase of decision making.*

■ Discuss the community, social, and financial services available through Social Services. *Social Services is the discipline with expertise in professional and community services.*

▲ Encourage the patient to verbalize concerns regarding health maintenance. *This enables the multidisci-plinary team to prioritize interventions based on the patient's perceptions. Teaching interventions can address items identified as concerns or problems by the patient.*

■ Discuss any inconsistencies between what the patient has or has not identified as health maintenance needs and the ability for self-care. *This helps the patient anticipate needs and make realistic and safe plans. This also gives the nurse an understanding of the patient's perception of his or her capabilities so that the patient's strengths can be maximized. A positive outcome expectancy is an attribute of optimism that "nurses can expect to have an impact on health-related behaviors, such as health-promotion activi-ties, attentiveness to symptoms, and likelihood of seeking health care."[9]*

Expected Outcome: The patient will actively participate in the decision-making process in determining appropriate support services—if in hospital, within 2 days of discharge and, if at home, by the second home visit.

▲ Communicate the expectation that the patient and family will be involved in decision making as appro-priate within cultural norms and expressed wishes. *This establishes a team approach to discharge plan-ning with the patient and family as active participants. Also, early communication of clear expectations helps prevent misunderstandings that may jeopardize a therapeutic relationship between the patient and family and the multidisciplinary discharge team.*

▲ Discuss the services that may be necessary such as meal preparation, Durable Medical Equipment (DME), and professional nursing services. *This provides the patient and family with specific information regarding the services they can expect following discharge.*

▲ Coordinate all referrals. *Miscommunications regarding specific needs can easily occur. The patient is then placed at risk for not having adequate supplies or services.*

▲ Provide the patient and family with a written discharge plan regarding medications to be taken, all refer-rals, and supplies. Include a date when they can expect services to begin, and provide the telephone number of their contact. *Written discharge instructions are a legal and professional responsibility.*

▲ Document all plans in the patient's medical record. *Written discharge instruction in the permanent record are a legal and professional responsibility.*

■ = nursing intervention; ▲ = collaborative intervention.

EVALUATION

Evaluation determines the effectiveness of the nursing interventions. The predicted changes specified in the expected patient outcomes are reviewed. Have the specific contributing factors of Altered Health Maintenance been reduced or eliminated? Ideally the expected patient outcomes are accomplished and the problem is resolved, but in actual practice some changes in the plan of care will most likely be needed, especially when the problem is complex and multidimensional.

Evaluation of the expected patient outcome that the patient will identify the need for assistance in obtaining appropriate referrals is usually accomplished by listening to the patient and family to determine if they agree with the referrals previously discussed. Sometimes negotiation among the patient, nurse, physician, social worker, and other health professionals is needed when the plan is not mutually acceptable. The ultimate goal is to maintain a safe environment for the patient. However, there may be a fine line between the patient's desire for independence and his or her safety. The nurse best evaluates the patient's active participation in the decision-making process when making plans for assistance by observing the patient's behavior and level of involvement.

◤ CASE STUDY WITH PLAN OF CARE

Mr. Marty M. is brought into the emergency department of a large city hospital. His friend tells the triage nurse that Mr. M.'s cough has become much worse in the last few days, and therefore he is unable to work. His friend reports, "Marty just isn't himself; he's lying around a lot and won't eat much either." Mr. M. was reluctant to seek medical attention, but his friend insisted. He is admitted to the hospital to rule out a diagnosis of upper respiratory infection, tuberculosis, anemia, or malnutrition. The patient's chief complaint is: "I get so tired these days, I can't catch my breath after walking a little bit. I can't work when I feel this bad, and lately my cough is worse. Maybe I just need some vitamins or something." The medical history indicates that Mr. M. drinks approximately four to six beers per day, and he has smoked one pack of cigarettes per day for 41 years. He was hospitalized 5 years before with acute GI bleeding and was told that he had the "start" of emphysema. He was advised to stop smoking and drinking. Mr.

M. has been divorced for 15 years. He has four adult children, none of whom he has seen or heard from in over 5 years. He lives in a boarding house and works as a temporary unskilled laborer for various local construction companies. If work is available, Mr. M. usually works 30 hours a week. He explains, "I make enough to live on," but admits that he worries about the time when he will be unable to work. He and his friends from the boarding house frequently get together to play cards or drink beer at a nearby tavern. When he is not working, Mr. M. usually stays around the lounge of the boarding house to watch television or visit with the other residents. A physical examination determines that Mr. M. is an alert 59-year-old white male with a blood pressure of 128/88 mm Hg, temperature of 100.2°F, pulse of 96 beats/min and regular, respirations of 32/min and shallow, productive cough of brownish colored sputum, coarse, moist breath sounds on auscultation, height of 5'8", weight of 132 pounds, and stool negative for blood.

◤ PLAN OF CARE FOR MR. MARTY M.
Nursing Diagnosis: Altered Health Maintenance Related to Lack of Perceived Threat to Health

---

Expected Outcome: Mr. M. will identify behaviors that contribute to an alteration in health maintenance.
- Discuss with Mr. M. his perception of his current health status, such as his diminished functional ability.
- Clarify misunderstandings or misinformation regarding probable reasons for his deteriorating health.

■ = nursing intervention; ▲ = collaborative intervention.

- Help Mr. M. examine the factors in his life that may contribute to acute or chronic illness. Initiate a tuberculosis history.
- Use active listening and encourage Mr. M. to verbalize his feelings about making a decision to change his lifestyle.

Expected Outcome: Mr. M. will verbalize the desire to participate in a health maintenance process to reduce or eliminate risk factors (alcohol and tobacco use and inadequate calorie intake).
- Assist Mr. M. in setting realistic and attainable short- and long-term goals, such as smoking one less cigarette per day.
- Help Mr. M. assess personal strengths and weaknesses.
- Discuss possible ways of using personal strengths to enhance health maintenance efforts.
- Explore with Mr. M. methods to modify the behaviors that impede health maintenance.
- Provide Mr. M. with emotional support and encouragement in making his own decisions.

Expected Outcome: Mr. M. will demonstrate the ability to manage health maintenance as evidenced by his participation in choosing appropriate referrals during hospitalization.
- Obtain referrals for social work and nutritional consultation.
- Communicate with contacts from all referrals to coordinate the plan of care and to support Mr. M.'s efforts to change his lifestyle.
- Provide Mr. M. with referrals to appropriate community resources such as public health services, veterans assistance, and local self-help groups.

Expected Outcome: Mr. M. will identify probable future health maintenance needs before hospital discharge.
- Help Mr. M. establish a self-monitoring follow-up plan to include a social support network.
- Reinforce the benefits of maintaining or improving health status (i.e., the ability to remain employed and live independently).

■■ CRITICAL THINKING EXERCISES

1. List Mr. M.'s strengths and limitations that support and impede his ability to manage his health adequately.
2. Excluding Altered Health Maintenance, discuss two other nursing diagnoses that may be appropriate for Mr. M.
3. Describe two questions to include in a focused assessment relative to a more individualized plan of care.
4. Mr. M. is found reading his bedside chart and he asks, "What is this thing I have called Altered Health Maintenance?" In layman's terms, how would you describe this nursing diagnosis to Mr. M.?

REFERENCES

1. American Psychiatric Association: *Diagnostic and statistical manual for mental disorders,* ed 4, Washington, D.C., 1994, The Association.
2. Boynton P: Health maintenance alteration: a nursing diagnosis of the elderly, *Clin Nurse Spec* 3(1):5–10, 1989.
3. Donley SR: Advanced practice nursing after health care reform, *Nurs Econ* 13(2):84–88, 1995.
4. Leininger M: Transcultural nursing education: a worldwide imperative, *Nursing & Health Care* 15(5):254–257, 1994.
5. National Center for Health Statistics: *Healthy People 2000 Review, 1993.* Hyattsville, Maryland, 1994, Public Health Service, pp. 139–140.
6. North American Nursing Diagnosis Association: *NANDA nursing diagnoses: definitions and classification, 1995–1996,* Philadelphia, 1994, The Association.
7. Rains J and Ray D: Participatory action research for community health promotion, *Pub Health Nurs* 12(4):256–261, 1995.

I

8. Shamansky SL: A longer-than-usual editorial about population-based managed care, *Pub Health Nurs* 12(4):211–212, 1995.

9. Stubblefield C: Optimism: a determinant of health behavior, *Nurs Forum* 30(1):19–24, 1995.

10. Swehla M: Identifying and validating nursing diagnoses in a gynecologic ambulatory-care setting, *JOGNN* 19(5):439–447, 1989.

11. Tripp SL and Stachowiak B: Health maintenance, health promotion: is there a difference, *Pub Health Nurs* 9(3):155–161, 1992.

12. U.S. Department of Health and Human Services: *Health United States 1994*, Department of Health and Human Services Pub No PHS 95-1232, Washington, D.C., 1995, U.S. Government Printing Office.

13. U.S. Department of Health and Human Services: *Healthy people 2000: national health promotion and disease prevention objectives*, Department of Health and Human Services Pub No PHS 91-50213, Washington, D.C., 1991, U.S. Government Printing Office.

14. Zink M: Nursing diagnosis in home care: audit tool development, *J Com Health Nurs* 11(1):51–58, 1994.

Health-Seeking Behaviors (Specify)

Health-Seeking Behaviors (Specify) *is the state in which a client with stable health actively seeks ways to alter personal health habits and/or the environment to achieve optimal health.*

OVERVIEW

Ellis[10] notes that although promoting human health has always been a goal of nursing, the concept of "health" is only gradually developing importance as more emphasis is placed on the health of individuals, families, groups, and communities. To work with clients who wish to strive toward optimal health, an understanding of health, health promotion, and factors related to the adoption of positive personal health habits is essential.

To date, the nursing literature offers no consensus definition of *health*. The nurse theorists' definitions of health differ and include stability,[20] adaptation,[15,28] wholeness or integrity,[22] and functional independence.[14] Health is also defined as a resource for everyday living.[11,23] Smith[29] identified four models of health: (1) the eudaemonistic model, in which health is self-actualization, (2) the adaptive model, in which health is flexible adaptation to the environment, (3) role performance, in which health is the ability to carry out social roles, and (4) the clinical model, in which health is the absence of signs or symptoms of disease or disability. When Smith's four models of health[29] are used to examine a client's progression toward health, the eudaemonistic model seems to most strongly espouse the client's potential to achieve total well-being. In the adaptive model, a need to gain or maintain stability motivates the person. In the role performance model, a need to gain mastery over a specific set of skills motivates the person. In the clinical model, prevention of disease motivates the person.

Stachtchenko and Jenicek[30] differentiate between health promotion and disease prevention. They note that reducing the risk of disease is the basis of disease prevention, whereas increasing well-being is the basis for health promotion. The essential aspects of health promotion include enabling the development of positive change in lifestyle behaviors and political action directed at creating "healthy" policy.[30] Other authors concur that health promotion focuses on well-being and use terms such as "actualization"[25,26] and "high-level wellness"[32] to define health promotion. Perhaps for nursing, the concept of health promotion as the process of enabling people to increase control over and improve their health[23] provides the clearest direction.

Meleis[19] notes that because nursing is practiced in many different clinical areas and in many different countries, each with its own cultural patterns, many definitions of health are required. In current literature, optimal health or wellness is defined as being unique to each client and dependent on his or her definition of health.[17] The uniqueness occurs because each person constantly interacts with the environment, and the relationship between the client and the environment (including family, peers, and the community) will affect the choice of a definition of health and the choice of health behaviors.[18]

Laffrey[17] emphasizes that although health is now viewed as a human right, individuals should assume the responsibility for their own health. Nurses can work as partners with clients while

I

assisting them to achieve health. The nurse's role in this partnership should include understanding the client's current definition of health and, when necessary, providing information about other dimensions of health, which may help the client to reach his or her potential.

Some health behaviors that affect health have been the focus of research studies. To date, research has mainly focused on health behaviors that significantly affect mortality. Breslow and Enstrom[7] studied seven health practices: never having smoked cigarettes, regular physical activity, moderate or no use of alcohol, 7 to 8 hours of sleep per day, maintaining proper weight, eating breakfast, and not eating between meals. The number of these health practices was inversely related to age-adjusted mortality rates. Belloc[6] found that five practices—smoking, weight control, drinking, hours of sleep, regularity of meals, and physical activity—also were inversely related to age-adjusted mortality rates. The link of smoking with lung cancer is well substantiated, and many authorities describe smoking as North America's greatest health risk. In developing a health habits scale, Williams and others[31] found smoking to be independent of other health behaviors. They concluded that health habits may not form a unitary construct.

A variety of social and psychological models have been proposed to describe the various factors associated with health-related behaviors.[1,2,4,5,26] Attitudes and beliefs are prominent factors in these models, along with factors such as self-efficacy (the belief in one's ability to perform a behavior) and the influence of significant others on behavior. Health-Seeking Behaviors may also be influenced by environmental and community characteristics.[9]

Several studies examine factors that influence health behaviors. There are published literature reviews of research related to health promotion and health-related behavior.[12,16,21,24] In a review of research related to health promotion and preventive health behavior since 1980, Kulbok and Baldwin[16] identified that factors such as health beliefs and values, personal concept of health, perceived locus of control, support systems and resources, and perceived difficulties in undertaking particular behavior were related to health behaviors. Norman,[21] in a review of current studies, notes that socioeconomic status is a particularly reliable indicator of how an individual will behave in health matters—the higher one's income, the more likely one is to engage in positive health practices. Age and educational level have also been highly correlated with positive health behaviors. Research suggests that the educational level underlying the socioeconomic status is the most likely reason for the positive health behavior. A meta-analysis of 23 studies published between 1983 and 1991[12] identifies self-efficacy as the strongest predictor of a health-supporting lifestyle, followed by factors such as definition of health, self-concept, support, and perceived barriers, as well as perceived benefits of engaging in the behavior. Palank[24] states that although various factors are shown to be related to health-promoting behaviors the percentage of variance explained by these factors remains low. Palank[24] suggests a need to explore situational and environmental factors that may impede or act as cues to engaging in unhealthy behaviors. Identification of the impact of societal factors on health-related behavior may facilitate interventions at the policy level rather than focus on behavioral approaches that separate people from their social, physical, and economic environments.

Most of the literature regarding Health-Seeking Behavior focuses on the behavior of individuals. However, recent literature is exploring health promotion at the community level. Robertson and Minkler[27] suggest that "full community participation occurs when communities participate in equal partnership with health professionals in defining their health problems and in developing solutions to address the health problems" (p. 305).

In summary, the literature identifies a number of factors that affect how the individual progresses toward optimal health, health behaviors that affect health, and significant factors that affect health behavior. The client who wishes to attain health may be an individual, a family, or a group. This chapter focuses primarily on Health-Seeking Behaviors at the individual level. Although most of the population could benefit from undertaking Health-Seeking Behaviors, the nurse may have to target his or her interventions toward those who are known to have fewer positive health practices or those whose health practices may compromise their health. These persons include, for example, people from lower socioeconomic groups, teens who smoke and drink or develop poor nutritional practices, adults with sedentary lifestyles, people under severe stress (such as single parents or elderly caregivers), and women whose children have left home and for whom, therefore, self-actualization has become important. However, programs that simply aim at changing personal behavior without recognizing the complex relationship of behavior to cultural, psychosocial, and environmental factors and public policy are unlikely to succeed.[3,13] The nurse's role may need to extend to advocacy and social action.[8]

ASSESSMENT

The nurse should assess the client's current health status. This includes a review of body systems; health beliefs, perceptions, and values; health practices; health risks; support systems; cultural factors; economic factors; and the environment. An assessment of family functioning and development is also important.

Many assessment tools are available. Some address specific health behaviors, whereas others are more comprehensive. The comprehensive tools have been developed for use in large-scale surveys. The nurse should select an assessment tool carefully because many tools address specific components of health status only, and most do not consider the client's definition of health, health values, and environmental factors that may affect health and Health-Seeking Behaviors. The tools, however, can help educate the client regarding practices that affect health. Pender's lifestyle and health habit assessment has ten sections that address general competence in self-care, nutritional practices, physical and recreational activity, sleep patterns, stress management, self-actualization, sense of purpose, relationships with others, and use of the health care system.[26] The nurse can use the client's score on this assessment tool to determine areas in which to encourage health-protecting or health-promoting behaviors.

Many clients who wish to progress toward optimal health will not have any medical diagnosis or condition. Often clients assume self-responsibility in reviewing their lifestyles, and they decide to change certain health behaviors to reduce health risks and move toward self-actualization. A client with a chronic health problem should be stabilized before undertaking difficult lifestyle changes. These clients will likely be unable to manage significant behavior changes because they are coping with illness-related stressors.

The major characteristic of the client seeking to move toward optimal health is a desire to seek a higher level of wellness. Observed behaviors that alert the nurse to the client's desire to seek a higher level of wellness include, for example, the client switching to nutritious snacks rather than eating doughnuts and drinking coffee. Joining a weight-control group or rising early to jog are also behavioral indicators of a desire to move toward optimal health—indicators that the nurse should explore with the client. Other behaviors that identify health-seeking clients include a request for information about community resources that could aid in the pursuit of health or a struggle with a difficult behavior change, such as stopping smoking without professional assistance.

An expressed desire to participate in decisions about health and to gain control of health practices, as well as behavior that implies such a desire (for example, questioning health care practices or requesting and clarifying information and alternatives), also identifies clients who are seeking to move toward optimal health. The expression of concern about environmental conditions, such as noxious fumes from a local chemical plant or inadequate recreational areas for children, also characterizes clients who may wish to lobby for changes in the environment that will affect health and move clients closer to optimal wellness.

Although some clients will be interested in reducing threats to health and request guidance to change old behavior patterns and maintain new ones, many clients will not be aware of how their behaviors affect their health. Persons with sedentary lifestyles, who have high-stress occupations, and whose high alcohol intake is associated with "business transactions" may see no reason to change their lifestyles until they are exposed to consciousness-raising information or suffer an assault to their health.

In summary, nurses need to be aware of the various ways in which clients communicate their desire to move toward higher levels of wellness. The nurse who notes only verbalized desires may overlook many clients. Behavioral clues, including behavior change and information-seeking behavior, can be excellent defining characteristics of health-seeking clients for the alert nurse.

To assist the client in moving toward higher levels of health, the nurse must understand the meaning of health for the client. The nurse needs to assess the client's values so that any changes in health practices will not conflict with these values. For example, the man who values time with his wife and family is unlikely to forfeit time with them to attend an exercise program, even though he is highly motivated to increase his physical activity.

To assist the client in achieving higher levels of health, the nurse may provide the client with information about specific health behaviors and environmental factors and their influence on health status. This information may assist the client in determining the behaviors he or she wishes to adopt or reduce. When the client is exposed to multiple risk factors, the nurse can assist the client in assigning priority to the choices so that he or she does not become overwhelmed.

Legislation has a major effect on health behaviors. Legislation on seat belts and children's car seats has enforced behavior change. Antismoking bylaws have also enforced reduction or elimination of smoking in the workplace. The nurse

should work with clients motivated to move toward higher levels of health by this type of legislation. The nurse can assist these clients to achieve their desired goals. When the behavior change is accomplished, it likely becomes its own motivator.

Several factors will affect the desire to move to a higher level of wellness. Confidence in one's ability to grow and change is a major one. The nurse can work with clients to increase self-efficacy or confidence in their ability to adopt and maintain the positive health behavior. The longer the client maintains a health-compromising behavior, the harder it is to change. Also, the client who suffers no noticeable ill effects may see no reason to change.

The nurse should assess the client's environment for support and stress. The nurse should determine the client's support systems, including the degree of support available to the client to initiate and maintain health-promoting behaviors. Family and friends can sabotage good intentions by encouraging old behaviors that they enjoyed with the client, such as drinking alcohol or smoking. Friends and family can also be positive forces, providing social interaction to reinforce positive health behaviors. Economic support is important because the low-wage earner may be unable to increase nutritious foods in the diet or take vacations from a stressful workplace.

Cultural factors may relate to behaviors that affect health. For example, dietary patterns associated with cultural identity may be difficult to change. Attending group programs that provide support for behavior change may be denied to women whose cultural norms do not encourage women to leave home alone.

The nurse should assess any factors that the client feels will interfere with the ability to engage in specific health-promoting behaviors. The nurse and client can then discuss strategies to reduce or eliminate these barriers. For example, time may also affect behavior change. For the single parent or the harassed executive, finding or taking the time for oneself is often difficult. Therefore behavior changes that can be worked easily into busy schedules are the most likely to be maintained.

- **Defining Characteristics**

The presence of the following defining characteristics indicates that the client may be experiencing Health-Seeking Behaviors:

- Desire to attain and maintain optimum physical capacity
- Desire to attain and maintain optimum psychological well-being
- Verbalized or otherwise expressed desire to initiate change or modify a health behavior

- **Related Factors**

The following related factors are associated with Health-Seeking Behaviors:

- Lethargy
- Reduced lung capacity
- Shortness of breath
- Excess body fat
- Degree of self-efficacy
- Anxiety related to risks to health
- Perceived control of health
- Self-concept
- Feeling stressed
- Age
- Educational level
- Socioeconomic status
- Definition of health
- Relating cultural practices to current environment
- Perceived lack of inner strength
- Perceived loss of contact with desired religion
- Social support

DIAGNOSIS

- **Differential Nursing Diagnosis**

A client with a diagnosis of Health-Seeking Behaviors is actively determining ways to change personal health behaviors or the environment to achieve optimal physical and psychological well-being. The client may recognize a need for change because of a recent illness, acquired knowledge of risk factors, a change in ability to fulfill roles, pressure from friends, or social norms. Unlike clients diagnosed with Ineffective Individual Coping, clients seeking to change behaviors and/or their environment have problem-solving abilities and are motivated to fulfill their social roles. However, clients with either diagnosis may suffer from stress overload in their lives. Unlike clients

suffering from Altered Health Maintenance, clients with a diagnosis of Health-Seeking Behaviors recognize the need for personal change. In Altered Health Maintenance the client is often unable to maintain basic health practices because of lack of knowledge or resources. Diversional Activity Deficit may be an appropriate diagnosis for clients seeking recreational activities to add some balance in their lives. However, for clients seeking to strengthen their health, the activities sought out would be diversional and health enhancing.

- **Medical and Psychiatric Diagnoses**

Medical or psychiatric problems or the perceived risk of these problems may precipitate health-seeking behaviors. A diagnosis of hypertension, angina pectoris, or myocardial infarction often is the impetus for clients to change their behavior in the areas of nutrition, exercise, and smoking. Actions to prevent or control obesity may include seeking information regarding healthy eating practices and developing an active lifestyle. Irritable bowel syndrome identifies the need for clients to seek sound dietary guidance and also to seek effective stress management techniques.

OUTCOME IDENTIFICATION, PLANNING, AND IMPLEMENTATION

The expected client outcomes should relate directly to specific goals established for a specific behavior (for example, quitting smoking by an agreed date).

These outcomes should be negotiated with the client along with the strategies to reach these outcomes. Both strategies and outcomes must be acceptable to the client and fit the client's lifestyle.

An important expected client outcome is: The client will initiate, reduce, or eliminate a specific behavior by a specific date. After the outcome is established the nurse will assist the client to establish a behavior pattern that the client finds acceptable and does not conflict with his or her values or cultural beliefs. The nurse should teach or reinforce skills that are required to carry out the

I

behavior. For example, the person who smokes cigarettes to reduce stress will need to learn other ways to manage stress. The client who wishes to eat nutritiously but is not aware of which foods to include in a balanced diet will require knowledge from a food guide and encouragement to develop skill in using food exchanges. The nurse may also provide information about potentially helpful community resources and make referrals if needed. For the client with a limited support system the nurse may enlist the support of significant persons in the client's life or refer the client to a

---

◢ NURSING CARE GUIDELINES
Nursing Diagnosis: Health-Seeking Behaviors (Specify)

Expected Outcome: The client will initiate (reduce or eliminate) a specific behavior by a specific date.
- Establish the pattern of behavior to be undertaken. *Client involvement is essential to ensure that the client is ready to make the change.*
- Determine that the pattern fits the client's values and cultural patterns. *Unless the behavior change matches the client's values and is acceptable in the client's culture it is very unlikely that change will occur.*
- Assist the client with the skill development required to carry out a chosen behavior. *Very often new skills are required for change to occur. The client who has a feeling of self-efficacy is likely to use the new skills effectively.*
- Address knowledge deficits related to resources to assist with behavior change. *Since behavior change is never easy, any available resources to assist the client with this process should be determined.*
- Provide information about anticipated consequences of behavior change. *Preparing the client for possible outcomes of the behavior change will assist the client to make positive responses when difficult situations arise.*
- Establish a supportive environment. *Helpful encouragement and confidence in the client's ability to change can be expressed by significant persons and/or organizations.*

Expected Outcome: The client will regularly engage in a specific behavior by a specific date and will integrate the chosen behavior into existing lifestyle practices.
- Assess the client's progress and motivation to continue with the behavior. *The interest and concern of the nurse will assist the client to pursue the behavior.*
- Provide support and encouragement to maintain progress. *Positive outcomes develop slowly, and clients may not initially perceive the benefits of the behavior change. Maintaining nursing support may assist in long-term commitment.*
- Identify the client's perceived barriers to engaging in the behavior. *This will allow the client to verbalize difficulties that have been encountered or anticipated.*
- Develop strategies with the client to reduce or eliminate barriers. *Negotiation with the client on how to address the barriers will be important for the client to incorporate the behavior successfully into existing lifestyle practices.*

Expected Outcome: The client will express satisfaction with behavior change and will verbalize feelings of increased well-being.
- Evaluate with the client perceived benefits of behavior change, including emotional responses. *It will be important for continuation of the behavior change that the client verbalize positive beliefs and attitudes about the outcomes of the behavior change. These may include perception of reduced health risks, satisfaction, and feelings of self-actualization.*

■ = nursing intervention; ▲ = collaborative intervention.

self-help or support group. The nurse should review anticipated consequences of the behavior change with the client.

A second important expected client outcome is: The client will regularly engage in a specific behavior by a specific date and will integrate the chosen behavior into existing lifestyle practices. The nurse will maintain contact with the individual to monitor progress and encourage the client to continue the behavior. Problems that are encountered can be discussed and strategies implemented to reduce or eliminate their effect. The nurse will also assist the client to articulate the benefits of the behavior pattern. Many clients find it difficult to maintain a behavior change over a long period. Continued efforts by the nurse to increase the client's self-efficacy and problem-solving skills will be important factors in behavior maintenance.

Finally, an important expected outcome is that the client will express satisfaction with behavior change and will verbalize feelings of increased well-being. The nurse and the client will evaluate feelings about the behavior and the benefits of the change. For the behavior to become integrated into the lifestyle of the client, the client will need to feel satisfied with the behavior and be able to articulate positive effects of the behavior change.

EVALUATION

The nurse will evaluate with the client the extent to which the established outcomes have been met. If the outcomes are fulfilled, the nurse will ask the client to evaluate his or her satisfaction with the planned strategies and whether other interventions could have helped. If the outcomes have not been met, the nurse will ask the client to determine why they were not met. The client should (1) feel satisfied with his or her move toward health, (2) feel competent to maintain chosen health behaviors, and (3) feel motivated to continue to grow toward or through self-actualization.

■ CASE STUDY WITH PLAN OF CARE

Mrs. Frances B. is a 30-year-old mother of two sons, 8 and 6 years of age. Mrs. B. has been separated from her husband for 1 year and works full-time to support herself and her family. Mrs. B.'s father recently suffered a myocardial infarction, and she has called the public health nurse because she is concerned about her potential risk of cardiovascular disease. On assessment, Mrs. B.'s health is stable, and she has never had any major health problems. She smokes one package of cigarettes per day and has recently felt she "needed a drink" when she arrived home every night from work. Mrs. B. works as a computer technician and has few social or recreational pursuits. She appears pale, with dark circles around the eyes; she stands 5'5" and weighs approximately 120 pounds. A review of her body systems does not reveal physical problems. However, Mrs. B. reports feeling overwhelmed by her responsibilities and not sleeping well. She also reports that she has recently started drinking two to four alcoholic beverages almost every night and, in the past 2 to 3 months, has increased her smoking to one and a half packages per day. Since her separation, she feels that old friends have ignored

her, and she has little interaction with peers except at work. Mrs. B. says that she used to enjoy golf but now finds she cannot afford this activity. Her family lives in a distant city, so Mrs. B. has no family support available. She recognizes that her children's behavior is normal but she sometimes finds that she is tired and impatient with them. Health to Mrs. B. means the ability to fulfill her various role expectations: employee, breadwinner, mother, and homemaker. She values her family and feeling confident in her roles. Together, the nurse and Mrs. B. identified several stressors that could affect Mrs. B.'s health: smoking one and a half packages of cigarettes per day, lack of social interaction, lack of time for self, her job as a computer operator, increased alcohol intake, lack of physical exercise, and lack of social support. The nurse and Mrs. B. discussed the relationship between stress and health. Mrs. B. expressed a desire to change her lifestyle. The nurse and Mrs. B. agreed that the stressors should be assigned priority as follows: lack of social support, lack of social interaction, lack of time for self, increased alcohol intake, smoking, and the computer job.

I

▶ **PLAN OF CARE FOR MRS. FRANCES B.**
Nursing Diagnosis: Health-Seeking Behavior (Seeking to Increase Personal and Community Supports) Related to Marital Breakup and Heavy Family Demands

Expected Outcome: Mrs. B. will express satisfaction with her ability to accept support from others.
- Determine Mrs. B.'s comfort in attending group meetings.
- Determine Mrs. B.'s perception of the support in her life.

Expected Outcome: Mrs. B. will attend meetings of support groups routinely.
- Assess Mrs. B.'s knowledge of community support groups for single parents, and inform Mrs. B. about Parents Without Partners (social activities, support programs, family activities, and emergency support network).
- Determine Mrs. B.'s level of comfort in attending meetings.
- Role-play situations that Mrs. B. might encounter at the first meeting.
- Refer Mrs. B. to the volunteer baby-sitting services for support programs.

Expected Outcome: Mrs. B. will express feelings of well-being.
- Perform ongoing assessment and counseling of stress and stress management.
- Perform ongoing assessment and counseling of unhealthy lifestyle behaviors, for example, alcohol and tobacco use.

Expected Outcome: Mrs. B. will express satisfaction with her role at work.
- Determine areas of work that are perceived stressful by Mrs. B.
- Discuss ways to reduce or manage the stress.

■ = nursing intervention; ▲ = collaborative intervention.

■ CRITICAL THINKING EXERCISES

1. How can the nurse work with a client to develop a realistic plan of care when the client wishes to engage in several different health-seeking behaviors?

2. What are the most important factors that the nurse should consider when negotiating a plan of care with a client seeking to engage in new health-seeking behaviors?

3. What are some of the environmental factors or policies that may make it easier or more difficult for the client to engage in specific health-seeking behaviors?

4. How can the nurse assist the client to modify the environment to support health-seeking behaviors?

REFERENCES

1. Ajzen I: *Attitudes, personality, and behaviour,* Bristol, Great Britain, 1988, Open University Press.

2. Ajzen I and Fishbein M: *Understanding attitudes and predicting social behaviour,* Englewood Cliffs, New Jersey, 1980, Prentice Hall Press.
3. Anderson ET and McFarlane JM: *Community as client,* Philadelphia, 1988, JB Lippincott Co.
4. Bandura A: *Social learning theory,* Englewood Cliffs, New Jersey, 1977, Prentice Hall Press.
5. Becker MH: The health belief model and personal health behaviour, *Health Ed Monographs* 2:326–473, 1974.
6. Belloc NB: Relationship of health practices and mortality, *Prev Med* 2:67–81, 1973.
7. Breslow L and Enstrom JE: Persistence of health habits and their relationship to mortality, *Prev Med* 9:469–483, 1980.
8. Butterfield PG: Thinking upstream: nurturing a conceptual understanding of the societal context of health behaviour, *ANS* 12(2):1–8, 1990.
9. Diehr P, Koepsell T, Cheadle A, Psaty B, Wagner E, and Curry S: Do communities differ in health behaviours? *J Clin Epidem* 46(10):1141–1149, 1993.
10. Ellis R: Conceptual issues in nursing, *Nurs Outlook* 30(7):406–410, 1982.
11. Epp J: *Achieving health for all: a framework for health promotion,* Ottawa, Canada, 1986, Supply and Services Canada.
12. Gillis, A: Determinants of a health-promoting lifestyle: an integrative review, *J Adv Nurs* 18:345–353, 1992.

13. Hancock T: Healthy women and the future, *Health Care Women Int* 8:249–260, 1987.

14. Henderson V: *Nature of nursing,* New York, 1966, Macmillan Publishing Co.

15. King IMA: *A theory for nursing: systems, concepts, processes,* New York, 1981, John Wiley & Sons, Inc.

16. Kulbok PA and Baldwin JH: From preventive health behaviour to health promotion: achieving a positive construct of health, *Adv Nurs Sci* 14(4):50–64, 1992.

17. Laffrey SC: Health promotion: relevance for nursing, *Top Clin Nurs* 7(2):29–38, 1985.

18. Laffrey SC, Loveland-Cherry CJ , and Winkler SJ: Health behaviour: evolution of two paradigms, *Public Health Nurs* 3(2):92–100, 1986.

19. Meleis AI: Being and becoming healthy: the core of nursing knowledge, *Nurs Sci Quart* 3(3):107–114, 1990.

20. Neuman B: *The Neuman systems model: application to nursing education and practice,* Norwalk, Connecticut, 1989, Appleton & Lange.

21. Norman R: Health behaviour: the implications of research, *Health Prom* 25(1,2):2–9, 1986.

22. Orem D: *Nursing: concepts of practice,* ed 5, St. Louis, 1995, Mosby–Year Book.

23. Ottawa Charter for Health Promotion: *Health Promotion* 1(4):iii–v, 1986.

24. Palank CL: Determinants of health-promotive behaviour: a review of current research, *Health Prom* 26(4):815–832, 1991.

25. Pender NJ: Health promotion and illness prevention. In Werley HH and Fitzpatrick JJ, editors: *Annual review of nursing research,* vol 2, New York, 1987, Springer Publishing.

26. Pender NJ: *Health promotion in nursing practice,* ed 2, Norwalk, Connecticut, 1987, Appleton & Lange.

27. Robertson A and Minkler M: New health promotion movement: a critical examination, *Health Ed Quart* 21(3):245–312, 1994.

28. Roy C: *Introduction to nursing: an adaptive model,* ed 2, Englewood Cliffs, New Jersey, 1983, Prentice Hall Press.

29. Smith JA: The idea of health: a philosophical inquiry, *ANS* 3(3):43–50, 1981.

30. Stachtchenko S and Jenicek M: Conceptual differences between prevention and health promotion: research implications for community health programs, *C J Public Health* 81(Jan/Feb):53–59, 1990.

31. Williams RL and others: Development of a health habits scale, *Res Nurs Health* 14:145–153, 1991.

32. World Health Organization: *Health promotion: a discussion document on the concept and principles,* Copenhagen, 1984, The Organization.

Risk for Infection

▶

Risk for Infection *is the state in which an individual has an increased susceptibility for invasion by pathogenic and/or opportunistic organisms.*

OVERVIEW

Risk for Infection is a nursing diagnosis that is pertinent for a broad spectrum of patients in varied settings. Depending on the degree of interaction between the host, the infectious organism, and the environment, any patient has the potential to develop an infection. Infectious organisms are present at all times in the atmosphere and in our bodies. For an infectious disease to develop, the delicate balance among host, organism, and environment must be upset. This imbalance can result from three factors: a change in the host that decreases existing defense mechanisms; an increase in the virulence of the infectious agent; or an environmental factor that influences the host, the disease-producing organism, or both. Therefore to identify patients who are at risk for infection, one most examine all three components of the triad.

Bacteria, viruses, chlamydiae, rickettsiae, fungi, protozoa, arthropods, and helminths are all organisms that can infect humans. Within these categories exist pathogenic and nonpathogenic organisms. Pathogenicity refers to the ability of an organism to cause disease. Nonpathogenic organisms include those that normally exist in or on the body. These organisms are referred to as normal flora. Normal flora usually do not cause disease unless host susceptibility increases. An infectious disease that develops in this manner is called an opportunistic infection. One example is the destruction of normal flora in the vaginal tract through the use of antimicrobial agents. These lactobacilli normally produce an environmental pH that is not conducive to the growth of yeast cells. When the normal flora is destroyed, *Candida albicans* can proliferate and cause a secondary, or opportunistic, vaginal infection. One must remember that almost all normally nonpathogenic organisms can become pathogenic.

Pathogens also can normally reside in the environment and the body without causing disease. One such organism is the varicella-zoster virus, which remains dormant in the nerve cells after recovery from chickenpox. These pathogens result in shingles when there is a change in virulence or in host susceptibility. *Virulence* is the degree to which an organism can cause disease. It is determined not only by the number of organisms present but also by the organism's ability to adhere to host cells, produce toxins, avoid phagocytosis, produce immunological injury, and mutate.[10,12]

An infectious disease occurs when a pathogen gains entry into a host and produces local, systemic, or focal effects. This process occurs through a sequence of events. First, the organism lives in a reservoir, living or nonliving, where it may multiply. It leaves the reservoir through a portal of exit and is transmitted to the host through a portal of entry. Transmission can occur by direct contact, as through touching or by droplet; by indirect contact, as through food or airborne organisms; or by vectors, such as mosquitos. After gaining access to the host, the pathogen multiplies, evades host defense mechanisms, penetrates and spreads through tissue by secreting enzymes, and may produce endotoxins or exotoxins. These enzymes and toxins, in combination with the host's response, are what cause the symptoms associated with the infectious disease.

Infection is resisted through the body's defense mechanisms. These include physical or mechanical barriers, chemical barriers, and cellular defenses. The skin and mucous membranes provide physical barriers as long as they remain intact. Mucous and ciliary action in the respiratory tract sweep organisms along to be eliminated by coughing or sneezing or through the gastrointestinal tract. Saliva, urine, and tears serve as barriers by washing organisms away. The acid pH of the skin and gastrointestinal and genitourinary tracts creates an environment that is unfavorable for the growth of certain microorganisms. Enzymes, fatty acids, and some protein substances in bodily secretions also create environments that are unfavorable for the growth of certain microorganisms.

If an infectious organism succeeds in breaking through these barriers, nonspecific and specific cellular defense mechanisms respond. As host cells are damaged, blood flow to the area increases through vasodilation in response to substances released by the destroyed cells. Vascular permeability also increases, allowing the release of fluid and phagocytic cells into the tissue. These actions result in the erythema, warmth, and edema that occur with infection. Phagocytic cells, which include both neutrophils and macrophages, engulf and digest or kill the invading organisms. In addition, the macrophages degrade destroyed host cells and function in the specific immune response described below. Debris of this phagocytic activity results in the formation of pus in localized infections.

Cell-mediated immunity and humoral immunity make up the body's specific immune response. Cell-mediated immunity involves T-lymphocytes. Macrophages present the foreign substance, or antigen, to the T-lymphocytes. In response, helper T-cells release lymphokines that stimulate B-cells, stimulate cytotoxic and suppressor T-cells, further activate the macrophage system, and help produce the nonspecific actions[5] described above.

Humoral immunity involves B-lymphocytes, the white blood cells that produce antibodies. Antibodies are protein substances that assist in fighting infection. They can act directly by causing agglutination, precipitation, or neutralization of the antigenic material present on invading organisms or by lysis of the organisms. Most of the activity against these infectious agents, however, is through activation of the complement system by antibody-antigen complexes. On activation, the complement system, which consists of enzyme precursors, produces lysis, agglutination, phagocytosis, and neutralization of invading organisms, as well as chemotaxis, activation of mast cells and basophils, and other inflammatory effects.[5]

The white blood cells involved in the different immune responses are produced, stored, and maturated in various body structures such as the bone marrow, thymus, spleen, and lymph nodes. During infection, these structures are stimulated to produce and release white blood cells. This action results in an overall increase in the white blood cell count above the normal 5,000 to 10,000 cells/mm³ and/or a shift in the differential cell count. A shift to the left in the differential is typically seen with bacterial infections where the increase in the number of white blood cells is due to an increase in the number of neutrophils, specifically immature cells or bands. Parasitic infections will cause an increase in the number of eosinophils. After production, the white blood cells depend on adequate blood and lymph circulation for transportation to the body sites where they are needed.

The possibility for infection to occur increases whenever any of the body's defense mechanisms are compromised. Compromised defense mechanisms occur with a break in the physical barriers of the skin and mucous membranes and also with alterations in pH, production of enzymes and protein substances, blood, blood-forming organs, and circulation.

The last component of the triad of infection is the environment. Weather can affect the ability of microorganisms to exist, proliferate, and be transmitted through the air. Reservoirs for pathogens include water and decaying materials. Hospitals specifically are breeding grounds for pathogenic organisms. Nosocomial, or hospital-acquired, infections pose a threat to all hospitalized patients.

Sanitation and hygiene practices are important safeguards against the proliferation and transmission of infectious organisms. This component involves many socioeconomic aspects. Education, economic status, culture, and religion can affect nutrition, hygiene, sanitation practices, willingness to seek information, access to agencies concerned with protection against and treatment for infections, and the ability to participate in programs that decrease Risk for Infection.

ASSESSMENT

Assessment and interventions must include all three components of the triad: pathogen, host, and environment. When assessing for Risk for Infection, one must first obtain a nursing history. Although all the Functional Health Patterns can provide pertinent data, those that are most important to assess are the following: Health-Perception—Health-Management Pattern, Nutritional-Metabolic Pattern, Sexuality-Reproductive Pattern, and Value-Belief Pattern. In addition, general information such as age, allergies, and even local address can contribute information for determining a Risk for Infection.

Assessment of the Health-Perception—Health-Management Pattern includes any existing health problems that could decrease resistance to infection. The nurse should note any treatments or medications that increase risk. These treatments include radiation therapy, chemotherapy, antimicrobial therapy, or any recent invasive procedures. The nurse should investigate recent contacts with infectious persons or environments, including travel to areas known to have certain diseases (such as malaria, cholera, or typhoid fever) endemic in the population. Past infectious diseases, as well as participation in immunization programs, should be documented.

Assessment of the Nutritional-Metabolic Pattern could identify nutritional deficits that decrease resources the body needs to produce the components that help resist infection. In addition, drug and alcohol use are associated with increased Risk for Infection.

Sexuality patterns and history of sexual abuse can help determine the risk for sexually transmitted diseases or past trauma. Multiple sexual partners or homosexual and bisexual lifestyles, as well as illicit drug use, are most important to assess in determining the risk for HIV transmission.

Assessment of the Value-Belief Pattern may indicate the potential for compliance or noncompliance with prescribed interventions that may be contrary to the patient's beliefs. For example, a person who fasts extensively and is prescribed a high-calorie diet may be reluctant to follow the prescribed diet. Particularly important is the assessment of a person's value system and religious affiliation.

After obtaining a history, the nurse should assess subjective and objective data within the Nutritional-Metabolic Pattern, the Elimination Pattern, the Activity-Exercise Pattern, the Sleep-Rest Pattern, and the Cognitive-Perceptual Pattern. Vital signs, condition of the skin, enlarged lymph nodes, breath sounds, any discharge, and complaints of pain, weakness, lethargy, or malaise are important to note. The complete blood count (CBC), electrolyte values, and urinalysis results are laboratory data to be evaluated as indicators of nutrition, immune function, and presence of infection. The nurse should observe personal hygiene, including cleanliness and condition of the mouth and teeth.

By gathering these data, the nurse can identify risk factors for the development of infection. Age is a risk factor. Normal skin changes that occur with aging, such as thinning, affect the skin's ability to act as a barrier against microorganisms. In addition, the production of secretions and blood flow and the rate of tissue regeneration decrease.[8] At the opposite end of the age continuum are infants, who are also at risk because of their immature immune systems and thin, easily damaged epithelial tissues.

Nutritional status can greatly increase a person's susceptibility to infection. For example, Vitamins A, B, and C all help in the maintenance of skin and mucous membranes, the healing of wounds, and the response to inflammation. Protein also contributes to these activities, in addition to being involved with the immune response. Production of bone marrow and liver, spleen, and lymphoid tissues depends on adequate stores of protein and iron. These are the tissues from which phagocytes and lymphocytes arise. In addition, an infectious state or other medical condition increases metabolic demands and further depletes nutritional stores.[5]

Medical conditions and treatments can compromise the body's defense mechanisms in other ways. Chemotherapy, radiation therapy, and any condition affecting the spleen, bone marrow, or liver can decrease the production of white blood cells. Diabetes mellitus, rheumatoid arthritis, and certain medications decrease the ability of white blood cells to reach the infection site. Phagocytosis may be ineffective in a person who has Hodgkin's disease, cirrhosis, or lupus erythematosus.[4] Renal insufficiency causes the accumulation of toxins, which may destroy the various defense mechanisms.

Cancer presents many problems leading to an increased Risk for Infection. Patients with cancer have increased nutritional needs and therefore are at risk for malnutrition and cachexia. Obstruction of lymph and blood circulation may decrease the ability to bring the necessary white blood cells and antibodies to the site of infection and also decrease drainage from these sites. All treatments for cancer, including surgery, radiation therapy, and chemotherapy, further compromise a person's ability to resist and combat infection. Some types of cancer can directly affect the body's ability to produce the cells involved in the immune response. These include leukemia, lymphoma, and myeloma.

Acquired immunodeficiency syndrome (AIDS) is caused by the human immunodeficiency virus (HIV). This virus affects the T-4 helper cells, which are lymphocytes involved in the immune response. The HIV causes these cells to replicate the virus, after which the T-4 helper cells die prematurely or are inactivated. Eventually the person develops an immunodeficiency state and is unable to resist infections and the growth of neoplasms.

Any type of invasive procedure, such as surgery, urinary catheterization, or central access lines, breaches the first line of defense, which is the skin and mucous membranes. This breach allows microorganisms access to the body. In addition, specific problems accompany each type of procedure.

Faulty surgical and aseptic technique, as well as the presence of an infection preoperatively, greatly increases the Risk for Infection in surgical patients. A decrease in the function of T-lymphocytes has been documented following the use of general anesthesia, and surgical procedures requiring more than 2 hours are associated with an increased risk for postoperative infection.[7]

Urinary catheterization may cause trauma to the urethra, thereby allowing microorganisms access. In addition, the catheter provides direct access to the bladder, a normally sterile environment. Microorganisms may travel along the catheter into the bladder and eventually to the kidneys. Urinary catheterization also bypasses the mechanical action of voiding, which usually sweeps bacteria through the urethra and provides an acid pH that is detrimental to the existence of microorganisms.

Endotracheal procedures tend to dry out the mucous membranes. They also provide direct access to the respiratory tract. By bypassing and damaging the cilia, the procedure does not allow foreign material and debris to be swept up and out of the lower airway.

Central access lines, venous and arterial, may contribute to infection in the body by allowing organisms to travel through the insertion site and along the catheter. These catheters further increase the risk for infection by promoting the formation of clots. Blood clots in and around the catheter, as well as the presence of moisture under the dressing, allow for the growth of bacteria.[2,9,11]

Also at risk are persons who are unable to protect themselves. This inability may result from physiological factors leading to hospitalization, where they must rely on others for care. It may also stem from a Knowledge Deficit. This deficit may be related to lack of knowledge regarding prevention of infection or an inability to understand or carry out instructions.

The presence of an infection increases the risk for further infection in a person who has decreased defense mechanisms. The clinician can identify an infection by an assessment of physiological signs and symptoms and laboratory data.

Hematological studies indicate the presence of an infection by an elevated white blood cell count and sedimentation rate. Other specimens and tests are specific to areas of infection. X-ray examination can indicate cysts, infiltrates, and bone abnormalities. Urinalysis and a culture and sensitivity test identify urinary tract infections. Cultures of sputum, stool, and blood indicate infections in their respective sites. Studies of cerebral spinal fluid can indicate bacterial and viral infections in the central nervous system.

Physiological signs and symptoms that indicate infection include subjective data such as complaints of pain or muscle aches, malaise, and lethargy. Objective data might reveal an elevated temperature, pulse, respiratory rate, and blood pressure; decreased urinary output indicative of dehydration; warm flushed skin; drainage; neck rigidity; rashes; and enlarged lymph nodes. These characteristics can result from the toxins produced by the organisms or the activities of the person's defense mechanisms.[1]

■ Risk Factors

The presence of the following behaviors, conditions, or circumstances renders the patient more vulnerable to Risk for Infection:

- Age (e.g., the very young, the very old)
- Inadequate physical barriers
- Inadequate chemical barriers
- Inadequate cellular response
- Inadequate acquired immunity
- Acute and chronic illnesses
- Invasive procedures
- Chemotherapy
- Lack of immunizations
- Radiation therapy

- Medications (e.g., antibiotics, steroids)
- Malnutrition
- Hospitalization
- Unsanitary living conditions
- Knowledge deficit

DIAGNOSIS

■ Differential Nursing Diagnosis

The diagnosis of Risk for Infection is closely related to Risk for Altered Body Temperature. Many of the risk factors for the two diagnoses are the same, and infection is one of the causes of an increase in body temperature. Risk for Infection has the higher priority diagnosis unless there is a problem with thermoregulation. It may also be difficult to discriminate between Risk for Infection and Altered Protection. These two diagnoses are seen frequently in the same patient, with Risk for Infection being the more specific diagnosis.

■ Medical and Psychiatric Diagnoses

Any medical condition that alters the immune system increases the Risk for Infection. These conditions include AIDS, cancer, and diabetes mellitus. Conditions affecting skin integrity, including peripheral vascular disease and burns, and psychiatric disorders interfering with nutrition, such as bipolar disorder and depressive disorder, also relate to Risk for Infection.

OUTCOME IDENTIFICATION, PLANNING, AND IMPLEMENTATION

Patient outcomes for an individual with the diagnosis Risk for Infection include freedom from infection, intact skin and mucous membranes, verbalization of risk factors for infection, identification of preventive measures to reduce infection, demonstration of a healthy lifestyle, and participation in immunization programs.

Freedom from infection is measured by continuously assessing for signs and symptoms of infection and identifying potential sites for infections.
Continued on p. 58

◢ **NURSING CARE GUIDELINES**
Nursing Diagnosis: Risk for Infection

Expected Outcome: The patient will be free of infection at every assessment as indicated by normal vital signs; normal white blood cell count; normal sedimentation rate; negative cultures; warm, dry skin; no flushing of skin; no drainage; no rash; no neck rigidity; clear breath sounds; clear, yellow urine; and no chills, pain, malaise, or lethargy.

- Wash hands between all patient contacts.
- Use universal blood and body fluid precautions and appropriate isolation techniques.
  Pathologic organisms are spread by direct contact through touching or by droplet.
- Monitor vital signs every shift.
- ▲ Monitor laboratory values for indications of infection.
- Monitor and document signs and symptoms of infection every shift.
  This information must be documented at least every shift or outpatient visit to identify changes from the baseline assessment.
- ▲ Collect specimens as needed. *Specimens assist in monitoring for the presence of an infection.*
- Encourage coughing and deep breathing or use of respiratory aids every hour.
- Encourage ambulation or position changes and extremity exercises every 2 hours.
  These activities decrease the pooling of secretions, improve circulation, and promote oxygen exchange.
- Use aseptic technique for all invasive procedures and dressing changes.
- Observe hospital guidelines for maintenance of intravenous and central lines.
  Aseptic technique and changing of intravenous and central lines assist in the prevention of nosocomial infections.
- Maintain urinary catheter systems closed and below the level of the bladder. *This prevents the contamination and backflow of urine into the bladder, which would increase the Risk for Infection.*
- Provide daily catheter care. *Daily catheter care prevents microorganisms from traveling along the catheter into the bladder and kidneys.*

Expected Outcome: The patient will have intact skin and mucous membranes at every assessment for previously intact tissues and at 7 days for wounds.

- Schedule and perform position changes every 1 to 2 hours. *Pressure impedes circulation and cellular metabolism, which results in skin breakdown.*
- Provide daily skin care and oral hygiene. *Promoting personal and oral hygiene helps to maintain the skin and mucous membranes.*
- Change soiled dressings.
- ▲ Use appropriate antimicrobial solutions and ointments for wound care.
  Clean, dry dressings and antimicrobial solutions and ointments provide an environment conducive to wound healing.

Expected Outcome: The patient will verbalize risk factors for infection after each teaching session.

- Teach risk factors for infection, including age, nutrition, defense mechanisms, chronic and acute illnesses, invasive procedures, medications, and sexual practices. *Knowledge of risk factors for infection can assist an individual to accept susceptibility for infection.*

Expected Outcome: The patient will demonstrate a lifestyle that promotes wellness, including no substance abuse, no smoking, adequate diet and fluid intake, proper skin care and oral hygiene, monogamous sexual relationships and/or the use of condoms, and the maintenance of a clean and safe environment at the time of the follow-up appointment.

■ = nursing intervention; ▲ = collaborative intervention.   *Continued*

◢ **NURSING CARE GUIDELINES — CONT'D**

- Develop and implement teaching plans regarding proper nutrition, the detrimental effects of smoking and substance abuse, safe sexual practices, personal hygiene, and sanitation.
- Participate in community programs for public sanitation, control of communicable diseases, and health promotion.
  Promotion of wellness is accomplished mainly through teaching. Hygiene, sanitation, and proper food handling are areas to be addressed to promote public health.

Expected Outcome: The patient will participate in immunization programs demonstrated by documented immunizations according to the schedules found in the current *Morbidity and Mortality Weekly Reports.*
- Encourage participation in immunization programs through individual and community teaching. *Immunizations protect individuals against certain diseases and decrease the potential for transmission of communicable diseases.*

Infection is prevented by promoting activities that support normal defense mechanisms. The current Centers for Disease Control and Prevention (CDCP) guidelines for universal blood and body fluid precautions should be strictly followed.[3] Proper isolation techniques should be used for persons at Risk for Infection and for those with an existing infection. All clinicians should carefully follow hospital policy for changing intravenous and central access tubings, solutions, and dressings. Aseptic technique must be used when performing any invasive procedure or dressing change. The risk for development of respiratory infections can be decreased through the use of incentive spirometers, coughing and deep breathing exercises, and early ambulation. If ambulation is contraindicated, position changes, extremity exercises, elevating the head of the bed, and sitting in a chair can be beneficial. Urinary drainage systems should be kept closed and below the level of the bladder. Cleansing with warm water and careful drying is suggested for patients with retention catheters.[4] Medications must be monitored for side effects that could depress patients' immune systems or promote growth of opportunistic organisms. The effectiveness of antimicrobials cannot be assured unless they are administered around the clock at equal time intervals and the dosage regimen is completed.

Promoting personal and oral hygiene helps maintain a patient's skin and mucous membranes. Skin care and oral hygiene should be done at least once every day. Daily baths should be carefully evaluated in elderly patients because of the drying effect that occurs with bathing. Skin creams and lubricants used on dry skin prevent cracking. Skin surfaces are to be kept dry, and contact between skin surfaces minimized. Hygiene also includes daily perineal care. Frequent position changes help prevent skin breakdown. Soiled dressings should be changed immediately, using antimicrobial solutions and ointments as ordered.

Patient verbalization of risk factors for infection and identification of preventive measures to reduce this risk serve to indicate patient understanding of these factors. Nurses should include teaching regarding risk factors and measures to prevent infection in their care of vulnerable patients.

Maintaining healthy lifestyles can assist patients to reduce their Risk for Infection. Promotion of wellness is accomplished mainly through teaching about behaviors that may lead to the inhibition or destruction of normal defense mechanisms, such as smoking, substance abuse, and unprotected sexual intercourse, and behaviors that help maintain the body's defense mechanisms, such as adequate hydration and a diet high in vitamin C, protein, and iron. Nurses should participate in developing community programs for health promotion that address areas such as maintenance of safe water supplies, proper food handling, and the control of communicable diseases.

Participation in immunization programs will assist individuals to decrease their risk for contracting communicable diseases. Nurses can be instrumental in the promotion of immunization programs for children and adults. Persons anticipating international travel should contact their local health departments to determine which vaccines are necessary. High-risk groups, such as children, the elderly, and the debilitated, should be assessed and educated regarding necessary immunizations. Nurses should provide instruction about potential side effects of vaccines and what to do if they develop, as well as the need to follow through on immunization series to receive full protection.

EVALUATION

Success of infection control programs can be evaluated by monitoring infection rates on individual, institutional, and community levels. Participation in community immunization and health promotion programs are also indicators that can be evaluated. The health care provider and the patient can measure individual progress regarding health practices against goals on which they have agreed. Areas to be addressed include lifestyle, personal hygiene, nutrition, and wound and skin care. Regardless of the method used for evaluation, accurate documentation of results is vital to ensure continuity of successful programs and accurate long-term planning and evaluation.

▶ CASE STUDY WITH PLAN OF CARE

Mrs. Lois S. is a 75-year-old woman who was admitted to the medical-surgical unit after a bowel resection for an obstruction resulting from a malignant lesion. She has a central line through which she receives hyperalimentation at 75 ml/hr. Mrs. S. also has a Foley catheter and a nasogastric tube connected to low intermittent suction. Her medical history reveals no other illnesses or previous surgeries. She does not smoke. Although she is widowed and living by herself, Mrs. S. does have a daughter living in the area. Presently Mrs. S. complains of incisional pain and weakness. Objective data includes a temperature of 98.6°F (37°C), pulse of 80 beats/min., respirations of 20/min., weight of 120 pounds, height of 5′4″, white blood cell count of 6000/mm³, hemoglobin of 14 g/dl, and hematocrit of 39%. Her lungs are clear; her skin is warm, dry, and intact; and she has an abdominal incision that has a dry dressing. Her urine is clear and amber colored.

▶ PLAN OF CARE FOR MRS. LOIS S.
Nursing Diagnosis: Risk for Infection Related to Surgery, Foley Catheter, Central Line, Age, and Cancer

Expected Outcome: Mrs. S. will be free of infections as indicated by T 98.6°F (37°C), P 60 to 68, R 16 to 25, BP 120/80, white blood cell count of 4,500 to 10,000/mm³; skin warm and dry; no flushing of skin; urine clear; no redness or edema at central line site; no tenderness, redness, or positive Homan's sign in lower extremities; and no complaint of chills.
- Wash hands and put on gloves before any direct contact with Mrs. S.
- Monitor and document vital signs every 4 hours.
- ▲ Monitor CBC for increase in white blood cell count, sedimentation rate, or decreased Hgb or Hct.
- Monitor and document skin condition, urine color, central line site, breath sounds, condition of lower extremities, and presence of chills every shift.
- ▲ Administer pain medication before ambulation or respiratory exercises.

■ = nursing intervention; ▲ = collaborative intervention.   *Continued*

I

▶ **PLAN OF CARE FOR MRS. LOIS S. — CONT'D**

- Encourage Mrs. S. to cough and deep breathe or use her incentive spirometer every hour.
- Assist Mrs. S. in ambulation at least every shift.
- ▲ Administer 500 mg of ampicillin every 6 hours around the clock. Assess for signs of superinfection or reaction.
- Change hyperalimentation bottle every 24 hours, using aseptic technique.
- Change hyperalimentation tubing and central line dressing every 48 hours, using aseptic technique.
- Maintain urinary drainage system closed and below the level of the bladder.
- Cleanse perineal area with warm water during bath and pat dry.
- Change nasogastric drainage container every 48 hours.

Expected Outcome: Mrs. S. will have a healed incision with no purulent drainage.
- Monitor and document condition of dressing and incision every shift.
- Using aseptic technique, change soiled or loose dressing.
- ▲ Culture any suspicious drainage, using aseptic technique.

Expected Outcome: Mrs. S.'s skin and mucous membranes will remain intact.
- Assist and instruct Mrs. S. to change her position every 2 hours when in bed.
- Assist Mrs. S. in washing with mild soap and water every morning. Ensure adequate towel drying. Apply lotion to areas of dryness.
- Assist Mrs. S. in brushing her teeth once each shift.
- Cleanse and lubricate nares around nasogastric tube at least every day.

Expected Outcome: Mrs. S. will have adequate nutrition as indicted by weight remaining 120 lb, intake equaling output, good skin turgor, Hgb 12 to 16 g/dl, Hct 37%, and blood sugar 70 to 115 mg/dl.
- ▲ Maintain hyperalimentation at 75 ml/hr.
- ▲ Assess and document blood sugar by finger-stick every 6 hours.
- Measure and record accurate intake and output every shift.
- Weigh Mrs. S. and record weight every morning at the same time and using the same scale.
- ▲ Monitor Hgb and Hct for anemia and dehydration.
- Instruct Mrs. S. on the need for a diet high in protein, vitamin C, and iron.
- Instruct Mrs. S. on the need for fluid intake of at lest 2400 ml/day.

▦ **CRITICAL THINKING EXERCISES**

1. It is Mrs. S.'s first postoperative day and you are preparing to assist her out of bed. She tells you that it is too difficult and she is in too much pain. She wants to wait until her IV and nasogastric tubes are removed. What explanation would you give to her regarding the need for early ambulation?

2. Mrs. S.'s nasogastric tube has been removed. A clear liquid diet has been ordered for her in addition to the hyperalimentation that she is receiving at 75 ml/hr. You overhear Mrs. S. tell her daughter that she doesn't need to drink anything because she is receiving enough fluid through the IV. What would be your response?

3. As you are preparing Mrs. S. for discharge, she asks you whether she should continue to receive her annual flu vaccination. Would you recommend that she receive the vaccination and why?

REFERENCES

1. Black JM and Matassarin-Jacobs E, editors: *Luckmann and Sorensen medical-surgical nursing: a psychophysiologic approach,* ed 4, Philadelphia, 1993, WB Saunders Co.
2. Bostrom-Ezrati J, Dibble S, and Ruzzuto C: Intravenous therapy management: who will develop insertion site symptoms? *Applied Nurs Res* 3(4):146–151, 1990.
3. Centers for Disease Control: Recommendations for prevention of HIV transmission in health-care settings, *Morbidity and Mortality Weekly Report,* Atlanta, 1987, U.S. Department of Health and Human Services.
4. Gurevich I and Tafuro P: The compromised host: deficit-specific infection and the spectrum of prevention, *Cancer Nurse* 9(5):263–275, 1986.
5. Guyton AC: *Textbook of medical physiology,* ed 8, Philadelphia, 1991, WB Saunders Co.
6. Keithley JK: Infection and the malnourished patient, *Heart Lung* 12(1):23–27, 1983.
7. Miller TA: *Physiologic basis of modern surgical care,* St. Louis, 1988, Mosby–Year Book.
8. Nagani P: Management of common infections in the elderly outpatient, *Geriatrics* 41(11):67–80, 1986.
9. Parsa MH and others: Intravenous catheter-related infection, *Infect Surg,* 789–798, Nov. 1985.
10. Patrick ML and others: *Medical-surgical nursing: pathophysiological concepts,* ed 2, Philadelphia, 1991, JB Lippincott Co.
11. Petrosino B and others: Infection rates in central venous catheter dressings, *Oncol Nurs Forum,* 15(6):709–711, 1988.
12. Porth CM: *Pathophysiology: concepts of altered health states,* ed 4, Philadelphia, 1992, JB Lippincott Co.

Risk for Perioperative Positioning Injury

▶

Risk for Perioperative Positioning Injury *is the state in which the patient is at risk for injury as a result of the environmental conditions in the perioperative setting.*[8]

OVERVIEW

Perioperative positioning is a basic component of preoperative nursing. The goal of positioning is to provide optimal surgical exposure while preventing injury and maintaining comfort and dignity. Although positioning may appear to be a simple process, desirable positions may have undesirable results. Careful positioning requires knowledge of the anatomical and physiological changes that accompany anesthesia, sedation, change in body alignment, and the operative procedure. Optimal positioning is crucial because the anesthetized or sedated patient is not fully able to alert the nurse to discomfort that is usually associated with improper body alignment.

The nursing actions for patients at Risk for Perioperative Positioning Injury may depend on the specific position and the individual patient, but certain elements are essential to all situations. These elements include: (1) maintenance of a correct and safe body position throughout the procedure; (2) access to the patient for the administration of medications and treatments; (3) protection of the skin and neuromuscular and skeletal structures; (4) prevention of interference with circulation and ventilation; and (5) consideration for patient privacy and dignity. Perioperative positioning injury can occur in any position. Therefore, in each position, safety must be maintained and proper body alignment must be

achieved with securing devices, adequate padding, and anatomical support.

The *supine* (dorsal recumbent) position is the most common procedural position. In this position areas such as the head, elbows, sacrum, and heels should be padded, and the arms and lumbar areas should be supported to reduce unnecessary strain. The most common sites for injury in the supine position are the brachial plexus and the ulnar nerve. To decrease the length of stretch to the brachial plexus, the arms should be placed at less than a 90° angle. In addition, the arms should be level with the body and with the palms turned up.[1,10] When the patient is supine and armboards are not used, the arms should be placed alongside the patient with the palms against the body or face down with the fingers extended.

The supine position produces minimal effects on respiration. Functional residual capacity declines about 800 ml when changing from a standing to a supine position. The administration of muscle relaxants further decreases lung capacity. Loss of skeletal muscle tone in the chest wall reduces opposition to the normal recoil of the lungs, further contributing to reduction in lung volumes.[5] Although the supine position has minimal effects on circulation, the presence of an abdominal mass (ascites, obesity, gravid uterus) or an anterior mediastinal mass that compresses the inferior vena cava can cause hemodynamic changes. This compression results in altered venous return, which leads to decreased cardiac output and hypotension.

In the supine position, the hips and the knees should be flexed slightly to facilitate venous drainage from the legs and decrease abdominal wall tension. Lumbar support from a pillow under the knees may decrease the incidence of postoperative back pain.[1] To prevent venous stasis and pressure on the tissue and nerves, the legs should remain uncrossed and the heels should be padded.

In the *prone* position the patient is face down, resting on the abdomen and the chest. Typically the patient is anesthetized on a stretcher and then turned and placed on the operative bed. A patient in the prone position may experience cephalad displacement of the diaphragm, which may interfere with the downward displacement of the diaphragm and cause pressure on the inferior vena cava and the aorta.[5] If the head is turned to one side, there may be obstruction of jugular venous drainage and vertebral artery blood flow. These circulatory changes may be responsible for postoperative neck pain or, in some cases, thrombosis.[5] For this reason, the neutral position of the head, placed on a foam ring (or doughnut), may be preferred. Facial structures such as the eyes, nose, or auricle of the ear can be injured by pressure or displacement. Care must be taken to ensure that these structures are free from pressure.

Structures such as the arms, legs, genitalia, and breasts are also at risk. The arms are placed at the side or extended alongside the head on armboards. Care should be taken to ensure that the ulnar nerves are not compressed. Firm rolls placed under the patient from clavicle to iliac crest can relieve abdominal pressure and facilitate venous return and lung ventilation. To prevent pressure on the toes, the legs may be slightly flexed at the knees, with the dorsum of the foot supported by a pillow. The legs should be uncrossed and placed slightly apart, allowing the genitals to be free from pressure. Fingers and toes, as in all positions, must be secured away from the bed joints, and no part of the patient's body should be resting on an unpadded surface.

The *Kraske* (jackknife) position is a modification of the prone position and is used for gluteal and anorectal procedures. The patient is placed in the prone position with the hips over the break in the table. The table is then flexed, raising the hips and lowering the upper portion of the body. A small

roll placed under each shoulder can prevent stretching of the brachial plexus. A pillow under the lower legs can prevent pressure on the toes. As in all positions, safety straps are used to secure the legs and arms.

In the *Trendelenburg* position the patient's head is positioned lower than the feet. This position is used for procedures on the lower abdomen because it causes the abdominal organs to be displaced toward the head, allowing improved visualization of the surgical area. To prevent sliding of the entire body, the patient may be braced at the shoulders. The shoulder braces are positioned away from the neck and against the acromion and the spinous processes of the scapula. This will prevent injury to the brachial plexus.[9]

Although this position is used to treat hypotension, it does not predictably improve cardiac output in hypotensive and hypvolemic patients.[5] In some patients, displacement of the abdominal organs pushes the diaphragm against the heart, causing a decrease in stroke volume. This change can cause accentuation of coexisting hypotension.[5] In addition, this position may hinder ventilation by causing lung compression from the abdominal organs. In some patients the Trendelenburg position can increase intracranial pressure by elevating venous pressure, leading to decreased venous outflow from the brain. Because blood pools in the upper body, movement from the Trendelenburg position should be gradual to allow the body to adjust to the accompanying hemodynamic changes.

The *reverse Trendelenburg* position is a modification of the supine position in which the head is tilted upward. This position is most often used for head and neck procedures and for procedures on the upper abdomen. Potential problems associated with this position include the following: venous pooling in the legs; misalignment of the arms, causing pressure on the radial, median, or ulnar nerves; and impaired skin integrity due to sheering forces if the patient slides downward.[6] A well-padded footboard and additional safety straps may be needed for stability. Pillows under the knees and the lumbar curve can assist in maintaining body alignment and comfort. If the patient is in the reverse Trendelenburg position for an extended period of time, antiembolectomy stockings will aid venous return.

The *lithotomy* position is used for procedures requiring a vaginal or perineal approach. The patient is supine with the legs raised and positioned in stirrups. The buttocks are near the lower break of the table with most of the patient's weight resting on the sacrum. To prevent pressure on the sacrum, additional padding may be required for obese patients or for patients undergoing lengthy procedures. A small lumbar pad may also help reduce back strain. The feet, which are in stirrups, should be covered to provide additional warmth and protection and to prevent shedding of skin. If the patient is to remain in the lithotomy position for more than 2 hours, ace bandages or antiembolectomy stocking should be applied.[9]

Peripheral nerve injuries to the sciatic, common peroneal, femoral, saphenous, and obturator nerves can occur in this position. Adequate padding can prevent direct pressure. Stretch and strain on the peripheral nerves can be prevented by elevating and flexing both legs simultaneously. The thighs should be flexed no more than 90° before rotating the stirrups to the side.[5]

A common problem in this position is unpadded or malpositioned stirrups, which may damage the saphenous and peroneal nerves and predispose the patient to venous thrombosis. In addition, peroneal nerve damage on the lateral aspect of the femoral head can cause foot drop. Excessive pressure on the femoral and obturator nerves in the groin can result from the stretching of nerves.[9] Such pressure can cause femoral artery compression and subsequent limb ischemia.

The *sitting* (modified Fowler's) position is most often used for a posterior fossa craniotomy because it allows for venous drainage and exposure to the operative site. The principal hazard in this position is venous air embolus. An air embolus is a threat because a negative pressure exists between the operative site and the right atrium. The possibility of air embolus is complicated by the fact that veins in the cut edges of the skull may not collapse

when transected. Air embolus can occur when air enters the right ventricle and interferes with blood flow into the pulmonary artery. Pulmonary edema and reflex bronchoconstriction may result from movement of air into the pulmonary circulation. Death can be caused by cardiovascular collapse.[5] To prevent air embolus, copious amounts of irrigation and wet sponges are used during the procedure to ensure that the irrigation solution rather than air is aspirated. If an air embolism is suspected, the anesthesiologist will attempt to aspirate it via the right atrial or pulmonary artery catheter.

In the *lateral recumbent* position, the patient is stabilized on the side. This position is used for procedures on the kidney, the chest, or the upper ureter. The patient is anesthetized in the supine position and then positioned on the unaffected side. The lateral recumbent position may be associated with circulatory and ventilatory changes. Compression of the inferior vena cava may occur, especially if the kidney rest (on the operative bed) is elevated under the patient's dependent iliac crest. The dependent lung may be poorly ventilated because of pressure from the abdominal contents and the mediastinum. The nondependent lung may be overventilated because of an increase in lung compliance. This is especially the case when the corresponding chest wall is opened. In this position gravity favors the distribution of the pulmonary blood to the dependent lung. The ventilation-perfusion mismatch that occurs in the lateral recumbent position may result in unexpected arterial hypoxia.[5]

Pressure on the dependent axilla is a potential problem. A roll placed under the chest just caudal to the axilla will prevent pressure on the neurovascular bundle of the axilla. Periodic checks of the radial pulse are useful to ensure that arterial compression has not occurred.[5] A pillow placed under the head will reduce stretching of the dependent brachial plexus. A pillow between the knees, with the dependent leg flexed at the knee, reduces pressure on the bony prominences and stretch on the nerves of the lower extremity. The nondependent arm can be positioned on an armboard that is elevated by pillows or suspended from a support bar, with measures taken to avoid stretch on the brachial plexus.[5]

In every position care must be given to the eyes, facial structures, and appendages. In anesthetized patients the eyes should be taped closed and, if desired, ointment can be applied to maintain moisture and prevent corneal damage. Pressure on the eyes may cause thrombosis of the central retinal artery that results in permanent blindness. The possibility of this complication is increased when the patient experiences hypotension during the surgical procedure. When positioning the patient, care must be taken to ensure that the orbit can be felt in its entirety.[5] Monitoring wires, tubing, and other equipment should be positioned away from the patient's head.

Injury to facial structures such as lips, nose, or ears can be caused by improper positioning, by pressure from equipment, or by members of the surgical team who inadvertently lean on the anesthetized patient. Care must be taken to ensure that such structures, for example, the auricle of the ear, are not folded and compressed between the patient and an immovable object. Pressure on the face can be avoided by vigilant monitoring and by placing a Mayo stand or bar over the patient's face to ensure that it is free from potential injury.

Whenever the patient or parts of the surgical bed are being repositioned, there is always the possibility that a finger or toe may be caught in one of the many gaps or structures of the operative table. A common occurrence for injury occurs when the foot of the bed is returned to the horizontal position from the lithotomy position. Vigilant monitoring of hands and fingers is necessary at this time.

ASSESSMENT

Assessment for Risk for Perioperative Positioning Injury should occur throughout the intraoperative period. During the preoperative phase, a minimal patient assessment should include the following: physical limitations, weight, height, nutritional status, skin condition, preexisting diseases, and type and length of procedure. In addition, the nurse must have knowledge of the selected perioperative position along with interventions to prevent common positioning injuries. During the intraoperative phase, the nurse should assess continually for proper body alignment and tissue integrity. The assessment should include but is not limited to the following systems: respiratory, circulatory, neuromuscular, and integumentary. This assessment is again conducted when the patient is discharged from the operating room and during the postoperative visit.

■ Risk Factors

The presence of the following conditions, behaviors, or circumstances renders the patient more vulnerable to Risk for Perioperative Positioning Injury:

External (environmental) factors
- Type and length of procedure
- Use of positioning devices
- Use of chemicals to cleanse the skin and the pooling of such solutions
- Absence of proper equipment or safety procedures (e.g., restraints)
- Inadequately trained personnel or inattentive staff
- External sheering forces or pressure from personnel
- Inattentive staff leaning on patient
- Administration of chemotherapy, immunosuppressive drugs, or radiation therapy
- Extremes in external temperature or humidity

Internal (environmental) factors
- Age extremes
- Presence of hypothermia or hypotension
- Disorientation or sensory-perceptual disturbances due to disease, medication, or anesthesia
- Muscle weakness or paralysis
- Altered nutritional status (obesity, emaciation, and malnutrition)

I

- Altered skin integrity due to edema, infection, moisture from draining wounds, or incontinence
- Preexisting conditions: trauma, pregnancy, diabetes, infection, incontinence, vascular insufficiency, low serum albumin, hepatic disease, steroid therapy, AIDS, cardiopulmonary disorders, or anemia
- Immobilization

DIAGNOSIS

■ Differential Nursing Diagnosis

The Risk for Preoperative Positioning Injury is closely related to other nursing diagnoses such as High Risk for Impaired Skin Integrity, High Risk for Injury, Altered Tissue Perfusion, and High Risk for Ineffective Breathing Pattern. Risk for Perioperative Positioning Injury differs from the above in that the anesthetized or sedated patient is unable to alert the nurse when such problems develop. In essence, Risk for Perioperative Positioning Injury is prevented by the members of the operative team. The external forces of the operative environment are complex and often dangerous. Only through vigilance and attention to detail can this risk be prevented.

■ Medical and Psychiatric Diagnoses

Medical diagnoses such as diabetes, obesity, and cardiac and respiratory diseases may put the patient at Risk for Perioperative Positioning Injury. Psychiatric disorders such as mental retardation, senile dementia, delirium tremens, and schizophrenic psychoses may also put the operative patient at risk for injury during the perioperative period.

OUTCOME IDENTIFICATION, PLANNING, AND IMPLEMENTATION

Although nursing goals and interventions for patients at Risk for Perioperative Positioning Injury depend on the specific position of the patient, the desired outcomes are the same. The overall plan focuses on five areas: (1) protection of

the skin and soft tissue, (2) protection of neuromuscular function, (3) maintenance of normal circulation, (4) maintenance of normal respiration, and (5) consideration for privacy and dignity. Each relates to a patient outcome.

The first outcome relates to assuring that the patient experiences no injury to the skin and soft tissue. Any area of the skin can become injured, and impaired skin integrity can be a problem for any patient who is immobilized for more than 1.5 hours. Many surgical procedures easily meet or exceed this time constraint. The effect of time coupled with improper positioning can result in changes in skin integrity because of ischemia and localized ulceration. Hypothermia and vasoconstrictive hypotension may enhance ischemic necrosis. The skin can be damaged by internal forces such as direct pressure from the patient's own weight or from the weight of some external force. Proper positioning and padding can protect these susceptible areas.

The second outcome relates to the maintenance of neuromuscular function. Nerve injury related to improper positioning can be a problem for a patient who is alert, sedated, or anesthetized. In the alert individual, correct body alignment is maintained by pain and pressure receptors that warn the person that muscles, ligaments, or tendons are being stretched. Although injury is not common in the alert patient, it can result from accidental trauma that occurs during the procedure. In the anesthetized patient, skeletal muscle tone is reduced, especially when muscle relaxants are administered. This relaxation leaves the patient vulnerable to unnatural positions. The relaxed patient loses the normal tone of opposing muscle groups that helps prevent stress and strain on the muscle fibers.[4]

The principal cause of peripheral nerve injuries in the anesthetized patient is ischemia.[5] Injury to the brachial plexus is common; therefore the arm should never be abducted more than 90°, and the palm should be supinated or in a natural position.[7] The radial or ulnar nerves may be injured if the arm strikes the table or if the nerve is compressed between the patient and the table surface. To

Continued on p. 68

◢ NURSING CARE GUIDELINES
Nursing Diagnosis: Risk for Perioperative Positioning Injury

Expected Outcome: The patient's skin and soft tissues will remain free from injury.
- Assess for evidence of internal and external risk factors associated with skin breakdown.
- Gather all positioning devices before placing the patient on the operative bed to ensure that *safe and clean devices are available to the patient.*
- Maintain body alignment and tissue integrity during positioning so that *tissues are not stretched or torn.*
- Assess for evidence of internal and external risk factors associated with skin breakdown.
- Reassess the patient after positioning by inspecting the entire body, checking pulses, and assuring that pressure points are padded. *Changes in patient status can occur after the desired position is achieved.*
- Secure the patient and continue to monitor patient position throughout the operative procedure. *Any movement of the patient can alter the desired position.*
- Document the patient's position and positioning devices used.

Expected Outcome: The patient's neuromuscular function will be intact.
- Assess for evidence of internal and external risk factors associated with neuromuscular injury.
- Use appropriate positioning devices (armboards, stirrups, pillows) to support bodily structures when appropriate *to prevent stretching and compression of nerves and to secure limbs in correct anatomical position.*
- Pad bony prominences *to prevent ulceration, ischemia, and pressure on peripheral nerves.*
- Retain legs in an uncrossed position *to avoid pressure on blood vessels and nerves.*
- Maintain normal body alignment *to prevent stretching of the nerves and resultant ischemia.*
- Document assessment and nursing care.

Expected Outcome: The patient's circulation will be optimized.
- Assess for evidence of internal and external risk factors associated with circulatory problems.
- ▲ Establish baseline values for blood pressure and heart rate and rhythm *to assess changes during the procedure.*
- ▲ Move the anesthetized patient in a gentle and slow fashion *to prevent circulatory depression.*
- ▲ Assist with the application of invasive monitors when appropriate *to assess changes during the procedure.*
- Document assessment and nursing care.

Expected Outcome: The patient's respiratory status will be optimized.
- Assess for evidence of internal and external risk factors associated with respiratory problems.
- Establish baseline values for respirations and oxygen saturation *to assess changes during the procedure.*
- ▲ Administer oxygen via nasal cannula or face mask.
- ▲ Never move the anesthetized patient without checking with the anesthesiologist. *Movement can displace the endotrachial tube.*
- ▲ The anesthetized patient is moved by the operative team in a gentle and slow fashion *to prevent circulatory depression.*
- ▲ When moving the patient, guard the head *to secure the airway and support the head and neck.*
- Document assessment and nursing care.

Expected Outcome: The patient's privacy and dignity will be maintained.
- ▲ Limit exposure of the body to the area required for the operative procedure.
- ▲ Ensure that adequate personnel are present when the patient is lifted into position. *The patient is never pushed or pulled.*
- ▲ Inform the patient of procedures before they are performed.
- ▲ Provide support and diversion through touch, conversation, and measures of distraction (e.g., listening to music).
- Document nursing care as appropriate.

▪ = nursing intervention; ▲ = collaborative intervention.

I

avoid injuries to the radial or ulnar nerves, the hand should be free from compression, padded at the elbow and wrist, and secured in correct anatomical position. To reduce stretching of the sciatic nerve, the patient should be positioned so that external rotation of the leg is minimized and the knees are flexed. Proper padding of the legs can reduce compression, which is manifested by (1) foot drop, (2) loss of extension of the toes, and (3) inability to evert the foot.[5] Padding of the knee between the medial aspect of the knee and the leg can prevent pressure on the saphenous nerve.

The third outcome relates to the maintenance of normal circulation. The cardiovascular system is affected by general, regional, and local anesthetic agents that can cause vascular dilation and constriction. The effects of body position, coupled with the effects of anesthesia, can cause several hemodynamic changes.

The Trendelenburg position has been shown to increase blood pressure slightly and should be used with caution in patients with coronary artery disease. These patients may be unable to tolerate the increased demand for myocardial oxygen as preload and heart rate increase.[3] In the prone position, proper positioning ensures unobstructed venous return from the inferior vena cava and the femoral vessels. This promotes cardiac filling and reduces the incidence of hypotension. In the sitting position, pressure gradients develop, which increase with the degree of elevation. Close monitoring and use of compression stockings can help prevent venous pooling and other circulatory complications.

The fourth outcome relates to the maintenance of normal respiration. Positioning can interfere with diaphragmatic movement, thereby limiting expansion of the lungs. This limitation may be due to mechanical restriction of the lungs or pressure on the diaphragm caused by the shifting of abdominal contents. A change from the vertical position to the horizontal position alters the airflow and the functional characteristics of the lungs. This change can alter the pulmonary capillary blood flow volume, thereby affecting the amount of blood available for oxygenation. In addition to these pulmonary changes, the horizontal position of the body may alter the normal flow of pulmonary secretions. In many perioperative positions the chest is compressed and the patient has to work harder to breathe. To reduce respiratory effort, the abdomen should remain unencumbered. This can be achieved by placing padding under the shoulders and pelvis, thereby allowing the abdomen to fall away from the diaphragm.

Although the goal of positioning is to provide optimal surgical exposure, this must be accomplished while maintaining patient privacy and dignity, the fifth expected outcome. This can be achieved by controlling unnecessary traffic, properly covering the patient at all times, controlling the occurrence of onlookers, monitoring conversation, and limiting the number of personnel in the operating room. Because the perioperative nurse has limited time with the patient, it is imperative that every effort be made to establish a relationship with the patient in a timely fashion. Through conversation, touch, and presence, the nurse can optimize efforts to provide emotional support, privacy, and dignity to the surgical patient.

EVALUATION

The overall indicator of the effectiveness of the patient position is that the patient is able to resume preoperative activities without any change in function. The patient should not show evidence of skin breakdown, especially over bony prominences. The patient should be able to resume a preoperative pattern of movement with no complaints of tingling, numbness, cramping, or pain. Cardiac and respiratory function should not be altered by positioning. Assess for conditions such as labored breathing, cyanosis, and abnormal arterial blood gases, which could indicate positioning injury.

◖ CASE STUDY WITH PLAN OF CARE

"I've been playing the trombone for almost 40 years. I wonder if that could have contributed to my hemorrhoid," states Mr. Roberto K. Mr. K., a musician with the San Francisco Symphony, is admitted to the Ambulatory Surgery Unit for removal of external hemorrhoids. Although the hemorrhoids have been troubling him for more than 3 years, a recent episode of acute thrombosis influenced his decision for surgery. Mr. K., an avid cyclist and runner, is an otherwise healthy 50-year-old.

He weighs 180 pounds and is 5′11″. His vital signs are blood pressure of 130/70, pulse of 64/min., respiration of 18/min., and temperature of 98.2°F. Because the acute episode has subsided, he is now a candidate for surgery. Following preoperative teaching and admission, he is taken to the operating room. A spinal anesthetic is delivered, and he is positioned for surgery in the jackknife position.

◖ PLAN OF CARE FOR MR. ROBERTO K.
Nursing Diagnosis Risk for Perioperative Positioning Injury Related to the Jackknife Position

Expected Outcome: Mr. K.'s skin and soft tissues will remain free from injury during and after surgery.
- Inspect the skin for redness, open wounds, drainage, lesions, and swelling.
- Gather all positioning devices: pillows, head rest, padding for bony prominences and dorsa of the feet, armboards, and safety straps.
- Place the patient's hips over the break in the bed and flex the table at 90°.
- Use pillows or padding to protect the ears, hips, groin, legs, knees, and feet from pressure.
- Ensure that the genitals are free from pressure.
- Position safety straps across the thighs.
- Apply hemorrhoid straps for optimal exposure and visualization. Protect the skin under these straps with tincture of benzoin.

Expected Outcome: Mr. K. will be free from numbness, paresthesia, and/or paralysis following surgery.
- Place the arms on padded armboards with the arms extended outward and upward, palms down, and elbows slightly flexed so that the head of the humerus is not stretching and compressing the axillary neurovascular bundle.
- Place a small roll under each shoulder.
- Pad the medial aspect of the elbows.

Expected Outcome: Mr. K. will be free from circulatory and respiratory distress during and after surgery.
- ▲ Monitor respirations with a precordial stethoscope.
- ▲ Monitor oxygen saturation with a pulse oximeter; monitor heart rate and rhythm with an EKG; monitor blood pressure to assess respirations and hemodynamic status.
- ▲ Administer oxygen via nasal cannula.

Expected Outcome: Mr. K.'s privacy and dignity will be maintained throughout the procedure.
- ▲ Ensure that only the surgical area is exposed.
- ▲ Ensure that adequate personnel are present when positioning Mr. K. after the spinal anesthetic is administered.
- ▲ Keep Mr. K. informed of activities in the operating room. Inform him of procedures before they are performed.
- ▲ Offer Mr. K. the use of headphones so that he may listen to music throughout the procedure.
- Document nursing care as appropriate.

■ = nursing intervention; ▲ = collaborative intervention.

■■ CRITICAL THINKING EXERCISES

1. How does the jackknife position affect the patient's respiratory status?
2. Discuss five external environmental factors that may predispose a patient to perioperative positioning injury.
3. Why is capillary pressure important when considering the effects of positioning?
4. What is the principal cause of peripheral nerve damage from positioning injury?
5. Discuss ways in which the cardiovascular system can be affected by the Trendelenburg, lateral recumbent, and prone positions.

REFERENCES

1. Association of Operating Room Nurses: Clinical issues, *AORN Journal* 58(6):1192, 1993.
2. Association of Operating Room Nurses: Recommended practices: positioning the surgical patient, *AORN Journal* 52(5):1035–1039, 1990.
3. Biddle C and Cannady M: Surgical positions: their effect on cardiovascular, respiratory systems, *AORN Journal* 52(2):350–359, 1990.
4. Fairchild SS: *Perioperative nursing—principles and practice,* Boston, 1993, Jones & Bartlett Publishers.
5. Groah LK: *Operating room nursing perioperative practice,* Norwalk, Connecticut, 1990, Appleton & Lange.
6. Gruendemann BJ and Meeker MH: *Alexander's care of the patient in surgery,* ed 8, St. Louis, 1987, The CV Mosby Co.
7. Martin JT: Patient positioning. In Barash PG, Cullen BF, and Stoelting RK: *Clinical anesthesia,* Philadelphia, 1989, JB Lippincott Co.
8. North American Nursing Diagnosis Association: *NANDA nursing diagnoses: definitions and classification, 1995–1996,* Philadelphia, 1994, The Association.
9. Perry SL: Positioning the patient. In Phippen ML and Wells MP: *Perioperative nursing practice,* Philadelphia, 1994, WB Saunders Co.
10. Stoelting RK and Miller RD: *Basics of anesthesia,* ed 2, New York, 1989, Churchill Livingstone.

Risk for Injury
▶ ─────────────────────────────────

Risk for Trauma
▶ ─────────────────────────────────

Risk for Poisoning
▶ ─────────────────────────────────

Risk for Suffocation
▶ ─────────────────────────────────

Risk for Injury *is the state in which the individual is at risk for injury as a result of the environmental conditions interacting with the individual's adaptive and defensive resources.*[14]

Risk for Trauma *is the accentuated risk for accidental tissue injury, including wounds, burns, and fractures.*[14]

Risk for Poisoning *is the accentuated risk for accidental exposure to or ingestion of drugs or dangerous products in doses sufficient to cause poisoning.*[14]

Risk for Suffocation *is the accentuated risk for accidental suffocation (inadequate air available for inhalation).*[14]

OVERVIEW

The diagnosis of Risk for Injury is classified by the North American Nursing Diagnosis Association as a higher level diagnosis that encompasses the five specific diagnoses of Risk for Trauma, Risk for Poisoning, Risk for Suffocation, Risk for Aspiration, and Risk for Disuse Syndrome.[14] This chapter presents an overview of injury in general

and addresses the diagnoses of Risk for Trauma, Poisoning, and Suffocation in particular.

Injury in the United States continues to remain a serious national health problem. In 1991 approximately 2.8 million Americans were hospitalized for injury or poisoning diagnoses.[7] The annual national cost of visits to emergency rooms for injury-related visits is $9.2 billion.[4] Healthy People 2000,[21] the health-related goals for the nation, addresses the need for injury prevention interventions, especially among high-risk populations. Nurses therefore must be aware of the many issues involved in injury and injury control as a prerequisite for implementing interventions for injury prevention and control.

Over the years the concept of injury has developed to replace the notion of "accident," which implied randomness and conveyed blame for reckless, thoughtless, or even sinful behavior. The term *accident* encouraged a fatalistic view that accepted accident and death as inevitable sequelae of chance encounters with external forces. In contrast, the concept of injury control encourages the outlook that reduction in harmful effects and morbidity can be expected as a result of study and intervention. *Injury* refers to tissue damage caused by exchanges of environmental energy that are beyond the body's resilient capacity.[9] Injury is amenable to investigation because it is viewed as having a distinct etiology—the inability to resist energy transfer.

In any injury there is an unfavorable relationship among the variables of host, agent, and environment. The agent-host-environment model may be used to understand injuries. The host is the injured person who is characterized by age, sex, developmental level, neuromuscular status, and coping ability. The agent is the form of energy (kinetic, gravitational, chemical, thermal, electrical, or lack of oxidation) that causes damage to the tissue. The environment includes the physical surroundings and the psychosocial situation.

Injury and its prevention have been recognized as an area of research requiring the interdisciplinary efforts of epidemiology, environmental studies, ergonomics, engineering, physical therapy, nursing, occupational medicine, and the social sciences. Haddon[9] developed a conceptual framework for the analysis of injury that incorporates a two-dimensional view of injury: event and event epidemiology. Along one dimension of the injury episode is time, a variable that consists of preevent, event, and postevent time frames. The second dimension of the injury episode is its epidemiology, which consists of four components: (1) human factors (characteristics of the individual), (2) agent or vehicle (proximal cause of injury), (3) physical environment (climate, geography, noxious gases, broken glass), and (4) sociocultural factors (laws, expectations, norms that affect injuries, and prevention strategies).[9, 15] In addition, Haddon[9] developed strategies or countermeasures to reduce injuries; these continue to serve as the basis of most injury prevention programs.

Unintentional injuries are the fifth leading cause of death in the United States.[10] Injury from trauma (crashes, falls, fires), poisoning, and drowning cause more than three fourths of all deaths from unintentional injury.[1] Moreover, trauma is the leading cause of death in children 1 to 4 years old and in adults 25 to 44 years old.[10] A recent study[18] estimated a national rate of nonfatal injuries. In this study injury rates varied by age, sex, and location. Boys had higher injury rates than girls for all locations (school, home, recreation, street) and for most of the causes (burns, bikes or skates, cuts, falls, sports, and motor vehicles).

Injury is one of the most urgent problems in urban minority communities.[17] Minority Americans have high rates of home-related injuries, especially house fires.[8] Residential fire deaths were the second leading cause of injury deaths among children 1 to 9 years old and the sixth leading cause of death among those 65 and older.[19]

Most fatal firearm deaths among children (including homicide, suicide, and unintentional injury) occur in a home environment.[2] Firearm deaths are present across the life span, grow in childhood, and increase dramatically throughout late adolescence, especially among African-American males.[6]

Poisoning occurs following exposure to a chemical agent. Poisoning causes 13,000 deaths per year. Poisoning occurs at all ages from infancy onward, but its incidence begins to increase at age 12 and peaks at age 38. After age 70, the incidence of poisoning rises with increasing age.[1] Young children are at risk for poisoning because of heightened curiosity and an inclination to experience new things by tasting and smelling. Accidental poisoning is the major cause of death in children under 5 years of age. The highest incidence occurs in the 2-year-old age group, followed by the 1-year-old age group. The major cause of nonsuicide deaths for poisoning in the 12 to 38-year-old group is attributed to narcotics use, especially heroin and cocaine.[1] Elderly persons are at risk for poisoning because they have failing vision and memory and are frequently required to take several medications daily.

Chronic lead poisoning continues to be a national health problem.[12] A national survey of blood–lead levels conducted from 1988 to 1991 indicated that the total number of lead-poisoned children decreased 8.9% during that period of time, reflecting the outlawing of leaded gasoline.

Yet almost 4 million children were estimated to have blood–lead levels of 10 µg or more per dl. In the survey, children from 1 to 5 years of age had a prevalence of lead poisoning that was 6.1% in Caucasians, 36.7% in African-Americans, and 17% in Hispanics.[3] Although the problem cuts across all socioeconomic levels, poor and minority children are disproportionately affected.[5,11]

Lead, a heavy metal with no known physiological use, is mainly present in industrial societies as a result of environmental pollution of air, dust, soil, food, and water. Lead-based paint is present in housing built before 1960 or in apartments or some housing built before 1978.[20] Lead in the environment may be readily absorbed through the respiratory tract and the gastrointestinal tract. Although the metal accumulates slowly, it is excreted extremely slowly from the body. Poisoning occurs after repeated exposure to small amounts of lead over a period of months. Children and pregnant women are most vulnerable to lead poisoning because it is toxic to fetal brain tissue and to rapidly developing brain cells of young children. In addition to its effects on the central nervous system, lead poisoning causes toxic effects on the hematopoietic, renal, gastrointestinal, musculoskeletal, and reproductive systems, resulting in severe anemia, weight loss, renal failure, joint pain, decreased fertility, miscarriages, premature births, diminished intelligence, behavioral problems, decreased hearing, growth impairment, mental retardation, seizures, coma, and possible death.[16]

Asphyxia or lack of oxygen may occur because of suffocation (obstruction of the airway by covering the nose and mouth or oxygen starvation through enclosure), strangulation, hanging, or choking (internal obstruction of the airway by food or a foreign body).[13] Causes of suffocation and strangulation deaths include plastic bags used as mattress covers; infants wedging between the mattress and the crib frame; cribs with widely spaced slats; abandoned refrigerators, dishwashers, and freezers; clothing with string at the neckline such as a hood; drape cords; and cave-ins of sand or earth.

ASSESSMENT

Risk for Injury

The role of the nurse in diagnosing Risk for Injury is to identify the host, the agent, and the environmental factors as they become evident in the course of a patient history interview and physical assessment. Data related to physiological and psychological status, including functional abilities and physical and mental integrity, are extremely important. The identification of any risk factors for Risk for Injury should alert the nurse to investigate for the presence of other factors that could result in trauma, poisoning, or suffocation for the purpose of modifying any preinjury risk factors that threaten the patient's physical integrity.

■ Risk Factors

The presence of the following behaviors, conditions, or circumstances renders the patient more vulnerable to Risk for Injury:

Host factors
- Developmental age: physiological and psychological
- Sensory or motor deficits
- Cognitive impairments
- Seizure disorder
- Integrative dysfunction
- Ambulatory devices
- Tissue hypoxia
- Malnutrition
- Fatigue
- Immune response impairment
- Abnormal blood profile
- Osteoporosis
- Central nervous system depressant drugs
- Impaired proprioceptive reflexes
- Children: number of injuries sustained before age 5, aggressive behavior, male sex
- Elderly: frail, restricted mobility, vertigo, orthostatic hypotension

Agent factors
- Energy: chemical, electrical, gravitational, mechanical, radiant, thermal

Environmental factors

- Physical: unsafe design, structure, or arrangement of home and community or unsafe mode of transportation
- Chemical: presence of pollutants, improperly marked or stored poisons or drugs, large supplies of drugs, and use of pesticides, preservatives, cosmetics, and dyes
- Sociocultural: presence of home remedies, religious practices involving products (e.g., peyote, mercury) that are harmful if ingested or become contaminants in the environment

Risk for Trauma

The very young and the very old who seem to be "accident prone" are at accentuated Risk for Trauma. Children who tend to run rather than walk, who like to climb, and who like to explore unfamiliar places may be especially prone to trauma. Parental awareness of safety factors, such as the use of a car seat appropriate for the child's age, gates to block steep stairways, and safety measures in kitchens and bathrooms, is especially important.

The elderly person with weakness, poor vision, or balancing difficulties is at Risk for Trauma because of falls (gravitational energy), burns (thermal energy), and cuts (mechanical energy). Normal aging processes and pathological processes increase the likelihood of trauma, especially when compounded by environmental factors such as slippery floors, unanchored rugs, and dimly lit stairways.

■ Risk Factors

The presence of the following behaviors, conditions, or circumstances renders the client more vulnerable to Risk for Trauma:

Host factors

- Weakness
- Poor vision
- Balancing difficulties
- Reduced hand-eye coordination
- Reduced tactile or temperature sensation
- Reduced coordination of large or small muscle groups
- Sensory or motor deficits
- Cognitive or emotional changes
- Insufficient use of safety precautions
- Insufficient finances to make safety repairs or changes
- History of previous trauma

Agent factors

- Energy: gravitational, mechanical, thermal, electrical, or radiant

Environmental factors

- Slippery floors
- Snow or ice on stairs or walkway
- Unanchored rugs
- Bathtub without hand grip or antislip surface
- Use of unsteady ladder or chair
- Entering unlighted room
- Unsturdy or absent handrails along a staircase
- Unanchored electrical wires
- Litter or liquid spills on floors or staircases
- High beds
- Children playing without gates at top or bottom of stairs
- Obstructed passageways
- Unsafe window protection in homes with young children
- Inappropriate or faulty call-aid devices for those on bed rest
- Pot handles facing the front of stove
- Bathing in very hot water
- Unsupervised bathing of young children
- Potential ignition of gas leaks
- Delayed ignition of gas burner or oven
- Experimenting with chemicals or gasoline
- Unscreened fireplaces or heaters
- Wearing plastic aprons or flowing clothing near open flame
- Playing with matches, candles, or cigarettes
- Inadequately stored combustibles, corrosives, acids, alkalis
- Highly flammable children's toys or clothing
- Overloaded fuse box

- Contact with rapidly moving machinery, belts, or pulleys
- Sliding on coarse linen or struggling with in-bed restraints
- Faulty electrical plugs, frayed wires, defective appliances
- Contact with acids or alkalis
- Playing with fireworks or gunpowder
- Contact with intense cold
- Overexposure to sun, sunlamps, or radiation therapy
- Use of cracked dishware or glasses
- Knives stored uncovered
- Guns or ammunition stored in unlocked cabinet
- Large icicles hanging from roof
- Exposure to dangerous machinery
- Children playing with sharp-edged toys
- High crime neighborhood
- Driving a mechanically unsafe vehicle
- Driving after drinking alcohol or using drugs
- Driving at excessive speed
- Driving without necessary visual aids
- Children riding in front seat of car
- Smoking in bed or near oxygen
- Overloaded electrical outlets
- Grease collected on stoves
- Use of thin or worn potholders
- Unrestrained babies riding in a car
- Failure to use automobile seat restraints
- Failure by cyclists to use head gear or improper use of head gear
- Young children carried on adult bicycles
- Unsafe road conditions
- Play or work near vehicle pathways or railroad tracks

Risk for Poisoning

The nurse assesses the patient and environment for risk factors that increase the likelihood of poisoning. Patients with cognitive limitations or emotional problems may not take proper precautions because they are not aware of the hazards of certain products or because they behave impetuously.

Characteristics of a child's developmental age, such as exploration associated with toddlers or peer pressure associated with teenagers, increase the likelihood of exposure to poisonous products or illicit drugs. The normal impulse of infants to put things in their mouths and children's tendency toward pica (ingestion of nonfood items) place them in danger of poisoning. In elderly populations, reduced vision, glaucoma, or cataracts may cause accidental poisonings if these patients cannot properly see the labeling on their medications.

■ Risk Factors

The presence of the following behaviors, conditions, or circumstances renders the patient more vulnerable to Risk for Poisoning:

Host factors
- Pica or mouthing of nonfood substances
- Reduced vision
- Cognitive or emotional difficulties
- Developmental age of child (crawling infant; exploring toddler; magical, egocentric thinking of preschooler; peer pressure of teenager) or adult
- Occupational setting that does not have adequate safeguards
- Lack of safety or drug education
- Lack of proper precautions
- Insufficient finances

Agent factors
- Chemical energy of the poison

Environmental factors
- Large supplies of drugs in the home
- Medicines stored in unlocked cabinets accessible to children or confused persons
- Availability of illicit drugs potentially contaminated by poisonous additives
- Flaking, peeling of lead-based paint or plaster in environment of young children
- Lead in dishes or cookware
- Lack of parental supervision
- Chemical contamination of food and water
- Unprotected contact with heavy metals, chemicals, or insecticides

- Paint in poorly ventilated areas or without proper storage
- Presence of poisonous vegetation
- Presence of atmospheric pollutants

Risk for Suffocation

Many of the risk factors for Risk for Suffocation are inherent in the developmental characteristics of infants, toddlers, and preschoolers. Children under 2 years of age commonly pick up items and place them in their mouths; this can be hazardous even if the child in is a "child-safe" environment. Young children, who have no fear of harm and do not understand safety precautions, and older children, who lack safety education, possess important host characteristics that place them at risk for suffocation, choking, aspiration, and submersion accidents. Numerous environmental risk factors place children, adults, and the elderly at risk for accidents that result in asphyxia.

■ Risk Factors

The presence of the following behaviors, conditions, or circumstances renders the patient more vulnerable to Risk for Suffocation:

Host factors
- Reduced olfactory sensation
- Reduced motor abilities
- Disease or injury processes
- Cognitive or emotional difficulties
- Lack of safety education or precautions
- Lack of awareness of hazards in environment

Agent factors
- Lack of oxygen

Environmental factors
- Pillow placed in infant's crib
- Vehicle warming in closed garage
- Children playing with plastic bags or inserting small objects into their mouths or noses
- Refrigerators or freezers discarded or left unused without removing doors
- Children left unattended in bathtubs or pools
- Household gas leaks
- Smoking in bed

- Use of fuel-burning space heaters not vented to outside
- Low-strung clotheslines
- Pacifier hung on cord around infant's neck
- Eating large mouthfuls of food
- Propped bottle placed in an infant's mouth
- Lack of parental supervision
- Lack of safety precautions

DIAGNOSIS

■ Differential Nursing Diagnosis

Risk for Injury encompasses the diagnoses addressed in this chapter (Risk for Trauma, Risk for Poisoning, Risk for Suffocation), as well as Risk for Aspiration and Risk for Disuse Syndrome. When a patient is determined to be at Risk for Injury, further assessment is required to specify the type of injury that may be a threat to the patient. Such specification will promote care planning directed toward the specific threat. The diagnoses classified under Altered Protection, that is, Impaired Tissue Integrity, Altered Oral Mucous Membrane, Impaired Skin Integrity, and Sensory/Perceptual Alterations, have implications for making the patient more susceptible to injury.

■ Related Medical and Psychiatric Diagnoses

The following are examples of commonly related medical and psychiatric diagnoses for Risk for Injury: arthritis, cataracts, blindness, blood dyscrasias, cerebrovascular accident, seizures, dementia, depression, and delusional paranoid disorder. Commonly related diagnoses for Risk for Trauma include Alzheimer's disease, anemia, bipolar disorder (manic episode), cataracts, glaucoma, cerebrovascular accident, delusional paranoid disorder, diabetes, seizures, osteoporosis, Parkinsonism. Risk for Poisoning may accompany depression, lead poisoning, mercury poisoning, organophosphate poisoning, or psychoactive substance use disorder. Risk for Suffocation may accompany the diagnoses of inhalation injuries, disorders affecting the ability to swallow or breathe such as asthma, status asthmaticus, myasthenia, and cerebrovascular accident.

OUTCOME IDENTIFICATION, PLANNING, AND IMPLEMENTATION

Risk for Injury

Selecting outcomes for planning and implementation to manage the cluster of diagnoses under Risk for Injury requires separate patient outcomes and interventions for each of the diagnoses addressed in this chapter. In planning interventions the nurse chooses actions that have the highest likelihood of preventing injury, trauma, poisoning, or suffocation. It is important to include the client and the family in stating appropriate outcomes and choosing interventions.

Risk for Trauma

Using the injury framework described earlier, the nurse must plan and implement strategies or countermeasures aimed at the agent causing the injury, so that the host is protected from the agent, or altering the environment, or both. To achieve the stated outcome of "no falls experienced while in the hospital," interventions must be aimed at strengthening the host, modifying the agent of gravitational energy, and manipulating the environment. The rationale for choosing a particular intervention to prevent trauma from falls in the toddler age group is very different from the rationale for choosing the same intervention in the elderly group, given the particular physical, psychological, and developmental features of each age group. Identification of outcome achievement is evaluated on a daily basis and at discharge. Fall prevention is an all-or-none outcome that has major implications for patient safety and survival.

Risk for Poisoning

The outcome of poison prevention has implications that are both time-specific for particular age groups and lifelong for all age groups. The ultimate expected outcome is that no poisoning of any kind occurs. It is important to note, however, that different medicines, chemicals, and pollutants have different hazard potentials and that some, such as carbon monoxide, have a highly rapid onset and fatal effects, whereas others, such as lead, have a more insidious onset and chronic effects. Achievement of the outcome of poison prevention requires awareness of the epidemiology of individual poisonous products and appreciation of the important role of anticipatory guidance and screening efforts.

Risk for Suffocation

The expected outcome of suffocation prevention also has implications that are both time-specific for various age groups and lifelong for all age groups. Achievement of the outcome requires awareness of the epidemiology of suffocation within age groups and an appreciation of the important role of anticipatory guidance, removal of sources of possible suffocation, and education of parents and community members regarding emergency rescue measures.

The planning and the implementation phases of the nursing process for Risk for Injury, Risk for Trauma, Risk for Poisoning, and Risk for Suffocation culminate with the documentation of completed actions and the patient's responses. Nursing Care Guidelines are presented for planning care for patients at risk for trauma, poisoning (lead), and suffocation. The focus of the expected outcome identified in each of the Nursing Care Guidelines is to prevent injury in the form of trauma, poisoning, or suffocation.

I

◢ **NURSING CARE GUIDELINES**
Nursing Diagnosis: Risk for Trauma

Expected Outcome: The patient will be free from injury from harmful agents in the hospital environment for the duration of stay.

Host

- Screen the patient for presence of risk factors for trauma from falls, cuts, or wounds:
- Assess patient characteristics of age, developmental level, mental ability, emotional state, socioeconomic status, mobility, strength, and capacity to carry out tasks. *The initial screening and assessment establishes essential baseline data with which to determine degree of risk for trauma.*
- Determine if history or presence of disease increases Risk for Trauma from falls. *Risk for Trauma is increased by a history of past trauma(s), certain medications, and sensory, mobility, and judgment impairments that accompany selected diseases.*
- Identify contributing factors. *Interventions may then be directed at removing or modifying factors that maintain or support the state of risk.*
- Educate the patient and family by explaining the risk factors that contribute to increased Risk for Injury and the necessary safety precautions to alleviate these. *Patients and their families need clear, precise information to improve their understanding of risk factors, with the aim of increasing compliance with injury prevention behavior.*
- Document findings and interventions on the patient's record. *Documentation provides a written record of teaching and safety measures employed for continuity of care, quality assurance, and legal considerations.*

Agent

- Identify agent of injury. Appropriate countermeasures may be employed.
▲ Implement countermeasures to prevent injury caused by agent of injury. *Countermeasures reduce the chance for a potential hazard, modify the rate of potential severity, and increase resistance of the host to damage by a hazard.*

Environment

- Identify and remove hazards in the environment that precipitate trauma. *Separate in time and space the hazard and the person to be protected.*
- Explain safety reasons for altering the environment, and prevent possible injury by providing general safety information. *Patients need clear, precise information that will encourage compliance with safety behaviors.*

- Provide specific anticipatory guidance about safety. *Provide individuals with safety information ahead of time so that trauma may be prevented.*
▲ Identify community resources for the elderly, for example, Meals on Wheels, Emergency Life Alarm, and the Telephone Reassurance Program. *The individual maintains support as needed over time.*

■ = nursing intervention; ▲ = collaborative intervention.

◢ **NURSING CARE GUIDELINES**
Nursing Diagnosis: Risk for Lead Poisoning

Expected Outcome: The client's venous blood will indicate absence of lead.

Host

- Screen for listlessness, anorexia, pallor, pica (eating or mouthing nonfood items). *Early identification of symptoms of poisoning will provide for prompt treatment.*
- Ask parents if the child eats well-balanced meals; complains of stomachaches; has hard, infrequent bowel movements; is irritable, distracted, or hyperactive; has change in sleep pattern; has forgotten any motor activities previously mastered. *Pointed questions help determine the extent of toxicity.*
- ▲ Refer children with positive screening to a physician for evaluation. *Appropriate laboratory and diagnostic tests will help determine if poisoning has occurred.*
- ▲ Monitor laboratory results for levels of hematocrit, hemoglobin, lead, FEP, and calcium in the urine to determine progress or deterioration.

Agent

- ▲ Determine the form of poison exposure responsible for the injury. *Appropriate countermeasures may be employed.*
- ▲ Implement countermeasures to prevent injury from lead through lead poison education programs and parent-child programs. *Educational programs alert parents to the dangers of lead hazards and encourage developmentally appropriate child-rearing behaviors by parents.*

Environment

- Assess and monitor family structure, passive parent, patterns of parent-child interaction, and family stressors. *Characteristics of the family may contribute to a delay in the reporting of symptoms.*
- Identify adults in the home who work in industries where lead exposure is likely and who may bring lead dust home via skin and clothing. *All potential sources of exposure must be identified.*
- Identify lead exposure in the home: old, flaking, chipped paint or plaster; colored newsprint; cigarette butts and ashes; water from lead-soldered pipes; soil with high lead content; food grown in soil contaminated by lead; leaded gasoline; foreign-made ceramic dishes or toys; and illegal moonshine manufactured in a still made from a lead-lined radiator. *Lead hazards are present in many forms.*
- ▲ Identify sources of lead in the air: exposure to a smelting factory, burning of leaded objects, living near a busy street or public garage, or living in older housing undergoing renovation. *Airborne lead dust may be inhaled through the respiratory tract and contribute to poisoning.*
- Assess parents' level of understanding of lead poisoning and educate them as needed. *Education about lead-poisoning prevention begins by building on familiar knowledge.*
- Provide anticipatory guidance on patterns of normal growth and development and the hazards for lead poisoning and their relationship to nutrition and development. *Parents need to be aware of patterns of normal growth and development and the hazards for lead poisoning and the role of nutrition.*
- Suggest activities for parents that promote parent-child interaction and decrease pica behavior in child. *Normal interaction with parents and family members will discourage opportunities for boredom and unobserved eating of nonfood items.*
- Refer to a community nurse for follow-up. *Growth and development and symptoms of lead poisoning must be assessed on an ongoing basis.*

■ = nursing intervention; ▲ = collaborative intervention.

I

◢ NURSING CARE GUIDELINES
Nursing Diagnosis: Risk for Suffocation

Expected Outcome: Suffocation will be prevented in the child at risk for the duration of hospital stay and beyond discharge.

Host

- Assess and monitor personal characteristics: age, developmental level, mental status, muscle strength, coordination, temperament, knowledge, and capacity to protect self from suffocation. *This establishes baseline data with which to determine the degree of Risk for Suffocation.*

Agent

- Determine possible causes of lack of oxygen supply that may result in airway obstruction and hypoxemia. *Common sources of airway obstruction and asphyxia vary by age level.*
- ▲ Use countermeasures to prevent or reduce injury from lack of oxygen, such as removing doors from discarded refrigerators and freezers; arranging for prompt removal of discarded refrigerators and freezers; placing fences around swimming pools; and child proofing surroundings. *Such countermeasures modify the potential severity of the hazard by altering the source.*
- Teach emergency rescue to parents, caregivers, siblings, and community. *Countermeasures provide for quick emergency response to offset damage already done.*
- Perform Heimlich maneuver or cardiopulmonary resuscitation if needed. *Countermeasures stabilize, repair, and rehabilitate the damaged host.*

Environment

- Identify environmental hazards that cause suffocation. *Hazards for suffocation may be removed or altered.*
- Alter the environment by removing hazards. *This reduces the chances of injury from existing hazards.*
- Determine parents' knowledge of safety precautions appropriate for the child's developmental level. *Common hazards vary by age group.*
- Inform parents of common items that pose safety problems. *Inform them about safety precautions and teach them to check and child proof the environment routinely to prevent the occurrence of existing hazards.*
- Work toward developing community support for environmental measures known to be effective in reducing injury. *This prevents the marshalling of the hazardous energy in the first place.*

■ = nursing intervention; ▲ = collaborative intervention.

EVALUATION

The nurse evaluates the plan of care during and following implementation. The nurse focuses evaluation on the patient's response to nursing interventions in relation to predetermined desired patient outcomes. The key determination to make when evaluating Risk for Injury, Risk for Trauma, Risk for Poisoning, and Risk for Suffocation is whether the patient suffered an injury.

One must determine whether the expected outcomes have been achieved completely, partially, or not at all. The following questions should be answered when evaluating the care for patients with these diagnoses: Were the desired outcomes of prevention of trauma, poisoning, or suffocation achieved and to what extent? What data support this? Were the interventions effective in preventing injury? If not, why? Is a different plan needed? What data support this decision? Was the plan of care communicated and carried out? Were the patient and significant others included in the planning? What obstacles prevent the plan from being executed? Is there a need for referral or collaboration? Is the diagnosis Risk for Injury valid for this patient, or is another diagnosis more appropriate? Is reevaluation of the data needed to confirm the diagnosis?

CASE STUDY WITH PLAN OF CARE

Mrs. Margaret S. is a 77-year-old Cuban-born widow with failing vision, who lives with her brother in an apartment in a major city. They emigrated to this country 20 years ago. Mrs. S. prides herself on her ability to remain independent and to provide a home for her brother and herself. Mrs. S. was getting out of the shower when she suddenly felt weak and fell backward, striking her head and her lower back on a heating pipe. There were no seizures or loss of consciousness. She was brought to the emergency room via ambulance. Physical assessment revealed the following findings: frail, elderly female with blood pressure of 140/90, pulse of 96 beats/min and regular, respirations of 24/min, and temperature of 98.5°F. Her skin was dry and pale. Swelling was noted on the right parietal surface of the skull, and bruising and swelling were noted over the right lumbar area. Mrs. S.

reports extreme pain in the lumbar area. Assessment revealed the following: chest clear on auscultation and percussion; peripheral pulses 1+, slight ankle edema; mental status—awake, disoriented to place; pupils 3 to 4 mm, equal, round, reactive to light and accommodation; spontaneous movement of all extremities with bilateral lower extremity quadricep weakness; and reflexes normal. Lab results and CT scan were normal.

Physician orders include transfer to nursing unit for observation; neurological checks every 2 hours; bed rest with commode privileges; and a soft diet. On the nursing unit Mrs. S. repeatedly tries to get out of bed to use the commode. Although she speaks and understands English, she now only communicates in Spanish. The following plan of care was developed for Mrs. S.

PLAN OF CARE FOR MRS. MARGARET S.
Nursing Diagnosis: Risk for Trauma Related to History of Falls and Disorientation

Expected Outcome: Mrs. S. will experience no trauma as evidenced by the absence of falls during her hospital stay.

Host
- Identify Mrs. S. as at Risk for Trauma (falls) and document.
- ▲ Assess and monitor her neurological status.
- Orient to time, place, and person at each encounter. Use Spanish language or interpreter.
- Explain procedures before initiating. Reassure Mrs. S. frequently, using a calm voice and unhurried manner.
- Instruct her to use the call bell for requesting assistance.
- Instruct her to remain in bed and remind her frequently.

Agent
- ▲ Implement countermeasures to prevent injury from falls caused by gravity such as altering floor surface characteristics by not waxing floors and by maintaining and increasing lower limb strength.

Environment
- ▲ Request an order for a family member, staff member, or companion to stay with her at all times while disorientation persists.
- Keep a night light on at night and keep bed rails up when Mrs. S. is unattended.
- Keep the bed in low position and wheels locked.
- Encourage voiding before retiring.
- Offer assistance to commode, as needed, around the clock.
- Use nonskid slippers.

■ = nursing intervention; ▲ = collaborative intervention.

I

Documentation of the usefulness of interventions in the achievement of outcomes and the answers to the questions listed above will guide the nurse in determining whether to (1) continue the plan of care with periodic reassessment, (2) modify the plan, or (3) terminate the plan if it is no longer needed. The process of planning appropriate care for patients diagnosed with Risk for Injury, Risk for Trauma, Risk for Poisoning, and Risk for Suffocation requires a foundation built on the concept of injury control and appreciation for the value of prevention in reducing injury.

■ CRITICAL THINKING EXERCISES

1. What might account for Mrs. S.'s use of her native tongue rather than English? How will her language preference influence her care requirements?
2. Which changes in neurological status would further increase the patient's risk for falls? What preventive measures should be employed?
3. Is the stated patient outcome of "no falls experienced for the duration of hospital stay" realistic? Why? Should you be concerned about Mrs. S. being at risk for falls when she is discharged to home? What are some of the consequences of failing to plan for discharge?

REFERENCES

1. Baker SP, O'Neill B, Ginsburg MJ, and Li G: *The injury fact book,* ed 2, New York, 1992, Oxford University Press.
2. Beaver BL, Moore VL, and Peclet M: Characteristics of pediatric firearm fatalities, *J Pediatr Surg* 25:97, 1990.
3. Brody DJ, Pirkle JL, Kramer RA, Flegal KM, Matte T, Gunter E, and Paschal D: Blood lead levels in the US population: Phase I of the third national health and nutrition examination Survey (NHANES III), 1988–1991, *JAMA* 272:277–283, 1994.
4. Burt CW: Injury-related visits to hospital emergency departments: United States, 1992, *Advance data from vital and health statistics,* no. 261, Hyattsville, Maryland, 1995, National Center for Health Statistics.
5. Environmental Defense Fund: *Legacy of lead: America's continuing epidemic of childhood lead poisoning,* Washington, D.C., 1990, Environmental Defense Fund.
6. Fingerhut LA: Firearm mortality among children, youth, and young adults 1–34 years of age, trends and current status: United States, 1985–1990. *Advance data from vital and health statistics,* no 231, Hyattsville, Maryland, 1993, National Center for Health Statistics.
7. Graves EJ: 1991 Summary: national hospital discharge survey, *Advance data from vital and health statistics,* no 227, Hyattsville, Maryland, 1993, National Center for Health Statistics.
8. Gulaid JA, Sattin RW, and Wazweiler FR: Deaths from residential fires, 1978–1984. CDC surveillance summaries, *Mortality and Morbidity Weekly* 37(SS-1):39–45, 1988.
9. Haddon W: On the escape of tigers: an ecologic note, *Am J Public Health* 74(12):2229–2334, 1970.
10. Kochanek KD and Hudson BL: Advance report of final mortality statistics, 1992, *Monthly vital statistics report* 43(6)(suppl), Hyattsville, Maryland, 1994, National Center for Health Statistics.
11. Needleman HL: Preventing childhood lead poisoning, *Prev Med* 23:634–637, 1994.
12. Needleman HL: The long-term effects of exposure to low doses of lead in childhood, *New Eng J Med* 32:83–88, 1990.
13. Nixon JW, Kemp A, Levene S, and Sibert JR: Suffocation, choking, and strangulation in childhood in England and Wales: epidemiology and prevention, *Arch Dis Child* 72:6–10, 1995.
14. North American Nursing Diagnosis Association: *NANDA nursing diagnoses: definitions and classification, 1995–1996,* Philadelphia, 1994, The Association.
15. Rivara FP and Alexander BH: Occupational injuries. In Rosenstock E and Cullen MR, *Textbook of clinical occupational and environmental medicine,* Philadelphia, 1994, WB Saunders Co.
16. Rosen JF: Adverse health effects of lead at low exposure levels: trends in the management of childhood lead poisoning, *Toxicology* 97:11–17, 1995.
17. Schwarz D and others: An injury prevention program in an urban African-American community, *Am J Public Health* 83(5):675–680, 1993.
18. Scheidt P, Harel Y, Trumble A, Jones D, Overpeck M, and Bijur P: The epidemiology of nonfatal injuries among US children and youth, *Am J Public Health* 85(7):932–938, 1995.
19. U.S. Department of Health and Human Services: Deaths resulting from residential fires—United States, 1991, *Morbidity and Mortality Weekly Report* 43(49):901–904, December 16, 1994.
20. U.S. Department of Health and Human Services, Public Health Service: *Questions parents ask about lead poisoning,* Atlanta, 1992, Center for Disease Control.
21. U.S. Department of Health and Human Services: *Healthy people 2000. National health promotion and disease prevention objectives,* DHHS Pub No (PHS) 91-50213, Washington, D.C., 1990, U.S. Government Printing Office.

Ineffective Management of Therapeutic Regimen (Individuals)

Ineffective Management of Therapeutic Regimen (Individuals) *is a pattern of regulating and integrating into daily living a program for the treatment of illness and the sequelae of illness that are* unsatisfactory *for meeting specific health goals.*

OVERVIEW

The first version of this diagnosis, Alteration in Management of Illness, was published in a diagnostic system by Lunney in 1982.[7] In 1986 the term *illness* was changed to *therapeutic regimen.* Therapeutic regimens are sets of rules, or habits, of diet, exercise, and manner of living that are intended to improve health and to treat or cure disease. An analysis and synthesis of the literature was done by Lunney to articulate the definition and defining characteristics of the diagnosis. This included a broad base of literature on managing specific types of regimens for health problems. The literature review served as a basis for a validity study conducted in 1990.[8] For this study, expert nurses who were working in community health were recruited at national public health conferences. The sample consisted of 58 nurses from 26 states, the District of Columbia, and Canada who agreed to participate. The findings provided empirical evidence for submission of the diagnosis to the North American Nursing Diagnosis Association (NANDA).

Nurses who participated in the validation study had an impressive amount of experience in helping patients to manage therapeutic regimens ($M = 18.8$

years), were educated at the baccalaureate degree or higher (77% had master's or doctor's degrees), and had a broad base of experience from working with all developmental stages and in many types of health care settings. According to Fehring's validation method, subjects rated each defining characteristic on a scale of 1 (almost never present) to 5 (almost always present).[3] The weighted means of these responses were computed to differentiate defining characteristics (DCs) as major, minor, and low relevance. One DC was identified as major with a validity index greater than .80. The remaining DCs were validated as minor, that is, the weighted means were between .50 and .79.

Individuals need to perform therapeutic regimens to produce positive health outcomes. To achieve health-related goals, therapeutic regimens must be incorporated with activities of daily living and family processes.[4,6] These can range from relatively simple regimens, such as taking Digoxin after assessing pulse rate, to complex regimens, such as performing peritoneal dialysis.

Making the diagnosis of ineffective or effective Management of Therapeutic Regimen (MTR) requires a high degree of collaboration between nurses and patients. Patients participate by making decisions about the fit of therapeutic regimens with their preferred lifestyle(s) and by acting on these decisions. The agent for MTR is the patient.

The concept of MTR includes the ability to regulate or integrate therapeutic regimens into lifestyle(s), the actions taken to do so, and the willingness to pursue improvements in management behaviors. After values clarification, if a patient does not wish to manage a therapeutic regimen, nurses should not use this diagnosis. Because interventions are focused on self-regulation, positive results will not occur unless the patient agrees with the diagnosis.

Use of this diagnosis assumes that the patient is able to manage a therapeutic regimen. If developmental status, cognitive deficits, physical handicaps, or other stable factors prevent patients from managing therapeutic regimens, the diagnosis does not apply, except perhaps to justify ongoing nursing care for management of therapeutic regimens such as long-term care and hospitalization.

The strength diagnosis should be used whenever a consumer has risk factors for ineffective MTR but assessment shows that a risk state does not actually exist. Making strength diagnoses reinforces that the nurse agrees with and supports the patient's MTR and helps nurses and others to prioritize interventions for other diagnoses.

A risk diagnosis pertaining to management of therapeutic regimen has not been submitted to NANDA, but an in-depth study of five patients with Congestive Heart Failure showed that the risk status diagnosis is useful to guide interventions for prevention.[5] In this study, Knowledge Deficit was a reliable contributing factor in four of the five cases. For example, one patient was taking eight medications and knew the rationale for only one of them.

A wellness diagnosis (e.g., Potential for Enhanced Management of Therapeutic Regimen) has not been submitted to NANDA but can be used for clinical cases in which the cues indicate less than optimum MTR but there is not a clearly defined problem state. Health promotion and health protection interventions can be used with the wellness diagnosis.[10,11]

ASSESSMENT

Assessment of the defining characteristics may be accomplished early in data collection or may require a broad base of data from the 11 Functional Health Patterns. Because the first of the Functional Health Patterns addresses Health Management, including management of therapeutic regimen, data collection in this pattern may yield sufficient cues to infer that MTR is effective or ineffective. However, data generated during assessment of other patterns should support or refute initial impressions. The diagnosis should be considered a hypothesis until integration of the therapeutic regimen with daily living is verified through other patterns. For example, an individual may first report that taking blood pressure medication is not a problem and later report that sleep patterns are disturbed by having to get up to go to the bathroom or that recreational trips cannot be made because of poor bladder control. Subsequent data that indicate difficulty integrating the therapeutic regimen into the individual's lifestyle suggests that MTR may need to be addressed and validated.

Making this diagnosis requires skill in taking health histories and establishing trusting relationships with patients. A nonjudgmental, caring approach will provide an environment for patients to reveal their everyday patterns of self-management. The diagnosis is based on patterns over time rather than on observable behavior; therefore the meaning of nonverbal behavior that is incongruent with verbal data should be validated (e.g., a woman who says she is on a low-salt diet but has a packaged coffeecake on the table).

The major defining characteristic, choices of daily activities are inappropriate for meeting the goals of a treatment or prevention program, reflects that desire and behavior are incongruent. The patient may agree to manage, or take charge of, the illness regimen and set goals accordingly, but such agreement does not mean that the goals are being met. When patients agree that behaviors can improve, it increases the need to focus on this diagnosis.

The defining characteristic, acceleration of illness symptoms, is a cue that the patient may need assistance from nurses to manage the regimen. Because the effectiveness of MTR is judged relative to specific health goals, defining characteristics include evidence that treatment goals are not being met. Treatment goals usually include controlling the negative effects of illness on daily living and the progression of illness; reducing risk factors for illness and its sequelae; and optimizing daily activities with consideration of health needs.

Because health goals should include the integration of illness regimens with daily routines, the defining characteristic, verbalized that did not take action to include treatment regimens in daily routines, indicates that consumer behaviors may be ineffective. Sources on management of chronic illnesses describe a multitude of factors that interfere with integration of treatment regimens in daily routines, including stigma, cultural traditions, and deficits in community resources.[6,9]

An expressed desire to manage the treatment of illness and prevention of sequelae may be a request for help in accomplishing these goals. At the very least, this cue should be assessed in making the diagnosis because improved MTR probably is not possible without the desire to do so.

The defining characteristic, verbalized difficulty with regulation/integration of treatment or prevention regimen, is a cue that the patient may need help to achieve treatment goals. If patients do not offer this information, nurses can seek the data when assessing for the diagnosis by asking appropriate questions (e.g., "How difficult has it been to change your diet?") or by validating the meaning of observations.

The defining characteristic, verbalized that did not take action to reduce risk factors for progression of illness and sequelae, indicates that health protection is not sufficient. Strategies in the categories of primary, secondary, and tertiary prevention may be indicated, depending on the health problem (e.g., managing stress, developing an exercise routine, and stopping smoking may prevent progression of heart disease).

Further research is needed to determine if other defining characteristics are appropriate for this diagnosis. Three additional defining characteristics—anxiety, reluctance to discuss the therapeutic regimen, and incongruence of verbal and nonverbal behaviors[8]—were recommended by nurse experts in the validation study for determining whether MTR is effective. These behaviors may reflect personal conflict between healthy behavior and values and/or unwillingness to share information about self-management. One explanation for unwillingness to share information is the overall emphasis in the health care system on compliance. If patients expect nurses to focus on compliance and perhaps to use power differences to coerce compliance, they may avoid discussing management issues.

Assessment of related factors requires knowledge of the health belief model.[10,11] Factors such as perceived seriousness, perceived susceptibility, perceived benefits, perceived barriers, and cues to action were explained by Pender.[10] The other related factors are explained in books on chronic illness.[6,9]

■ Defining Characteristics

The presence of the following defining characteristics indicates that individuals may be experiencing Ineffective Management of Therapeutic Regimen:

Major
- Choices of daily living are inappropriate for meeting the goals of treatment or prevention

Minor
- Acceleration (expected or unexpected) of illness symptoms
- Verbalized desire to manage the treatment of illness and the prevention of sequelae
- Verbalized difficulty with regulation/integration of one or more prescribed regimens for the treatment of illness and its effects or the prevention of complications
- Verbalized that did not take action to include treatment regimens in daily routines
- Verbalized that did not take action to reduce risk factors for progression of the illness and its sequelae

I

The diagnosis Effective Management of Therapeutic Regimen: Individual can be made when the individual exhibits strengths in all or most of the above factors.

■ Related Factors

The following related factors are associated with Ineffective Management of Therapeutic Regimen: (Individuals):

- Complexity of the health care system
- Complexity of the therapeutic regimen
- Decisional conflicts
- Economic difficulties
- Excessive demands made on the individual or family
- Family conflict
- Family patterns of health care
- Inadequate number and types of cues to action
- Knowledge deficits
- Mistrust of the regimen and/or health care personnel
- Perceived seriousness
- Perceived susceptibility
- Perceived barriers
- Perceived benefits
- Powerlessness
- Social support deficits

DIAGNOSIS

■ Differential Nursing Diagnosis

This diagnosis overlaps significantly with the diagnosis of Noncompliance. The concept of MTR is more comprehensive than the concept of compliance because its focus is self-regulation and integration based on the consumer's values and goals, not merely compliance with the instructions of others. The concept of MTR was developed, studied, and submitted to NANDA by Lunney to serve as an alternative to the concepts of compliance and adherence. Ineffective MTR can be used for many of the clinical situations for which nurses would use Noncompliance. The article by Bakker and others is recommended for a more thorough explanation of differences between these two diagnoses.[1] Noncompliance may be more useful than Ineffective MTR with medical diagnoses such as Tuberculosis because patient-initiated changes in the medication regimen can lead to drug-resistant TB, a serious problem for both individuals and society. Other nursing diagnoses that may be considered in differential diagnosis are Altered Health Maintenance and Health-Seeking Behaviors (Specify). Altered Health Maintenance is more general than Ineffective MTR and is not specific enough when the major concern is MTR. The diagnosis Health-Seeking Behaviors is an alternative to the strength diagnosis Effective MTR. The choice of which diagnosis to use depends on which one best provides direction for interventions.

■ Medical and Psychiatric Diagnoses

Any medical or psychiatric diagnosis that requires patients to initiate and maintain changes in lifestyle based on prescriptions for the health problem may be associated with his nursing diagnosis. Diagnoses that require complex changes in living patterns, such as taking medications more than once a day, making significant changes in eating habits, or avoiding behaviors that previously were habits (e.g., smoking), are particularly important. These include medical diagnoses such as diabetes mellitus, coronary artery disease and psychiatric diagnoses such as schizophrenia and depression.

OUTCOME IDENTIFICATION, PLANNING, AND IMPLEMENTATION

The expected outcomes for this diagnosis are ones that represent improvements in health behaviors. The expected outcomes stated here are generic to any illness. In actual situations the expected outcomes can be stated according to specific changes in health behavior (e.g., MJ will describe integration of an 1800-calorie ADA diet with daily lifestyle by 2/01).

The outcome that the consumer will describe medication-taking, nutrition, activity-exercise, and/

or sleep-rest patterns that are consistent with health-related goals demonstrates that patients have sufficient knowledge to integrate therapeutic regimens with daily living. Interventions that facilitate achievement of this outcome are ones that require a high degree of interpersonal skills. The trusting relationship that was begun during the diagnostic process needs to continue as the patient and nurse *work together* to improve health behaviors. The nurse should demonstrate respect and trust in the patient's decisions through verbal and nonverbal behaviors. For example, if a patient refuses to follow particular advice, the nurse should avoid showing anger or hurt feelings. Words, voice control, and body language should continue to show awareness that the power of self-management is with the patient, not the nurse, and that the nurse is there as a helper. Knowledge of cultural variations in health management and tolerance for decisions based on cultural factors will help nurses to work with patients on self-management.[2] Types of interventions that are frequently used with this diagnosis are active listening, contracting, values clarification, and culture brokerage.

Nursing interventions to accomplish this expected outcome are those that help patients to change patterns. A need to integrate therapeutic regimens (e.g., diet, exercise, and rest) into lifestyle is a challenge for all patients because previous habits have already been established based on values and lifestyle. The nurse's acknowledgement of the challenge may be perceived as supportive. Other types of social support should be identified and mobilized. Values clarification can be used to identify values that are inconsistent with current behaviors; for example, the value of controlling blood pressure may be inconsistent with the patient's usual ways of responding to stress. Other methods to increase self-awareness (e.g., body scanning for symptoms) should be taught.

The goal for improvements in medication-taking requires sufficient knowledge bases and changes in daily habits so the goals of taking medications are met and the dangers are minimized.

Although the intention of taking medications is to achieve positive outcomes, self-management practices, such as changing dosages or times and mixing with over-the-counter drugs, may defeat the purpose of taking medications. At other times, self-management practices that differ from medical and nursing prescriptions may be better for the patient than what was prescribed. In these instances, the nurse can act as advocate for the patient or, preferably, help the patient with self-advocacy in reporting this information to the provider who prescribed the drug.

If medication-taking has been accomplishing the patient's goals and differs from the prescription (e.g., a patient takes a lower dosage of antihypertensive drugs) it is probably best to report this to the provider rather than suggest that the patient take the prescribed dosage. Nursing advice on medication-taking should be based on a thorough understanding of the drugs that the patient is taking now and others that are in the home (i.e., knowledge of each drug, drug interactions, and possible side effects and adverse effects). Drug dosages that the patient has been taking for a few days or more should not be increased or decreased, even to follow a previous prescription, without consulting the health provider who prescribed the drug.

Nursing interventions for the outcome that the patient will verbalize a feeling of power and control for management of therapeutic regimens should focus on enhancement of the patient's power for self-management. A useful model for helping patients to attain and maintain a sense of power is Miller's model for coping with chronic illness.[9] Using this model, the nurse fosters the patient's resources for power, which are physical strength, psychological stamina–social support, positive self-concept, energy, knowledge and insight, motivation, and belief system–hope. Although knowledge is important, it is only one of the power resources. Supporting the patient's coping style (approach, avoidance, or nonspecific) and effective coping strategies also enhances a sense of power.

I

◢ **NURSING CARE GUIDELINES**
Nursing Diagnosis: Ineffective Management of Therapeutic Regimen

---

Expected Outcome: The patient will describe medication-taking, nutrition, activity-exercise, and/or sleep-rest patterns that are consistent with desired health goals.

- Clarify the health-related values and goals of the patient. *Awareness of values and goals will help patients make subsequent decisions and will help nurses understand patient behaviors.*
- Identify perceptions of illness progression, and match these perceptions with the illness trajectory. *Because therapeutic regimens are performed in the context of an illness, this intervention will provide the nurse and the patient with shared visions of what is occurring and what is expected to occur.*
- Explore symptom awareness and beliefs; analyze the relationships of symptoms and patient actions to ameliorate symptoms; provide correct information in respect to symptoms. *Symptom awareness and beliefs may be inaccurate; patient actions to ameliorate symptoms may be inappropriate; knowledge provides a basis for changes in behavior. Knowledge is necessary but not sufficient.*
- Encourage the patient to talk about difficulties with MTR. *In a mutually trusting relationship a person can share perceived difficulties, successes, and failures.*
- Acknowledge the difficulty of changing daily habits and provide support for the patient's efforts. *Perceptions of being supported by others are associated with meeting health-related goals.*
- Analyze current medication-taking practices, including prescribed and over-the-counter drugs. Review knowledge of and beliefs about drugs and drug interactions. With the patient, determine changes needed in current practices (e.g., dosage, time, and methods of taking medicine). *Medications are foreign substances, many of which are harmful or have unwanted side effects and adverse effects.*
- Assist with repatterning through use of schedules and reminders and by associating medication-taking with other activities such as meals. *Aids for remembering when to take medications are needed to integrate medication routines with lifestyle.*
- In the home, ask to see all drugs the patient has, even drugs not currently taking; discuss the advisability of discarding old drugs. *There may be drugs in the home that should not be taken with prescribed medications.*
- Use formal or informal contracting to facilitate desired changes, and consider the use of rewards as positive reinforcement. *Contracting provides succinct, specific, and measurable goals and increases the probability of achieving them.*
- ▲ Work with the patient to select changes that are possible, considering factors such s lifestyle (homeless, drug addiction, 12-hour work shifts, single parent, etc.), culture, and family dynamics. *Collaboration with providers on these changes may be the impetus that makes change possible; discussion provides a cue to act.*
- ▲ Identify community resources that will help the patient repattern (e.g., self-help groups and home care). *Consumers need ongoing support after interactions with providers.*

Expected Outcome: The patient will verbalize a feeling of power for management of therapeutic regimens.

- Analyze the status of each of the seven resources for power, and assist the patient to optimize each resource. *Maximizing power resources facilitates the ability to cope with illness and MTR.*
- Discuss and plan energy conservation. *Energy is needed for MTR and for coping with illness.*
- Reinforce feelings of competence, mastery, and self-efficacy for self-advocacy. *Self-advocacy promotes the ongoing ability to negotiate with health providers for services and resources that are needed.*
- ▲ Do a genogram or other analysis to identify social networks and supports, to help the patient mobilize supports, and to support psychological stamina. *Often patients do not realize the number and types of supports that they have and do not know how to mobilize them. Doing a genogram clarifies social support status and methods for improving it.*

■ = nursing intervention; ▲ = collaborative intervention.

▲ Treat the patient with the utmost respect and dignity at all times to support self-esteem; show recognition of other aspects of personhood besides the illness; and assist with changes in body image and role performance. *Self-esteem, a power resource, can be adversely affected by the attitudes and approaches of providers.*

▲ Teach positive self-talk. *Negative self-talk can jeopardize MTR.*

▲ Provide information, verbally and in writing, on all aspects of illness regimen, including the rationale for all changes in behavior. *Knowledge is an important resource for power.*

▲ Identify and support coping strategies within the usual coping style that are working to maintain control. *Coping with illness includes many specific tasks, including modifying daily routines to accommodate therapeutic regimens.*

EVALUATION

The expected outcomes related to this diagnosis are evaluated by maintaining continued relationships with patients and by speaking to them, in person or by phone, regarding improvements in management strategies. With shortened hospital stays, hospital nurses may have to refer individuals to home care for follow-up and evaluation. For persons with chronic illnesses, ongoing connections with self-help groups and support groups are excellent ways to facilitate continued management, especially when there are changes in health status. If the patient is unable to report improvements in health behaviors as planned, the nurse and the patient should consider whether their goals and objectives are still plausible considering current health potentials and whether additional assistance is needed from the nurse or others.

◤ CASE STUDY WITH PLAN OF CARE

Mrs. Sarah E. is a 74-year-old woman who has been hypertensive for 15 years and was admitted 3 days ago for hypertensive crisis. A review of health patterns before hospitalization reveals that most of the time she took medications as prescribed, but at times she did not get new prescriptions filled in time and omitted some dosages. She has a low-salt diet and understands it but often does not follow it. Since her husband's death 2 years ago, she has been living with her son and her daughter-in-law, Jane. She has not spoken with Jane about her health-related needs because she thinks that Jane does not want her to live with them, and she does not have experience in relationships with younger women. Jane does all the shopping and cooking in the family. Jane has not approached Mrs. E. about the illness regimen.

◤ PLAN OF CARE FOR MRS. SARAH E.

Nursing Diagnosis: Ineffective Management of Therapeutic Regimen Related to Communication Gap Between Patient and Family

Expected Outcome: Mrs. E. will set up a meeting of herself, her daughter-in-law, and the nurse for planning.

■ After validating the diagnosis, discuss the rationale with Mrs. E. for ongoing effective management and discharge planning, including taking medications, low-salt diet, weight control, and stress management.

■ Assess and support her power resources, such as her physical strength, self-esteem, and belief system.

■ Provide information as needed for stress management (e.g., dealing with family conflict).

■ = nursing intervention; ▲ = collaborative intervention.   *Continued*

■ PLAN OF CARE FOR MRS. SARAH E. — CONT'D

- Review the various ways that Mrs. E. can communicate her needs to Jane.
- Assist Mrs. E. to select a specific means of asking Jane to meet with her for planning future strategies. For example, ask Mrs. E. to rehearse what she would say, and offer ideas as needed.

Expected Outcome: Mrs. E. will plan strategies for future management with her daughter-in-law and perhaps her son.
- During the meeting, support Mrs. E. as she tells her daughter-in-law about her illness regimen and problems solves with her regarding the best ways to manage.
- Consider ways of increasing the independence of Mrs. E.
- Discuss the role of the son in helping the mother with MTR.
- Refer Mrs. E. to home care if the nursing diagnosis is not resolved.

■ CRITICAL THINKING EXERCISES

1. What are six possible hypotheses other than the actual diagnosis for Sarah E. that could have been considered during the diagnostic reasoning process?
2. Identify a common assumption that should be challenged when the cues are similar to those presented by Mrs. E.
3. What are three types of specialized knowledge that are needed to implement the nursing interventions for Mrs. E.?

REFERENCES

1. Bakker RH, Kastermans MC, and Dassen TWN: An analysis of the nursing diagnosis ineffective management of therapeutic regimen compared to Noncompliance and Orem's self-care deficit theory of nursing, *Nurs Diagnosis* 6:161–166, 1995.
2. Degazon C: Cultural diversity and community health nursing practice. In M Stanhope and J Lancaster: *Community health nursing: promoting health of aggregates, families, and individuals,* ed 4, St. Louis, 1996, Mosby–Year Book.
3. Fehring R: Methods to validate nursing diagnoses, *Heart Lung* 16:625–629, 1987.
4. Friedman MM: *Family nursing: theory and practice,* ed 3, Norwalk, Connecticut, 1994, Appleton & Lange.
5. Fujita LY and Duncan J: High risk for ineffective management of therapeutic regimen: a protocol study, *Rehab Nurs* 192):75–79, 1994.
6. Lubkin IM: *Chronic illness: impact and interventions,* ed 3, Boston, 1994, Jones & Bartlett Publishers.
7. Lunney M: Nursing diagnosis: refining the system, *Am J Nurs* 82:456–459, 1982.
8. Lunney M: *The concept of management of therapeutic regimen: validation of four nursing diagnoses,* unpublished paper submitted to NANDA, 1991.
9. Miller JF: *Coping with chronic illness: overcoming powerlessness,* ed 2, Philadelphia, 1992, FA Davis.
10. Pender NJ: *Health promotion in nursing practice,* ed 3, Norwalk, Connecticut, 1996, Appleton & Lange.
11. Swanson JM and Albrecht M: *Community health nursing: promoting the health of aggregates,* Philadelphia, 1993, WB Saunders Co.

Ineffective Management of Therapeutic Regimen: Families

Ineffective Management of Therapeutic Regimen: Community

Effective Management of Therapeutic Regimen: Individual

Ineffective Management of Therapeutic Regimen: Families *is a pattern of regulating and integrating into family processes a program for the treatment of illness and the sequelae of illness that are unsatisfactory for meeting specific health goals.*

Ineffective Management of Therapeutic Regimen: Community *is a pattern of regulating and integrating into community processes programs for the treatment of illness and the sequelae of illness that are unsatisfactory for meeting health-related goals.*

Effective Management of Therapeutic Regimen: Individual *is a pattern of regulating and integrating into daily living a program for the treatment of illness and the sequelae that are satisfactory for meeting specific health goals.*

OVERVIEW

A *therapeutic regimen* is broadly defined as a systematic activity plan designed to improve or maintain health. Goals of therapeutic regimens include effective treatment and prevention of specific health problems. Evaluating therapeutic regimens assumes the existence of more than one approach to effective illness management and health promotion. The approach selected depends on the client's choices, based on their individual circumstances. *Management* refers to the skillful direction of necessary activities, and *client* refers to an individual, family, or community. *Families* and *communities* are aggregate units defined as a group or population of people sharing common personal or environmental characteristics. This nursing diagnostic cluster separately addresses the family and community's ineffective management and the individual's effective management of therapeutic regimens.

The theoretical framework is based on Bronfenbrenner's social ecological model and the theory of reasoned action.[4,6] The social ecological model focuses on the relationships among individuals and the contexts in which they function. Within this framework, there are four levels of nested concentric structures: the microsystem, mesosystem, exosystem, and macrosystem. Microsystems refer to interpersonal relationships among the individual, family, peer group, and school or work. At this level the individual—the client, as referred to in nursing—is central to analysis, with family, school, work, and peer groups as the context or environment. Mesosystems, the second level, entail interrelated microsystems, in which families are one of several aggregate units. The third level is the exosystem, comprised of larger social units such as the community within which the family exists and functions. The fourth level consists of the macrosystem—the pervasive cultural context in which individuals, families, and communities interact. This level is central to understanding client-selected activities constituting management of the therapeutic regimen.

Understanding clients' management requires exploration of multiple levels of relationships extending from the individual through the family to the community. Microsystem, mesosystem, or exosystem levels may be central or contextual, depending on which client is the focus of analysis. This perspective assumes that clients, whether individuals, families, or communities, cannot function in isolation. This view is concordant with nursing's holistic approach to the client.

The theory of reasoned action is based on the premise that the client's verbalized intent to perform the behavior is the best predictor of that behavior. Intent is potently influenced by the client's attitude and subjective norms. Attitudes are presumed to result from the product of the client's belief that the behavior will lead to a certain outcome and the client's expectation that the outcome will be positive or negative.

Subjective norms are defined by this theory as the product of the client's belief that important referents think the client should perform the behavior and the degree of the client's motivation to adhere to the referents' perceived view. Interventions then, from this perspective, should be directed toward influencing the client's beliefs and evaluations.

A commonly accepted definition of the *family* is a group of people who love and care for each other. This definition is independent of biological or legal relationships. These persons share emotional resources but perhaps not physical resources. For the purposes of this chapter, individual members comprising the family unit must reside in close proximity to each other if not in the same household. Proximity is required for family members to be available to manage the therapeutic regimen. The family as client presumes that, as a unit, the family is more than the sum of its individual members. It is the focus on the aggregate family unit that distinguishes family health care from family-centered care. the focus of family-centered care is on individual members, but with the family accorded careful consideration in planning and implementing care.

As the primary caregiver for its members, the family is the basic system where therapeutic regimens are managed. The effectiveness of family functioning often affects the skill with which those regimens can be managed. Family health behaviors are a product of family members' beliefs, attitudes, and values, as well as the multiple social systems with which they are involved.

Community is defined as a group of interacting persons with multiple, shared characteristics that may include geographic location, social status, and similar norms and values. Community includes individuals, families, and organizations as its integral parts. Like the family, the community as an aggregate is considered more than the sum of its parts. It is assumed that significant determinants of changing health behavior are embedded within community relationships.[1]

Assessing and evaluating the effectiveness of the client's therapeutic regimen requires the nurse to determine the client's available resources and capacity to manage those resources. Including assessment and evaluation of resources relieves the client of total responsibility for management.

The goal of community assessment is to establish a diagnosis addressing a population at risk. Assessment is predicated on the assumption that each community has a unique pattern of health services that are rarely developed with substantial coordination, leading to an overabundance of some health services and a scarcity of others.

To date, scant published research and conceptual writing exists on Ineffective Management of Therapeutic Regimen. Fujita and Dugan conducted a protocol study to evaluate the usefulness of the nursing diagnosis High Risk for Ineffective Management of Therapeutic Regimen.[2] The study focused on five individuals with congestive heart failure who experienced a specific nursing protocol related to their prescribed medication regimens. This nursing management strategy was judged by evaluating the subjects' self-care behaviors for 1 to 2 weeks after discharge. In this study the individuals were central to analysis, with the family as context. This diagnosis was observed to be reliable for all individuals but one, who refused follow-up care.

ASSESSMENT

Complete and accurate assessment is the critical basis for determining accurate nursing diagnoses and planning appropriate care. Planning assumes continuous assessment, allowing for necessary revisions as new client information is discovered. Comprehensive assessment is premised on the trusting relationship the nurse develops and maintains with the client.

Assessing management of therapeutic regimens begins with an evaluation of the client's health status, comparing the actual status with what would be expected given the recommended therapeutic regimen. The nurse identifies the responsible activities currently employed by the client, permitting the determination of the extent to which the therapeutic regimen is effectively managed by the client. Concomitantly, the requisite knowledge of the regimen and the desire to manage it effectively are also assessed. At minimum, assessment includes the client's educational needs, personal and community resources, and client attitudes. These arenas are significantly influenced by the client's cultural values and health beliefs and the opinions of significant persons who may be the sources of subjective norms influencing the client's behavior.

Ineffective Management of Therapeutic Regimen: Families

The major defining characteristic, inappropriate family activities for meeting treatment or pre-vention goals, reflects family choices made on the basis of their capacity to manage, knowledge of the illness, resources utilized, and daily pattern of living. These factors, potently influenced by the family's cultural health beliefs and attitudes, provide the basis for the subjective norms influencing the family's health care behaviors. It is necessary not only to determine the resources available to the family but to determine which resources are utilized and under what conditions.

The defining characteristic, acceleration of illness symptoms of a family member, provides the initial clue to the family's ineffective management of the regimen. The presence of illness symptoms may be expected or unexpected. Symptoms also may or may not be recognized by the family. Consequently this characteristic serves as a cue that the family needs the nurse's assistance to meet the client's goals for therapeutic management.

Lack of attention to the illness and its sequelae could result from a knowledge deficit or a situational crisis that distracts the family from effective illness management. Knowledge deficits may originate from prior health teaching never completely understood by the family, teaching based on information originally learned but forgotten, or teaching misinterpreted over time. Such instances are often influenced by the prevailing cultural norms and attitudes. Additionally, the family may have previously adjusted to chronic strains (e.g., low income), but these may now be exacerbated, jeopardizing effective illness management. The presence of a situational crisis or exacerbated chronic strain stresses personal resources utilized by the family, compromising the family's capacity to manage. These life stressors often take precedence over optimum illness management.

All the above characteristics occur while the family verbalizes a desire to manage the treatment of illness and prevention of sequelae. Ineffective management therefore is not a result of lack of motivation. These verbalizations can be interpreted as a request for assistance and are often accompanied by a verbalized difficulty with regulation or integration of one or more effects of illness or prevention of complications. This verbalization may also be precipitated by situational crises, exacerbated chronic strains, or knowledge deficits. A decrease in the number or quality of social support persons who have assisted with the regimen may also be a primary reason for the inability to perform necessary activities. These situations expedite ineffective management as the complexity of the regimen increases. As a culmination of the above defining characteristics, the family may verbalize that it did not take action to reduce risk factors for progression of illness and its sequelae. This verbalization may occur before or subsequent to illness symptom acceleration. All of these characteristics are influenced by overall family function. Family function, if ineffective in other areas of daily living, is likely to affect management of the therapeutic regimen.

■ Defining Characteristics

The presence of the following defining characteristics indicates that the family may be experiencing Ineffective Management of Therapeutic Regimen: Families:

Major
- Inappropriate family activities for meeting the goals of a treatment or prevention program

Minor
- Acceleration (expected or unexpected) of illness symptoms of a family member
- Lack of attention to illness and its sequelae
- Verbalized desire to manage the treatment of illness and prevention of the sequelae
- Verbalized difficulty with regulation or integration of one or more effects or prevention of complications
- Verbalization that the family did not take action to reduce risk factors for progression of illness and its sequelae

■ Related Factors

The following related factors are associated with Ineffective Management of Therapeutic Regimen: Families:

- Complexity of the regimen
- Knowledge deficit

- Exacerbated chronic strains
- Family dysfunction
- Situational crisis

Ineffective Management of Therapeutic Regimen: Community

The defining characteristic, illness symptoms above the norm expected for the number and type of population, is often the first manifestation of the community's ineffective management of a therapeutic regimen. This is commonly based on recorded community statistics such as mortality and morbidity rates. These statistics reflect illness distribution, determinants, and frequency in a given population. Alternatively, evaluation of illness symptoms may be based on the health care provider's personal observations.

A common statistic to assess community health is disease or cause-specific morbidity rates. Cause-specific morbidity rates are the number of new cases in the total population at risk within a specified time period.[3] Rates can be category specific (i.e., calculated considering characteristics such as age, ethnicity, or sex). These rates are then referred to as adjusted or standardized rates, which enable valid comparisons among communities. Use of standardized rates establishes that illness symptoms are beyond those expected for the community.

Information on cause-specific morbidity rates can also be appraised through clinical experience derived from self-reporting measures or the outcome of screening programs. However, both approaches are susceptible to a high percentage of false negatives (when the targeted clinical indicator is actually present but is interpreted as absent) and false positives (when the indicator is interpreted as being present but is actually absent).

The defining characteristic, unexpected acceleration of illness, is observed consequent to the unexpected increase in illness symptoms. Although analysts may continue to rely on cause-specific morbidity rates, mortality rates are more frequently employed to measure the end point of illness. *Cause-specific mortality rates* are the number of deaths in the total population during a defined time period.[3]

Availability, accessibility, and the acceptance of community health care resources largely determine the community's ability to manage the therapeutic regimen effectively. Health care resources are categorized as human or system resources. Human resources include the number, type, and distribution of health care providers, health care advocates, and administrative officials. System resources include the community's health care programs and physical facilities to provide the care.

Unavailability is the essence of two defining characteristics: (1) the number of health care resources is insufficient for the incidence or prevalence of illness and (2) health resources are unavailable for illness care. The presence of either characteristic precludes the community's ability to manage the therapeutic regimen effectively. When health care resources are available, such resources would still be inadequate if they were not accessible and acceptable to community members.

The defining characteristics, deficits in persons and programs to be accountable for illness care of aggregates and deficits in advocates for aggregates, reflect inaccessible and unacceptable health care resources. To assess accessibility, it is necessary to evaluate the personal resources of the community, including factors such as the percentage of the community with adequate health insurance and reliable transportation. Health care resources may be available and accessible yet not acceptable to community members. The existence of health resources for the health problem is less effective if not appropriately utilized by the community members in need of those resources. Knowledge of cultural health beliefs and attitudes is likely to reveal reasons why such resources are unacceptable.

Specifically, identification of important referent persons and their beliefs discloses subjective norms and probable reasons why the existing health care resources are considered unacceptable. Recognition of these persons will rarely be obvious, yet they are likely to become evident over time. When health care resources are deemed unacceptable, the likelihood increases that community members will not participate in those activities designed to minimize illness symptoms

and acceleration of illness. The defining characteristic that develops is deficits in community activities for secondary and tertiary prevention.

Any of the defining characteristics given above can lead to overburdened or crowded health care facilities. This situation could result from a chronically inadequate budget or be precipitated by a situational crisis (e.g., a natural disaster resulting in urgent needs in areas superseding illness management). Additionally, these characteristic could be related to the multiple risk factors present in the community such as numerous community members with inadequate health insurance or members ineligible for government assistance.

Community assessment must focus on illness problems of large numbers of individuals. Unlike families, these individuals are likely to be dissimilar and have a greater diversity of health beliefs and cultural attitudes. Assessment requires evaluation of not only the individuals and families experiencing accelerated illness but the institutions designed to provide secondary and tertiary care. Effective assessment necessitates examination of health policies as implemented in the community.

■ Defining Characteristics

The presence of the following defining characteristics indicates that the community may be experiencing Ineffective Management of Therapeutic Regimen: Community:

- Illness symptoms above the norm expected for the number and type of population
- Unexpected acceleration of illness(es)
- Deficits in persons and programs accountable for illness care of aggregates
- Deficits in community activities for secondary and tertiary prevention
- Deficits in advocates for aggregates
- The number of health care resources is insufficient for the incidence or prevalence of illness(es)
- Unavailable health care resources for illness care

■ Related Factors

The following related factors are associated with Ineffective Management of Therapeutic Regimen: Community:

- Multiple risk factors in the community
- Inadequate health care facilities
- Overburdened or crowded health care facilities

Effective Management of Therapeutic Regimen: Individual

The major defining characteristic, appropriate choices of daily activities for meeting the treatment or prevention goals, is the primary criterion distinguishing Effective from Ineffective Management of Therapeutic Regimen: Individual. The individual who makes appropriate choices is likely to have sufficient support services and resources available when necessary. As a result of these appropriate choices, illness symptoms are within the normal range of expectation. It cannot be assumed, however, that this individual has an accurate base of knowledge about the illness. If misperceptions exist, the individual may be at high risk for Ineffective Management of Therapeutic Regimen. It also cannot be assumed that if illness symptoms are within the expected range that appropriate choices of daily activities occur. The period during which the individual is being evaluated may be a quiescent period when illness symptoms are inapparent. Stability of a support system, including family and community resources, is also critical to determine the individual's risk for undesirable treatment outcomes.

Effective illness management is further supported by a verbalized desire to manage the treatment of illness and prevention of sequelae and the verbalized intent to reduce risk factors for progression of illness and its sequelae. Thus the individual is motivated to continue effective management. If knowledge deficits are present, the individual is most likely ready to learn. This is an ideal situation for health teaching because anxiety is probably lower than it would be during an acute crisis such as accelerated illness symptoms.

This diagnosis is distinguished from diagnoses involving family and community by its emphasis on a single person versus an aggregate of persons. Consequently, assessment is narrower, with consideration of family and community factors as influences and essential aspects of the individual's resources and support system. For this diagnosis emphasis is on the identification of factors that support continued meeting of health goals in contrast to reducing barriers that prevent health goals from being met.

■ Defining Characteristics

The presence of the following defining characteristics indicates that the individual may be experiencing Effective Management of Therapeutic Regimen: Individual:

Major

- Appropriate choices of daily activities for meeting the goals of a treatment or prevention program

Minor

- Illness symptoms are within a normal range of expectation
- Verbalized desire to manage the treatment of illness and prevention of sequelae
- Verbalized intent to reduce risk factors for progression of illness and sequelae

■ Related Factors

The following related factors are associated with Effective Management of Therapeutic Regimen: Individual:

- The individual is motivated to manage the treatment of illness
- Supportive family and friends
- Adequate resources are available

DIAGNOSIS

■ Differential Nursing Diagnosis

The principal means to differentiate among the nursing diagnoses in this cluster relates to the client focus, that is, whether the client is the individual, the family, or the community. The cluster is differentiated from other nursing diagnoses such as Noncompliance because the emphasis of Noncompliance is on the prescribed regimen as recommended by the health care provider and the factors preventing the client from complying. Ineffective Management of Therapeutic Regimen, however, focuses on difficulty the client experiences integrating illness treatment or prevention into activities of daily living, thus requiring ongoing interaction between the client and the nurse.[1]

It is also differentiated from diagnoses such as Caregiver Role Strain, Altered Parenting, Altered Family Processes, and Knowledge Deficit. These diagnoses are likely contributors to ineffective management. However, it is possible that these diagnoses, while present, may be compensated for by the client and may not necessarily lead to Ineffective Management of Therapeutic Regimen. This cluster can also be differentiated from Family Coping when a usually supportive person provides inadequate support necessary for effective illness management. Although this situation may be a primary or sole contributing factor, it does not obviate the comprehensive evaluation required to confirm the diagnosis of Ineffective Management of Therapeutic Regimen.

■ Medical and Psychiatric Diagnoses

Examples of related medical and psychiatric diagnoses for Ineffective Management of Therapeutic Regimen include Alzheimer's disease, depression, and manic depression. These examples share the common feature that affected individuals are cognitively less able to manage the therapeutic regimen effectively. The significance of these diagnoses is that the health care provider may not yet be aware of them. Consequently, these conditions are not being medically managed. In fact, Ineffective Management of Therapeutic Regimen may be the initial manifestation of these disorders. Other examples of related medical diagnoses include diabetes mellitus and chronic renal failure. The common relevant feature relates to the complexity of the medical regimen necessary for effective management. Finally, related medical diagnoses may include coronary artery disease, chronic obstructive pulmonary disease, and tuberculosis, with the commonality being that individuals comprising the family or community

may lack the energy to physically carry out the necessary therapeutic regimen.

OUTCOME IDENTIFICATION, PLANNING, AND IMPLEMENTATION

Expected outcomes focus on improvement of the client's health status, including positive health behaviors and decreased incidence and prevalence of health problems. Outcome identification for this nursing diagnostic cluster begins with a review of therapeutic goals for the health problem with the client. Given the goals, subsequent planning and implementation consider the client's ability to plan, organize, implement, and evaluate the regimen.

Ineffective Management of Therapeutic Regimen: Family

The first expected outcome for Ineffective Management of Therapeutic Regimen: Family involves the family identifying and participating in activities necessary to attain stated goals of the treatment program. This outcome is critical to effective management of the regimen. To achieve this end, it is necessary to evaluate the family's customary routines, identify problematic areas related to the therapeutic regimen, and determine the family's rationale for the activities chosen. This allows the nurse to understand and identify the underlying reasons for ineffective management. Once understood, the nurse can discuss with the family reasons why prior activities were not effective. After discussion, alternative approaches can be explored, with the anticipated result of Effective Management of Therapeutic Regimen. Alternatives selected consider the family's cultural influences and normal daily routine. The alternative approaches may not be the ideal management strategy from the nurse's perspective, although the alternatives would likely yield greater success for meeting treatment goals.

The second outcome focuses on family identification of initial signs and symptoms of accelerated

illness in a family member, which indicates ineffective management. Once noted, the family will
contact a health provider as necessary. This outcome is a critical cue presented by the family that
alerts the nurse to probable illness complications.
Once identified, adjustments to the therapeutic
regimen can be made on a timely basis. Ideally this
will prevent long-term sequelae. Assessing the
family's comprehension of the health problem is
necessary to evaluate the adequacy of the family's
data base. This is particularly important for families that have a member with a chronic illness for
which health teaching occurred some time ago.
Once evaluated, the family can be reeducated, and
correct knowledge can be reinforced. The nurse
identifying potential barriers to contacting a health
care provider and determining alternatives will
consider factors other than the family's apparent
willingness or unwillingness to manage the regimen effectively. This strategy also discourages
blaming the family as the sole cause of illness
acceleration.

Ineffective Management of Therapeutic Regimen: Community

The first expected outcome for Ineffective
Management of Therapeutic Regimen: Community involves community participation in activities
necessary to attain treatment goals. This outcome
is a critical prerequisite for Effective Management
of Therapeutic Regimen. It requires the nurse to
meet with community members who are influential or responsible for the therapeutic regimen.
These individuals are important for setting priorities and allocating resources appropriately, including the addition and expansion of services. It is
crucial to include not only the community members formally responsible (i.e., administrative officials), but also the leaders with informal but
substantial community influence. The latter group
may include businesspeople, community advocates, and nonmedical persons responsible for the
prevalent subjective norms. Discussions with
community representatives should include identification of various approaches that can be used
to share information with community members

(e.g., bulletin boards, television commercials, and
posters) to inform the public of available resources
and how to access them. Strategies such as incentives should also be identified to encourage active
community participation. These discussions should
particularly consider those cultural influences that
discourage acceptance of necessary activities and
approaches that will increase community acceptance. The activities to be promoted should be as
consistent as possible with prevailing cultural
health beliefs.

The second outcome focuses on having an adequate number of community health care resources
to participate fully in necessary activities for the
treatment program. This outcome is critical because it is impossible to have community participation without the necessary health care
resources. Meetings with formal and informal
community members should be arranged for the
purpose of acquiring new or maximizing existing
available health care resources. As with the activities addressed in the first outcome, these resources should be acceptable to the targeted community members. Selection of an approach should
be primarily the community's decision. This increases the likelihood that the resources and
activities chosen are accessible and acceptable.

Effective Management of Therapeutic Regimen: Individual

The outcomes identified aim to maintain and
support the individual's Effective Management of
Therapeutic Regimen. The first outcome relates
to the individual's continuing involvement in the
activities necessary to attain therapeutic treatment
goals. This outcome emphasizes the selection of
and participation in appropriate activities by the
individual. It is critical to assess the individual's
comprehension of the rationale for the activities
because the selection of activities may not be
based on accurate knowledge of the illness. If the
selection of activities is based on inaccurate knowledge, the individual could be at high risk for ineffective management. Consequently, the person's
knowledge base is either reinforced or corrected.

Continued on p. 100

■ NURSING CARE GUIDELINES
Nursing Diagnosis: Ineffective Management of Therapeutic Regimen: Family

Expected Outcome: The family will identify and participate in the necessary activities to attain the stated goals of the treatment program within 4 weeks.

- ▪ Discuss with the family reasons that prior activities were not effective *to encourage the family's understanding of how those activities contribute to Ineffective Management of Therapeutic Regimen.*
- ▪ Evaluate the family's customary routines, identifying problematic areas as they relate to the therapeutic regimen *to determine reasons that prior management was ineffective within the context of the family's life.*
- ▲ Explore alternative approaches that should result in Effective Management of Therapeutic Regimen, considering the family's normal daily routines and including pertinent cultural considerations. *Developing alternative approaches suited to the family expands their options, increases their preparedness in the event of situational crises or exacerbated chronic strains, and improves the likelihood of long-term management success.*

Expected Outcome: The family will identify initial signs of accelerated illness of a family member, indicating ineffective management, and will contact a health provider as necessary within 1 week.

- ▪ Assess the family's comprehension of the health problem *to determine the specific educational needs of the family.*
- ▪ Educate the family on early signs and symptoms and the value of prevention *to increase chances of long-term adherence to the necessary management activities.*
- ▪ Identify potential barriers to contacting a health care provider and determine alternatives *to assure timely assistance as necessary.*

▪ = nursing intervention; ▲ = collaborative intervention.

■ NURSING CARE GUIDELINES
Nursing Diagnosis: Ineffective Management of Therapeutic Regimen: Community

Expected Outcome: The community will participate in the necessary activities to attain the stated goals of the therapeutic treatment program within 15 months.

- ▲ Discuss with responsible community representatives various approaches (e.g., bulletin boards and other media) to inform the public of available resources. *This will publicize resources of which community members may be unaware.*
- ▲ Discuss incentives or similar alternatives *to encourage community participation.*

Expected Outcome: The community will have the necessary number of health care resources to attain the stated goals of the treatment program within 1 year.

- ▲ Meet with influential community representatives to identify critical resources *to facilitate the community's participation in the necessary activities.*
- ▲ Discuss with responsible community representatives various approaches to attain critical resources *to identify alternatives if the first and ideal choice proves infeasible.*
- ▲ Together with the community, select the approach to be implemented *to encourage community decision making that is consistent with their unique approach to problem solving.*

▪ = nursing intervention; ▲ = collaborative intervention.

◢ **NURSING CARE GUIDELINES**
Nursing Diagnosis: Effective Management of Therapeutic Regimen: Individual

Expected Outcome: The individual will continue to engage in the necessary activities to attain the therapeutic treatment goals.
- Determine the individual's understanding of the rationale for necessary activities *to determine specific educational needs.*
- Reinforce critical activities *to reinforce long-term success and to minimize the risk of Ineffective Management of Therapeutic Regimen.*
- Assess current health resources available to develop alternative management approaches with the individual. *It is important to have another plan ready in the event the current one cannot be implemented.*

Expected Outcome: The individual will identify signs and symptoms indicating accelerated illness and, if identified, will contact a health care provider within 1 week.
- Evaluate the individual's knowledge of the health problem, correcting misperceptions as needed *to decrease the probability of Ineffective Management of Therapeutic Regimen.*
- Discuss with the individual the early signs and symptoms of accelerated illness *to avoid illness complications.*
- With the individual, identify potential barriers to contacting a health care provider and develop alternative plans *as a method of secondary prevention, decreasing the risk of ineffective management.*

■ = nursing intervention; ▲ = collaborative intervention.

Health resources utilized by the individual must be identified to determine the strengths of the individual's support system. If the support system is less than ideal, alternative resources should be identified with the individual client.

Similarly, the second outcome focuses on the individual's identifying early signs and symptoms that indicate accelerated illness. When noted, the client will contact a health care provider. This creates the opportunity to reinforce and reeducate as needed, an ideal setting for secondary prevention. The success of this outcome is predicated on the individual having an accurate knowledge base of the illness.

EVALUATION

Evaluation should reflect the client's ability to manage the therapeutic regimen effectively after implementing the nursing plan. It is assumed that the regimen was designed according to the client's capabilities. Achievement of outcomes for the family should be met within 4 weeks unless there is substantial family dysfunction or an unusual, extensive situational crisis. If achievement of the outcomes is not possible, the nurse needs to reevaluate the therapeutic regimen and reassess the family's understanding of it.

Implementation and subsequent evaluation for the community require longer time periods because of the plan's complexity and the involvement of multiple individuals and groups. If specified outcomes cannot be met, the most likely reason is that additional time is needed. Alternatively, the nurse should reexamine the individuals involved in planning and implementation, particularly if informal leaders are inadequately represented.

Outcomes should be easily achieved within the given time frame for individuals diagnosed with Effective Management of Therapeutic Regimen because correct choices are already being made. If not, the most likely reason is that more education is needed.

▶ CASE STUDY WITH PLAN OF CARE

Midtown, America, is an urban city of 100,000 people of diverse cultures. Compared to the state, Midtown has 50% more adolescents, single women, and African-Americans than the state average. Mean years of education is 11, whereas the state's average is 12, and the median income is $20,000 per year, $10,000 less than the state average. For the past 5 years, Midtown has had 40% more preterm births and low-birth-weight infants than the state average. During the same time period, 50% of the city's pregnant women began prenatal care in the first trimester, compared with 75% of pregnant women in the state as a whole. In a recent study conducted in Midtown, the three most common reasons that women gave postpartum for delaying prenatal care were (1) not knowing they were pregnant, (2) being unable to obtain a timely appointment, and (3) inadequate transportation to keep their appointments.

▶ PLAN OF CARE FOR MIDTOWN, AMERICA

Nursing Diagnosis: Ineffective Management of Therapeutic Regimen: Community, Related to 40% More Preterm Births and Low-Birth-Weight Infants

Expected Outcome: At least 80% of the pregnant women in Midtown will begin prenatal care in the first trimester within 1 year.

▲ Discuss with Midtown's public health administrators and obstetric health care providers approaches to inform pregnant women of the available clinics, private medical providers, and methods of access.

▲ Apply for financial grants to enable expansion of obstetric services.

▲ Utilize a mobile van to reach pregnant women with transportation problems.

▲ Encourage bus tokens, on-site child care services, and flexible clinic hours, including Saturdays and evenings.

▲ Seek to expand Medicaid eligibility to the federal limit (i.e., 150% of the federal poverty level) to increase financial aid for prenatal care.

▲ Plan educational programs with the community on health behaviors to decrease preterm births and low-birth-weight infants, taking cultural beliefs and behaviors into consideration.

▲ Encourage health care advocacy among support persons and persons responsible for subjective norms.

▲ Consider home visiting and other alternative approaches to care.

▲ Encourage coordination of services and "one-stop shopping," and consider nontraditional health care sites such as churches.

▲ Determine which services are culturally unacceptable and discuss alternatives that still meet treatment goals and that accept, respect, and attend to differences in health beliefs, values, and customs.

▲ Consider incentives such as coupon books, which provide free services or desired items that can be redeemed after each visit.

▲ Assess, evaluate, and treat social causes of ill-health (e.g., physical abuse and living deficiencies) and create linkages with other social departments.

▲ Employ outreach efforts, using informal community leaders, to reach pregnant women.

Expected Outcome: Within 1 year, Midtown will have an additional clinic site, four more prenatal health care providers, and a mobile van to deliver care.

▲ Meet with Midtown's public health administrators and obstetric health care providers to identify necessary resources.

■ Determine who the lay midwives are and facilitate their education to allow them to practice legally.

■ Collaborate with communities to develop a plan jointly.

■ = nursing intervention; ▲ = collaborative intervention.

I

■ CRITICAL THINKING EXERCISES

1. According to Bronfenbrenner's social ecological model, which level is central to analysis?
2. What components of data collection are necessary to make this diagnosis?
3. Why is it so important to have the participation of Midtown's informal leaders in planning for the community?

REFERENCES

1. Eng E, Salmon ME, and Mullan F: Community empowerment: the critical base for primary care, *Fam Commun Health* 15(1):1–12, 1992.
2. Fujita LY and Dugan J: High risk for ineffective management of therapeutic regimen: a protocol study, *Rehab Nurs* 19(2):75–79, 1994.
3. Hennekens CH and Buring JE: *Epidemiology in medicine*, Boston, 1987, Little, Brown & Co.
4. Kazak AE: Families with physically handicapped children: social ecology and family systems, *Family Process* 25:265–281, 1986.
5. North American Nursing Diagnosis Association: *NANDA nursing diagnoses: definitions and classification, 1995–1996*, Philadelphia, 1994, The Association.
6. Zotti ME and Kozlowski LA: Promoting prenatal care: what do community leaders know and believe about it?, *Public Health Nurs* 11(4):206–213, 1994.

Noncompliance (Specify)

▶

Noncompliance (Specify) *is the state in which an individual who has expressed the desire and intent to adhere to therapeutic recommendations does not adhere to the recommendations.*

OVERVIEW

Use of the terms *compliance* and *noncompliance* was frequently debated in the 1970s and early 1980s. Some health care providers felt that the terms were judgmental and that they automatically placed blame on a patient who failed to comply with or adhere to a therapeutic recommendation. Haynes, Taylor, and Sackett[10] attempted to dispute the "unhealthy connotations" of the terms and presented a definition of compliance that they believed was nonjudgmental. Compliance was defined "as the extent to which a person's behavior (in terms of taking medications, following diets, or executing lifestyle changes) coincides with medical or health advice."[9] It was further noted that the term *adherence* could be used interchangeably with the term *compliance*.

The debate about the use of the term *noncompliance* continues. Keeling and colleagues[13] argue that the term should not be used as a nursing diagnosis because "it implies coercion and dominance by health professionals." The concern may arise in part from the North American Nursing Diagnosis Association's definition of *Noncompliance:* "A person's informed decision not to adhere to a therapeutic regimen."[16]

The definition around which this overview of Noncompliance is developed is the alternative definition presented above. This definition implies that although a person has expressed the intention to comply with therapeutic recommendations, he or she does not comply. This definition recognizes *Noncompliance* as a neutral term, and supports the contention that the term is used to describe "one aspect of patient behavior that may be either appropriate or inappropriate to the patient's best interests."[14]

Compliance with therapeutic recommendations can vary in degree. The extent to which a person's behavior coincides with a therapeutic recommendation may range from not following any of the aspects of the recommendation to following the total therapeutic plan. The challenge to health care providers is to identify the variables or factors that will contribute to or interfere with a person's ability or readiness to comply with therapeutic recommendations. To meet this challenge, several models that focus on health behavior and compliance have been proposed. Specific models that have been used in nursing practice and research are presented; these models attempt to identify specific variables and their relationship to compliant behavior.[5–7,10,15,20]

Interaction Model of Client Health Behavior

Cox[5] specifies three elements in the interaction model of client health behavior: (1) client singularity, (2) client-professional interaction, and (3) health outcomes, one of which is adherence to the recommended care regimen. Client singularity includes four background variables (demographic characteristics, social influence, previous health care experience, and environmental resources) and three internal personal variables (intrinsic motivation, cognitive appraisal, and affective response). These background and personal variables interact and influence one another and also interact with and have an effect on client-professional interaction.

Client-professional interaction involves affective support, health information, decision control, and professional and technical competencies. These elements also interact with one another and, with the personal variables, influence all aspects of health outcome. Health outcome comprises the use of health care resources, clinical health status indicators, the severity of the health care problem, adherence to the recommended care regimen, and satisfaction with care. This model offers direction for the initial assessment, which may indicate that attainment of a desired health outcome is jeopardized, or for a reassessment, which is performed to determine why the intended health outcome was not achieved. Cox has applied the interaction model of client health behavior to a study of community-based elders.[6]

Interactionist Model for Compliance or Noncompliance

Dracup and Meleis[7] have proposed an interactionist model for compliance/noncompliance based on role theory that is founded on three assumptions: (1) "the act of compliance or noncompliance is an outcome of a health transaction"; (2) three conditions should be present before behavior can be analyzed in terms of compliance or noncompliance: (a) the patient is a partner in any attempt to increase compliance, (b) the diagnosis must be correct, and (c) the proposed therapy must benefit the patient; and (3) compliance is a result of the patient's interaction with significant others and the environment.

Within the model, four components are identified and their relationship to compliance and noncompliance is delineated:

1. *Compliance role enactment.* Compliance involves behaviors and activities that are demanded by the performance of a new role (e.g.,

participating in regular exercise or omitting the consumption of certain foods).
2. *Self-concept.* The sick role or the at-risk role must be incorporated into the patient's self-concept for compliance to occur.
3. *Counter-roles.* To enhance compliance, health professionals, spouses, and significant others should reinforce the compliance role of the patient and assume roles that are congruent to or complementary with all of the patient's roles.
4. *Evaluation.* The patient's roles (behaviors related to the therapeutic recommendations) and the counter-roles that others have assumed should be periodically evaluated to promote behaviors of compliance.

In essence, "the individual who complies with health regimens must identify with a compliance role, have access to cues and behaviors of the proposed role, receive cues from others to enact such a role, and evaluate self and others vis-a-vis that role."[7] This interactionist model of compliance or noncompliance can guide the nurse in assessing the degree of success a patient may have in assuming and maintaining behaviors reflecting compliance.

Health Belief Model

The health belief model (HBM), like the models discussed above, is an interactive model in which each variable affects the others. The original HBM was developed to predict preventive health behavior (i.e., health-promoting behavior) and was later revised to explain and predict compliance behavior.[2,20] The revised HBM (see Figure 2) provides a conceptual framework for examining the multiple variables, their interaction, and their effect on compliance behavior. It can be used as a guide for assessing and evaluating a patient's readiness to undertake the recommended compliance behavior and for determining the presence of factors that can hinder or assist the patient's adherence to the therapeutic recommendation.

To determine a patient's readiness to undertake the recommended compliance behavior, three areas should be examined: the patient's health-

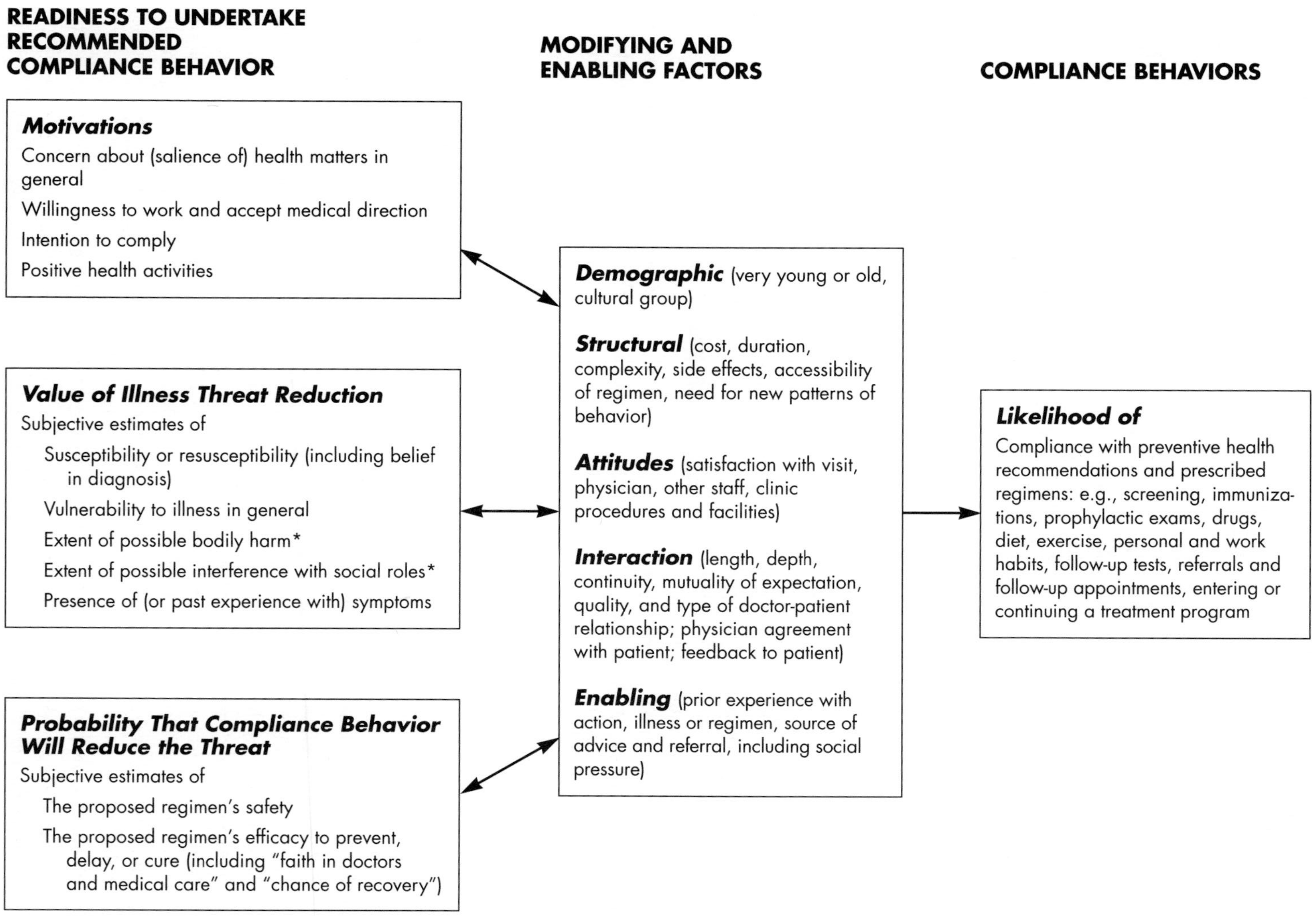

READINESS TO UNDERTAKE RECOMMENDED COMPLIANCE BEHAVIOR

MODIFYING AND ENABLING FACTORS

COMPLIANCE BEHAVIORS

Motivations

Concern about (salience of) health matters in general

Willingness to work and accept medical direction

Intention to comply

Positive health activities

Value of Illness Threat Reduction

Subjective estimates of

Susceptibility or resusceptibility (including belief in diagnosis)

Vulnerability to illness in general

Extent of possible bodily harm*

Extent of possible interference with social roles*

Presence of (or past experience with) symptoms

Probability That Compliance Behavior Will Reduce the Threat

Subjective estimates of

The proposed regimen's safety

The proposed regimen's efficacy to prevent, delay, or cure (including "faith in doctors and medical care" and "chance of recovery")

Demographic (very young or old, cultural group)

Structural (cost, duration, complexity, side effects, accessibility of regimen, need for new patterns of behavior)

Attitudes (satisfaction with visit, physician, other staff, clinic procedures and facilities)

Interaction (length, depth, continuity, mutuality of expectation, quality, and type of doctor-patient relationship; physician agreement with patient; feedback to patient)

Enabling (prior experience with action, illness or regimen, source of advice and referral, including social pressure)

Likelihood of

Compliance with preventive health recommendations and prescribed regimens: e.g., screening, immunizations, prophylactic exams, drugs, diet, exercise, personal and work habits, follow-up tests, referrals and follow-up appointments, entering or continuing a treatment program

* At motivating, but not inhibiting, levels.

Figure 2   Revised Health Belief Model for Predicting and Explaining Compliance (From Weiss SM, editor: *Proceedings of the National Heart and Lung Institute Working Conference on Health Behavior*, DHEW Pub No (NIH) 76-868, Bethesda, Maryland, 1976, National Institutes of Health.)

I

oriented motivations, the value the patient places on reducing the illness threat (perceived susceptibility and severity), and the patient's belief that compliance behavior can reduce the illness threat (perceived benefits and costs). Rosenstock[18] proposes that self-efficacy should be added to the beliefs necessary for compliance behavior. "The belief in one's personal self-efficacy is the conviction that one is capable of carrying out the health recommendation. Patients may believe in the effectiveness or benefits of a regimen but still not comply with it if they do not believe they have the ability to follow it."

Although the nurse may determine that a patient is ready to undertake compliance behaviors, factors may be present that will prevent the internalization of such behaviors. Demographic and personal factors can have such an effect. For example, the very young and the very old may have difficulty understanding and performing specific behaviors, or a specific cultural heritage may make it difficult to accept certain compliance behaviors.[12] Additional factors that can enhance or hinder the patient's readiness to follow the therapeutic recommendation have been categorized as structural factors (e.g., the complexity, side effects, and duration of the proposed therapeutic regimen), attitudinal factors (e.g., satisfaction with health care providers and facilities), personal interaction factors (e.g., the quality and type of relationship with the health care providers), and enabling factors (e.g., previous experience with the illness or illness threat and actual compliance behaviors).

Fishbein's Model of Reasoned Action

Fishbein's model was designed for two purposes: (1) to predict volitional behavior and (2) to assist in understanding psychological determinants of the behavior. The model focuses on a patient's intention to perform a behavior as being the immediate determinant of the patient's behavior. "Behavioral intention, in turn, is a function of attitude (the value to the individual, favorable or unfavorable, of performing the behavior) toward a behavior and subjective norm."[15] The personal beliefs of others and the motivation to comply with the behavior comprise the subjective norm.

Using the model as a guide for assessment directs the nurse to focus data collection on four areas: (1) the patient's attitude toward the compliance behavior; (2) the patient's intention to perform the behavior; (3) the patient's motivation to comply with the therapeutic recommendation; and (4) the patient's perception of the beliefs of significant others regarding the therapeutic recommendation.

In summary, models focusing on health behaviors and compliance reflect the complexity inherent in attempting to identify the variables that influence whether or not a person adopts compliance behaviors. The nurse can use a single model or a combination of models to guide the collection of data that will help determine why a person who has been an informed, willing participant in the identification of therapeutic goals and indicates a desire to comply does not comply with the therapeutic recommendation.

ASSESSMENT

To make the nursing diagnosis of Noncompliance, the nurse must collect subjective and objective data that indicate the patient's nonadherence to the recommended therapeutic regimen. Suggested in the definition of the diagnosis is that the patient must be aware of the recommendations and express an intention to follow them. This means that the patient's abilities, inabilities, desires, and intentions must be assessed before the therapeutic recommendation is made. The patient's perception of the benefits and barriers associated with the recommendation must be considered also.[17] Although it may seem that such an assessment would determine whether or not a patient will comply, it is important to acknowledge that a patient's motivation, the estimate of susceptibility to an illness, or the estimate of the efficacy of the therapy may change. Factors that initially promoted compliance, such as a positive nurse-patient relationship, can also change.

Thus when caring for a patient who has willingly assumed the responsibility of following a particular therapeutic recommendation, the nurse must provide ongoing assessment to determine whether characteristics indicating Noncompliance become apparent. Two defining characteristics directly indicate that the patient is not adhering to the therapeutic recommendation: (1) the nurse observes noncompliance behavior, and (2) the patient or significant others make statements that describe the patient's noncompliance behavior. Other defining characteristics include (1) the results of objective tests that reflect noncompliance behavior (e.g., drug assays, physiological measures, or detection markers), (2) evidence of the development of complications or exacerbation of symptoms that the recommended therapy should prevent or control, (3) failure to progress or to achieve therapeutic goals, and (4) failure to keep appointments or follow through on referrals.

After the nurse determines that the patient is not complying with therapeutic recommendations, the nurse must seek to identify the factor or factors contributing to the behavior. The contributing or related factors for Noncompliance can be categorized into four groups: personal factors, interpersonal factors, environmental factors, and treatment-related factors.

Personal factors are factors intimate to the patient. These include the following: one's values; one's beliefs about health, the illness threat, and the therapy; one's ability to implement the recommended therapy; and one's ability to integrate the compliance role into one's existing repertoire of roles. The nurse assesses whether the therapeutic recommendation is compatible with the patient's general health motivations, cultural influences, and spiritual beliefs. The patient's developmental level in terms of age, physical ability, and emotional maturity must also be considered.[11] The patient's appraisal of the illness threat and the costs and benefits of the therapeutic recommendation will also affect a patient's willingness to initiate or continue to incorporate compliance behaviors into a daily routine.

Interpersonal factors refer to factors involving relationships with others. The helpfulness of the support offered by others, including health care providers, and the satisfaction gained from it are critical to enhancing compliance behavior. If relationships are nonsupportive or unsatisfactory and messages that are meant to support the patient in assuming compliance behaviors are unclear, the patient may feel inadequate and not attempt to comply with the therapeutic recommendation.

Environmental factors can create barriers to the patient's desire and intent to comply. Such barriers can be in the home (e.g., inadequate food storage and preparation facilities to provide a special diet), the community (e.g., unsafe streets that interfere with participating in prescribed exercise), and the health care facility (e.g., noisy, crowded waiting rooms that cause an already anxious patient to become more anxious). The distance the patient must travel to keep appointments or to have prescriptions for medications refilled and the availability and costs of transportation can have an adverse effect on the patient's initial intention to participate in follow-up care.

Burke and Walsh[4] identify four *treatment-related factors* that may influence an elderly patient's willingness to adhere to a prescribed medication regimen: (1) the prescribed medication may be too expensive; (2) the medication, in terms of administration requirements or therapeutic or side effects, may interfere with usual daily activities; (3) the medication may make the patient feel ill; and (4) the patient may view the medication as ineffective.

These same factors can also be applied to other age groups and expanded to incorporate therapeutic recommendations other than medication. For example, prescribed activity-exercise and dietary recommendations may be perceived as (1) expensive (e.g., the cost involved in special diets or exercise equipment), (2) ineffective (e.g., the actual weight lost when on a weight reduction diet is not as much as anticipated), (3) interfering with usual daily activities (e.g., the need to change one's usual routine to incorporate new activities or an exercise program), and (4) causing one to feel worse than before (e.g., the soreness experienced when embarking on a new exercise regimen or the constant feelings of hunger resulting from dietary restrictions).

The identification of defining characteristics and related factors of Noncompliance depends on a thorough health assessment.[10,14,16,21] The nurse must employ well-developed intellectual, interpersonal, and technical skills to elicit the data needed to make the diagnosis Noncompliance and to plan, implement, and evaluate care that will enhance the patient's ability to adopt compliance behaviors for optimal wellness.

■ **Defining Characteristics**

The presence of the following defining characteristics indicates that the patient may be experiencing Noncompliance:

- Objective tests indicating noncompliance behavior (physiological measures or the detection of markers)
- Evidence of the development of complications
- Evidence of the exacerbation of symptoms
- Display of noncompliance behavior
- Statements by the patient or significant others describing noncompliance behavior
- Failure to keep appointments or follow through on referrals
- Failure to progress or to achieve therapeutic goals

■ **Related Factors**

The following related factors are associated with Noncompliance:

Personal factors
- Incongruence between the therapeutic recommendation and the patient's personal value system
- Conflicts with general health motivations, cultural influences, or spiritual beliefs
- Developmental level (very young or very old)
- Perception that self is nonsusceptible or invulnerable to the illness threat
- Knowledge or skill deficit
- Not identifying self with a compliance role

Interpersonal factors
- Nonsupportive family or significant others
- Unsatisfactory relationship with health care providers
- Confusion resulting from the unsuccessful communication of health information

- Lack of confidence in the professional and technical capabilities of health care providers

Environmental factors
- Nontherapeutic environment of the home, community, or health care facility
- Distance or lack of transportation prevent the patient from keeping appointments or following through on referrals

Treatment-related factors
- Perception that the costs outweigh the benefits of the therapeutic recommendations
- Perception that the therapeutic recommendations are ineffective
- Previous unsuccessful experience with a therapeutic recommendation
- Experiencing the side effects from therapy

DIAGNOSIS

■ **Differential Nursing Diagnosis**

The nursing diagnosis Noncompliance is conceptually different from Ineffective Management of Therapeutic Regimen.[1] The distinction between the two diagnoses relates to the focus of each diagnosis. An assumption made when making the diagnosis of Noncompliance is that the patient is not adhering to the therapeutic recommendation. The focus is on the therapeutic recommendation and the factors interfering with patient compliance. Ineffective Management of Therapeutic Regimen implies that the patient is having difficulty integrating a program of treatment into daily life. As such, Ineffective Management of Therapeutic Regimen can be considered a treatment-related factor that puts the patient at risk for Noncompliance.

When making the diagnosis of Noncompliance the nurse should identify the specific therapeutic recommendation that the patient is not following. Saba[19] developed a classification of home health care nursing diagnoses and interventions. The nursing diagnosis category of Noncompliance includes six subcategories: diagnostic (laboratory test), dietary regimen, fluid volume, medication regimen, safety precaution, and therapeutic regimen.

■ Medical and Psychiatric Diagnoses

Patients with medical and psychiatric diagnoses that require an incorporation of therapeutic recommendations into their present life patterns may experience Noncompliance. The health problems may be chronic or acute in nature, and they may incorporate therapeutic recommendations that are intended to prevent the development of or progression of the medical or psychiatric problem. Medical and psychiatric diagnoses of chronic health problems, with their associated treatments (which are often complex and need to be continued over a long period of time), can challenge the patient's usual coping behaviors and lifestyle. Examples of these diagnoses include diabetes, hypertension, and substance abuse disorders.

OUTCOME IDENTIFICATION, PLANNING, AND IMPLEMENTATION

In planning care for the patient with the diagnosis of Noncompliance, the nurse and the patient should focus attention on the long-term goal of patient compliance with the therapeutic recommendation. If this goal is mutually acceptable, nursing interventions will be directed toward eliminating or reducing the factors that contribute to the Noncompliance behavior. The nurse and the patient must work together in identifying patient outcomes and nursing interventions that will support achievement of this long-term goal. Specifically, the nurse can guide the patient in (1) appraising readiness to incorporate the therapeutic recommendations into the present life pattern, (2) enacting strategies for change, and (3) integrating the change into the existing life pattern.[8] Educational strategies are used to enable patients to integrate therapeutic recommendations into their lifestyle, and behavioral modification strategies are used to enhance compliance behavior.[3]

To address the personal factors that contribute to Noncompliance, expected outcomes reflect one or more of the following areas: the patient's motivation to protect or restore health; the patient's acceptance of susceptibility to the illness threat or acceptance of actual disease; the patient's belief that the benefit of following the therapeutic recommendation outweighs its associated costs and inconvenience; and the patient's belief in the capability to follow therapeutic recommendations (i.e., the ability to assume the compliance role).[18]

To achieve such outcomes, the patient's unique needs, beliefs, and preferences about the therapeutic recommendation must be addressed. It is also essential that the patient understand the principles of the recommended therapy and be able to perform procedures required by the recommendations. If the recommended therapy is complex, the patient should be taught elements or components of the therapy gradually and allotted adequate time to incorporate each component into the newly acquired compliance role.

For the patient whose Noncompliance derives from interpersonal factors, the expected outcomes must focus on eliminating or controlling nonsupportive and unsatisfactory relationships with significant others and health care providers. The nurse should work with the patient in determining how these relationships can be improved so that they will support the patient's compliance. Providers and significant others can enhance compliance by being responsive to the patient's needs, by acknowledging the patient's successful efforts, and by reinforcing the "what, why, and how" of the therapeutic recommendation. If a patient expresses a lack of confidence in health care providers, the nurse should explore the situation and give the patient information that will correct misconceptions or offer the needed support to correct the situation.

Environmental factors that impede a patient's intention and desire to comply should be addressed by controlling or eliminating the environmental conditions that create barriers to compliance behavior. Treatment-related factors are often intertwined with environmental factors. For example, the nurse can explore the options available to the patient who lacks the facilities to prepare a prescribed diet. Guidance might be provided about simplifying the purchase, storage, and preparation of required foods. Other options, such as eating out

I

◢ NURSING CARE GUIDELINES
Nursing Diagnosis: Noncompliance

Expected Outcome: The patient will resolve conflicts between personal values and beliefs and the therapeutic recommendation.
- Explore with the patient the incongruence between his or her values (e.g., general health beliefs and spiritual and cultural values and beliefs) and the therapeutic recommendation.
- Examine with the patient specific existing conflicts between personal values and the therapeutic recommendation.
- Explore with the patient and other members of the health care team the possibility of altering or revising the therapeutic recommendation so that it is compatible with the patient's personal values.
  The patient's values and beliefs must be considered in identifying therapeutic recommendations with which the patient will comply; if the patient's values and beliefs are in conflict with the recommendations, the therapeutic recommendations must be altered or changed.

Expected Outcome The patient will acknowledge susceptibility to the illness threat.
- Explore with the patient the factors that put the patient at risk for illness or that indicate the presence of illness or disease.
- ▲ Explain to the patient the signs, symptoms, and risk factors for the illness threat; compare these to ones the patient is experiencing.
  The patient's awareness of susceptibility as it relates to the illness threat is necessary for the patient to recognize the benefits that the therapeutic recommendation can provide.

Expected Outcome: The patient will identify the benefits of the therapy that outweigh the costs and inconveniences.
- Explore what the patient identifies as benefits and costs of the therapeutic recommendation.
- ▲ Explore with the patient ways to reduce the costs of the therapeutic recommendation (e.g., side effects, inconveniences, changing a comfortable lifestyle, or actual financial costs).
- ▲ Discuss with the patient the benefits of the therapeutic recommendation, emphasizing the benefits in terms of maintaining or regaining health and a sense of well-being.
  Providing information about the benefits and costs of the therapeutic recommendation assists the patient in realistically evaluating the desirability of the recommendation. Educating about the therapeutic recommendation provides the patient with a sense of control and makes him/her a partner in care.

Expected Outcome: The patient will feel capable of adhering to the therapeutic recommendation.
- ▲ Explain to the patient the underlying principles and any procedures related to the therapeutic recommendation.
- Provide the patient an opportunity to describe and demonstrate the "what, why, and how" of the therapeutic recommendation.
- Explain ways that the recommendation can be incorporated into the patient's daily routine.
- ▲ Include the patient's significant others in explanation of the recommendation.
  Providing the patient with information about the therapeutic recommendation and ways it can be implemented is critical to enhancing compliance.[14]

■ = nursing intervention; ▲ = collaborative intervention.

---

and having meals delivered to the home, should be explored also.

For the patient who lacks the transportation necessary for keeping appointments, the nurse should explore public and private transportation services. If cost is a factor, the nurse may refer the patient to social services so that adequate transportation arrangements can be made. When the factors threatening compliance exist in the health care facility, the staff should be realistic in their assessment of the situation and creative in determining an appropriate solution. For example, an alternative waiting area could be found for the patient who is bothered by a noisy, crowded waiting room.

Because the variables that influence whether a person will comply with a therapeutic recommendation are numerous and their interaction complex, the nurse must consider the specific needs of the patient in planning and implementing care. The Nursing Care Guidelines focus on personal factors that can interfere with a patient's desire to comply and are intended to provide general examples of patient outcomes and nursing interventions.

EVALUATION

The patient's achievement of identified outcomes should be a reliable indicator that the contributing or related factors have been controlled or eliminated. However, it is necessary for the nurse to maintain an ongoing assessment. The patient's actual and potential compliance behavior must be continually evaluated.

The presence of characteristics that reflect continuing Noncompliance should be investigated. If the patient continues to have difficulty adhering to the therapeutic recommendations, the nurse must seek to validate the related factors that were initially identified as contributing to Noncompliance. If the related factors are assessed as accurate, the chosen nursing interventions should be reviewed and evaluated.

Such an evaluation may indicate that the interventions were inadequate for a particular patient. For example, a patient seen in an outpatient clinic and diagnosed with Noncompliance related to a skill deficit could have a learning disability of which the nurse is unaware. The patient may have been attentive to the explanation of principles and the demonstration of a procedure but is unable to recall the steps when attempting to perform the procedure on the following day. Although the nurse and the patient may have been confident that the expected outcome was achieved before the patient left the clinic the previous day, it becomes obvious that evaluating the patient's attainment of new information must continue over time. This situation emphasizes the importance of collecting assessment data that reflects the uniqueness of each patient and planning care that is tailored to each patient.

▛ CASE STUDY WITH PLAN OF CARE

Mrs. Rita L. is a 38-year-old African-American woman who considers herself to be in good health. Last month she visited a women's health clinic for her annual physical examination and Papanicolaou smear. Initial evaluation at the clinic revealed the following data: blood pressure of 154/92 supine and 149/98 standing, height of 5'3", and weight of 172 pounds. History, physical examination findings, and laboratory results were negative except for obesity and mild hypertension. The clinic notes indicate that "Mrs. L. was counseled about dietary restrictions and the need for weight loss; a daily diet low in fat (30 g) and high in fiber (20 g) with controlled calorie and sodium intake is recommended." Mrs. L. reports that her mother had high blood pressure, and her mother had to take medication that made her feel worse. Mrs. L.'s mother died at the age of 64 following a cerebral vascular accident. The prospect of controlling her blood pressure through dietary restrictions appears to appeal to Mrs. L. She states that she really wants to lose weight because she is uncomfortable and unhappy with herself.

Mrs. L. lives with her husband and three daughters, ages 18, 17, and 15. The entire family is overweight, and their meals consist mainly of convenience foods. Mrs. L. returned to the clinic 1 month after her initial visit to have her blood pressure and weight monitored. Her blood pressure remained the same as the previous visit, and she had lost $\frac{1}{2}$ pound. Mrs. L. stated that she had hoped she would be able to lose weight and that she feels very discouraged by her lack of progress. She admitted that her diet continued to consist mainly of convenience foods. Although she attempted to prepare low-calorie meals for herself, she found that she was "tempted" to eat the food she prepared for her family. When asked why she prepared separate meals for the family, she responded, "They told me that they don't want to eat diet food and that I shouldn't diet because they love me the way I am."

I

► PLAN OF CARE FOR MRS. RITA L.

Nursing Diagnosis: Noncompliance with Dietary Recommendation Related to Lack of Support by Family Members

Expected Outcome: Mrs. L. will adhere to prescribed dietary recommendations.

▲ Provide Mrs. L. a listing of foods with fat and fiber content identified; review the list with Mrs. L.

▲ Discuss with Mrs. L. foods that she should avoid because of high sodium content (e.g., processed luncheon meats, pickles, and canned foods).

▲ Demonstrate to Mrs. L. how to interpret "nutrition facts" included on most food labels.

▲ Review with Mrs. L. what foods and beverages could be included on a daily diet of 1300 calories that allows 30 g of fat and 20 g of fiber.

▲ Work with Mrs. L. and her family to prepare a weekly meal plan that (1) is appealing, (2) provides essential nutrients, (3) is low in fat and high in fiber, (4) provides the appropriate number of calories, and (5) reduces sodium intake.

■ Recommend to Mrs. L. that she maintain a food diary and that she bring the diary with her when she has an appointment.

■ Emphasize to the family the importance of their role in supporting Mrs. L. in losing weight.

▲ Discuss with Mrs. L. a daily routine that incorporates exercise.

■ Assess Mrs. L.'s need for support through a group that focuses on good nutrition and weight loss; review with her the support groups in the area (e.g., Weight Watchers); if needed, assist Mrs. L. in contacting the group she feels would be the most helpful.

■ = nursing intervention; ▲ = collaborative intervention.

■■ CRITICAL THINKING EXERCISES

1. Prepare a week of menus for Mrs. L. that address her dietary restrictions. Analyze the food and beverage intake on 1 day, identifying the calorie, fat, and fiber content.

2. Develop an assessment guide that could be used for patients such as Mrs. L. Specify questions and areas to observe that would provide data about the personal, interpersonal, environmental, and treatment-related factors that could enhance or hinder the patient's compliance.

3. Develop a patient education booklet for persons who are newly diagnosed with hypertension. What information would be most helpful to promoting compliance in such patients?

REFERENCES

1. Baker RH, Kastermans MC, and Dassen TWN: An analysis of the nursing diagnosis ineffective management of therapeutic regimen compared to noncompliance and Orem's self-care deficit theory of nursing, *Nurs Diagnosis* 6:161–166.

2. Becker MH and others: Patient perceptions and compliance: recent studies of the health belief model. In Haynes RB, Taylor DW, and Sackett DL, editors: *Compliance in health care,* Baltimore, 1979, The Johns Hopkins University Press.

3. Burke LE and Dunbar-Jacob J: Adherence to medication, diet, and activity recommendations: from assessment to maintenance, *J Cardiovasc Nurs* 9:62–79, 1995.

4. Burke MM and Walsh MB: *Gerontologic nursing: care of the frail elderly,* St. Louis, 1992, Mosby–Year Book.

5. Cox CL: An interaction model of client behavior: theoretical perspectives for nursing, *Adv Nurs Sci* 5:41–56, 1982.

6. Cox CL: The interaction model of client behaviors: application to the study of community based elders, *Adv Nurs Sci* 9:4–57, 1986.

7. Dracup KA and Meleis AI: Compliance: an interactionist approach, *Nurs Res* 31:31–36, 1982.

8. Fleury JD: Empowering potential: a theory of wellness motivation, *Nurs Res* 40:286–291, 1991.

9. Haynes RB: Introduction. In Haynes RB, Taylor DW, and Sackett DL, editors: *Compliance in health care,* Baltimore, 1979, The Johns Hopkins University Press.

10. Haynes RB, Taylor DW, and Sackett DL, editors: *Compliance in health care,* Baltimore, 1979, The Johns Hopkins University Press.

11. Hussey LC: Overcoming the clinical barriers of low literacy and medication noncompliance among the elderly, *J Geront Nurs* 17(3):27–29, 1991.

I

12. Hymovick EP and Hagopian GA: *Chronic illness in children and adults: a psychosocial approach,* Philadelphia, 1992, WB Saunders Co.

13. Keeling A and others: Noncompliance revisited: a disciplinary perspective of a nursing diagnosis, *Nurs Diagnosis* 4(3):91–98, 1993.

14. Kern DE: Patient compliance with medical advice. In Barker LR, Burton JR, and Zieve PD, editors: *Textbook of ambulatory medicine,* Baltimore, 1994, Williams & Wilkins.

15. Miller P, Wikoff R, and Hiatt A: Fishbein's model of reasoned action and compliance behavior of hypertensive patients, *Nurs Res* 41:104–109, 1992.

16. North American Nursing Diagnosis Association: *NANDA nursing diagnoses: definitions and classification, 1995–1996,* Philadelphia, 1994, The Association.

17. Richardson MA, Simons-Morton B, and Annegers JF: Effect of perceived barriers on compliance with antihypertensive medication, *Health Ed Quart* 20(4):489–503, 1993.

18. Rosenstock IM: Enhancing compliance with health recommendations, *J Pediatr Health Care* 2(2):67–72, 1988.

19. Saba VK: Diagnosis and interventions: the classification of home health care nursing, *Caring* 11(3)50–57, 1992.

20. Weiss SM, editor: *Proceedings of the National Heart and Lung Institute Working Conference on Health Behavior,* DHEW Pub No (NIH) 76-868, Bethesda, Maryland, 1976, National Institutes of Health.

21. Whitley GG: Noncompliance: an update, *Iss Ment Health Nurs* 12:229–238, 1991.

Altered Protection

▶

Altered Protection *is the state in which an individual experiences a decrease in the ability to guard the self from internal or external threats, such as illness or injury.*[7]

OVERVIEW

Protection refers to the ability to guard oneself from danger or injury and the ability to provide a safe environment. Altered Protection as a nursing diagnosis can be applied to many diseases, injuries, and therapies in diverse patient populations in acute and chronic settings across the life span. These include those with cancer (particularly lymphoma, leukemia, and multiple myeloma), immune diseases such as acquired immunodeficiency syndrome (AIDS), diseases requiring the use of immunotherapeutic agents, burns over more than 20% of the body surface, and coagulation disorders such as disseminated intravascular coagulopathy. Also at risk are patients undergoing general surgery (particularly with the use of general anesthesia), radiation therapy, or organ transplantation. Age (under 2 or over 60 years of age), nutritional status (e.g., those who suffer from malnutrition), lifestyle (e.g., those who experience stressful situations), the use of drugs (e.g., allergic reactions to prescribed drugs, side effects of drugs, abusive use of drugs) put patients at risk for Altered Protection also.[6]

The immune response is a normal protective mechanism that functions in several ways, including destroying the threatening agent and preparing an area to make it less vulnerable to attack. Immunity protects the body against foreign materials, invasion by microbial agents, and prolifera-

tion of mutant cells. When it is deficient, inappropriate, or misdirected, the response can cause disease.[8]

The immune system does not originate in any one organ or area of the body but instead can be found in various organs and cells. The organs of the immune system are the lymph nodes, the thymus, the spleen, and the tonsils. The lymphoid tissues are present throughout the body and include the lymphocytes and the plasma cells. The cells of the immune system include the macrophage, the B-lymphocyte, and the T-lymphocyte. The types of immunity are antibody-mediated immunity and cell-mediated immunity.[2,8]

Macrophages are mature monocytes that surround, engulf, and dispose of microorganisms and cellular debris. They are active at the site of injury and remove foreign waste products from the body. Macrophages have a cooperative role in the immune response by processing antigens and transferring them to the lymphocytes. Lymphocytes originate in the bone marrow and make up 25% to 30% of the total white blood cell count. The two types of lymphocytes are B-cells and T-cells.

The T-lymphocytes are thought to originate in the stem cells of the bone marrow and to mature under the influence of the thymus gland. These long-living cells (from a few months to the duration of an individual's life) account for 70% to 80% of the blood lymphocytes. When the T-cells are exposed to an antigen, they divide rapidly and produce new T-cells sensitized to that antigen. Types of T-cells include killer cells, helper cells, and suppressor cells.[2] Killer T-lymphocytes adhere to the surface of the invading cell and disrupt the membrane, killing it by altering its intracellular environment. Helper T-cells stimulate B-lymphocytes to differentiate into antibody producers. Suppressor cells reduce the humoral response.

The B-lymphocytes originate in the bone marrow and mature in the bone marrow or another part of the body. B-cells have a life span of about 7 days, have on their surface antigens and immunoglobulins (causing antibody formation), and appear larger than the T-cells. The B-cell population is high in certain tissues of the tonsil and the spleen and low in the circulating blood volume. B-cells proliferate and differentiate into plasma cells and memory cells when exposed to an antigen. Plasma cells synthesize and secrete copious amounts of antibodies. Memory cells develop into antibody-secreting cells when reexposed to a specific antigen.

Antibody-mediated (humoral) immunity refers to immunity mediated by antibodies in body fluids such as plasma or lymph. Such antibodies are secreted and synthesized by the B-lymphocytes. Cell-mediated immunity results from an activation of the sensitized T-lymphocytes. Immunity refers to all these mechanisms used by the body with the purpose of preventing harm.[2,8] Through examination of this immune response, the practitioner can identify patients at risk for Altered Protection.

Patients with cancer, especially lymphoma, leukemia, and multiple myeloma, and patients receiving cancer chemotherapy and radiation therapy are at high risk for impaired immune function. Patients with lymphoma experience malignancies in the lymphocytes, thus affecting the immunological defense. Leukemia invades the bone marrow, replacing healthy white blood cells with malignant, immature cells. A multiple myeloma is a malignant neoplasm of the bone marrow. Cancer treatments, particularly chemotherapy and radiation therapy, cause damage to both the healthy cells and the malignant cells. Particularly susceptible are bone marrow cells, which reproduce rapidly.

Acquired immunodeficiency syndrome (AIDS) destroys the cell-mediated immune system. AIDS is caused by the human immunodeficiency virus (HIV), which affects the helper T-lymphocytes and the macrophages. These cells are responsible for cell-mediated immunity and contribute various opportunistic infections when weakened. Patients with blood dyscrasias, such as disseminated intravascular coagulopathy (DIC), are also at risk for Altered Protection through excessive stimulation of the body's clotting response, predisposing the patient to disseminated thrombosis and bleeding.

The systemic effects of pharmocological interventions, such as corticosteroids, immunotherapeutic agents, antibiotics, anticoagulants, and thrombolytic medications, should be considered in relation to Altered Protection. Corticosteroids cause an increase in susceptibility to infection and immunosuppression. Anticoagulant therapy and thrombolytic enzymes increase the risk of injury and bleeding by delayed coagulation of the blood. Penicillin and cephalosporin antibiotic therapy can cause superinfections, whereas tetracycline and chloramphenicol can cause an inhibition of cellular immunity.[5]

The patient with a history of alcoholism can experience anemia, difficulty in counteracting infection, and interference with clotting mechanisms, all predisposing factors for Altered Protection. Alcohol also interferes with the delivery of folate to the bone marrow precursors. Malnutrition can also cause a secondary immunosuppression because of the loss of or inadequate synthesis of the immunoglobulins.[2]

Stress may be considered a risk factor for Altered Protection because of its effects on the immune system. Stress causes an increase in the production of corticosteroids, which in turn can lower the body's defense mechanisms. Stress can cause a decrease in the production of T-cells and macrophages, thereby decreasing the body's ability to recognize antigens, permitting the spread of infection. The patient with full-thickness burns greater than 10% or partial-thickness burns greater than 20% of the total body surface area burned is also at risk for Altered Protection. Normal skin function is compromised or lost, causing a loss of protective barriers, loss of temperature control, fluid volume imbalance, and susceptibility to infection.

The immune system is poorly developed in the very young (less than 2 years of age) and somewhat compromised in the older, mature adult (more than 60 years old), thus predisposing these individuals to an increased incidence of infections and autoimmune diseases. Homelessness can also be considered a predisposing factor for Altered Protection. In addition to increased exposure to the hazards of the environment, homeless persons do not usually have routine care providers or easy access to health care facilities, resulting in delay of treatment for illness.

ASSESSMENT

Assessment of the patient with Altered Protection begins by obtaining a thorough health history. After obtaining demographic data, information is gathered concerning the reason for seeking health care, history of present complaint, past health history, family history, a functional assessment, and the patient's perception of health. Special attention should be given to childhood illnesses, surgery or injuries, and the immunization record. Nutritional assessment can be completed by asking the patient what food and alcohol was consumed in the last 24 hours, and a family history assessment for the incidence of cancer, anemia, and autoimmune disease is helpful. Functional assessment should include an assessment for the incidence of unanticipated change or crisis in the home environment, as well as a summary of health maintenance activities used by the individual. This information often can be easily obtained by asking for a description of a typical day for the patient, including activities, exercise, stressors, and sleep patterns.

The nurse should obtain information about the patient's chief complaint, recording the complaint using the patient's own words and including a description of the patient's perception of the problem. It is important to explore the presenting problem according to the "PQRST" method: (1) provocative and palliative—what initiates the complaint and what makes it better; (2) the quality and quantity of discomfort; (3) the region and radiation of the complaint; (4) the severity based on a scale of 1 to 10; and (5) the timing—when does it start, how long does it last, and how often does it occur.[1]

The next step in assessment is an objective review of the systems. The patient's height, weight, and vital signs are recorded, and any history of weakness or fatigue is noted. The assessment of the eyes, ears, nose, and throat is useful in revealing the incidence of nosebleeds, bleeding from the gums, headaches, frequent colds, and frequent sore throats. The lymph nodes in the head and the neck are examined for swelling and pain. The respiratory and cardiovascular systems are assessed, with particular attention to the occurrence of a productive or nonproductive cough; the presence, color, odor, and consistency of sputum; the presence of orthopnea and dyspnea; and complaints by the patient of palpitations, wheezing, and dependent edema. The patient may complain of anorexia, dehydration, nausea, and vomiting. Genitourinary assessment might demonstrate frequent urination with complaints of burning and the presence of blood in the urine. The integumentary system, particularly the skin and the mucous membranes, should be included in the assessment. Surgical or traumatic wounds, burn injuries, or pressure sores breach the body's physical defenses.[5] The patient at risk for Altered Protection should be examined additionally for muscle or joint pains and signs of easy bruising or bleeding. The surgical patient may demonstrate signs of impaired healing.

Laboratory data to be evaluated include the complete blood count (CBC) with differential (emphasis is placed on the white and red blood cell count, the hemoglobin, and the hematocrit), urinalysis, and blood culture. The CBC is evaluated to determine the presence of acute diseases and infections, to track the progress of diseases, and to monitor for the side effects of certain drugs that may cause blood dyscrasias. The white blood cell count is generally increased in infection and decreased in acquired immune deficiency syndrome, lupus, leukemia, bone marrow depression, and as a side effect to certain medications (antibiotics, antineoplastics, and immunosuppressives are specific to Altered Protection). The red blood cell count may be increased due to burns and dehydration and decreased in the presence of anemia, bone marrow suppression, and leukemia. Drugs that can decrease the red blood cell count include ampicillin, antineoplastics, and tetracycline. The hemoglobin and hematocrit may be increased in any condition that increases the red blood cell count and decreased in anemia and bone marrow suppression.

Blood cultures, normally negative, will be positive in the presence of bacteremia or septicemia. The urine culture, usually demonstrating the normal type and amount of cells of the urinary tract, will be increased in urinary tract infections and inflammation.[3]

The prothrombin time, coagulation studies, and partial thromboplastin time may be altered in the presence of a blood dyscrasia. The chest X ray is performed, but changes may be subtle in the patient with Altered Protection. No one diagnostic tool, but rather a combination of several, is necessary to make the diagnosis of Altered Protection. The nurse must assess the trends in the data and combine them with the clinical assessment findings.

■ Defining Characteristics

The presence of the following defining characteristics indicates that the patient may be experiencing Altered Protection:

- Impaired healing
- Altered clotting mechanism
- Neurosensory alterations
- Impaired or lost skin barrier
- Chilling
- Perspiring
- Dyspnea
- Cough
- Itching
- Fatigue
- Anorexia
- Weight loss
- Weakness
- Immobility
- Pressure sores
- Frequent infections
- Altered CBC, coagulation profile, blood culture, urinalysis
- Maladaptive stress response
- Restlessness
- Insomnia

■ Related Factors

The following related factors are associated with Altered Protection:

- Nutritional status (undernourished or malnourished)
- Abnormal blood profiles (leukopenia, thrombocytopenia, anemia, coagulation)
- Drug therapies (antineoplastic, corticosteriod, anticogulant, thrombolytic)
- Treatments (surgery, radiation)
- Diseases (cancer, immune disorders)
- Immunization status
- Developmental level (under 2 or over 60 years of age)
- Patterns of sleep, exercise, and rest
- Alcohol and drug use or abuse
- Healthy and nonhealthy coping mechanisms
- Environmental safety and security factors (e.g., shelter, urban or rural dwelling, exposure to pollution)

DIAGNOSIS

■ Differential Nursing Diagnosis

The nursing diagnoses Risk for Infection and Risk for Injury are closely related to and sometimes difficult to discriminate from Altered Protection. One method of differentiation may include the recognition of Altered Protection as an actual problem and Risk for Infection and Risk for Injury as potential problems. On inspection, Altered Protection appears more global in its application and includes physiological, psychological, and social issues for consideration in application to nursing practice.

■ Medical and Psychiatric Diagnoses

The medical diagnoses most commonly related to Altered Protection include disorders of the connective tissues (rheumatoid arthritis, lupus erythematosus, and local inflammatory disorders), disorders of the immune system (AIDS, drug- and radiation-induced immunodeficiencies, and allergy-induced immunodeficiencies), disorders of altered cell growth and development (leukemia and cancer), infection, and disorders of the integumentary system (pressure sores and burns). Alterations in the immune function have an impact on the overall protective status of the patient. Connective tissue disorders affect over 37 million people in the United States and require an interdisciplinary approach to care. Cancer has the potential to develop in any organ or tissue,[4] and burns present the patient with multiple physiological and psychological concerns. Clearly, multiple physiological internal and external threats to the patient's protective functions exist.

OUTCOME IDENTIFICATION, PLANNING, AND IMPLEMENTATION

Expected patient outcomes and nursing interventions for the patient with Altered Protection will differ based on the related factors involved but should include the following: (1) monitoring and assessing for the defining characteristics of Altered Protection; (2) maintaining adequate nutrition; (3) promoting adequate rest, safety, and control of physiological and psychological stressors; (4) promoting and maintaining intact skin integrity; and (5) education regarding factors related to problems of protection.

Vital signs, laboratory values, and physical assessment within normal limits indicate adaptation to physiological stressors. Vital signs are taken and recorded at least every 4 hours, with emphasis on heart rate, respiratory rate, and body temperature. Laboratory data on the complete blood count, coagulation studies, urinalysis, and chest X ray are obtained and observed for abnormalities. The nurse should perform the guaiac test on stools and gastric secretions and assess for signs of acute infection (i.e., sore throat, tender and swollen lymph nodes, weakness, fatigue, and diarrhea).

Adequate and balanced hydration and nutrition enhance inherent and acquired protective mechanisms. Monitor the patient's intake, output, calorie count, and weight daily. The nurse, in collaboration with the dietitian, should help to promote the maintenance of a regular diet based on the patient's food preferences with cultural and religious considerations. Offer small, frequent meals

if helpful. Supplemental feedings, vitamins, fluids, tube feedings, and total parenteral nutrition may be necessary.

Adequate rest, control of physiological and psychological stressors, and freedom from injury are desired objectives for the patient with Altered Protection. Narcotics are administered, if ordered, to control pain and to promote rest but not to interfere with mobility, coughing, and deep breathing. Measures such as back rubs and position changes promote relaxation and comfort. Control of physiological and psychological stressors begins with the patient's recognition of the stress and the factors that precipitate it. Stress management can be supported in the hospital setting with medication, deep breathing, meditation exercises, diversional activities, and relaxation tapes. The environment should be examined for unsafe conditions.

Intact skin functions as a protective barrier against harmful microorganisms. Promotion of wound healing is essential in the patient with burns, pressure sores, or a surgical incision. Aseptic technique during all dressing changes and wound care prevents contamination. Continuous observation and care of wounds with monitoring of color, odor, and amount and consistency of the drainage assures early detection of a wound infection. The patient's position is changed every 2 hours. Use of bed cradles and egg crates and pressure mattresses prevents pressure sores. The site of all invasive procedures, such as central lines and arterial lines, are examined routinely.

Verbalization of the related factors and health measures utilized for maintenance of protective functioning partially signifies successful patient education. The patient's knowledge base regarding the disease and the treatment plan should be assessed. Education is offered to the patient, family, and significant others. Recognition of the signs and symptoms of bleeding is taught, and the patient is encouraged to maintain a safe environment and to avoid trauma. Blood and body fluid precautions should be taken in the hospital and the home. The patient should avoid people with viral and bacterial infections and crowds in indoor places. Guidelines that address prevention and transmission of communicable diseases should be included.

◢ **NURSING CARE GUIDELINES**
Nursing Diagnosis: Altered Protection

Expected Outcome: The patient will achieve and maintain adaptive protection by the hospital discharge date as measured by temperature, heart rate, and respiratory rate within normal limits; complete blood count, coagulation profile, urinalysis, and chest X ray within normal limits; absence of swollen lymph nodes, weakness, and fatigue; and intact skin.
- Record vital signs every 4 hours, or as indicated.
- Monitor blood work, observing trends.
- Observe the patient's activity level, documenting the presence of weakness and fatigue.
- Change the patient's position every 2 hours, if bedridden.
- Apply egg crate or foam mattress to the patient's bed, if indicated.
- Assess the patient's wounds and/or skin for signs of redness, breakdown, and discharge.
  Accurate and continuous monitoring promotes early diagnosis and appropriate nursing interventions for Altered Protection.

Expected Outcome: The patient will demonstrate adequate hydration within 24 hours and adaptive nutrition by the hospital discharge date as measured by the following:
- Record intake and output every 8 hours.
- Perform orthostatic vital signs, if indicated.
- Encourage the patient to drink fluids frequently.
- Record the patient's weight every 24 hours.
▲ Record caloric count for 3 days.
▲ Determine the patient's cultural, religious, and personal food preferences, and provide them if diet and circumstances permit.
- Offer small, frequent meals, avoiding an excess of hot, spicy, high-fiber foods.
- Examine the patient's prescribed and over-the-counter medications for possible gastrointestinal side effects.
  A regular, spontaneous diet promotes vitamin, mineral, and positive nitrogen balance.

Expected Outcome: The patient will achieve and maintain adequate rest, freedom from injury, and control of stressors within 1 month of hospital discharge as measured by self-reports of adequate sleep, absence of injury, and moderate control of stress response through the use of positive coping mechanisms.
- Monitor the patient's sleep patterns.
- Space nursing care activities to allow several rest periods during the day and several 2-hour rest periods at night.
- Observe the patient for signs of fatigue.
- Provide a quiet environment, enhanced by relaxation techniques such as back rubs.
▲ Assist the patient in recognizing stress and in identifying coping strategies for dealing with stress.
▲ With patient's approval, implement stress-reduction techniques such as relaxation therapy and meditation.
- Assess the patient's environment for safety hazards.
  Control of pain, recognition of stressors, and promotion of rest enhance inherent protective functioning. Recognition of safety hazards prevents accidents and trauma.

Expected Outcome: The protective function of the patient's skin will be maintained throughout hospitalization, and the skin will appear intact by the date of discharge, as measured by the absence of redness, swelling, pain, and purulent discharge from wounds; the absence of redness and breakdown in pressure areas.
- Assess wounds every shift for signs of infection.
- Assess the skin for signs of reddened or blanched areas.
- Change the patient's position every 2 hours, massaging all bony prominences. Massage the skin with lubricant or lotion, if indicated.

■ = nursing intervention; ▲ = collaborative intervention.   *Continued*

I

■ **NURSING CARE GUIDELINES — CONT'D**

- Maintain aseptic technique during treatments, dressing changes, and invasive procedures.
- ▲ Institute active and passive range-of-motion exercises.
  Aseptic technique prevents contamination. Continuous observation and care of wounds, and monitoring of drainage assures early detection of wound sepsis. Position change prevents skin breakdown.

Expected Outcome: The patient will have adequate knowledge of methods that enhance protective functions by the hospital discharge date as measured by verbalization of actions that foster adaptive functioning.
- Assess the patient's level of knowledge and readiness to learn.
- Assess the environment for distractions that might hinder learning.
- Identify family members and significant others who should participate in learning.
- Assess the patient's and significant others' motivation and anxiety level.
- Provide verbal and written information on methods of enhancing inherent protective functions.
- ▲ Promote wellness through instruction, example, and referrals after discharge.
  Patient and family education provides the information necessary to foster adaptation to an illness and promotes participation by and a sense of control in the patient.

EVALUATION

Patients with Altered Protection should demonstrate optimal nutrition, fluid, and electrolyte balance and be free from infection by the hospital discharge date. The patient should experience adequate sleep patterns and be free from injury. Skin integrity will be maintained. The patient and significant others will verbalize information that is essential for maintenance of adaptive protection. If the expected outcomes are not achieved within the designated time frame, the plan should be reassessed and revised as necessary, taking into consideration the specifics of the patient situation. With the early-discharge trend evident in inpatient facilities, many of the expected outcomes will require follow-up interventions by the home health nurse.

■ **CASE STUDY WITH PLAN OF CARE**

Mr. Christopher T. is a 38-year-old clinical psychologist who was diagnosed as HIV positive 2 years ago. Mr. T. has a successful independent practice composed mostly of clients recovering from alcoholism. In his free time, he enjoys the opera, old movies, racketball, and vegetarian cooking. Mr. T. owns a condominium where he lives with his partner Bob. Mr. T. and Bob are active in the Episcopal church. Mr. T. is one of three children; his parents are alive and well.

Mr. T. has been experiencing periods of low-grade temperature and chills for about 3 months. Two weeks ago he developed a markedly elevated temperature of 103°F, night sweats, intermittent chest pain, a persistent nonproductive cough, and profound anorexia. Bob encouraged Mr. T. to seek help at a nearby clinic, where the tentative diagnosis of pneumocystis carinii pneumonia was made. He was admitted to a medical floor at the nearby medical center.

Mr. T. was anxious and upset on admission. Initial physical assessment reveals a mildly undernourished, diaphoretic male. His chief complaint is tightness in his chest. Rales are auscultated one third up the right lung. Initial laboratory data reveals a Hbg of 10.1, Hct of 35, Po_2 of 76, and T-cell count of 250 cells/μL. Admission orders include complete bed rest, an IV infusion of 5% dextrose in 0.45% saline to be infused at 125 cc/hr, and blood and body fluid precautions. Nasal oxygen is initiated at 3 L, and Mr. T. is scheduled for a chest X ray and bronchoscopy. His medications include Bactrim IV, Pentamidine IV, and Tylenol by mouth for temperature greater than 101°F. The primary nursing diagnosis for Mr. T. is Altered Protection related to immunosuppressed status and inadequate nutrition. Other possible nursing diagnoses include Impaired Gas Exchange, Social Isolation, and Ineffective Coping.

◤ PLAN OF CARE FOR MR. CHRISTOPHER T.

Nursing Diagnosis: Altered Protection Related to Immunosuppressed Status and Inadequate Nutrition

Expected Outcome: Mr. T. will regain adaptive protective mechanisms as measured by temperature less than 99.8° Hbg, Hct, and T-cell count increasing to within normal limits; and absence of weakness and fatigue.
- Monitor vital signs, especially temperature, at least every 4 hours.
- Monitor Hbg, Hct, and WBC count daily.
- Institute blood and body fluid precautions.
▲ Instruct Mr. T. and Bob about infection control.
- Administer antibiotics and antipyretics as ordered.
- Encourage fluid intake.
- Space nursing activities to assure that Mr. T. gets adequate rest.
- Initiate relaxation techniques.

Expected Outcome: Mr. T. will demonstrate adequate nutrition and hydration as measured by the ability to eat 75% of a meal, no further weight loss, intake that equals output, and electrolytes within normal limits.
- Measure Mr. T.'s weight daily.
- Monitor intake and output.
- Monitor electrolytes, particularly potassium, sodium, and chlorides.
▲ Calculate Mr. T.'s 3-day calorie count to identify nutritional needs.
▲ Encourage Bob and Mr. T.'s family to bring his favorite foods.
- Offer nutritional snacks between meals.
▲ Consult with the dietitian for a specific diet prescription.

Expected Outcome: Mr. T. will acquire sufficient knowledge to foster protective mechanisms as measured by verbalization about transmission of the HIV virus, signs and symptoms of opportunistic infections, and infection-control precautions.
- Assess Mr. T.'s knowledge of the HIV virus and how it affects protective mechanisms.
- Determine Mr. T.'s level of anxiety and the effect it has on his readiness to learn.
▲ Instruct Mr. T. and Bob on the signs and symptoms of opportunistic infections, when to seek help, and infection-control precautions.
- Evaluate the effect of the instruction and reinforce it, if needed.
▲ Provide Mr. T. with methods of acquiring additional information after discharge.

■ = nursing intervention; ▲ = collaborative intervention.

▦ CRITICAL THINKING EXERCISES

1. After being hospitalized for 2 weeks, Mr. T. is being discharged. He expresses concern regarding the future and begins to cry. What other data would support a diagnosis of Ineffective Individual Coping? Describe how you would respond to Mr. T.

2. Mr. S., a patient in the room next to Mr. T., is receiving an infusion of platelets when you notice a temperature of 101.8°F. What should be administered to lower the temperature? Why?

3. Mr. T. is readmitted to the hospital in 1 month with a dangerously low white blood cell count, and protective isolation is instituted. Prioritize outcomes for Mr. T., and describe your nursing interventions.

I

REFERENCES

1. Bates B: *A guide to physical examination and history taking,* Philadelphia, 1991, JB Lippincott Co.
2. Bullock D and Rosendahl P: *Pathophysiology: adaptations and alterations in function,* ed 3, Philadelphia, 1992, JB Lippincott Co.
3. Chernecky C, Krech R, and Berger B: *Laboratory tests and diagnostic procedures,* Philadelphia, 1993, WB Saunders Co.
4. Cooper G: *Elements of human cancer,* Boston, 1992, Jones & Bartlett Publishers.
5. Hudak C, Gallo B, and Benz J: *Critical care nursing: a holistic approach,* ed 6, Philadelphia, 1994, JB Lippincott Co.
6. Ignataviticius D, Workman M, and Mishler M: *Medical-surgical nursing: a nursing process approach,* ed 2, Philadelphia, 1995, WB Saunders Co.
7. North American Nursing Diagnosis Association: *NANDA nursing diagnoses: definitions and classification, 1995–1996,* Philadelphia, 1994, The Association.
8. Porth C: *Pathophysiology: concepts of altered health status,* ed 4, Philadelphia, 1994, JB Lippincott Co.

Risk for Aspiration

▶

Risk for Aspiration *is the state in which an individual is at risk for entry of gastrointestinal secretions, oropharyngeal secretions, or solids or fluids into tracheobronchial passages.*[21]

OVERVIEW

Aspiration occurs when there is a disruption in the defenses that normally protect the tracheobronchial tree and may result in lung tissue damage, pneumonia, respiratory distress syndrome, and death. However, aspiration has been reported to occur frequently in healthy individuals without resulting in adverse pulmonary sequelae. Huxley and others[9] found that 45% of normal adults aspirate oropharyngeal secretions during sleep. Factors contributing to the development of pulmonary complications secondary to aspiration relate to the frequency, volume, and character of the aspirated material. Aspiration of gastrointestinal contents results in a severe chemical pneumonitis when the aspirate has a pH of 2.5 or less and the volume of the aspirate in the adult exceeds 50 ml. Oropharyngeal secretions contain bacteria that reside in the upper airways and can cause pneumonia when aspirated. Aspiration of solid material results in partial or complete airway obstruction and may or may not be a medical emergency, depending on the level of obstruction.[2]

Developmentally, individuals are at Risk for Aspiration across the life span. Infants and young children are at Risk for Aspiration when they are fed in a lying position, when they are force fed,[3] or when they are unable to suck and swallow effectively because of prematurity. Children age 1 to 3 are at Risk for Aspiration of solid materials. During this stage of development, children explore and manipulate their environment and assert their independence. They frequently play with objects and then insert them into their mouths, thereby becoming at Risk for Aspiration. Almost any object children place in their mouths may be aspirated. Some of the most commonly aspirated materials in this age group include toy parts, coins, crayons, pop-tops, uninflated balloons, safety pins, eggshells, pills, peanuts, and popcorn.[8] Children who are at Risk for Injury secondary to child abuse may also be at Risk for Aspiration. Nolte[20] reported a case of death secondary to aspiration of coins in a 5½-month-old infant. Autopsy findings revealed three pennies in the esophagus and other injuries consistent with child abuse.

Adults who aspirate solid material may present with symptoms similar to those of a myocardial infarction when in fact they are choking. This condition is known as "cafe coronary" and requires prompt intervention of either manual extraction or use of the Heimlich maneuver. If the intervention is unsuccessful, an immediate tracheotomy followed by hospitalization and bronchial lavage are indicated.[11]

Approximately 90% of drowning and near-drowning accidents result in aspiration.[19] Children age 4 and younger, men age 15 to 34, and black males are at highest risk for drowning and near-drowning accidents and, therefore, at Risk for Aspiration. In children age 4 and younger, drowning and near-drowning accidents usually occur in residential pools. Therefore it is essential that safety measures be instituted to prevent these accidents and thus contribute to decreasing the child's Risk for Aspiration. Drowning and near-drowning accidents in men age 15 to 34 are related to boating and water activities and alcohol use combined with these activities. The causes of drowning and near-drowning accidents in black males are unknown and virtually unstudied, as are measures to decrease the risk of aspiration in this population.[31]

Pregnant women are at Risk for Aspiration during labor and delivery. Aspiration occurs as a result of an increase in gastric pressure because of the enlarged uterus and from relaxation of the gastroesophageal sphincter by progesterone.[29]

The elderly are at Risk for Aspiration for several reasons. First, normal changes with aging result in a decrease in salivation, oral sensation, motility, lower esophageal sphincter pressure, and response of the protective laryngeal reflexes and an increase in motor response time for chewing. The decrease in salivation and peristalsis results in a delay in gastric emptying.[5,23] These occurrences, coupled with the decrease in lower esophageal sphincter pressure and in pharyngeal reflexes, place the elderly at Risk for Aspiration. Second, the elderly may have a decreased gag reflex caused by the repeated insertion and removal of dentures. Individuals with a decreased gag reflex are at Risk for Aspiration.[15] Third, the elderly frequently take a variety of medications that increase the gastric pH, which fosters bacterial growth in the oropharynx and the stomach.[22] Fourth, the elderly frequently are prescribed tranquilizers, phenothiazines, and psychotropic medications. These medications may cause a drug-induced dysphagia; therefore individuals who take these medications are at Risk for Aspiration[27]

In addition to developmental risk factors, many other conditions may predispose a patient to be at Risk for Aspiration. These include those causing (1) reduced levels of consciousness resulting in compromise of glottic closure and the cough reflex; (2) dysphagia from neurological deficits, esophageal disorders, or the use of psychotropic medications; (3) mechanical disruption of the glottic closure or the lower esophageal sphincter because of the presence of a tracheostomy tube, an

endotracheal tube, or a nasoenteral feeding tube; (4) increased intragastric pressure; (5) increased gastric residuals; (6) delayed gastric emptying; (7) facial, oral, or neck surgery or trauma; (8) wired jaws; (9) protracted vomiting and gastric outlet obstruction; and (10) pharyngeal anesthesia.[2,21]

Early discharge from the hospital with home health care nursing is increasing in an attempt to control health care costs. As a result, more complex home health care services are being offered. One of these services includes providing care to patients discharged from the hospital who continue to receive enteral nutrition through feeding tubes. Caregivers need specific instructions regarding ways to prevent aspiration and a plan of action if aspiration occurs.[22]

ASSESSMENT

Identification and observation of the patient at Risk for Aspiration may prevent its occurrence. Assessment of a patient at Risk for Aspiration should center on the examination of subjective and objective data. In gathering subjective data the nurse should focus on whether the patient has a history of aspiration or any condition that may predispose him or her to aspiration (see risk factors). The nurse should ascertain whether the patient has difficulty swallowing food and fluids, controlling saliva, food sticking in the throat, food or fluids escaping from the mouth or nose, coughing while eating, or episodes of choking.[1,13] A history of smoking and alcohol use should be ascertained because these activities compromise activity of the respiratory epithelial cilia, which help in clearing secretions. A dental history, including daily care of the mouth, teeth or dentures, and gums, should be obtained because poor oral hygiene results in an increase in the concentration of anaerobic bacteria in oropharyngeal secretions.[30] A review of the patient's current medications will provide information regarding the use of medications that may predispose a patient to aspiration, such as medications that may cause drug-induced dysphagia, decreased gastric emptying, decreased gastrointestinal motility, decreased lower esophageal sphincter pressure, and increased gastric pH.[5,22,27]

In obtaining objective data, the nurse should first assess the patient's mental status. A reduced or altered level of consciousness can lead to choking and aspiration, with slowing of the swallowing response as the patient becomes less alert. Lethargy, fatigue, and cognitive, perceptual, and behavioral deficits place a patient at Risk for Aspiration. When overly weary or fatigued, the patient may lack motivation to use compensatory swallowing strategies or may fall asleep with food in the mouth. Patients with attention deficits may have difficulty focusing on eating and swallowing and may forget to swallow. Food remaining in the mouth may be aspirated. Patients with impulsive eating behaviors may place large amounts of food in the mouth without swallowing between bites.[1,15]

Assessment of cranial nerves V, VII, IX, X, and XII will provide information regarding the swallowing response, the quality of the patient's voice, the gag reflex, the cough reflex, and muscle strength in the face, neck, throat, and mouth. The act of swallowing is a highly coordinated activity involving cranial nerves V, VII, IX, X, and XII in conjunction with the oral and facial muscles. Assessment of the swallowing reflex should be performed in patients with impaired swallowing or dysphagia before starting food or fluids.[1,13,15]

Assessment of the quality of the patient's voice (cranial nerves IX and X) will provide information regarding closure of the vocal cords. Incomplete closure of the vocal cords during swallowing may place a patient at Risk for Aspiration. Patients with incomplete closure of the vocal cords during speech may have a hoarse, breathy, or gurgly voice. Patients with soft palate weakness or inadequate closure of the nasal passageway while swallowing may have a nasal voice.[1]

The gag reflex (cranial nerves IX and X) and the cough reflex (cranial nerve X) are upper airway protective mechanisms. The gag reflex should not be tested unless an intact cough and swallow response have been demonstrated. However, findings of a sufficient voluntary cough on physical examination

should be interpreted with caution because a patient with an adequate voluntary cough may not be able to cough reflexively. A more accurate assessment of a patient's reflexive coughing ability, although not applicable to all care settings, can be observed when a nasogastric tube is being passed or during oropharyngeal suctioning.[1,15]

The nurse should assess the patient for signs of muscle weakness in the face, neck, throat, and mouth (cranial nerve VII). Drooling of secretions from the mouth or facial dropping suggest weakness of the facial muscles and lips. Patients with cheek and lip muscle weakness may pocket food in the space between the teeth and cheek or lose food and liquid from the mouth. Patients with impaired tongue strength and mobility (cranial nerve XII) may have difficulty forming and manipulating a bolus of food and controlling liquid in their mouths. Decreased strength or excursion of the muscles of mastication (cranial nerve V) may result in the inability to bite adequately or to chew food sufficiently.[1,15]

Patients with mechanical disruption of the glottic closure secondary to the presence of a tracheostomy tube or an endotracheal tube are at Risk for Aspiration. Patients with tracheostomy tubes are more likely to aspirate than those with endotracheal tubes. The use of a cuffed tracheostomy tube or a cuffed endotracheal tube does not prevent aspiration of saliva or gastric contents and may facilitate aspiration by compressing the esophagus, thereby resulting in a partial or functional esophageal obstruction. Cuffed endotracheal tubes should be small in relation to the size of the trachea. Large cuffs may develop invaginations when they cannot be completely inflated and thus increase the patient's Risk for Aspiration.[5]

Patients with nasoenteral tubes are at Risk for Aspiration secondary to mechanical disruption of the lower esophageal sphincter. Tube placement should be ascertained before the start of feedings. Patients receiving nasoenteral feedings may develop increased gastric residual volumes, which places them at Risk for Aspiration. These patients should be monitored for residual volumes.

■ Risk Factors

The presence of the following behaviors, conditions, or circumstances renders the patient more vulnerable to Risk for Aspiration:

Reduced or altered level of consciousness secondary to

- Alcoholic intoxication
- Cerebrovascular accident
- Delirium
- Dementia
- Diabetic coma
- Drug overdose
- General anesthesia
- Seizures

Dysphagia secondary to esophageal disorder

- Achalasia
- Bowel obstruction
- Diverticula
- Foreign body, tumor adenopathy
- Gastroesophageal reflux
- Hiatal hernia
- Neoplasm
- Scleroderma
- Stricture
- Tracheoesophageal fistula

Dysphagia secondary to neurological disorder

- Multiple sclerosis
- Myasthenia gravis
- Parkinson's disease
- Amyotrophic lateral sclerosois
- Pseudobulbar palsy
- Depressed cough and gag reflex
- Impaired swallowing
- Debilitating conditions
- Poor dentition or oral hygiene
- Presence of tracheostomy or endotracheal tube
- Incomplete lower esophageal sphincter
- Presence of gastrointestinal tubes
- Tube feedings
- Increased intragastric pressure
- Increased gastric residual volume
- Decreased gastrointestinal motility
- Delayed gastric emptying
- Situations hindering elevation of the upper body

- Drowning and near-drowning accidents
- Facial, oral, or neck surgery or trauma
- Wired jaws
- Pregnancy, labor, emergency cesarean section
- Medication administration
- Drugs such as tranquilizers, phenothiazines, and psychotropic medications
- Preexisting pulmonary disease
- Cognitive deficits
- Perceptual deficits
- Attention deficits
- Impulsive eating behavior
- Premature birth
- Cardiopulmonary arrest

DIAGNOSIS

■ Differential Nursing Diagnosis

The nursing diagnosis Risk for Aspiration can be applied whenever an individual is in jeopardy of having gastrointestinal secretions, oropharyngeal secretions, solids, or fluids enter the tracheobronchial passages. Patients with Impaired Swallowing are at Risk for Aspiration, although the nursing diagnosis Impaired Swallowing is used specifically to address the needs of individuals who have a decreased ability to pass fluids or solids from the mouth to the stomach. Nursing interventions for the diagnosis Risk for Aspiration are directed toward preventing aspiration in healthy and ill individuals in various settings across the life span. Nursing interventions for the diagnosis Impaired Swallowing are primarily directed toward minimizing the effects of a swallowing impairment and providing care to resolve it. Measures to prevent aspiration are specific to this population.

■ Medical and Psychiatric Diagnoses

The diagnosis Risk for Aspiration is unique to nursing, although the medical literature is replete with specific diagnoses that predispose an individual to aspiration (see risk factors). Prevention of aspiration is a collaborative effort among nurses, physicians, dietitians, and speech therapists, especially in the care of patients with Impaired Swallowing, those receiving enteral nutrition, and those requiring cardiopulmonary resuscitation. Physicians usually insert narrow-bore feeding tubes. However, nurses may insert wide-bore nasogastric tubes for feeding or decompression, depending on hospital policy. Nurses and physicians collaborate to determine a plan of care to prevent aspiration when the patient receiving enteral feedings has an abnormality on gastrointestinal examination or excessive gastric residual volumes. Advanced practice nurses, in time, may assume the physician's role in the prevention of aspiration.

OUTCOME IDENTIFICATION, PLANNING, AND IMPLEMENTATION

The expected outcome for the patient with a diagnosis of Risk for Aspiration is that the patient will not aspirate food, fluids, or secretions. Nursing interventions are developed to meet the specific needs of patients who are at Risk for Aspiration.

Aspiration Prevention for the Patient with a Reduced or Altered Level of Consciousness

If not medically contraindicated, the nurse should position the patient with a reduced level of consciousness on his or her side, with the head of the bed elevated, and should make certain that the tongue does not occlude the airway.[30] Confused and agitated patients may require restraints. Vest and wrist restraints may be harmful if the patient cannot sit up or turn to the side in the event of vomiting. If it is necessary to use restraints, also position the patient on his or her side, with the head of the bed elevated whenever possible. Always use the least restrictive type of restraint.[15] Good oral hygiene should be provided, and secretions should be cleared from the mouth and throat with suctioning if necessary.[30]

Aspiration Prevention for the Patient with an Endotracheal or Tracheostomy Tube

To prevent aspiration in a patient with an endotracheal or tracheostomy tube, the nurse should

suction secretions using sterile technique at least every 2 hours, or more frequently if necessary, to maintain airway patency and to clear secretions. After suctioning the endotracheal or tracheostomy tube, the nurse should remove secretions from the mouth and pharynx. The nurse should provide good oral hygiene. To help in making a diagnosis of aspiration, the nurse can place a small amount of blue food coloring on the posterior portion of the patient's tongue every 4 to 6 hours.[6] However, this practice should not be performed in patients who are allergic to FD&C yellow no. 5, an ingredient in most green or blue colorings.

Aspiration Prevention for the Patient Receiving Enteral Nutrition

Enteral feedings may be delivered through a nasogastric, nasointestinal, gastrostomy (surgical or percutaneous), jejunostomy, or gastrostomy/jejunostomy feeding tube.[26] Metheny and others[17] reported that aspiration occurs less frequently with small-bore nasointestinal tubes than with large-bore nasogastric tubes. However, Sands[24] noted that the incidence of pulmonary aspiration in endotracheally intubated patients receiving enteral nutrition through wide- and narrow-bore nasogastric feeding tubes was not significant.

To prevent aspiration in the patient receiving enteral nutrition, the nurse should first make certain that the nasoenteral tube is positioned correctly. The most accurate method for ascertaining tube placement is radiography, although pH testing of tube aspirates has been found to be useful. The auscultatory method, the bubbling-under-water method, and observing for respiratory symptoms are unreliable and should not be used to assess tube placement.[16] Metheny and others[18] reported that the visual appearance of aspirates is helpful in distinguishing between gastric (cloudy and green, tan or off-white, or bloody or brown) and intestinal (clear and yellow to bile-colored) tube placement but is of little value in excluding respiratory placement. Research is under way to develop a model for testing tube placement in which pH, visual characteristics of feeding tube aspirates, and bilirubin and enzyme content of the aspirate can be used to predict feeding tube location.[18]

After the tube is correctly placed, the exit site should be marked to monitor for changes in tube position. Although marking the tube is useful in detecting the extent of tube migration, the distal portion of the tube may become displaced with severe coughing, retching, or vomiting without disruption to the tube marking.[16]

A gastrointestinal assessment should be performed before the start of enteral feedings and every 4 hours during continuous feedings. Patients should be assessed for abdominal distention, nausea, vomiting, and hypoactive or absent bowel sounds. Enteral feedings should be discontinued when there is an increase in abdominal girth from 8 to 10 cm above the baseline.[12,16]

Pulmonary aspiration is often a silent event; therefore the nurse should check pulmonary secretions for the presence of glucose. Ideno and Dedo[10] maintain that glucose testing is a more accurate and safer method for detecting carbohydrate presence in secretions than the blue dye method. Food dye in enteral tube feedings may cause contamination of the enteral feeding and may affect the accuracy of occult blood and gastric pH tests. In addition, most green or blue colorings contain FD&C yellow no. 5, which can potentially induce serious allergic reactions.

Methany noted (1) that several recommendations exist regarding the frequency with which gastric residual volumes should be measured and (2) that there is little agreement as to what constitutes an excessive residual volume. Therefore a conservative and cautious approach is suggested. The nurse should assess the gastric residual volume before beginning enteral feedings and every 4 hours during continuous feeding.[12] Intermittent tube feedings should not be given when the gastric residual volume is greater than 100 ml. If this occurs, the gastric residual volume should be reassessed at the next scheduled feeding. If the gastric residual is greater than 100 ml on the second assessment, the nurse should discontinue the feeding and notify the physician.[4] Continuous tube feedings should be discontinued when the gastric residual volume is greater than 200 ml in patients with nasogastric tubes and 100 ml in patients with surgically or endoscopically placed gastrostomy tubes.[14]

The nurse should administer intermittent tube feedings slowly with the head of the patient's bed elevated 30° to 45° during the feeding. The patient should also remain in this position for 1 to 2 hours after the feeding.[16,22] Continuous feedings should be administered via an infusion pump, with the head of the bed elevated at all times.

Aspiration Prevention for the Patient with Impaired Swallowing

The nurse should assess the patient's cough and gag reflexes and the ability to chew and swallow. The patient's position during eating should be determined by the specific swallowing impairment.[1,25] Patients should be observed for signs of aspiration during eating. Single-textured soft foods that retain their shape, such as blenderized foods and cooked cereals, in amounts of $\frac{1}{4}$ to $\frac{1}{2}$ teaspoon should be given. Particulate foods (e.g., hamburger and crunchy foods), foods containing more than one texture (e.g., beef stew), sticky foods (e.g., peanut butter, bananas, and white bread), and stringy foods (e.g., fruits and vegetables) should be avoided.[1,15]

Thin liquids are difficult to control in the mouth and are easily aspirated. Thick liquids (e.g., tomato juice and apricot nectar) or very thick liquids (e.g., pudding and yogurt) in amounts of 5 to 10 ml should be given to prevent aspiration. Thickening agents may be applied to thin liquids to increase their consistency. Gelatin, sherbet, ice chips, and ice cream may become thin liquids when held in the mouth and may be contraindicated for some patients. Medications should be crushed and mixed with a food such as yogurt or pudding so that it can be formed easily into a bolus. Enteric-coated tablets and sustained-release capsules should not be altered because crushing may affect the absorption or action of the drug. Oral hygiene should be performed after meals because food that may be lodged in the mouth can be aspirated.[1]

Continued on p. 130

◢ **NURSING CARE GUIDELINES**
Nursing Diagnosis: Risk for Aspiration

II

Expected Outcome: The patient will not aspirate food, fluids, or secretions.

For the patient with a reduced or altered level of consciousness
- If not medically contraindicated, position the patient on the side, with the head of the bed elevated. *Gravity reduces the likelihood of regurgitation of gastric contents from a distended stomach.*
- Maintain airway patency and make certain that the tongue has not occluded the airway.
- Clear secretions from the mouth and throat with a tissue or by suctioning.
- Provide good oral hygiene. *Poor oral hygiene promotes bacterial growth, which may be aspirated via secretions.*

For the patient with an endotracheal or tracheostomy tube
- Using sterile technique, suction the patient's airway every 2 hours, or more frequently if necessary, to maintain adequate airway patency and to remove secretions. *Excessive secretions may be aspirated.*
- Maintain good oral hygiene for the patient and remove secretions from his or her mouth and pharynx as necessary. *Poor oral hygiene promotes bacterial growth.*
- Place a small amount of blue food coloring on the posterior portion of the patient's tongue every 4 to 6 hours, then assess the patient's pulmonary secretions for the presence of blue dye. *The presence of blue dye in pulmonary secretions is a positive sign of aspiration.*

For the patient receiving enteral nutrition
- ▲ Assess placement of the feeding tube. *It is crucial that the feeding tube be placed in the gastrointestinal tract and not in the tracheobronchial passages.*
- After the tube is correctly placed, mark the exit site. *Marking the exit site is useful in assessing changes in tube position.*
- Perform a gastrointestinal assessment before the start of enteral feedings and every 4 hours during continuous feedings. *Feedings should not be administered when the patient has hypoactive or absent bowel sounds, abdominal distention, nausea, or active vomiting because these findings indicate decreased motility.*
- Check the patient's tracheal aspirate every 6 hours for the presence of glucose. *The presence of glucose in the tracheal aspirate is a positive sign of aspiration.*
- Position the patient so that he or she is in a sitting position, with the head of the bed elevated 30° to 45° during the feeding. Maintain the patient in this position for 1 to 2 hours after the feeding. The head of the bed should be elevated at all times during continuous feedings. *The head of the bed should not be raised to a 90° angle because this position causes an increase in intraabdominal pressure and subsequent gastroesophageal reflux.*
- Check the patient's gastric residual volume before intermittent tube feedings and every 4 hours with continuous feedings. *Excessive gastric volumes increase the risk of vomiting and subsequent aspiration.*
- Tube feedings should be administered at room temperature; intermittent feedings should be administered slowly; continuous feedings should be administered via an infusion pump and the infusion rate should be checked hourly.

For the patient with impaired swallowing
- ▲ Collaborate with the speech therapist in caring for the patient with impaired swallowing.
- Assess the patient's cough and gag reflexes. *The cough and gag reflexes are upper airway protective mechanisms.*
- Assess the patient's ability to chew. *Inability to masticate food adequately may result in choking and subsequent aspiration.*

■ = nursing intervention; ▲ = collaborative intervention.   *Continued*

II

- Assess the patient's swallow response before food or fluids are placed in the mouth. *Abnormalities in the swallowing response may result in aspiration.*
- The patient's position during eating should be based on the patient's specific swallowing impairment. The upright, chin-tuck position is useful in patients with vallecular defects. *Use of this position helps gravity to keep food in the middle to the anterior part of the mouth and thus prevents food particles and liquid from falling over the base of the tongue into the open airway. Flexing the neck also helps elevate the larynx into its protective position under the base of the tongue.* The patient with unilateral weakness should rotate the head toward the weaker side of the pharynx. *Use of this position helps direct the bolus down the stronger side.* Patients with gastroesophageal reflux should be fed in an upright sitting position, and this position should be maintained for 2 hours after eating. *These interventions help prevent aspiration of refluxed material.*
- Provide foods that are easy to chew and swallow, such s a mechanical soft diet, pureed foods, and thick liquids. Offer solids and liquids separately. *The Risk of Aspiration decreases with single textured foods and liquids with a thicker consistency.*
- Observe the patient eat, and assess for signs of aspiration; suction equipment should be readily available in the event that aspiration occurs. *Feedings should be discontinued if there are signs of aspiration.*
- After the patient eats, provide good oral hygiene. *Food that may be lodged in the mouth may be aspirated.*

For the patient requiring cardiopulmonary resuscitation

- If the patient vomits during cardiopulmonary resuscitation, clear the mouth and pharynx of any regurgitated material.
- ▲ Decompress the patient's stomach during or after cardiopulmonary resuscitation as necessary. Hospital policy will determine whether this is a nursing function. *Gastric distention occurs frequently during cardiopulmonary resuscitation.*
- After cardiopulmonary resuscitation, assess the patient for signs and symptoms of aspiration.

Aspiration Prevention for the Patient Requiring Cardiopulmonary Resuscitation

During cardiopulmonary resuscitation, the patient may vomit and thus be predisposed to aspiration. If vomiting occurs during cardiopulmonary resuscitation, turn the patient to the side and sweep out the mouth before continuing resuscitative efforts. The patient's stomach should be decompressed during or after cardiopulmonary resuscitation as necessary. After cardiopulmonary resuscitation, the nurse should assess the patient for signs and symptoms of aspiration.[28]

Aspiration Prevention for the Patient Requiring Home Health Care

Caregivers of discharged patients at Risk for Aspiration may have a knowledge deficit regarding the causes of aspiration and ways to prevent it. The nurse should develop a plan of care with the caregiver that addresses (1) the causes of aspiration in the patient being discharged, (2) ways to prevent it, and (3) a specific course of action if it occurs.[22]

Developmental Considerations in Aspiration Prevention

To prevent aspiration, infants should be held upright for feedings, and young children, adults, and the elderly should be fed while sitting upright. Forced feeding in infants should be discouraged. Meals should be eaten slowly and small bites should be taken to prevent choking and aspiration. Activities such as talking, running, and playing should not be performed while eating or with food in the mouth. Children should be taught not to put objects in their mouths. Measures should be taken to identify children and others who are at Risk for Aspiration secondary to abuse. Good oral hygiene, including brushing and flossing after meals and regular dental checkups, should be practiced by all individuals across the life span. Dentures, complete or partial, if needed, should be fitted securely. Safety should be of concern to all age groups in swimming and boating activities, and alcohol should not be used in combination with these activities. Children should have an adult escort in residential pools and at beaches and lakes.

EVALUATION

Aspiration can occur across the life span in many clinical and nonclinical settings. It may be a silent event and difficult to detect; therefore the nurse must have a high degree of suspicion in patients who are at risk. Nursing interventions are successful when the patient does not aspirate food, fluids, or secretions into the tracheobronchial passages. The absence of dyspnea, tachypnea, tachycardia, wheezing, rales, rhonchi, fever, unusual restlessness, confusion (elderly), impaired cognitive functioning (elderly), tube feedings in the oropharynx of patients receiving enteral nutrition, a positive reaction on the glucose oxidase reagent strip in patients receiving enteral nutrition, blue food coloring in tracheal aspirates of patients with endotracheal or tracheostomy tubes, or a diffuse alveolar infiltrate on a chest X ray are indications that aspiration has not occurred.[2,6,7,10]

◤ CASE STUDY WITH PLAN OF CARE

Mr. Fred B., a 74-year-old male, was admitted to the hospital for evaluation of exertional angina. Cardiac catheterization revealed a critical stenosis in the left main coronary artery as well as severe, triple-vessel coronary artery disease. He elected coronary artery bypass grafting. He was extubated on the first postoperative day and transferred to the intermediate surgical care unit on the second postoperative day. The afternoon of the second postoperative day he had an expressive aphasia and dysphagia. The result of a computed tomographic scan of the head was unremarkable. The cerebrovascular accident was attributed to a small embolus. It was necessary to place a Dobbhoff tube to supplement his oral nutrition with tube feedings. Mr. B. is currently recuperating satisfactorily from his surgery and the cerebrovascular accident after being transferred to the general floor. His past medical history includes gastritis, past surgical history includes right-sided inguinal herniorrhaphy, transurethral prostatectomy, and hemorrhoidectomy. Mr. B. has no known allergies. Medications given were dipyridamole USP (Persantine), 75 mg three times a day; digoxin, 0.25 mg daily; metoprolol tartrate (Lopressor), 50 mg twice a day; and ranitidine hydrochloride (Zantac), 150 mg twice a day. Mr. B. is a retired sheet metal worker. He bowls once a week in a league and plays softball in the spring and the summer. Mr. B. lives with his wife, who is in good health. His only son died of a cerebrovascular accident. Three daughters and 18 grandchildren are alive and well. His father died at age 45 of carcinoma of the larynx, and his mother died at age 55 of a myocardial infarction.

Results of physical examination were as follows: temperature, 98.8°F; heart rate, 82 beats/min and regular; blood pressure, 140/86 mm Hg; height, 5'11"; weight, 212 pounds; head, normocephalic; cranial nerves, gag reflex absent (cranial nerve IX); heart, regular rhythm with no murmurs; lungs, clear to auscultation and percussion, neck, grade II/VI right carotid bruit, none on the left; abdomen, bowel sounds present, no palpable masses, no tenderness; liver and spleen, not palpable; musculoskeletal, freely movable joints; pulses, 2+ femoral, popliteal, posterior tibial, and dorsalis pedal pulses bilaterally; no peripheral edema.

II

▶ PLAN OF CARE FOR MR. FRED B.
Nursing Diagnosis: Risk for Aspiration Related to Multiple Factors

Expected Outcome: Mr. Fred B. will receive adequate nutrition to maintain bodily functions, and he will not aspirate food, fluids, or secretions.
- ▲ Consult speech therapy.
- ■ Assess Mr. B.'s abdomen for bowel sounds and abdominal distention; inquire as to the presence of gastrointestinal discomfort, particularly nausea, vomiting, diarrhea, or constipation.
- ■ Assess Mr. B.'s cough and gag reflexes.
- ■ Assess Mr. B.'s ability to chew and swallow.
- ■ Position Mr. B. in the upright, chin-tuck position while he is eating.
- ■ Before giving tube feedings, check the gastric residual volume; if it is greater than 100 ml do not give the tube feeding.
- ▲ Collaborate with a registered dietician so that foods are served at the proper temperature and are easy to chew and swallow. Use thickening agents as necessary to increase the consistency of thin liquids.
- ■ Observe Mr. B. for aspiration while he is eating and during tube feedings.
- ▲ Maintain calorie count with the registered dietitian; monitor daily weights and intake and output measurements.
- ■ Provide good oral hygiene after Mr. B. eats.

Expected Outcome: Mr. Fred B. will have a patent airway and an effective breathing pattern.
- ■ Assess Mr. B.'s respiratory status: check the rate and depth of his breathing; auscultate and percuss the lung fields; assess for dyspnea, tachypnea, tachycardia, wheezing, rales, rhonchi, cyanosis, fever, unusual restlessness, confusion and/or cognitive impairment, and leukocytosis; and check a chest X ray for the presence of an infiltrate.

■ = nursing intervention; ▲ = collaborative intervention.

▦ CRITICAL THINKING EXERCISES

1. Mr. B. has several risk factors that predispose him to aspiration. What are these?
2. You assess Mr. B. before giving his supplemental enteral feeding and find that he is restless, confused, disoriented, and short of breath. What nursing actions would you perform?
3. Mr. B. is progressing satisfactorily and is now ready for discharge. He continues to have a swallowing impairment and remains on aspiration precautions. He will be discharged with the Dobbhoff tube in place so that his nutrition can be supplemented with enteral feedings. Develop a plan of care for him that will be instituted at discharge. Would you include his wife or other family members in developing his care plan? What referrals to other health care providers would you consider for his home care?

REFERENCES

1. Baker DM: Assessment and management of impairments in swallowing, *Nurs Clin North Am* 28(4):793–805, 1993.
2. Bartlett JG: Aspiration pneumonia. In Baum GL and Wolinsky E, editors: *Textbook of pulmonary diseases,* ed 4, Boston, 1994, Little, Brown & Co.
3. Buffin A: Force-feeding of infants in North Cameroon. A harmful tradition—preventive approach, *Arch Pediatr* 1(12):1138–1143, 1994.
4. Eisenberg P: Enteral nutrition. Indications, formulas, and delivery techniques, *Nurs Clin North Am* 24(2):315–338, 1989.
5. Eisenberg PG: Pulmonary complications from enteral nutrition, *Crit Care Nurs Clin North Am* 3(4):641–649, 1991.
6. Elpern EH, Jacobs ER, and Bone RC: Incidence of aspiration in tracheally intubated adults, *Heart Lung* 16(5):527–531, 1987.
7. Fein, AM and Niederman MS: Severe pneumonia in the elderly, *Clin Geriatr Med* 10(1):121–143, 1994.
8. Haines JD: Wheezing as a sign of foreign-body aspiration in infants and children, *Postgrad Med* 90(6):153–154, 1991.

9. Huxley EJ and others: Pharyngeal aspiration in normal adults and patients with depressed consciousness, *Am J Med* 90(6):564–568, 1978.

10. Ideno KT and Dedo YL: Alternatives to food coloring in enteral feeding, *Crit Care Nurse* 13(5):20–21, 1993.

11. Jacob B and others: Laryngologic aspects of bolus asphyxiation-bolus death, *Dysphagia* 7(1):31–35, 1992.

12. Kohn CL and Keithley JK: Enteral nutrition. Potential complications and patient monitoring, *Nurs Clin North Am* 24(2):339–353, 1989.

13. Luggar KE: Dysphagia in the elderly stroke patient, *J Neurosci Nurs* 26(2):78–84, 1994.

14. McClave S and others: Use of residual volume as a marker for enteral feeding intolerance: prospective blinded comparison with physical examination and radiographic findings, *J Parenter Enteral Nutr* 16(2):99–105, 1992.

15. Meehan M: Nursing Dx: potential for aspiration, *RN* 55(1):30–34, 1992.

16. Metheny N: Minimizing respiratory complications of nasoenteric tube feedings: state of the science, *Heart Lung* 22(3):213–223, 1993.

17. Metheny N, Eisenberg P, and Spies M: Aspiration pneumonia in patients fed through nasoenteral tubes, *Heart Lung* 15(3):256–261, 1986.

18. Metheny N and others: Visual characteristics of aspirates from feeding tubes as a method for predicting tube location, *Nurs Res* 43(5):282–287, 1994.

19. Modell JH: Drowning, *N Eng J Med* 328(4):253–256, 1993.

20. Nolte KB: Esophageal foreign bodies as child abuse. Potential fatal mechanisms, *Am J Forensic Med Path* 14(4):323–326, 1993.

21. North American Nursing Diagnosis Association: *NANDA nursing diagnoses: definitions and classification, 1995–1996,* Philadelphia, 1994, The Association.

22. Ouellette F: Pulmonary aspiration of enteral feedings: a model for prevention, *J Home Health Care Prac* 7(2): 45–55, 1995.

23. Saleh KM: The elderly patient in the post anesthesia care unit, *Nurs Clin North Am* 28(3):507–518, 1993.

24. Sands JA: Incidence of pulmonary aspiration in intubated patients receiving enteral nutrition through wide- and narrow-bore gastric feeding tubes, *Heart Lung* 20(1): 75–80, 1991.

25. Shanahan TK and others: Chin-down posture effect on aspiration in dysphagic patients, *Arch Phys Med Rehabil* 74(7):736–739, 1993.

26. Shuster MH: Enteral feeding of the critically ill, *AACN Clin Issues Crit Care Nurs* 5(4):459–475, 1994.

27. Sliwa JA and Lis S: Drug-induced dysphagia, *Arch Phys Med Rehabil* 74(4):445–447, 1993.

28. Sommers MS: Potential for injury: trauma after cardiopulmonary resuscitation, *Heart Lung* 20(3):287–291, 1991.

29. Thappa V and Sicilian L: Respiratory changes in pregnancy. Distinguishing between physiologic alterations and true disease, *Consultant* 32(6):136–140, 1992.

30. Vincent MT and Goldman BS: Anaerobic lung infections, *Am Family Physician* 49(8):1815–1820, 1994.

31. U.S. Department of Health and Human Services: *Healthy people 2000: national health promotion and disease prevention objections,* Boston, 1992, Jones & Bartlett Publishers.

II

Risk for Altered Body Temperature
▶

Hypothermia
▶

Hyperthermia
▶

Ineffective Thermoregulation
▶

Risk for Altered Body Temperature *is the state in which the individual is at risk for failure to maintain body temperature within normal range.*[15]

Hypothermia *is the state in which an individual's body temperature is reduced below his or her normal range.*[15]

Hyperthermia *is the state in which an individual's temperature is elevated above his or her normal range.*[15]

Ineffective Thermoregulation *is the state in which an individual's temperature fluctuates between hypothermia and hyperthermia.*[15]

OVERVIEW

The North American Nursing Diagnosis Association has approved four diagnoses related to potential and actual problems a person may experience with thermoregulation. This chapter presents an overview of body temperature regulation (i.e., thermoregulation) and specifically addresses the diagnoses of Risk for Altered Body Temperature, Hypothermia, Hyperthermia, and Ineffective Thermoregulation.

Changes in body temperature affect virtually all biochemical processes in the body. Most of the body's heat is produced by metabolic processes that occur within deeper core structures (muscles and viscera) of the body. A balance of heat load (gain) and heat dissipation (loss) is required to maintain proper body temperature. *Heat load* is the sum of metabolic and environmental heat. Heat dissipation occurs at the body's surface when heat from core structures is transported to the skin by the circulating blood. If heat were not lost by the body at rest, the temperature of the body would rise 1.8°F per hour; with light work, the temperature would rise 2.6°F per hour.[9] The dynamic process of heat dissipation occurs through conduction, convection, radiation, and evaporation.[3,12,17]

Conduction is the direct transfer of heat from the body to noncirculating cooler objects (e.g., from cells and capillaries to skin and onto clothing or from the body to still water, as in ice water immersion). Body temperature can be significantly affected by exposure of the body's vascular surfaces, especially the head, face, hands, and feet, to environmental temperature extremes. When environmental temperatures are low, body heat is conducted from the blood vessels to the skin to the air and cold is conducted from the air to the skin to the blood vessels.

The conduction of heat to the body's surface is influenced by blood volume. In hot weather, the body compensates by increasing blood volume as a means of dissipating heat. Mild ankle swelling can be a result of blood volume expansion in hot weather. Exposure to cold, whether by snow, rain, or contact with cold surfaces or objects, results in diuresis with a consequent reduction in blood volume; this is the body's way of reducing the amount of heat that needs to be transferred from the inner body to the body's surface. In an operating room, heat loss by conduction can occur when a normothermic patient is placed on a cold operating room table and exposed to cold prep solutions and instruments.

Convection is the transfer of heat to circulating fluids or gas. Heat moves from warmer body core areas to the skin to the cooler moving air next to the skin. The effect of the moving air is referred to as the windchill factor, which combines the effect of convection caused by the wind with the actual temperature of the air when still. Significant heat loss via convection can occur outdoors on a cold windy day when a hat, gloves, and jacket are not worn or during a surgical procedure when the patient is exposed to cool circulating air moving across body parts.

When the environmental temperature is less than that of the body, *radiation* is involved in the transfer of heat from the skin to the environment. Heat loss through radiation varies with the temperature of the environment. The very young and very old are more sensitive to environmental temperatures and can lose heat rapidly through radiation. Heat loss by radiation is exacerbated by exposure to a cold environment, inappropriate protective clothing, inadequate shelter, and alcohol intake, which produces vasoconstriction and then vasodilation.

When the ambient temperature becomes greater than the skin temperature, the body rids itself of heat through *evaporation*. Evaporation involves the use of body heat to convert water on the skin and in the respiratory tract to water vapor. Sweating occurs through the sweat glands and is controlled by the sympathetic nervous system. Sweat glands are found on all body surfaces with the exception of the margin of the lips, the glans penis, and the inner surface of the prepuce. Water vapor also can diffuse through the skin rather than being secreted by sweat glands; this is termed *insensible perspiration* or *insensible sweating*. Conditions that prevent evaporative heat loss will cause the body temperature to rise by preventing the loss of heat through moisture into the environment.

Thermoregulation

Fluctuations in core body temperature among individuals would be much greater without thermoregulation.[17] Heat accumulation occurs through three mechanisms. Heat is produced within the body through metabolism, through muscular activity during exercise, and through absorption of heat from the environment when the environmental temperature rises above body temperature. Hyperthermia occurs when the thermoregulatory balance is overtaxed and heat accumulation outweighs heat dissipation. Hypothermia occurs when heat loss exceeds the body's ability to produce heat.

The hypothalamus acts as the internal thermostat to govern thermoregulation. The efficient operation of this heat regulatory center of the body relies on skin temperature sensors and heat sensitive neurons in the hypothalamus to receive stimuli from the environment and to transmit this information to the thermostatic center in the hypothalamus. This center regulates core body temperature, rather than surface body temperature, by controlling the rate of heat production in the body and the rate of heat loss from the body.

The thermostatic "set point" of the thermoregulatory center is set so that the temperature of the body is regulated within the normal range. When the core body temperature falls below the normal range, heat production behaviors are initiated; when the core temperature begins to rise above the normal range, heat dissipating behaviors are initiated. Heat production is mediated through secretion of thyroid-stimulating hormone–releasing hormone (TSH-RH), which initiates physiological responses that result in the production and conservation of heat. The hypothalamus can reverse the process by shutting down the TSH-RH pathways, thus stimulating the heat-loss mechanisms.

The cardiovascular system comes into play with the heat-conservation, heat-production, and heat-loss mechanisms that are controlled by the hypothalamus. Normally cardiac output increases and decreases proportionally to the rise and fall in core body temperature. When cardiac output cannot increase enough to maintain blood pressure (e.g., after a massive myocardial infarction), peripheral vascular resistance increases to compensate. Although this results in vasoconstriction and restoration of blood pressure, heat loss can be severely impaired. For the patient with compromised cardiac output who has an infection resulting in a high body temperature, this could create a life-threatening situation.

When the body becomes too cold, cutaneous vessels contribute to temperature control by vasoconstriction. The skin becomes pale and cool as blood is shunted toward warm internal organs.[2] Shivering plays an integral role in maintaining the "set point."[11] When body temperatures begin to fall, shivering provides a heat-generating defense against the cold. Shivering, characterized by rhythmic isotonic contractions of the flexors and extensors against a constant load, mimics aerobic activity. This process increases oxygen consumption. Although shivering can generate significant amounts of heat, it interferes with heat conservation. In febrile states, shivering is not caused by an actual heat deficit but rather by a "perceived" one. Shivering during the "chill phase" of fever is mediated by the same mechanisms responsible for cooling, despite rising body temperature.

Conversely, sweating occurs when the body temperature exceeds the parameters of the set point. Metabolic heat produced during exercise causes the temperature of the blood perfusing the hypothalamus to rise. The hypothalamus responds with signals that stimulate cutaneous vasodilation and the onset of sweating. Increased perfusion of cutaneous vessels delivers heated blood to the skin, where it is cooled by a transfer of heat to the environment, primarily through convection and evaporation.

Measurement of Body Temperature

Temperatures differ in various parts of the body. Core temperatures (measured with esophageal, tympanic, and rectal thermometers) are higher than temperatures of the extremities or the body surface (usually measured by oral or axillary thermometers).[8] Esophageal temperatures are measured during general anesthesia by a sensor attached to the esophageal stethoscope. The tympanic temperature, an indirect measure of hypothalamic temperature, can be measured noninvasively with a digital thermometer placed in the external ear canal. Tympanic thermometers are easy to use, comfortable for patients, reflect an accurate core body temperature, and take only 1 to 2 seconds to register. The use of rectal thermometers provides a traditional method of measuring core temperature.

Before the availability of affordable tympanic thermometers, oral thermometers were commonly used. This method was practical, economical, and generally satisfactory for most purposes. The oral temperature measurement can be up to 1°F lower than the rectal temperature. Oral temperatures can be lowered by tachypnea (rapid breathing) and after drinking ice water or cold drinks. Inaccurate measurements may occur also as a result of drinking hot liquids, chewing gum, and smoking, necessitating a 15-minute wait before taking the temperature.[18] A 30-minute wait is recommended for patients over 60 years of age for accurate oral readings.

Determining the route of temperature measurement depends on several factors. The presence of localized infections involving the ear canal, oral cavity, axillary region, or rectal area requires that the nurse identify a route not involving the infected area. Oral measurement is contraindicated in patients who are unconscious, disoriented, or seizure-prone; in young children and infants; and in patients who mouth breathe to facilitate respirations. Oxygen therapy via nasal canula is not a contraindication for an oral temperature measurement; temperature elevations secondary to oxygen administration account for a rise of only about 0.3°F.[18]

Rectal measurement is contraindicated in patients with diarrhea; in patients who have had recent rectal or prostatic surgery or injury; and in patients who have cardiac problems (anal manipulation may stimulate the vagus nerve, causing a cardiac rhythm disturbance). Additionally, rectal temperatures are contraindicated in the newborn until anal patency is determined; the presence of meconium is an indicator.

ASSESSMENT

Diagnostic Factors

Assessment of disorders in thermoregulation includes a careful investigation of factors that may contribute to a diagnosis of Risk for Altered Body Temperature, Hypothermia, Hyperthermia, or Ineffective Thermoregulation. Seven factors are common to the four diagnoses and must be considered for each.

Age. Temperature variations are of particular concern for those at either end of the age continuum. Temperature-regulating mechanisms in infants and young children are not well developed, and dramatic fluctuations can occur. Development of the muscles necessary for shivering increases with age, as does the amount of adipose tissue necessary for insulation against heat loss.[10] Infants have underdeveloped sweat glands, less subcutaneous fat, poor vasomotor control, and lower metabolic rates and greater heat loss through convection and radiation than older children and adults.

Older adults are also at risk for thermoregulatory problems. Complex, multifactorial changes occur in the elderly that influence temperature maintenance. Many of the same mechanisms influencing temperature instability in the very young are also operative in the very old, but for different reasons. The elderly have lost their ability to respond to temperature change. Sweat glands have atrophied, blood vessels have lost elasticity and do not dilate and constrict as readily, and metabolic rate is generally lowered. The low metabolic rate results partially from a decrease in physical activity and a resulting decrease in heat production.

Weight. Persons who are more than 20% underweight or overweight are more prone to alterations in body temperature. In general, those who are overweight are at greater risk for Hyperthermia because excess fat inhibits the release of heat. Heavyset military recruits have a threefold increase in the incidence of experiencing heat illness during basic training.[9] Those who are underweight are at risk for Hypothermia because of decreased body insulation and lower metabolism.

Exposure to Extremes of Temperature. Short-term exposure to moderate changes of external ambient temperature is generally of little consequence to the healthy individual. Prolonged exposure to extremes of environmental temperature can severely tax the body's thermoregulatory mechanisms and leave a person at higher risk for Ineffective Thermoregulation. Exposure to temperature extremes can also aggravate existing pathological conditions. Wearing inadequate protective clothing and failure to take measures to control exposure in extremely hot or cold environments put the person at Risk for Altered Body Temperature and can contribute to the development of Hyperthermia or Hypothermia.

Activity or Exercise. Activity tends to increase body temperature. Vigorous exercise for an individual who is not properly conditioned, compounded by the presence of additional risk factors such as being overweight or exercising during hot weather, places a person at high risk for a heat-related disorder. For an elderly person, too little activity or exercise in an environmental temperature that is cold, cool, or even normal can result in a below-normal body temperature.

Illness, Disease, and Trauma. Acute and chronic illnesses and their treatments (e.g., surgical procedures or prescribed medications) can increase the risk for developing Hyperthermia or Hypothermia. Persons with hypertension, cardiovascular and respiratory diseases, central nervous system disorders, thyroid imbalances, autoimmune conditions, infections, and psychological disorders can be especially vulnerable for disorders of thermoregulation.

Major trauma also can have an effect on temperature regulation. Serious central nervous system injury usually causes a sustained temperature elevation (central Hyperthermia), which is challenging to treat. Other types of trauma (e.g., accidental injury accompanied by hemorrhaging, burns, and surgery) can cause Hypothermia.

Drugs and Alcohol. Certain medications, alcohol, and anesthetics can result in temperature regulation problems. Drug groups that contribute to Hyperthermia or Hypothermia are diuretics, phenothiazides, antihypertensives, and antidepressants. Many of these drugs cause vasomotor and neurological changes, altered metabolic rates, sedation, and decreased alertness, thereby compromising the body's ability to adapt to environmental changes.

Socioeconomic Status. Low socioeconomic status is a common feature among patients with temperature disorders, especially among the elderly. A large number of elderly persons live alone or at a level of near-poverty; many live in substandard conditions and attempt to conserve resources by severely limiting the amount of money spent on food, heat, and clothing. Additionally, elderly individuals may be unaware that they are at greater risk for Hypothermia and therefore do not take precautions. Because of sensory deficits, the elderly may be less alert to symptoms of impending temperature disorders.

Risk for Altered Body Temperature

The preceding discussion of factors related to disorders of thermoregulation are especially useful as a guide in determining if a patient is at Risk for Altered Body Temperature. Assessment should focus on the following areas: the patient's developmental age, weight, and nutritional status; usual or unusual exposure to extremes of temperature; activity and exercise patterns; recent history of illness, disease, or trauma; use of drugs (prescribed and recreational) and alcohol; and socioeconomic status (focusing on living conditions).

■ Risk Factors

The presence of the following behaviors, conditions, or circumstances renders the patient more vulnerable to Risk for Altered Body Temperature:

- Extremes of age
- Extremes of weight
- Exposure to cold/cool or warm/hot environments
- Dehydration
- Inactivity or vigorous activity
- Medications causing vasoconstriction or vasodilation
- Altered metabolic rate
- Sedation
- Inappropriate clothing for the environmental temperature
- Illness or trauma affecting temperature regulation

Hypothermia

Unfortunately, Hypothermia is often unrecognized, yet the significance of the problem remains impressive. The majority of severely hypothermic patients die before reaching the hospital. For those who reach the hospital alive, survival depends on immediately initiating the appropriate treatment and on the patient's status related to the factors that put him or her at risk for Ineffective Thermoregulation resulting in Hypothermia.[3,12]

Hypothermia is generally diagnosed when the core body temperature (esophageal, rectal, or tympanic) is less than 95°F. Below this core temperature, the human body becomes less capable of producing heat. When a core temperature is below 86°F, the body assumes the temperature of the environment (i.e., becomes poikilothermic).[12,14] Summers[19] described and validated three distinct types of Hypothermia: inadvertent, accidental, and intentional.

Inadvertent Hypothermia can result from a surgical patient's exposure to a cold operating room environment. The patient's core temperature is 96.8°F or lower. Shivering, pale skin, or pale mucous membrane color, cyanotic nail beds, capillary refill greater than 5 seconds, and increased metabolism (because of the stress response for tissue repair when the incision is made) are defining characteristics of this type of Hypothermia.

Accidental Hypothermia occurs as a result of accidental exposure to environmental factors, leading to heat loss.[16] The patient's temperature is less than or equal to 95°F. Other defining characteristics that should be assessed include blood pressure, pulse, and respiratory rate lower than normal; cardiac arrhythmia; evidence of tissue damage or frostbite; decreased metabolism; shivering; piloerection; drowsiness; and confusion.

Intentional Hypothermia is a result of the purposeful cooling of a patient for surgical procedures (e.g., bypass grafting or cardiac transplants). The patient's core body temperature will usually range between 80° and 85°F, with shivering, cyanotic nail beds (despite 98% to 100% oxygen saturation on pulse oximetry), pale skin or pale mucous membrane color, slow capillary return, and increased metabolism (because of the stress response initiated by making the surgical incision).[19]

Generally considered a problem secondary to an exposure to extreme cold, Hypothermia can occur in any season or climate. It can occur when someone is exposed to a moderate environmental temperature (e.g., 60°F) that exceeds an individual's clothing, shelter, or thermogenic situation. Water immersion and high wind magnify this effect.[10] Although one might think that living in a moderate climate, such as North Carolina's, for example, would decrease the risk for Hypothermia, it is interesting to note that, during the period of 1979 to 1991, North Carolina ranked second among the 50 states in number and ninth in rate of deaths associated with hypothermia.[4]

Manifestations of Hypothermia are related to the degree of Hypothermia the patient experiences (see Table 1). As might be expected, lowering the body's core temperature below 95°F has a wide range of physiological consequences. The diagnosis of Hypothermia can be missed if temperatures are not routinely taken. Surface or core temperatures below 95°F should be remeasured to ensure accuracy. The patient may present a myriad of neurological, psychiatric, cardiovascular, and metabolic signs and symptoms, all of which

TABLE 1 Manifestations of Hypothermia[10,14]

Stage	Core Temperature	Potential Effects
Mild	33°–35°C (91.4°–95°F)	Tachypnea, tachycardia Ataxia, dysarthria Lethargy, apathy Poor judgment Pale, cold, numb skin Hyperactive reflexes Shivering to generate heat
Moderate	27°–32°C (80.6°–89.6°F)	Atrial fibrillation→undetectable pulse Stupor, progressive decrease in level of consciousness 25%–50% decrease in oxygen consumption Decreased ventricular fibrillation threshold Pulmonary edema Poikilothermy Loss of reflexes Loss of shivering response
Severe	15.2°–26°C (59.4°–78.8°F)	Pulse 20% of normal→asystole Coma Significant hypotension 75% decrease in oxygen consumption Major acid-base disturbances

II

may be attributed to other conditions if Hypothermia is not considered.

Once the diagnosis of Hypothermia is made, it is important to identify factors that may have contributed to the patient becoming hypothermic. The related factors associated with Hypothermia can be categorized according to personal factors (e.g., age, health status, physical fitness, lack of appropriate shelter), environmental factors (i.e., prolonged exposure to cold air or water and sudden change in environmental temperature from high to low), and factors interfering with the thermoregulation response (e.g., injury to the hypothalamus, hypothyroidism, and use of alcohol or medications causing vasodilation).

■ Defining Characteristics

The presence of the following characteristics indicates that the patient may be experiencing Hypothermia:

Major
- Reduction in body temperature below normal range
- Shivering (mild)
- Cool skin
- Pallor (moderate)

Minor
- Slow capillary refill
- Tachycardia
- Cyanotic nail beds
- Hypertension (early response)
- Piloerection

■ Related Factors

The following related factors are associated with Hypothermia:

- Exposure to cool or cold environments
- Age extremes
- Illness or trauma
- Damage to hypothalamus
- Inability or decreased ability to shiver
- Malnutrition
- Inadequate clothing
- Consumption of alcohol

- Medication causing vasodilation
- Decreased metabolic rate (e.g., hypothyroidism)
- Inactivity

Hyperthermia

Hyperthermia is the state in which an individual's body temperature is elevated above the normal range. Heat illnesses occur when the body is unable to dissipate heat adequately. Heat exhaustion, heat stroke, and malignant hyperthermia are examples of heat illnesses. *Heat exhaustion* is a common disorder caused by excessive loss of body fluids, resulting in hypovolemia. The patient may complain of headache, nausea, vomiting, lightheadedness, fatigue, and muscle cramps.[20] Core body temperature is usually normal or slightly elevated (to as high as 100°F).[7] In addition, a weak, rapid pulse, orthostatic hypotension, and cold, clammy, diaphoretic skin is noted. With the replacement of fluids, recovery is usually rapid. An exception would be the patient experiencing severe hypotension with consequent decreased profusion to the heart, kidneys, or brain.

Heat stroke is a life-threatening, progressive, multisystem disorder reflecting collapse of the thermoregulatory system.[8,12] There are two distinct types of heat stroke:[5] (1) nonexertional or classic heat stroke, which is a consequence of intense exposure to a hot environment, and (2) exertional heat stroke, which develops during vigorous exercise.

The clinical hallmarks of classic heat stroke are elevated body temperature (105° to 106°F), central nervous system dysfunction, and the absence of sweating (anhidrosis). The presence of this constellation of characteristics requires immediate emergency treatment. A 70% mortality rate has been reported for those who experience a 2-hour delay in treatment.

Whereas elevated core body temperature is usually a critical indicator of heat illnesses, it is unreliable for exertional heat stroke. Also, although classic heat stroke is associated with the absence of sweating, this is not a consistent finding in exertional heat stroke. Diagnosis of exertional heat stroke must be made on the basis of neurological alterations and evidence of organ damage or dysfunction.[3,5,7,9] Neurological alterations can range from lethargy, confusion, bizarre mentation, and disorientation to delirium and coma. Organ damage or dysfunction usually manifests as circulatory collapse; coagulopathy with tissue hemorrhage and disseminated intravascular coagulation; metabolic acidosis; renal and hepatic failure; muscle necrosis; and coma. The amount of organ damage depends on the degree of temperature elevation and the duration of the hyperthermic state.

Many patients who experience heat stroke, whether exertional or nonexertional (i.e., classic), have identifiable predisposing factors that impair normal thermoregulation.[5] Patients with classic (nonexertional) heat stroke often have a predisposing medical illness. The most common illnesses are cardiopulmonary disease, which limits the ability to profuse the peripheral vessels adequately, limiting cutaneous vasodilation, and diabetes, which is associated with peripheral neuropathy. Predisposing factors for exertional heat stroke include the use of medications that impair heat loss, poor physical conditioning, concomitant or recent diarrheal or febrile illness, obesity, the use of protective gear (e.g., firefighters), sleep deprivation, and dehydration. Persons not acclimatized to increasing environmental temperatures are also predisposed to exertional heat stroke.

Malignant Hyperthermia (MH), a third type of heat emergency, is a familial myopathy precipitated by the administration of inhalant general anesthesia and depolarizing muscle-blocking agents. It is a rare, life-threatening disorder, most often seen in children and adolescents.[1,5,6] This disorder may occur any time during or shortly after the anesthesia experience. It is characterized by a dramatic onset of severe and sustained masseter muscle rigidity, and most patients exhibit whole body rigidity.[5,6] Characteristics of the syndrome include cellular hypermetabolism resulting in hypercarbia, tachypnea, tachycardia, hypoxia, metabolic and respiratory acidosis, and elevated temperature. Although the rise in body core temperature (at the rate of about 1.8°F every 5 minutes[4]) is the hallmark of MH, it is one of the late manifestations.[6]

Cardiovascular clinical signs of MH include tachycardia, which could progress to ventricular fibrillation and unstable blood pressure. The patient develops a generalized erythematous flush, peripheral mottling, and cyanosis secondary to generalized vasoconstriction and accelerated by oxygen consumption by muscles. If left untreated, this hypermetabolic disorder of the skeletal muscles can result in death.

■ Defining Characteristics

The presence of the following characteristics indicates that the patient may be experiencing Hyperthermia:

Major
- Increase in body temperature above the normal range

Minor
- Flushed skin
- Skin warm to the touch
- Increased respiratory rate
- Tachycardia
- Alterations in mental status
- An absence of or limited sweating
- Seizures or convulsions

■ Related Factors

The following related factors are associated with Hyperthermia:

- Exposure to a hot environment
- Vigorous activity
- Physically unfit
- Medications or anesthesia
- Inappropriate clothing
- Increased metabolic rate
- Illness or trauma directly or indirectly affecting the body's thermoregulatory mechanisms
- Dehydration
- Inability or decreased ability to perspire

Ineffective Thermoregulation

Ineffective Thermoregulation tends to occur in premature or newborn infants whose usual temperature control mechanisms are not yet fully de-

II

veloped. The frail elderly are also prone to inadequate thermoregulatory control, especially when the usual temperature regulatory mechanisms are no longer functioning adequately as a result of degeneration or disease. In all age groups, toxic agents, trauma, tumors, infection, or vascular disease can impair the hypothalamus and alter its temperature regulatory response when the body's core temperature shifts above and below normal.[2] In addition to noxious agents directly affecting the hypothalamus, alterations of the skin, peripheral nerves, and autonomic nervous system can result in Ineffective Thermoregulation. Thus usual environmental temperature fluctuations can result in Ineffective Thermoregulation for patients whose thermoregulatory response is impaired, whether due to premature developmental level, age extremes, or physiological impairment of the hypothalamus and its related responses.

Ineffective Thermoregulation results in the fluctuation of temperature between hypothermic and hyperthermic states. Therefore, in assessing the patient for Ineffective Thermoregulation, the nurse should direct the assessment focus to the defining characteristics of Hyperthermia and Hypothermia.

■ Defining Characteristics

The presence of the following characteristics indicates that the patient may be experiencing Ineffective Thermoregulation:

- Fluctuations in body temperature above and below the normal range
- Refer to the defining characteristics for Hypothermia and Hyperthermia

■ Related Factors

The following related factors are associated with Ineffective Thermoregulation:

- Trauma and illness affecting the thermoregulatory system
- Immature development of the thermoregulatory system (e.g., prematurity)
- Extremes of age (i.e., very young and very old)
- Fluctuating environmental temperature

DIAGNOSIS

■ Differential Nursing Diagnosis

When making diagnoses related to an actual or potential alteration in body temperature, the effectiveness of the patient's thermoregulatory system must be considered. There are other nursing diagnoses that by definition encompass defining characteristics or related factors for the diagnoses of Risk for Altered Body Temperature, Hyperthermia, Hypothermia, and Ineffective Thermoregulation. For example, a premature infant diagnosed with Disorganized Infant Behavior might also be diagnosed with Risk for Altered Body Temperature or Ineffective Thermoregulation. Likewise, an adult experiencing Fatigue, Fluid Volume Deficit, or Altered Tissue Perfusion may also be experiencing Hyperthermia. In infants, the diagnosis of Disorganized Behavior implies that the thermoregulatory system of an infant may be immature. In adults, the initial diagnoses, when considered with other signs and symptoms, may indicate that the patient is at Risk for Altered Body Temperature. A comprehensive assessment is critical to making correct diagnoses and prioritizing them.

■ Medical and Psychiatric Diagnoses

Examples of related medical and psychiatric diagnoses for Risk for Altered Body Temperature include major trauma affecting the skin (e.g., burns) or the central nervous system (e.g., closed head injury); diseases (e.g., brain tumor, diabetes, cardiovascular diseases, and cerebrovascular diseases); infections (e.g., pneumonia); and substance abuse (e.g., alcoholism). Patients with these diagnoses may be at Risk for Altered Body Temperature and should be assessed frequently for the presence of defining characteristics indicating that they are experiencing Ineffective Thermoregulation, Hyperthermia, or Hypothermia. Open communication among the nurses, physicians, clinical pharmacologists, and other members of the health care team enhances early identification of characteristics and factors related to alterations in thermoregulation.

OUTCOME IDENTIFICATION, PLANNING, AND IMPLEMENTATION

The desired outcome for each of the diagnoses in this cluster is to maintain or achieve a core body temperature within the patient's normal range. The normal range for most adults is 98.6° to 100.4°F, measured by rectal or tympanic thermometers, and the normal range for most infants is 97.7° to 99.5°F.[17] Desired outcomes specific to each diagnosis relate to eliminating (if possible) or controlling the related factors. These outcomes are achieved through the involvement of the patient and/or significant others and therefore depend on the quality of patient education.

Risk for Altered Body Temperature

The nursing care for a patient diagnosed with Risk for Altered Body Temperature focuses on preventing any deviation from the patient's normal range of core body temperature. This is accomplished through continuous monitoring and patient education. Patient education should include (1) an overview of the risk factors, (2) measures the patient can take to incorporate risk reduction strategies into the daily routine, and (3) discussion of the defining characteristics of Hyperthermia, Hypothermia, and Ineffective Thermoregulation. It is important that the patient participate in his or her care, if able, by being alert to symptoms that may indicate an alteration in body temperature and by introducing changes in lifestyle that will reduce risk factors.

Hypothermia

To support a return of the body's core temperature to the patient's normal range, the nurse must continuously monitor, carefully rewarm, and give supportive care to the patient. Special attention is given to electrocardiogram (ECG) monitoring because the heart muscle is especially vulnerable to the effects of Hypothermia. Fluid balance, urinary output, blood gases, and blood chemistry are important indicators of circulatory status and the presence of hypoxia and acidosis. Supportive care

may include intubation to maintain a patent airway and careful administration of prescribed drugs. The decrease in body metabolism can delay absorption and excretion of medications, resulting in the bolus effect when circulation returns to normal.

Hyperthermia

In severe Hyperthermia or heat stroke, the immediate objective is to reduce the patient's temperature, which can be as high as 106°F, to 102°F as rapidly as possible to prevent damage to vital organs.[12] Fluid balance should be maintained through intravenous infusions to replace fluid loss and to maintain adequate circulation and urine output. Infusion rates must be monitored carefully to prevent heart and kidney damage as a result of overloading the circulatory system. Electrolytes are monitored continuously to detect acidosis, hypocalcemia, and hypokalemia so that appropriate treatment can be started immediately. Oxygen may be administered to supply tissue needs because of increased metabolic rate and to prevent heart and respiratory failure. The patient's mental status must be monitored for changes in affect and cognition. Such changes can be an early indicator of heat stroke.

Careful monitoring throughout the cooling process is important because a sudden drop in temperature could cause dysrhythmias and circulatory collapse. After the acute phase, attention is directed to reducing the risk of future episodes. Patients should be advised to avoid reexposure to high temperatures because they will be hypersensitive to heat for an extended period of time.

Ineffective Thermoregulation

Patients with this diagnosis can experience episodes of Hypothermia and Hyperthermia. The patient's normal range of core body temperature is exceeded at both ends. Nursing interventions are directed toward controlling and treating the hyperthermic and hypothermic episodes to promote a normothermic state. The respective nursing care guidelines for Hypothermia and Hyperthermia should be implemented when the patient becomes hypothermic or hyperthermic.

II

II

◢ NURSING CARE GUIDELINES
Nursing Diagnosis: Risk for Altered Body Temperature

Expected Outcome: The patient will maintain a core body temperature within his or her normal range.
- Monitor temperature and other vital signs on a regular schedule.
- Determine baseline data for the neurological and cardiovascular systems; initiate regularly scheduled assessments of these systems and compare them to baseline data. *Ongoing assessment is necessary to detect any change in the patient's status so that interventions for treating Hyperthermia or Hypothermia can be instituted immediately if necessary.*
- Review with the patient and/or significant others guidelines for maintaining (1) adequate nutritional and fluid intake; (2) adequate protection in relation to the environment (i.e., adequate clothing and shelter and the adjustment of environmental temperature when possible); and (3) an appropriate balance of exercise-activity and rest. *Instituting measures that support maintenance of the patient's temperature within the normal range can assist in preventing the development of Hyperthermia or Hypothermia.*

Expected Outcome: The patient and/or significant others will identify the risk factors associated with Altered Body Temperature and take appropriate preventive measures in relation to those risk factors.
- ▲ Discuss with the patient and/or significant others the patient's risk factors that may predispose him or her to experience Altered Body Temperature; encourage questions.
- ▲ Explain appropriate preventive measures as they relate to the risk factors over which the patient has some control.
- Reinforce information about risk factors and preventive measures during interactions with the patient and/or significant others. *Education of the patient and/or significant others provides the necessary information to support changes in lifestyle that reduce the risk for developing alterations in body temperature.*

■ = nursing intervention; ▲ = collaborative intervention.

◢ NURSING CARE GUIDELINES
Nursing Diagnosis: Hypothermia

Expected Outcome: The patient will become normothermic as evidenced by a core body temperature maintained within normal limits and will have no signs or symptoms of hypothermia (i.e., shivering; cool, pale skin; piloerection; cyanotic nail beds; tachycardia; and hypertension).
- ▲ For slow-onset hypothermia, the body should be rewarmed gradually, using blankets and warm environmental temperature.
- ▲ For abrupt-onset hypothermia, rapid warming should be done using a hyperthermia blanket and immersion in warm water; rapid body core warming should be done using heated intravenous fluids, hemodialysis, peritoneal dialysis, or gastric and colonic irrigations as ordered. *External and internal warming interventions are necessary to compensate for the body's Ineffective Thermoregulation.*
- ▲ Maintain patent airway.
- ▲ Monitor core body temperature continuously until it is stable and within normal limits.
- ▲ Monitor vital signs continuously; maintain continuous ECG monitoring; and note any dysrhythmias.
- ▲ Monitor laboratory studies (e.g., ABG, serum electrolytes, BUN, blood glucose) and report abnormalities.
- ▲ Monitor urine output every 2 hours and report output of less than 1 ml/kg/hr.
- ▲ When moving or turning the patient, use gentle handling because cold tissue is susceptible to injury. *Continuous monitoring of the patient provides opportunities for immediate intervention if the patient's condition becomes life threatening.*

■ = nursing intervention; ▲ = collaborative intervention.

Expected Outcome: The patient and/or significant others will identify factors related to the development of Hypothermia and use measures to counteract those factors.

▲ When the patient's physiological status stabilizes, discuss with the patient and/or family (1) factors that contribute to the development of Hypothermia (e.g., malnourishment, acute and chronic illnesses, and inadequate shelter and clothing) and (2) specific measures to counteract those factors (e.g., dietary changes that should be made, avoidance of factors contributing to acute illnesses, interventions to counteract the effects of chronic illness, and dressing for protection against extremes in environmental conditions).

■ Emphasize that previous episodes of Hypothermia predispose the patient to subsequent attacks.
Education of the patient and/or significant others provides the necessary information to support changes in lifestyle that reduce the risk for developing Hypothermia.

NURSING CARE GUIDELINES
Nursing Diagnosis: Hyperthermia

Expected Outcome: The patient will become normothermic as evidenced by a core body temperature maintained within normal limits and will have no signs or symptoms of hyperthermia (i.e., skin flushed and warm to the touch; increased respiratory rate; tachycardia; hypotension; and central nervous system manifestations such as delirium, seizures, and coma).

▲ Apply internal and external cooling measures as ordered (e.g., cold water bath, hypothermia blanket, ice packs, cold compresses, and a spray of lukewarm water blown over the patient by a fan, which results in heat loss through evaporation) *to promote cooling and to lower the core body temperature.*

▲ Maintain a patent airway.

▲ Administer intravenous fluids as necessary.

▲ Monitor mental status for changes.

▲ Monitor temperature and other vital signs continuously.

▲ Monitor laboratory studies (e.g., ABG and blood and urine tests).
Continuous monitoring of the patient provides opportunities for immediate intervention if the patient's condition becomes life threatening.

▲ Discontinue the cooling process at a core body temperature of 101° to 102°F *to prevent the development of clinical Hypothermia.*

Expected Outcome: The patient and/or significant others will identify factors related to the development of Hyperthermia and use measures to counteract those factors.

▲ When the patient's physiological status stabilizes, discuss with the patient and/or family (1) factors that contribute to the development of Hyperthermia (e.g., dehydration, vigorous activity, certain medications, and inappropriate clothing) and (2) specific measures to counteract those factors (e.g., increasing fluid intake, exercise appropriate to physical conditioning, alertness to effects of medications, and dressing for protection against extremes in environmental conditions).

■ Emphasize that previous episodes of Hyperthermia may increase the patient's susceptibility to subsequent attacks.
Education of the patient and/or significant others provides the necessary information to support changes in lifestyle that reduce the risk for developing Hyperthermia.

■ = nursing intervention; ▲ = collaborative intervention.

II

■ **NURSING CARE GUIDELINES**
Nursing Diagnosis: Ineffective Thermoregulation

Expected Outcome: The patient will maintain a core body temperature within normal limits.

- ■ Assess to determine whether the patient is hyperthermic or hypothermic; institute nursing interventions specific to Hyperthermia or Hypothermia as the patient's condition warrants (refer to the Nursing Care Guidelines for Hyperthermia and Hypothermia).
- ▲ During cooling or warming procedures, monitor core temperature and other vital signs continuously until the patient is stabilized.
- ▲ Adjust environmental temperature and conditions to meet the patient's needs.
- ▲ Monitor skin temperature and relate it to ambient air temperature.
- ▲ Monitor lab values for evidence of instability (e.g., elevated BUN, hypoglycemia, hyperkalemia, and acidosis).
  Continuous monitoring of the patient provides opportunities for immediate intervention if the patient's condition becomes life threatening.

Expected Outcome: The patient and/or significant others will identify factors related to Ineffective Thermoregulation and use measures to counteract those factors.

- ▲ When the patient's physiological status stabilizes, discuss with the patient and/or significant others those factors that predispose the patient to Ineffective Thermoregulation (e.g., developmental immaturity or prematurity, aging, fluctuating environmental temperature, trauma, or illness).
- ▲ Review with the patient and/or significant others measures to counteract these factors. Examples include keeping the premature infant sufficiently warm (i.e., controlling clothing and the environment) and making sure that the aged patient has appropriate clothing and shelter to protect from environmental conditions (e.g., contacting community services if patient needs help in paying heating bills in winter). The patient and family must be vigilant to the effects of trauma or illnesses and their treatments that may interfere with effective thermoregulation.
  Education of the patient and/or significant others provides the necessary information to support changes that support effective thermoregulation.

■ = nursing intervention; ▲ = collaborative intervention.

EVALUATION

The primary outcome for each of the four diagnoses related to altered body temperature is the maintenance of core body temperature within the normal range for the patient. Immediate treatment of the actual or potential temperature alteration should contribute to achieving a core body temperature within the normal range. To maintain this normothermic temperature, risk and related factors should be modified or eliminated. Management of the risk and related factors may depend on the effectiveness of patient education and the consequent involvement of the patient and/or significant others in the plan of care.

If the patient with Hypothermia, Hyperthermia, or Ineffective Thermoregulation does not achieve a normothermic temperature, the effectiveness of interventions must be quickly assessed and revised as necessary. If the patient achieves a normothermic temperature but does not maintain it over time, the effectiveness of the interventions directed at patient education must be reviewed and revised as necessary.

▶ CASE STUDY WITH PLAN OF CARE

Mrs. Mary S., an 82-year-old widow who lives alone in a small city in northern Florida, arrives by ambulance at the emergency department of the local hospital. The admitting nurse notes that Mrs. S. appears to be drowsy, confused, and disoriented. A neighbor who accompanied Mrs. S. to the hospital reported that she found Mrs. S. at about 11:00 A.M. lying on her kitchen floor in her nightgown with her newspaper in her hand. Her back door was open. The neighbor surmised that Mrs. S. must have collapsed after going outdoors earlier in the morning to get her newspaper off the porch. The weather was unseasonably cold for January, with early morning temperatures dipping into the 30s.

Mrs. S.'s medical history includes hypertension treated with diuretics, arteriosclerosis, congestive heart failure, and progressive weight loss caused by poor appetite. The initial assessment reveals a temperature of 93°F by tympanic thermometer; blood pressure 90/60; pulse 45/min; respirations 12/min; weight 90 pounds; height 5′2″; skin pale and cold; reflexes decreased; pupils sluggish and slightly constricted. Mrs. S.'s neighbor stated that Mrs. S. is on a very limited budget. The neighbor offers to take Mrs. S. shopping once a week, but Mrs. S. often says she does not feel well enough to go.

▶ PLAN OF CARE FOR MRS. MARY S.
Nursing Diagnosis: Hypothermia Related to Cold Environmental Temperature, Cardiovascular Disease, and Malnutrition

Expected Outcome: Mrs. S.'s temperature and other vital signs will be maintained within normal limits in 3 to 4 hours, and no dysrhythmias will be present.
▲ Monitor Mrs. S.'s temperature continuously until stable and within normal limits.
▲ Monitor Mrs. S.'s blood pressure, pulse, and respirations continuously until stable and within normal limits.
▲ Maintain continuous monitoring of Mrs. S.'s ECG until her blood pressure and pulse are stable.
▲ Slowly rewarm Mrs. S., using thermal blankets, to increase her body temperature 1° to 2° per hour.
▲ Monitor Mrs. S.'s neurological status and mental status; note changes.

Expected Outcome: Mrs. S.'s skin will be warm and pink.
■ Support Mrs. S. in a warm, comfortable environment with room temperature maintained between 70° and 75°F.

Expected Outcome: Mrs. S. will identify related factors contributing to the development of Hypothermia.
■ Discuss with Mrs. S. factors that can predispose her to the development of Hypothermia (i.e., her age, inadequate nutrition, inactivity, exposure to cold and inadequate clothing, and the presence of cardiovascular disease).
■ Encourage Mrs. S. to ask questions she may have about the predisposing factors.

Expected Outcome: Mrs. S. will implement appropriate measures to prevent Hypothermia from occurring again.
▲ Assist Mrs. S. in planning preventive measures.
■ Contact the utility company regarding discounts for low-income senior citizens on their utility bills; discuss with Mrs. S. maintaining indoor temperature at between 70° and 75°F.
▲ Arrange a dietary consultation to support Mrs. S. in planning a diet that would support her reaching an ideal body weight of 100 to 120 pounds.
■ Identify warm clothing that Mrs. S. has and sources for additional clothing at reasonable costs (e.g., the community thrift shop).
■ Describe and discuss simple, moderate exercises Mrs. S. can perform three to four times a week to stimulate her metabolism (walking, going up and down stairs, or a light exercise program at the senior citizen's center).
■ Discuss a schedule for developing and maintaining daily contacts with neighbors and friends.

■ = nursing intervention; ▲ = collaborative intervention.

■ CRITICAL THINKING EXERCISES

1. What additional information is needed about Mrs. S. to assess her existing support system adequately. How would you get this information?

2. If Mrs. S. lived in your city, what organizations (agency- and community-related) could be contacted to get information or support for Mrs. S.? Specify names, addresses, phone numbers, and contact persons for these organizations.

3. What specific physiological factors put Mrs. S. at Risk for Altered Body Temperature in the future? Discuss the physiological responses to these factors as they relate to thermoregulation.

REFERENCES

1. Beck CF: Malignant hyperthermia: are you prepared?, *AORN Journal* 59(2):367–390, 1994.
2. Black JM and Matassarin-Jacobs E: Nursing care of clients with a loss of protective function. In *Luckman and Sorensen's medical surgical nursing: a psychophysiological approach*, ed 4, Philadelphia, 1993, WB Saunders Co.
3. Bross MH, Nash BT, and Carlton FB: Heat emergencies, *Am Family Physician* (50)2:389–399, 1994.
4. Butts JD: Hypothermia-related deaths—North Carolina, November 1993–March 1994, *Morbidity and Mortality Weekly Report* 43(46):849–856, 1995.
5. Delaney KA: Heat stroke: underlying processes and lifesaving management, *Postgrad Med* (91)4:379–388, 1992.
6. Donnelly AJ: Malignant hyperthermia: epidemiology, pathophysiology, treatment, *AORN Journal* 59(2):393–405, 1994.
7. Drake DK and Nettina SM: Recognition and management of heat-related illness, *Nurs Practit* (19)8:43–47, 1994.
8. Erickson R and Yount S: Comparison of tympanic and oral temperatures in the surgical patient, *Nurs Res* 40(2):90–93, 1991.
9. Gardner JW, Kark JA, and Gastaldo E: Management and prevention of exertional heat illness in healthy young adults, Unpublished manuscript, February 4, 1994.
10. Hector MG: Treatment of accidental hypothermia, *Am Family Physician* 45(2):785–792, 1992.
11. Holtzclaw BJ: The shivering response. In Fitzpatrick JJ and Stevenson JS, editors: *Annual review of nursing research*, vol II: focus on patient/client symptoms, New York, 1993, Springer.
12. Iseke RJ: Heat-related illnesses. In Noble J, editor: *Textbook of primary care medicine*, ed 2, St. Louis, 1996, Mosby–Year Book.
13. Jackson L: Quick response to hypothermia and frostbite, *Am J Nurs* 95(3):52, 1995.
14. Jolly BT and Ghezzi KT: Accidental hypothermia, *Emergency Med Clin No Am* 10(2):311–327, 1992.
15. North American Nursing Diagnosis Association: *NANDA nursing diagnoses: definitions and classification, 1995–1996*, Philadelphia, 1994, The Association.
16. Nozaki R and others: Accidental profound hypothermia, *N Eng J Med* 315:1680, 1986 (letter).
17. Porth CM: Alterations in temperature regulation. In: *Pathophysiology—concepts of altered health states*, ed 4, Philadelphia, 1994, JB Lippincott Co.
18. Quinless FW and Blauer RE: Fundamental procedures. In: *Nursing procedures*, Springhouse, Pennsylvania, 1992, Springhouse.
19. Summers S: Hypothermia: one nursing diagnosis or three?, *Nurs Diagnosis* 3(1):2–11, 1992.
20. Tek D and Olshaker JS: Heat illness, *Emergency Med Clin No Am* 10(2):299–310, 1992.

Ineffective Breastfeeding

▶

Ineffective Breastfeeding *is the state in which the mother, infant, or family experiences dissatisfaction or difficulty with the breastfeeding process.*

OVERVIEW

Lactation is a normal physiological process.° However, the art of breastfeeding is more than a method of feeding. It involves a dyadic relationship that is synchronous in nature and requires maternal sensitivity to the infant's cries. Mother's decision to breastfeed her infant is influenced by her cultural background, socioeconomic status, support systems, role models, and previous experience with breastfeeding.[25] "Breastfeeding is important for maternal and child health in every culture, and it is essential that women who choose to breastfeed are given the assistance necessary for doing so successfully and exclusively . . ."[4,10,12,15]

The American Academy of Pediatrics, the Association for Women's Health, Obstetric and Neonatal Nurses, and the College of Obstetricians and Gynecologists support breastfeeding as the method of choice for infant feeding. It is the ambition of United States National Health Promotion and Disease Prevention objectives to increase the proportion of mothers who breastfeed in the early postpartum period to at least 75% and to increase the proportion of mothers who continue to breastfeed until their infants reach 5 to 6 months to 50%.[1]

Human breast milk is the ideal and only food necessary for the human infant in the first 4 to 6 months of life.[1] Why then are mothers discontinuing breastfeeding in the first few days, weeks, or months after they give birth? An authoritative study reveals that one of the most common reasons for discontinuing breastfeeding is a perceived or actual insufficient supply of breast milk.[17] Other reasons cited include returning to work outside the home, little or no support from the partner or significant members of the extended family, nipple soreness, and a lack of knowledge about breastfeeding.°

ASSESSMENT

The major defining characteristic of Ineffective Breastfeeding is expressed dissatisfaction with the breastfeeding process. In the mother, this may manifest as a desire to stop breastfeeding or anxiety about the infant's well-being. In the partner or family, it may manifest as an actual lack of support for the mother's efforts or lack of confidence that the mother can adequately feed the child. The infant may not be gaining weight adequately and may be apathetic or extremely fussy.

Several minor defining characteristics may reveal Ineffective Breastfeeding. An inadequate milk supply can influence breastfeeding behavior. Evidence is increasing that certain anatomical and hormonal factors affect lactation.[17] A subsequent pregnancy has been known to decrease the maternal breast milk supply markedly.[17]

Recognition of the infant's contribution to breastfeeding success is increasing. The nurse must assess the infant's breastfeeding behavior along with the mother's.[9,16,21]

The infant's ineffective suck may cause an inability to attach to the mother's nipple correctly,

---

°References 4, 10, 11, 12, 19.

°References 1, 5, 6, 7, 15, 23, 24.

II

which is another defining characteristic.[9,16,21] Also, the infant may be unable to attach to the mother's nipple correctly because of genetic, iatrogenic, or positioning problems; and anatomical problem in the mother, such as an inverted nipple or one tends to retract; or an anatomical problem in the infant, such as a cleft lip or palate. Breast shape seems to have some effect on lactation.[15]

Oxytocin release, stimulated in the mother by thoughts of her infant or by the infant suckling at her breast, is responsible for the ejection of breast milk.[12] When oxytocin stimulates the release of milk, the milk may leak from the breast that is not being used. Studies have shown that it may take 2 or more minutes of sucking for a continuous flow from the milk-producing cells.[12] If oxytocin release is inadequate, then mothers will have Ineffective Breastfeeding.

The infant may demonstrate nonsustained suckling at the breast, that is, sucking for short periods of time and then stopping. The infant prefers continuous feeding without a break for the mother, and he or she may cry when put down. There is slow or no weight gain. However, one must remember that breastfeeding infants do not regain their weight as rapidly as bottle-fed infants. Related factors may include a premature infant or an infant with a heart defect; both of these conditions will cause the infant to be fatigued easily.[12]

Occasionally infants will only suck from one breast, although both may be offered. Observation of both breasts may reveal that one nipple is retracted or inverted. The infant will find that sucking from the normal nipple produces more milk with less work, so he or she will then show a definite preference for it. Also, the mother may offer only one breast to suck because of a sore nipple on one side.[7,22]

The nurse may consider a diagnosis of Ineffective Breastfeeding when observing a newborn infant who is breastfeeding less than seven times in 24 hours. The successfully breastfed infant will sleep for periods of 2 to 3 hours[12] between feedings and breastfeed with eyes closed. The emptying time of the stomach for breast milk is about 1½ hours. The nurse should encourage feedings every 2 to 3 hours until a breastfeeding routine is established, especially in the newborn.

Nipple soreness is quite common in the first 2 weeks of breastfeeding.[7,12,14,22] Bleeding, cracks, or fissures in the nipple, and pain for the duration of breastfeeding may accompany prolonged, persistent soreness. The nurse can assess the actual condition of the nipple by observation and the presence of pain by careful questioning of the mother. Assessing the positioning of the infant at the breast will reveal whether incorrect positioning is the primary cause.[7,12,15]

In the absence of physiological causes, such as sore nipples, the mother may show reluctance to breastfeed her baby because she has internalized some of the North American culture's ambivalent feelings about breastfeeding.[12,15,22]

It may also be overwhelming to a woman to find herself now committed to her infant for 6 to 12 feedings a day for months.[12] Mother's perception of her role and perception of the use of the breasts for feeding her infant influence her ease and satisfaction with breastfeeding as her infant-feeding method of choice.

Although breastfeeding is now believed to be the method of choice for infant feeding, the female breast is still seen as a sexual object that is often the partner's exclusive domain. Discussing how she made her decision to breastfeed, her partner's feelings and those of her extended family will be a part of the assessment process.

The nurse may consider a diagnosis of Ineffective Breastfeeding when the infant exhibits fussiness and crying within the first hour after breastfeeding and does not respond to other comfort measures or when the infant arches and cries at the breast and resists latching on. Infants who wake within the first hour may not have had sufficient milk. Usually breast milk is not totally digested for at least 1½ hours.[12] The infant needs to suckle at each breast for a sufficient length of time to receive the hind milk, which is rich in fat and comes at the end of the feeding. The fat content of breast milk not only provides the calories infants need but also satiates them. Sucking time should not be limited.[7] The nurse needs to consider variables specific to each infant. Some infants may stretch, extending their heads and arching their backs as they resist latching on to the breast. These infants may actually seem to be pulling away from the mother and her breast. In these circumstances, assessment includes a check for a neurological defect.

Perceived inadequate milk supply may influence breastfeeding behavior. For a variety of reasons that may be psychological, a mother may believe that her milk cannot be as nutritious for her child as a scientifically prepared formula.[12,15] Because the present cultural norm in some communities is to breastfeed, a mother may discover that an insufficient milk supply is a socially acceptable reason for ceasing breastfeeding when she has no true personal commitment to breastfeed. Issues to consider when determining whether the mother perceives inadequate milk supply and factors to consider in terms of their effect on the volume of milk supply include (1) inadequate knowledge of breast milk production,[21] (2) socioeconomic status of the mother (which may correlate to her nutrition intake), (3) drug use by the mother (prescribed by the physician or self-prescribed),[12] and (4) inadequate knowledge of the growth spurts that all babies have at different times in the first 6 months of life.[15]

Studies by Atkinson and associates[12] show that the milk of mothers who have premature infants is higher in protein nitrogen than milk of mothers with full-term infants. The protein requirement of premature infants is higher than full-term infants.[12,20] The other advantages of breast milk, such as the immunological factors, will be of value to the premature infant too. However, the premature infant may not be sufficiently strong to suck to initiate milk production. This situation will require that the mother learn hand expression, storage, and how to maintain an adequate milk supply at the time she is adjusting to the fact that she has an infant at risk.

An infant anomaly, such as a cleft lip or cleft palate, may interfere with the sucking reflex. Observation of the infant will include making sure that the infant's tongue is around the mother's

nipple and areola, using the mother's breast to secure adequate suction. A cardiac defect may decrease the infant's energy level so that sucking for a period long enough to obtain sufficient milk may be difficult. Assessment includes the amount of time the infant sucks at each breast and how frequently the infant feeds. An infant with Down syndrome or a neurological impairment may have poor muscle tone, which may interfere with the sucking reflex.

Maternal breast anomaly, infections, or previous breast surgery may influence the mother's ability to breastfeed. Breast anomalies include nipples that are flat, inverted, or, in rare situations, completely absent. Sucking for the infant is quite difficult because the infant has nothing to grasp in its mouth. Occasionally a breast is so very large and pendulous that it is too heavy for the baby's mouth to hold. The nipple is lost, and the infant becomes frustrated. A physical assessment of the nipple and areola, especially prenatally, is imperative. Interference with breastfeeding may occur after cosmetic surgery, including breast augmentation and reduction, but this depends on the type of surgery performed.[17,18] What has to be assessed is interference with milk production and its delivery to the nipple for the infant to suck.

Interruption of breastfeeding related to maternal or infant needs will influence successful breastfeeding. Temporary interruptions in breastfeeding may result if the infant develops milk jaundice; if the mother develops sore, cracked nipples;[15,20] if the mother or infant becomes ill; or if a mother with mastitis develops an abscess and needs medical intervention.[12] If medical intervention includes a prescription for medication, the effect of the medication on breastfeeding should be determined.[3] If the infant develops a preference for the breastfeeding substitute the resumption of breastfeeding becomes difficult. Assessing the length of the interruption and keeping it to a minimum is most important.[22] Mothers returning to work outside the home may temporarily interrupt the rhythm established by the breastfeeding dyad.[1,6]

The influence of previous breastfeeding failure will depend on the reason for the failure, how the

II

mother accepted the situation, and the support she received from her support system in dealing with resultant feelings of guilt. Her level of self-esteem in the mothering role will contribute to her success or lack thereof. A detailed history of previous births will elicit this information.

The use of supplemental feedings with an artificial nipple may impair breastfeeding. Two barriers to successful breastfeeding are introduced with this one action—the infant will not continue to suck for a sufficient length of time on the breast to increase milk supply,[12] and nipple confusion occurs. An infant has to work harder to receive breast milk than to receive a breast milk substitute. The infant will learn to prefer the latter and refuse to nurse at the breast.[12] It is well documented that early and frequent supplementation of breastfeeding and introduction of bottles and pacifiers leads to early discontinuation of breastfeeding.[20]

A poor reflex, which may be caused by genetic or developmental problems in the infant, will influence breastfeeding. Genetic or developmental problems will be recognizable by observation. Some infants are ineffective sucklers because of illness, prematurity, or sedation.[12,15] To assist in making this diagnosis the nurse needs to understand the sucking reflex and to know that not all infants are born with an instinctive and correct sucking pattern.

North American families may not have role models who exemplify breastfeeding success. Most extended family members, especially the infant's grandmothers, did not breastfeed their babies. Studies have demonstrated that partner and family support and encouragement directly affect breastfeeding success. Conversely, lack of support, jealousy of the partner for the mother-infant dyad, and doubt about the mother's ability to nourish the infant adequately will all contribute to breastfeeding failure.[12,15] The availability of support from the family and partner will influence breastfeeding success.

Closely related to support is the realization that breastfeeding is a learned process for the mother and the infant both.[11] In the second half of the century, new mothers have moved away from their traditional sources of assistance. Women in the middle part of the century lost the knowledge and skills to assist breastfeeding mothers. The American Academy of Pediatrics and the Canadian Paediatric Society stated that schools should provide education for the public and health professionals to increase breastfeeding success.[4,19] Knowledge deficits about milk composition, the milk ejection reflex, proper sucking, and frequency of breastfeeding adversely affect the duration of breastfeeding.[12]

Few medical diagnoses should interfere with the breastfeeding process. Mothers with breast cancer should not breastfeed their infants; they should receive treatment immediately.[12,18] With the advent of AIDS, questions have arisen about infected mothers breastfeeding their infants. In countries such as Canada and the United States mothers infected with the human immunodeficiency virus (HIV) have been advised against breastfeeding their infants when safe alternatives are available. HIV has been isolated in breast milk.[25] The nurse should determine the source of breastfeeding substitutes as part of an assessment strategy. Discussion continues regarding the best advice for breastfeeding women.[25]

Several assessment tools that assist in measuring breastfeeding success are recorded in the literature:

Jensen[9]: Documentation tool for identifying breastfeeding problems (LATCH, The Latch Scoring Table).
Lawrence[12]: Parameters for evaluation for breastfed infants.
Matthew[13]: Instrument to measure maternal satisfaction and neonates' feeding behaviors (IBFAT, Infant Breastfeeding Assessment Tool).
Mulford[16]: Assessment method for rating the progress of a mother and baby learning to breastfeed (MBA, Mother-Baby Breastfeeding Assessment Tool).
Riordan[20]: Assessment forms for indicating nipple function and breastfeeding evaluation, and a hospital breastfeeding teaching checklist.
Shrago and Bocar[21]: Systematic Assessment of Infant at Breast (SAIB).

■ Defining Characteristics

The presence of the following defining characteristics indicates that the mother may experiencing Ineffective Breastfeeding:

- Unsatisfactory breastfeeding process
- Actual or perceived inadequate milk supply
- Inability of the infant to attach to maternal nipple correctly
- No observable signs of oxytocin release
- Nonsustained sucking at the breast
- Suckling at only one breast per feeding
- Breastfeeding less than seven times in 24 hours
- Persistence of sore nipples beyond the infant's first week of life
- Infant exhibiting fussiness and crying within the first hour after breastfeeding
- Unresponsiveness of the infant to other comfort measures
- Infant arching and crying at the breast
- Resistance of the infant to latch on to the breast
- Maternal reluctance to put infant to breast[11]

■ Related Factors

The following related factors are associated with Ineffective Breastfeeding:

- Prematurity or infant anomaly
- Maternal breast anomaly
- Previous breast surgery
- Infant receiving supplemental feedings with artificial nipple
- Poor infant sucking reflex
- History of breastfeeding failure
- Knowledge deficit
- Nonsupportive partner or family
- Interruption in breastfeeding
- Medical conditions (e.g., AIDS or breast cancer)
- Incongruent cultural norms and expectations

DIAGNOSIS

■ Differential Nursing Diagnosis

Ineffective Breastfeeding can be differentiated from the diagnosis Ineffective Infant Feeding Pattern when carefully considering the related factors and defining characteristics that apply to each diag-nosis. Ineffective Breastfeeding encompasses the difficulty and the dissatisfaction with breastfeeding that the mother and the infant both experience. Most importantly, nursing observation, assessment, and interventions are centered around enhancing the mother's milk supply and improving her breast-feeding positioning and technique. Ineffective Breastfeeding may or may not involve the infant's ability to initiate, sustain, or coordinate the suck, swallowing, and breathing pattern required to feed effectively. The infant may simply resist latching on to the mother's breast. Ineffective Infant Feeding can be the result of a physical condition, an inap-propriate food choice, a maladaptive parent-feed-ing interaction, or a combination of these.

■ Medical and Psychiatric Diagnoses

Physiological conditions experienced by the mother that impair the ability to breastfeed are anxiety, postpartum depression, substance abuse, fibrocystic breast disease, breast augmentation, breast cancer, infection of nipples, and mastitis. For the infant, the nurse must consider medical conditions such as, prematurity, low birth weight, poor suck reflex, cardiovascular anomalies, cleft palate, cleft lip, and neurological dysfunction. Psy-chiatric diagnoses for the mother include condi-tions such as major depression and schizophrenia. Nursing care focuses on the observation and assessment of the mother and the infant to pro-mote optimal and satisfying breastfeeding and bonding experiences

OUTCOME IDENTIFICATION, PLANNING, AND IMPLEMENTATION

The ultimate expected outcome is successful breastfeeding in which the adult members of the family are satisfied with the process and are having minimal difficulty. The defining characteristics and related factors in the individual family situa-tion will influence the nursing response to assist families to reach this outcome. A discussion of interventions associated with various related fac-tors follows.

Families, the public at large, and health professionals need information about the advantages of breastfeeding, the physiology of lactation, and the emotional and social factors that influence lactation.[4,8,11] The majority of issues and related factors surrounding the diagnosis Ineffective Breastfeeding could be prevented by education and skills development at appropriate intervals during the prenatal period. Some nursing interventions are appropriate in the prenatal period, whereas others are appropriate in the immediate postpartum period in the hospital and immediately after discharge.

Research supports the observation that the maternity nurse has not significantly increased his or her breastfeeding knowledge over the past 10 years. Studies consistently demonstrate low mean scores (approximating 50%) on questionnaires designed to test breastfeeding knowledge.[1]

Duration of breastfeeding does not cause sore nipples.[20] Many mothers have soreness in the first week of breastfeeding when the ductules are not yet filled with milk.[12] Mothers need reassurance and information at this time. The following technique is recommended.[4,12,15]

Sitting upright in bed, with her back and arms supported, the mother positions the infant across her abdomen on the side so that the infant's face, chest, genitals, and knees are all facing her. The infant should not have to turn the neck to feed. If the mother brings her knees up, she will support the infant in this position (and relieve the strain on her back). A pillow under the infant and across the mother's abdomen will assist a mother who has had a cesarean delivery. Once the baby is positioned, the mother gives attention to her nipple and areola. The mother should spread her fingers around the breast, with her thumb above the breast and the four fingers below and supporting it.

The mother may then be instructed to tickle the infant's upper lip gently. The infant will present a wide open mouth. The mother will then draw the infant's whole body toward her own until the infant's nose is just touching her breast. The mother may need to support her breast during feedings until the infant's suckling is stronger. The mother needs to be sure that the infant is not pulling down on her breast and that the infant has all of the nipple and at least some of the areola in the mouth. Positioning of the infant on the breast can vary so that pressure is distributed more evenly all around the nipple and areola. Observation of the baby's sucking pattern will confirm if the baby's position is correct.[7] Air-drying of nipples for up to fifteen minutes after each feeding can be encouraged. Nipple shields should not be used unless other interventions are not working.[12] Pumping without a shield has been demonstrated to yield statistically larger milk volumes.[20]

Situations that may be linked to faulty sucking include prematurity or infants with congenital oral anomalies, cardiac defects, or neurological impairments. If the infant has difficulty with the sucking reflex, the nurse should observe the position of the infant's tongue. The wide open mouth should latch on to the breast with the tongue below the nipple and extended over the lower gum and the lower lip extended out rather than in over the lower gums. The nipple and the areola are drawn well into the infant's mouth so that the gums compress the areola behind the nipple, forcing the milk gathered in the breast's sinuses into the back of the infant's mouth. "In the absence of audible swallowing, a digital suck assessment can be performed . . . To perform a digital suck assessment, the nurse uses a finger covered with a well-fitting glove or finger cot and gently tickles the infant's lips to elicit mouth opening. The finger is then inserted into the infant's mouth. Normally the infant's tongue curls around the examining finger, forming a trough beneath the finger. The tongue and the lips form a complete seal around the finger, with noticeable negative pressure exerted on the finger in a rhythmic pattern . . ."[21]

If the infant has an oral defect, suction may be achieved by bringing the infant closer and having the soft breast tissue fill in for the absence, such as occurs with a cleft lip. Because the infant may tire more quickly from this very hard work, "switch" breastfeeding may be recommended.[22] The infant

II

◢ NURSING CARE GUIDELINES
Nursing Diagnosis: Ineffective Breastfeeding

Expected Outcome: The family will have the knowledge and skills to ensure breastfeeding success.
- Provide education and hands-on practical demonstrations. *Families need information about the advantages of breastfeeding, the physiological of lactation, and the emotional and social factors that influence breastfeeding success and prevent complications.*[1,4,8,11]

Expected Outcome: The mother's soreness will be contained or eliminated.
- Demonstrate proper positioning of the infant at the breast and educate the mother about nipple care (e.g., air drying, no special preparation before feeding, and as a last resort, nipple shields). *Continuing soreness of the nipple is thought to result from incorrect positioning of the infant at the breast.*[4,12,15,24]

Expected Outcome: The infant will suck correctly with the tongue in proper position and suction being achieved.
- Observe the infant sucking and demonstrate technique for effective latching on and methods to ensure suction. *Observation of the baby's sucking pattern will confirm if the baby's position is correct.*[7]
- Encourage "switch" breastfeeding. *Switch the infant back and forth from breast to breast to maximize the volume of milk received per feeding.*[22]
- Perform digital suck assessment if audible swallowing not heard. *Milk is being ingested if the infant is swallowing.*[15]

Expected Outcome: The mother will understand the relationship of the milk ejection reflex to milk production, and she will be relaxed enough to allow the milk ejection reflex to occur.
- Explain the physiology of the milk ejection reflex, including the importance of frequency and adequacy of feeding time. *Interference with the milk ejection reflex may produce a crying infant a short time after feeding, an actual reduction in milk production, or weight loss, or slow weight gain in the infant.*[21] *Oxytocin, which activates the milk ejection reflex, may require 2 or more minutes of sucking to get the full response, which peaks after 6 to 10 minutes.*[21]
- Support and encourage the mother in building confidence.

Expected Outcome: The mother will have sufficient milk to satisfy the infant's needs, and the infant will gain weight at a pace congruent with established growth charts.
- Assess techniques used by the mother. *Milk production is directly related to the complete emptying of both breasts at each feeding.*[22]
- Chart the infant's weight gain. *Distinction must be made between an infant who normally gains weight slowly and one who is not thriving because of an insufficient milk supply.*
- Do a family history. Help the mother eliminate breastfeeding substitutes. *Breastfeeding substitutes cause nipple confusion for the infant and interfere with the prolactin reflex, which influences milk production.*[20]
- Review the maternal diet, well-being, and lifestyle habits, and adjust these if necessary. *The mother's diet and general well-being affect the volume of milk produced.*[5,6]
- Demonstrate the use of supplemental feeding device. *Nursing supplementation devices may be used to supply breast milk pumped from mother's breast to an infant who needs extra nourishment and did not empty the breast at a previous feeding.*[2]

■ = nursing intervention; ▲ = collaborative intervention.

may be switched back and forth from breast to breast so that the volume of milk received per feeding is maximized. Milk collects in both breasts at several times during a feeding and can pool in the sinuses in the "off" interval.

The milk ejection reflex is "a nerve reflex from the breast to the hypothalamus causing the release of oxytocin by the posterior pituitary gland. Elicited by the infant's suckling, or sometimes even by the mother's thoughts of her baby, this reflex initiates the flow of milk." Limiting the breastfeeding time on each breast to less than 5 minutes does not allow sufficient time to stimulate milk production.

The foremilk, which collects in the lactiferous sinuses immediately behind the areola between feeds, is more dilute and less than the hind milk. The hind milk is stored in the milk ducts of the breast until oxytocin secreted by the pituitary gland stimulates the myoepithelial cells to contract and eject the milk from the ducts.[13] The infant will not be satisfied until he or she receives the milk with the higher protein and fat content. This milk also supplies most of the calories to ensure weight gain. Milk production is directly related to the complete emptying of both breasts at each feeding. The mother should be encouraged to be as comfortable and relaxed as possible before she breastfeeds. Initially, at least, she should be encouraged to feed every 2 or 3 hours or on demand if the infant does not sleep for long periods. The infant's crying may stimulate oxytocin release, causing milk ejection.

Several of the problems previously discussed will influence the milk supply. Inhibited milk ejection reflex, incomplete emptying of the breasts, the mother's ingestion of certain drugs, and the mother's diet and smoking behaviors all directly affect the volume of breast milk produced. Initially, a distinction may be made between an infant who normally gains weight slowly and one who is not thriving because of an insufficient milk supply. If the infant appears satisfied, even though he or she is thin and gains weight slowly, the infant probably is a slow weight gainer. An assessment of the family's history may reveal that one of the parents was also thin.

Breast milk substitutes should be avoided, at least in the first month of life. The early introduction of bottles and pacifiers should be avoided because their use interferes with the prolactin reflex, which influences milk production.[20]

The mother's diet and general well-being affect the volume of milk produced.[5,6] Malnutrition seems to reduce the quantity of milk. Further research is necessary to assess the value of maternal diet supplementation because studies to date have produced some conflicting results.[13] Health professionals and families who encourage and support the new mother will help her by increasing her confidence in her body's ability to feed the infant. The nurse should encourage the extended family to offer practical assistance to the mother so the mother can rest, establish her breast milk, and look after her infant. A nursing supplementation device may be used to supply breast milk pumped from the mother's breast to an infant who needs the extra nourishment and did not empty the breasts at a previous feeding.[2]

EVALUATION

Expected outcomes have been achieved when the mother and family are satisfied with the breastfeeding experience. Families will have sufficient, relevant, correct, and appropriate information to sustain breastfeeding.

Mothers will have confidence in their ability to nurture their infants. Nipple or breast soreness will be eliminated, and infants will suckle effectively. Milk production and ejection will be sufficient so that the family is happy and the baby is thriving (demonstrating an adequate weight gain appropriate to the age and birth weight).

▶ CASE STUDY WITH PLAN OF CARE

Mrs. Joanne B. is a 23-year-old primiparous mother who attended prenatal childbirth classes. She learned the importance of breastfeeding for herself and her baby. Although she knew of other friends who recommended breastfeeding her newborn, she was a bit ambivalent in her decision making. She expressed concerns about "feeling embarrassed to feed in public" and really having "no role model." She stated that she "wanted to try." After the delivery, she attempted to feed her new son, but he preferred to listen to her voice and only licked at her nipples. Mrs. Joanne B. was encouraged by the staff to continue to breastfeed. However, by the second day after the birth, her baby is still not latching on properly. The baby is continuing to lose weight and is becoming dehydrated. Mrs. B. is engorged; she complains that her breasts are "so hard and sore" and that her episiotomy "hurts awful." She is thinking about allowing the baby to begin formula feedings.

▶ PLAN OF CARE FOR MRS. JOANNE B.

Nursing Diagnosis: Ineffective Breastfeeding Related to Positioning of Mother, Engorgement of Breasts, Inadequate Sucking Reflex of Baby, and Insecure Mother

Expected Outcome: Mrs. B. will maintain a position that is comfortable and supportive.
- Change the height of the bed, and support Mrs. B. with pillows.
- Educate Mrs. B. about the various positions for holding the baby at the breast.

Expected Outcome: Mrs. B.'s breasts will no longer be engorged and sore as evidenced by infant's ability to breastfeed. Mother's pain will be relieved.
- Demonstrate hand expression of some milk to soften breasts sufficiently to allow the infant to grasp the nipple and areola and establish suction.

Expected Outcome: Mrs. B.'s baby will establish effective sucking as evidenced by audible swallowing and a content baby.
- Properly position the baby's body in relation to Mrs. B.'s body.
- Demonstrate the proper technique; e.g., the baby's tongue should be under the nipple; the nipple and some of the areola should be in baby's mouth.
- Observe the infant to assess for proper suction and swallowing.

Expected Outcome: Mrs. B. will adjust her lifestyle to promote a satisfying breastfeeding experience.
- Encourage Mrs. B. to drink an adequate amount of fluids and eat a balanced diet.
- Encourage Mrs. B. to get adequate rest and sleep.

Expected Outcome: Mrs. B. will be confident in her ability to breastfeed her baby as evidenced by her expression of same on hospital discharge.
- Encourage, support, and praise Mrs. B. for her efforts.
- Reassure Mrs. B. that the difficulties she is experiencing are not unusual.
- Chart the infant's weight gain and inform Mrs. B. as progress is made.
- Refer Mrs. B. to community nursing agency.
- Provide Mrs. B. with educational materials as desired.

■ = nursing intervention; ▲ = collaborative intervention.

II

■■ CRITICAL THINKING EXERCISES

1. Mrs. Joanne B. has expressed her discomfort to her nurse. Her breasts are "so hard and sore" and her episiotomy "hurts awful." What would be the most positive response by the nurse to encourage Mrs. B. to continue breastfeeding her baby?

2. Based on nursing assessment of Mrs. B. and observations of the dyad during feeding, what are the corresponding defining characteristics, associated related factors, and examples of medical diagnoses that confirm the nursing diagnosis of Ineffective Breastfeeding?

3. What educational materials and interventions should be included in a teaching plan to assist Mrs. B. with breastfeeding her baby?

REFERENCES

1. American Academy of Pediatrics, Committee on Nutrition: Follow-up of weaning formulas, *Pediatrics* 89:1105, 1992.
2. Anderson E and Geden E: Nurses' knowledge of breastfeeding, *J Obstet Gynecol Neonat Nurs* 20(1):58–63, 1991.
3. Briggs GC, Freeman RK, and Yaffee SJ: *Drugs in pregnancy and lactation,* ed 3, Baltimore, 1990, Williams & Wilkins.
4. Chute GE: Promoting breastfeeding success: an overview of basic management. In Chute GE, editor: Breastfeeding, *Clin Issues Perinat Women's Health Nurs* 3:570–582, 1992.
5. Driscoll JW: Breastfeeding success and failure: implications for nurses. In Chute GE, editor: Breastfeeding, *Clin Issues Perinat Women's Health Nurs* 3:565–569, 1991.
6. Duckett L: Maternal employment and breastfeeding. In Chute GE, editor: Breastfeeding, *Clin Issues Perinat Women's Health Nurs* 3:701–712, 1992.
7. Erkin M, Keirse MJ, and Chalmers I: *A guide to effective care in pregnancy and childbirth,* New York, 1989, Oxford University Press.
8. Huggins K: *The nursing mother's companion,* Boston, 1990, Harvard Common Press.
9. Jensen D and others: LATCH: A breastfeeding charting system and documentation tool, *J Obstet Gynecol Neonat Nurs* 23:27–32, 1994.
10. Komuvesh M: *Infant nutrition: a guide for health professionals,* Toronto, 1984, Ontario Ministry of Health.
11. La Leche League International: *The womanly art of breastfeeding,* ed 5, Franklin Park, Illinois, 1991, The League.
12. Lawrence RA: *Breastfeeding: a guide for the medical profession,* ed 4, St. Louis, 1994, Mosby–Year Book.
13. Matthew MK: Mothers' satisfaction with their neonates' breastfeeding behaviors, *J Obstet Gynecol Neonat Nurs* 20(1):49–55, 1991.
14. Minchin M: *Breastfeeding matters,* North Sydney, Australia, 1985, George Allen & Unwin.
15. Minchin MK: Positioning for breastfeeding, *Birth* 16(2):67–80, 1989.
16. Mulford C: The mother-baby assessment (MBA): an "Apgar score" for breastfeeding, *J Hum Lact* 8:79, 1992.
17. Neifert MR and Seacat JM: Lactation insufficiency: a rational approach, *Birth* 14(4):182–188, 1987.
18. Neifert M: Breastfeeding after breast surgical procedure or breast cancer. In Chute GE, editor: Breastfeeding, *Clin Issues Perinat Women's Health Nurs* 3:673–682, 1991.
19. Renfrew M, Fisher C, and Arms S: *Bestfeeding: getting breastfeeding right for you,* Berkeley, California, 1990, Celestial Arts.
20. Riordan J and Auerbach K: *Breastfeeding and human lactation,* Boston, 1993, Jones & Bartlett Publishers.
21. Shrago L and Bocar D: The infant's contribution to breastfeeding, *J Obstet Gynecol Neonat Nurs* 19(3):209–215, 1990.
22. U.S. Department of Health and Human Services: *Report of the Surgeon General's Workshop on Breastfeeding and Human Lactation,* Rockville, Maryland, 1985, Government Printing Office.
23. U.S. Department of Health and Human Services: *Healthy people 2000: full report with commentary,* Department of Health and Human Services Pub No 91-50212, Washington, D.C., 1991, Government Printing Office.
24. Ziemer MM and Pigeon JG: Skin changes and pain in the nipple during the first week of lactation, *J Obstet Gynecol Neonat Nurs* 22:247–256, 1993.
25. Ziegler JB and others: Postnatal transmission of AIDS-associated retrovirus from mother to infant, *Lancet* 1:896, 1985.

Effective Breastfeeding

Effective Breastfeeding *is the state in which a mother-infant dyad or a family exhibits adequate proficiency and satisfaction with breastfeeding behaviors.*[4]

OVERVIEW

Breastfeeding is an interactive process with psychological and physiological dimensions. The benefits to the mother and the infant have been documented.[1,10,15] The most effective measure of successful breastfeeding is its intended outcome; that is, the development of a healthy infant. With successful breastfeeding, assessment of the infant demonstrates an infant with adequate weight gain as well as daily stools and urine output. The mother's milk production and effective nursing techniques must meet the newborn's needs for adequate caloric and fluid intake.

Each female breast is divided into 15 to 20 glandular lobes. Each lobe contains many alveoli, which are the milk-producing structures. Muscle tissue surrounding the alveoli squeezes the alveoli and causes milk to enter ducts and be carried to the sinuses behind the nipple. During pregnancy, estrogen and progesterone have effects on the breast tissue. Estrogen causes the duct system to expand, whereas progesterone stimulates increases in alveolar size. After birth, separation of the placenta causes the anterior pituitary to release prolactin, which stimulates milk production by the alveoli. When sucking occurs, the posterior pituitary releases oxytocin, which acts on the muscle tissue around the alveoli, causing the muscle tissue to contract and milk to be released into the ducts and sinuses behind the nipple for the infant. The let-down reflex is an involuntary reflex that causes the pituitary to release oxytocin; sucking and the smell, cry, and touch of the infant initiate the reflex. Inhibitors of the reflex are pain, stress, fear, and anxiety. Interventions, such as making the mother more comfortable and the room quieter and less bright, gentle stroking of the breast, and warm compresses or showers, may stimulate the let-down reflex.

The infant's ability to "latch on" and suck is crucial to effective breastfeeding. Immediately after the birth the infant has a period during which it is quietly alert. During this period breastfeeding may be begun as the infant searches the environment for sounds and voices. Rooting may be stimulated to encourage the infant to latch on and nurse. The presence in the infant of maternal sedatives within several hours of birth may affect an infant's readiness to nurse in the early postpartum period.[6,17] If this is the case the mother should be encouraged to try to initiate nursing after a short time. The infant's sucking controls the amount of milk produced. Putting the baby to the breast on demand supports continued production of an adequate milk supply.[10]

Three types of milk are produced in the initial process of establishing lactation. Colostrum, a thick yellowish fluid, contains more protein, fat-soluble vitamins, and minerals than the milk produced later. This early form of milk contains high levels of immunoglobulin, which impart immunity to factors to which the mother has been exposed. The colostrum is expressed during pregnancy and is replaced by transitional milk several days after birth. Transitional milk contains lactose, high levels of fat, and water-soluble vitamins and is high in calories to enhance growth, which is rapid in early infancy. Mature milk, which appears after 2 weeks, is thin and watery. Mothers often question its nutritive ability based on its appearance.[7,16] Mature breast milk, however, contains adequate calories for the baby.

Infant formulas have been developed to deliver the same calorie-to-fluid intake ratio as the breast milk standard. Infant formulas may contain a higher percentage of calories from protein and stress immature kidneys with the metabolism of the waste products of protein breakdown. Infant nutritional needs include 50 to 55 calories per pound of weight each day and 64 to 73 millimeters per pound of weight each day to produce a weight gain of 1 ounce per day for the first 6 months, and half of that amount the last 6 months of the first year.[1]

The American Academy of Pediatrics[1] recommends the use of breast milk exclusively for the first 6 months of life. The advantages to the infant are nutritional, immunological, and psychological. Breast milk contains easily digested fatty acids, amino acids, lipids, and lactose. The whey-protein-to-casein-protein ratio helps the infant to use all the formula by complete digestion. The more easily absorbed breast milk leaves the stomach sooner, and the infant may require more frequent feeding than a formula-fed infant.[5] The iron content of breast milk is related to the mother's nutritional state. If the mother's iron stores are sufficient, the breast milk will contain adequate amounts of iron for the developing infant. Although the levels of iron in breast milk are lower than in iron-fortified formulas, the iron in breast milk is more readily absorbed. The mother's nutritional state affects her ability to produce milk that is nutritionally adequate for the baby.[7,19]

The mother's immunological factors are transferred to the infant in breast milk. The early milk contains high levels of antiviral, antibacterial, and antigenic-inhibiting factors. The infant uses the benefit of this inheritance during the first year of life.[10,17,19]

Breastfeeding has psychological advantages in the promotion of the attachment of mother to infant and infant to mother. The direct skin-to-skin contact of breastfeeding and the frequency of this contact facilitate the development of the relationship.[15] Breastfeeding experience helps the mother reconcile the differences between the fantasized infant of pregnancy and the reality of the newborn.[7,9,15]

The decision to breastfeed is usually made by the end of the second trimester based on the family needs, advice of relatives, and cultural norms, and less on basis of knowledge about breastfeeding.[7,9,10,13] The role of family and friends and the experiences communicated to the new mother on selection of feeding methods have been described. Difficulty in establishing effective breastfeeding may occur when a mother chooses to nurse solely on the advice of a support person and never examines her own feelings concerning this method of feeding.[8,13,21] The development of problems, such as nipple tenderness and engorgement, may affect the desire to nurse.[6,10,15] The mother's knowledge level about the common problems of breastfeeding and the self-care measures that may remedy them may indicate the need for additional support through education about nursing.[14,19]

Cultural norms and expectations play a role in the development of effective breastfeeding.[9,10] A culture that encourages breastfeeding may assist the mother in continuing to nurse if difficulties arise in achieving the success valued by the culture. Western societies encourage the mother to nurse soon after birth and to continue as long as desired. The hospital environment may not facilitate the early initiation of nursing, and nursing past the first year often draws frowns.[2,3] In Western societies babies may be nursed as long as 4 years, but most have been weaned by several months after birth.[3,9] The social pressure to wean a child may be felt through stares and polite suggestions concerning the welfare of the mother and the baby. Mothers in Asian cultures are also subject to the influences of culture. Often these mothers do not nurse their infants until the mature milk has begun because they believe that colostrum cannot nourish the baby. Many women supplement breastfeeding with formula and do not pump their breasts for relief of engorgement or for the storage of milk for their infant.[11,12,15] Early introduction of solid foods is encouraged in some rural Western cultures based on the desire for healthy infants. The myth that a fat infant is a healthy infant supports this practice. The American Academy of Pediatrics[1] recommends that no solids be introduced until the fifth to sixth month. Understanding the culturally prescribed beliefs about breastfeeding may help the nurse address needs and concerns in a culturally appropriate manner.

ASSESSMENT

By gathering historical data and by physically examining the breasts, the nurse may assess the physical capability to breastfeed effectively. Historical information related to previous breastfeeding experiences and any history of breast disorders can be collected during a prenatal visit if the mother seeks prenatal care. This information is placed on the prenatal record, and the nurse assisting at the time of birth may refer to it. If prenatal access to the mother is limited because of delayed prenatal care or other reasons, this information should be collected on admission to the birthing area. Information related to prenatal education, knowledge of breastfeeding, and support from significant others for nursing may be assessed.

Information about previous pregnancies and postpartum experiences may provide insight into the postpartum course. Mothers may have elected to change the method of feeding with subsequent pregnancies and may be novices at nursing, although multiparous. A previous history of breast disease can be obtained, including recent or current episodes of acute mastitis and chronic fibrocystic breast disease. Although neither of these precludes breastfeeding entirely, the extent and severity of symptoms may affect the mother's ability to nurse effectively. Review of the breast changes associated with pregnancy in preparation for nursing includes the increased size of the breast (usually noted at 20 weeks), nodular texture of the breast, darkness of the areola and nipple, and tingling of the breast. Physical examination of the breast includes inspection of the surface of the breast for irregularities of shape and size, nonsymmetrical dimpling of the skin, venous pattern

prominence associated with pregnancy, and hyperpigmentation of the areola and nipple. Palpation of the breast is done for irregularities of texture (the breast normally feels nodular as tubercles of Montgomery enlarge), unilateral masses, pain in the breast, colostrum that may be present after the twelfth week of the pregnancy, and striae on the breasts. In addition, the size, shape, and ability of the nipple to become erect for latching-on can be determined. After feedings, nipples may be assessed for redness or cracking.

Psychosocial factors may affect a mother's readiness for nursing and potential for success. Personal factors, such as maturity level, dependency needs, anxiety, and low self-esteem, have been associated with breastfeeding difficulty.[5,6,15] Personal attitudes related to the advantages and disadvantages of breastfeeding may lead to the establishment of effective breastfeeding. Beliefs that the breastfeeding is demanding, inconvenient, embarrassing, and uncomfortable and that bottle feeding is more convenient have been associated with difficulty in breastfeeding. The attitudes and beliefs of family, friends, and spouse can affect the ability to breastfeed successfully.[9,10] Stress and conflict within the changing marital relationship can affect the mother's ability to nurse successfully.

The infant's behavior may affect the success of breastfeeding. Weak or ineffective sucking affects the establishment of lactation. The infant's excessive crying, irritability, and passivity have been associated with breastfeeding difficulties.[10,15] After breastfeeding has been initiated, assessment of infant growth, urinary output, quantity and characteristics of stools, and contentment with feeding provides indicators of the effectiveness of breastfeeding.

■ Defining Characteristics

The presence of the following defining characteristics indicates that the patient may be experiencing Effective Breastfeeding:

For mother
- Signs or symptoms of oxytocin release (let-down or milk ejection reflex)

II

- Infant correctly positioned at breast and stimulation of rooting reflex
- Nursing infant on demand
- Continued nursing of infant after early postpartum period
- Comments about satisfaction with breastfeeding

For infant

- Adequate weight gain
- Soft stools
- More than six wet diapers per day of unconcentrated urine
- Latches onto nipple
- Sucks vigorously
- Regular and sustained suckling at the breast (8 to 10 times in 24 hours)
- Eagerness to nurse
- Content after feeding

■ Related Factors

The following related factors are associated with Effective Breastfeeding:

For mother

- Normal breast structure
- Basic breastfeeding knowledge
- Maternal confidence
- Support sources

For infant

- Normal infant oral structure
- Infant gestational age greater than 34 weeks

DIAGNOSIS

■ Differential Nursing Diagnosis

Effective Breastfeeding can be differentiated from the diagnosis Ineffective Breastfeeding when carefully considering the relative factors and defining characteristics that apply to each diagnosis. Successful and satisfying breastfeeding produces an infant eager to nurse, who gives evidence of adequate weight gain, and remains contented after feeding. The mother confidently nurses her infant on demand, comments about feeling satisfaction with her breastfeeding experiences and continues to nurse after the early postpartum period. Ineffective Breastfeeding encompasses difficulty and dissatisfaction with the breastfeeding process for the mother and her infant and requires nursing interventions that relate exclusively to increasing the mother's milk supply and improving her breastfeeding positioning and technique.

■ Medical and Psychiatric Diagnoses

The unlikely occurrence of advanced fibrocystic disease of the breast, treatment for carcinoma of the breast and the absence of major depression, schizophrenia, and bipolar disorder (manic-depression), lend to effective maternal breastfeeding. The infant born full-term, without cardiac, oral (cleft lip or cleft palate), or other neurological congenital anomalies will feed at the breast without difficulty latching on and learning easily. Nursing care provides basic breastfeeding knowledge to the mother and builds her confidence in her ability to feed and nourish her infant.

OUTCOME IDENTIFICATION, PLANNING, AND IMPLEMENTATION

Nursing planning and care affect a mother's ability to achieve Effective Breastfeeding.[3,4] Planning nursing care to assist the mother to maintain Effective Breastfeeding involves the collaboration of the mother, the spouse or support person, and other nurses caring for the mother. The nurse performs an initial assessment of knowledge and experiences of breastfeeding. Based on these data, the nurse begins to teach the mother and support person, if desired, the techniques of breastfeeding, including nipple stimulation, latching-on of infant to nipple, stimulation of let-down reflex, infant positioning for feeding, alternation of breasts for initiation of each feeding, removal of infant from the breast by breaking suction, breast care, and cleaning of hands and breasts before nursing. After the teaching of these techniques through demonstrations or media, the nurse observes the mother-infant couple breastfeeding to determine the use of information in the performance of breastfeeding and proficiency. Mothers have reported concerns about their privacy when nursing during hospitalization. Placing signs on the door or curtains within the room may ensure privacy.

II

■ **NURSING CARE GUIDELINES**
Nursing Diagnosis: Effective Breastfeeding

Expected Outcome: The mother will communicate knowledge of breastfeeding techniques, breastfeed the infant successfully, and be satisfied with the experience.

- ■ Determine mother's knowledge and experience with breastfeeding. *Assessment data provides for the development of a teaching plan to promote breastfeeding that is physically effective and satisfying to the mother and infant.*[6]
- ▲ Teach the mother and significant others about techniques of breastfeeding: positions for feeding, positions to enable infant to grasp most of areola, need to change positions to avoid or reduce nipple tenderness, use of both breasts at each feeding, stimulation of let-down response, removal from breast by breaking suction, the fact that time limits no longer are recommended in early breastfeeding, cleaning of hands and breasts before nursing, and breast care.
- ▲ Teach techniques for stimulating the let-down response: warm shower, warm compresses, relaxation, imagery, closeness with infant, cry of the infant, and infant suckling.
  Teaching and demonstrating techniques provides baseline breastfeeding knowledge and allows the nurse to determine the use of the information in the performance of breastfeeding and proficiency.[6]
- ▲ Teach mother about her nutritional needs: an extra 500 calories a day, increased fluid intake (extra two glasses of fluids a day), limited caffeine, well-balanced diet, and avoidance of foods that make mother uncomfortable (such as highly seasoned foods). *Successful nursing requires that mother's nutritional intake is adequate.*
- ■ Encourage mother to describe her feelings about breastfeedings. *Planning care to assist the mother to maintain Effective Breastfeeding involves the collaboration of the mother, the spouse, and support persons.*
- ■ Encourage discussion of accommodation of infant feeding and other demands on mother's time.
- ■ Encourage discussion of cultural and familial influences on success of breastfeeding.
- ■ Encourage discussion of concerns related to energy level, need for rest, and physical strength.
  Discussion with the mother about concerns related to energy level, the need for rest, relief from discomfort, physical strength, and lifestyle changes helps identify factors that may affect the mother's ability to nurse more successfully.[2,3,5]

Expected Outcome: The infant will grow and develop within developmental expectations.

- ▲ Teach mother and significant others the expectations for breastfed infants: 8 to 12 stools a day or as few as one a day, soft to liquid nonodorous stools, habit of nursing every 2 to 3 hours, 6 to 8 wet diapers a day, restful after nursing, need for nonnutritive sucking, generally healthy appearance. *Determine if the infant is growing as expected with breastfeeding.*

Expected Outcome: Mother-infant dyad will continue breastfeeding after early postpartum period.

- ■ Assist mother and family in planning for home care: need to rest when infant sleeps, assistance with infant care by significant others, need for self-care to regain energy, maintenance of family relationships, techniques for expression and storage of breast milk, signs of engorgement and infection, and planning for nursing and working. *Assists mother in the continuation of breastfeeding after the early postpartum period.*[6]
- ■ Provide a quiet, private environment for nursing. *Mothers have reported concerns about privacy when nursing during hospitalization.*[14]
- ■ Encourage mother to verbalize her concerns and feelings about breastfeeding and her abilities to breastfeed. *Identifies factors that may affect mother's ability to continue nursing successfully.*[6]
- ■ Provide written information about sources of support within the community for the breastfeeding mother. *Resources help answer questions, address concerns, and assist mother to continue to breastfeed after the early postpartum period.*[17]

■ = nursing intervention; ▲ = collaborative intervention.

II

Successful nursing requires that the mother's nutritional intake be adequate. The nurse teaches the mother about the need to consume an extra 500 calories a day, increase fluid intake an extra two glasses a day, and limit caffeine and foods that are highly seasoned or make the mother uncomfortable. The nurse should initiate teaching that includes scheduling of mother's rest when the infant sleeps, planned assistance with infant care, plans for self-care, strategies to maintain family relationships, techniques for expression and storage of breast milk, signs of engorgement and infection, and techniques for returning to work and continuing to nurse.[15,16]

The infant is continually assessed for normal growth and development. The mother learns how to determine if the infant is thriving on breastfeeding. Expectations for the infant include 8 to 12 soft to liquid nonodorous stools per day, 6 to 8 wet diapers a day, a tendency to quiet after nursing, vigorous suck, a need for nonnutritive sucking, and generally healthy appearance. The nurse provides sources of support within the community for the breastfeeding mother.

The mother who is unable to breastfeed the baby because of infection, infant prematurity, or maternal illness uses the breast pump to stimulate lactation.[11,12,16,18] The milk may be stored (if not contraindicated because of infection or medications) and used to feed the baby later.

EVALUATION

The nurse will evaluate with the mother the extent to which the expected outcomes have been met. If the outcomes have been met, data to support this evaluation will include subjective statements of the mother, observations of the mother and infant, and observations and statements of the family members. The mother should continue to (1) demonstrate successful latching-on, let-down of milk, positioning of infant, and removal from the breast, (2) verbalize satisfaction with breastfeeding, (3) nurse the infant after postpartum hospital discharge, (4) plan for assistance at home, and (5) have an infant whose growth is consistent and within norms. If outcomes have not been met, the nurse will ask the mother to discuss her perceived reasons for not being able to meet goals.

◤ **CASE STUDY WITH PLAN OF CARE**

Mrs. Angie C., a 40-year-old primigravida, has just given birth via cesarean delivery for failure to progress to an 8-lb 7-oz girl after a 14-hour labor. Prenatal records indicate that it is the mother's desire to breastfeed her infant after delivery. Knowing this, the staff placed the baby at the mother's breast in recovery. Mrs. C. laid her daughter on her chest and stroked and spoke to her. An alert baby girl C. gazed up at her mother as her cheek was stroked with mother's erect nipple. Baby girl C. rooted, latched on, and suckled at her mother's breast. Mrs. C. smiled. After a short stay in the recovery room, Mrs. C. and baby were transferred to the mother-baby unit. Within 2 hours, Mrs. C. inquired about putting her daughter to the breast again.

◤ **PLAN OF CARE FOR MRS. ANGIE C. AND BABY**
Nursing Diagnosis: Effective Breastfeeding Related to Initiation of Breastfeeding with Demonstrated Beginning-Level Proficiency and Satisfaction with Breastfeeding Behaviors

---

Expected Outcome: Mrs. C. will describe techniques of breastfeeding, such as positions for nursing, rotation of nursing positions, and on-demand feeding.
- Educate Mrs. C. regarding techniques of breastfeeding after assessing her knowledge level, including the following: positions for nursing (cradle-hold, football hold, side-lying); assisting infant to grasp entire areola;

■ = nursing intervention; ▲ = collaborative intervention.

rotation of nursing positions to prevent nipple soreness; offering alternate breasts initially at each feeding; on-demand feeding to establish milk supply; stimulation of the let-down reflex with nipple stimulation, sucking, warm compresses, and relaxation; information that limiting nursing time is not recommended.

Expected Outcome: Mrs. C. will breastfeed her infant successfully as evidenced by let-down, latching on, alternating nipples, on-demand nursing, rotating positions of infant, and normal weight gain of infant.
- Teach Mrs. C. about factors that indicate her infant has been breastfed successfully: normal weight gain by newborn; demonstration of successful latching-on, removal from the breast, and let-down of milk.
- Observe infant to determine whether she nurses at each breast at each feeding and the infant is restful after each feeding.
- Observe mother and infant for successful breastfeeding: let-down, latching-on, alternating nipples, on-demand nursing, and rotating positions of infant.
- Assess Mrs. C.'s cultural and familial supports for successful breastfeeding.

Expected Outcome: Breastfeeding will be a satisfactory experience for Mrs. C. as evidenced by expressions of satisfaction with choice made to nurse her baby and by continued breastfeeding when difficulties arise, such as sore nipples.
- Provide a quiet, private environment for nursing.
- Provide positive feedback.
- Assist Mrs. C. in addressing problems as they arise and planning actions to address them. For example, for problems with let-down when nipples are sore, use warm shower, warm compresses, relaxation, imagery, closeness with the infant, continued sucking, and vitamin E.

Expected Outcome: Infant's growth will be within normal developmental expectations: baby loses no more than 10% of body weight within 3 days of delivery, weight is within the 10th and 90th percentiles.
- Educate Mrs. C. about nutritional needs of the nursing mother: extra 500 calories/day, increased fluid intake, limited caffeine, and well-balanced diet; avoidance of foods that affect mother, such as beans, which produce gas.
- Encourage Mrs. C. to feed baby on demand to establish a balance between milk production and the infant's needs.

Expected Outcome: Mrs. C. and her baby will continue to nurse after the early postpartum period.
- Teach Mrs. C. about expectations for the breastfed baby after returning home: as many as 8 to 12 stools/day or as few as one stool/day; soft to liquid nonodorous stools; nursing at least every 2 to 3 hours unless sleeping; 6 to 8 wet diapers/day; tendency to quiet after nursing; and need for nonnutritive sucking.
- Assist mother to plan help at home.
- Assist mother to plan for rest at home.
- Provide resources in the community for help with breastfeeding problems.

▪▪ CRITICAL THINKING EXERCISES

1. What are key nursing interventions to ensure successful breastfeeding for Mrs. C. and her daughter after transfer to the mother-baby unit?
2. Based on nursing assessment of the initial breastfeeding experience, what are the corresponding defining characteristics and associated related factors that confirm the nursing diagnosis of Effective Breastfeeding?
3. What educational materials should be included in a teaching plan to assist Mrs. C. with her confidence and her abilities to continue breastfeeding her daughter after the early postpartum period?

II

REFERENCES

1. American Academy of Pediatrics, Committee on Fetus and Newborn: *Guidelines for perinatal care,* ed 2, Elk Grove Village, Illinois, 1988, The Academy.
2. Anderson E: Nurses' knowledge of breastfeeding, *J Obstet Gynecol Neonat Nurs* 20(1):58–64, 1991.
3. Barness LA: Bases of weaning recommendations, *J Pediatr* 117:S84, 1990.
4. Carroll-Johnson RM, editor: *Classification of nursing diagnoses: proceedings of the Ninth Conference,* Philadelphia, 1991, JB Lippincott Co.
5. Chapman J, Macey M, and Keegan M: Concerns of breastfeeding mothers from birth to four months, *Nurs Res* 24(6): 374, 1985.
6. Chute GE: Promoting breastfeeding success: an overview of basic management. In Chute GE, editor: Breastfeeding, *Clin Issues Perinat Women's Health Nurs* 3:570–582, 1992.
7. Eggert JV and Rayburn WF: Nutrition and lactation. In Sciarra JJ, editor: *Gynecology and obstetrics,* vol 2, Philadelphia, 1994, Harper Collins.
8. Janke JR: Development of the breast-feeding attrition prediction tool, *Nurs Res* 43:100–104, 1994.
9. Lawrence RA: Will it become American to breastfeed?, *Birth* 18:226–227, 1991.
10. Lawrence RA: Breastfeeding: a guide for the medical profession, ed 4, St. Louis, 1994, Mosby–Year Book.
11. Neifert M and Seacat J: Practical aspects of breastfeeding the premature infant, *Perinatol Neonatal* 12:24, 1988.
12. Neifert M: Breastfeeding standards of care for low-risk infants, Denver, 1989, St. Luke's Hospital.
13. O'Campo P and others: Prenatal factors associated with breastfeeding duration: recommendations for prenatal interventions, *Birth* 19:195–201, 1992.
14. Renfrew M, Fisher C, and Arms S: *Bestfeeding: getting breastfeeding right for you,* Berkeley, California, 1990, Celestial Arts.
15. Riordan J and Auerbach K: *Breastfeeding and human lactation,* Boston, 1993, Jones & Bartlett Publishers.
16. Riordan J and Countryman B: Basics of breastfeeding, part V: self-care for continued breastfeeding problems and solutions, *J Obstet Gynecol Neonat News* 9:357, 1980.
17. Weiss ME and Armstrong M: Postpartum mothers' preferences for nighttime care of the neonate, *J Obstet Gynecol Neonat Nurs* 20:290–295, 1991.
18. Woldt EH: Breastfeeding support groups in the NICU, *Neonat Net* 9(5):53–56, 1991.
19. Worthington-Roberts B and Williams SR: *Nutrition in pregnancy and lactation,* ed 5, St. Louis, 1993, Mosby–Year Book.

Interrupted Breastfeeding

▶

Interrupted Breastfeeding *is a break in the continuity of the breastfeeding process as a result of the inability or inadvisability of putting the baby to the breast for feeding.*[15]

OVERVIEW

More and more mothers wish to breastfeed and consider it central to their relationship with their new babies. Certain conditions can lead to a temporary interruption in breastfeeding, however. Most common is the mother's return to work. Various maternal or neonatal conditions can lead also to Interruption in Breastfeeding. When this occurs, mothers are often advised to discontinue nursing. In fact, some argue that efforts to continue breastfeeding may compromise the health of the mother or the baby. This perspective ignores the natural aspects of the process and focuses on negative aspects of the situation. In most cases, the interruption need only be very brief, and breastfeeding can be successfully resumed in a short time. If the mother wishes to continue lactation, the professional nurse can provide information about ways to maintain lactation and to store expressed milk so that it can be fed to the baby until breastfeeding can be resumed.

ASSESSMENT

The major defining characteristic of Interrupted Breastfeeding is that the infant does not receive nourishment at the breast for some or all feedings. Other defining characteristics come into play as well. Basic among these is the mother's wish to maintain lactation and to breastfeed her baby after the interruption. The decision to breastfeed, as well as the degree of commitment to maintaining it, is often influenced by the attitudes and opinions of friends, relatives, and the significant other and by cultural customs. In view of the availability of infant formulas, it is important to assess the commitment and support available to the mother in maintaining breastfeeding when it is interrupted.

The nurse must be alert to any of the conditions that may lead to a temporary interruption in lactation. In the case of the mother, breastfeeding is often interrupted because of an illness or a condition that requires medication or hospitalization or because the mother returns to work and breastfeeding is interrupted during work hours.[8,11] For the neonate, illnesses, impairments, and prematurity often lead to Interrupted Breastfeeding.[13]

Exacerbations of preexisting medical conditions of the mother may result in Interrupted Breastfeeding. By scrutinizing the mother's history, the nurse can identify potential problem areas. In addition to assessing for the development of problems, the nurse needs to determine the effect of ongoing medications on the nursing neonate. It is often the nurse who recognizes which medications would or would not adversely affect the neonate when nursing.

With more diabetic women now able to reproduce, there has been a growing number who desire to breastfeed. In addition to benefitting the neonate, breastfeeding helps the mother because it heightens normalcy in an otherwise high-risk pregnancy. Because women with diabetes are more prone than other mothers to infections that may lead to interruptions in breastfeeding, assess-

167

II

ment of symptoms indicating such infections and interventions to prevent them are warranted. Assessment of the diabetic state, including dietary intake, can often ward off the development of abnormal metabolic states that can influence breast milk and potentially interrupt lactation. Frequent breastfeedings and assessment of neonatal hypoglycemia help avoid interruptions that occur when the infant needs to be bottlefed because of hypoglycemia.[16]

Allergic diseases of the mother, especially asthma, often require medications that can affect the nursing neonate. Careful attention to the type of medication and assessment of allergic symptoms can lessen the likelihood of Interrupted Breastfeeding.[16]

Whether a mother with kidney disease experiences an interruption in breastfeeding or not depends on the degree of kidney impairment before pregnancy. If the impairment is mild to moderate, breastfeeding can often be maintained without any interruption. If there is severe kidney impairment, mothers are typically advised not to breastfeed. In addition, mothers are usually advised to avoid breastfeeding if hypertension accompanies the kidney impairment. Attention to a diagnosis of kidney disease necessitates careful postpartum assessment of blood pressure, urinary output, and any symptoms of complications. Because mothers who have had a renal transplant receive immunosuppressants, many physicians advise these mothers not to breastfeed because these medications affect the infant's immune system.[16]

Mothers who have chronic hypertension may experience difficulties in controlling blood pressure during pregnancy and right after birth. Breastfeeding may be interrupted while the mother receives medications to maintain or regain blood pressure control. Often, however, medications can be altered and breastfeeding can be continued.

Whether previous breast surgery leads to cessation or merely a temporary interruption of breastfeeding seems to depend on the location and type of procedure. Studies indicate that mastectomies,

breast reductions, or even biopsies can lead to problems with milk supply.[1,14] In particular, women with periareolar incisions are five times more likely to have lactation insufficiency. Careful scrutiny of the patient's history and assessment of the breast itself can provide cues to potential problems. Vigilance in adhering to breastfeeding protocols that foster success in the face of altered breast tissue can help avoid an interruption in breastfeeding. Particularly important is assessment of the sufficiency of the milk supply so that the nutritional well-being of the infant is assured.

Certain conditions associated with pregnancy can lead to Interrupted Breastfeeding. Primary among these is pregnancy-induced hypertension. In particular, administration of magnesium sulfate often interrupts lactation because it is a central nervous system depressant for the baby as well as the mother. Assessment of signs indicating worsening of pregnancy-induced hypertension (i.e., elevated blood pressure, protein in the urine, edema, hyperactive reflexes, and reduced output) and side effects of magnesium sulfate (i.e., depressed respirations and reflexes) is warranted. Some allow breastfeeding to continue while magnesium sulfate is being administered. If so, the infant's behavior should be assessed for effects of the drug.[13]

Infections or the development of a fever also can lead to Interrupted Breastfeeding until the source of the infection or fever is identified and pharmacological treatment is initiated or completed. Common infections are mastitis, endometritis, and cystitis. Careful assessment for infection of the breast (warm, reddened, tender area and fever), uterus (fever, lower abdominal tenderness, and foul-smelling lochia), or urinary tract (frequency, urgency, dysuria, and retention) is advocated.[4,16]

Maternal medications often lead to an interruption in breastfeeding because they can stimulate or inhibit lactation, change the milk composition, or pass into the breast milk, thereby affecting the infant. Most drugs do pass into the breast milk. The actual effect of these drugs on the baby depends on many factors. Some of these factors are the amount or dose, the sucking activity of the infant, functional changes in the gastrointestinal tract of the infant over time, and the gastrointestinal tract pH of the baby. Most antimicrobials do not pose any risk to the baby, but a few (e.g., chloramphenicol) may result in temporary interruption of breastfeeding. Neurotropic drugs, which are often prescribed for epilepsy, anxiety, depression, and psychoses, are often a concern to health care providers. In reality, however, these drugs are typically of little significance to the nursing infant unless the baby has hepatic insufficiency or immature kidneys. Definitely contraindicated during breastfeeding are anticancer drugs, radioactive drugs, lithium, phenylbutazone, atropine, and ergot alkaloids. In addition, high doses of prednisone necessitate Interrupted Breastfeeding until 4 hours after each dose. Careful attention to the mother's history and medications prescribed for her can alert the nurse to the necessity for interruptions in lactation and can provide a basis for assessment of effects on the nursing neonate.[13]

Neonatal illnesses and conditions can lead to Interrupted Breastfeeding. Primary among these is prematurity of the infant. Many advocate the use of expressed breast milk (in gavage feedings) until actual breastfeeding of the preterm neonate can be initiated. Social support is particularly important during the time breastfeedings are interrupted. During this time, assessment of pumping techniques and milk storage is necessary so that the milk supply is adequately stimulated and safe breast milk is provided for the baby. With proper education and assistance, initiating breastfeeding of the preterm neonate can be eased considerably and the nutritional status of the infant maintained. In the past, progressing from gavage feeding to bottle feeding before starting breastfeeding was recommended, based on the idea that breastfeeding was the most fatiguing way for the preterm neonate to feed. More recently breastfeeding has been determined to be less stressful than bottle feeding. Progressing from gavage feeding to breastfeeding is therefore advocated. Assessment of signs indicating that the preterm neonate is ready for breastfeeding allows initiation of the process at a time when the baby is capable and when the physiological status of the preterm neonate is stabilized. Monitoring physiological responses during breastfeedings, maternal and infant feeding behaviors, and adequacy of milk supply can then help ensure the success of lactation.[9,12]

Other neonatal conditions besides prematurity can also lead to Interrupted Breastfeeding. These include neonatal anomalies (e.g., cleft lip or palate),[2] neonatal illnesses (e.g., neonatal sepsis or necrotizing enterocolitis),[5] neurological impairments that affect sucking,[13] respiratory problems (e.g., respiratory distress syndrome or meconium aspiration),[7] or common surgical problems (e.g., gastroschisis, omphalocele, tracheal esophageal fistula, meconium ileus, imperforate anus, diaphragmatic hernia, meningocele, and hydrocephalus).[17] The alarming increase in the number of mothers who abuse alcohol or other drugs has contributed to an increase in the number of infants who have fetal alcohol syndrome or who experience the effects of withdrawal. Both of these affect sucking and therefore can interrupt breastfeeding.[6,13] After the neonatal conditions are resolved or the infant is stabilized, breastfeeding can be resumed. Assessing the progress of breastfeeding is then warranted.

Jaundice is relatively common in neonates, occurring in up to 60% of infants in the first week. Recent research indicates that breastfed babies typically have fewer stools than bottle fed babies in the first few days. As a result, some of the conjugated bilirubin in the small bowel is reabsorbed instead of being excreted in the stool, resulting in an increased load of bilirubin that needs to be conjugated in the hepatic system. In addition, breastfed babies take in fewer calories than bottle fed babies in the first few days; this contributes to decreased clearance of bilirubin. To counteract these two effects, early, frequent breastfeeding is advocated to hasten early stools and to provide calories. In the past, many health care providers advocated interrupting lactation and supplementing breastfeedings with bottle feedings of sterile water or glucose water. It was thought that supplementation would increase the number of stools and the intake of calories. It has been found, however, that babies who receive supplemental bottles have fewer stools rather than more stools and higher bilirubin levels than those who are breastfed and are not supplemented.[3,19]

There is a condition called true breast milk jaundice that often leads to an interruption in breastfeeding. It occurs in 1% to 5% of breastfed babies. This type of jaundice is characterized by bilirubin levels that rise between 4 and 7 days, that peak around 2 weeks (at 20 to 25 mg/dl), and that require 4 to 16 weeks to resolve. Etiology of this condition remains elusive. A currently accepted theory suggests that breastfeeding leads to higher levels of free fatty acids than bottle feeding. These higher levels inhibit enzymes involved with conjugation of bilirubin in the liver.[3,13]

Interruption of breastfeeding is often advocated during phototherapy treatment for jaundice. In the past, formula feedings during treatment were advocated because they were thought to complement the phototherapy by increasing stool excretion and by increasing hepatic clearance of bilirubin. Some health care providers, however, have suggested more frequent breastfeeding with a supplementation device rather than interrupting breastfeeding for these purposes.[3,19]

Relatively common difficulties that contribute to Ineffective Breastfeeding may result in interrupted lactation. These include breast engorgement, sore nipples, inadequate let-down, inadequate suck, or temporary insufficiencies of milk supply (which often necessitate supplementation).[10,20] Assessment includes observation of feeding patterns (frequency and duration) and feeding behaviors. In addition, signs of let-down, indicators of adequacy of milk supply, and signs of infant growth are assessed.[13]

Cesarean birth, breastfeeding multiples, and the father's feelings of separation have also been associated with Interrupted Breastfeeding. For some, merely having a cesarean birth may result in pain that interrupts breastfeeding. At times, breastfeeding is interrupted to allow the father an opportunity to lessen feelings of separation by feeding the baby. Breastfeeding multiples can lead to interruption in the process for one baby.[18] One infant may suck less vigorously than the other and

need supplementation; or there may be a brief insufficiency of supply for several babies.

■ Defining Characteristics

The presence of the following characteristics indicates that the patient may be experiencing Interrupted Breastfeeding:

- Infant not receiving nourishment at the breast for some or all feedings
- Separation of mother and infant
- Maternal desire to maintain lactation and provide (or eventually provide) her breast milk for her infant's nutritional needs
- Lack of knowledge regarding expression of milk, maintenance of milk supply, or storage of breast milk

■ Related Factors

The following related factors are associated with Interrupted Breastfeeding:

Maternal factors
- Previous breast surgery
- Infection
- Illness
- Pain
- Fever, etiology undetermined
- Medication contraindicating breastfeeding
- Conditions of the breast (e.g., sore or cracked nipples, mastitis)
- Admission to hospital
- Employment
- Breastfeeding multiples

Infant factors
- True breast milk jaundice
- Prematurity
- Illness
- Anomaly

DIAGNOSIS

■ Differential Nursing Diagnosis

There are two nursing diagnoses that are closely related to Interrupted Breastfeeding. Most closely related is Ineffective Breastfeeding. In comparing and contrasting the nursing diagnoses of Interrupted Breastfeeding and Ineffective Breastfeeding, it is noted that there are differences in the definitions. Interrupted Breastfeeding focuses on an actual interruption in breastfeeding, whereas Ineffective Breastfeeding focuses on dissatisfaction or difficulty in the ongoing process of breastfeeding. With Ineffective Breastfeeding, the process is not interrupted or stopped; breastfeeding continues, but there are difficulties or dissatisfaction with it.

In comparing and contrasting the nursing diagnoses of Interrupted Breastfeeding and Ineffective Infant Feeding Pattern, the differences in the definitions are noted. Interrupted Breastfeeding implies a break in the continuity of the breastfeeding process, whereas Ineffective Infant Feeding Pattern focuses on the infant's inability or impaired ability to suck or coordinate the suck-swallow response that occurs with breastfeeding or bottle feeding. Thus with Ineffective Infant Feeding Pattern, the infant may be fed by breast or by bottle. The ineffectiveness of feeding is characterized by the infant's inability to suck or to coordinate the suck-swallow response. When breastfeeding is interrupted, the infant may be able to suck and coordinate the suck-swallow response. The breastfeeding process may be effective and only interrupted for a time because of maternal and infant health factors.

■ Medical and Psychiatric Diagnoses

Various medical diagnoses are commonly related to Interrupted Breastfeeding. These conditions and diagnoses can occur in the mother or the infant. Common maternal diagnoses include breast surgery (e.g., simple mastectomy or breast reduction), diabetes mellitus, cardiovascular diagnoses (e.g., hypertension, pregnancy-induced hypertension, or heart disease), respiratory diagnoses (e.g., asthma), infections (e.g., mastitis), and psychological diagnoses (e.g., depression requiring medications that are incompatible with breastfeeding). Most of these diagnoses render the mother unable to breastfeed for a time because of pain or debility, or they require medications that cannot be taken while breastfeeding. Infant diagnoses include respiratory diagnoses (e.g., pneumonia or respiratory distress syndrome), hypoglycemia associated with being an infant of a diabetic mother, oral defects or anomalies (e.g., cleft palate), jaundice, and sepsis.

OUTCOME IDENTIFICATION, PLANNING, AND IMPLEMENTATION

Overall the expected outcomes after a temporary interruption in breastfeeding are successful resumption of breastfeeding and assurance of adequate neonatal intake. To accomplish this, more specific outcomes need to be achieved. These include breasts and nipples that are adequate for breastfeeding, a quiet and comfortable environment for breastfeeding, maintenance of the milk supply, safety of the milk supply, successful resumption of breastfeeding, and adequate maternal nutritional and fluid intake.

Breast tissue must be sufficient to produce milk. It is rare that it is not, but certain conditions (such as breast surgery) may affect the ability of the breasts to produce milk and may cause a temporary interruption.[1,14] The nurse should review the patient's medical history to identify past breast surgery. In addition, other factors that may hinder lactation should be noted. These include mastitis, engorgement, flat nipples, nipple pain, and bruising or cracking of the nipples.

Emotional factors and anxiety may influence let-down. Therefore, assuring a comfortable and relaxing environment during breastfeeding or pumping is essential. This may be difficult because in the hospital space is often limited; and later, when the patient returns to work, it may be difficult to find a quiet, private place to pump the breasts. A great deal of ingenuity is required on the part of the nurse and the patient to identify comfortable and relaxing places for breastfeeding or pumping.[11]

Maintenance of the milk supply requires consistent stimulation of the breasts at regular intervals, initially every 2 to 3 hours and then at 3 to 4-hour intervals. While breastfeeding is interrupted, each breast cust be pumped for at least 5 to 10 minutes per session; many health care providers recommend at least 10 minutes per

Continued on p. 174

II

II

◢ NURSING CARE GUIDELINES
Nursing Diagnosis: Interrupted Breastfeeding

Expected Outcome: The mother's breasts will be adequate for breastfeeding as evidenced by: breasts soft immediately after pumping; breasts filling, with ropy texture, after pumping; breasts symmetrical; absence of noninfectious or infectious mastitis; and absence of engorgement.
- Assess the breasts by observation and palpation for indications of breast milk and for factors that may hinder breastfeeding (e.g., noninfectious and infectious mastitis). *Breast fullness and mastitis can be painful and can discourage the mother from breastfeeding.*
- For mastitis, teach the mother to pump the breasts frequently, massaging above the tender area while pumping. *Pumping frequently enhances let-down, empties the breast, and minimizes stasis and the growth of microorganisms.*
- If the breasts are engorged, teach the mother to pump the breasts frequently, around the clock. Also instruct her to massage the breasts, to apply warm compresses before pumping, and to pump long enough to empty the breasts. *Heat softens the breast, and pumping empties the breasts so that stasis is prevented.*

Expected Outcome: The mother's nipples will be favorable for breastfeeding as evidenced by: nipples everted (not flat or inverted); absence of bruising, cracking, or bleeding of nipples; minimal soreness of nipples with discomfort occurring only with latch-on or at the beginning of pumping.
- Assess nipples for ease of latch-on or indications of trauma. *Asymmetry of the baby's mouth or palate or high pump pressure can cause discomfort.*
- Do the "pinch" test to determine if the nipples are flat or inverted. *Flat or inverted nipples make it difficult for the baby to "latch-on."*
- If the nipples are flat, instruct the mother how to use breast shells between pumpings. *Pumping will help nipples evert. Breast shells apply pressure behind the nipple to help it become more prominent.*
- If nipples are sore, teach the mother how to use the pump correctly. *Soreness and pain inhibit let-down. In addition, trauma makes the breast more prone to infection.* Advise the nursing mother to pump frequently with low pressure and to apply a small amount of breast milk or Lonsinoh to lubricate and soften the nipples after pumping. *Breast milk lubricates and softens the nipples. Lonsinoh creates a moist, healing environment for crusted nipples that is safe for babies, does not have to be removed, and does not have additives or perfumes. It creates a semiocclusive moisture barrier over the nipple that slows evaporation of natural moisture.*
- Instruct the mother to avoid soap on the nipples because *it can dry the epithelium and cause soreness and make the nipples more prone to infection.*
- Instruct the mother how to air dry the nipples after pumping; *this helps toughen nipples.*
- If the nipples are bruised, check pumping techniques. *High pressure can traumatize nipples.*
- If nipples are cracked, check pumping techniques, and when the baby nurses again, position the infant correctly. *If the baby is positioned correctly, nipple trauma should not occur.*

Expected Outcome: The mother will have a comfortable environment for pumping as evidenced by: a private room; a comfortable chair with arm supports; and time for pumping.
- Assist the mother to find a comfortable environment for pumping. *Anxiety can inhibit let-down.*

Expected Outcome: The mother will adequately stimulate and empty her breasts on an ongoing basis as evidenced by: breasts pumped every 2 to 3 hours for at least 10 minutes per breast; handheld pump or electric pump used correctly; a similar quantity of breast milk expressed each time; breasts becoming soft after pumping, filling, and becoming firm again after pumping; and absence of symptoms of infectious or noninfectious mastitis.

■ = nursing intervention; ▲ = collaborative intervention.

- Instruct the mother to pump the breasts every 2 to 3 hours. *The impetus for breast milk production is the sucking of the infant, which stimulates the prolactin and let-down reflexes. Maintenance of the milk supply requires consistent stimulation of the breast at regular intervals of 2 to 3 hours at first and then at 3- to 4-hour intervals. Longer intervals between feedings can result in engorged stasis and possible mastitis.*
- Relay information about types of pumps (handheld and electric), advantages and disadvantages, costs, and where to purchase. *Factual information aids in making informed choices.*
- Demonstrate in detail how to use the selected pump. *Demonstration of psychomotor skills aids learning.* For an electric pump, teach the mother to assemble the sterile or clean container, tubing, and equipment; to wash her hands and breasts; to massage the breasts to stimulate let-down; to place flange on the breasts; to turn on and regulate suction so it is gentle, starting with low suction.
- For the handheld cylinder pump, teach the mother to slide outer cylinder of pump away from the breast to create suction.
- Instruct the mother to pump every 2 to 3 hours or 3 to 4 hours for at lest 10 minutes per breast. *Longer intervals do not stimulate sufficient milk supply.*
- Instruct the mother to feed or pump exclusively for the first 4 to 6 weeks. *This ensures a well-established milk supply and avoids nipple confusion. It is well documented that sucking at the breast is quite different from sucking on an artificial nipple. Many believe that these differences confuse the infant, which leads to difficulty in sucking at the breast.*
- Instruct the mother to pump at intervals at a low pressure. *Continuous pumping or too high a pressure can result in trauma with subsequent infection.*

Expected Outcome: The mother will maintain the safety of expressed milk (so it can be fed to the baby by bottle or other means) as evidenced by: hands washed before pumping; milk stored in an appropriate plastic bottle or disposable liner labeled with the date and time of expression; expressed milk appropriately cool even during transportation; milk frozen at proper temperature; refrigerated milk fed within 48 hours; pump equipment sterilized every day or placed in dishwasher at proper temperature; milk thawed by placing in gradually warmer water until milk liquefies.

- Inform the mother about the type of container appropriate for storing expressed milk (*not glass because immunological factors adhere to glass*). Most mothers use a small plastic container rather than plastic liners. Store milk in single-use containers *because once thawed or heated, milk should not be refrozen or stored.*
- Instruct the mother how to label expressed milk *so it can be used in proper sequence to minimize contamination.*
- Instruct on proper cooling *to minimize bacterial growth.* Keep milk in a cooler on ice, or use ice packs during transport.
- Teach how to freeze milk properly if necessary; *freeze at 0°C. Use within 2 weeks if in a refrigerator or within 6 months if in deep freeze.*
- Teach how to sterilize pump equipment and milk containers if necessary. Premature babies, for example, require a greater degree of concern about cleanliness to prevent bacterial growth. *Boil equipment for 5 minutes or wash it in a dishwasher with the water temperature at 180°F.*
- Teach how to thaw milk appropriately in gradually warming water.
- Caution against boiling milk (*it destroys immune properties*) or heating it in a microwave (*it can burn the baby*).

Expected Outcome: The mother will have an adequate intake of nutrients and fluids for lactation as evidenced by: dietary recall reflecting adequate intake of fluid per day and adequate intake of dairy products, meat, poultry, fish, whole grain products, fruits, and vegetables.

- Obtain typical 24-hour dietary recall. Analyze recall for adequacy; compare intake with requirements for lactation. *Nutrients and fluids are necessary to meet energy, growth, and physical activity needs of the infant.*

Continued

◢ NURSING CARE GUIDELINES — CONT'D

- Instruct on changes needed to meet nutritional requirements for lactation. *New mothers are often unaware of nutritional requirements for lactation.*
- Individualize teaching to include preferences. *Merely providing information on nutrition requirements is often not sufficient to ensure compliance. Paying attention to food preferences helps individualize teaching so mothers can translate requirements into action.*
- Instruct about adequate fluid intake.

Expected Outcome: The mother will be able to breastfeed when she and the infant are able as evidenced by: adequate latch-on; correct position at the breast; adequate, vigorous, rhythmic nutritive suck; adequate let-down; and adequate weight gain of baby.

- Assess for and assist with adequate latch-on behaviors (infant's mouth wide open, tongue under nipple, lips everted or flared out, nipple and $\frac{1}{4}''$ to $\frac{1}{2}''$ of the areola in mouth, and a complete seal).
- Assess for and assist with the correct position at the breast (ventral surface of baby to ventral surface of mother; mouth at the level of the nipple; no sideways turning of head or extension of trunk or neck so the baby does not come off the breast); changing holds from cradle hold to football hold *to change the area of greatest pressure. The correct position at the breast minimizes nipple soreness and aids let-down.*
- If let-down is a problem, teach the mother to massage her breasts before nursing, to use warm compresses before nursing, to avoid fatigue, and to allow sufficient time to stimulate let-down.
- Assess for and assist with adequate suck. Instruct the mother to avoid artificial nipples, pacifiers, or breast shields that cause nipple confusion. *The suck differs on breasts and on artificial nipples.*
- Observe for nutritive suck (rhythmic with swallowing after about three sucks, or about one suck/second; cheeks hollow; no smacking or clicking sounds).
- For facial nerve problems, use a football hold, then present the nipple by stroking it down over midline of the upper lip and then the lower lip. In the cradle hold, place the unaffected side down and stroke the lower corner of the mouth. Use oral stimulation before the feeding: gently stroke around the baby's lips and gums, then allow baby to suck on mother's finger.
- For cleft lip, place the nipple to one side of cleft and use the mother's thumb to fill the gap and create a seal. For cleft palate, position the nipple to one side of the cleft; keep areola soft so that latch-on is easier. Hold baby in upright position for feeding. Burp baby frequently. Have mother use a pump or nipple roll to elongate the nipple.
- For a high palate or groove, teach the mother to use a supplementer device, and try the side-lying position.
- Use an incentive of breast milk on the infant's lower or upper lip just before latch-on.
- Assess for adequate let-down (milk dripping from other breast; areolar fullness; tingling sensation; nutritive suck).
- Assess for adequacy of the milk supply to *assure that the infant has appropriate weight gain; six wet diapers per day; regular bowel movements; no fussiness after a feeding; awake during feeding; stays on breast; nurses eight or more times per day.*

breast. For those who pump at work, more frequent breastfeeding at home is advised. Exclusive breastfeeding or pumping for the first 4 to 6 weeks (rather than offering bottles) is also advocated.[7,11] Other interventions by the nurse include providing information about the frequency and duration of pumping and citing advantages, disadvantages, and costs of various pumps. It is also important to demonstrate use of the pump selected and to caution about potential trauma that can be inflicted by pumping.[8,16]

If expressed breast milk is to be fed to the infant by bottle or gavage, the nurse must help the mother focus on assuring the safety of the milk. This involves education about the importance of general cleanliness, of sterilizing or cleaning pump equipment, of clean milk storage containers, and of proper storage of milk. The nurse can help the mother decide on a convenient method for storing her milk. Information about labeling milk containers needs to be provided. Discussion of the proper temperatures for the refrigerator or freezer, the length of time that milk can be stored, and the proper thawing of milk is also necessary.[11,16]

After the need for the temporary interruption of breastfeeding no longer exists, the nurse assists the mother in resuming breastfeeding. Careful assessment of all aspects of breastfeeding (e.g., position, latch-on, and sucking behavior) is essential. The nurse should offer guidance for breastfeeding babies with particular problems (e.g., a baby with cleft palate). Discussing indicators of let-down as well as the baby's unique sucking behaviors is also important.[16] An ongoing assessment to determine whether the baby is receiving adequate nutrition is essential.

It is important for the nurse to pay attention to the patient's dietary recall and individualize teaching about nutritional and fluid requirements for lactation. If the patient has difficulty maintaining an appropriate nutritional intake, a consultation with a dietitian is recommended. Stressing the importance of maintaining adequate nutritional intake to the mother and the breastfeeding infant should enhance the mother's motivation to meet nutritional needs.

EVALUATION

Mothers who had their breastfeeding temporarily interrupted by maternal or infant conditions, medications, or difficulties contributing to Interrupted Breastfeeding will decide on a method of pumping their breasts, will successfully stimulate an adequate milk supply through pumping, will maintain the safety of expressed breast milk, will have an adequate nutrition and fluid intake for lactation, and will have resumed breastfeeding as soon as the mother and the infant are able. Nursing information, instruction, and support should assist the mother in being successful with breastfeeding even though it was temporarily interrupted.

Case Study with Plan of Care

Monica S. is a 25-year-old, married, primigravida woman who attended childbirth education classes. Long before becoming pregnant, she decided that she wanted to breastfeed. Mrs. S. started reading books about breastfeeding relatively early in her pregnancy and was looking forward to the experience. At 34 weeks gestation, her membranes ruptured prematurely; she went into labor and delivered a premature baby girl. Mrs. S. was disappointed about not being able to breastfeed right away and inquired whether she would be able to breastfeed at all. The nursing staff helped Mrs. S. by supporting her intentions to breastfeed and by teaching her how to pump and store breast milk, which was fed to her baby by gavage feedings.

Plan of Care for Mrs. Monica S.

Nursing Diagnosis: Interrupted Breastfeeding Related to Prematurity

Expected Outcome: Mrs. S. will initiate breastfeeding at appropriate time as evidenced by: infant weight gain; infant's sucking organized into bursts of four or five sucks with ability to swallow secretions; infant is clinically stable (absence of ventilatory support, parenteral fluids, neurological problems); infant tolerates enteral feedings; and infant maintains body temperature when outside incubator.

- ▪ Assess preterm neonate for ability to initiate breastfeeding (organized suck and swallow, clinical stability, maintenance of body temperature outside incubator).

▪ = nursing intervention; ▲ = collaborative intervention.

Continued

II

▶ PLAN OF CARE FOR MRS. MONICA S. — CONT'D

Expected Outcome: Mrs. S. will maintain breastfeeding of her preterm infant as evidenced by: infant nurses with nutritive suck for as along as possible and empties the breasts completely.

- Provide an environment that is comfortable and private.
- Assist Mrs. S. to a comfortable position for breastfeeding, providing pillows to support the arms.
- Assist Mrs. S. to position the infant at the breast in a semiupright position with mouth at nipple.
- Instruct Mrs. S. to initiate let-down by using a pump before starting the infant at the breast.
- Instruct Mrs. S. to allow the infant to do licking and nonnutritive sucking.
- Assist by exerting gentle downward pressure on the infant's mandible as the infant opens mouth.
- Help Mrs. S. move the infant's head onto nipple when infant opens mouth; maintain gentle pressure behind head.
- Assist Mrs. S. to recognize signs of satiety to know when to terminate feeding.
- If breast is not empty, have Mrs. S. pump breasts.

Expected Outcome: Mrs. S.'s infant will have adaptive infant response to breastfeeding as evidenced by: maintains adaptive temperature and exhibits adaptive indices of oxygenation; lengthens nutritive suck at each feeding; terminates feeding when tired or satiated; and can be fed on demand at the breast.

- Assess and monitor temperature and oxygenation of infant. Terminate feeding if either becomes abnormal.
- Assess for signs of satiety (falling asleep or ceasing to suck) and then terminate feeding.

Expected Outcome: Mrs. S.'s infant will have adequate nutrition and fluid intake as evidenced by: adequate weight gain; at least six wet diapers per day; regular bowel movements; and without signs of dehydration.

- Test weigh the infant at each feeding (weigh before and after feeding; subtract pre-fed weight from post-fed weight to obtain the amount of breast milk obtained by the infant at that feeding).
- Supplement breastfeeding with nasogastric tube if necessary to maintain intake at amount it was when the infant was exclusively tube fed.
- Monitor the infant's weight gain.
- Monitor the infant's feeding patterns, demand schedule, sleep-wake cycle, and fussiness.

▦ CRITICAL THINKING EXERCISES

1. Describe how to assess Mrs. S. and her infant for the adequacy of Mrs. S.'s breast milk supply.
2. Compare and contrast interventions that prevent Ineffective Breastfeeding with those that prevent Interrupted Breastfeeding.
3. Compare and contrast interventions that foster Effective Breastfeeding with those that prevent Interrupted Breastfeeding.

REFERENCES

1. Boyce KM: Case study: breastfeeding following mastectomy, *Midwives Chronicle* June:173–174, 1991.
2. Curtin G: The infant with cleft lip or palate: more than a surgical problem, *J Perin Neonat Nurs* 3(3):80–89, 1990.
3. deSteuben C: Breastfeeding and jaundice, *J Nurse-Midwifery* 37(1):59S–66S, 1992.
4. Foxman B, Schwartz K, and Looman SJ: Breastfeeding practices and lactation mastitis, *So Sci Med* 38(5):755–761, 1994.
5. Gerdes JS: Clinicopathologic approach to the diagnosis of neonatal sepsis, *Clin Perinatol* 18(2):361–379, 1991.
6. Gosse G: Neonatal abstinence syndrome, *Canadian Nurse* May:17–22, 1992.
7. Graves BW: Differential diagnosis of respiratory distress, *J Nurse-Midwifery* 37(2):27S–35S, 1992.
8. Greenberg CS and Smith K: Anticipatory guidance for the employed breastfeeding mother, *J Pediatr Health Care* 5(4):204–209, 1991.
9. Holditch-Davis D, Borham LN, O'Haley A, and Tucker B: Effect of standard rest periods on convalescent preterm infants, *JOGNN* 24(5):424–432, 1995.
10. Huml SC: Cracked nipples in the breastfeeding mother, *Adv Nurse Prac* 3(4):29–31, 1995.
11. Humphrey N: Breastfeeding: working moms can make it work, *Adv Nurse Prac* 2(6):21–23, 1994.

II

12. Kavanaugh K, Mead L, Meier P, and Mangurten HH: Getting enough; mothers' concerns about breastfeeding a preterm infant after discharge, *JOGNN* 24(1):23–32, 1995.

13. Ladewig PW, London ML, and Olds SB: Essentials of maternal-newborn nursing, ed 3, Redwood City, California, 1994, Addison-Wesley.

14. Neifert M and others: The influence of breast surgery, breast appearance, and pregnancy-induced breast changes on lactation sufficiency as measured by infant weight gain, *Birth* 17(1):31–38, 1990.

15. North American Nursing Diagnosis Association: *NANDA nursing diagnoses: definitions and classification, 1995–1996,* Philadelphia, 1994, The Association.

16. Olds SB, London ML, and Ladewig PW: *Maternal-newborn nursing,* ed 4, Menlo Park, California, 1992, Addison-Wesley.

17. Shaw N: Common surgical problems in the newborn, *J Perin Neonat Nurs* 3(3):50–64, 1990.

18. Sollid DT, Evans BT, McClowry SG, and Garrett A: Breastfeeding multiples, *J Perin Neonat Nurs* 3(1):46–65, 1989.

19. Tan KL: Phototherapy for neonatal jaundice, *Clin Perinatol* 18(3):423–439, 1991.

20. Ziemer MM, Paone JP, Schupay J, and Cole E: Methods to prevent and manage nipple pain in breastfeeding women, *West J Nurs Res* 12(6):732–744, 1990.

Fluid Volume Excess

▶ ─────────────────────────────────────

Fluid Volume Deficit

▶ ─────────────────────────────────────

Risk for Fluid Volume Deficit

▶ ─────────────────────────────────────

Fluid Volume Excess *is the state in which an individual experiences increased fluid retention and edema because of an increase in interstitial and vascular volumes. This condition is the result of excessive sodium and water intake or inadequate sodium and water losses.*[11,12]

Fluid Volume Deficit *is the state in which an individual experiences vascular, cellular, or intracellular dehydration because of inadequate fluid intake or excessive fluid losses.*[11]

Risk for Fluid Volume Deficit *is the state in which an individual is at risk of experiencing vascular, cellular, or intracellular dehydration.*[11]

OVERVIEW

Body fluids comprise water, electrolytes, proteins, and other dissolved substances. These fluids are distributed between two body compartments: the intracellular compartment and the extracellular compartment. Fluids in the intracellular compartment, which account for about two thirds of the body's water, are contained in the billions of cells that make up the body. Fluids in the extracellular compartment, which contains the remaining one third of body water, are found in the interstitial spaces surrounding the cells, in the circulatory system, in the cerebrospinal fluid, and in

body spaces. Fluid homeostasis is maintained through the osmotic properties and electrolyte concentrations of the body fluids.[12]

Body water has many functions. It provides a medium for the transport and exchange of nutrients, oxygen, carbon dioxide, and other wastes to and from cells; it also serves as the medium in which chemical reactions occur. Body water also helps in the regulation of body temperature, provides structure and insulation, and acts as a lubricant.

Total body water accounts for almost 60% of total body weight in adults, but this figure differs depending on age, gender, and the amount of body fat. In a full-term infant, water accounts for as much as 75% to 80% of total body weight. Aging results in a decrease in total body water; after the age of 65, body water may decrease to 45% to 50% of total body weight.[15] Because fat cells contain little water, the slender person has a higher proportion of body water to total body weight, whereas the obese person has a lower proportion. Women with a higher ratio of fat to lean muscle mass than men have a lower percentage of body water content.

The adult normally has a balanced gain and loss of 2500 ml of body water in a 24-hour period. Water is gained through oral intake and in food and through metabolic oxidation. Water is lost through urine, in the feces, and through insensible losses from the lungs and the skin. All healthy people require about 100 ml of water per 100 calories metabolized.[12] Increased body water is lost when a person has an elevated body temperature with resultant increased metabolic rate. Infants are more likely to experience fluid volume alterations because they have a higher metabolic rate and a larger surface area in relation to body mass than children and adults. The infant is also less able to concentrate urine because kidney structures are still immature.

Body fluid volume is regulated by a complex interaction of the renal, neuroendocrine, and vascular systems. These systems maintain plasma osmolality within a narrow range of 280 to 300 mOsm/kg.[8] The primary solutes that determine plasma osmolality are sodium, glucose, and urea; intracellular osmolality is primarily determined by potassium, glucose, and urea. The plasma solute content remains relatively stable in healthy people, with changes in osmolality most often the result of alterations in water balance. For example, Fluid Volume Deficit from dehydration secondary to vomiting and diarrhea is manifested as an increase in plasma osmolality from extracellular water losses rather than from solute gains.[14]

The mechanisms that control body water balance are thirst and antidiuretic hormone (ADH). Thirst, which is the desire to drink water, is stimulated by cellular dehydration sensed by osmoreceptors and by volume depletion sensed by baroreceptors. Cellular dehydration, the result of conditions that cause water to shift out of the cells, is seen in disorders that cause an increase in the extracellular solute concentration or a decrease in extracellular water. The hyperosmolar state that results is usually associated with hypernatremia, an increase in plasma osmolality, and intracellular water losses. Conditions that may cause cellular dehydration include diabetes insipidus and hypokalemia.[14] The stimulus for thirst may be impaired by increasing age and by disorders such as cerebral vascular accidents and head trauma. The ability to respond to thirst is compromised in people with alterations in mobility and in those who have altered levels of consciousness or are confused.

ADH (also called vasopressin), a water-conserving hormone, is synthesized in the hypothalamus and stored in the posterior pituitary. Its most important function is renal control of osmolality. ADH release is stimulated by increased plasma osmolality and inhibited by a hypoosmolar state. Levels of ADH are controlled by extracellular volume, sensed by stretch receptors in the great veins, the atria, and the carotid sinus, and by osmolar changes, sensed by osmoreceptors in the pituitary. An increase in ADH levels produces an increase in water reabsorption from the renal distal tubules and collecting ducts. A decrease in ADH levels inhibits reabsorption, and increased water is eliminated in the urine.

ADH levels are altered by various pathological conditions and chemicals. Stress, severe pain, nausea, trauma, surgery, nicotine, and certain drugs (e.g., acetaminophen, morphine, meperidine, chlorothiazide, and tricylic antidepressants) increase ADH levels. Of these conditions, nausea is the most potent in increasing ADH. ADH release is inhibited by alcohol, glucocorticoids, lithium carbonate, norepinephrine, phenytoin, and reserpine.[8,12]

Diabetes insipidus and the syndrome of inappropriate ADH (SIADH) are disorders of ADH regulation.[7,8] Diabetes insipidus may be neurogenic (caused by a defect in the formation or release of ADH) or nephrogenic (the result of an inability of the kidneys to respond to ADH). These defects result in an inability to concentrate urine and increased serum osmolality.[1] Diabetes insipidus may be the result of cerebral disease or injury, potassium depletion, or chronic hypercalcemia. SIADH is the result of the failure of the negative feedback mechanism that normally controls ADH levels. ADH secretion continues, despite decreased serum osmolality, leading to the retention of water in excess of sodium and dilutional hyponatremia.[12] SIADH may result from cerebral disease or injury, renal disease, stress, pain, intrathoracic conditions, or drugs. These two conditions may be transient or permanent.

Aldosterone, the primary mineralocorticoid hormone produced by the adrenal cortex, and

II

atrial natriuretic peptide (ANP) are also critical elements in fluid balance. Aldosterone is released in response to plasma volume changes sensed by stretch receptors in the renal afferent arterioles. In response to a decrease in volume and blood pressure, the juxtaglomerular cells of the kidney secrete renin. Renin is converted to angiotensin I by angiotensinogen from the liver. Angiotensin I is then converted to angiotensin II by an enzyme from the lungs. Angiotensin II stimulates the release of aldosterone, which increases sodium transport in the renal tubules. This action facilitates sodium and water reabsorption. Primary adrenal deficiencies are the result of Addison's disease, adrenal hemorrhage, sepsis, or AIDS. Secondary adrenal deficiencies are associated with decreased pituitary ACTH secretion from long-term exogenous glucocorticoid administration, pituitary tumors, and surgery or radiation of the pituitary gland.[6]

ANP is released by the atria in response to increased atrial pressure. It increases renal excretion of sodium and water; causes a decrease in the synthesis of renin and release of aldosterone; decreases ADH release; and is a vasodilator. ANP is released in conditions that cause an increase in plasma volume or elevated cardiac filling pressures, such as congestive heart failure, chronic renal failure, atrial tachycardia, or vasoconstricting drugs.[8]

As a result of these complex physiological mechanisms, alterations in fluid volume balance may result from several causes. Fluid Volume Excess may result from excessive sodium and water intake or from inadequate sodium and water losses and may be manifested by circulatory overload or interstitial edema. Patients receiving intravenous fluids of any type are always at risk for Fluid Volume Excess; those receiving hypertonic or colloid oncotic solutions, are older adults, and have heart disease are at even greater risk. Severe mental illness may lead to excessive oral water intake, leading to water intoxication and even death.[3]

Fluid Volume Deficits are primarily the result of an increased loss of fluid or an inadequate intake of water and are manifested by decreased circula-

tory volume and dehydration of cells and tissues. The Risk for Fluid Volume Deficit is greatest in patients who are unconscious, unable to swallow, taking potent diuretics, have surgery, or have severe vomiting and diarrhea. The very young and the very old who are community-dwelling are at even greater risk in situations of increased environmental temperatures. Other patients at Risk for Fluid Volume Deficit are those with large, open, draining wounds and those who have third-space fluid losses.[2]

ASSESSMENT

To assess the patient's fluid status accurately, the nurse collects and analyzes both subjective and objective data. The nursing history considers physiological, psychological, developmental, spiritual, and sociocultural factors. Objective data collected by the clinical assessment includes intake and output, weight, vital signs, and assessment of the skin, the cardiovascular system, the neurological system, and the gastrointestinal system. Other Functional Health Patterns to assess that influence fluid volume status include the Health-Perception—Health-Management Pattern, the Nutritional-Metabolic Pattern, the Elimination Pattern, the Cognitive-Perceptual Pattern, the Coping—Stress-Tolerance Pattern, and the Value-Belief Pattern.

Fluid Volume Excess

The nursing history conducted for the patient with Fluid Volume Excess includes questions about the presence of localized infections and chronic diseases, such as heart disease, renal disease, liver disease, or endocrine diseases. The patient is also asked about the oral intake of fluids and the use of table salt and high-sodium foods, over-the-counter medications that may contain sodium, and prescribed steroids. Symptoms that indicate Fluid Volume Excess are shortness of breath; difficulty sleeping with the head flat (orthopnea); scanty, dark urine; weight gain; and cough. The patient should also be asked about significant stressful life events, belief about the value of current treatment (e.g., the patient may not be taking diuretics because of nighttime wakening), and availability of resources to buy low-sodium foods or medications.

Daily assessment of weight and intake and output are important means of monitoring fluid volume status. Sudden weight gain is usually an indicator of acute fluid gain, with each kg gained equivalent to 1 L of fluid retained. To be accurate, weight should be taken at the same time each day (usually before breakfast), wearing the same clothes and using the same scales. Intake and output is measured and recorded on a regular basis, with trends monitored across time. Urine output of less than 30 ml to 50 ml per hour or a positive fluid balance on a 24-hour total of intake and output are critical indicators of Fluid Volume Excess.[10]

Vital signs and hemodynamic monitors provide data for Fluid Volume Excess. Fluid accumulation in the lungs is assessed by auscultating crackles, gurgles, or wheezes. Bounding pulses and an elevated blood pressure are often indications of circulatory fluid volume overload. Hemodynamic monitoring of the patient with Fluid Volume Excess will demonstrate increased central venous pressure (CVP) of greater than 6 mm Hg or 12 cm H_2O and pulmonary artery pressure (PAP) of greater than 30/15 mm Hg.[8]

Physical assessment of the integument of the patient with Fluid Volume Excess will reveal edema. Local areas of edema are usually the result of inflammation. When sodium and water balance is altered, capillary function is impaired, and the collection of fluid in the interstitial spaces is generalized (called *anasarca*), manifested by edema in the periorbital, sacral, or pretibial areas. Edema is classified as pitting or nonpitting. Pitting edema is assessed by pressing the skin over a bony surface such as the tibia and rating the degree of indentation from 1+ (for only a slight indentation) to 4+ (for deep, long-lasting indentation).

Cardiovascular assessment for Fluid Volume Excess reveals a gallop heart rhythm, jugular vein distention (greater than 3 cm), and an increased time to empty the hand veins (more than 3 to 5 seconds). Changes in mental status include anxiety, restlessness, lethargy, and confusion; disorienta-tion and coma may follow as a result of the effect of fluid overload on the brain. Other assessments that may be made in the patient with Fluid Volume Excess include ascites and pleural effusion.

Laboratory data that support a diagnosis of Fluid Volume Excess include serum sodium, serum osmolality, urine osmolality, and hematocrit. Hyponatremia and decreased serum osmolality are seen in patients who ingest or are administered more water than the kidneys can excrete, who have abnormal kidney function, or who have elevated ADH levels. Urine osmolality is decreased in fluid volume overload. The hematocrit is decreased from hemodilution. Fluid accumulation in the lungs may be seen on chest X ray.

■ Defining Characteristics

The presence of the following defining characteristics indicates that the patient may be experiencing Fluid Volume Excess:

- Edema
- Anasarca
- Intake is greater than output
- Decreased hematocrit
- Weight gain
- Increased CVP
- Dyspnea
- Increased PAP
- Orthopnea
- Hyponatremia
- Rales, gurgles, and wheezes
- Decreased serum and urine osmolality
- Pulmonary congestion (seen in X ray)
- Scanty, concentrated urine (<30 ml/hr)
- Gallop rhythm (S3)
- Increased blood pressure
- Restlessness and anxiety
- Jugular distention
- Decreasing levels of consciousness
- Positive hepatojugular reflex
- Effusion and ascites

■ Related Factors

The following related factors are associated with Fluid Volume Excess:

- Compromised regulatory mechanisms
- Excess fluid intake
- Excess sodium intake

Fluid Volume Deficit

The nursing history conducted for the patient with a Fluid Volume Deficit includes questions about the presence of chronic illnesses, such as gastrointestinal tract disorders that cause persistent diarrhea, renal disorders, or endocrine disorders. The patient is also asked about the oral intake of fluids, the use of medications such as diuretics or laxatives, or the presence of draining wounds. Symptoms that indicate Fluid Volume Deficit are thirst, weakness, fatigue, weight loss, a dry mouth and dry skin, and decreased urine output. Environmental factors are determined by asking about exposure to high temperatures without adequate cooling. Developmental considerations are important; infants and older adults more commonly have Fluid Volume Deficit. The nurse also explores the patient's belief about the value of current treatment (e.g., the patient with diabetes who continues to eat high-calories foods and has hyperglycemia), spiritual beliefs that may affect treatments (e.g., the replacement of whole blood), and resource availability (e.g., ready access to clean water).

Fluid Volume Deficit may also be assessed and monitored by measuring daily weight and intake and output. Sudden weight loss may indicate fluid loss, with a 2-kg (4.4-lb) weight loss equaling 2 L of fluid. However, fluid may shift from one space to another and the patient will have Fluid Volume Deficit without a loss of weight. Intake is less than output in dehydration. Output records should include measurements of urine, liquid feces, vomitus, nasogastric drainage, wound drainage, fistula drainage, and diaphoresis. Although increased urine output may precipitate Fluid Volume Deficit, the patient who is dehydrated will have decreased urine output.

Vital signs and hemodynamic findings provide data for Fluid Volume Deficit. The body temperature is often lower than normal, with rectal temperature falling as low as 35°C (95°F).[8] The respiratory rate may become more rapid, while the heart rate increases as a compensatory mechanism to maintain cardiac output. The pulse is often weak and thready, and the blood pressure decreases. Hemodynamic monitoring for the patient with a Fluid Volume Deficit will demonstrate a decreased CVP (less than 2 mm Hg or 5 cm H_2O) and a PAP of less than 20/8 mm Hg.[8]

Physical assessment of the skin and the mucous membranes of the patient with Fluid Volume Deficit will reveal dry mucous membranes and flushed, dry skin. Turgor is decreased; however, this assessment must be made with caution in the older adult who may normally have decreased skin elasticity. The furrows of the tongue may be deeper, and there is less fluid in the oral cavity between the cheek and gums. The eyes are sunken and the eyeballs may be soft. The fontanelles of infants will be depressed.

Cardiovascular assessment for Fluid Volume Deficit reveals an increased time for the filling of hand veins. The patient may be restless and confused, have anorexia, and be thirsty. Severe Fluid Volume Deficit may cause dehydration of cerebral neurons, causing generalized muscle weakness, rigidity, and tremors; hallucinations; and maniacal behavior.

Laboratory data that support a diagnosis of Fluid Volume Deficit include serum sodium, serum osmolality, urine osmolality and specific gravity, and hematocrit. Hypernatremia and high serum osmolality may be present, accompanied by an increase in urine osmolality and specific gravity. The hematocrit often increases as a result of hemoconcentration.

■ Defining Characteristics

The presence of the following defining characteristics indicates that the patient may be experiencing Fluid Volume Deficit:

- Dry skin
- Dry mucous membranes
- Weight loss
- Thirst

- Decreased skin turgor
- Decreased blood pressure
- Tachycardia
- Rapid respirations
- Increased temperature
- Sunken, soft eyeballs
- Increased venous filling time
- Increased serum and urine osmolality
- Decreased urine output
- Increased hematocrit
- Sunken fontanelles
- Weakness
- Fatigue
- Restlessness
- Hallucinations

■ Related Factors

The following related factors are associated with Fluid Volume Deficit:

- Failure of regulatory mechanisms
- Active fluid volume loss

Risk for Fluid Volume Deficit

The nursing history reveals factors that increase the risk for Fluid Volume Deficit. Questions should be asked about renal disease, ulcerative colitis, Crohn's disease, diabetes mellitus, or diabetes insipidus. Other conditions that may cause Fluid Volume Deficit include persistent fever, draining wounds, draining abscesses, burns, hyperemesis gravidarum, and previous surgery that removed a large part of the large intestine. Decreased oral intake of fluids may result from an inability to swallow, persistent nausea, or oral pain. Extremes of age and extremes of weight increase the Risk for Fluid Volume Deficit, as do extremes of environmental temperature. The patient who is physically immobile, has neurological deficits, has psychological impairments, or is homeless may be unable to access water or to respond to the need for water.

Other patients at Risk for Fluid Volume Deficit are those who have an increased output from any source. This includes nasogastric suction, urinary frequency from diuretic administration, and a chronic use of laxatives and enemas. These factors may be the result of the patient's lack of knowledge about the use and effects of medications.

■ Risk Factors

The presence of the following behaviors, conditions, or circumstances renders the patient more vulnerable to the Risk for Fluid Volume Deficit:

- Extremes of age
- Extremes of weight
- Loss through normal routes: vomiting, diarrhea, urine, and perspiration
- Loss through abnormal routes: gastrointestinal suction and wound drainage
- Deviations affecting access to intake or absorption: physical immobility, coma, homelessness, ulcerative colitis, and colectomy
- Factors influencing fluid needs: hypermetabolic states, diabetic ketoacidosis, hyperosmolar hyperglycemic nonketotic coma (HHNC), and diabetes insipidus
- Knowledge deficit

DIAGNOSIS

■ Differential Nursing Diagnosis

The diagnosis Fluid Volume Excess may be used in error when an illness is not responsive to independent nursing interventions. For example, the client with cerebral edema and increased intracranial pressure requires collaborative interventions to reduce the cellular fluid overload. Risk for Fluid Volume Deficit can be used when the patient is NPO for an extended period of time and should not be used when the patient is NPO for a short period of time (e.g., 24 hours or less) and has adequate parenteral fluid replacement.

■ Medical and Psychiatric Diagnoses

Medical diagnoses commonly related to Fluid Volume Excess involve the regulatory mechanisms, the heart, and the endocrine system. Congestive heart failure, with changes in cardiac output and the failure of homeostatic mechanisms, results in peripheral and pulmonary edema. Renal failure leaves the nephrons unable to excrete fluids. Cushing's syndrome results in hypersecretion of glucocorticoids with sodium and water retention. SIADH leads to overhydration and decreased serum osmolality. Cancer and lymphedema may prevent the flow of lymphatic fluid, resulting in peripheral edema.

Medical diagnoses commonly associated with Risk for Fluid Volume Deficit and Fluid Volume Deficit focus on disorders of hormones and inflammatory disorders. Diabetes insipidus results in a defect in the release of ADH, followed by the excretion of large amounts of dilute urine. Diabetes mellitus, a disorder of chronic hyperglycemia caused by a defect in the production or utilization of insulin, is manifested by increased osmolality and urine output. Disorders such as ulcerative colitis and Crohn's disease result in chronic diarrhea with resultant fluid loss.

OUTCOME IDENTIFICATION, PLANNING, AND IMPLEMENTATION

The primary expected outcome for the patient with Fluid Volume Excess, Fluid Volume Deficit, or Risk for Fluid Volume Deficit is that a balanced fluid state will be achieved or maintained. Other specific outcome criteria focus on an increased or decreased intake of fluids and sodium, the prevention of complications, and teaching the patient self-management of fluid status.

Fluid Volume Excess

The outcomes for the patient with Fluid Volume Excess are that the patient will regain fluid balance as evidenced by weight loss, balanced intake and output; decreasing edema, normal vital signs and hemodynamics, and normal urine specific gravity (1.010 to 1.030); the patient will experience less dyspnea and will maintain intact skin and mucous membranes. To reach these outcomes the patient is weighed daily; has vital signs, breath sounds, intake and output, and urine specific grav-

ity assessed on a regular schedule; has fluids restricted and follows a low-sodium diet as prescribed; has the head of the bed elevated 30° to 40°; is turned every 2 hours; and has regular skin care and oral care. These planned interventions are especially important for patients who are older, who have chronic or debilitating illnesses, and who have excessive ADH secretion in response to stressors. In addition, all patients receiving intravenous therapy require close monitoring for the development of Fluid Volume Excess.

The patient and significant others require appropriate teaching, based on the underlying cause of the fluid excess. Topics include sodium restriction, the use of salt substitutes, fluid restriction, the use of over-the-counter and prescription medications, and manifestations to report to the primary health care provider such as peripheral edema, acute weight gain, easy fatigability, shortness of breath, or persistent cough. It is important to assess cultural or ethnic dietary patterns and the use of folk medicines before initiating teaching about diet and medications.

Fluid Volume Deficit and Risk for Fluid Volume Deficit

The outcomes for the patient who is at risk for or has an actual Fluid Volume Deficit are that the patient will maintain or regain fluid balance as evidenced by weight within normal range; balanced intake and output; normal vital signs, hemodynamics, and urine specific gravity; good skin turgor; moist mucous membranes; and normal mental status. To reach these outcomes, the patient is weighed daily and has careful assessment of vital signs, intake and output, peripheral pulses, skin turgor, hydration of mucous membranes, and mental status on a regular schedule. Patients who are most at risk require more frequent assessment; including those who are comatose or disoriented and those with gastrointestinal suction, draining wounds, severe infections, and hyperthermia. A critical consideration is dehydration of the older adult as a result of hospitalization, institutionalization, existing chronic illnesses, age-related alterations in regulatory mechanisms, and surgery.[9]

Continued on p. 187

◀ NURSING CARE GUIDELINES
Nursing Diagnosis: Fluid Volume Excess

It is difficult to estimate an exact time for achieving expected outcomes for patients with Fluid Volume Excess. The length of time necessary depends on the age and general health of the patient, the underlying cause, and the severity of the abnormal response.

Expected Outcome: The patient will regain and maintain fluid balance.
- Take and record intake output on a regular basis. If urine output is less than 30 ml to 50 ml per hour, measure urine hourly. *Inadequate cardiac output and renal perfusion may result in fluid retention and decreased urinary output.*
- Assess for edema in the periorbital, pretibial, and sacral areas. *Periorbital edema indicates anasarca. Localized edema tends to accumulate in dependent areas of the body and is assessed in the feet and lower legs of the patient who is ambulatory and in the sacral area of the patient who is on bed rest.*
- Assess vital signs, heart sounds, peripheral pulses, and hemodynamic indicators such as CVP. *Fluid Volume Excess is indicated by hypertension, crackles and gurgles, an S3 gallop rhythm, and an elevated CVP.*
- Weigh the patient daily at the same time, wearing the same clothing, and using the same scales. *Acute weight gain is often caused by fluid retention. Each kg of increased weight represents 1L of fluid.*
- ▲ Restrict oral fluids to prescribed levels. Mutually develop a 24-hour schedule for times and amounts of fluids allowed. *Oral fluids are usually restricted to facilitate regaining a normal fluid balance.*
- ▲ Provide a sodium-restricted diet as prescribed. *Excess sodium intake in foods contributes to fluid retention.*
- ▲ Administer diuretics as prescribed. *Diuretics are often prescribed to increase urinary output and to decrease Fluid Volume Excess.*
- ▲ Monitor and report abnormal laboratory and X-ray findings: serum sodium, serum osmolality, urine osmolality, hematocrit, pH, $PaCO_2$, bicarbonate, blood urea nitrogen (BUN), and chest X ray. *Patients with Fluid Volume Excess often have decreased serum sodium, osmolality, hematocrit and BUN; fluid retention in the lungs is indicated by changes in arterial blood gases and is seen on chest X ray.*

Expected Outcome: The patient will maintain intact skin and mucous membranes during episodes of Fluid Volume Excess.
- Assess tissues over bony prominences and in areas of edema. *Edematous tissue is more prone to tissue breakdown.*
- Reposition the patient at least every 2 hours. Avoid moving the patient in such a way that shearing forces are exerted. *Changing positions decreases the length of time pressure is applied to one area. Shearing forces precipitate tissue breakdown.*
- Institute measures to prevent tissue pressure, such as using eggcrate mattresses and foot cradles. *Devices to distribute pressure or to reduce pressure are useful in preventing tissue breakdown in edematous areas.*
- Keep the patient's skin clean and dry. *Clean, dry skin is less likely to develop tissue breakdown.*
- Provide oral care on a regular schedule. *Oral care increases comfort, helps maintain intact mucous membranes, and relieves thirst if fluids are restricted.*

Expected Outcome: The client will verbalize an increased ability to breathe while Fluid Volume Excess is present.
- Elevate the head of the bed 30° to 40°. *Elevating the head of the bed allows better expansion of the lungs, thus facilitating respirations.*
- Assess the respiratory rate and breath sounds on a regular schedule. *Respiratory rate is often increased in Fluid Volume Excess. If the patient is hypervolemic, pulmonary congestion may occur, as evidenced by crackles and gurgles.*

■ = nursing intervention; ▲ = collaborative intervention. *Continued*

◢ NURSING CARE GUIDELINES — CONT'D

Expected Outcome: The patient or the patient's significant others will verbalize an adequate knowledge base of measures to manage fluid balance.
- Assess the knowledge base, cultural and ethnic background, and use of folk medicine of the patient and significant others.
- Provide information about the cause of the fluid excess and how to prevent its recurrence; the rationale for treatment; the dietary and pharmacological sources of sodium, the use of salt substitutes, and who to contact for questions or problems. *Providing information for self-management is an essential component of continuity of care between health care settings.*

◢ NURSING CARE GUIDELINES
Nursing Diagnosis: Fluid Volume Deficit and Risk for Fluid Volume Deficit

It is difficult to estimate an exact time for achieving expected outcomes for patients with Fluid Volume Deficit. The length of time necessary depends on the age and general health of the patient, the underlying cause, and the severity of the abnormal response.

Expected Outcome: The patient with a Fluid Volume Deficit will regain fluid balance.
- Take and record intake and output on a regular basis. If urine output is less than 30 ml to 50 ml per hour, measure urine hourly.[5] *Inadequate renal perfusion, cardiac failure, fluid shifts, decreased oral fluid intake, or increased fluid output may contribute to oliguria or anuria.*
- Assess vital signs, peripheral pulses, and hemodynamic indicators on a regular schedule. *Hypotension, tachycardia, weak pulses, and a decreased CVP indicate Fluid Volume Deficit and dehydration.*
- Weigh the patient daily at the same time, wearing the same clothing, and using the same scales. *Acute weight loss is often caused by fluid loss. Each kg of decreased weight represents 1L of fluid.*
- Assess the patient's mental status during neurological assessment. *Fluid Volume Deficit may cause dehydration of cerebral neurons, resulting in changes in mentation and behavior.*
- Increase oral fluid intake as tolerated. *Oral fluids facilitate regaining normal fluid balance. The nurse and the patient should mutually develop a plan for the types, amounts, and times for fluid intake.*
- ▲ Monitor and report abnormal hematocrit levels. *Patients who have Fluid Volume Deficit often have increased hematocrit levels.*
- ▲ Administer intravenous fluids as prescribed. *The patient with severe Fluid Volume Deficit will require intravenous fluid replacement. Carefully monitor all patients receiving intravenous fluids for fluid volume overload.*
- ▲ Administer prescribed medications. *Medications may be prescribed to correct the failure of fluid volume regulatory mechanisms. The medications may include vasopressin for the patient with diabetes insipidus, insulin for the patient with diabetic ketoacidosis and HHNK, and steroids for the patient with primary adrenal insufficiency.*

Expected Outcome: The patient will maintain intact skin and mucous membranes during episodes of Fluid Volume Deficit.
- Assess skin turgor, mucous membranes, and skin moisture. *Skin folds will remain in a raised position for several seconds, mucous membranes are dry, and the skin is dry in patients who are dehydrated.[10] In addition, infants will have depressed fontanelles and may be unable to cry tears.*
- Provide skin care and oral care. *Dry skin and mucous membranes are prone to develop tissue breakdown.*

■ = nursing intervention; ▲ = collaborative intervention.

Expected Outcome: The patient at Risk for Fluid Volume Deficit will maintain fluid balance.
- Monitor the fluid status of all patients with nasogastric suction, draining wounds, burns, or increased urinary output for an imbalance in intake and output.
- Monitor the fluid status of all patients who are unconscious, disoriented, have physical limitations, or have vomiting and diarrhea.
- Monitor the fluid status of the very young and the very old. *All of these conditions increase the risk of the development of Fluid Volume Deficit.*

Expected Outcome: The patient or the patient's significant others will verbalize an adequate knowledge base of measures to manage fluid balance.
- Assess the knowledge base, cultural and ethnic background, and living environment of the patient and significant others.
- Provide information about the cause of the fluid deficit and how to prevent its recurrence; the rationale for treatment; and safety measures to prevent falls from postural hypotension, fluid replacements for vomiting and diarrhea, and who to contact for questions or problems. *Providing information for self-management is an essential component of continuity of care between health care settings.*

The very-low-birth-weight infant is also at greater risk as a result of body fluid composition, skin and renal immaturity, and environmental stressors.[13]

Client and family teaching is provided to prevent Fluid Volume Deficit. Before teaching, it is important to assess the patient's usual living environment and resources. Topics for teaching include the amount and type of fluids that should be consumed each day, the importance of increasing fluid intake and decreasing activity in hot weather, and the types of fluids to take when experiencing vomiting and diarrhea. Fluid Volume Deficit often causes postural hypotension; teaching safety measures when rising from a supine or sitting position is therefore important in preventing falls.

The older adult is at greater Risk for Fluid Volume Deficit as a result of multiple factors. These factors include a general decrease in thirst perception, a decreased fluid reserve, decreased renal glomerular filtration, and impaired thermoregulation. The older adult may have physical disabilities from chronic illnesses such as arthritis that limit the ability to access fluids, or the older adult may have cognitive impairments that interfere with the recognition of thirst. In addition, the older adult may resist the use of air-conditioners or fans in extreme heat and may limit fluid intake to prevent incontinence. Teaching the older adult

about preventing Fluid Volume Deficit includes the regular intake of preferred fluids, the use of alternate sources of liquid (such as gelatin or broth), and ways to monitor intake and output.

EVALUATION

The following indicators provide evidence of the effectiveness of nursing interventions.

Fluid Volume Excess

The patient has normal fluid balance, intact skin and mucous membranes, verbalizes an increased ability to breathe, and verbalizes an adequate knowledge base to self-manage fluid balance. The patient's weight is within his or her normal range, vital signs and hemodynamic parameters are within normal limits, and electrolytes and arterial blood gases are within normal ranges. Breath sounds and chest X ray are clear. Edema is decreasing or absent. The patient verbalizes causes and self-management of the fluid volume imbalance and the rationale for treatment and knows who to contact with questions or problems.

Indicators of the need to reevaluate the plan are abnormal breath sounds, abnormal vital signs and hemodynamics, an acute weight gain, and increasing dyspnea or orthopnea. Consultation by a clinical specialist may be necessary if skin care becomes a problem. Collaboration with the primary health care provider is necessary to redesign the plan of care for changes in fluid restrictions, diet, and medications.

Fluid Volume Deficit and Risk for Fluid Volume Deficit

The patient regains or maintains normal fluid balance, has intact skin and mucous membranes, and verbalizes an adequate knowledge base of measures to manage fluid balance. The patient has good skin turgor, normal weight, and normal vital signs. Hemodynamic parameters, urine specific gravity, and laboratory data are within normal limits. Intake and output are balanced over a 24-hour period for several days. The patient is fully oriented. Skin is intact and mucous membranes are moist. The patient verbalizes causes and self-management of the fluid volume imbalance and the rationale for treatment and knows who to contact with questions or problems. The patient at risk identifies measures to prevent the development of a Fluid Volume Deficit.

If the outcomes are not achieved, collaboration with the primary health care provider is necessary. This is indicated by an acute weight loss, poor skin turgor, abnormal vital signs and hemodynamic parameters, an imbalance in intake and output, and changes in mental status. Patients at risk who develop an actual Fluid Volume Deficit may require additional teaching.

▶ CASE STUDY WITH PLAN OF CARE

Mrs. Ann T., a 77-year-old woman, came to the local health clinic with increasing dyspnea on exertion and three-pillow orthopnea. She also states that her feet and ankles have become so swollen that she can no longer wear her shoes. Mrs. T. has previously been diagnosed with congestive heart failure, for which furosemide (40 mg each morning), digoxin (0.025 mg each morning), and a low-sodium diet were prescribed. However, Mrs. T. says that she "just hasn't had the money to buy her medications this month." The physical assessment includes abnormal findings of 3+ pitting edema bilaterally in her feet and lower legs, distended neck veins, a positive hepatojugular reflex, bounding pulses, an S3 on cardiac auscultation, and respiratory crackles. Mrs. T. has gained 10 pounds since her last clinic visit 2 weeks ago. A chest X ray illustrates pulmonary congestion. Laboratory tests show a serum sodium level of 130 mEq/l with decreased osmolality. Mrs. T. was sent to the hospital for evaluation and treatment. At the hospital, her vital signs included a pulse of 115 beats/min and a respiratory rate of 30/min. Hemodynamic monitoring revealed a CVP of 16.

▶ PLAN OF CARE FOR MRS. T.
Nursing Diagnosis: Fluid Volume Excess Related to Congestive Heart Failure Secondary to Cardiac Pump Failure

---

Expected Outcome: Mrs. T. will regain and maintain a normal fluid balance.
- Weigh Mrs. T. each morning at 7 A.M., using the same scales.
- Monitor intake and output and record each shift. If output falls to less than 30 ml/hr to 50 ml/hr, measure urine output every 1 to 2 hours.
- Measure urine specific gravity.
- ▲ Maintain fluid restriction of 200 ml from 7:00 A.M. to 3:00 P.M., 200 ml from 3:00 P.M. to 11:00 P.M., and 100 ml from 11:00 P.M. to 7:00 A.M. Mrs. T. prefers cold water and tea.
- ▲ Administer prescribed diuretics.

■ = nursing intervention; ▲ = collaborative intervention.

▲ Provide a restricted sodium diet as prescribed. Ask the dietitian to consult with Mrs. T. about preferred foods.
▲ Monitor the results of laboratory tests of serum sodium and osmolality.

Expected Outcome: Mrs. T. will regain and maintain a stable hemodynamic balance.
■ Take and record her vital signs every 4 hours.
■ Assess jugular distention and hepatojugular reflex every 8 hours.
▲ Monitor and record CVP every 4 hours.
▲ Monitor the results of laboratory data.
▲ Administer prescribed cardiotonic glycoside.

Expected Outcome: Mrs. T. will verbalize less dyspnea and increasing comfort.
■ Elevate the head of the bed 30° to 40°.
■ Assess respiratory rate and breath sounds every 4 hours.
■ Encourage coughing, deep breathing, and incentive spirometry every 2 hours and as needed.
▲ Administer oxygen as prescribed.
▲ Monitor the results of laboratory tests of arterial blood gases (ABGs) and chest X ray.

Expected Outcome: Mrs. T. will maintain intact skin and mucous membranes.
■ Keep the skin dry and clean; do not massage edematous areas.
■ Use a bed cradle to keep covers off edematous feet and legs.
■ Encourage Mrs. T. to change position every 1 to 2 hours while in bed and while sitting in the chair.
■ Assist Mrs. T. with oral hygiene every 4 hours and as needed.

Expected Outcome: Mrs. T. will verbalize knowledge of the disease process, the rationale for treatment, and self-care measures to prevent Fluid Volume Excess.
■ Explain the role of the heart in maintaining fluid balance in the body.
■ Describe the changes that occur in the body in congestive heart failure.
■ Describe the effects of diuretics and digoxin and why it is important to take these medications as prescribed.
■ Discuss the types of foods and fluids that may be consumed on a low-sodium diet and compare these to Mrs. T.'s usual dietary intake.[4] Ask Mrs. T. to keep a record of the foods and fluids she consumes during the next week and to bring this to her return appointment at the clinic.
■ Discuss methods to help prevent dependent edema, such as avoiding constricting clothing, wearing support stockings, changing positions frequently, avoiding crossing the legs when sitting, and elevating the legs when sitting.
■ Discuss economic and personal resources and make referrals as necessary to a social worker.

■ CRITICAL THINKING EXERCISES

1. You are developing plans of care for two patients. One patient is 82 years old and has non-insulin-dependent diabetes; the other patient is a 24-year-old who just completed a long-distance run in temperatures of over 90°. Both patients have Fluid Volume Deficit. How would the plans of care differ for these two patients?

2. Mrs. J., a 70-year-old woman, fell in her bathtub and has a closed head injury. She is unconscious. What assessments would indicate the onset of SIADH and resultant Fluid Volume Excess?

3. When making a home visit, you discover that Mr. M., who has chronic renal failure, is continuing to take multiple over-the-counter medications that are high in sodium. Mr. M. proudly tells you that he is following his low-

sodium diet. On assessment you note increasing bilateral pulmonary rales, a weight gain of 5 pounds in 2 weeks, an increase in blood pressure, and 2+ pitting edema in his feet and ankles. What would you do now?

4. The J. family, consisting of a mother, father, and an 8-month-old infant, are homeless. They have been living in their car. Mrs. J. has weaned the baby from the bottle and has been withholding oral fluids because the baby has diarrhea. Describe the risk factors for Fluid Volume Deficit in the baby, and develop a teaching plan to minimize the risk.

REFERENCES

1. Bell TN: Diabetes insipidus, *Crit Care Nurs Clin North Am,* 6(4):675–685, 1994.
2. Bove L: How fluids and electrolytes shift, *Nursing 94* 24(8): 34–39, 1994.
3. Boyd M and others: Target weight procedure for disordered water balance in long-term care facilities, *J Psychosoc Nurs* 30(12):22–37, 1992.
4. Bridle R: Drink problem . . . Fluid and electrolyte replacement ability of commercially prepared canned drinks, *Nursing Times* 90(29):46–47, 1994.
5. Bulechek GM and McCloskey JC: *Nursing interventions: essential nursing treatments,* ed 2, Philadelphia, 1992, WB Saunders Co.
6. Epstein CD: Adrenocortical insufficiency in the critically ill patient, *AACN Clin Iss Crit Care Nurs* 3(3):705–713, 1992.
7. Gildea JH: High and dry—low and wet: the key to DI and SIADH, *Pediatr Nurs* 19(5):478–481, 1993.
8. Home MM and Swearingen PL: *Fluids, electrolytes, and acid-base balance,* ed 2, St. Louis, 1993, Mosby–Year Book.
9. Martin J and Larsen P: Dehydration in the elderly surgical patient, *AORN Journal* 60(4):666–671, 1994.
10. Metheny NM: *Fluid and electrolyte balance: nursing considerations,* Philadelphia, 1992, JB Lippincott Co.
11. North American Nursing Diagnosis Association: *NANDA nursing diagnoses: definitions and classification, 1995–1996,* Philadelphia, 1994, The Association.
12. Porth CM: *Pathophysiology: concepts of altered health states,* ed 4, Philadelphia, 1994, Lippincott-Raven.
13. Poulsen N: Fluid and electrolyte management of the very-low-birth-weight infant, *J Perin Neonat Nurs* 8(4):59–70, 1995.
14. Toto KH: Regulation of plasma osmolality: thirst and vasopressin, *Crit Care Nurs Clin North Am* 6(4):661–674, 1994.
15. Welty NJ: *Body fluids and electrolytes,* ed 6, St. Louis, 1992, Mosby–Year Book.

Ineffective Infant Feeding Pattern

▶

Ineffective Infant Feeding Pattern *is a state in which an infant demonstrates an impaired ability to suck or coordinate the suck-swallow response.*[9]

OVERVIEW

The development of functional feeding for the infant is an intricate physiological process compounded by neurological maturation and learned behaviors. Essential to the process of normal feeding and swallowing is adequate nutrition and airway competence.[15] The infant who demonstrates dysfunctional feeding or swallowing is often malnourished and experiences respiratory symptoms with significant Risk for Aspiration. Nurses often regard circumoral cyanosis, duskiness, and tachypnea as indicators of respiratory changes during feeding.[6,11] Other clinical manifestations of dysfunctional feeding include gagging, choking, coughing, apnea, bradycardia, wheezing, and chronic congestion.[6,7,12]

Providing nourishment and caring for the infant is central to the parent-infant relationship. Parent-infant bonding is enhanced by the parents' ability to provide pleasurable, relaxed, and satisfying feedings for their infant. Parents influence their infant's feeding behavior, but the infant also exerts a substantial influence on the parents and other family members.

Classic studies by Ainsworth and Bell[1] suggest that infant feeding is most successful when parents are sensitive to the infant cues elicited. Important to note are the timing, amount, preference, pacing, and eating capabilities of the infant. Parents and infants reciprocally refine the feeding process,

acquiring skill and regulating their adaptability. Feeding begins with an in-and-out pattern of moving the tongue or suckling and the reflexive suck-swallow and breathing responses in the newborn. The suck consists of an up-and-down motion, the dorsum of the tongue in harmony with the mandible. The lips are tightly closed around the nipple to draw out liquid from the breast or bottle. The suckle/suck-swallow response continues in the infant until approximately 4 to 6 months of age.[15]

The infant's breathing pattern is coordinated with swallowing. Respiration ceases during the pharyngeal stage of swallowing.[5] The presence of a nipple, coupled with the infant's small oropharynx, requires nose breathing. The infant who experiences any type of respiratory difficulty does not feed well. Infants with prematurity, neurological impairment, central nervous system dysfunction, severe gastrointestinal disease, or congenital anomalies may demonstrate an uncoordinated suck-swallow response and require prolonged enteral or parenteral feedings.

The literature supports the concept of a critical period related to feeding development.[1,7,8,11] Infants receiving enteral or parenteral feedings are precluded from opportunities to practice suck, swallow, and breathing patterns in relation to their satiety and self-regulation of dietary intake.[11] Prolonged gavage feedings present the infant with repeated and unpleasant stimulation of the mouth, pharynx, and esophagus. Oral hypersensitivity places the infant at risk for defensive and resistant feeding. Infants at risk for an ineffective feeding pattern require a plan of care that includes an oral

II

stimulation program to prevent feeding resistance and to acquire positive oral-feeding skills.

ASSESSMENT

Each infant must be assessed individually regarding the ability to initiate, sustain, and coordinate sucking with swallowing and breathing. The appropriate feeding schedule and method are an essential part of nutritional management for the infant. Feeding times and methods may have to be changed or adjusted several times before the correct combination is determined.

Chatoor and others[4] report that feeding disturbances occurring during the first 3 months may be due to the infant's physical limitations, such as poor coordination of the oropharyngeal musculature; congenital anomalies of the gastrointestinal tract (cleft lip, cleft palate, esophageal atresia, and tracheoesophageal fistula); or a liable autonomic nervous system (oral hypersensitivity in an infant difficult to calm). These problems may be further compounded by limited parental sensitivity and responsiveness to the infant's feeding cues.

The assessment of infant feeding interactions can be readily attained with the use of the Chatoor Observational Scale for mother-infant/toddler interaction during feeding,[5] the Barnard Nursing Child Assessment Feeding scale,[2] or the Price AMIS Scale of sensitivity in mother-infant interactions.[10]

Feeding the premature infant presents a particular challenge for the nurse. Gestational age, physical condition, and neurological status must be assessed. Severe mental retardation presents Risk for Aspiration to the infant who has difficulty sucking or who has an uncoordinated suck, swallow, and breathing response. Apnea during feeding may occur in the premature infant when milk or formula flows too quickly for a swallow. Other signs and symptoms of difficulty during feeding include tachypnea, coughing, choking, cyanosis, bradycardia, and sleepiness.[6,7,12]

Intermittent gavage feeding is the method of choice for the infant with an uncoordinated suck-swallow response or who tires easily while nip-

pling.[7,11] One complication of long-term gavage feeding is that the infant is deprived of the pleasures and comforts of sucking. Infants who experience sucking during gavage feedings are better prepared for nutritive sucking.[3,7,8,11]

The nursing process is of particular importance in the management of Ineffective Infant Feeding Pattern because of the amount of time the nurse is engaged in the observation, handling, and feeding of the infant.[7,11] The nurse continually revises and modifies the plan of care until the infant is tolerating feedings and thriving.

▪ Defining Characteristics

The presence of the following defining characteristics indicates that the infant may be experiencing Ineffective Infant Feeding Pattern:

- Inability to initiate or sustain an effective suck
- Inability to coordinate sucking, swallowing, and breathing

▪ Related Factors

The following related factors are associated with Ineffective Infant Feeding Pattern:

- Prematurity
- Poor coordination of the oropharyngeal musculature
- Congenital anomalies
- Surgery of the gastrointestinal tract
- Neurological impairment or delay
- Weight loss
- Hyperirritability
- Oral hypersensitivity
- Lethargy
- Sedation
- Prolonged NPO status
- Force feeding
- Delayed feeding
- Failing to feed to satiety

DIAGNOSIS

▪ Differential Nursing Diagnosis

Ineffective Infant Feeding Pattern can be differentiated from the diagnoses Altered Nutrition:

Less Than Body Requirements and Ineffective Breastfeeding when the related factors and defining characteristics that apply to each diagnosis are carefully considered. Infant feeding problems can be the result of a physical condition, an inappropriate food choice, a maladaptive parent-infant feeding interaction, or a combination of these factors. The infant is unable to initiate or sustain the suck or to coordinate the suck, swallow, and breathing pattern required to feed effectively. In contrast, the infant diagnosed with Altered Nutrition: Less Than Body Requirements is able to coordinate the suck, swallow, and breathing pattern and has an adequate food intake. The difficulties lie in the digestion or absorption of nutrients as evidenced by the infant's weight loss. No problem exists with initiating or sustaining the suck and coordinating it with breathing. Ineffective Breastfeeding, although encompassing difficulty and dissatisfaction with the breastfeeding process for the mother and infant, involves nursing interventions that exclusively relate to the mother's milk supply and breastfeeding technique. The problem may or may not involve the infant's ability to initiate, sustain, or coordinate the suck. The infant may simply resist latching on to the mother's breast.

■ Medical and Psychiatric Diagnoses

The premature infant presents a particular challenge to the nurse in terms of feeding. Conditions frequently encountered by the preterm infant, such as apnea, bradycardia, asphyxia, sepsis, cardiac defect, and intraventricular hemorrhage, may impair the infant's ability to suck. Intermittent or continuous gavage feedings are the method of choice for infants with these medical conditions. Nursing care is of particular importance because of the amount of time required for observing, handling, and feeding the infant.

OUTCOME IDENTIFICATION, PLANNING, AND IMPLEMENTATION

Nursing care for the infant with an Ineffective Feeding Pattern fosters normal growth and development for the infant and encourages positive parental interaction. Nursing goals ensue the prevention of fatigue and aspiration with feedings and provide for adequate nutrition.[6,7] Research indicates that optimizing parent-infant interaction facilitates effective feeding.[13]

Gavage feeding is the method of choice for the ill or premature infant. Eventually, as the infant demonstrates consistent weight gain and tolerance of gavage feedings (without apneic spells or the presence of residuals), an oral stimulation program is begun. The infant is offered a pacifier with gavage feedings.

As the infant grows and matures, as evidenced by weight gain, length increase, and other increases in body measurements (e.g., head circumference and chest circumference) and continues to tolerate gavage feeding with nonnutritive sucking, a nipple feeding program is instituted. During feedings, the infant is fed in a semisitting position and observed for possible respiratory difficulty and the presence of exhaustion or fatigue.

The neonatal and pediatric nurse can lend guidance and support to parents learning to feed their ill or premature infant. Unlike more primitive societies, our culture provides limited support to parents during the infant's early months.[13] Parents need nursing assistance to learn and initiate effective feeding techniques that are pleasurable to the infant.

The primary goal of infant feeding is to provide the infant with congenial and satisfying feedings. Effective feeding is a dynamic process that depends on the abilities of the infant and the caretaker and that requires much more than getting nutrition into the infant.

II

◢ **NURSING CARE GUIDELINES**
Nursing Diagnosis: Ineffective Infant Feeding Pattern°

Expected Outcome: The infant will ingest adequate amounts of breast milk or formula by nipple or gavage feeding to meet growth needs, as evidenced by no more than a 15% weight loss within the first 3 days of life; steady weight gain of 6 to 8 oz per week; normal fontanelle size and shape; good skin turgor; moist mucous membranes; urine output of 1 to 3 cc per kilogram per hour; and specific gravity less than 1.013.
- Perform A.M. daily weights and document weight gain. *Nipple feedings require energy and calories expenditure; fluctuations in weight are highly sensitive indicators of fluid balance.*
- ▲ Weigh all diapers and record urine specific gravity. *Comparison of intake and output over a 24-hour period provides an accurate indicator of fluid balance.*
- ▲ Supplement nipple feedings with intravenous therapy, as ordered. *This provides additional calories for growth per day.*

Expected Outcome: The infant will tolerate nipple or gavage feeding as evidenced by the absence of respiratory difficulty; no regurgitation; and no emesis.
- ▲ Maintain regular feeding times, and feed the infant for a maximum of 20 to 30 minutes. *This avoids excessive tiring.*
- Observe for and document evidence of tachypnea, choking, coughing, cyanosis, apnea, bradycardia, and sleepiness with feeds. *Indicates feeding difficulty and potential aspiration.*
- Gently burp infant after feeding and position on right side with support. *Prevents gas build-up; enhances gastric emptying and decreases risk of aspiration.*

Expected Outcome: The infant will experience oral gratification and emotional satiety during feeding times as evidenced by calmness, the absence of crying, readiness to suck on the nipple, and cuddling.
- ▲ Hold the infant and provide a pacifier during feedings as tolerated. *These interventions comfort and relax the infant and encourage the sucking reflex.*
- ▲ Initiate nipple feedings with a smaller, more pliable nipple until the sucking reflex becomes strong. *This conserves energy and calories and avoids infant tiring.*
- ▲ Increase nipple feeds slowly and progressively as tolerated. *This provides positive feeding experience.*
- Monitor infant strength and ability to tolerate a regular-size nipple. *This avoids exhaustion, conserves calories, and prevents aspiration.*
- ▲ Involve parents in infant feeding and teach them the appropriate goals, techniques, and behaviors as necessary. *Parent involvement in infant's care promotes infant growth and development and facilitates the parent-child bond.*

■ = nursing intervention; ▲ = collaborative intervention.
°References 1, 3, 13, 14, 15

EVALUATION

The nursing care plan for the infant with an Ineffective Feeding Pattern is successful when the infant demonstrates adequate and consistent weight gain for growth and an improved or normal suck-swallow response during feeding times. The need for gavage feedings will be eliminated, and the infant will tolerate nipple feedings without evidence of exhaustion or fatigue. Parents will have an understanding of feeding dynamics and feel confident in their abilities to provide for the infant's emotional needs during feeding. Together the nurse and the infant's parents address goals, interventions, and modifications for the plan of care to benefit the infant and the family.

II

CASE STUDY WITH PLAN OF CARE

Baby Joey, born at 38 weeks and weighing 7 lb, 9 oz, is the product of a full-term normal pregnancy. Joey's mother is a 25-year-old Gravida 1, Para 1. Apgars were 8 at 1 minute and 9 at 5 minutes. Joey had a vigorous cry and alert appearance. A physical exam revealed no obvious congenital anomalies but diagnosed the presence of a loud, harsh, pansystolic murmur and a palpable thrill. A cardiology follow-up and echocardiogram gave evidence of a small, ventricular septal defect.

The primary nurse noted that Baby Joey was tiring easily when given formula by nipple and was losing more than 2% of his weight each day. Baby Joey's mother was passionately involved in his care and had many concerns about her infant's heart problem and his ability to tolerate nippling. "His pretty blue eyes look so stressed now. I don't want to push him. I can give him all the time he needs to finish. I don't want to lose him."

PLAN OF CARE FOR BABY JOEY

Nursing Diagnosis: Ineffective Infant Feeding Pattern Related to Presence of a Congenital Heart Defect and Prolonged Feeding

Expected Outcome: Baby Joey will tolerate adequate amounts of formula for growth through intermittent nipple and gavage feedings.
- Maintain Joey in a neutral thermal environment.
- Perform daily weights and document weight gain.
- Weigh all diapers and record urine specific gravity.
- Measure abdominal girths, note the presence of distention, and aspirate for gastric residuals before feedings.
- Decrease environmental stress and sensory overload during feedings.
- Supplement nipple and gavage feedings with intravenous therapy as ordered.

Expected Outcome: Baby Joey will demonstrate an improved tolerance of nipple feedings without fatigue.
- Monitor Joey's strength and ability to tolerate a regular-sized nipple with feedings.
- Observe and report any evidence of exhaustion, respiratory distress, or emesis during feeding time.

Expected Outcome: Baby Joey's mother will feel confident in her ability to feed him.
- Encourage the mother to avoid overbundling and excessive cuddling during the baby's feedings.
- Teach the mother to feed Joey in a semisitting position.
- Gently burp Joey after feeding and position him on his right side with support.
▲ Encourage, praise, and reassure Joey's mother as to her feeding technique and effort; reteach appropriate feeding goals and behaviors as necessary.
▲ Provide Joey's mother with additional educational materials as needed.

■ = nursing intervention; ▲ = collaborative intervention.

CRITICAL THINKING EXERCISES

1. Baby Joey's mother has expressed reluctance to continue nipple feeding her infant. "His eyes seem so stressed; I don't want to push him." How can the nurse best respond to assist his mother in understanding key concepts necessary to feed her infant effectively?

2. Based on the nurse's initial observation and assessment of Baby Joey's feeding, what are the corresponding defining characteristics, related factors, and examples of medical diagnoses that

II

support the nursing diagnosis of Ineffective Infant Feeding Pattern?

3. What educational interventions should be included in a teaching plan to assist Baby Joey's mother with her confidence and her ability to feed her infant?

REFERENCES

1. Ainsworth MDS and Bell SM: Some contemporary patterns of mother-infant interaction in the feeding situation. In Ambrose A, editor: *Stimulation in early infancy*, New York, 1969, Academic Press.

2. Barnard KE and others: Measurement and meaning of parent-child interaction. In Morrison F, Lora C, and Keating D, editors: *Applied developmental psychology*, vol 3, New York, 1991, Academic Press.

3. Bragdon D: A basis for the nursing management of feeding the premature infant, *JOGNN* supplement, May/June: 51–57, 1983.

4. Chatoor I, Dickson L, and Schaefer S: A developmental classification of feeding disorders associated with failure to thrive: diagnosis and treatment. In Drotar D, editor: *New directions in failure to thrive: implications for research and practice*, New York, 1986, Plenum Press.

5. Chatoor I, Menville E, Getson P, and O'Connell R: *Observational scale for mother-infant/toddler interaction during feeding*, Washington, D.C., 1989, Children's Hospital Medical Center.

6. Hill AS: Preliminary findings: maximum oral feeding time for premature infants, the relationship to physiological indicators, *Maternal-Child Nurse* 20(2):105–109, 1992.

7. Kinner MD and Beachy P: Nipple feeding premature infants in the neonatal intensive care unit: factors and discussions, *JOGNN* 23(2):81–95, 1994.

8. McCain GC: Promotion of pre-term infant nipple feeding with nonnutritive sucking, *J Pediatr Nurs* 10(1):3–8, 1995.

9. North American Nursing Diagnosis Association: *NANDA nursing diagnoses: definitions and classification, 1995–1996*, Philadelphia, 1994, The Association.

10. Price GM: Sensitivity in mother-infant interactions: the AMS Scale, *Infant Behav Dev* 6:353–360, 1983.

11. Pridham K, Sondel S, Chang A, and Green C: Nipple feeding for pre-term infants with broncho-pulmonary dysplasia, *JOGNN* 22(2):147–155, 1993.

12. Richard ME: Feeding the newborn with cleft lip and/or palate: the enlargement, stimulate, swallow, rest (ESSR) method, *J Pediatr Nurs* 6(5):317–320, 1991.

13. Satter EM: The feeding relationship: problems and interventions, *J Pediatr* 117:184, 1990.

14. Satyshur RD: Ineffective infant feeding pattern. In *Clinical nursing*, St. Louis, 1993, Mosby–Year Book.

15. Stevenson RD and Allaire JH: The development of normal feeding and swallowing, *Pediatr Clin North Am* 38:1450, 1991.

Altered Nutrition: Risk for More Than Body Requirements

▶

Altered Nutrition: More Than Body Requirements

▶

Altered Nutrition: Less Than Body Requirements

▶

Altered Nutrition: Risk for More Than Body Requirements *is the state in which an individual is at risk of experiencing an intake of nutrients that exceeds metabolic needs.*[17]

Altered Nutrition: More Than Body Requirements *is the state in which an individual is experiencing an intake of nutrients that exceeds metabolic needs.*[17]

Altered Nutrition: Less Than Body Requirements *is the state in which an individual experiences an intake of nutrients insufficient to meet metabolic needs.*[17]

OVERVIEW

Nutrition can be described as an end product resulting from the ingestion, digestion, absorption, transportation, utilization, and excretion of nutrients and their metabolites. Alterations in nutrition, either more than or less than body requirements, may be the result of various physiological, psychological, sociocultural, and environmental factors.

Altered Nutrition: Risk for More Than Body Requirements or Altered Nutrition: More Than Body Requirements is a human response prevalent in the United States today. Twenty-four percent of adult men and 27% of adult women are overweight. This health problem is worsening in spite of the numerous commercial diets and exercise facilities available. Excess body weight is more prevalent in African-Americans and Hispanic-Americans than in the European-American population. The incidence of overweight increases with age but is more prevalent in women than men.[24]

All activities require energy in the form of calories derived from carbohydrates, protein, and fat. A state of energy balance can be calculated by comparing energy intake with energy output. Body fat is formed and weight increases when one consumes more calories than are expended. For example, if a person consumes 500 extra calories a day for 7 days with no increase in exercise, 1 pound of body fat will be gained, which is equal to 3500 calories.[6] *Overweight* can be described as weight in excess of one's recommended weight for one's age; *obesity* is an excess of body weight. Obesity is categorized as follows:

- Mild obesity: 120% to 140% of ideal body weight
- Moderate obesity: 141% to 200% of ideal body weight
- Severe or morbid obesity: more than 200% of ideal body weight

Overeating was long believed to be the main cause of weight gain and obesity, but several alternative theories have recently been formulated to attempt to explain the etiology of this problem. The theories can be grouped into four categories: (1) hereditary, (2) environmental (family, culture, and community), (3) physiological, and (4) psychological.

Heredity is a major factor in determining whether an adult will be obese. Successions of family generations tend to show the same amount of weight gain and body configuration, supporting heredity as a strong influence in obesity. Obese children tend to have parents who are also overweight or obese.[21] Research indicates that adopted children have different patterns of weight gain than their adoptive parents and siblings.[10] The "fat cell" theory supports the belief that obese individuals of all ages tend to have more fat cells than children and adults of normal weight. Although cell size can decrease with dieting, the number of fat cells remains constant, making weight loss difficult because of the energy needed by these cells.[4]

Family, culture, and community also influence the type and amount of food one consumes and the activity in which one participates. Fatness tends to be passed from generation to generation, making the eating habits and customs of a family important environmental factors when considering a risk for obesity. For example, unattended bottle feeding of infants, using food as a comfort measure, overfeeding, and valuing chubbiness in babies are contributors to early development of obesity.[22] Using food as a reward for good behavior and allowing children to eat nutritionally inadequate foods can result in excess weight in later years.[2,16] A correlation also exists between the number of hours of television viewed and obesity in adolescents.[5] Other environmental factors that influence weight gain are level of income and educational level. For women, the lower the income and education, the greater the incidence of obesity. For men, obesity is more common in higher income brackets and with higher educational levels.[10]

Physiological bases for obesity include the set point theory, thermogenesis, and endocrine imbalances. The set point theory states that each person

has an ideal biological weight, established by biological or genetic factors and controlled by the hypothalamus. When fat stores fall below a certain level, the body adjusts its metabolic rate to maintain its adipose tissue, making it impossible for some people to lose weight.[4] *Thermogenesis* is heat production that rids the body of excess energy. People of normal weight have an increase in thermogenesis after eating, whereas obese people tend to have a lower thermogenic response to eating. This may be due to a lower availability of adenosine diphosphate–burning sites, which are responsible for utilizing energy not associated with physical activity.[21] An insufficiency of thyroid hormone may lower the basal metabolic rate, leading to weight gain. Obesity is also related to adipose and muscle cell insulin resistance, contributing to non-insulin-dependent diabetes mellitus.

Psychological causes for obesity are more difficult to identify. Research shows that persons with strong support systems, positive self-esteem, and healthy relationships participate in lifestyles and eating habits that promote health.[12,15] Positive correlations are found between depression and weight gain,[18] and between negative body image and obesity in females.[19]

Altered Nutrition: Less Than Body Requirements occurs in all age groups, at any point on the health-illness continuum, and in all sociocultural and economic classes. Persons most at risk for nutritional deficits are those with low income, the elderly, and hospitalized patients. Asian-American elderly are often underweight and are especially at risk for poor nutritional status related to poor calcium intake.[13]

When the intake of nutrients is less than body requirements, certain adaptive changes take place. Glycogen stores are depleted during starvation, and the fasting body begins to break down proteins and fats to maintain blood glucose levels. As the body loses its protein and fat stores, a negative nitrogen balance results. Healthy individuals of normal weight can lose only 35% to 40% of their normal weight. This figure represents about one third of total body protein, and losses exceeding this amount are fatal. If the person is deficient in nutrients and weight, a smaller loss is critical.[7]

Nutritional deficits may be classified as primary or secondary. Primary deficiencies are the result of failure to meet normal nutritional needs because of an inadequate food intake. The deficit may result from poor food habits, lack of knowledge about selecting and preparing foods, inadequate economic resources, or lack of facilities to prepare and store food. Secondary nutritional deficits occur when other physiological factors interfere with the utilization of nutrients, even though the diet is sufficient. These factors include but are not limited to growth spurts, pregnancy, chemical dependency, anorexia nervosa, disease, and pharmacotherapeutic treatments.

ASSESSMENT

The nurse must collect subjective and objective data to assess the patient's nutritional metabolic pattern effectively. Subjective data includes a dietary history. A 24-hour recall of food intake or a 3- to 7-day eating and activity diary is a useful tool in determining nutritional status. A food diary should contain the following information: time of day food is eaten, minutes spent eating, activity while eating, location of meals, type and quantity of food eaten, food preferences and intolerances, people present, and feelings while eating. Objective data include height, daily weights, arm circumference, skin fold measurements, and caloric intake. Other Functional Health Patterns that influence the patient's nutritional status and that should be assessed are the Elimination Pattern, the Activity-Exercise Pattern, the Role-Relationship Pattern, the Self-Perception—Self-Concept Pattern, and the Value-Belief Pattern.

Altered Nutrition: Risk for More Than Body Requirements

The objective defining characteristics of this diagnosis include the presence of related physiological or psychological problems or a body weight that is in the upper limits of the normal range for that individual. Two subjective defining characteristics considered critical for this diagnosis are (1) reported overweight or obesity of one or both parents and (2) reported accelerated growth in infancy and childhood. If a patient has always been larger than most of his or her peers, there is a high risk for that trend to continue in adulthood.

In addition, a 1-week food diary of the amount and types of food eaten, where it was eaten, activities accompanying eating, and the time required to finish eating is useful. Consumption of a high-fat diet can predispose one to obesity.[3] Obese people do not eat more per meal than nonobese people, but they tend to eat at a steadier pace without slowing their intake as satiety occurs.[9] Eating while engaging in other activities such as reading or watching television can contribute to weight gain because these activities tend to reduce awareness of the amount of food being eaten. Eating more calories at the end of the day can promote weight gain because calorie utilization is reduced during sleep. Eating for reasons other than hunger, such as at a particular time of day, in a social situation for which eating is customary, or at times of anxiety or loneliness can also promote weight gain.[23] Finally, a history of weight retention after pregnancy can predispose a patient to obesity. Therefore a history of the amount of weight gained with each pregnancy should be ascertained, and the length of time required to return to baseline weight should be calculated.

■ Risk Factors

The presence of the following behaviors, conditions, or circumstances renders the patient more vulnerable to Altered Nutrition: Risk for More Than Body Requirements:

- Obesity in one or both parents
- Rapid growth in infants or children
- History of weight retention after pregnancy
- History of consuming a high-fat diet[3]
- Dysfunctional eating patterns
- Eating in response to cues other than hunger
- Using food for rewards
- Low self-esteem

Altered Nutrition: More Than Body Requirements

In addition to assessing food intake and anthropometric measurements the nurse needs to assess the patient's level of motivation. Does the patient want to lose weight? What value does the patient see in weight loss? Does the patient feel capable of losing weight? What are the reasons the patient wants to lose weight? If the patient's reasons are based on social or family pressures, the patient probably will not succeed.[4]

The patient's body image and level of self-esteem should also be assessed. What is the patient's level of socialization? Does this patient have meaningful personal goals and feel accepted by others, including family and society? Social and family support is essential for a dieter to succeed in weight loss. Lack of understanding, jealousy, and negative attitudes regarding weight loss by significant others impede success.

A history of the patient's age at onset and the duration of the weight gain, as well as a description and the results of diets and exercise used in the past, are also pertinent. Daily activities should be assessed along with any regular exercise patterns because a sedentary lifestyle lends itself to obesity. Ask the patient about reasons for not dieting and not exercising. Also determine if the patient has had any associated medical diseases (cardiovascular, respiratory, endocrine, or neuromuscular).

■ Defining Characteristics

The presence of the following defining characteristics indicates that the patient may be experiencing Altered Nutrition: More Than Body Requirements:

- Weight 10% to 20% over ideal for height and body frame
- Triceps >15 mm in males, >25 mm in females
- Dysfunctional eating patterns
- Sedentary lifestyle

■ Related Factors

The following related factors are associated with Altered Nutrition: More Than Body Requirements:

- Intake greater than metabolic need
- Heredity; obesity in parents
- Lower metabolic rate
- Income
- Educational level
- Eating patterns
- Family customs
- Family values
- Thermogenetic response
- Stress
- Depression
- Lack of support systems
- Low self-esteem

Altered Nutrition: Less Than Body Requirements

The defining characteristics for Altered Nutrition: Less Than Body Requirements are focused on weight loss, interest in and availability of food, and body functions. The characteristics are (1) loss of weight with adequate food intake, (2) body weight 20% or more under the ideal for height and frame, and (3) reported inadequate intake of nutrients falling below Recommended daily Allowances (RDA).[17] Defining characteristics specific to food interest and availability are (1) reported or evident lack of food, (2) lack of interest in food, (3) perceived inability to ingest food, and (4) aversion to eating. Functional defining characteristics are (1) weakness of muscles required for swallowing or mastication, (2) reported altered taste sensation, (3) satiety immediately after ingesting food, (4) abdominal pain with or without pathological conditions, and (5) a sore, inflamed buccal cavity.[9]

Physical assessments that indicate undernutrition are summarized in Table 2. Anthropometric measurements (obtained with skin calipers, scales, and a measuring tape) include height and weight; circumference of the triceps, subscapular area, and midarm; and triceps skinfold. Data supporting this diagnosis are a weight 20% or more below the ideal for a specific height and frame and measurements of arm circumference and skinfolds less than 90% of the reference standard.[7]

Biochemical data, such as serum albumin (normal = 4 to 5 g/dl) and transferrin (normal =

205 to 410 mg/dl), are especially useful for assessing nutritional deficits. A low total lymphocyte count is also commonly found when nutrition is less than body requirements. Nitrogen balance can be measured and used as an indicator of anabolism or catabolism of protein. A negative nitrogen balance indicates a catabolic state in which protein is lost from muscles and other tissues and metabolic demands are not being met.[9]

Questions specific to this diagnosis relate to the ability to chew and swallow; appetite; food likes, dislikes, and intolerances; and bowel habits. The dietary guides used are the 24-hour food recall and a diary of all food and beverages consumed over a specific period of time (usually 3 to 7 days). Information obtained with these guides is highly subjective and depends on normal cognitive function.

■ Defining Characteristics

The presence of the following defining characteristics indicates that the patient may be experiencing Altered Nutrition: Less Than Body Requirements:

- Inadequate food intake
- 10% to 20% below ideal body weight

- Low serum albumin
- Low serum transferrin
- Triceps skinfold or arm circumference <60% standard
- Sore, inflamed buccal cavity
- Weak chewing or swallowing muscles
- Abdominal cramping and pain
- Poor muscle tone
- Altered taste sensation
- Aversion to food
- Lack of interest in food
- Lack of information
- Perceived inability to ingest food

■ Related Factors

The following related factors are associated with Altered Nutrition: Less Than Body Requirements:

- Lack of knowledge
- Pregnancy
- Stress
- Peer pressure
- Poor living conditions
- Inadequate income
- Homelessness
- Social influences
- Lack of transportation

TABLE 2 Physical Assessments Indicative of Altered Nutrition: Less Than Body Requirements

Body Area Assessed	Abnormal Data
Hair	Dull, dry, brittle, sparse
Eyes	Zerophthalmia; Bitot's spots; increased vascularity; kerkeratomalacia
Lips, buccal cavity	Cheilosis; angular fissures; red, swollen lesions
Tongue	Smooth, swollen, beefy red, atrophic papillae
Gums	Spongy, recessed, bleed easily
Skin	Rough, dry, pale, petechiae; lacking subcutaneous fat; loss of turgor
Muscles	Wasted, flaccid; tenderness; weakness; loss of tone
Nervous system	Decreased or absent knee and ankle reflexes; lethargy; irritability
Cardiovascular	Cardiomegaly; bradycardia at rest and tachycardia with exercise; hypotension
Skeletal	Prominent ribs, scapula; bowed legs or knock-knees
Abdomen	Enlarged, hepatomegaly

DIAGNOSIS

■ Differential Nursing Diagnosis

Altered Nutrition: More Than Body Requirements may be used inappropriately if the patient's main problem is more closely related to the diagnoses Altered Health Maintenance Management, Ineffective Management of Therapeutic Regimen, or Ineffective Individual Coping. The patient needs to be assessed carefully to explore the possibility of one of these other underlying related nursing diagnoses. Altered Nutrition: More Than Body Requirements can be used when the weight gain is related to a physiological, metabolic, or chemical change. This diagnosis may require more collaborative medical interventions to treat the underlying physiological etiology. However, the nurse has a major role in assisting the patient with understanding and maintaining a plan of care to promote weight reduction. Altered Nutrition: Risk for More Than Body Requirements is used when the patient is at risk for gaining excessive weight related to past history or a recent change in chemical or metabolic processes.

Altered Nutrition: Less Than Body Requirements may also be used inappropriately if the patient's problem is actually Impaired Swallowing or Altered Oral Mucous Membranes. It is important to determine the etiology of the problem to use this diagnosis correctly.

■ Medical and Psychiatric Diagnoses

Medical diagnoses commonly related to the nursing diagnosis Risk for More Than Body requirements include non-insulin-dependent diabetes mellitus, Cushing's syndrome, thyroid deficiencies, and hypothalamic abnormalities. Utilization of carbohydrates is decreased in diabetes, which can lead to weight gain. In Cushing's syndrome, increased cortisone increases the process of gluconeogenesis and decreases the action of insulin, which leads to weight gain in addition to that caused by fluid retention. Psychological diagnoses such as depression and low self-esteem may also predispose a patient to weight gain.

Patients who have the nursing diagnosis Altered Nutrition: More Than Body Requirements are at risk for developing several cardiovascular complications because, as body weight rises, serum cholesterol rises. These complications may include coronary artery disease, hypertension, and hypercholesterolemia. Adipose cells in obese patients may develop insulin resistance and result in non-insulin-dependent diabetes. Severe obesity can also lead to a premature death. Obesity often has an even greater effect on the psychological status of the patient. Overweight individuals are often influenced by social pressures in a society that emphasizes the advantages and beauty associated with being thin. Obese children and adults may feel rejected by society when they are viewed as being unclean or lazy. Prolonged psychological stress may lead to depression in the obese patient.

Several medical diagnoses predispose the patient to Altered Nutrition: Less Than Body Requirements. These include but are not limited to Crohn's disease, achlorhydria, acquired immunodeficiency syndrome (AIDS), metastatic diseases, hepatic cirrhosis, burns, endocrine disorders, gastrointestinal surgery, and parasitic infestation. Medical treatments associated with Altered Nutrition: Less Than Body Requirements include gastrointestinal surgery, chemotherapy, and radiation therapy. Psychological diagnoses that lead to weight loss include anorexia nervosa, bulimic eating disorder, substance abuse disorders, and often major depression. Infectious disease is often the precipitating factor of weight loss with the elderly.[25]

OUTCOME IDENTIFICATION, PLANNING, AND IMPLEMENTATION

Altered Nutrition: Risk for More Than Body Requirements

The implications of obesity for health are an important component in teaching the patient with Altered Nutrition: Risk for More Than Body Requirements. Education should include an explanation of what obesity is and what specific factors increase the potential for its development. The implications for health include a discussion of the effects of excess body weight on the cardiovascular system, on longevity, and on mental health. The patient should be able to understand and discuss this information.

Behavioral modification begins with self-monitoring. By keeping a daily eating diary, the patient can identify patterns of food intake that result in obesity. This diary is an effective way to help patients develop an awareness of dietary patterns to keep them actively involved in the plan of care.

The patient must know how to make proper food choices to develop effective menu plans. The nurse should teach about the food pyramid; the distribution of proteins, carbohydrates, and fats in foods that are a part of the patient's normal diet; and the caloric requirements for this specific patient.

The nurse can help the patient identify and plan modifications of behaviors associated with excess food intake. This may include such modifications as eating only when sitting at the table with a complete place setting, eliminating reading or watching television while eating, taking small bites and chewing thoroughly, placing the fork on the plate between bites, drinking water before and during meals, and learning the difference between appetite and hunger. The patient needs to be actively involved in selecting behaviors to be modified.

Physical activity is an essential component in any weight-control program. The exercise program should be based on activities that the patient enjoys and be tailored to the patient's tolerance level.

Individuals who become overweight or obese often have lower self-esteem than those of normal weight. Once goals have been established and weight loss begins, the patient should begin to show evidence of a positive self-image through discussion and actions. The nurse should include a teaching plan mutual goal setting that is realistic in terms of actual food intake, a change in eating behaviors, and an exercise program.

Altered Nutrition: More Than Body Requirements

An individual's eating behaviors are influenced by people with whom he or she interacts daily.[8]

People who influence food choices include the spouse, family members, co-workers, colleagues, and peers. Other influences on eating behaviors include ethnic and cultural backgrounds, family traditions, age group, and environmental factors such as type of employment and hours worked. The spouse and family must understand and be involved in the patient's weight-loss program for success in meeting goals. Patients should be encouraged to participate in weight-loss competitions at their place of employment, and to join community programs such as Weight Watchers or Take Off Pounds Sensibly (TOPS).

Monitoring patient activities will identify behaviors that can be changed or that increase caloric expenditure. For example, the patient may decide to park the car a longer distance from work and walk the remaining distance or take stairs rather than ride elevators. The patient may also become involved in a regular exercise program at a community recreation center. Before participating in any exercise program, the patient should have a thorough health assessment, following the recommendations of the American College of Sports Medicine. The behavior changes that are mutually agreed on should be written in contract form; allowing some type of reward for each successful behavior change may facilitate patient compliance.

The nurse has an important role in teaching the patient how to restrict calories and maintain a nutritionally sound diet. Calories should come from all four food groups and not fall below 1000 to 1200 calories per day for women and 1200 to 1500 calories per day for men.[14] To calculate calorie restriction, determine the recommended caloric requirement for ideal body weigh and subtract the necessary number of calories per day for desired weight loss (e.g., 500 calories per day results in a weight loss of 1 pound per week; 1000 calories per day results in a weight loss of 2 pounds per week.)[7] Encourage patients to read food labels and to be aware of the calorie and fat content of foods. The patient should plan to reduce calories by 500 calories for each pound of body weight he or she desires to lose.

◢ **NURSING CARE GUIDELINES**
Nursing Diagnosis: Altered Nutrition: Risk for More Than Body Requirements

Expected Outcome: The patient will identify risk factors and defining characteristics that promote the potential for weight gain by the end of the first teaching session.
- Teach the patient hereditary, environmental, physiological, and psychological factors that predispose the individual to weight gain.
▲ Discuss the patient's current health status in relation to defining characteristics and risk factors of this diagnosis. *Patient health education is the teaching-learning process of influencing patient and family behavior through changes in knowledge, attitudes, and beliefs.*

Expected Outcome: The patient will self-monitor eating habits and activities for 1 week, then identify behaviors that need modification to prevent weight gain.
- Explain the process of keeping a daily diary.
- Contact the patient midweek to determine compliance and offer assistance.
- Analyze the diary with the patient, and assist with identification of needed behavioral changes. *Analysis of the log by the patient and the nurse will reveal eating patterns, including which stimuli lead to eating, the types of foods eaten, what precipitates eating, the most likely times and places for eating, and amount of exercise.*

Expected Outcome: The patient will develop 1-week menus based on the individual's own caloric and nutritional needs.
- Teach the patient his or her normal weight range, the food pyramid, recommended caloric intake, and use of food substitution and exchanges. *By knowing basic body requirements, the patient can make informed choices for meals and snacks.*

Expected Outcome: The patient will change two eating-related behaviors per week that might cause weight gain.
- Discuss the effects on intake of concurrent activities, a rigid eating schedule, rapid eating, and varied eating locations.
- Assist the patient in choosing behaviors to be changed.
- Positively reinforce each successful behavior change.
- Support the patient through each failure. *All of these behaviors are helpful in controlling the amount of food intake.*

Expected Outcome: The patient will establish a physical activity routine reaching 20 to 30 minutes' duration four or five times per week.
- Teach the patient initial steps to take, such as using stairs instead of the elevator or walking to destinations.
- Encourage the patient to initiate a regular walking program, with gradually increasing distances.
- Investigate more vigorous activities with the patient, following the advise of a physician. *Exercise, when part of a diet program, increases weight loss through loss of fat rather than muscle and also improves muscle tone, cardiopulmonary status, and mental attitude.*[20]

Expected Outcome: The patient will show evidence of improved self-image by making positive statements about self and taking the initiative in setting goals once he or she begins to lose weight.
- Use a nonjudgmental approach toward the patient's behavior.
- Avoid critical comments when the patient fails to meet specific goals. *A higher level of self-esteem may enhance the motivation to lose weight.*[1]
- Encourage realistic short-term goals.
- Establish a reward system with the patient.

■ = nursing intervention; ▲ = collaborative intervention.

■ Encourage the patient to make choices and take responsibility for actions. *Unrealistic expectations about weight loss or exercise capability may lead to feelings of defeat and failure, which in turn can cause the patient to give up and return to previous weight-increasing behaviors.*

◀ **NURSING CARE GUIDELINES**
Nursing Diagnosis: Altered Nutrition: More Than Body Requirements

Expected Outcome: The patient will identify some form of social support for dieting and exercise.
■ Inform the patient of the significance of social support in influencing eating and exercise habits.
■ Provide information on community programs.
■ Inform the family of their role in the patient's success. *Counseling and referrals for social support are essential in promoting successful, long-lasting, healthy eating habits.*

Expected Outcome: The patient will monitor weight, diet, and exercise activities for 2 weeks to identify those activities and eating habits that can be changed to reduce caloric intake and to increase energy expenditure.
■ Teach the patient the methods and significance of self-assessment and rewards in promoting weight loss. *Eating and exercise habits are learned behaviors and can be modified by specific behavioral strategies.*

Expected Outcome: The patient will reduce caloric intake by 500 calories a day for each pound of weight loss per week.
■ Teach the patient how to calculate ideal body weight and calorie restriction.
■ Teach the patient methods of decreasing caloric intake. *The patient should consume only enough calories to promote a 1- to 2-pound weight loss each week. Limiting fat intake can greatly decrease calorie intake.*

Expected Outcome: The patient will participate in a plan of exercise for 20 to 30 minutes three to four times a week.
■ Assist the patient with developing an individualized exercise plan. *Exercise increases metabolic rate, suppresses appetite, reduces fat percentage, lowers blood pressure, lowers serum glucose and lipid levels, relieves tension, and improves self-concept.*

■ = nursing intervention; ▲ = collaborative intervention.

Obese people often resist exercise because of embarrassment caused by poor body image or the discomfort caused by excess weight. The patient should start any exercise program slowly and build up to 20 to 30 minutes of exercise three to four times a week. Elevating the resting heart rate to 40% to 60% of its maximum rate will burn up stored fat as energy.

Altered Nutrition: Less Than Body Requirements

The plan of care to improve nutrition for patients with Altered Nutrition: Less Than Body Requirements must include activities to meet sev-eral physical and psychosocial needs. In most instances, expected patient outcomes are long-term, with improvement taking 6 to 8 months. Despite this long time period, nursing interventions are beneficial in meeting nutritional needs and in coordinating nutritional care activities at any level of deficiency.

The reasons for nutritional deficits and significant risk factors should be discussed with the patient. The patient needs to be able to identify risk factors that cause the nutritional deficit in order to take an active role in planning effective interventions to promote weight gain. Interventions to facilitate improved nutrition are independent and

II

◀ **NURSING CARE GUIDELINES**

Nursing Diagnosis: Altered Nutrition: Less Than Body Requirements

---

Expected Outcome: The patient will identify the factors that cause nutritional deficits.
- Discuss significant risk factors with the patient.
- Document nutritional status with physical assessments, anthropometric measurements, nursing history, and food history and patterns. This provides a baseline assessment to determine outcome goals for the patient. *Understanding the cause of problems often helps reduce anxiety and facilitates compliance with the plan of care.*

Expected Outcome: The patient will improve and maintain food intake to meet metabolic demands.
- Encourage verbalization by the patient and the family of preferred mealtimes, meal locations, and food likes and dislikes.
- Encourage personal care and an environment conducive to enhanced appetite, including oral hygiene, clean surroundings, and encouragement of family members to bring food from home and visit during mealtimes.
- Schedule procedures so they do not conflict with meals.
- Administer ordered medications for pain or nausea. *Good oral hygiene improves the taste of food, making it more palatable, and also helps prevent oral infections. Proper positioning is necessary for chewing and swallowing. Foods that are palatable and have the correct texture and temperature can improve appetite. Procedures should be scheduled so they do not interfere with mealtimes.*
- Teach the patient to prepare or buy high-protein, high-calorie supplements. *Liquid supplements can help meet the patient's metabolic needs when intake is difficult.*
- Encourage the patient to vary food textures and tastes. *A variety of food can stimulate one's appetite.*
- Encourage the patient to eat with others in a pleasant, relaxed atmosphere. *Social isolation, excessive noise, and noxious stimuli can decrease one's appetite.*

■ = nursing intervention; ▲ = collaborative intervention.

---

collaborative. Independent interventions include oral hygiene, positioning, food service, and schedule coordination. Environmental interventions to improve appetite and food intake include the elimination or reduction of unpleasant sights, sounds, and odors to make eating more pleasurable.

Psychosocial support can be provided by therapeutic communications, by encouraging participation in meals by family members or other significant others, and by referrals to community agencies, therapists, or other health care providers (such as social workers, dietitians, or ministers). The patient should always be involved to increase self-esteem and to promote psychological security.

Teaching about diet involves the nurse, the patient, the family, and other members of the health care team. Included in the teaching plan should be nutritional guidelines, risk factors, and self-care activities to improve nutrition. If nutritional status does not improve, referrals should be made for sup-plemental or parenteral feedings, psychological counseling, or community support systems.

EVALUATION

The nurse and the patient must meet frequently at planned times to assess the patient's nutritional status. These meetings should include a review of the patient's diary or log of eating patterns, Activity-Exercise Patterns, and Elimination Patterns. Regular measurements of skinfold, arm circumference, and caloric intake should also be reviewed. The patient and nurse will mutually determine which outcomes have or have not been met.

Altered Nutrition: Risk for More Than Body Requirements

The patient's knowledge of risk factors and defining characteristics of Altered Nutrition: More Than Body Requirements can be evaluated by asking the patient questions at the end of the first teaching session to determine the need to provide more information. Consideration needs to be given to an alternative teaching method if the patient is not able to identify personal risk factors at this time. Review and evaluate weekly the patient's daily diary of eating and activity patterns. Praise and encourage patterns that will prevent weight gain. Discuss those eating and activity patterns that promote weight gain for the patient to understand which goals are not being met. Explore reasons for the ineffective eating and activity patterns. Assist the patient to find reasonable alternatives to prevent weight gain. Perhaps the planned physical activity is too strenuous for the patient and a less vigorous exercise plan is needed as a starting point. Other menu plans may need to be examined to meet the patient's needs and preferences better. Ask the patient how he or she feels about self and the plan of care. If the patient does not make positive comments about self, reevaluate short-term goals to plan more achievable outcomes to enhance the patient's self-esteem.

Altered Nutrition: More Than Body Requirements

Evaluate the patient's social support systems that will facilitate proper dieting and exercise to promote weight loss. Encourage the patient to continue to be a part of any support systems that promote a healthy Nutritional-Metabolic Pattern and Activity-Exercise Pattern. However, if the patient is not an active participant in the support group, explore other supportive alternatives that may be more meaningful to the patient. Review a 2-week dietary and activity diary kept by the patient to identify dysfunctional eating and activity patterns. Reevaluate the patient's dietary intake and activity diary and daily weights 1 week after an activity and dietary plan is agreed on by the nurse and the patient. If the patient's weight loss goal has not been met, determine if caloric intake has been reduced by 500 calories per day for each desired pound of weight loss. Discuss any discrepancies with the patient to reset more realistic outcomes and to increase patient understanding of the importance of reduced caloric intake and a planned activity-exercise schedule.

Altered Nutrition: Less Than Body Requirements

Evaluate the patient's understanding of the cause of the nutritional deficit, the defining characteristics, and the risk factors by the end of the first teaching session. Continue to discuss and explain any unclear areas. Monitor daily caloric intake and body weight. If there is no improvement in food intake, explore other food preferences and alternatives (supplements) with the patient and family. Determine if the mealtime atmosphere and the company are conducive to stimulating one's appetite.

■ CASE STUDY WITH PLAN OF CARE

Mr. Tom P., a 63-year-old African-American, was admitted to the hospital with the chief complaint of weight loss. Mr. P.'s last admission was 6 months earlier, when a diagnosis of cancer of the colon was made. A colon resection was done, and chemotherapy was started with doxorubicin hydrochloride (Adriamycin). Since that time, Mr. P. has become progressively anorexic and nauseated and has lost 23 pounds. At 132 pounds his body weight is 22% below ideal. The following admission physical assessment data were noted: appears cachectic; skin pale with poor turgor; hair dry and brittle; oral cavity shows red, swollen mucosa and tongue; gums spongy and bleed easily; fissures present at corner of mouth; decreased skinfold and midarm circumference; decreased strength and tone in extremity muscles; ankle edema present; and liver palpable 4 cm below costal margin. Mr. P. was accompanied by his wife, who states, "I'll do anything I can to help him get better."

II

◤ PLAN OF CARE FOR MR. TOM P.

Nursing Diagnosis: Altered Nutrition: Less Than Body Requirements Related to Stomatitis Caused by Chemotherapy

Expected Outcome: Mr. P. will identify the side effects of chemotherapy affecting his ability to ingest food.
- Discuss goals and side effects of chemotherapy with Mr. P. and his wife.
- Assess and document physical status, based on admission findings: weigh and record daily at 7:00 A.M.; monitor and report abnormal laboratory data; and assess condition of oral structures twice a day.
- Reinforce previous teaching.

Expected Outcome: Mr. P. will improve and maintain his food intake to meet metabolic needs, as evidenced by a weight gain of 1 to 1 ½ pounds per week; eating 80% to 100% of food; normal laboratory data; skinfold and arm circumference 90% to 100% of ideal; and body weight 80% to 100% of ideal.
- Facilitate self-care and independence by allowing Mr. P. to choose oral care methods and having him choose foods.
- Encourage Mrs. P. to bring food from home and to visit at mealtime (if possible, eat meals in the dayroom).
- Suggest soft, bland foods at moderate temperature.
- ▲ Give antiemetic every 4 hours as ordered, monitor and document effectiveness.
- Give oral care every 2 hours when Mr. P. is awake and before and after meals according to these guidelines: use a toothette or soft toothbrush; use solution of half hydrogen peroxide and half normal saline solution or water; lubricate lips with agent of choice; do *not* use lemon, glycerin, or mouthwash; and give popsicles (ask Mr. P. his flavor preference).
- Give snacks every 2 hours between meals.
- Be sure room is clean and odorless.
- Refer to dietitian.
- Reinforce teaching for Mr. and Mrs. P. about nutritional guidelines.
- Monitor food intake and physical status weekly.
- ▲ If no improvement in 1 to 2 weeks, refer to physician for supplemental or alternate feeding methods.

■ = nursing intervention; ▲ = collaborative intervention.

▦ CRITICAL THINKING EXERCISES

1. How would you begin to assess a patient's Nutritional-Metabolic Pattern?
2. Describe situations when each of the following diagnostic categories is appropriate to use in cases of patient obesity:
   - Altered Nutrition; More Than Body Requirements
   - Altered Health Maintenance Management
   - Ineffective Management of Therapeutic Requirements
   - Ineffective Individual Coping
3. What psychosocial nursing interventions are most important to assist a patient with a weight reduction plan of care?

REFERENCES

1. Allan JD: Women who successfully manage their weight, *Western J Nurs Research* 11(6):657–675, 1989.
2. Anderson JJ: The status of adolescent nutrition, *Nutr Today* 26(2):7–10, 1991.
3. Astrup A and others: Obesity as an adaptation to a high-fat diet: evidence from a cross-sectional study, *Am Soc Clin Nutr* 59:350–355, 1994.
4. Bronwell KD: The psychology and physiology of obesity: implications for screening and treatment, *J Am Dietet Assoc* 84:406, 1984.
5. Dietz WH: You are what you eat—what you eat is what you are, *J Adolesc Health Care* 11:76–81, 1990.
6. Eckstein-Harmon M: Eating disorders: the changing role of nutrition intervention with anorexic and bulimic patients during psychiatric hospitalization, *J Am Dietet Assoc* 93(9):1039–1040, 1993.

7. Escheleman MM: *Introductory nutrition and diet therapy,* ed 2, Philadelphia, 1991, JB Lippincott Co.

8. Farthing MC: Current eating patterns of adolescents in the United States, *Nutr Today* 26(2):35–39, 1991.

9. Food and Nutrition Board, National Academy of Sciences–National Research Council: *Recommended daily allowances,* Washington, D.C., 1980, The Academy.

10. Garn SM, Bailey SM, Cole PE, and Higgins ITT: Level of education, level of income, and level of fatness in adults, *Am J Clin Nutr* 30(5):721–725, 1977.

11. Greenwood MR: *Genetic and metabolic aspects in obesity,* New York, 1983, Churchill-Livingston.

12. Hubbard P, Muhlenkamp AF, and Brown N: The relationship between social support and self-care practice, *Nurs Res* 33:266, 1984.

13. Kim KK and others: Nutritional status of Chinese-, Korean-, and Japanese-American elderly, *J Am Dietet Assoc* 93(12):1416–1422, 1993.

14. McBride AB: Fat: a woman's issue in search of a holistic approach to treatment, *Holistic Nurs Prac* 3(1):9–15, 1988.

15. Muhlenkamp AF and Sayles JA: Self-esteem, social support, and positive health practices, *Nurs Res* 35:334, 1986.

16. National Dairy Council: Children's health issues, *Dairy Council Digest* 61(6):31–36, 1990.

17. North American Nursing Diagnosis Association: *NANDA nursing diagnoses: definitions and classification, 1995–1996,* Philadelphia, 1994, The Association.

18. Polivy J and Herman CP: Clinical depression and weight change: a complex relation, *J Abnorm Psych* 85:338, 1976.

19. Popkess-Vawter S: Assessment of positive and negative body image in normal weight and overweight females. In Carroll-Johnson RM, editor: *Classification of nursing diagnoses: proceedings of the Eighth Conference,* Philadelphia, 1989, JB Lippincott Co.

20. Pratt C: Weight reduction: its role in health promotion, *Family Community Health* 12(1):67–71, 1989.

21. Schultz LO: Brown adipose tissue: regulation of thermogenesis and implications for obesity, *J Am Dietet Assoc* 87:761, 1987.

22. Sherman JB and Alexander MA: Obesity in children: a research update, *J Pediatr Nurs* 5(3):161–167, 1990.

23. Stunkard A and others: Obesity and eating style, *Arch Gen Psychiatry* 37:1127, 1980.

24. Williamson DF: Descriptive epidemiology of body weight and weight change in U.S. adults, *Ann Int Med* 119(7):646–649, 1993.

25. Wright BA: Weight loss and weight gain in a nursing home: a prospective study, *Geriatr Nurs* 14(3):156–159, 1993.

II

Altered Oral Mucous Membrane

▶

Altered Oral Mucous Membrane *is the state in which an individual experiences change or damage to the oral mucous membrane.*

OVERVIEW

Striated squamous cells make up the epithelium of the oral cavity. Although the tissue type is the same as that of the skin, it lacks the keratin (the tough, fibrous protein formed from flattened, dead cells) typically found on the epidermis. These flattened, platelike cells of the oral mucous membrane are easily shed and replaced by cell division in the deeper germinative epithelial layer.[21] The entire surface of the mucous membrane is replaced approximately every 7 days.[3] When the balance is upset between the cells that are lost and those that replace them, the integrity of the tissue may be compromised.

Like any body tissue, the mucous membranes are subject to changes at the cellular level in response to alterations in the environment. Cellular loss or changes may result from many factors. Mechanical trauma or injury, such as may result from broken or jagged dentition, habitual cheek biting, a surgical procedure, or an accident from a child placing items in the mouth, may be the cause.[9,21] Physical injury of the oral mucous membrane also may occur because of the drying effect of certain risk factors (e.g., mouth breathing, a continuous flow of oxygen, intermittent suctioning, certain medications, and metabolic changes).[7,16] Physical injuries also may result from significant thermal changes. Extreme heat from hot foods or fluids may cause burns of the oral cavity and destruction of the epithelium. This may be especially frequent in the elderly if sensory perception is decreased, and the tissues may be more fragile. Extreme cold may cause cellular injury and has a profound drying effect.

Chemical injury of the oral mucous membrane may be the direct result of contact with some irritating substances as in the case of ingestion of alcohol, use of tobacco, intake of acidic food, or the body's production of toxins (e.g., the mucosa becomes inflamed and ulcerated in patients with renal dysfunction when the levels of ammonia and uremic toxins are elevated). Damage to oral tissue also may have an indirect cause; for example, certain drugs (such as chemotherapeutic agents, antibiotics, steroids, and antidepressants) may produce side effects observed in the oral cavity.[13]

Radiation injury also may be a factor in the cellular damage of the oral mucous membranes. Radiation may have a direct effect if the tissues are within the field of treatment, as in radiation therapy for head and neck cancers, or it may have an indirect and potentially permanent effect by decreasing saliva production if the salivary glands are included in the field.[25] The tissue of the lips is subject to the long-term effects of ultraviolet radiation, as occurs to patients in occupations requiring much time outdoors.

Biological agents also are responsible for changes at the cellular level. Microorganisms, such as *Candida albicans* (fungus), *Herpes simplex* (virus), *Streptococcus* (gram-positive bacteria), and *Pseudomonas* (gram-negative bacteria), can injure the mucous membranes through a number of mechanisms, such as interference with cellular production of adenosine triphosphate or the release of endotoxins. In addition, these organisms have the ability to replicate, thereby continuing the injurious process.[19] In the case of periodontal disease, a chronic inflammatory disease that occurs most frequently in adults, a combination of bacteria and the mucus that forms dental plaque is responsible for the initiation of the disease process.

Finally, cellular injury of the oral mucous membrane may result from nutritional imbalance. Specifically, deficiencies of several of the B vitamins (riboflavin, niacin, folic acid, vitamin B_{12}, and pyridoxine) or iron may lead to changes in the tissue of the oral cavity.

The effect of these alterations on the tissue of the oral mucous membranes may vary. Atrophy (a decrease in size) of the epithelium may result from the aging process, a disease process, or nutritional deficiency.[18] Hyperplasia (an increase in the number of cells) may occur. An example is the gingival hyperplasia that occurs in response to inflammation or to fibrous changes, as occurs as a side effect of diphenylhydantoin (Dilantin).[20] Hypertrophy (an increase in the amount of functioning tissue mass of an organ or part) also may occur; for example, mumps causes hypertrophy of the acinar cells of the parotid gland.[14, 20] Leukoplakia (a thickened white patch that does not rub off) is an example of the dysplasia (deranged cell growth with a variation of size, shape, and appearance) that may occur in response to chronic irritation or inflammation of the oral mucous membranes. Although dysplasia is an adaptive process, its progression may lead to neoplastic (abnormal new growth) disease.[14, 20]

In the presence of one or more of these factors related to cellular injury, the patient may demonstrate the defining characteristics leading to the nursing diagnosis of Altered Oral Mucous Membrane. It is important to note that an interruption in the integrity of the tissue or underlying structures of the oral cavity will increase the patient's risk for infection because of a break in the body's first line of defense. Alteration in the oral mucous membrane can also influence the patient's level of comfort, nutritional status, ability to communicate, fluid balance, sense of taste, and body image.

ASSESSMENT

The nurse may begin the assessment by obtaining subjective information concerning any sensory changes in the oral cavity, such as pain or discomfort, burning, numbness, paresthesia, sensitivity to temperature changes, or impaired taste (dysgeusia). It is important to include the exact location and duration of the identified changes. Ear pain (otalgia) occasionally is experienced as referred pain in patients with lesions in the posterior oral cavity (pharynx, tonsillar region, posterior tongue, or hypopharynx). Other information to obtain includes current medications; a history of trauma (including previous infections or lesions), tobacco use, alcohol ingestion, ingestion of highly seasoned or hot foods, usual dental practices, and any difficulty chewing or swallowing (dysphagia); oral sexual practices; and speech changes or voice impairment (dysphonia).

Physical assessment is conducted by means of inspection and palpation with the use of the following equipment: gloves, a light, a tongue blade, $4'' \times 4''$ gauze, and a dental mirror, if available. A systematic physical assessment of the oral cavity should include data about the following: saliva, lips, buccal mucosa (internal cheeks), teeth, gingivae, tongue, hard and soft palates, pharynx, and regional lymph nodes. Some general characteristics of the mucous membranes in the oral cavity are that they are moist, smooth, and pink or coral in color.

One of the first things observed during inspection of the oral cavity is the amount of saliva (moisture) on the mucosa. Saliva cleans the mouth, regulates the pH, maintains the integrity of the tissue (through glycoproteins that bind to the surface) and the teeth, fights bacteria (through immunoglobulins and enzymes), and begins the process of digestion of carbohydrates.[14, 21] Approximately 1.5 L of saliva are produced daily, primarily from the parotid, submandibular, and sublingual glands and to a much lesser degree from minor salivary glands, such as the labial, palatal, and buccal glands.[16] The consistency of saliva normally is similar to that of water, and saliva

II

has a pH of 6.0 to 7.0. A decrease in the amount of saliva and the symptom of xerostomia (dry mouth) may be the result of dehydration, anxiety, glandular disease (such as an infection or obstruction of the duct), drug therapy (especially antihistamines, narcotics, antidepressants, and chemotherapeutic agents), radiation therapy, or an endocrine disorder.[16] In response to a decrease in amount, the consistency of the saliva may change from thin and watery to being viscous and ropy. Along with subjective information and visual inspection of the saliva for clarity and consistency, the amount of moisture in the oral cavity can be assessed by running a gloved finger over the surfaces to evaluate the stickiness of the mucous membranes. Because of saliva's functions in the oral cavity, a decrease in saliva has a profound effect on the other structures.

The color of the mucosa changes with anemia (pallor), hypoxia (cyanosis), or other pathological conditions. Peutz-Jeghers syndrome, associated with multiple intestinal polyps, may be manifested by pigmented spots on the lips. It is important to note, however, that pigment changes may occur in dark-skinned individuals who have no disease. Purple discoloration of the oral mucosa caused by extravasation of blood in the area is present in purpura. Increased redness and edema of the oral cavity is indicative of stomatitis, an inflammation of the oral mucosa. The term *mucositis* also is used in conjunction with this inflammation, but unless location is specified, it could mean an inflammation of any mucosal surface.[4] (See Table 3 for a suggested scale to use in assessing stomatitis.) Desquamation, a shedding of the epithelial layer, also may occur.

Lesion or ulcers, which may be considered pathological and appear on mucosal surfaces, include *Herpes simplex,* which is characterized by vesicular eruptions that break and crust over; aphthous ulcers (chancre sores), which may be solitary or multiple, small, round or oval, painful, white ulcers surrounded by a halo of reddened mucosa; chancres associated with syphilis, appearing as firm, buttonlike lesions that ulcerate and crust when external; a mucocele, which is a round, reg-

TABLE 3 Gradings of Oral Stomatitis

Grade	Description
I	Mild; generalized erythema of oral mucosa
II	Moderate; generalized erythema of oral mucosa and isolated, small ulcerations and/or white patches
III	Severe; confluent ulcerations with white patches covering more than 25% of oral mucosa
IV	Severe; hemorrhagic ulcerations

From Goodman J and Stoner C: Mucous membrane integrity, impairment of, related to stomatitis. In McNally JC and others, editors: *Guidelines for oncology nursing practice,* ed 2, Philadelphia, 1991, WB Saunders Co. Reproduced with permission of the Oncology Nursing Society.

ular, translucent, or blue nodule; leukoplakia, a white, thickened plaque over a small area or large patch that has a tendency to progress to malignant growth; or a verrucous (warty) growth. Any plaque, ulcer, or warty growth that does not heal is considered suspicious for cancer and should be evaluated. In addition, the oral mucosa is frequently the site of candidiasis (moniliasis or thrush), a yeast infection characterized by removable, white plaques that resemble milk curds and, less frequently, a shiny erythema. Clinically this may appear on any or all mucosal surfaces in the oral cavity, and *Candida albicans* is frequently the organism identified when cultured.[19,20,21] Because of the opportunistic nature of fungal infections such as candidiasis, the incidence increases in patients receiving antibiotics (which destroy the normally inhibitory bacterial flora) or immunosuppressive agents (such as corticosteroids or cytotoxic drugs)[30] or in those who are immunocompromised, such as patients with acquired immunodeficiency syndrome (AIDS). Other microorganisms that cause infections and the clinical manifestations that may occur include gram-positive bacterial, which produce a dry, brownish yellow, circular, raised eruption; gram-negative bacteria, which cause a creamy white, raised, moist, glistening, nonpurulent, painful ulcer with a reddened base; and *Pseudomonas*, which produce a yellow, dry, painless ulcer with defined borders that may progress to the necrotic center.[12]

The lips should be symmetrical in movement. The inner lip is covered by the mucous membrane. Normally the faint vertical lines on the surface of the outer lip become more prominent with age or with the absence of teeth or dentures.[21] It is important to assess the lip from commissure to commissure and from outer border to inner mucosal surface. Edema of the lip may be in response to injury or may be an allergic reaction. In addition to the previously mentioned lesions and ulcers, abnormalities of the lips may be manifested as fissures, dry crusts, scales, and cracking (angular stomatitis or cheilosis if the angle of the mouth is involved), which may be indicative of dehydration, nutritional deficiency, overclosure of the mouth, or sensitivity to cosmetics or dentifrice[19] or may be in response to extreme cold or dryness of the environment.

With the aid of a light and a tongue blade for retraction, an inspection of the buccal mucosa is possible. A bimanual (gloved finger internally and other finger externally) examination is useful for palpation and to detect changes in tissue consistency. The Stensen ducts (opening of the parotid gland) can be seen bilaterally on the surface of buccal mucosa adjacent to the upper second molar. Fordyce spots (yellow granules on the buccal mucosa and the inner lip) are sebaceous glands that are visible in most adults and are considered normal. An occlusion line may also be apparent on the mucosa adjacent to the point where the teeth meet.

The crown of the tooth is usually the only part of the tooth visible. Normally the teeth appear shiny and white (although the color may range to yellow or gray), with smooth edges and no debris. Dental caries may appear first as chalky, white deposits on the tooth surface; if caries is allowed to advance, these lesions then become brown or black, soft, and cavitary. Attrition (flattening of the biting surfaces) may be seen in the older adult. If the patient has dentures, the nurse should assess them for tightness of fit and should determine the condition of the mucosa on the

underlying alveolar ridge because this is frequently a site of irritation.

The gingivae (gums) are normally coral pink in color and moist, with a stippled surface and a tight margin with the tooth surface. Increased melanin pigment (patchy, brown discoloration) of the gingivae is normal in some adults but also may be associated with Addison's disease. A bluish-black line on the gingivae approximately 1 mm from the margin may indicate lead or bismuth poisoning. Swelling and redness of the gums (gingivitis) occurs in response to irritation. With severe gingivitis the stippling is decreased, the gums may bleed easily, and the interdental papilla (gingiva between the teeth) becomes bulbous. This may occur in periodontal disease, in which the inflammation process (in response to calculus formation) progresses to involve the deeper supporting structures of the teeth. Pockets may form, and the gums are recessed. Halitosis frequently is associated with periodontal disease but also is related to infection and tissue necrosis elsewhere in the cavity. Gingival changes also are common in the patient with leukemia caused by the presence of leukemic infiltrates. These changes may include gingivitis, gingival hyperplasia, hemorrhage, petechiae, and ulcerations.[20]

Movement of the tongue should be symmetrical and mobile in all directions. The dorsal and lateral surfaces are slightly rough with papillae and moist, and they occasionally glisten with slight fissures, whereas the ventral surface is smooth, with a prominent venous system. With age the papillae become less distinct and the ventral veins may become varicose. Wharton's ducts of the submaxillary gland can be identified under the tongue on the floor of the mouth near the midline on either side of the frenulum (the vertical fold under the tongue that attaches it to the floor of the mouth). Gauze and a dental mirror may aid in the retraction of the tongue during the inspection and palpation of all surfaces. The facial nerve innervates the anterior two thirds of the tongue and should be evaluated for the ability to distinguish sweet, sour, salty, and bitter tastes. It also innervates certain salivary glands. Sour and bitter are the primary tastes associated with the posterior one third and lateral surfaces of the tongue, which is innervated by the glossopharyngeal nerve. Moisture (saliva) in the oral cavity is essential for the person to perceive the taste of a given substance. The sense of taste is generally thought to decrease with age. Taste alteration may be associated with certain medications or radiation therapy and, in the presence of cancer, may result from tumor byproducts. Mouth blindness (ageusia) is associated with the lack of a sense of taste, whereas dysgeusia refers to aberrant taste sensation. The tongue may become inflamed (glossitis) in response to leukoplakia, ulcers, lesions, or a vitamin B deficiency. The tongue also may become smooth in appearance as a result of vitamin deficiencies. Other abnormalities of the tongue include hairy tongue (elongated papillae on the dorsum, usually in response to antibiotic therapy, but also seen in patients with AIDS), geographic tongue (scattered, red, smooth areas on the dorsum), coated tongue (white, excessive appearance caused by keratinization of the papillae in response to an irritant, tobacco, candies, or drugs), and furrowed tongue (deep fissures in the surface that may be the result of dehydration, chronic irritation, or vitamin deficiency).[19,20,21]

The mucous membrane covering the hard palate is paler and has an irregular texture. The transverse rugae are the ridges on the anterior surface on either side of the linear raphe (the center line of union between the palatine bones). A common abnormality of the hard palate is torus palatinus. This is defined as a bony midline outgrowth that may vary in size. The mucous membranes of the soft palate and uvula are moist, smooth, pink, movable, and symmetrical.

The nurse can examine the pharynx during the assessment of the palate, and examination includes the inspection of the uvula, retromolar trigone, anterior and posterior tonsillar pillars, and the posterior pharynx. A tongue blade and light are needed. The tonsils normally may have clefts (crypts) in the surface.

Finally, assessment of the oral cavity should include palpation of the lymph nodes of the neck, especially the tonsillar, submaxillary, and submental nodes, because these are the primary routes of internal drainage from the mouth. The presence of palpable nodes (lymphadenectasia) will lend supporting data to clinical findings of inflammation or possible malignancy but may also help to identify areas needing further assessment.

■ Defining Characteristics

The presence of the following defining characteristics indicates that the patient may be experiencing Altered Oral Mucous Membrane:

- Sensory changes: pain, burning taste, paresthesia, numbness, and temperature sensitivity
- Decreased moisture: xerostomia, viscous saliva, and fissures
- Color changes: erythema, pallor, pigmentation, coated tongue, and exudate
- Lesions or ulcers: vesicles, aphthous ulcers, chancres, mucoceles, leukoplakia, and erythroplakia
- Oral plaque or dental caries
- Bleeding, hyperemia, or hemorrhage
- Induration of tissue or lymph nodes
- Inflammation or edema: mucositis, stomatitis, gingivitis, glossitis, and desquamation
- Halitosis

■ Related Factors

The following related factors are associated with Altered Oral Mucous Membrane:

- Mechanical trauma
- Physical injury or drying effect
- Chemical trauma
- Radiation injury
- Injury from biological agents
- Nutritional imbalance
- Psychosocial factors
- Surgery, broken teeth, cheek biting, and pressure from oral tubes or improperly fit dentures
- Mouth breathing, oxygen therapy, decreased salivation, and temperature extremes
- Alcohol, tobacco, acidic foods, and side effects of medications
- Radiation therapy to the area or prolonged exposure to ultraviolet rays

- Ineffective oral hygiene and overgrowth of microorganisms (bacterial, viral, and fungal)
- Malnutrition and vitamin deficiency
- Lack of economic resources for preventive or restorative treatment

DIAGNOSIS

■ Differential Nursing Diagnosis

The diagnosis of Altered Oral Mucous Membrane may be closely related to several other nursing diagnoses, and in some situations it may be difficult to select the diagnostic label that best reflects the patient's major problem. Because the oral cavity has so many important functions, other relevant diagnoses may include Altered Nutrition, Pain, Airway Obstruction, Impaired Communication, Impaired Swallowing, and Self-esteem Disturbance. The diagnosis of Impaired Tissue Integrity probably most closely correlates with this diagnosis. Differentiating between diagnoses is based on the ability to specify the alteration. Interventions for alteration in the oral cavity are unique compared to interventions for other tissue surfaces because of the structure and function of the oral mucous membrane.

■ Medical and Psychiatric Diagnoses

Related medical diagnoses for Altered Oral Mucous Membrane include fractured mandible, leukoplakia related to chronic tobacco use, and squamous cell carcinoma of the retromolar trigone. These diagnoses may lead to surgical interventions. Medical interventions would be prescribed for the diagnosis of *Herpes simplex* viral infection. The collaborative care path developed for each of these diagnoses will identify the responsibilities of each member of the health care team.

OUTCOME IDENTIFICATION, PLANNING, AND IMPLEMENTATION

The primary outcome of nursing interventions is to maintain or attain intact tissue integrity within the oral cavity. Basic oral hygiene, including brushing with a soft or medium-soft brush and nonabrasive fluoride toothpaste, daily flossing, and oral rinsing, is the most important intervention in the maintenance of a healthy mucous membrane.[3,5,10,23] The timing of the prescribed mouth care regimen is important and should take into account patient preferences. Mouthwashes frequently are used before meals to help freshen the patient's mouth and to stimulate the appetite, and brushing and rinsing after meals and at bedtime will remove debris and plaque from teeth. Omission of oral hygiene for longer than 6 hours will nullify past benefits attained.[9] Research indicates that oral hygiene measures administered every 4 hours are the most effective in improving salivation, moisture of the tongue, moisture of the palate, condition of the mucous membrane, and texture and moisture of the lips.[5]

The nursing decision concerning the equipment to be used for cleansing the oral cavity should include assessment data, specifically, information about the patient's age, the present condition of the mouth, and platelet and white blood cell counts. A soft-bristle brush is especially important for the patient with thrombocytopenia and for the older adult because of age-related changes of the oral mucosa that may be present, such as thinning of the epithelium, a decrease in saliva, and increased susceptibility to injury.[5,21] In the edentulous patient, oral hygiene can be accomplished with thorough cleansing of the removed dentures, the use of mouthwashes, and cleansing of the mucosal surface with a sponge or soft toothbrush before a denture or bridge is reinserted. Sponge sticks are ineffective in removing debris from tooth surfaces.[4] In patients with severe stomatitis, thrombocytopenia, or neutropenia, a toothbrush may be contraindicated because of the potential for further damage. Gauze (4″ × 4″), moistened with normal saline and wrapped around a gloved finger, may be used to remove dental debris.[9] If oral irrigations are ordered or oral rinsing is problematic for reasons related to the patient's condition, such as altered level of consciousness or wired jaws, additional equipment may be needed. A Water-Pic, power sprayer, Asepto syringe, or elevated enema bag with a catheter tip may be used. Suction with a Tonsil Tip

II

may also be needed if the patient is unable to expectorate. Lemon and glycerin swabs should never be used on inflamed or broken mucous membrane because of the irritating effects of the lemon and the drying effect of the glycerin.[4]

When the integrity of the mucous membrane is altered, additional interventions are required for cleansing. If stomatitis is present or if the risk of it occurring is high, additional use of mouthwashes with normal saline after and between brushings will soothe inflamed mucosa. Warm saline mouthwashes frequently are ordered for the patient who has had oral surgery. Sterile normal saline (0.9% sodium chloride) should be used in the presence of mouth ulcers, severe neutropenia, or recent oral surgery. However, if the sterility of the solution is not a concern, it can be prepared by mixing 1 teaspoon of salt in 1000 ml (1 quart) of water. Most commercial mouthwashes contain alcohol, which may irritate already inflamed mucosal surfaces. If thick mucus, crust, or debris are present, an oxidizing agent is necessary for mechanical debridement. Two commonly used solutions are hydrogen peroxide and normal saline, in a 1:4 ratio, or sodium bicarbonate, 1 teaspoon in 8 ounces of water. Use of these solutions should be followed by rinsing with warm water or normal saline.[12] Use of hydrogen peroxide in the presence of granulation tissue is usually contraindicated, because it may destroy the new tissue. It also may cause overgrowth of papillae on the tongue and an increased susceptibility to candidiasis if it is not diluted and rinsed properly.[4,22] Other agents that may be used in cleansing the oral cavity are dilute acetic acid, dilute chlorhexidine gluconate (Peridex), dilute providone-iodine (Betadine), sodium perborate (Amosan), carbamide peroxide (Gly-oxide), or the enzyme combination of glucose oxidase and lactoperoxidase (Bioténe). The frequency of the oral hygiene regimen may be increased to every 2 hours and once or twice during the night if more severe (grade IV) stomatitis is observed. This is imperative in the immunocompromised patient; for example, in the patient who is receiving an antimetabolite chemotherapeutic agent. Because of the ability of chlorhexidine to bind with the surface of the mucous membrane, using it twice

a day is sufficient to provide the desired antibacterial protection.[7] A denture or bridge should not be reinserted if a lesion or severe stomatitis is present.

The maintenance of moisture in the oral cavity is another expected outcome that will contribute to unimpaired tissue integrity. Maintaining fluid balance and avoiding dehydration are essential. Oral rinsing every 2 to 4 hours (as has been described) also will help prevent xerostomia. Additional agents available for the prevention or treatment of xerostomia include artificial saliva preparations, which may contain sorbitol, sodium carboxymethylcellulose or mucins,[8] fluoride, and electrolytes (or enzymes) normally found in saliva, or a solution of calcium and phosphate; sugar-free gum or candies to stimulate saliva production; water-soluble emollient for the lips and mucous membrane; and humidification. Oil-based lubricants should be avoided because of the danger of aspiration pneumonia and they are highly flammable in the presence of oxygen therapy.[4] High-moisture foods, those prepared with gravy or sauces, and extra fluids (if not contraindicated) should be included in the meal planning of patients with xerostomia.

The prevention of infection is an expected outcome of interventions when dealing with any tissue with impaired continuity. Cultures should be obtained at the first sign of a possible infection. If viral infection is suspected, a culture should be obtained using viral transport medium (a calcium alginate swab can inactivate the virus) and kept cold. Antifungal, antiviral, or antibacterial agents then may be ordered, depending on the results of culturing. Such agents also may be ordered prophylactically in patients at risk for infection. Antifungal agents (chlotrimazole troches or nystatin suspension) usually are applied topically and also should be applied to any dentures. The patient should avoid eating or drinking for 30 minutes after application.[2]

Interventions targeted for the patient outcome of the absence of discomfort include using topical or systemic analgesics, especially before meals, and altering the diet to avoid acidic or spicy foods, extremes in temperature, and foods that are rough

II

◢ NURSING CARE GUIDELINES

Nursing Diagnosis: Altered Oral Mucous Membrane Related to Chemical Injury (Decreased Mucosal Cellular Replacement) as a Result of Chemotherapy

Expected Outcome: The patient will exhibit unimpaired tissue integrity of oral mucosa as evidenced by moist, pink, smooth mucosal surfaces and the absence of debris on dental surfaces within 2 weeks after the administration of chemotherapy.

- Assess all surfaces of oral cavity at least once a day, including color, moisture, presence of lesions or ulcers, discomfort, debris on and odor of all surfaces, and presence of palpable lymph nodes *to identify alterations.*
- Assist the patient to perform oral hygiene very 4 hours (if self-care is difficult) while awake; this consists of brushing with soft-bristle brush and nonabrasive toothpaste; rinsing with normal saline after brushing and every 2 hours between; flossing with unwaxed dental floss every morning; and moisturizing lips with water-soluble gel or lip balm *to cleanse and lessen further damage to oral mucosa.*
- ▲ Monitor laboratory values daily, especially white blood cell and platelet counts *to anticipate duration of increased risk for oral mucous membrane breakdown.*

Expected Outcome: The patient will experience no oral discomfort as evidenced by verbalization of same, the ability to communicate needs verbally, and an oral intake of 2 to 3 L of fluid per day and at least 75% of patient's usual diet, within 2 weeks after chemotherapy.

- Assess the patient's ability to communicate, and monitor amounts of food and fluid intake; avoid acidic and highly seasoned food, rough textures, and extremes in temperature; consult with dietitian *to identify alterations.*
- Discourage use of alcohol or tobacco, *which could cause further damage.*
- ▲ Medicate with topical or systemic analgesics, as ordered, 30 to 40 minutes before meals *to lessen discomfort.*
- Encourage frequent dental evaluations. Provide information about low-cost community dental services, if needed, *to prevent alterations in the future.*

Expected Outcome: The patient will state signs and symptoms of tissue alterations and the purpose of an oral hygiene regimen and will demonstrate proper technique within 2 days.

- Assess the patient's current knowledge regarding oral hygiene *to develop an appropriate teaching plan.*
- Discuss changes that may occur (stomatitis, ulcers, or infections) related to specific chemotherapeutic agents and the oral hygiene regimen suggested *to prepare the patient for potential problems.*
- Request that the patient demonstrate the oral regimen and correct technique when appropriate *to determine if learning has taken place.*
- ▲ Discuss possible diet changes and use of medications *as part of teaching plan.*

■ = nursing intervention; ▲ = collaborative intervention.

in texture. Patients with more severe, generalized oral alterations (e.g., grade IV hemorrhagic ulcerations) may require parenteral narcotics (morphine sulfate, meperidine hydrochloride) and nasogastric or parenteral feedings to relieve oral discomfort and provide nutrition. In addition, pressure or topical thrombin (Thrombostat) may be needed if bleeding persists.

Topical analgesics may vary and frequently are used in combination, which may include drugs from two or more of the following classifications: antihistamine (diphenhydramine hydrochloride); antacid (Milk of Magnesia or Maalox); antiinflammatory (hydrocortisone); topical anesthetic (dyclonine hydrochloride 0.5%, Xylocaine viscous 2%, or benzocaine 20%); and agents used to form a protective coating (kaolin/pectin or Sucralfate).[2] Many of these have systemic side effects, which should be taken into consideration. For example, diphenhydramine hydrochloride (Benadryl) can cause drowsiness and cardiovascular effects. Lidocaine hydrochloride (Xylocaine) can affect the pharyngeal stage of swallowing, causes numbness, and normally should be limited to 120 ml every 24 hours because of its cardiovascular side effects. Antifungal and antibacterial agents frequently are added when hydrocortisone is used because of the propensity for superinfections to occur. An example of one of these combinations is "stomatitis cocktail," which is a mixture of equal parts of lidocaine hydrochloride, diphenhydramine hydrochloride (12.5 mg/ml), and Maalox, with 30 ml to be swished and swallowed every 2 to 4 hours as needed.[12] Anesthetic agents have also been combined with carboxymethylcellulose (Orabase) or hydroxpropylcellulose (Zilactin) to form a film that adheres to mucosal surfaces, thereby extending the relief obtained in patients with oral ulcers (grade II to grade IV).

Finally, interventions also should be focused on patient knowledge of factors affecting the oral mucosa and on oral self-care techniques as an expected outcome. The teaching plan should include daily oral self-examination, the oral hygiene regimen, suggested diet changes, the importance of dental evaluations, the risks associated with tobacco and alcohol use, pain control, medication administration, and side effects.

EVALUATION

Evaluation of the interventions will center on the appearance of the oral mucous membranes, including the absence of defining characteristics; the level of comfort; and the ability of the patient to communicate orally, to consume nutrients, and finally, to incorporate effective oral hygiene techniques into the daily routine.

▪ CASE STUDY WITH PLAN OF CARE

Mr. Joe W., a 76-year-old man, was admitted to the hospital for evaluation and treatment of a superior right nasal mass. He had sought treatment a week earlier from his private physician for a complaint of a dull, constant headache posterior to his right eye, an increase in lacrimation of the right eye over the past 6 to 7 weeks, and two episodes of epistaxis in the previous week. He was given a prescription of amoxicillin and referred to University Hospital. His medical history included coronary artery bypass grafting 3 years ago, colectomy for left colon cancer 15 months earlier, and non-insulin-dependent diabetes mellitus diagnosed 9 months earlier. On admission he was alert and oriented, his pupils were equal in size, round, and reactive to light, and extraocular movements of the right eye were decreased on the lateral and medial gaze, with proptosis of the right eye. The oral assessment revealed pink, slightly dry, smooth mucous membranes, teeth in a good state of repair, and tongue with increased rugosity (folds, wrinkles) but supple and with a full range of motion. With the exception of an irregular pulse rate of 64 beats per min and an elevated glucose level of 366 mg/dl, all other physical findings and laboratory data were within normal limits. Mr. W. had been living with his wife, who

was very concerned and supportive, in their own home about 25 miles from the hospital. A magnetic resonance imaging (MRI) scan done the next day revealed an extensive intracranial tumor from the floor of the frontal fossa to the corpus callosum, filling the sphenoid and both ethmoids with erosion of the medial half of the right orbital roof. The tumor was inoperable, and chemotherapy and radiation for palliation were discussed. Mr. W.'s physical condition quickly declined. Within 3 days he became increasing somnolent and developed left-side weakness. He was started on dexamethasone, 24 mg every 6 hours, and phenytoin, 200 mg twice a day. Radiation therapy was begun on day 5 of his hospitalization. His blood glucose had to be controlled with sliding-scale insulin coverage after administration of dexamethasone began. Nutrition and hydration became a problem because of his decreased level of consciousness. His albumin dropped to 3.4 gm/dl, and his blood urea nitrogen increased to 33 mg/dl by the fifth day. His diet was changed to a pureed-consistency, 2000-calorie (American Diabetes Association) diet, and an intravenous line was inserted for hydration. An oral assessment on the seventh day revealed generalized stomatitis, the lips were dry and cracked, his tongue had increased fissures, and there was a white, curdlike plaque covering the entire buccal mucosa bilaterally and the lateral surfaces of the tongue.

The following plan of care was instituted: The alteration in nutrition was dealt with in a separate nursing diagnosis. When the effectiveness of the nursing interventions in meeting the identified patient outcomes was evaluated, the daily oral assessment indicated gradual improvement. By the time of discharge, 5 days later, Mr. W.'s oral mucosa still had slight erythema, but the can-

didiasis had subsided. His tongue was moist and without fissures, and his lips were still slightly dry but no longer cracked. The radiation therapist had approved the use of a water-soluble lip balm because that area was not in the direct field of treatment. Mr. W.'s level of oral comfort remained good, and his wife was able to state the rationale and demonstrate the ability to provide oral hygiene for her husband before discharge. Radiation therapy continued at the local hospital.

II

▶ PLAN OF CARE FOR MR. JOE W.
Nursing Diagnosis: Altered Oral Mucous Membrane*

Expected Outcome: Mr. W. will exhibit a return to moist, pink, smooth, mucosal surfaces without plaque or debris within 7 days.
- ▲ Send culture of oral plaque.
- ■ Assess oral cavity every shift, and obtain laboratory values daily.
- ■ Perform oral hygiene every 4 hours (beginning at 9 A.M.) and once during the night, consisting of brushing with a soft-bristle brush; using a sponge on mucosal surfaces; swishing with a solution of 1 teaspoon baking soda and 8 ounces water; rinsing with normal saline; and flossing once a day.
- ▲ Spray mouth with artificial saliva between oral hygiene procedures.
- ▲ Have Mr. W. swish with 5 ml nystatin (500,000 units) for 2 to 3 minutes and swallow four times a day.
- ■ Institute aspiration precautions (if level of consciousness decreases) during oral hygiene, including Sims' position, tonsil suction at bedside, and use of toothbrush with built-in vacuum tip, large syringe for rinsing, and cotton or sponge applicator for applying medication.
- ▲ Consult with radiation therapy personnel before applying lip moisturizers; this will be contraindicated if lips are with the treatment field.

Expected Outcome: Mr. W. will not exhibit signs or symptoms of discomfort, as evidenced by no complaints (dependent on level of consciousness) and no grimacing or restlessness during oral care or swallowing.
- ■ Assess for discomfort.
- ■ Monitor intake and output.
- ■ Maintain intake (by mouth and intravenous) of 2 to 3 L per day.
- ▲ Monitor dietary intake to ensure adequate calorie and protein intake.

Expected Outcome: Mr. W.'s wife will identify contributing factors and be able to state the purpose and demonstrate techniques of the oral hygiene regimen, by time of discharge.
- ■ Institute a teaching plan with Mr. W.'s wife for home care (include oral hygiene measures).

■ = nursing intervention; ▲ = collaborative intervention.
*Related to physical injury—the drying effect of mouth breathing and dehydration; chemical injury—possible gingival hyperplasia; injury from biological agent—overgrowth of *Candida albicans* secondary to recent antibiotic therapy, immunosuppressive nature of dexamethasone, and increased blood glucose with uncontrolled diabetes mellitus; and radiation injury resulting from radiation therapy to nasal-frontal tumor.

II

▪▪ CRITICAL THINKING EXERCISES

1. Mr. Joe W.'s condition worsens and he has a seizure, during which he bites his tongue, creating a 1-inch laceration with bleeding. How will this change your plan of oral care?

2. Mr. W. became nauseated with each dose of nystatin. How will this alter your plan of care?

3. As the radiation therapy continued, Mr. W. developed grade III oral stomatitis involving the soft and hard palate. He rated his pain as 7 on scale of 1 to 10 (10 being the worst). How would you plan for his care?

4. Mrs. W. shares with you that because of financial constraints she and her husband have not visited the dentist in 3 years. How would you assist Mrs. W. and her husband to receive regular checkups?

REFERENCES

1. Addems A and others: The lack of efficacy of a foam brush in maintaining gingival health: a controlled study, *Special Care in Dentistry* 12(3):103, 1992.

2. Bavier A: Nursing management of acute oral complications of cancer, *NCI Monographs* 9:123, 1990.

3. Beck S: Impact of a systemic oral care protocol on stomatitis after chemotherapy, *Cancer Nurs* 2:185, 1979.

4. Daeffler R: Oral hygiene measures for patients with cancer, *Cancer Nurs* 3:347, 1980 (Part I); 3:427, 1980 (Part II); 4:29, 1981 (Part III).

5. DeWalt E: Effect of timed hygienic measures on oral mucosa in a group of elderly subjects, *Nurs Res* 24:104, 1975.

6. DeWalt E and Haines S: Effects of specified stressors on healthy oral mucosa, *Nurs Res* 18:22, 1969.

7. Feretti G and others: Oral antimicrobial agents—Chlorhexidine, *NCI Monographs* 9:51, 1990.

8. Greenspan D: Management of salivary dysfunction, *NCI Monographs* 9:159, 1990.

9. Kim MJ, McFarland GK, and McLane AM: *Pocket guide to nursing diagnoses*, ed 6, St. Louis, 1995, Mosby–Year Book.

10. Klocke J and Sudduth A: Oral hygiene instruction and plaque formation during hospitalization, *Nurs Res* 18:124, 1969.

11. Kusler DL and Rambur BA: Treatment for radiation-induced xerostomia, *Cancer Nurs* 15(3):191, 1992.

12. McNally JC and others: *Guidelines for oncology nursing practice*, ed 2, Philadelphia, 1991, WB Saunders Co.

13. Niehaus CS, Peterson DE, and Overholser CD: Oral complications in children during cancer therapy, *Cancer Nurs* 10:15, 1987.

14. Ofstehage JC and Magilvy K: Oral health and aging, *Geriatr Nurs* 7(5):238, 1986.

15. Passos J and Brand L: Effects of agents for oral hygiene, *Nurs Res* 15:186, 1966.

16. Porth CM and Erickson M: Physiology of thirst and drinking: implication for nursing practice, *Heart Lung* 21(3):273, 1992.

17. Resio MJ: Nursing diagnosis: alteration in oral/nasal mucous membrane related to trauma of transsphenoidal surgery, *J Neurosci Nurs* 18:112, 1986.

18. Roth PT and Creason NS: Nursing administered oral hygiene: is there a scientific basis? *J Adv Nurs* 11:323, 1986.

19. Schaaf M and Carl W: Dental oncology. In Holleb AI, Fink DJ, and Murphy GP, editors: *Clinical oncology*, Atlanta, 1991, American Cancer Society.

20. Schweiger J and others: Oral assessment: how to do it, *Am J Nurs* 80:654, 1980.

21. Squier CA: Mucosal alterations, *NCI Monographs* 9:169, 1990.

22. Tombes MB and Gallucci B: The effects of hydrogen peroxide rinses on the normal oral mucosa, *Nursing Res* 42(6):332, 1993.

23. Trevelyan J: Oral traditions, *Nursing Times* 90(14):24, 1994.

24. Turner G: Oral care for patients who are terminally ill, *Nurs Standard* 8(4):49, 1994.

25. Zerbe MB and others: Relationship between oral mucositis and treatment variables in bone marrow transplant patients, *Cancer Nurs* 15(3):196, 1992.

Risk for Impaired Skin Integrity

▶
─────────────────────────────────────

Impaired Skin Integrity

▶
─────────────────────────────────────

Risk for Impaired Skin Integrity *is a state in which the individual's skin is at risk of being adversely altered.*

Impaired Skin Integrity *is a state in which the individual's skin is adversely altered.*

OVERVIEW

The functions of the skin are to provide a tough, protective covering for the internal environment of the body, to act as a barrier to the loss of water and electrolytes, to regulate temperature, and to function in excretion, absorption, and sensation.[12] Care of the skin requires diligence and advanced assessment skills on the part of the practicing nurse for prevention and adequate treatment.

Several risk factors thought to predispose an individual to skin breakdown and to interfere with the healing process of an existing skin impairment have been identified. These are organized into intrinsic and extrinsic factors. Intrinsic factors relate to the internal physiological functions that have an effect on skin integrity (e.g., nutritional status). Extrinsic factors generally represent any external force that may adversely affect the skin (e.g., prolonged pressure and shearing forces).

The development of impaired skin integrity usually includes multiple factors acting on the individual at a given time. The individual's ability to respond to the threat to or, in the case of actual disruption of skin integrity, the ability to heal varies in relation to the intrinsic and extrinsic factors present. The nurse's responsibility is to identify individuals at Risk for Impaired Skin Integrity so that more effective preventive steps can be taken.

The terms *pressure ulcer, decubitus ulcer,* and *bedsore* often are used interchangeably to describe an area of cellular necrosis affecting the skin. The ulcer represents a break in skin integrity that can progress in severity to affect the epidermis, the dermis, the subcutaneous tissue, and even the muscle. Incidence rates for decubitus ulcers vary depending on the population studied and the surveying methods used. With respect to the hospitalized patient population, many rates have been reported, but they generally range from 3% to 10% of all hospitalized patients.[10] Actual skin impairments have serious financial, psychological, and social ramifications for the individual and the community at large. Therefore it is imperative that prevention be the primary goal and that individuals with skin impairments be identified and treated promptly.

ASSESSMENT

Risk for Impaired Skin Integrity

Assessment of individuals at Risk for Impaired Skin Integrity is a complex process. Many factors contributing to skin health must be considered. In addition, analysis of the individual level of resis-

221

II

tance to the development of impairment and the ability to heal a lesion must be completed as part of a comprehensive assessment. Intrinsic factors include altered nutritional states such as malnutrition, emaciation, and obesity. Poor nutrition interferes with the normal tissue integrity and impairs proper wound healing. Specifically, disturbances such as hypoproteinemia; ascorbic acid, iron, and zinc deficiencies; fat and carbohydrate insufficiency; and vitamin A, B, C, D, and K deficiencies may result in impaired tissue rehydration and repair.[9] Chronic malnutrition results in weight loss (emaciation) and decreased padding from loss of subcutaneous tissue and muscle mass, thereby predisposing the individual to skin impairments or compounding existing ones. The presence of a negative nitrogen balance, which is associated with some nutritional disturbances, predisposes an individual to edema formation, and this makes the skin more vulnerable to injury. Obesity may result in decreased sensation and possibly decreased circulation related to the effects of the additional adipose tissues[1,2]

Altered circulation, which accompanies peripheral vascular disease and diabetes, will result in less than optimal blood flow carrying oxygen and nutrients to the skin, thus increasing the likelihood of skin breakdown. Altered sensation results in decreased or absent response to various stimuli, such as heat, pressure, and pain, that serve as a warning of potential damage to the skin integrity.

Specific age-related changes in the skin, such as loss of dermal thickness, reduction of circulation through the dermis, or decreased or altered pressure perception and light touch response, render the elderly population at Risk for Impaired Skin Integrity.[8] Alterations in skin turgor related to loss of collagen and elastic fibers with aging may impair skin integrity. Itching, burning, and cracking of the skin can result from dry skin, medications, communicable diseases, or psychogenic reactions.[1,8] Itching followed by frequent or intense scratching may result in disruption in skin integrity.

Extrinsic factors also may affect skin integrity. Shearing forces and friction injuries to the epider-

mis are sustained as the individual slides up or down in bed. Scratching represents a potential extrinsic cause of impaired skin, although the initiating process may be internal (e.g., histamine release or dryness). Prolonged pressure from physical immobilization, fractures, or restraint impairs circulation. When the external pressure exerted on an area of skin is greater than the capillary hydrostatic pressure, capillary obstruction occurs, which produces ischemia, resulting in a nutritional deficit. Pressure sustained for more than 1 to 2 hours may result in pathological changes that lead to necrosis. Maceration of the epidermis because of the presence of moisture on a chronic basis (urine, perspiration, or humidity) reduces the skin's effective ability to resist destruction from other forces.[1,9] Poor hygiene provides an ischemic environment that attracts and fosters the growth and proliferation of bacteria, thus contributing to skin breakdown. Heat, exhibited as fever, raises the metabolic needs and the demand for oxygen; this can potentiate tissue ischemia, especially if an individual is already in a compromised condition.[2] Fecal incontinence may contribute to skin impairment through exposure of the skin to bacteria and toxins in the stool and through skin maceration.[2,9] Similarly, infants and small children may be at increased risk for skin breakdown because of excessive skin exposure to urine, which can lead to maceration of the skin.

The literature describes several assessment tools that attempt to predict or identify individuals at Risk for Impaired Skin Integrity.[6] Three scales will be discussed here. The best-known pressure ulcer assessment tool is the Norton Scale. Norton and associates pioneered this clinical area with the formation of a scale that determines scores based on five categories: mobility, activity, incontinence, mental status, and physical condition. Some find the categories used by Norton to be confusing, and the tool tends to overpredict some situations.[4] Gosnell in 1973 introduced a tool that built on Norton's work, and in 1987 Gosnell again released a revised tool. An extended application of this tool included a more detailed assessment of the skin, nutrition, and hydration status, and it provided room for documentation of interventions. A third tool, the Braden Scale for Predicting Pressure Sore Risk, was developed in 1987 by Berstrom and associates. This tool measures six factors: sensory perception, activity, mobility, moisture, friction, and nutrition. Many institutions modified the tools described above to develop their own risk assessment scale but lack adequate clinical testing and usage of these tools for proven worth.

■ Risk Factors

The presence of the following behaviors, conditions, or circumstances renders the patient more vulnerable to Risk for Impaired Skin Integrity:

External (environmental) factors

- Hyperthermia or hypothermia
- Chemical substance
- Mechanical factors: shearing forces, pressure, restraints
- Radiation
- Physical immobilization
- Excretions and secretions
- Humidity

Internal (somatic) factors

- Medications
- Altered nutritional state: obesity, emaciation, and malnutrition
- Altered circulation
- Decreased sensation
- Skeletal prominence
- Developmental factors
- Immunological deficit
- Alterations in skin turgor (change in elasticity)
- Excretions and secretions
- Psychogenic factors
- Edema

Impaired Skin Integrity

The defining characteristics for Impaired Skin Integrity include disruption of skin integrity, destruction of skin layers, and invasion of body structures.[11]

The plan of care of the decubitus ulcer should be based on the specific stage as described in the literature. Although many different staging systems are described in the literature, a staging system devised by the International Association of Enterostomal Therapists (IAET) will be described here because of the leadership of enterostomal therapy nurses in skin care.

Stage 1: Erythema not resolving within 30 minutes of pressure relief. Epidermis remains intact. Reversible with intervention.

Stage 2: Partial thickness loss of skin layers involving epidermis and possibly penetrating into but not through the dermis. May present as blistering with erythema or induration; wound base moist and pink; painful; free of necrotic tissue.

Stage 3: Full-thickness tissue loss extending through dermis to involve subcutaneous tissue. Presents as shallow crater, unless covered by eschar. May include necrotic tissue, undermining, sinus tract formation, exudate, or infection. Wound base is not usually painful.

Stage 4: Deep tissue destruction extending through subcutaneous tissue to fascia and may involve muscle layers, joint, or bone. Presents as deep crater, unless covered by eschar. May include necrotic tissue, undermining, sinus tract formation, exudate, or infection. Wound base is not usually painful.[7]

■ Defining Characteristics

The presence of the following defining characteristics indicates that the patient may be experiencing Impaired Skin Integrity:

- Disruption of skin surface
- Destruction of skin layers
- Invasion of body structures

■ Related Factors

The presence of the following behaviors, conditions, or circumstances are related to Impaired Skin Integrity:

External (environmental) factors

- Hyperthermia or hypothermia
- Chemical substance
- Mechanical factors: shearing forces, pressure, restraints
- Radiation
- Physical immobilization
- Excretions and secretions
- Humidity

Internal (somatic) factors

- Medications
- Altered nutritional state: obesity, emaciation, malnutrition
- Altered circulation
- Decreased sensation
- Skeletal prominence
- Developmental factors
- Immunological deficit
- Alterations in skin turgor (change in elasticity)
- Excretions and secretions
- Psychogenic factors
- Edema

DIAGNOSIS

■ Differential Nursing Diagnosis

Risk for Impaired Skin Integrity should be contrasted with the diagnosis Altered Protection. Risk for Impaired Skin Integrity more often is related to internal factors such as general nutrition, immobility, impaired circulation to and nutrition of the skin, hydration, or the external factors such as skin exposure to macerating moisture or excessive heat. Altered Protection refers to the ability to guard oneself from danger or injury and to the ability to provide a safe environment. The existence of a medical diagnosis of cancer, acquired immunodeficiency syndrome (AIDS), or leukemia results in the patient being at risk for Altered Protection because the internal resources are impaired. The lack of internal protective mechanisms may make the patient vulnerable to disruption in skin integrity also. However, the diagnosis Risk for Impaired Skin Integrity relates to those factors specifically threatening the external protective barrier of the body.

■ Medical and Psychiatric Diagnoses

Medical and psychiatric diagnoses most commonly related to the nursing diagnosis, Impaired Skin Integrity, include conditions such as chicken pox, measles, dermatitis, burn injury, stomatitis, oral cancer, or herpes simplex. Other generalized conditions that can have serious effects on skin integrity and create Risk for Impaired Skin Integrity include diabetes mellitus, chronic renal failure, diarrhea and dehydration, cirrhosis, dermatitis, or immobility caused by paralysis or a coma state. Psychiatric conditions such as hallucinations or delusion may cause the patient to scratch the skin in self-mutilation efforts or to wash excessively in response to an obsessive-compulsive disorder, thereby removing protective skin oils.

OUTCOME IDENTIFICATION, PLANNING, AND IMPLEMENTATION

Risk for Impaired Skin Integrity

The expected outcome of the plan is the maintenance of intact skin integrity, and the nurse achieves this by performing nursing interventions aimed at reducing or eliminating the risk factors that contribute to impaired skin integrity.[3,13,14] The overall plan focuses on (1) conducting a thorough assessment, (2) providing adequate general skin care, (3) preventing unnecessary trauma to the skin, (4) optimizing circulatory status, and (5) optimizing nutritional status.

First, assess the individual's integument and determine the presence of risk factors, as previously identified, to develop appropriate strategies. Inspect the skin for its integrity and absence or presence of redness, blisters, warmth, swelling, and drainage. Capillary refill should also be checked. Monitor laboratory values, as ordered, that have an effect on the integument, albumin, uric acid, bilirubin, arterial blood gases, blood urea nitrogen, hemoglobin, and hematocrit.[1,9] Report the results to the physician.

The second step in the plan is to provide good general skin care. Keep the skin clean and dry to prevent breakdown of the epidermis from maceration and to limit bacterial growth.[9] Identify incontinent patients and keep them as dry as possible. Assess for incontinent episodes with each position change, apply protective creams to the affected area, and, in collaboration with the physician, institute measures to control the problem. The expected outcome is that the skin will remain intact throughout the health care admission.

Third, avoid unnecessary injury to the patient's skin. Friction and shearing forces act on the skin as the patient slides in bed.[1,9] To lessen the trauma of these forces, the nurse should move the patient up in bed by means of a pull sheet to avoid dragging the person. The use of a footboard or knee gatch is sometimes useful to keep patients from sliding in the bed. The 30° Fowler's position should be limited to less than an hour because this position has been found to destroy tissues.[5] Avoid the 90° lateral position because it may hasten the development of trochanteric and malleolar ulcers. Use occlusive dressings to act as a second layer of skin, and use powders applied to the skin to reduce the trauma in high-risk body areas.[5] The expected outcome is that the skin will remain intact throughout the health care admission.

Fourth, increase circulation to all areas of the body to allow intake of nutrients and removal of waste. Ambulate patients, if possible, and limit the sitting position to less than 2 hours. Reposition bedfast patients every 1 to 2 hours and provide range-of-motion exercises with each position change. Use pressure relieving or reducing mattresses (water mattress, air-fluidized bed, or alternating air mattress) as indicated.[5] The expected outcome is that adequate circulation will be maintained to all areas of the body and that the skin will remain intact throughout the health care admission.

Nutritional deficits are a common problem in hospitalized patients and are a major cause of skin breakdown.[9] Collaborate with the physician to identify nutritional deficiencies and to implement strategies to improve patient status. Collaborate with the dietitian to provide the patient with a sufficient intake of calories, protein, and fluids. Be aggressive and prompt in reporting inadequate nutrition to the physician so that supplements or alternative feeding methods can be instituted. Monitor problems by assessing weekly weights, dietary intake, and albumin levels. The expected outcome is that the patient will receive adequate nutritional intake to maintain a positive nitrogen balance throughout the health care admission.

Impaired Skin Integrity

The outcomes for the individual with Impaired Skin Integrity are (1) to regain intact skin integrity by the time of discharge, (2) to reduce or eliminate factors that contribute to the development or extension of the skin impairment, (3) to increase comfort if pain or itching is present, and (4) the individual or family will participate in the plan of care as appropriate. The plan must incorporate the following principles: provide adequate general skin care, prevent unnecessary trauma to the skin, optimize circulation status, and optimize nutritional status.

First, assess the skin impairment for location, size, depth, presence of redness or drainage, signs of infection, presence of granulation tissue, presence of necrotic tissue, and presence of sinus tract.[6] If possible, identify the contributing causes to lessen the extent of the impairment. Document the ulcer stage according to a standard staging system if the impairment is a pressure ulcer. Accurate assessment and regular documentation of skin impairments will improve the quality of care and the evaluation of treatments.[6]

Treatment of decubiti, often the responsibility of the nurse, includes determining appropriate treatment. Many hospitals employ an enterostomal therapy (ET) nurse, who is a specialist in skin care. The ET nurse should collaborate with the nursing and medicine departments to recommend an appropriate treatment plan for individual patients. Much of the literature on topical treatments for decubitus ulcers lacks a scientific research base and should be reviewed carefully. Treatment of decubitus ulcers includes the following principles: (1) the decubitus ulcer heals slowly, and therefore time must be allowed for a given treatment to take effect before evaluating the treatment; (2) continuity of treatment throughout all shifts is essential for healing and for proper evaluation of the treatment; (3) the choice of treatment should consider the stage, location, cause, and status of the ulcer, whether it is secreting or nonsecreting, and the presence or absence of necrotic tissue.

All wounds must be cleansed before and as part of the treatment. Some of the commonly used antimicrobial cleaning agents are providone-iodine, hydrogen peroxide, chlorhexidine gluconate, and acetic acid.[5] Their value and effectiveness is questioned because they are thought to delay wound healing in some cases.[4] If these products are used, they must be diluted (especially the providone-iodine) before cleaning an open wound. Some practitioners find cleaning superficial ulcers and abrasions with soap and water to be superior to topical antiseptics. Another recommendation is the use of water-based surfactant cleaners, which contain wetting agent beads that break down the surface action between water and oil and do not impair healing. Nursing research on topical therapies for decubitus ulcers is more rigorous and now includes the use of control groups, which should improve treatment modalities in the future.

In stage 3 and stage 4 ulcers, the necrotic tissue must be removed, or debrided, before healing will begin. Debridement can be achieved by mechanical scrubbing, use of sharp instruments, and by enzymatic agents such as sutilains (Travase) and fibrinolysin. Skin-barrier creams and ointments are available to protect the skin from excessive moisture and breakdown. These can also be applied to stage 1 ulcers (reddened areas) to prevent extension.[3, 13] For almost a decade, significant developments have occurred in topical therapy based on the principles of moist wound healing. A moist environment is maintained by applying an occlusive, adhesive, moisture vapor film or wafer over the wound and surrounding skin. Because there is no scab formation, the moist environment speeds epithelialization and allows the individual's white blood cells to phagocytize the debris and microorganisms in the wound.[5] These adhesive dressings increase patient comfort, reduce friction, can remain in place 1 to 7 days, and have demonstrated success in the treatment of stage 1, 2, and 3 ulcers.[4] For deeper stage 3 and stage 4 ulcers, absorptive dressings such as gauze, karaya powder, and dressings composed of dextranomer beads or copolymer starches are recommended. The outcome of the above measures will be a clean, healing lesion before patient discharge from the health care setting.

To reduce itching and scratching, minimize the patient's dry skin if possible by limiting the frequency of baths, using a mild soap sparingly, blotting skin dry after bathing, applying lotion to skin when wet,[12] and maintaining adequate hydration status. Administer physician-ordered antipruritics to control itching. Remind the patient about the dangers of scratching (e.g., damage to the epidermis and the potential for infection). Keep fingernails short and free of rough edges to reduce damage by scratching. Use distraction techniques to remove the individual's focus from the itching sensation. Use mitts and other restraints when needed for young children or confused adults to prevent scratching. The outcome is that relief of itching will reduce damage induced by scratching and preserve the integument before patient discharge from the health care setting.

Patient and family involvement in the plan of care is the fourth goal. The patient or the family should be knowledgeable about general skin care and assessment, the use of lubricants, protocols for increasing circulation, the importance of nutrition, the mechanism of action for topical treatments, the causes of pruritus, interventions that relieve itching, and factors that increase itching.

◢ **NURSING CARE GUIDELINES**
Nursing Diagnosis: Risk for Impaired Skin Integrity

Expected Outcome: The patient's risk factors will be identified early in the admission process.
- Assess for the presence of intrinsic and extrinsic risk factors.
- Inspect the skin for redness, lesions, blisters, swelling, and drainage and document them.
- ▲ Monitor laboratory values that have an effect on the skin: hematocrit, hemoglobin, bilirubin, blood urea nitrogen, albumin, uric acid, and arterial blood gases. Report them to the physician.
  Assessment of risk factors is essential to establishing an appropriate plan of care.

Expected Outcome: The patient's skin will remain intact throughout admission.
- Keep skin clean and dry.
- Cleanse the skin with mild soap promptly after incontinence.
- Apply protective creams if reddened areas develop from incontinence.
- Consult enterostomal therapy nurse.
- Assess patient and family knowledge regarding skin breakdown and preventive care.
  Effective care will minimize skin breakdown.

Expected Outcome: The patient's skin will be free from trauma throughout care.
- Use assistive devices and techniques to facilitate dependent and independent movements, leg trapeze, lifts, turning sheets, transfer boards.
- Use powder judiciously on surfaces contacting the skin.
- Place footboard on bed.
- Use knee gatch when head of bed is elevated.
- Limit Fowler's position to less than 1 hour.
- Apply clear occlusive dressing to high-risk areas of the skin.
  Physical trauma from friction and shearing forces contributes to skin breakdown.

Expected Outcome: The patient's circulation will be maximized.
- Get the patient out of bed and ambulating if possible.
- Limit the sitting position to less than 2 hours.
- Reposition the patient every 1 to 2 hours, using all four sides.
- Provide range-of-motion exercises every 2 hours.
- Avoid massaging reddened areas when repositioning patient.
- Use pressure-relieving device for patients who cannot tolerate turning.
- Use pressure-reducing device in conjunction with turning schedule.
  Necrosis may occur from high pressure over short periods of time or from low pressure over long periods of time.

Expected Outcome: The patient's nutritional status will be optimized.
- ▲ With the physician, monitor and assess nutritional parameters: oral or parenteral intake of protein, calories, and fluids; albumin and total protein levels; and weekly weights in relation to ideal weight.
  Optimum tissue hydration and a positive nitrogen balance are critical elements in total body health and wound healing.

■ = nursing intervention; ▲ = collaborative intervention.

◾ **NURSING CARE GUIDELINES**
Nursing Diagnosis: Impaired Skin Integrity

Expected Outcome: The patient will attain intact skin by the time of discharge.
- Assess and eliminate (if possible) etiological factors contributing to skin breakdown.
- Assess the impairment and document the location, size, depth, and presence of redness, drainage, or necrotic tissue; the presence or absence of granulation tissue; and symptoms of infection.
  Accurate assessment and regular documentation of skin impairments will improve the quality of care and the evaluation of treatments.
- Consult enterostomal therapy nurse.
▲ In collaboration with ET nurse and physician, institute a topical therapy to create a favorable environment for healing.
- Use topical therapy to keep the wound surface clean, moist, and free from infection (transparent adhesive, hydrocolloid, gel, or moist gauze dressings).
  Science-based therapy will hasten healing and the restoration of skin integrity.

Expected Outcome: The patient will achieve comfort through relief of itching within 24 hours.
- Assess causative factors of itching.
- Prevent excessive dryness of the skin: bathe only as necessary, use mild soap, lubricate skin after bathing, and maintain adequate hydration status.
- Teach patient about the need to refrain from scratching.
- Trim and file nails to limit damage from scratching.
▲ Administer antihistamines and antipruritics as ordered, as needed.
- Use distraction techniques to keep patient from scratching.
- Provide mitts or restraints for confused individuals to prevent scratching.
  Relief of itching will reduce skin damage induced by scratching and help preserve the integument.

Expected Outcome: The patient and family will participate in the plan of care throughout the patient's stay.
- Teach the patient and family about general skin care, the mechanism of action and application of treatments, the importance of providing an adequate dietary intake, and measures to prevent skin impairments.
- Encourage patient and family self-care when appropriate.
  The patient and family's participation in the plan of care increases knowledge and skill in self-care and the plan's potential for success.

◾ = nursing intervention; ▲ = collaborative intervention.

EVALUATION

The overall indicator that demonstrates the effectiveness of the nursing interventions for the nursing diagnosis of Risk for Impaired Skin Integrity is the presence of intact skin. By maintaining clean and dry skin, avoiding trauma to the skin, and maximizing circulatory and nutritional status, the nurse increases the patient's resistance to skin breakdown.

The first patient outcome for the patient with impaired skin integrity is to regain skin integrity. Data indicating improvement in this condition are (1) the skin impairment is clean and free of secondary bacterial infection; (2) the impairment decreases in size; and (3) the skin is warm, dry, and intact. The next expected outcome is that the individual will demonstrate increased comfort through the relief of itching. Data indicating improvement in this status are subjective reports from the individual of relief of itching and the presence of intact skin. The last expected outcome is that the individual or family will participate appropriately in the plan of care. This is achieved through follow-up observation of a demonstration of skin care by the patient or family.

⌐ CASE STUDY WITH PLAN OF CARE

Mrs. Vicki W., a 75-year-old widow, was admitted to the medical unit for treatment of severe dehydration. The daughter reported that Mrs. W. had experienced decreased appetite for about 3 weeks and that during the past week she often refused to eat. Furthermore, during the week she began to stay in bed most of the day, getting up only to use the bathroom. Initial assessment revealed a frail, slightly lethargic but oriented elderly woman. Body weight was 90 pounds for a frame of 5'1"; skin was flaking off her arms; a 10-cm stage 2 pressure ulcer was located on her left hip; albumin level was 2.7 gm/dl (low); and blood urea nitrogen was 68 mg/dl. One nursing diagnosis was that of Impaired Skin Integrity related to immobility and malnutrition.

⌐ PLAN OF CARE FOR MRS. VICKI W.

Nursing Diagnosis: Impaired Skin Integrity Related to Immobility, Malnutrition, and Dehydration

Expected Outcome: Mrs. W. will retain skin integrity throughout admission.
- Assess, monitor, and document the characteristics of the wound.
- Cleanse the wound with soap and water and pat dry.
- Apply Op-Site clear occlusive dressing to wound and surrounding tissue.
- Consult the enterostomal therapy nurse.

Expected Outcome: Mrs. W. will demonstrate absence or control of factors that contribute to the formation of the impairment—poor nutrition and immobility—throughout admission.
- Monitor nutritional status.
- Follow daily weights, albumin levels, and tolerance to feedings.
- Maintain nasogastric tube feedings as ordered.
- Maintain hydrating intravenous line as ordered.
- Place Mrs. W. on alternating air mattress.
- Remove Mrs. W. from her bed and ambulate as tolerated.
- Reposition Mrs. W. every 2 hours if necessary.
- Add lubricating oil to bath water, apply body lotion after bath, and limit frequency of baths.
- Monitor blood chemistries that affect skin and report these: blood urea nitrogen, albumin, hematocrit, hemoglobin, arterial blood gases, uric acid, and bilirubin.

■ = nursing intervention; ▲ = collaborative intervention.

⊞ CRITICAL THINKING EXERCISES

1. Discuss various means for assessment of the wound and documentation that best describes the stage, the progress, and the treatment of Mrs. W.'s wound. Give examples.
2. What nutritional elements need to be included in Mrs. W.'s diet that will aid in healing her stage 2 lesion? Develop a 24-hour meal plan that includes these elements.
3. Discuss the role of activity in the healing of Mrs. W.'s lesion. How can the effects of activity on Mrs. W.'s total well-being be assessed and documented? What will be the focus of teaching regarding activity for the patient and family? Prepare a teaching plan for Mrs. W. and her family that includes activity.
4. A patient is admitted to the acute care setting from a foster home care setting. The patient suffers from dehydration and has multiple stage 1 and stage 2 decubiti. The personal relationship between the foster care provider and the patient is very good, and the foster care provider is the only visitor the patient has.

The patient will return to the foster home setting. How would you approach the foster home care provider to teach her how to improve the quality of care she provides?

5. If you were a nurse manager responsible for evaluation of a new product used in the care of the skin, what would be your criteria for evaluation? Who would you involve in the evaluation process? How would you implement the evaluation process?

6. If you were responsible for designing a policy for delegation of certain aspects of skin care to certified nursing assistants (CNAs), what tasks would you allow to be delegated? What is your rationale for delegating these tasks? How would you monitor and evaluate the quality of delegated skin care the CNA provides?

REFERENCES

1. Agency for Health Care Policy and Research (AHCPR): *Pressure ulcers in adults: prediction and prevention, Clinical Practice Guidelines No 3, AHCPR Bulletin No 92-00047,* Rockville, Maryland, Agency for Health Care Policy and Research, Public Health Services, U.S. Department of Health and Human Services, 1992.

2. Agency for Health Care Policy and Research (AHCPR): Clinical guidelines: how to predict and prevent pressure ulcers, *AJN* 92(7):54–56, 1992.

3. Bolton L and van Rijswijk L: Wound dressings: meeting clinical and biological needs, *Dermatol Nurs* 3:146–161, 1991.

4. Cuzzell JZ: Test your wound assessment skills, *AJN* 94(4):34–35, 1994.

5. Erwin-Toth P and Hocevar BJ: Wound care: selecting the right dressing, *AJN* 95(2):46–51, 1995.

6. Halpin-Landry JE: Documenting wounds through the camera's eye, *Nursing 94* 24(12):58–60, 1994.

7. International Association of Enterostomal Therapists: Standards of care—dermal wounds: pressure sores, *J Enterostom Ther* 15(1):4–17, 1987.

8. Kelley L and Mobily P: Iatrogenesis in the elderly: impaired skin integrity, *J Geront Nurs* 17(9):24–29, 1991.

9. Kosiak M: Prevention and rehabilitation of pressure ulcers, *Decubitus* 4(2):60–68, 1991.

10. Kuhn BA and Coulter SP: Balancing the pressure ulcer cost and quality equation, *Adv Nurs* 17(10):353–359, 1992.

11. Maklebust J: Impact of AHCPR pressure ulcer guidelines on nursing practice, *Decubitus* 4(2):46–50, 1991.

12. Phipps NJ and others: *Medical surgical nursing concepts and clinical practice,* ed 4, St. Louis, 1991, Mosby–Year Book.

13. Van Etten NK, Sexton P, and Smith R: Development and implementation of a skin care program, *Ostomy Wound Manage* 27(3):40–54, 1990.

14. Wound Care Update 91, *Nurs 91* 21(4):47–50, 1991.

Impaired Swallowing

▶

Impaired Swallowing *is the state in which the individual has decreased ability to pass fluids or solids voluntarily from the mouth to the stomach.*[17]

OVERVIEW

Impaired Swallowing is a human response that crosses virtually all age groups and is associated with a broad range of medical illnesses. Impaired Swallowing historically has been associated primarily with medical diagnoses such as stroke and cancer of the head and neck. However, the literature indicates that Impaired Swallowing exists as an actual or risk diagnosis for a much larger patient population than that previously identified.[8, 20] Discussion of the normal swallowing process is an essential first step in the discussion of this impairment.

Swallowing results from a series of complex actions that reflect the intricate anatomy of the oral and pharyngeal structures, multiple neural mechanisms, characteristics of the bolus, and factors specific to the patient (e.g., the physical, cognitive, and emotional level of function).[1] A complete swallowing cycle lasts an average of 5 to 10 seconds and occurs in four stages: oral preparatory, oral, pharyngeal, and esophageal.[11]

In the oral preparatory stage, food or liquid is masticated or manipulated. Lip closure keeps the bolus within the oral cavity, and lingual lateralization maneuvers the bolus to and from the teeth and mixes it with saliva. The oral stage begins when the tongue propels the bolus in an upward and backward motion and ends when the bolus enters the pharynx. These two stages are under

voluntary control. The pharyngeal stage begins with the triggering of the pharyngeal swallow, which is mediated by the action of the medulla and characterized by a series of neuromuscular events.[11] The esophageal phase is marked by peristaltic wave action of the esophagus that moves the bolus through it to the stomach. Table 4 details the nerves that support the activities in each of the swallowing stages.[13]

Impaired Swallowing often is seen in patients with an inadequate cough or gag reflex, a speech disorder, abnormal oral secretions, musculoskeletal deficits, or impaired neurological functioning. A diverse group of medical diagnoses includes Impaired Swallowing as a symptom or outcome. Rubin and others[18] classify such diagnoses as structural or neuromuscular in nature. Impaired Swallowing resulting in aspiration is common in patients sustaining strokes. DePippo, Holas, and Reding[3] have focused on risk management of patients following strokes. Their work appears to validate a dysphagia screening test that identifies patients in the rehabilitation phase after the stroke at risk for pneumonia, recurrent upper airway obstruction, and death.

In children congenital anomalies such as cleft palate, cerebral palsy, and Down syndrome can contribute to Impaired Swallowing. Many traumatically brain-injured individuals have problems with oral intake associated with Impaired Swallowing. Lazarus and Logemann[10] examined the frequency of swallowing disorder in 53 traumatic brain-injured individuals ranging from 4 to 69 years of age. Among the nine different types of disorders identified, delayed triggering of the pha-

TABLE 4 Cranial Nerve Functions in Swallowing

Stage	Structure	Nerves	Function
Oral preparatory	Lips	V, VIII	Keeps bolus in oral cavity
Oral	Tongue	VII, IX	Manipulates bolus
	Soft palate	VII, IX, X	Separation of oral and nasal cavity
	Cheeks	V, VII	Controls bolus when chewing
	Tongue	VII, IX	Collects and moves bolus
Pharyngeal	Oropharynx	IX, X	Moves bolus to hypopharynx
	Hypopharynx	X, XI	Moves bolus into esophagus
Esophageal	Esophagus	X	Moves bolus into stomach

ryngeal swallow and reduced tongue control occurred most frequently. Impaired Swallowing is increasingly identified as related to medical problems found in the multihandicapped, mentally retarded population,[14] where the leading cause of death is asphyxia, often related to the aspiration of food.[2]

Weiden and Harrigan[21] caution that the presence of Impaired Swallowing should not be dismissed as relating to an emotional disturbance. In discussing patients with drug-induced Impaired Swallowing, they note that both Parkinson's disease and tardive dyskinesia can cause eating and swallowing disturbances. Psychotropic medications and most anticholinergic agents may impair the gag reflex and thus contribute to Impaired Swallowing.

Health professionals are increasingly expected to treat clients outside of health care facilities. This is most true in rural areas, where multidisciplinary support staff are unavailable or insufficiently trained in identification and management of swallowing disorders. Kohler[8] has proposed a three-stage Impaired Swallowing management model for patients residing in rural areas. The model focuses on training home health care providers to observe, record, and report Impaired Swallowing problems. This approach has resulted in significant improvements in care delivery and the strategic targeting of resources.

The nurse must have a clear and complete knowledge of normal swallowing to be effective in identifying impairments. The timely and accurate identification of the patient with or at increased risk for Impaired Swallowing is the focus of the nursing assessment.

ASSESSMENT

Meerhoff[15] notes that detailed patient history can assist greatly in formulating the causes of Impaired Swallowing and offers a detailed history and assessment algorithm to guide this process. Such a systematic approach also can be used by the nurse to pinpoint related factors. Loustau and Lee[13] suggest that reflexes, speech and voice, secretions, supporting muscles, and orientation are five broad areas around which to organize nursing assessment of patients having or suspected of having Impaired Swallowing.

Assessment begins with identification of existing health deficits that increase the patient's risk of having or developing Impaired Swallowing. Patients who have had cerebrovascular accidents are often the most severely affected group; other high-risk populations may not be as obvious. Loustau and Lee[13] address this problem, proposing a five-dimensional approach to assessment. Similarly, Gordon[5] proposes assessment based on 11 areas applicable to all patients. Because of their relevance to clinical practice and their ability to provide conceptual direction for patient assessment, Gordon's Functional Health Patterns can be used to guide the nursing assessment.

Assessment of the Health-Perception—Health-Management Pattern includes determination of the patient's perception of swallowing ability and what measures are used to assist swallowing. The quality of the patient's diet along with a history of weight changes, body temperature, and skin integrity provide important assessment data for the Nutritional-Metabolic Pattern. Discussing favorite foods or having the patient list the types of food and fluids consumed in an average day gives important clues as to the presence of a swallowing disorder.

Patients with Impaired Swallowing also may demonstrate changes in their Elimination Pattern. A careful history of bowel and bladder habits can help determine the duration and intensity of a swallowing impairment. Similarly, identifying changes in the patient's Activity-Exercise Pattern permits discussion of the patient's goals and level of satisfaction with his or her current health status.

Assessment of the patient's Cognitive-Perceptual pattern is especially important when the potential for Impaired swallowing exists. The status of the patient's senses and perception of pain aid in defining the level of impairment. Memory, judgment, ability to concentrate, and decision-making skills will determine the appropriateness of self-care-focused educational interventions.

Assessment of the Sleep-Rest Pattern provides valuable information for the appropriate timing of care interventions and for identifying when the patient is at an optimum ability to participate in care. Similarly, the patient's emotions and feelings associated with the Self-Perception—Self-Concept pattern provide important information on the effect a change in swallowing ability has had on personal identity and body image. These assessment data are vital, especially if interventions such as the placement of a nasogastric or other alimentary system tube is being considered.

The quality and size of the patient's social sup-port system can be identified through assessment of the Role-Relationship Pattern. Information about resources for support and assistance in the home is vital to planning for meeting recovery and rehabilitation goals of patients recovering from strokes, closed head injuries, or other long-term illnesses that frequently include Impaired Swallowing among their side effects.

Assessment of the Sexuality-Reproductive Pattern in the patient with or at risk for Impaired Swallowing most often focuses on the effects of the impairment on physical energy and psychological well-being. Similarly, assessment data related to the patient's Coping—Stress-Tolerance Pattern can identify the degree to which actual or risk for Impaired Swallowing is of concern to the patient, what other stressors are contributing to this effect, and what patient-directed versus assisted-coping mechanisms are appropriate.

Finally, assessment of the patient's Value-Belief Pattern focuses on identifying the spiritual and philosophical principles that guide the way the patient views life. Assessment data from this pattern can provide invaluable insight into the potential for patient participation in the management of Impaired Swallowing.

Defining characteristics of this diagnosis include subjective and objective findings. Subjective data collection includes a detailed health history, with a focus on the patient's view of changes in nutritional status (e.g., weight loss or anorexia), oral health (e.g., changes in the quality or quantity of secretions, pain, and bleeding), and speech and voice quality. Objective data are obtained from interdisciplinary assessment,[7] including assessment of the quality of reflexes, head and neck structures, general health status, psychosocial status, and speech and voice quality.

In gathering subjective data the nurse must determine the patient's ability to recall, describe, and discuss past and present health status. If the patient displays significant memory impairment, is easily confused, or appears to be expressively or receptively aphasic, subjective data may be limited or may have to be obtained by interviewing a family member or friend. In all cases the nurse should take all necessary steps to maximize the patient's participation in this phase of the assessment process.

Objective data collection begins with a detailed physical assessment, with attention to clues about overall nutritional health (e.g., oral mucous membranes, height to weight ratios, skin turgor) and neurological and musculoskeletal status. Identification of the status of the gag, cough, and swallowing reflexes and assessment of the quality of mouth and upper airway structures are critical activities in the performance of a comprehensive evaluation of the patient's health. Inspection and palpation are key assessment behaviors.

■ Defining Characteristics

The presence of the following defining characteristics indicates that the patient may be experiencing Impaired Swallowing:

- Cough when eating or drinking
- Reduced buccal or facial tone
- Reduced soft palate function
- Delayed or absent swallowing reflex
- History of declining oral intake
- Pain on swallowing
- Avoidance of favorite foods
- Limited socialization
- Reduced tongue control
- Weight loss
- Choking
- Fear of choking
- Severe depression
- Denial of changes in health
- Avoidance of eating with others

■ Related Factors

The following related factors are associated with Impaired Swallowing:

- Neuromuscular dysfunction
- Reddened or irritated oropharyngeal cavity
- Neurological deficits
- Depression over current changes in health
- Absence or loss of social support system

- Loss of cultural incentives related to eating
- Loss of valuing life and survival
- Mechanical obstruction
- Developmental disability

DIAGNOSIS

■ Differential Nursing Diagnosis

Impaired Swallowing is similar to but can be differentiated from six other NANDA-approved nursing diagnoses. For example, for the diagnosis Altered Oral Mucous Membrane, although physical assessment findings may be similar, outcome interventions will be primarily focused on the structural condition of the oral cavity. In Impaired Swallowing, this diagnosis may be discussed as a relational factor (i.e., that Altered Oral Mucous Membrane interferes with performance of the oral phase of swallowing). Similarly, for the diagnosis Risk for Aspiration, the presence of dysphagia from neurological or esophageal disorders is one of several risk factors that can predispose a patient to aspiration. However, because the mortality rate for this diagnosis is high (50% to 70%), nursing interventions are directed at prevention. This contrasts with the treatment focus of interventions for Impaired Swallowing. Four other diagnoses may be viewed as possible outcomes of unsuccessful management of Impaired Swallowing. They are Altered Nutrition: Less Than Body Requirements; Risk for Fluid Volume Deficit; and Fluid Volume Deficit. For these diagnoses, altered intake is the consistent risk factor, and Impaired Swallowing is one of many possible etiologies. Finally, assessment resulting in determination of the diagnosis Self-Care Deficit: Feeding may result in identification of the diagnosis of Impaired Swallowing. However, this diagnosis is distinguished from Impaired Swallowing in its focus on the type and degree of impact of an inability to perform the self-care behavior of feeding oneself.

■ Medical and Psychiatric Diagnoses

Numerous medical and psychiatric diagnoses are associated with Impaired Swallowing. The five

II

most common examples are cerebrovascular accident, esophageal cancer, myasthenia gravis, Parkinson's disease, and developmental disablement. Although each is defined by a specific set of physical or behavioral findings, they share commonality in the treatment or management of Impaired Swallowing. Consistent with current trends in collaborative care, a comprehensive, multidisciplinary approach to treatment, planning, and implementation is the standard of practice today.

OUTCOME IDENTIFICATION, PLANNING, AND IMPLEMENTATION

Nursing interventions for patients with Impaired Swallowing can be grouped into three major areas:

(1) assessment of the patient for changes from the initially assessed baseline function or competency regarding swallowing; (2) implementation and evaluation of specific treatment measures designed to eliminate or minimize the diagnosis and its effects; and (3) teaching the patient and family about the diagnosis.

The first expected patient outcome listed in the Nursing Care Guidelines focuses on the quality and degree of understanding by the patient and family of the specific characteristics of the patient's swallowing impairment. The second expected patient outcome focuses on the patient's and family's ability to perform care behaviors in support of successful swallowing. The third expected patient outcome focuses on the degree of resolution of the impairment in swallowing.

◢ **NURSING CARE GUIDELINES**
Nursing Diagnosis: Impaired Swallowing

Expected Outcome: No later than the time of discharge, the patient and family will state correct information regarding the swallowing impairment.
▲ Perform and document patient assessment.
▲ Explain findings to the patient and family and discuss them.
▲ Validate understanding of information.
 Interventions associated with this outcome ensure that the patient and family will be provided accurate and timely information about the nature of the impairment.

Expected Outcome: No later than the time of discharge, the patient and family will demonstrate correct performance of care behaviors such as the selection and preparation of foods, positioning, oral care, and use of assistive devices.
▲ Teach care behaviors to the patient and family.
■ Observe and document patient and family performance of care behaviors and reinstruct as necessary.
 Interventions associated with this outcome ensure that the patient will attain a level of self-care ability that will sustain an acceptable level of health regarding management of swallowing.

Expected Outcome: No later than the time of discharge, the patient will be able to swallow selected foods and fluids without evidence of choking, coughing, or aspiration.
▲ Observe performance of the patient's swallow, and evaluate problems.
▲ Reteach care behaviors as necessary.
▲ Request consultation by adjunctive specialties (e.g., dietitian, speech therapist, etc.) as necessary.
 Interventions associated with this outcome ensure the patient will be able to manage the impairment alone or will be able to manage it with additional guidance and/or support.

 ■ = nursing intervention; ▲ = collaborative intervention.

EVALUATION

The degree of achievement of expected patient outcomes will vary depending on the nature and intensity of the impairment, the ability of the patient to participate in care, and the presence of other acute or chronic health problems that tax resources and capabilities. The nurse can determine if the first outcome is achieved by questioning the patient and family directly or by discussing the patient's hospitalization in general and then focusing discussion on the patient's views regarding his or her Impaired Swallowing. Incorrect or incomplete patient or family statements will require further discussions and explanations regarding the impairment. If the patient does not achieve this outcome, the nurse must act to ensure that at least one significant other is able to state correct information.[6]

The nurse can determine the attainment of the second listed expected outcome by having the patient or family respond to "what if" scenarios in discussions of post–hospital care and by direct observation of the patient's self-care behaviors.[4,12] If the patient cannot perform his or her self-care or needs assistance, the nurse must act to ensure that a significant other is knowledgeable and available to assist the patient or family in identifying private or public sources of assistance (e.g., a public health nurse or home health aide).

The degree of achievement of the third expected outcome, being able to swallow selected foods and fluids without problems, will vary based on the amount of success possible within the limitations of the impairment and the existence of complicating health problems. The nurse can determine the quality of achievement of this outcome by direct observation of the patient under various swallowing conditions. A corollary to this outcome is that the patient must consume sufficient quantities of food and fluids to maintain acceptable levels of nutrition and hydration. If this condition is not met, the nurse should consider discussion of the use of assistive systems to support the patient's intake for short-term or long-term use.[9,16]

▶ CASE STUDY WITH PLAN OF CARE

Mr. Carl M. is being evaluated in the ENT clinic. He is accompanied by his wife, who gives the following medical history: Mr. M. is a 64-year-old black male, a retired carpenter, who was in reasonably good health until 2 years ago when he suffered a mild stroke. Initially he lost the function of his left side and had left facial drooping and moderate expressive aphasia. Mrs. M. states that since the stroke her husband regained the use of his left side but continues to have some facial drooping and occasional confused speech. He has lost 20 lbs in the last 2 months, and she has noticed that his voice is hoarse. Mr. M. states that "it hurts sometimes when I swallow" and that he is more tired lately. Today the doctor told him that he has a "small cancer" in his throat, and he advised radiation therapy as treatment. The couple has two grown sons who live with their families in nearby cities. Mrs. M. is a retired schoolteacher who does church work but otherwise is home with her husband. She describes her health as very good.

Progress notes indicate significant resolution of Mr. M.'s stroke-related side effects. The patient smoked 1 to 2 packs of cigarettes per day for 40 years but quit 2 years ago (after the stroke). He has mild hypertension and drinks no alcohol. His blood pressure is 150/90 mm Hg, respirations are 22/min, temperature is 98.2°F, and pulse is 84 beats/min. He is 73 inches tall and weighs 152 lbs (his life average is 175 to 180 lbs; down to 170 to 175 lbs after his stroke). His voice is hoarse, but his speech is intelligible. The physician's note states that Mr. M. has a 3 cm lesion of the left true vocal cord and moderate pharyngeal erythema and tenderness. The tentative medical diagnosis is squamous cell carcinoma of the left true vocal cord. The medical plan is for a full medical workup followed by a 6-week course of radiation therapy. Mr. M.'s cough and gag reflexes are intact, and there is no other evidence of oral disease.

Mr. M. teaches basic carpentry part-time at the local high school (now in summer recess) and does odd jobs around the house. He enjoys visits from his students, who often come by to discuss carpentry projects. He describes his wife as "my companion"; their interaction appears very warm and loving. Mr. M. describes having frequent contact with his sons and their families and says that they come to see him more often since he has not been feeling well. Mr. and Mrs. M.'s combined retirement incomes are described as sufficient with "a little extra." Mr. M.'s routine mealtimes are 8 A.M., 1 P.M., and 6 P.M. He noticed increased difficulty eating fried foods and most meats and now eats mostly soups, stews, custards, and mashed potatoes ("easier to get down than steak"). His appetite has progressively decreased over the last 2 to 3 months. Mr. M. is generally quiet during the interview but responds verbally in an appropriate manner when spoken to. He says he feels "anxious but hopeful" that treatment will be effective, and he indicates a desire to participate actively in his care and health management.

▶ PLAN OF CARE FOR MR. CARL M.

Nursing Diagnosis: Impaired Swallowing Related to Residual Stroke-Related Side Effects, Presence of Vocal Cord Lesion, and Common Effects of Radiation Therapy

---

Expected Outcome: By the end of the preradiation evaluation period, Mr. M. and his family will accurately identify and describe his current status related to the side effects of stroke as evidenced by the consistency of the patient's description with clinical facts.
- Discuss the patient's health history related to current activities of daily living and self-care ability.
- Identify and agree on the areas where help is needed and by whom.
- ▲ Discuss and assess the effect of stroke on Mr. M.'s ability to chew, swallow, control secretions, and maintain weight.

Expected Outcome: By the end of the preradiation evaluation period, Mr. M. will accurately describe his current health limitations and abilities related to new health problems as evidenced by the consistency of the patient's description with clinical facts.
- ▲ Discuss and assess the effect of new health problems on Mr. M.'s ability to chew, swallow, speak, control secretions, and maintain weight.

Expected Outcome: Not later than the day of his first radiation treatment (RXT), Mr. M. will accurately identify and describe the common side effects of radiation therapy and the measures used to prevent or minimize these effects.
- ▲ Explain RXT (e.g., the purpose, use, and side effects).
- Provide a copy of patient education literature on RXT and set aside time to discuss content.
- Discuss and demonstrate care measures Mr. M. can use to prevent or minimize RXT effects related to swallowing: oral care procedures, use of analgesics, secretion supplements, daily oral exams, dietary supplements, activity and rest needs, and symptoms and emergencies.
- Consult to speech therapy for assessment and treatment.

Expected Outcome: Throughout the period of RXT, Mr. M. will maintain adequate nutritional and hydration status (as evidenced by a weight loss of no more than 8 lbs from start to end of treatment), balanced intake and output, and stable physiological parameters (e.g., electrolytes).
- Have Mr. M. weigh himself daily.
- Have Mr. M. keep intake, output, and calorie count records.
- Teach Mr. M. how to assess oral and pharyngeal health.
- Consult to oral hygienist for assessment and fluoride treatments.
- Monitor systemic signs of hydration (e.g., skin turgor, temperature, and blood chemistries).

■ = nursing intervention; ▲ = collaborative intervention. *Continued*

II

▶ **PLAN OF CARE FOR MR. CARL M. — CONT'D**

Expected Outcome: Within 1 week of completion of RXT, Mr. M. will demonstrate stabilized or improved ability to swallow food and fluids as evidenced by demonstrated swallowing ability and the patient's perception of the quality of that ability.

▲ Encourage Mr. M. to expand and build swallowing skills, and encourage family to provide verbal support and encouragement.

Expected Outcome: Not later than the day of discharge, Mr. M. will participate in making plans regarding his care and future as evidenced by the content of conversations with family, friends, and health care staff.

- Encourage Mr. M. to make plans regarding the resumption of work and hobbies.
- Compliment Mr. M. on his ability to participate in care.
- Encourage Mr. M. to be active in self-care, and praise his efforts.

■ **CRITICAL THINKING EXERCISES**

1. In today's managed care environment, inpatient stays continue to be of short duration and in some cases are discontinued in favor of outpatient management. Consider how to provide necessary teaching and other support to Mr. M. if all his care for this illness is done as an outpatient. What community resources could be used? What support groups could be used?

2. What measures can be taken to ensure continuity of care across illness events and treatment settings? What role will Mr. M.'s health insurance play in this process?

3. How can Mr. M.'s wife and family be best assisted or facilitated in supporting Mr. M.'s care needs?

REFERENCES

1. Bach DB and others: An integrated team approach to the management of patients with oropharyngeal dysphagia, *J Allied Health* 18(5):4459–4468, 1989.
2. Carter G and Jancar J: Mortality in mentally handicapped: fifty year survey of stroke park hospitals, *J Ment Defic Res* 27:143–156, 1983.
3. DePippo KL, Holas MA, and Reding MJ: The Burke Dysphagia Screening Test: validation of its use in patients with stroke, *Arch Phys Med Rehab* 75:1264–1266, 1994.
4. Donahue PA: When it's hard to swallow: feeding techniques for dysphagia management, *J Geront Nurs* 16(4):6–9, 41–42, 1990.
5. Gordon M: *Nursing diagnosis: process and application,* ed 3, St. Louis, 1994, Mosby–Year Book.
6. Hutchins BF: Establishing a dysphagic family intervention program for head-injured patients, *J Head Trauma Rehab* 4(4):64–72, 1989.
7. Krafting I and others: A retrospective analysis of interdisciplinary dysphagia assessment data, *Phys Occup Ther Geriatr* 9(2):79–95, 1991.
8. Kohler ES: A dysphagia management model for rural elderly, *Phys Occup Ther Geriatr* 10(1):81–95, 1991.
9. Lazarus BA, Murphy JB, and Culpepper L: Aspiration associated with long-term gastric versus jejunal feedings: a critical analysis of the literature, *Arch Phys Med Rehab* 71:46–52, 1990.
10. Lazarus C and Logemann J: Swallowing disorders in closed head trauma patients, *Arch Phys Med Rehab* 68:79–84, 1987.
11. Lazarus CL: Swallowing disorders after traumatic brain injury, *J Head Trauma Rehab* 4(4):34–41, 1989.
12. Logemann JA and others: The benefits of head rotation on pharyngoesophageal dysphagia, *Arch Phys Med Rehab* 70:767–771, 1989.
13. Loustau A and Lee K: Dealing with the dangers of dysphagia, *Nursing 85* 15(2):47, 1985.
14. Lust CA, Fleetwood DE, and Molteler EL: Development and implementation of a dysphagia program in a mental retardation residential facility, *Occup Ther Health Care* 6(2/3):153–172, 1989.
15. Meerhoff JC: Diagnosis of dysphagia, *Hosp Prac:* p. 162, April 15, 1985.
16. Mochizuki RM and others: Heparin lock for nighttime intravenous fluid management in a dysphagic patient, *Rehab Nurs* 15(6):322–324, 1990.
17. North American Nursing Diagnosis Association: *NANDA nursing diagnoses: definitions and classification, 1995–1996,* Philadelphia, 1994, The Association.

18. Rubin M and others: Dysphagia: a clinical guide, *Hosp Med* 20:231, 1984.

19. Schwaab LM, Niman CW, and Gisel E: Tongue movements in normal 2-, 3-, and 4-year-old children: a continuation study, *Am J Occup Ther* 40:180, 1986.

20. Stratton M: Clinical management of dysphagia in the developmentally disabled adult, *Occup Ther Health Care* 6(2/3):143–152, 1989.

21. Weiden P and Harrigan M: A clinical guide for diagnosing and managing patients with drug-induced dysphagia, *Hosp Comm Psychiatry* 37:396, 1986.

II

Impaired Tissue Integrity

▶ ─────────────────────────────────────

Impaired Tissue Integrity *is the state in which an individual experiences damage (reversible or irreversible) to mucous membrane, corneal, integumentary, or subcutaneous tissue.*

OVERVIEW

Tissue impairment is characterized by an inflammatory response to tissue damage regardless of the etiology, duration, or extent of the injury. Tissue type and severity of damage determine how healing proceeds. Damage is reversible if cells remain intact, as with a stage I pressure ulcer. Injured epidermal tissues (the outer skin layer and cornea) regenerate in a relatively short time; however, damage to the dermis (the inner skin layer) or subcutaneous tissues involving the vasculature requires complex reparative processes.

Irreversible damage resulting from cell death is characterized by the appearance in the wound of soft yellow, white, or dry brown necrotic tissue. This tissue is an excellent medium for bacterial growth.[21] It also acts like a foreign body, prolonging the normal inflammatory response and preventing the easy migration of epithelial cells across the wound bed. Necrosis of deeper tissues may not be immediately visible.

There are many mechanisms of tissue injury. Pressure ulcers are caused by the effects of anaerobic metabolism resulting from the lack of oxygen suffered by tissues subjected to extrinsic pressure. Radiation therapy interrupts the DNA strands in cells, causing tissue impairment, the extent of which is determined by the depth and the dose of radiation.[22] Exposure to chemical and thermal

agents also results in tissue impairment and subsequent inflammation.

On injury, hemostatic mechanisms of reflex vasospasm and platelet aggregation prevent excessive blood loss and, by isolating the wound from the rest of the body, provide initial protection against bacterial invasion.[10] Injured tissues then release histamine, prostaglandins, and serotonins, which cause surrounding capillary walls to leak, making the injured area accessible to the immune system cells. This inflammation is an immediate immune system response to the injury that protects against infection and sets the stage for healing. The complement system begins destroying bacteria first, followed by polymorphonuclear leukocytes (PMNs), which begin to phagocytize bacteria within 24 hours. Macrophages also enter the wound to phagocytize bacteria and are essential to the following repair processes.[1] If inflammation is suppressed, wound healing is delayed or prevented.[7]

Wounds characterized by vascular and connective tissue damage must build new granulation tissue before the wound can be covered with new skin, or reepithelialized. During this stage of repair, new blood vessels are formed and collagen-based tissue grows in the base of the wound. Hypoxic conditions in the wound base stimulate granulation tissue growth. The presence of necrotic tissue in the wound delays the proliferation of granulation tissue and prolongs the inflammatory process. A moist wound bed allows the immune system cells to remain in the wound and digest necrotic tissue. This process is called *autolytic debridement*. The wound edges also contract during this period, producing a smaller wound and necessitating less production of granulation tissue and epithelialization. After a healthy vascular wound bed has developed, epithelial cells migrate from the wound edges until the wound is covered.

The final stage of healing is remodeling of the wound. For up to a year after the wound has been closed, collagen bundles are rearranged along the lines of mechanical stress to create stronger tissue. With the most efficient, normal wound healing, final tissue strength reaches only 70% to 80% of the strength of uninjured tissue.

ASSESSMENT

Interpretation of data gathered during assessment determines the plan of care. The nurse must consider the location of tissue impairment and its depth, etiology, and related factors in choosing systemic and topical care and equipment. Assessment data can be focused in two major areas: defining characteristics and related factors. In relation to defining characteristics, erythema is indicative of the inflammatory response to tissue injury. Non-blanchable erythema over a bony prominence is considered a stage I pressure ulcer.[15] Erythema, induration, edema, exudate, and pain are associated with wound infections. The nurse must be aware, however, that exudate and odor without other signs of infection do not always indicate an infection. Other possible causes are the desirable autolytic debridement, or digestion, of necrotic tissue by white blood cells, which occurs with moist wound–healing techniques. The nurse should clean the wound before complete assessment.

The nurse must consider the type of tissue disruption. The appearance of the impairment is important in differentiating the etiology. A discrete lesion over a bony prominence could be a pressure ulcer. A red, raised, itchy rash with eroding skin in the same location may indicate a fungus infection.

The patient's complaints of pain and itching are very helpful cues. Superficial pressure ulcers where nerves are intact can be painful as compared to deeper, potentially less painful lesions.

Increased pain in a wound is also an important clue for diagnosing wound infection. Itching of the axilla or the skin under an ostomy appliance could indicate a *Candida* fungal infection.

Many factors are related to the development of tissue impairment. Because tissues cannot heal without removal of tissue irritants and amelioration of contributing conditions, the success of the treatment plan depends on the correct identification of the related factors. Research is ongoing to establish strong scientific support for many of the factors listed at the end of this section. Indications are that no one factor can be identified in an individual case of tissue impairment. For example, the immobile patient may be receiving steroids for chronic obstructive pulmonary disease (COPD) and be unable to get out of bed when experiencing of diarrhea.

Tissues must receive oxygen via the circulatory system to remain healthy. Extrinsic pressures can close vessels caught between a hard surface and a bony prominence, resulting in a pressure ulcer. The immobile patient is at risk for tissue impairment. Intrinsic developments such as peripheral vascular disease or diabetes can cause venous stasis or arterial ulcers.[18,19]

Trauma to tissues, whether accidental or deliberate, arises from three sources: physical, chemical, or biological agents. Tissue can be damaged by sharp or hard objects such as bed rails, slider boards, or fingernails. Friction against bed sheets will eventually abrade skin. Shearing causes deeper damage when muscle rubs against bony prominences as the head of a bed is raised.

Chemical agents are anything that causes topical irritation to the skin, the eyes, or mucous membranes, such as soaps or insecticides. Medications are intrinsic chemical agents that may cause tissue reactions. Chemotherapeutic agents (e.g., 5-fluorouracil or cyclophosphamide) are associated with mucous membrane lesions and skin erythema. Steroids suppress the inflammatory response necessary for wound healing.[2,11] Skin also atrophies and becomes very susceptible to extrinsic damage (e.g., stripping by tape) after long-term use of steroids. Allergic reactions to medications such as antibiotics are sometimes manifested by skin rashes.

Contact with biological agents such as stools or wound drainage can cause erosion of skin and deeper tissues. Tissues become macerated, increasing susceptibility to trauma. Incontinence and moisture on the skin also increase susceptibility to opportunistic skin infections such as *Candida*.[14,20]

Other microorganisms cause tissue impairment. Herpes lesions may look like pressure ulcers. Lack of healing after treatment has been instituted, severe pain at the wound site, or a history of a "cold sore" in an immunosuppressed patient may be clues to consider herpes. The nurse may be the first to see these infections and must be astute.

Radiation from the sun or radiation therapy damages tissues. Radiation therapy damage can vary from superficial dry skin to deep, open, draining wounds as tumor cells necrose.[22] In many cases the damage from radiation therapy must run its course. Radiation therapy can damage tissues permanently, leaving them more susceptible to pressure damage and slowed, weakened wound healing.

Nutrition is important in keeping tissues healthy and supporting the repair process. Severe visceral protein depletion results in interstitial edema. Tissue edema may prevent efficient tissue oxygenation.[12] Lack of protein, zinc, and vitamins inhibits the repair process. Several studies have found a possible link between malnutrition, tissue breakdown, and impaired wound healing.[5,13,17]

Lack of knowledge or misinformation may be a factor related to Impaired Tissue Integrity. People at risk must know how to prevent tissue problems. A new paraplegic needs to learn how to care for the skin. A person receiving radiation therapy or medications needs information on side effects and tissue-protective strategies. The nurse should assess a patient's knowledge and beliefs about wound healing to identify potential inconsistencies between prescribed care and the patient's beliefs about wound healing. Knowledge about a person's social and financial situation may also assist the nurse to develop the treatment plan most likely to be effective. A person without money or physical assistance will not be able to accomplish a complex or expensive wound care plan.

Emotional states sometimes have a serious effect on self-care ability, even for a person with adequate knowledge of proper skin care. The depressed person may not eat. The hopeless paraplegic may not take the trouble to shift weight frequently.

■ Defining Characteristics

The presence of the following defining characteristics indicates that the patient may be experiencing Impaired Tissue Integrity:

- Erythema
- Edema
- Ecchymosis
- Induration
- Rashes, blisters, or lesions
- Eschar
- Exudate
- Odor
- Pain
- Itching

■ Related Factors

The following related factors are associated with Impaired Tissue Integrity:

- Altered circulation
- Immobility
- Pressure
- Disease (e.g., diabetes)
- Trauma
- Incontinence
- Shearing and friction
- Nutritional deficits
- Thermal extremes
- Radiation (including therapeutic)
- Microorganisms
- Medications (e.g., steroids)
- Depression
- Knowledge deficit
- Hopelessness
- Poverty

DIAGNOSIS

■ Differential Nursing Diagnosis

In the North American Nursing Diagnosis Association's taxonomy of approved nursing diagnoses

Altered Oral Mucous Membrane and Impaired Skin Integrity are subcategories of Impaired Tissue Integrity.[16] Although these diagnostic subcategories may be clearly differentiated by the tissue type involved, they share the general characteristics of the more abstract, higher order category of Impaired Tissue Integrity. Impaired Tissue Integrity is a subcategory of the diagnosis Altered Protection and thus shares some of the general characteristics of this higher order category.[16] Determining the diagnostic level of abstraction when selecting a label to define a human response is similar to the process of differential diagnosis. Identifying the defining characteristics of a diagnosis is important to choose the most specific and useful label. For example, the diagnosis Impaired Tissue Integrity captures the situation in which the oral mucous membranes, the skin, and the subcutaneous tissues are all disrupted related to the same factor of therapeutic radiation exposure for head and neck cancers. In contrast, the diagnoses Altered Mucous Membrane and Impaired Skin Integrity each defines only part of the situation, whereas a diagnosis of Altered Protection is too broad and may not define the problem with enough precision to be useful clinically.

■ Medical and Psychiatric Diagnoses

Numerous medical and psychiatric conditions can be associated with Impaired Tissue Integrity. Of particular significance are conditions that compromise the delivery of oxygen and nutrients to the tissues. These include cardiovascular and pulmonary diseases and diabetes. Infections and autoimmune responses can result in tissue impairment in the form of rashes and lesions. Conditions that limit mobility also are of great importance in considering the etiology of conditions such as pressure ulcers. Decreased ability to move can result from injuries, surgeries, aging, debilitating chronic diseases, and terminal disease. Psychiatric diagnoses such as depression often adversely affect a person's self-care ability, potentially resulting in pressure ulcers in patients at risk. Self-inflicted tissue injury is sometimes seen with psychotic patients. Given the multifactorial etiology of

Impaired Tissue Integrity, successful wound healing may require an interdisciplinary team of nurses and other clinicians (e.g., wound care nurse specialists, physicians, dietitians, physical therapists, and orthotists). Topical care, mobility, nutrition, and systemic illness can all be addressed to give the individual the best conditions for healing.

OUTCOME IDENTIFICATION, PLANNING, AND IMPLEMENTATION

Adequate circulation and tissue perfusion are necessary for the transport of oxygen and nutrients to healing tissues. External pressures on tissues must be reduced below capillary closure. Pressure relief may be needed for patients while in bed or in a chair—the type of equipment determined by the patient's individual characteristics.[8] Other types of equipment, such as cervical collars, tubing, splints, braces, and compression stockings, may be sources of pressure and need careful management. Increased mobility decreases the risk of pressure ulcer development. Active movement by the patient who is oriented and physically capable may be enhanced through exercise programs tailored for an individual's age, general health, and freedom of movement. When moving is problematic, assistance or passive movement by the nurse or physical therapist, with or without assistive devices, may be necessary. Patients with poor circulation related to endogenous causes, such as peripheral vascular disease, will also require medical management. Compression stockings and elevation of extremities may be prescribed to improve venous circulation. Therapeutic compression must be monitored to assure proper fit and prevention of restriction of circulation, especially for patients who may have impaired arterial circulation also.

Wounds need a moist, protected environment to support granulation and reepithelialization of tissues.[9] The nurse should carefully select dressings based on the wound's characteristics and the goal of the topical care. Wound size, location, amount and type of exudate, and presence or absence of necrotic tissue should be considered.

II

Necrotic tissue must be removed before healing can proceed easily. This can be accomplished by a clinician skilled with a scalpel. A slower but effective method is autolytic debridement, using hydrocolloid wafers, gels, foam pads, or transparent dressings. Mechanical debridement by whirlpool treatment or gauze dressings can remove necrotic tissue but may also damage granulation tissue. Whirlpool treatment should be used only for a short time to remove extensive necrotic tissue. After necrotic tissue has been removed from the wound, moist wound–healing methods should be continued to support optimal healing and to prevent the development of new necrotic tissue caused by a dry environment. If exudate needs to be removed from a wound during a dressing change, the wound can be gently irrigated with normal saline or surfactant-based wound cleansers. Use of antiseptic solutions such as povidone-iodine and hydrogen peroxide should be avoided because of their toxic effects on granulation tissue.[3,4]

Nutritional intervention may be needed. This may take the form of patient education or more active intervention, depending on the patient's ability and motivation to accept a diet that will support wound healing. A high-protein, high-carbohydrate, moderately low-fat diet with adequate calories is needed; supplemental vitamins (especially A and C) and minerals also may be indicated.[5,6] Consultation with a dietitian is helpful if diet is a major factor in individual cases. Frequent small meals or snacks may be a way to provide the increased nutrients needed for wound healing. Fluid intake should be increased also, especially for the patient with a burn or a draining wound. In addition to water, fluids with nutritional value will provide extra calories and nutrients.

Patients, families, and other caretakers need to be provided with information about factors related to healing, their specific wound care needs, prevention of recurrence, and, if needed, general hygienic instruction. Learners' feedback will guide the pace of teaching. Teaching should proceed from the simple, less threatening aspects of care to the more complex, with time allowed for the patient or family to practice and demonstrate competency in care.

◢ **NURSING CARE GUIDELINES**
Nursing Diagnosis: Impaired Tissue Integrity

Expected Outcome: The patient will have maximal circulation as evidenced by appropriate skin temperature and color, brisk capillary refill in surrounding tissues, pulses present, and resolving edema when initially present. The patient with peripheral vascular disease may show improvement in these parameters without achieving the normal characteristics described above.

- Provide pressure relief while in bed, chair, or wheelchair by using pressure relief devices; frequent, small, body repositionings; and turning the patient at least every 2 hours (side-back-side) *to prevent capillary closure and to maintain maximal blood flow to the tissues.*
- ▲ Prevent or relieve pressure from medical devices by using padding or by periodically loosening equipment when appropriate. Monitor and adjust devices to fit well or consult with physician regarding possible removal if unable to maintain proper fit *to prevent restriction of circulation.*
- Keep edematous extremities elevated *to decrease resistance to venous circulation.*
- ▲ Consult with physician regarding application of compression stockings when appropriate *to prevent or reduce edema in extremities.*
- ▲ Consult with physician regarding possible medical or surgical treatment of impaired systemic circulation *to maximize blood flow to the tissues.*
- ▲ Consult with physical therapist, if needed, *to maximize patient's mobility.*

Expected Outcome: The patient will show evidence of tissue healing by a decrease of necrotic tissue; development of red or pink, moist, granulation tissue in the wound bed; and progressively reduced diameter and depth of the wound. Superficial tissue impairment, without the development of necrotic tissue,

---

■ = nursing intervention; ▲ = collaborative intervention.

will show evidence of healing within 3 to 5 days. Deeper damage will take more time, depending on the extent of the wound.

- Cover wounds with the appropriate dressings *to promote moist wound healing, debridement of necrotic tissue, and absorption of excess wound drainage while keeping surrounding unimpaired tissues dry.*
- Adjust the type of dressing as the wound changes *to fit evolving wound characteristics.*
- Cleanse wounds with biocompatible solutions and minimal mechanical force *to remove necrotic tissue, excess wound exudate, and dressing residue.*
- Avoid diapers and use a fecal pouch or moisture barrier ointments *to protect tissues from further damage related to fecal and urinary incontinence.*
- ▲ Collaborate with physician *to identify and treat bacterial, fungal, and viral tissue infections.*
- ▲ Collaborate with dietitian *to provide high-protein diet of sufficient calories to support healing.*

Expected Outcome: The patient or family will demonstrate correct care for impaired tissues and describe a knowledgeable understanding of factors related to tissue impairment and healing by the time of discharge from the health care setting.

- Teach patient and family about factors that adversely affect tissues, such as immobility, medications, other medical treatments, and poor diet *to enlist their cooperation with treatment and prepare for self-care.*
- Teach patient and family how to protect tissue from pressure, excessive moisture, and incontinence *to promote self-care.*
- Teach patient and family appropriate wound care techniques *to assure competent self-care.*
- Teach patient and family signs and symptoms of Impaired Tissue Integrity, infection, and evidence of normal healing *to provide a framework for decision making after the patient assumes total self-care regarding the need for nursing or medical consultation.*

EVALUATION

Systematic evaluation focuses on specific outcomes expected as a response to treatments for Impaired Tissue Integrity. The frequency of observations should be timed to detect positive and negative changes in impaired tissues, depending on the phase of healing and the extent to which the related factors have been eliminated or controlled.

When oxygen saturation levels and transport are normal, circulation to tissues can be observed in the symmetrical color, brisk capillary refill time (less than 3 seconds), and skin temperature that is slightly cool or warm within expected variations related to the area observed. With adequate circulation, as tissues repair, swelling (edema) will resolve. The size, shape, and turgor of tissues will change and normalize as swelling decreases. Watch for erythema over bony prominences when repositioning the patient to determine whether pressure relief is adequate.

Wounds heal in a constant trajectory over time under optimal conditions. Tissue regeneration in wounds is evidenced by decreasing necrotic tissue

as the wound fills with red or pink, moist granulation tissue. Drainage will change in color, consistency, and amount, depending on the etiology of the wound. Pain will decrease, especially in a wound with a resolving infection. Regular serial measurements of open wounds by tracings on acetate paper or photographs should reveal progressively reduced diameter and depth (plumbed by Q-tip). Percentage of wound contraction can be calculated to take into account wound size and allow comparison of healing rates over time:

$$\text{Percent contraction} = 100 \times \frac{\text{Original area} - \text{Later area}}{\text{Original area}}^{[4]}$$

Patient and family knowledge and skills related to self-care need to be confirmed as teaching progresses by observing their ability to perform care correctly and consistently. It is also important to determine their perceptions of self-care efficacy. As self-care capacity increases, patients may be involved in caring for their wounds in preparation for total self-care when that is indicated.

▶ CASE STUDY WITH PLAN OF CARE

Ms. Helen W. is a 74-year-old woman with a 15-year history of Chronic Obstructive Pulmonary Disease. She has taken Prednisone for 10 years to control her respiratory symptoms. In the 2 weeks before admission to the hospital she had increasing difficulty breathing. She slept in a recliner chair because she "couldn't get her head high enough to breathe in bed." She reported losing 10 pounds in the last 6 weeks. She was admitted to the hospital 7 days ago for increasing respiratory distress and pitting edema of her lower extremities. On examination, respirations are 40/min and labored with rhonchi heard in both lungs. Pitting edema is present on lower legs and feet. Her skin is thin, dry, and scaly. She has multiple ecchymotic areas on her arms, with a 2-cm skin tear on her right forearm. Her coccyx area has a 2 cm by 3 cm shallow open lesion covered with a thin layer of yellow necrotic tissue. Tube feedings were begun 2 days ago. She now has diarrhea that she cannot control. She is unable to get out of bed without assistance. Her buttocks are erythematous and an itchy, red, raised rash with satellite lesions is beginning to appear.

▶ PLAN OF CARE FOR MS. W.

Nursing Diagnosis: Impaired Tissue Integrity Related to Pressure, Diarrhea, Steroid Use, Malnutrition, Edema, and Fungal Infection

Expected Outcome: Ms. W. will exhibit wound healing as evidenced by disappearance of rash within 7 days; dissolution of necrotic tissue; development of granulation tissue and epithelialization in 3 to 4 weeks; closure of skin tear within 2 weeks.
- Place fecal pouch around anus as long as diarrhea continues.
- Cover coccyx wound with hydrocolloid dressing. Use adhesive remover to remove dressing gently, and replace every 2 to 3 days. As drainage decreases, lengthen the time between hydrocolloid dressing changes. Place hydrogel dressing over skin tear. Change every day.
- ▲ Collaborate with physician to treat fungal infection and diarrhea.
- ▲ Collaborate with dietitian to provide high-protein diet, including tube feeding and oral intake. Assist patient to eat as needed.

Expected Outcome: Ms. W. will have maximized circulation as evidenced by decreased edema in extremities and the absence of erythema over bony prominences.
- Place airflow overlay on bed.
- Assist Ms. W. to stay off her back as much as possible.
- ▲ Place compression stockings on legs. Remove for 30 minutes every 4 hours.
- ▲ Collaborate with physician regarding fluid management and monitoring the expected shift of fluids from the interstitial tissues to the intravascular system.
- Keep legs elevated.
- ▲ Collaborate with physical therapist regarding maximizing patient mobility.

Expected Outcome: Ms. W. will demonstrate knowledge of how to prevent damage to her tissues.
- While performing skin and tissue care, show Ms. W. how to prevent damage from pressure and friction.
- Teach signs and symptoms of tissue damage.
- Teach which equipment and skin care products to use.
- Explain the importance of good nutrition and hydration to the maintenance of tissue integrity.

■ = nursing intervention; ▲ = collaborative intervention.

■ CRITICAL THINKING EXERCISES

1. How has each related factor contributed to Ms. W.'s Impaired Tissue Integrity?

2. What rationale underlies each dressing selected for Ms. W.'s Impaired Tissue Integrity?

3. What is the nurse's role in the collaborative process of care for Ms. W.'s Impaired Tissue Integrity?

REFERENCES

1. Barbul A: Immune aspects of wound repair, *Clin Plastic Surg* 17(3):433–442, 1990.

2. Baxter JD: The effects of glucocorticoid therapy, *Hosp Prac* 15:111–134, September 1992.

3. Bergstrom N and others: *Treatment of pressure ulcers*, Clinical Practice Guideline No 15, Pub No 95-0652, Rockville, Maryland, 1994, Agency for Health Care Policy and Research, Public Health Service, U.S. Department of Health and Human Services.

4. Bolton L and van Rijswijk L: Wound dressings: meeting clinical and biological needs, *Dermatol Nurs* 3(3):146–160, 1991.

5. Breslow RA, Hallfrisch J, and Goldberg AP: Malnutrition in tubefed nursing home patients with pressure sores, *J Parenter Enteral Nutr* 15(6):663–668, 1991.

6. Breslow RA and others: The importance of dietary protein in healing pressure ulcers, *J Am Geriatr Soc* 41(4):357–362, 1993.

7. Carrico T, Mehrhof A, and Cohen I: Biology of wound healing, *Surg Clin North Am* 64:721–733, 1984.

8. Counsell C, Seymour S, Guin P, and Hudson A: Interface skin pressures on four pressure relieving devices, *J Enterostom Ther* 17(4):150–153, 1990.

9. Dyson M and others: Comparison of the effects of moist and dry conditions on dermal repair, *J Investigat Dermatol* 91(5):434–439, 1988.

10. Gogia PP: The biology of wound healing, *Ostomy/Wound Management* 38(9):12–22, 1992.

11. Hotter AN: Wound healing and immunocompromise, *Nurs Clin North Am* 25(1):193–203, 1990.

12. Hunt TK, Rabkin J, and von Smitten K: Effects of edema and anemia on wound healing and infection, *Curr Stud Hematol Blood Transfus* 53:101–111, 1986.

13. Kemp MG and others: Factors that contribute to pressure sores in surgical patients, *Res Nurs Health* 13:293–301, 1990.

14. McMullen D: *Candida albicans* and incontinence, *Dermatol Nurs* 3(1):21–24, 1991.

15. National Pressure Ulcer Advisory Panel: Pressure ulcers' prevalence, cost and risk assessment: consensus development conference statement, *Decubitus* 2(2):24–28, 1989.

16. North American Nursing Diagnosis Association: *NANDA nursing diagnoses: definitions and classification, 1995–1996*, Philadelphia, 1994, The Association.

17. Pieper B and others: Visceral protein nutritional assessment of patients placed on a high- or low-air-loss bed, *J Enterostom Ther* 17(4):145–149, 1990.

18. Phillips TJ and Dover JS: Leg ulcers, *J Am Acad Dermatol* 25(6, part 1):965–987, 1991.

19. Rosenberg CS: Wound healing in the patient with diabetes mellitus, *Nurs Clin North Am* 25(1):247–261, 1990.

20. Roth RR and James WD: Microbiology of the skin: resident flora, ecology, infection, *J Am Acad Dermatol* 20(3):367–390, 1989.

21. Rodeheaver G and others: Wound healing and wound management: focus on debridement, *Adv Wound Care* 7(1):22–36, 1994.

22. Strunk B and Maher K: Collaborative nurse management of multifactorial moist desquamation in a patient undergoing radiotherapy, *J Enterostom Ther* 10(4):152–157, 1993.

ELIMINATION PATTERN

Constipation
▶ _____

Perceived Constipation
▶ _____

Colonic Constipation
▶ _____

Diarrhea
▶ _____

Bowel Incontinence
▶ _____

Constipation *is the state in which an individual experiences a change in normal bowel habits characterized by a decrease in the frequency of stools or the passage of hard, dry stools.*[8]

Perceived Constipation *is the state in which an individual makes a self-diagnosis of Constipation and ensures a daily bowel movement through abuse of laxatives, enemas, and suppositories; the expected passage of a stool at the same time every day.*[8]

Colonic Constipation *is the state in which an individual's pattern of elimination is characterized by hard, dry stools, which results from a delay in passage of food residue.*[8]

Diarrhea *is the state in which an individual experiences a change in normal bowel habits characterized by the frequent passage of loose, fluid, unformed stools.*[8]

Bowel Incontinence *is the state in which an individual experiences a change in normal bowel habits characterized by the involuntary passage of stools.*[8]

OVERVIEW

Use of the diagnostic labels Diarrhea, Constipation, Perceived Constipation, Colonic Constipation, and Bowel Incontinence indicates that a patient is experiencing a problem related to altered bowel elimination. The normal bowel pattern of individuals varies because of the influences of age, gender, activity level, emotional state, medication use, and the presence of disease. To understand the factors that affect bowel elimination, an understanding of the normal processes of fecal continence and defecation is necessary.

The anatomy and physiology of defecation and continence can be described as a set of complex, interrelated processes that depend primarily on the coordination of the pelvic floor, anal sphincters, rectum, anal canal, and colon.[11] The acquisition of continence seen in children depends primarily on the maturation of the nerve pathways in the anorectal structures as well as the social awareness of the child. During the aging process, a deterioration of the intestinal muscles, decreased peristalsis, and decreased activity may lead to an alteration in bowel elimination.[13] Continence also depends on (1) the orderly passage of stools of the appropriate volume and consistency into the distal gastrointestinal tract; (2) a compliant rectum that serves as an adequate storage compartment; (3) intact sensation in the pelvic floor that alerts the individual to the need for defecation; (4) the type of rectal content; and (5) an adequate sphincter mechanism that can maintain anal canal pressures higher than pressures in the rectum.[11]

Defecation is the process of eliminating wastes and undigested food from the body in the form of feces (stool) within an appropriate period of time. Expulsive forces, such as increasing abdominal pressures, via the Valsalva maneuver, are necessary to propel the intraluminal contents into the rectum and subsequently the anal canal, while the anal sphincter relaxes and allows the feces to pass.[11] Individuals delay defecation for several reasons: childhood training practices, socially unacceptable timing, uncomfortable or unclean toilet facilities, fear of pain from previous defecation, lack of privacy, and confinement to bed because of illness or other disabilities.[1] The individual may reinstate the urge to defecate by bearing down and breathing deeply; however, this secondary urge is less efficient than the original urge.[5]

The normal defecation pattern in the United States varies widely among individuals, as demonstrated by a survey of young adults, which indicated that 90% of respondents reported a stool frequency of two to seven stools per week, with the passage of one stool per day being the most common bowel elimination pattern.[12] Defecation patterns have been reported to be affected by gender—males tend to report more frequent defecation patterns than females. Cultural factors also influence the pattern of defecation. For example, Senegalese people normally defecate twice a day and consider themselves constipated if they pass only one stool a day. Americans report an average of at least three stools a week. Other bowel elimination patterns observed in the United States are that whites tend to defecate more often than African-Americans (race); young people defecate

more than older adults (age); and persons who consume more fruits and vegetables defecate more often than those who eat less fiber (diet).[12]

When a patient is diagnosed as having Constipation, it should be recognized that Constipation is a symptom that may indicate various metabolic or endocrine disorders. Examples of such disorders include diabetes mellitus, hypothyroidism, hypercalcemia, and panhypopituitarism. Some colonic and rectal disorders associated with Constipation include tumors, irritable bowel syndrome, diverticular disease, inflammatory strictures, hemorrhoids, and anal fissures. Neuromuscular disorders (e.g., intestinal pseudoobstruction, autonomic neuropathy, multiple sclerosis, Parkinson's disease, and Hirschsprung's disease) also have been associated with Constipation.[4] Malnutrition, dehydration, chronic pain, immobility, and anxiety are conditions that also have been related to Constipation.

No common definition exists for the term *constipation.*[13] Some health care practitioners base their diagnosis of Constipation on a stool frequency of less than three per week, straining to have a bowel movement, and dry, hard stools. The patient may report symptoms such as painful defecation, feelings of incomplete evacuation, changes in stool consistency, and decreased frequency.

Children often experience Constipation. This results from painful passage of stool, after which the child will withhold stool in an attempt to avoid discomfort. Boys are more commonly affected than girls. Fecal soiling, or *encopresis,* is often what brings the child to medical attention. Even though children with chronic Constipation may develop lax anal muscles, the possibility of child sexual abuse must be considered when examining the anal area.[1]

Elders are more prone to have Constipation as a result of age-related factors such as decreased peristalsis, altered activity, and weakening of the intestinal muscles.[13] The elderly especially need to be assessed for bowel habits, diet, hydration, level of activity, psychological status, and medication use.[6] It is important to note that decreased intake of fiber and fluids is the most common cause of Constipation in the elderly.

The patient with Perceived Constipation may have a normal bowel elimination pattern but may perceive it as abnormal. The factors contributing to this diagnosis may be a lack of knowledge about normal bowel function as well as variations in the bowel elimination pattern. Other factors contributing to Perceived Constipation are cultural and family health beliefs and impaired thought processes. Laxative abuse is a common problem of patients who perceive themselves to be constipated. Laxative abuse is associated with morphologic damage to the intestinal mucosa and erosion of villi, colonic smooth muscle atrophy, fluid and electrolyte disturbances, malabsorption of such nutrients as vitamin D and calcium, and dilated cathartic colon.[13]

Colonic Constipation is a direct result of lack of dietary intake of fluids and fiber, inadequate physical activity, and the chronic use of enemas. Other causative factors include lack of privacy during defecation, a change in daily routine (e.g., traveling), stress, immobility, narcotic use, psychogenic disease, and metabolic problems (e.g., hypothyroidism, hypocalcemia, or hypokalemia).

Diarrhea is characterized by the frequent passage of loose, liquid, and unformed stools.[8] Diarrhea occurs when the colon is unable to absorb ileal effluent. Four types of diarrhea are identified: motility disturbance, secretory diarrhea, osmotic diarrhea, and malabsorption diarrhea.[2] Motility diarrhea may be related to a decreased motility caused by bacterial overgrowth or fecal impaction (in which liquid stool moves around a hard stool). This type of diarrhea may be a result of stress, irritable bowel syndrome, diabetic visceral neuropathy, scleroderma, or postvagotomy. Secretory diarrhea is characterized by increased intestinal secretions resulting from enterotoxins, fluid-secreting tumors, and hypersecretion of endogenous hormones. Osmotic diarrhea results from a decrease in the ability of the colon to absorb fluids because of ingestion of nonabsorbables such as lactulose, sorbitol, citrates, and hyperosmolar enteral feedings. The last type

of diarrhea, malabsorption diarrhea, occurs when the intestine cannot absorb fluids because of an enzyme deficiency (pancreatic insufficiency and bile salts) or because of morphological and structural changes that cause a decrease in the absorptive space. Such changes can be a result of radiation, enteritis, inflammatory bowel disease, chemotherapeutic agents, severe malnutrition, or short bowel syndrome.[3]

Diarrhea is common in childhood. The average American child experiences 6 to 11 episodes of diarrhea before age 6, and 1 in 15 American children will be hospitalized for a diarrhea-related episode before the age of 6. Risk factors for childhood fatalities resulting from diarrhea-induced dehydration include being less than 1 year of age, living in the South, and contracting an illness between the months of October and February.[10] Studies show that early oral rehydration therapy for children, using a rehydration solution containing salt, sugar, and water, can decrease the mortality rate.

Bowel Incontinence is an embarrassing disorder that may be difficult to identify without a thorough patient history. Continence is maintained by a balance between neurological and muscular activity of the lower bowel. Continence requires the ability to sense rectal filling and to distinguish the nature of rectal contents; the ability of the rectum and the distal colon to store feces; and the ability of the internal and external anal sphincters to control defecation.

Two common causes of fecal incontinence are fecal impaction and neurogenic factors. Other causes include neoplasms, inflammatory bowel disease, diverticular disease, gastroenteritis, weakness of the pelvic floor, rectal prolapse, anorectal procedures, and injuries sustained during childhood.

Fecal impaction is an easily treated cause of fecal incontinence. Fecal impaction is the main cause of fecal incontinence among older people living in long-term care facilities.[9] Severe Constipation leads to impaction of feces; consequently, overdistention of the rectum results in fecal incontinence as liquid stool passes around the impacted fecal mass.

Neurogenic influences on the bowel are similar to those affecting the bladder. A neurogenic bowel occurs in persons with a damaged cerebral cortex by dementia or focal lesions. Injury of spinal cord segments T1 to T12 results in incontinence because voluntary control of abdominal muscle contraction and the subsequent contraction of the rectal wall may be lost. If the injury involves cord segments S3 to S5, incontinence will result because of the loss of sphincter tone and reflex activity.

Dementia accompanied by personality changes or altered mental functions may result in temporary or chronic Bowel Incontinence. Patients with dementia may be unable to communicate the need to defecate. An unconscious patient will also be incontinent because of the inability to recognize the urge to defecate and the loss of muscular control.

ASSESSMENT

Data collection serves as the basis for identifying defining characteristics and related factors, for formulating the nursing diagnoses, and for planning interventions. Defining characteristics of altered bowel elimination can be indicated by subjective and objective data. A thorough history of the patient's past and present bowel elimination patterns provides subjective data. Objective data is obtained during the physical examination and from diagnostic tests. Obtaining an accurate history is crucial because treatment measures are determined by the cause of the problem. Some patients may need education only, whereas others will require more extensive interventions.

How the physical examination and diagnostic tests are conducted is important. Privacy must be maintained to minimize embarrassment and to ensure patient cooperation. The physical examination should begin with the vital signs. An increased temperature and heart rate may indicate infection, whereas decreased blood pressure may signal fluid losses. The abdomen should be assessed for bowel sounds, distention, ascites, or the presence of a mass. A rectal examination is also important because many rectal cancers and other lesions lie low

in the rectum and may be missed by a barium enema. A rectal examination may reveal a common cause of Diarrhea, namely, fecal impaction. Normally the rectum is free of stool. The presence of stool in the rectum indicates Constipation. At the time of the rectal examination, the perianal region should be examined for fissures, abscesses, fistulas, and hemorrhoids. Any stool that remains on the examiner's glove should be assessed for blood (including occult blood), color, odor, and consistency. Diagnostic tests and procedures include stool examination, measurement of serum electrolytes, proctosigmoidoscopy, barium enema, and colonoscopy.

Constipation

Constipation may be considered a symptom rather than a disease; as such, subjective data collected from the patient is important. Collecting objective data from the patient with Constipation includes stool examination, rectal examination, sigmoidoscopy, and bowel transit studies. Anorectal manometry, which involves insertion of a small balloon into the rectum, can provide an estimation of rectal sensation, quantify sphincter tone, and measure bowel elasticity.[4] Stool examination may reveal the presence of a small, dry fecal mass. The stool should be examined for the presence of blood or mucus. A digital examination of the rectum may reveal fecal impaction or a rectal or pelvic tumor. The rectum may contain large amounts of stool, even immediately after defecation. During the rectal examination, the perineal region should be examined for any fissure, abscess, fistula formation, rectal prolapse, or hemorrhoids because these are complications of chronic Constipation.

The sigmoidoscopy and barium enema usually reveal no abnormalities. The presence of blood or mucus or a mucosal abnormality should be investigated further. A barium enema is indicated for individuals with intractable symptoms, for older patients, or for those with a recent change in bowel habits.

Bowel transit studies are indicated if there is no response to a high-fiber diet. Radiopaque markers are administered with breakfast, and an abdomi-

III

nal X-ray examination follows within 2 to 5 days. Normal subjects excrete some of the markers within 2 days and at least 80% of the markers in 5 days.

It is important to remember that childhood Constipation initially may be recognized as encopresis. Frequently a child will withhold defecation because of a past experience with painful defecation, and a formed, soft stool will leak around the outside of a hard mass inside the rectum. Soiling occurs most often during the day, when the child is in the upright position and is exercising or walking.[13]

■ Defining Characteristics

The presence of the following defining characteristics indicates that the patient may be experiencing Constipation:

- Decreased frequency of stool passage
- Hard, dry, small stools
- Decreased weight of stools
- Difficulty passing stools
- Straining to defecate
- Abdominal distention
- Pain with defecation
- Pruritis ani
- Feeling of incomplete bowel evacuation
- Feeling of rectal fullness
- Weak abdominal muscles
- Failure to respond to the urge to defecate
- Decreased appetite

■ Related Factors

The following related factors are associated with Constipation:

- Pregnancy and menstruation
- Postmenopause
- Prolonged immobility
- Impaired neuromuscular function
- Medications (e.g., opiates, aluminum-based antacids, and anticholinergics)
- History of poor eating habits
- Lack of or inadequate dietary fiber
- Inadequate fluid intake
- Inability to chew high-fiber foods
- Inattention to the defecation reflex
- Laxative abuse
- Overuse of enemas

- Lack of physical exercise
- Travel
- Lack of acceptable toilet facilities
- Lack of privacy for defecation
- Anorexia
- Stress
- Grief or anger

Perceived Constipation

When assessing the patient for Perceived Constipation, the same objective data that is obtained for a patient with a diagnosis of Constipation will be used. The patient with Perceived Constipation may have normal results for these diagnostic procedures, depending on the duration of the problem. The nurse must review the patient's usual food intake, fluid intake, and bowel movements to identify potential causes. The prolonged use of laxatives may necessitate bowel retraining along with dietary modification. If possible, encourage the patient to keep a diary recording intake, bowel movements, and activities and exercise over a 1-week period. This will assist in gathering accurate data.

■ Defining Characteristics

The presence of the following defining characteristics indicates that the patient may be experiencing Perceived Constipation:

- Regular use of laxatives, enemas, or suppositories
- Expectation of a daily bowel movement
- Expectation of stool passage at the same time every day

■ Related Factors

The following related factors are associated with Perceived Constipation:

- Lack of knowledge of normal bowel function
- Faulty appraisal of bowel elimination pattern
- Cultural and family health beliefs
- Impaired thought processes

Colonic Constipation

When assessing a patient for Colonic Constipation, the patient's activity level and dietary intake of fluids and fiber must be assessed. Patients should be asked if lack of privacy during defecation, an increase in stress, or a change in daily routine has recently occurred. A medication history, including the use of enemas, should also be obtained. The patient's medical history plays an important role in diagnosing Colonic Constipation. For example, patients with hypothyroidism, hypocalcemia, or hypokalemia are at risk for Colonic Constipation.

■ Defining Characteristics

The presence of the following defining characteristics indicates that the patient may be experiencing Colonic Constipation:

- Decreased frequency of stool passage
- Hard, dry stool
- Straining to defecate
- Painful defecation
- Abdominal distention
- Palpable mass
- Rectal pressure
- Headache
- Abdominal pain
- Appetite impairment

■ Related Factors

The following related factors are associated with Colonic Constipation:

- Inadequate fluid, dietary, or fiber intake
- Inadequate physical activity
- Metabolic problems (e.g., hypothyroidism, hypocalcemia, or hypokalemia)
- Immobility
- Lack of privacy for defecation
- Emotional disturbances
- Regular use of medications and enemas
- Stress
- Change in daily routine

Diarrhea

When Diarrhea is suspected, a stool examination should be done using a fresh stool specimen. The goal is to identify a causative agent so that an appropriate plan of intervention can be developed. The stool is analyzed for the presence of bacteria, ova, parasites, blood, leukocytes, fat, and meat fibers. In addition, a stool smear may be com-

pleted using Wright's stain to identify the presence of leukocytes, which indicates inflammation. The stool also should be tested for the presence of occult blood on at least three samples.

Serum electrolytes (sodium, potassium, chloride, and bicarbonate) are assessed to determine the presence of fluid and electrolyte imbalances. A complete blood count, including levels of hemoglobin, hematocrit, white blood cells, differential white blood cells, red blood cells, and platelets, helps to identify inflammation and anemia. Evaluation of calcium, total protein, and blood sugar levels and prothrombin time also is recommended.

A proctosigmoidoscopy is recommended to identify the presence of Crohn's disease, ulcerative colitis, rectal neoplasms, or laxative abuse. Stool specimens can be obtained and biopsies completed during the proctosigmoidoscopy. A biopsy identifies the presence of inflammatory disease and neoplasms.

A barium enema assists in the identification of mucosal abnormalities such as ulceration and edema; abnormalities of the bowel lumen such as narrowing or dilation; and the presence of masses, diverticula, and fistulas. Colonoscopy allows for the visualization of the colon proximal to the area reached by sigmoidoscopy. Finally, abdominal X-ray examinations identify the presence of distention and bowel obstruction.

■ Defining Characteristics

The presence of the following defining characteristics indicates that the patient may be experiencing Diarrhea:

- Increased urgency and frequency of stool passage
- Increased frequency of bowel sounds
- Loose, liquid stools
- Change in color and odor of stools
- Anal irritation
- Abdominal pain or cramping
- Fluid and electrolyte imbalances

■ Related Factors

The following related factors are associated with Diarrhea:

- Gastrointestinal disorders

III

- Metabolic disorders
- Nutritional disorders
- Endocrine disorders
- Medications (e.g., ampicillin)
- Change in dietary intake
- Fecal impaction
- Tube feedings
- Antibiotic treatment
- Magnesium-based antacids
- Cathartic abuse
- Ingestion of contaminants
- Ingestion of heavy metals
- Inflammation or irritation of bowel or malabsorption by bowel
- Bacterial or viral toxins
- Protozoa
- Stress and anxiety

Bowel Incontinence

Obtaining objective data related to Bowel Incontinence begins with a rectal examination. During the digital examination, muscle strength (or weakness) can be assessed. To test muscle strength, the patient is asked to cough while the examiner observes the anal area. If stool leakage occurs during coughing, the problem is related to weak muscles. An electromyogram (EMG) is useful in locating specific areas of anal muscle weakness.

Loss of sensation in the anal area is a related factor of Bowel Incontinence. Stroking the skin near the anus with a piece of cotton should result in a local contraction (the anal wink). If contraction does not occur, the defecation reflex is damaged. The presence of surgical scars in the anal area may provide clues to sphincter abnormalities. Assessment of the neurological system also provides valuable information, especially when the patient has a generalized neurological disorder or a disorder affecting the spinal cord or brain. A barium enema is indicated to determine whether the incontinence is linked to inflammatory bowel disease.

■ Defining Characteristics

The presence of the following defining characteristics indicates that the patient may be experiencing Bowel Incontinence:

- Fecal soiling of underwear
- Involuntary passage of stool
- Lack of awareness of urge to defecate

■ Related Factors

The following related factors are associated with Bowel Incontinence:

- Anal surgery
- Colostomy
- Gastrointestinal disorders
- Neuromuscular disorders
- Loss of rectal sphincter control
- Anal-rectal muscle weakness
- Laxative abuse
- Stress and anxiety
- Cognitive impairment

DIAGNOSIS

■ Differential Nursing Diagnosis

It is important to differentiate nursing diagnoses within the cluster of alteration of bowel elimination to determine a correlation with other nursing diagnoses. For example, the person with a nursing diagnosis of Activity Intolerance may also have a nursing diagnosis of Constipation related to decreased activity. The person with a diagnosis of Anxiety or Fluid Volume Deficit may also have a nursing diagnosis of Diarrhea. A person with the nursing diagnosis Fluid Volume Excess may be confused and restless and consequently may experience Bowel Incontinence.

Another widely used nursing diagnosis is Knowledge Deficit, which can be applied readily to the person with Perceived Constipation who expects to have a daily bowel movement; in this case the person needs to be taught what is "normal" and how to avoid the inappropriate use of laxatives. Alternatively, the person with a nursing diagnosis of Altered Nutrition: Less Than Body Requirements may be diagnosed with Colonic Constipation related to inadequate fluid, dietary, or fiber intake. It is important to remember that in most cases when a person experiences an alteration in bowel elimination, there will likely be several other applicable nursing diagnoses.

■ Medical and Psychiatric Diagnoses

The most common medical and psychiatric diagnoses related to Constipation and Colonic Constipation are cerebrovascular accident, depression, diabetes mellitus, hypothyroidism, and spinal cord injury. When a person has the nursing diagnosis Perceived Constipation, the most common related medical and psychiatric diagnoses are dementia and depression. The nursing diagnosis Diarrhea should be specified as acute or chronic when discussing the most common related medical psychiatric diagnoses. Acute Diarrhea is most closely linked with the medical diagnoses diverticulitis, drug reactions, lactose intolerance, lead poisoning, and infections related to *Shigella, Salmonella, Campylobacter*, or *Giardia lamblia*. Chronic Diarrhea is most closely associated with acquired immune deficiency syndrome (AIDS), colon cancer, Crohn's disease, hyperthyroidism, irritable bowel syndrome, and ulcerative colitis.

OUTCOME IDENTIFICATION, PLANNING, AND IMPLEMENTATION

The desired patient outcomes and nursing interventions for individuals experiencing altered bowel elimination focus on assisting the patient to regain a normal pattern of bowel elimination. For patients with pathophysiological or psychological alterations, the nursing care supports treatment of the illness or disease. Whether the problem in bowel function is illness- or disease-related or symptomatic or an alteration in self-care behaviors, the nurse uses educational strategies to support and guide the patient in controlling factors contributing to the problem.

Constipation, Perceived Constipation, and Colonic Constipation

The specific outcomes for each of the diagnoses involving Constipation are developed to support the patient's achievement of a regular bowel elimination pattern. Patients with Constipation, Perceived Constipation, or Colonic Constipation should spend at least 10 minutes after one meal each day—preferably breakfast—seated on the toilet. The nurse should explain the importance of responding to the urge to defecate, provide privacy, and allow adequate time for defecation. When the urge to defecate is ignored, water is reabsorbed from the fecal mass, resulting in stool that is dry, hard, and difficult to pass. Attention to privacy creates a more relaxed atmosphere for the normal process of stool elimination. Lack of privacy may result in avoidance of defecation and persistent Constipation, especially in adolescents and older adults.

The patient's diet should be modified to include adequate amounts of bulk and fluids. Bulk can be added to the diet by increasing fiber. Fiber is the unabsorbable element of food, found most abundantly in fruits and vegetables. Bacterial degradation of fiber enhances colonic motility. Bran is a recommended source of dietary bulk. Bran can be mixed with applesauce, juice, yogurt, or other foods to make it more palatable. Highly refined foods such as pastries and "fast food" should be avoided. In addition to bulk, an adequate fluid intake is necessary for proper bowel function. Fluid should be increased to 1 to 2 quarts per day.

Physical activity and exercise is important to the establishment and maintenance of a regular bowel elimination pattern. At least 15 to 20 minutes per day should be allotted to activity and exercise. The nurse should explain the importance of muscle tone for defecation and the relationship between exercise and intestinal motility. Walking is a good exercise that most people can do. Activity levels should be increased gradually, and the patient should be encouraged to focus on strenthening the abdominal muscles.

As strategies are introduced, the pattern of elimination and the consistency of stools are monitored. Ongoing assessment affords the nurse the opportunity to adjust the plan of care in a timely manner in response to the patient's progress. Outcomes and interventions specific to each of the Constipation-related diagnoses are addressed in the Nursing Care Guidelines.

Diarrhea

Nursing care for the patient with Diarrhea focuses on decreasing the number and frequency

III

of stools passed and on preventing or correcting fluid and electrolyte imbalances. Although most cases of diarrhea are mild, the patient with Diarrhea is at risk for developing dehydration, cardiac dysrhythmias, and hypovolemic shock. Expert nursing care is required to avoid these life-threatening complications.

Fluids and electrolytes should be monitored—and treated, if necessary—to assure they are maintained within normal limits. This can be accomplished through oral rehydration therapy or, if necessary, through intravenous administration of fluids and electrolytes. The type of oral fluids administered to the patient is determined by the severity of the diarrhea and the age of the patient. Adults respond to Gatorade or nondiet, decaffeinated soft drinks alternated with nonfat chicken broth. Children may respond to lemonade or Kool-Aid. Prune juice, milk, milk products, and concentrated sweets should be avoided. When Diarrhea subsides, soft foods such as bananas, rice, applesauce, toast, and soda crackers can be introduced.

Patients who have an emotional basis for their Diarrhea need to establish an effective pattern of coping. The nurse should assist the patient in identifying stressful life situations. The patient can then be taught stress-reduction techniques such as deep breathing exercises, meditation, and relaxing, diversional activities.

Assessment of the patient's status and his or her response to interventions continues until Diarrhea is eliminated and the patient's elimination pattern returns to normal. The nurse should monitor serum electrolyte values; asses skin turgor and mucous membranes for signs of dehydration; and monitor the patient for altered vital signs, particularly heart rate and rhythm. Daily weights should be taken to determine fluid gains and losses.

Bowel Incontinence

The desired outcome of care for the patient with Bowel Incontinence is to maintain control over bowel elimination. This outcome is unrealistic when the patient is unconscious or mentally incompetent. A bowel-training program can be supportive of the alert, conscious patient's achieving this outcome. A bowel-training program includes increased fluid intake, warm or hot liq-

Continued on p. 258

■ **NURSING CARE GUIDELINES**
Nursing Diagnosis: Constipation

Expected Outcome: The patient will demonstrate improved bowel elimination as evidenced by three soft stools a week.

- Record date and time of the patient's bowel movements. *This record helps to monitor compliance and to allow appropriate adjustments in the treatment program by the patient and staff.*[7]
- Encourage the patient to maintain a regular exercise program; assist the patient in planning such a program. *Regular physical exercise is required for maintaining normal bowel function and increases muscle tone that is needed for fecal expulsion.*[5]
- Monitor the consistency of the patient's stools. *Although the patient may be having three stools a week, they may not be of normal consistency.*

Expected Outcome: The patient will alter his or her diet to include adequate amounts of fiber and fluids as evidenced by a diary kept by the patient.

- Encourage daily intake of foods high in fiber. *A diet high in fiber will stimulate peristalsis.*
- Encourage the patient to drink at least eight glasses of water a day. *At least eight to ten glasses of water are necessary to maintain bowel patterns and to promote proper stool consistency.*
- Teach the patient to avoid highly refined cereals and breads (e.g., pastries and pasta). *Diets that are low in fiber and high in concentrated refined foods produce small, hard stools.*

■ = nursing intervention; ▲ = collaborative intervention.

NURSING CARE GUIDELINES
Nursing Diagnosis: Perceived Constipation

Expected Outcome: The patient will identify the importance of avoiding laxative use.
- Teach the patient the hazards of laxatives. *Laxatives cause muscular atony and provide only temporary relief from Constipation.*
- Explain that bowel movements are needed every 2 to 3 days, not daily. *Often patients have a faulty appraisal of what is a "normal" bowel movement.*

Expected Outcome: The patient will verbalize the causes of perceived constipation.
- Discuss with the patient those factors contributing to the Constipation. *Contributing factors such as cultural and family beliefs about defecation affect the patient's perception of Constipation. The patient may have an inadequate diet or a lack of exercise that is dictated by a cultural belief system.*
- Assess the patient's regular time for elimination. *Frequently a time for defecation may need to be determined and included in the patient's regular routine, or a stimulus such as drinking a glass of warm water may be added to the morning routine.*

■ = nursing intervention; ▲ = collaborative intervention.

NURSING CARE GUIDELINES
Nursing Diagnosis: Colonic Constipation

Expected Outcome: The patient will verbalize an intent to increase fiber, fluids, and exercise in daily routine.
- Review with the patient a list of foods high in bulk. *Foods high in bulk are necessary for peristalsis.*
- Determine with the patient a regular schedule for fluid intake. *A routine is necessary to maintain adequate fluid intake; eight to ten glasses of fluid are necessary for soft stools.*
- Determine with the patient a regular schedule for exercise. *Some patients need to establish a routine to increase activity and exercise.*

■ = nursing intervention; ▲ = collaborative intervention.

NURSING CARE GUIDELINES
Nursing Diagnosis: Diarrhea

Expected Outcome: The patient will describe factors contributing to the Diarrhea.
- Teach the patient about factors that may be contributing to the Diarrhea (e.g., tube feedings, contaminated foods, dietetic foods, food allergies, or foreign travel). *Patients often need education about what is causing their diarrhea; knowledge and understanding enhance the likelihood of complying with the plan of care.*
- Assess the patient's level of stress. *Stress contributes to diarrhea; stress reduction may be needed.*

Expected Outcome: The patient will take appropriate actions to reduce Diarrhea.
- Encourage the patient to drink liquids high in glucose and electrolytes (e.g., fruit juices and Gatorade). *By replacing fluid and electrolytes lost in Diarrhea, the patient prevents dehydration.*
- Teach the patient to avoid milk products, whole grains, fat, fresh fruits, and vegetables. *These items increase peristalsis.*
- Teach the patient to add gradually the appropriate solid foods to the diet (e.g., crackers, yogurt, rice, bananas, and applesauce). *These items help decrease peristalsis.*
- Teach the patient to avoid large quantities of dietetic foods containing sorbitol, hexitol, and mannitol. *These substances have a laxative effect.*

■ = nursing intervention; ▲ = collaborative intervention.

III

III

◢ **NURSING CARE GUIDELINES**
Nursing Diagnosis: Bowel Incontinence

Expected Outcome: The patient will have decreased episodes of soiling.

- Offer the patient the bedpan or beside commode after each meal. *Timing the evacuation after a meal takes advantage of the gastrocolic stimulus.*
- Position a functionally able patient in a sitting position. *This position helps the patient achieve the proper angle between the rectum and the anal canal that is necessary for defecation.*
- Instruct the patient to use abdominal muscles, Valsalva's maneuver, and abdominal massage. *These maneuvers increase abdominal pressure and assist in defecation.*

Expected Outcome: The patient will regain a regular pattern of bowel elimination.

- Assess the patient's neurological status and functional ability to *determine if the patient is able to participate in care.*
- With the patient, plan a daily routine incorporating times to defecate. *With routine, a pattern develops that is predictable.*
- Provide the patient with privacy and a nonstressful environment. *Privacy is reassuring to the patient and provides protection against embarrassment while establishing a bowel program.*
- Implement a bowel-training program, if feasible. *Such a program provides a coordinated effort to establish a regular pattern of bowel elimination.*

■ = nursing intervention; ▲ = collaborative intervention.

---

uids, high-fiber foods, low-fat or fat-free foods, increased physical activity, abdominal and rectal strengthening exercises, establishing a regular time for defecation, and biofeedback. Laxatives and suppositories may be indicated for the patient with a spinal cord injury. The patient should be encouraged to keep a daily record of bowel elimination and dietary intake.

To assist the patient in decreasing the episodes of soiling, the nurse should encourage the patient to use the commode or, if necessary, the bedpan after each meal. Adequate time and privacy should be provided for defecation. The patient who is continent should have stool that is of normal consistency. This outcome is accomplished by dietary modification as discussed for the patient with Constipation.

EVALUATION

The effectiveness of the plan of care for the patient with Constipation, Perceived Constipation, Colonic Constipation, Diarrhea, or Bowel Incon-

tinence can be measured by the patient's success in establishing a normal pattern of bowel elimination. Regardless of the diagnosis, successful treatment or intervention should result in stool that is normal in color, odor, frequency, and consistency.

The nurse and the patient together should evaluate the achievement of identified and desired outcomes. During the review of the plan of care, the nurse can elicit input as to the patient's perception of the effectiveness of each strategy the nurse or other members of the health care team introduced. If the desired outcomes were not achieved, such a review with the patient can result in a revised plan of care.

Of special importance during the evaluation phase of the nursing process is the determination of the effectiveness of patient education strategies. When reviewing the plan of care with the patient, the nurse can assess whether or not the teaching strategies used were as effective as intended. The patient should be queried about his or her perceptions of the strengths and limitations of the teaching strategies and other interventions.

▶ CASE STUDY WITH PLAN OF CARE

Sam H. is a 4-year-old who lives at home with his parents and siblings (one sister, age 8, and two brothers, ages 10 and 12). He attends day care from 9 A.M. to 5 P.M. while his parents are at work and his siblings are in school. Sam was born with a myelomeningocele and experiences neurogenic bowel dysfunction. Sam's parents have set in place a scheduled toileting regimen that is carefully followed by the day care providers and by Sam's two older brothers. Sam is brought to the pediatric nurse practitioner by his mother, who states that 2 days ago Sam started having bloody, mucousy stools that smelled like sulfur. A physical examination revealed a temperature of 101°F, heart rate of 140/min, respiratory rate of 26/min, and blood pressure of 100/60 mm Hg.

Sam appears lethargic and has poor capillary refill and poor skin turgor. A urinalysis reveals a specific gravity of 1.035 and a pH of 4.3. Results of blood work reveal a potassium value of 3.3 mEq/L, sodium value of 134 mEq/L, and chloride value of 45 mEq/L. A stool culture indicates a bacterial infection with *Salmonella*.

Further discussion with Sam's mother reveals that the day care center recently had a picnic and that four other children also became ill. Sam's mother reports that he looks thinner, and when he is weighed, Sam is 3 pounds lighter than he was a month ago. Sam's mother also reports that Sam is the only member of the family that is ill.

▶ PLAN OF CARE FOR SAM M.
Nursing Diagnosis: Diarrhea Related to Bacterial Infection

Expected Outcome: Sam's parents will take steps to decrease the number of diarrhea stools in a 24-hour period.
- Instruct Sam's mother to encourage him to drink liquids high in glucose and electrolytes (ginger ale, diluted Jell-O water, sugar water, and apple juice) and to provide chilled (but not cold) liquids.
- Instruct Sam's mother to introduce gradually nonstimulating foods (e.g., toast, rice, bananas, and crackers) to Sam's diet.
- Instruct Sam's mother to administer his antibiotics as ordered and to notify the nurse practitioner if diarrhea persists for more than 3 days.
- Instruct Sam's mother to eliminate milk, caffeine, and raw vegetables from Sam's diet.

Expected Outcome: Sam's skin will remain intact without redness or breakdown.
- Instruct Sam's family and day care personnel to provide Sam with meticulous skin care using a mild soap.
- During acute episodes of diarrhea, encourage Sam's mother to use a pull-up type of diaper and to change Sam's diaper frequently.
- Instruct Sam's mother to apply petroleum jelly or A&D ointment to protect the skin.
- Explain to Sam's mother that scheduled toileting can resume as stools become firm.
- Teach Sam's mother to observe his skin for signs of breakdown.

Expected Outcome: Sam's fluids and electrolytes will be maintained within normal limits for a child (sodium [Na] = 135–145 mEq/L, potassium [K] = 3.5–5.5 mEq/L, and chloride [Cl] = 98–105 mEq/L).
- Assess serum, electrolytes, skin turgor, and mucous membranes.
- Instruct Sam's mother to encourage him to drink fluids high in potassium and sodium (orange and grapefruit juices and bouillon) and to weigh Sam daily.
- Explain to Sam's mother the signs of dehydration and when to seek further medical attention.
- Instruct Sam's mother to replace lost fluids with products high in electrolytes (e.g., Pedialyte).

■ = nursing intervention; ▲ = collaborative intervention.

Continued

III

▶ PLAN OF CARE FOR SAM M. — CONT'D

Expected Outcome: Sam's family will list actions that will reduce future episodes of diarrhea.
- Teach Sam's family how to prevent the transmission of bacteria by frequent hand washing, especially after cleaning Sam after a diarrheal episode.
- Teach Sam's family about the importance of properly storing and cooking food.
- Teach Sam's family to avoid fresh fruit, salads, and milk and to drink only bottled beverages if traveling to a foreign country.

■ CRITICAL THINKING EXERCISES

1. What effect can Sam's Diarrhea have on Sam's self-esteem? Describe interventions supportive of Sam's maintaining his self esteem.
2. Describe home and day care environmental factors that could contribute to Sam developing another episode of Diarrhea related to bacterial infections. What specific questions would you ask Sam's mother about his home environment and about his day care environment?
3. Describe Sam's developmental stage as a 4-year-old. How could Sam participate in the implementation of interventions suggested to his mother and family?

REFERENCES

1. Almond P: Constipation: a family-centered approach, *Health Visitor* 66:404–405, 1993.
2. Fruto LV: Current concepts: management of diarrhea in acute care, *J Wound Ostomy Contin Nurs* 21:199–205, 1994.
3. Glass R and others: Estimates of morbidity and mortality rates for diarrheal diseases in American children, *J Pediatrics* 118(4):S27–S33, 1991.
4. Haines S: Treating constipation in the patient with diabetes, *Diabetes Ed* 21:223–232.
5. Hall GR, Karstens M, Rakel B, and Swanson E: Managing constipation using a research-based protocol, *Med-Surgical Nursing* 4(1):11–20.
6. Karam S and Neis D: Student/staff collaboration: a pilot bowel management program, *J Geront Nurs* 20(3):32–40, 1994.
7. Loening-Baucke V: Assessment, diagnosis, and treatment of constipation in childhood, *J Wound Ostomy Contin Nurs* 21:49–58.
8. North American Nursing Diagnosis Association: *NANDA nursing diagnoses: definitions and classification, 1995–1996*, Philadelphia, 1994, The Association.
9. Norton C and Fader M: Continence management, *Elderly Care* 6(6):23–27, 1994.
10. Rice KH: Oral rehydration therapy: a simple, effective solution, *J Pediatr Nurs* 9:349–356, 1994.
11. Rothenberger D and Orrom W: Anatomy and physiology of defecation. In Doughty DB, editor: *Urinary and fecal incontinence: nursing management*, St. Louis, 1991, Mosby-Year Book.
12. Sandler RS, Jordan MC, and Shelton BJ: Demographic and dietary determinants of constipation in the U.S. population, *Am J Pub Health* 80:185–189, 1990.
13. Van der Horst ML, Skyula JA, and Lingley K: The constipation quandary, *Canad Nurse* 90(1):25–30, 1994.

Altered Urinary Elimination

▶ ——————————————————————————————

Functional Incontinence

▶ ——————————————————————————————

Stress Incontinence

▶ ——————————————————————————————

Reflex Incontinence

▶ ——————————————————————————————

Urge Incontinence

▶ ——————————————————————————————

Total Incontinence

▶ ——————————————————————————————

Urinary Retention

▶ ——————————————————————————————

Altered Urinary Elimination *is the state in which an individual experiences a disturbance in urine elimination.*[27]

Functional Incontinence *is the state in which an individual experiences an involuntary, unpredictable passage of urine that occurs because of a nonurinary problem.*[27]

Stress Incontinence *is the state in which an individual experiences a loss of urine of less than 50 ml with increased abdominal pressure.*[27]

Reflex Incontinence *is the state in which an individual experiences an involuntary loss of urine that occurs at somewhat predictable intervals when a specific bladder volume is reached.*[27]

Urge Incontinence *is the state in which an individual experiences involuntary passage of urine soon after a strong sense of urgency to void.*[27]

Total Incontinence *is the state in which an individual experiences a continuous and unpredictable loss of urine.*[27]

Urinary Retention *is the state in which an individual experiences incomplete emptying of the bladder.*[27]

OVERVIEW

Urinary elimination starts with the complex blood-filtering and regulatory system of the kidneys. Ureters convey the urine from the kidneys to

III

the bladder. The lower urinary tract is composed of a storage receptacle (the bladder) and a drainage mechanism (the urethra and two sphincters). Structurally the bladder is composed of mucous membranes, connective tissue, and the detrusor muscle, which has the ability to expand and contract. Two sphincters, one internal and involuntary and the other external and voluntary, control the expulsion of urine into and through the urethra. The muscles of the pelvic floor surround part of the external sphincter. When the detrusor is relaxed and the sphincter closed, urine is stored. When the detrusor contracts and the sphincter relaxes, urine is eliminated.

This reciprocal relaxation and contraction relationship is controlled by a complex system of nerves. In an infant, voiding is a reflex action. Stretch receptors in the bladder stimulate a sacral reflex that causes detrusor contraction. This is coordinated with sphincter relaxation through a micturition center in the pons area of the brain. Later the cerebral cortex develops an inhibitory center that allows for voluntary control of voiding. Therefore, after toilet training, and given no unusual circumstances, a person can maintain voluntary control over urinary elimination.

Normal voiding is a cyclical event. As the bladder fills, tension increases on the walls. Threshold stretch receptors in the bladder wall and the proximal urethra send a signal to the sacral spinal cord micturition center. Parasympathetic impulses are sent back to the detrusor muscle, causing it to contract and the internal sphincter to relax. Meanwhile, this contraction causes nerve impulses to move up the spinal cord to the brain, signaling a need to void. If circumstances allow the person to void, the external sphincter is relaxed to allow the expulsion of urine; if not, the urge to void is suppressed. In the latter case, the external sphincter remains closed and, if the bladder is not overly full, the contractions may cease and the basal bladder tone pattern returns. If voiding does not occur, this cycle is repeated any time from a few minutes to an hour later. With each round of the cycle, the urge becomes more powerful.

Normal urine output varies with the amount of input over any given time period. On average,

most persons urinate five or six times per day for a total of 1500 ml, but there is a wide range of what is considered normal. The term *oliguria* is used to describe urine output of less than 400 ml per day. *Anuria* refers to urine output of 100 ml or less over 24 hours. *Polyuria* describes a large volume of urine with frequent urination.

On average, urine is acidic with a pH of 6.0, although it can range from 4.5 to 8.0 in the normal adult. The concentration of the urine, or its specific gravity, depends on fluid intake and the amount of solutes in the urine; on average it is 1.010, but it can vary widely. Small amounts of protein may be excreted in the urine, but excess protein is abnormal. Glucose and ketones also are not normally found in the urine.

Normal urination is a painless process, beginning with the urge to void. The stream of urine begins easily, flows with a steady pressure, and ends with the bladder nearly completely empty. Urine is clear yellow with a slight ammonia odor. Any deviation from the average is a suspected problem until some normal set of events, such as fluid depletion or excess, can explain the deviation.

Men and women differ slightly in urinary structures and voiding styles. The urethra is much shorter in women. The prostate gland in men, while not directly part of the urinary structures, is posterior to the bladder neck and, when enlarged, can exert pressure against the internal sphincter and urethra. In women, the uterus, located above and behind the bladder, can exert pressure on the bladder. Men usually urinate standing up, whereas women squat or sit. A woman's urethral meatus is located in proximity to the vagina and anus, sometimes making the migration of bacteria a problem.

Of the seven urinary elimination diagnoses, Altered Urinary Elimination is the least specific. Because most of the urinary elimination problems for which nurses provide care relate to incontinence or retention, the more general diagnosis of Altered Urinary Elimination will be used infrequently. When a patient's signs and symptoms support a more specific nursing diagnosis, such as Urge Incontinence or Urinary Retention, the specific label should be used. When a patient exhibits a urinary problem that is neither incontinence nor retention, the nurse should consider devising a specific non-NANDA label or using the general label of Altered Urinary Elimination.

Many problems could fall into this broad category. Pregnant women often have altered patterns (frequency) because of uterine pressure on the bladder. Men who cannot stand to void because of medical problems may have altered patterns. Children being toilet trained may hold urine for long periods, urinate more frequently, or resist wearing a diaper, thus exhibiting Altered Urinary Elimination.

Nurses must also be alert to situations in which a factor indicating an obvious alteration in elimination might actually be another type of problem. For example, patients who have indwelling urinary catheters may experience discomfort, embarrassment, or a knowledge deficit, and they always have high risk for urinary tract infections. Although this situation clearly indicates an alteration in urinary elimination, the overall problem is often better described using accepted nursing diagnoses such as Risk for Infection, Risk for Injury, Knowledge Deficit, or Body Image Disturbance. In such cases the indwelling catheter, rather than being the problem, causes other problems.

Beginning nurses may find it easier to use the broader diagnosis of Altered Urinary Elimination, but with increasing expertise they will be able to discriminate between specific urinary problems and describe them concretely, using more specific diagnoses.

Incontinence is a very common problem, especially among elderly patients. There are wide differences in the reported figures on the prevalence of this problem. Most figures show that 40% to 60% of institutionalized patients and 9% to 30% of community-dwelling persons are incontinent.[1,16,22,23] Regardless of the diverse figures, however, it is clear that incontinence is a psychologically distressing, socially disruptive problem, especially for the elderly.

Incontinence has been studied extensively in recent years. The surge of interest in the topic is prompted by many factors, not the least of which is that incontinence is a common reason for nursing home admission.[18,28] Another factor is the cost

of incontinence care, which amounts to approximately $10 billion per year,[17,23] with the federal government paying $8 billion of that bill.

Because of the cost and importance of this problem, the federal government is devising new policies. Federal guidelines now require standards of incontinence care for nursing home facilities. These guidelines specify assessment time and require the facilities to set up retraining programs or other care for incontinent patients.[37] Urinary incontinence in the adult continues to gain attention. It was the focus of early clinical guidelines developed by the Agency for Health Care Policy and Research (AHCPR), which can be used to guide care.[1]

Incontinence, the involuntary loss of urine, is a complex problem. Many different types of incontinence have been described. You will recall from the preceding discussion on normal voiding that continence depends on pressure in the urethra being higher than pressure in the bladder. Conversely, incontinence can occur when pressure in the urethra is lower than pressure in the bladder. Several factors can influence these pressures, such as bladder volume, intraabdominal pressure, and detrusor muscle tone. Urethral pressure depends on pelvic muscle tone, intraabdominal pressure, urethral and bladder neck muscle condition, and the thickness of the urethral mucosa. Each of these factors depends on an intact nervous system and a functional environment that allows for toileting.

In the cycle of (1) a felt need to void, (2) holding urine, and (3) an increasing need to void, voiding is the inevitable outcome. Eventually, if voiding is not allowed, the bladder will distend so far that the intravesicular (bladder) pressure will overcome the intraurethral pressure and the external sphincter will relax; incontinence will result. In the normal person who is past toilet-training age, voiding is voluntary and urine is expelled only at appropriate times in appropriate receptacles. When this does not occur and voiding becomes involuntary, incontinence occurs.

There are many classifications of incontinence, a variety of labels for each type, and lack of agreement on terms. The five types of incontinence presently in the NANDA taxonomy are Functional

Incontinence, Stress Incontinence, Reflex Incontinence, Urge Incontinence, and Total Incontinence.[27] The essential differences among the five types of incontinence are presented in Table 5. This table can serve as a tool for determining which type of incontinence is present. It should be noted that some patients have a combination of types of incontinence: for example, persons with Urge Incontinence also may have Functional Incontinence if their mobility is decreased. Recently, Woodtli proposed a new diagnosis, Mixed Incontinence, because Stress Incontinence and Urge Incontinence are often seen together.[48]

Urinary Retention is diagnosed when a person has problems with bladder emptying. It may be manifested as a total inability to void, difficulty starting a stream of urine, or incomplete bladder emptying. The difficulty may be transient, lasting for hours or days; long-term, lasting weeks or months; or permanent. The extreme variability of signs and symptoms of Urinary Retention has been supported in research.[15,46] Urinary Retention is potentially very serious; when the bladder is overdistended, urine may reflux through the ureters into the kidneys, causing renal damage. Persistent bladder overdistention also causes the detrusor muscle to decompensate. Incomplete bladder emptying allows urine to stagnate in the bladder, which predisposes to urinary tract infections and stone formation.

Urinary Retention is often described as a type of incontinence because when the bladder does not empty completely urine may eventually overflow without control. Other terms that describe patterns associated with Urinary Retention include *obstructive incontinence, overflow incontinence, paradoxical incontinence, flaccid bladder, atonic bladder, detrusor hyporeflexia,* and *lower motor neuron incontinence. Neurogenic bladder* is a term often used to describe a variety of neurological dysfunctions of the bladder, including incontinence and retention. Diagnosing the retention rather than the incontinence is more specific because the incontinence is actually a sign of the retention.

Nurses should be aware of the various terms used to describe Urinary Retention and its associated phenomena. They need to evaluate their clinical practice and literature on the subject with openness to these variations. It is also important to have a clear idea of the definition of Urinary Retention to avoid confusing it with other urinary disorders. For example, in oliguria the kidneys produce less than normal urine volume, and in anuria no urine; therefore there is no urine in the bladder to be retained. When retention occurs, urine cannot be expelled because the bladder, the urethra, or the surrounding structures are malfunctioning.

It is difficult to determine the actual incidence of Urinary Retention in the general population. However, retention can be a problem for many patients, especially those with neurological or muscular problems or those who have undergone surgery. The onset of urinary retention may occur suddenly, or it may develop gradually over time. It may or may not be linked to a specific event such as surgery.

ASSESSMENT

Altered Urinary Elimination

Because normal urinary elimination encompasses varied individual patterns, an assessment should begin with baseline data on the patient's usual urinary elimination pattern.[31] Ask the patient about usual urinary patterns, including timing and frequency of voiding; the amount, color, and odor of urine; usual position during voiding; and any discomfort with voiding. Combine this description with patient data on usual fluid intake, including the type, amount, and timing of input. All forthcoming data about the present or future situation can then be compared with this normal urinary pattern.

After this baseline has been established, determine if changes have occurred and, if so, what may have caused them. Very often the patient's own perspective will guide the nurse into logical areas of assessment, therefore saving time in data collection. Sometimes patients have perfectly simple reasons for Altered Urinary Elimination. For example, decreased urinary output with more concentrated urine may be the result of the patient's not drink-

TABLE 5   Comparison of Characteristics of Five Types of Incontinence

Characteristic	Functional	Stress	Reflex	Urge	Total
Character of voiding urge	Usually strong	Sudden and associated with increased abdominal pressure	None	Very strong	None
Amount voided	Moderate to large	Small	Moderate	Small or moderate to large	Constant leakage
Nocturia	May be present	Possible, not usual	Always	Common	Always
Precipitating factors	Inability to reach receptacle	Increased intraabdominal pressure	Full bladder, unhibited bladder contraction or spasm	Sensation of full bladder, inability to reach toilet in time	Unpredictable
Awareness of incontinence	Aware	Aware	Unaware	Aware	Unaware
Frequency of urination	Variable	Increased	Regular intervals related to volume	Increased	Unpredictable and constant
Anatomical problem	Not urinary, but sensory, cognitive, mobility, or environmental defects	Increased urethrovesicular angle, sagging support structures, weak sphincter tone	Nerve pathway problems	Stretch receptor changes, reduced bladder capacity, detrusor overactivity	Sensorimotor nerve damage, no neuron control, fistulas
Related factors and causes	Altered environment, sensory deficits, cognitive deficits, mobility deficits, drug use, stool impaction, closed head injury, emotional illness	Obesity, gravid uterus, increased age, incompetent bladder outlet, weak pelvic muscles, overdistention between voiding, jolting exercise (e.g., jogging)	Spinal cord injury, multiple sclerosis, spinal cord tumors, spondylosis, cerebral lesions	Abdominal surgery, catheter use, bladder infections, alcohol intake, caffeine use, increased fluid intake, increased urine concentration, overdistention of bladder, neurological disorders (cerebrovascular accident, incomplete supraspinal cord injury, multiple sclerosis, Parkinson's disease, brain tumors, trauma), Alzheimer's disease, cancer of bladder, urethritis	Neuropathy, neurological misfiring, surgery, trauma, spinal cord diseases, anatomical problems (fistula), severe neurological diseases

III

ing cola because the vending machine at work was out of order. When there is no such simple explanation, ask for descriptions of the change by prompting the patient to consider the following aspects: pain or discomfort on urinating; frequency, hesitancy, or urgency of voiding; incontinence or retention; amount, color, odor, and concentration of urine; or edema in any part of the body.

For a complete assessment, the nurse must consider any family and patient history of urinary problems. Inquire about a history of renal disease, hypertension, diabetes, infectious diseases, congenital disorders, connective tissue diseases (such as lupus erythematosus), urinary or renal calculi, gout, urinary tract infections, or trauma. Ask women about their history of pregnancies and any associated urinary problems. A history of any of these can indicate risk factors or problems in urinary elimination. Because sexual and urinary structures are anatomically combined, the nurse must also obtain a sexual profile of the patient, including the amount and type of sexual activity, any discomfort, and vaginal or penile infections. A significant question for women patients is whether they have any difficulty voiding after sexual intercourse.

Hygiene measures must also be considered. Women should be asked about their method of wiping after urination and bowel movements. A front-to-back wiping technique decreases the likelihood of fecal bacteria entering the urinary tract. Drug intake is another important assessment. Ask the patient about all drug intake, including over-the-counter medications. Some drugs are toxic to the kidneys; others can change the characteristics of urine or cause urinary incontinence or retention.

After collecting subjective data, the nurse should gather objective data on the patient's urination pattern. Percuss and palpate the abdomen to determine abdominal muscle tone and to check for bladder distention. Observe the patient voiding to determine the necessity of any special positions, appliances, or procedures and to note the patient's ability to use them appropriately. Note fluid intake, including the amount, timing, and type of intake. Compare this intake with output. Check the patient for edema, especially in dependent body parts.

Finally, the urine itself should be examined for amount, color, odor, specific gravity, and pH. When the results of laboratory urinalysis and cultures are available or indicated, check them. The box on page 267 provides a summary of these assessment guidelines. It should be used as a guide for a broad, baseline assessment of urinary elimination patterns.

■ **Defining Characteristics**

The presence of the following defining characteristics indicates that the patient may be experiencing Altered Urinary Elimination:

- Dysuria
- Hesitancy
- Nocturia
- Urgency
- Edema
- Bladder distention
- Inability to urinate without special assists
- Frequency
- Incontinence
- Retention
- Change in amount, color, or odor of urine
- Decreased or increased force of stream

■ **Related Factors**

The following related factors are associated with Altered Urinary Elimination:

- Changes in fluid intake
- Anatomical obstruction
- Fecal impaction
- Indwelling urinary catheters
- Use of commode, bedpan, or urinal
- Mechanical trauma
- Immobility
- Pregnancy
- Drug therapies
- Motor impairment
- General or spinal anesthesia
- Psychological disorders
- Age-related or developmental factors
- Cognitive or sensory impairments
- Emotional stress
- Lack of privacy
- Strange environment

All Types of Incontinence

The nurse's goal in assessing patients for incontinence is to identify the specific signs or symptoms that are critical to differentiating the type of incontinence. The general guidelines for assessing urinary elimination patterns presented in the previous section should be used. If incontinence is found, then a more specific assessment is in order. The nurse must first assess how long the incontinence has existed and consider any obvious change in the patient's health that correlates with the onset. If there is no clear correlation, the next set of questions or observations should be directed at assessing for critical characteristics of one or two types of incontinence. Stress Incontinence is perhaps one of the easiest to rule out. Does the incontinence occur only with an increase in intraabdominal pressure, such as sneezing, coughing, or strenuous exercise? If so, then Stress Incontinence is very likely. If not, the second easiest characteristic to eliminate is the patient's sense of urgency to void. If the urge is very strong, sudden, and usually uncontrollable, Urge Incontinence can be suspected. If there is no strong urge, Reflex Incontinence or Total Incontinence can be suspected.

The nurse also must assess the voiding intervals. If urine is expelled at regular intervals with dry periods interspersed and without the patient's awareness, incontinence is of the reflex type. If urine is leaked constantly, Total Incontinence is likely. If there is no clear-cut pattern to the incontinence, Functional Incontinence should be suspected. In that case, look for answers to such questions as why the patient is not able to reach a receptacle appropriate for voiding. If there are problems associated with more than one type of incontinence, the nurse must consider the possibility that a combination of types exists. These key initial assessment parameters are summarized in the box on page 268.

III

GUIDELINES FOR ASSESSING URINARY ELIMINATION

SUBJECTIVE DATA

Usual urinary elimination pattern
Timing, frequency
Amount, color, odor of urine
Position during voiding
Discomfort with voiding
Special assists (commode, bedpan, catheters, etc.)
Usual fluid intake
Timing, amount, type of fluids
Recent changes in pattern
Known related factors
Pain, discomfort
Frequency, hesitancy, urgency
Incontinence, retention
Urine amount, color, odor, concentration
Edema
Family and personal history
Renal disease, hypertension, diabetes
Infectious diseases
Congenital disorders
Connective tissue diseases (e.g., lupus erythematosus)
Neurological diseases (e.g., multiple sclerosis)
Urinary or renal calculi, gout
Urinary tract infections
Trauma
Sexual problems, related infections, discomfort
Drug intake (over-the-counter and prescription)
Women: history of pregnancies and associated
    urinary problems; hygiene practices; method
    of wiping perineal area
Men: history of prostate problems

OBJECTIVE DATA

Abdominal muscle tone
Bladder distention
Amount, color, odor, specific gravity, pH of urine
Force of stream
Timing, frequency
Position during voiding
Special assists, ability to use
Fluid intake, amount, timing, type
Edema
Laboratory data: urinalysis, cultures

III

KEY INITIAL ASSESSMENT PARAMETERS AND SUSPECTED TYPE OF INCONTINENCE

- Does incontinence occur only with an increase in intraabdominal pressure? (Stress Incontinence)
- Is the urge to void before an incontinent episode always extremely strong and uncontrollable? (Urge Incontinence)

- Is urine expelled at regular intervals, with dry periods between, without the patient's awareness? (Reflex Incontinence)
- Is urine leaked continuously? (Total Incontinence)
- Is there no clear pattern of response to the questions presented above? (Functional Incontinence)

After the possibilities are narrowed, a more detailed assessment is needed. Most authors and clinicians advocate the use of a voiding record or an incontinence chart that can be kept by the patient who is cognitively able or by the nurse.[1,12,24,32,41] This record allows for documentation of voiding times and attempts; indications of incontinent or continent episodes; the amount of urine (large, medium, small, or dribbling); the nature of the urge before voiding; and what the person was doing at the time the incontinence occurred. Although these types of records provide a good picture of incontinence patterns, such records may call attention to the problem and allow patients or nurses to change their behaviors before a true picture of the usual pattern emerges. This poses less of a problem for the clinician than for the researcher. Therefore in clinical situations the voiding record is definitely a valuable tool for assessment. This record should be kept around the clock for several days until a clear pattern is established. From data on a voiding record the nurse will know the pattern of incontinent episodes.

Although nurses may diagnose types of incontinence independently, in many cases the definitive diagnosis is made in collaboration with others, usually the physician. Ideally, after incontinence is identified, a thorough urological, gynecological, neurological, and medical history and a physical exam are done. Cystometry, urethral pressure profilometry, uroflowmetry, and pressure flow studies are examples of specific tests that typically differentiate types of incontinence.[1,8] There is not yet a consensus as to which patients should have these detailed medical assessments for incontinence.[1,36] Therefore nurses, who often are the first to notice incontinence, should see that their role encompasses thorough assessments and differentiation of the types of incontinence.

Functional Incontinence

With the nursing diagnosis Functional Incontinence, the line between defining characteristics and related factors is not clear cut because the related factors help to define the "functional" part of the label or problem. Functional disease is an organ problem in which there is no apparent impairment or structural change. Therefore, in assessing for Functional Incontinence, the nurse assumes there is no apparent impairment of the urinary system itself; rather, some other problem is causing incontinence in a potentially continent person. Functional Incontinence often is diagnosed by eliminating factors that might point to other types of incontinence. After establishing that no overt urinary problem is causing the incontinence, the nurse focuses on secondary problems that might be interfering with normal voiding and toileting practices. What is it that keeps the patient from reaching a toilet, bedpan, commode, or urinal in time to void? Therefore the assessment of Functional Incontinence focuses largely on related factors or causes. To narrow the possible factors, the nurse should look for obvious problems not related to urinary function. Williams and Gaylord[45] advocate a functional assessment of the following areas: (1) physical functional ability (transfer ability, mobility, balance, arm strength, torso flexibility, manual dexterity, toileting, and vision), (2) mental functional ability, (3) social functional considerations, and (4) environmental considerations (access from bed, chair, or sofa, toileting distance, availability of bedside commode, lighting, supports such as grab bars and rails, access to bathroom, and toilet height). Any of these could prevent timely voiding.

It also is important to look at data collected in other functional patterns.[45] Bowel elimination often is a problem area because a stool impaction can exert enough pressure on the bladder and urethra to prevent normal urinary elimination. Similarly, because drug treatments produce incontinence, the nurse should always assess drug use in an incontinent patient. Anticholinergic drugs (e.g., atropine and some cold remedies) may cause relaxation of the detrusor muscle; this results in urinary retention and overflow of urine. Alpha-sympathetic blockers (antihypertensives such as methyldopa and phenoxybenzamine) may cause relaxation of the internal sphincter. Drugs that are beta sympathetic in action (e.g., isoproterenol and metaproterenol) may cause relaxation of the detrusor muscle. Skeletal muscle relaxants (e.g., baclofen and diazepam) also can cause relaxation of the external urinary sphincter. Diuretics (e.g., furosemide and hydrochlorothiazide) obviously increase urine output.[1,12,32] Nothing should be overlooked in an attempt to identify functional or environmental problems that could cause incontinence. Sometimes the simplest of things, such as a cluttered room or a new garment with complicated fasteners, can prevent normal toileting. In institutional settings, a major factor contributing to Functional Incontinence may be a nurse's busy schedule. If a patient's call for toileting is delayed, incontinence can result from the lack of available assistance.

■ **Defining Characteristics**

The presence of the following defining characteristics indicates that the patient may be experiencing Functional Incontinence:

- Variable frequency of incontinent episodes

- No overt urinary problem found (other types of incontinence ruled out)
- Presence of some obstacle to normal voiding pattern (see Related Factors)

■ **Related Factors**

The following related factors are associated with Functional Incontinence:

- Stool impaction
- Sensory deficits
- Mobility deficits
- Drug use
- Cognitive deficits
- Emotional problems (e.g., anger or hostility)
- Altered environment
- Lack of available assistance for voiding

Stress Incontinence

The classic characteristic of Stress Incontinence, which is much more common in women than in men, is involuntary leakage of urine when there is an increase in intraabdominal pressure. This may occur consistently or may vary, depending on the amount of pressure exerted. The bladder does not really empty during these episodes, which may occur frequently or infrequently and may be accompanied by a need to hurry to the toilet.[47] The severity of this problem initially can be assessed from a voiding record. A complete assessment of Stress Incontinence to determine severity would be a collaborative effort of the physician and the nurse. The nurse often is the first person to identify this problem. A nursing assessment identifies the frequency of the incontinence, the circumstances precipitating the incontinence, and the timing of the episodes.

Objective assessment measures include direct observation of the urinary meatus to check for leakage. The patient should be instructed to cough when the person has a full bladder and is in the lithotomy position. If there is no leakage, raise the head of the bed or the examination table to 45° and repeat the process. If there is still no leakage, have the patient stand with feet apart and cough again.

III

III

This procedure points to the severity of the problem. Leakage when the patient is in the lithotomy position generally indicates more severe Stress Incontinence than that seen only when a patient is in a standing position.

With these data a diagnosis of Stress Incontinence can be made. The patient's physician should be consulted to determine if further diagnostic tests are in order. There are several tests that physicians and nurses may use collaboratively to determine the severity and causes of Stress Incontinence. A pelvic examination will rule out a cystocele or rectocele and establish the size and position of the uterus. A cystoscopic examination and a urethral pressure profile may be done. Other tests involve lifting the anterior wall of the vagina with a finger against one side of the urethra while having the patient exert pressure. Various laboratory tests may be ordered to rule out precipitating factors.

Assessment of related factors should begin with a look for weakened muscles of the pelvic floor. When these muscles are weakened or traumatized, a misalignment of the bladder and the urethra can occur and can cause Stress Incontinence. Weakened pelvic floor muscles can be caused by traumatic pregnancies and births, obesity, increased age, or neurological problems. One study found that vaginal births, an episiotomy or tear during delivery, multiple urinary tract infections, and having a mother with Stress Incontinence were risk factors for Stress Incontinence.[38] Therefore the nurse should assess for a history of pregnancies, a family history of incontinence, pelvic trauma or surgery, and patient age and weight. Objective data on pelvic muscle strength can be collected with a digital test in which a woman squeezes the perivaginal muscles around the examiner's fingers. Brink and others have been working on a measurement scale to accompany such an examination.[4]

Stress Incontinence in women also can be caused by an estrogen deficiency.[32] Estrogen is important for urethral tissue tone; if there is a deficiency, urethral tissue is flaccid and loses its contractility. Such a problem may be a suspected condition in elderly, postmenopausal women or in women whose uterus and ovaries have been removed surgically. Women should be questioned about menopause, hysterectomies, and any felt changes in vaginal tissue that might indicate estrogen deficiency.

Another category of related factors is damage to the sphincters, which can occur after fractures of the pelvis, transurethral resection of the prostate, or other genitourinary surgical procedures. The nurse should assess for a history of any such problems

Other functional variables in a person with Stress Incontinence may make the problem even worse. An overdistended bladder will increase the ratio of bladder pressure to urethral pressure. Therefore it is important to assess how often the patient voids and how much.

■ Defining Characteristics

The presence of the following defining characteristics indicates that the patient may be experiencing Stress Incontinence:

- Sudden urine leakage associated with activities that cause increased intraabdominal pressure (e.g., coughing, laughing, lifting, standing, and jogging)
- Small volume of urine loss
- Little or no nocturia
- Need to hurry to toilet
- Feeling that bladder is not empty after voiding

■ Related Factors

The following related factors are associated with Stress Incontinence:

- Chronic increase in intraabdominal pressure
- Weak pelvic muscles
- Multiple pregnancies
- Traumatic vaginal infant deliveries (tears)
- Episiotomies
- Bladder overdistention between voidings
- Obesity
- Estrogen deficiency
- Weak sphincter tone
- Increased urethrovesicular angle

- Sphincter damage caused by transurethral resection of the prostate, other genitourinary surgeries, or pelvic trauma

Reflex Incontinence

Reflex Incontinence is a voiding pattern much like that seen in an infant whose bladder emptying occurs at regular intervals without any inhibitions. It occurs in individuals who have damage to spinal nerve pathways to and from the brain but have intact sacral spinal reflexes. The spinal reflex arc allows for voiding, but there is no mechanism to inactivate the reflex. This type of incontinence is sometimes called *automatic incontinence, spastic incontinence, hypertonic incontinence, upper motor neuron incontinence,* or *suprasacral bladder incontinence.*

Assessment for this type of incontinence involves looking for a pattern of regular voiding without the patient having a sensation of voiding. This pattern usually will occur equally day and night, depending on the timing of fluid intake. Percussion over the bladder area will reveal a distended bladder before incontinence. After the patient voids, the nurse can check for urine left in the bladder by catheterizing the patient. Often Reflex Incontinence is accompanied by increased residual urine. This is important in assessing for the problem and for planning interventions. A large postvoiding residual urine volume can indicate a second problem, Urinary Retention, and predispose the patient to urinary tract infections.

Even though a sensation of a full bladder is not felt before voiding, some patients may report other body sensations. Often, especially with spinal cord injuries, a full bladder may trigger a sympathetic response that the patient can identify. These responses differ from person to person. Therefore the nurse should ask the patient to identify sensations felt before voiding. These responses often can be seen objectively. In mild forms the sympathetic response may produce diaphoresis, flushing, pilomotor responses (gooseflesh), or nausea. In extreme form, such a response can be life threatening and is called *autonomic dysreflexia.* This is seen most commonly in patients with high thoracic

and cervical spinal cord lesions and can occur when a distended bladder or bowel triggers an exaggerated automatic or sympathetic nervous system response. Signs of autonomic reflexia include severe hypertension, severe throbbing headache, bradycardia, profuse diaphoresis, blurred vision, nausea, flushing of the skin above the lesion level, severe pilomotor spasms, shortness of breath, and anxiety.[2]

■ Defining Characteristics

The presence of the following defining characteristics indicates that the patient may be experiencing Reflex Incontinence:

- Voiding occurs without urge being felt
- Regular intervals between incontinent episodes
- Nocturia
- Probable increased postvoiding urine residual
- Sympathetic response (e.g., diaphoresis, flushing, or nausea) before voiding

■ Related Factors

Because related factors for Reflex Incontinence are always medical problems, the related medical diagnoses become the related factors.

Urge Incontinence

Urge Incontinence is the most common type of incontinence in elderly patients.[32] It is characterized by a sudden, uncontrolled loss of urine preceded by a strong urge to void. Because patients are aware of the need to urinate but cannot hold urine long enough to reach a toilet or another appropriate receptacle, it sometimes can be misdiagnosed as Functional Incontinence. The signs and symptoms of Urge Incontinence are frequent voiding, nocturia, loss of urine in any position (standing, sitting, or lying), low postvoiding residual volume, and suprapubic discomfort with voiding.

Much of these data come from a voiding or incontinence record (refer to the discussion under All Types of Incontinence). Along with that information the nurse looks for the classic symptom of a strong urge to void preceding the incontinent episodes. In addition, the nurse should check the

III

amount of postvoiding residual to make sure that the patient is fully emptying the bladder. If not, a secondary problem of Urinary Retention is present.

Assessment of related factors or causes will tell the nurse if this problem can be cured or only managed for symptoms. In some patients no cause is evident. More frequently the cause is detrusor overactivity, also termed *detrusor instability* or *hyperreflexia*. With this condition the bladder contracts reflexively while the central nervous system inhibitory mechanism malfunctions. The bladder contracts but cannot be controlled adequately. Reduced bladder capacity is a related factor; it may be caused by abdominal surgery, bladder tumors, or long-term use of an indwelling catheter. Other related factors are those that directly cause the bladder to be overactive or irritable, such as cystitis (bladder infection) or urethritis. Less severe irritants to the bladder are alcohol, caffeine, and increased urine concentration. Overdistention of the bladder caused by increased fluid intake, decreased voicing frequency, or use of diuretics also can cause Urge Incontinence.

From the long list of related factors one can see that this assessment often is a collaborative effort of physicians and nurses. Physicians who assess for medical problems may diagnose Urge Incontinence and its related factors. Nurses who focus on patient responses to illness may diagnose Urge Incontinence and its related factors.

Nurses should be especially aware of related factors such as overdistention of the bladder, decreased voiding frequency, increased urine concentration, intake of bladder-irritating substances, and patient responses after the removal of indwelling catheters. A thorough assessment involves a search for any of these related factors, even in the presence of an obvious medical cause.

■ Defining Characteristics

The presence of the following defining characteristics indicates that the patient may be experiencing Urge Incontinence:

- Sudden, uncontrolled loss of urine preceded by strong urge to void

- Increased frequency of voiding
- Nocturia
- Loss of urine in any position (standing, lying, sitting)
- Suprapubic discomfort with urination
- Small, moderate, or large amount of urine voided
- Low postvoiding residual volume

■ Related Factors

The following related factors are associated with Urge Incontinence:

- Decreased bladder capacity after long-term indwelling catheter use or abdominal surgery or from bladder tumors
- Increased bladder irritability from cystitis, urethritis, use of alcohol or caffeine, or increased urine concentration
- Overdistention of bladder from increased fluid intake, decreased voiding frequency, or use of diuretics

Total Incontinence

Total Incontinence is rare. It is sometimes referred to as *true incontinence* or *constant incontinence* because of its characteristic nearly continuous flow of urine without a predictable cycle of the bladder filling and emptying. Total Incontinence also is used to describe incontinence that does not respond to treatments. It often is diagnosed by ruling out all other types of incontinence.

The key assessment finding for this diagnosis is the unpredictable, constant leakage of urine that occurs day and night. The nurse should collect other data to validate this diagnosis and rule out other possible problems. Sometimes Urinary Retention with urine overflow initially can appear to be Total Incontinence because there is frequent leakage of small amounts of urine. Therefore the bladder area should be palpated and percussed to check for distention, and the patient should be catheterized to check for urine in the bladder. If there is a large volume of urine in the bladder, other assessment is needed, but directed toward Urinary Retention, not Total Incontinence.

It also is important to check the patient's awareness of incontinence. Most patients with Total Incontinence have no sensation of the bladder filling and emptying. Cognitively aware patients will, of course, feel the wetness of the leaked urine but may not feel it being expelled. Patients with severe neurological deficits may be aware of nothing.

Total Incontinence is caused by a disease process, anatomical problems, or damage resulting from surgery, trauma, or radiation treatments. The most common related factor in male patients is prostate surgery, where damage may be done to the external sphincter or to the nerves of the bladder. Other surgeries, such as abdominoperineal resection for rectal cancer, may result in Total Incontinence. Other related factors are fistulas that develop from trauma, radiation treatments to the pelvis, obstetrical injuries, and surgery. There also are rare congenital anomalies (such as exstrophy of the bladder, where the bladder is exposed on the abdomen, or ectopic ureters that are misplaced into the vagina) that cause total incontinence.[14] Disease processes that produce Total Incontinence usually are those that destroy nerves, such as spinal cord infarction or demyelinating diseases. Neurological diseases may prevent the bladder reflex transmission or may cause misfiring of nerve signals, resulting in voiding at unpredictable times.

Some surgical procedures are done to produce Total Incontinence when normal bladder emptying must be bypassed. Ileal conduits (urinary diversions where the ureters are attached to a segment of ileum brought through the abdominal wall) or cystostomies (urinary diversion where the bladder is opened and drained through an abdominal opening) are examples of normal cyclic emptying of the bladder being replaced by a constant, uncontrolled flow of urine. Although patients with these urinary diversions technically have Total Incontinence, it does not usually warrant the nurse making this diagnosis because the diversion itself is not a problem but a treatment. In such cases other nursing diagnoses, such as Impaired Skin Integrity, might well be made with the Total Incontinence as a related factor.

■ Defining Characteristics

The presence of the following defining characteristics indicates that the patient may be experiencing Total Incontinence:

- Continuous or nearly continuous flow of urine
- No predictable cycle of the bladder filling and emptying
- Nocturia
- Little or no residual urine in the bladder
- No patient awareness of incontinence

■ Related Factors

The following related factors are associated with Total Incontinence:

- Surgical procedures that damage nerves or sphincters, such as transurethral resection of the prostate and abdominoperineal resection
- Fistulas developed from trauma, radiation treatments, obstetrical injuries, or surgery
- Congenital anatomical anomalies such as exstrophy of bladder and ectopic ureters

Urinary Retention

Any decrease in urine output should be considered a diagnostic cue for Urinary Retention. If the patient can talk about it, difficulty with voiding may be reported. This difficulty may be expressed as a problem in starting a stream of urine, interruptions of the stream or a decrease in its force, a sensation of bladder fullness after voiding, painful voiding, or actual inability to void at all. Even without a patient report of symptoms, the nurse should suspect Urinary Retention when a patient voids frequently in small amounts or has frequent dribbling of incontinent urine. Frequent dribbling is easily misdiagnosed as incontinence rather than retention. Further assessment is needed when frequent dribbling of urine occurs. A most critical sign is a distended bladder. Percuss and palpate the lower abdominal area to detect bladder fullness. Percussion of a full bladder will produce a dull or nonresonant sound in the suprapubic area that is different from the somewhat hollow sound found in the normal, intestine-filled lower abdomen. A full bladder may be felt during palpation

III

III

of the lower abdomen. Pressure over the bladder area may cause discomfort or dribbling of urine when the bladder is very full.

Catheterization is usually performed to determine the amount of urine in the bladder. This is best done after the patient voids to determine the amount of residual urine in the bladder. A large postvoiding residual urine volume (generally more than 100 ml) is indicative of retention. Patients with severe retention may have very large amounts of urine in the bladder.

Recently bladder ultrasonography has enabled nurses to assess urinary retention without unnecessary catheterizations.[29,34] An ultrasound scanner, when passed over the bladder, can "read" the amount of urine inside. It is likely that this assessment technique will become more widely available because of its usefulness.

The nurse should suspect Urinary Retention when a patient is restless or diaphoretic. In this case the amount of recent urine output should be checked immediately. Patients with any risk for Urinary Retention or those who have some signs of retention should be monitored or intake and output. If the patient is receiving a regular diet, fluid intake is usually about equal to output. Nonmeasurable fluids in foods will usually balance out the insensible fluid loss through the lungs, the skin, and the intestines. If the patient is receiving fluids only, urine output will be somewhat less than intake. If output is significantly less than intake, Urinary Retention should be suspected.

Many factors may contribute to Urinary Retention. After the long-term use of an indwelling catheter, some patients have problems with incomplete emptying.[35] Postoperative Urinary Retention is fairly common, especially in elderly patients and in those who have had spinal anesthesia. Postoperative assessment should always include assessment of urine output. After giving birth, mothers should also be assessed for Urinary Retention caused by swelling of the meatus or the perineal area, hemorrhoids, or spasms of the perineal muscles. Women who have had traumatic vaginal deliveries may fear pain with voiding and may have difficulty relaxing the external sphincter.

Another group of related factors includes bladder outlet obstructions (e.g., prostatic hypertrophy), urethral strictures, fecal impaction, hemorrhoids, tumors, or perineal edema. Obstructions are more common in men than in women.[36] Many obstructions, such as fecal impaction, hemorrhoids, or edema, may be detected through nursing assessment; others are detected by medical examination.

Resnick[36] reported a newly discovered common phenomenon—detrusor hyperactivity with impaired contractility (DHIC)—which was associated with Urinary Retention. With DHIC the bladder contracts slowly and inefficiently, resulting in Urinary Retention. Patients may also have Stress Incontinence or overflow incontinence, so a definitive diagnosis must be made urodynamically.[1]

Side effects of some medications produce Urinary Retention. Anticholinergic medications such as atropine, propantheline bromide, or belladonna preparations; cold remedies such as pseudoephedrine; tranquilizers such as the phenothiazines or butyrophenone; calcium channel blockers; and narcotic analgesics are but a few examples of such medications.[1,12,32] All medications, including over-the-counter products such as cold remedies, should be evaluated for this side effect before they are administered to a patient with Urinary Retention.

Environmental or psychosocial problems may also contribute to Urinary Retention. Events that cause anxiety or muscle tension may produce temporary retention. Lack of privacy, inability to assume a usual voiding position, timing difficulties, or the use of different receptacles (bedpans, urinals, or commodes) are potential contributors to this problem and are easily overlooked in an assessment that is focused too narrowly on the urinary system. As with any assessment, the patient's total response must be considered in searching for problems' related factors.

■ **Defining Characteristics**

The presence of the following defining characteristics indicates that the patient may be experiencing Urinary Retention:

- Cessation or decrease in urinary output
- Reported difficulty starting urine stream
- Inability to start urine stream
- Decrease in force of urine stream
- Interruptions in urine stream
- Sensation of bladder fullness
- Painful voiding
- Frequent voiding of small amounts
- Dribbling incontinence
- Distended bladder
- Pressure, discomfort in lower abdomen
- Postvoiding residual urine volume more than 100 ml
- Restlessness
- Diaphoresis
- Output less than input

■ Related Factors

The following related factors are associated with Urinary Retention:

- Previous use of indwelling urinary catheter
- General or spinal anesthesia
- Postpartum condition such as swelling of meatus or perineum; hemorrhoids; perineal muscle spasms; or fear of discomfort with voiding
- Bladder outlet obstruction such as urethral strictures, fecal impaction, hemorrhoids, or perineal edema
- Side effects of medications, especially anticholinergic drugs, cold remedies, and tranquilizers
- Environmental or psychological factors such as anxiety, muscle tension, lack of privacy, inability to assume usual voiding position, timing difficulties, and use of different toileting receptacles.

DIAGNOSIS

■ Differential Nursing Diagnosis

Altered Urinary Elimination incorporates all diagnoses indicating a change from the baseline in urinary elimination. As such, the defining characteristics are broad. Whenever possible, the nurse should examine the data to determine if a more specific diagnostic label could be applied. Each of the incontinence diagnoses and the diagnosis of Urinary Retention should be considered if the problem is a lack of control over voiding. In cases where incontinence or retention are not obvious problems, consideration of the cause of the alteration will often point to a more appropriate specific diagnosis, such as Impaired Physical Mobility, Fluid Volume Excess or Deficit, Toileting Self-Care Deficit, or Altered Thought Processes.

All incontinence diagnoses should be differentiated from Functional Incontinence. Any of the related factors associated with this diagnosis could be considered differential diagnoses. Because of the wide range of factors contributing to Functional Incontinence, it is easy to focus on the incontinence and miss the more prominent underlying issues. For example, Constipation, Impaired Mobility, Impaired Adjustment, Chronic Confusion, Acute Confusion, and Social Isolation could be appropriate for a patient with Functional Incontinence.

Once Stress Incontinence has been differentiated from other types of incontinence (refer to Assessment), the nurse should consider if one of the related factors for the incontinence should be the primary care focus. If a patient is obese, the diagnosis Altered Nutrition: More Than Body Requirements should be made so that a weight reduction plan can be started. The Stress Incontinence might be alleviated with such an approach. Diagnoses related to muscle function, such as Impaired Mobility or Activity Intolerance, also might be considered if muscle weakness underlies the Stress Incontinence. Increasing muscle tone would alleviate the problem and might be a more inclusive focus for nursing care.

True Reflex Incontinence must be differentiated from the other types of incontinence. Because Reflex Incontinence usually cannot be eliminated by nursing interventions, the nurse must decide if it is more critical to focus on reducing the risks associated with Reflex Incontinence. If so, the diagnosis Risk for Infection or Dysreflexia might be made so that prevention of those problems can be the primary focus of care.

Urge Incontinence and Functional Incontinence often are seen simultaneously in elderly patients who have other mobility or sensory deficits. Therefore, in patients who appear to have Functional Incontinence, the nurse should assess other signs and symptoms indicating Urge Incontinence. A case has been made by Woodtli for a new nursing diagnosis, Mixed Incontinence, because Urge Incontinence and Stress Incontinence were found to occur in one third of the subjects in one study and in one fourth of the subjects in another study.[48] The AHCPR *Guidelines* also list Mixed Incontinence as a combination of Stress Incontinence and Urge Incontinence.[1] It is also important to determine that Urinary Retention is not masked by symptoms of Urge Incontinence. This can be determined by checking postvoiding residual volume through catheterization.

Total Incontinence often cannot be alleviated, only managed through nursing interventions; therefore to make an appropriate differential diagnosis, the nurse should think "forward" to nursing care planning and implementation. Many interventions are focused on preventing skin problems that often accompany Total Incontinence. In such cases the diagnosis Risk for Impaired Skin Integrity (related to Total Incontinence) could provide a more accurate reflection of the problem under care. Because such incontinence can be devastating to the cognitively aware person, diagnoses more reflective of the patient's functional problems might be a better label for those responses. Examples of these are Body Image Disturbance, Impaired Adjustment, and Ineffective Individual Coping.

Urinary Retention can be manifested as incontinence and vice versa (refer to the Assessment section). It is critical to make this distinction because undiagnosed Urinary Retention has the potential for causing serious problems. Another important distinction to make is the difference between Fluid Volume Deficit and Urinary Retention. If urinary output is low because of low fluid intake, cardiovascular and renal function could be at high risk. Misdiagnosing low output as Urinary Retention therefore could result in the patient not receiving necessary treatment for other health problems.

■ Medical and Psychiatric Diagnoses

Neurological disorders such as cerebrovascular accidents, spinal cord injuries, and multiple sclerosis often result in Altered Urinary Elimination. Patients with diabetes mellitus often have urinary frequency as an early sign of high glucose levels. Men with enlarged prostates caused by prostatic hypertrophy or cancer often have changed patterns of urination as a first clue to the problem. Changed patterns of elimination often are the first signs of several disease processes, and it is important to make the appropriate medical diagnosis.

Almost any illness can produce Functional Incontinence. Diseases or injuries affecting cognitive function (e.g., dementia, depression, or traumatic brain injuries) can affect the patient's control over toileting. The effects of the disease or injury may decrease the ability to recognize the socially appropriate method of voiding or directly affect neurological pathways necessary for voiding. Owen and others found that post-CVA patients whose incontinence was not controlled had more difficulty with orientation, memory, and problem solving.[30] Diseases affecting mobility (e.g., arthritis, fractures, and multiple sclerosis) also frequently interfere with toileting ability.

People with diabetes mellitus, multiple sclerosis, Parkinson's disease, and cerebrovascular accidents are especially at risk for Stress Incontinence. Similarly, persons with diseases that affect their muscle tone, either directly or indirectly, can have this nursing diagnosis. Sometimes a long, debilitating illness can weaken a person to the point that control of the micturition muscles is lost.

Reflex Incontinence is always related to a medical problem. Because of this, Reflex Incontinence usually is diagnosed by the physician and the nurse. Reflex Incontinence often is seen in patients with spinal cord injuries that result from auto accidents, sports accidents, or trauma from bullet wounds. Spinal cord tumors or degenerative changes in the spine (spondylosis) also can result in Reflex Incontinence. It is sometimes seen with multiple sclerosis and certain cerebral lesions.

Neurological diseases, such as dementia, brain tumors, cerebrovascular accidents, Parkinson's disease, brain or spinal cord injuries or tumors, and spondylosis, often are accompanied by Urge Incontinence. In addition, diseases directly affecting bladder capacity or irritability, such as bladder tumors and urinary tract infections, are prime conditions for this nursing diagnosis.

Total Incontinence is specifically related to disease processes, physiological alterations, and surgery. Examples of these include fistulas; spinal cord diseases and injuries; neurological diseases and injuries; congenital anatomical anomalies affecting anatomical structures concerned with urinary elimination; and surgical procedures that damage nerves or the sphincter muscles (e.g., abdominoperineal resection).

In general, postsurgical and postpartum patients are at risk for Urinary Retention. Diseases of the nervous and muscular systems may also affect bladder contractility or the sphincter muscle, causing Urinary Retention. Examples of these diseases include autonomic neuropathy associated with diabetes or alcoholism; tabes dorsalis; spinal cord injuries, lesions, tumors, or herniated disks, especially in S2 to S4 spaces; cauda equina syndrome; multiple sclerosis; myelomeningocele; and cerebral lesions.[12,46] Even osteoporosis, which causes vertebral fractures, may lead to Urinary Retention.[46] Patients with direct bladder problems (such as tumors, stones, or infections) and bladder proximity problems (such as prostatic hypertrophy) often exhibit Urinary Retention.

OUTCOME IDENTIFICATION, PLANNING, AND IMPLEMENTATION

There are some general approaches to care for urinary problems. Some persons find urinary problems embarrassing. They may be reluctant to discuss them and may look for ways to take care of the problems themselves. Nurses must establish rapport with patients to promote easy and open communication about urinary concerns. Many people do not know that incontinence can be treated.[13]

Nurses must teach patients about treatment options and debunk the myth that urinary prob-

lems are the natural result of aging. Patients, families, and health care providers often believe this myth. Any urinary problem should be seen as an abnormal phenomenon for which care approaches should be planned. Urinary elimination is a complex physiological phenomenon, and lay persons are often confused about it. Nurses must take care to use language that patients can understand when care, especially teaching, is provided.

When the urinary problem is incontinence, nurses often focus on managing the soiling rather than on managing the incontinence. However, most incontinence can be cured or at least significantly improved.[9] Health care providers often reflect society's stereotyped beliefs about incontinence. Nurses must focus care on eliminating or controlling incontinence rather than accepting the incontinence and soiling as inevitable.

Incontinence care needs an interdisciplinary approach. It is a problem that crosses disciplines and cannot be treated in a multidisciplinary manner when each provider does a piece of the care. Many care approaches to incontinence require consistency and collaboration from several providers.

Altered Urinary Elimination

Because the diagnostic label Altered Urinary Elimination is so broad, a standard plan of care is difficult to describe. As noted earlier, this diagnostic label should not be used when one of the more specific types of incontinence or retention is applicable. Ideally, if a cluster of data does not fit one of the incontinence or retention diagnoses, the nurse should devise a label that is more specific than Altered Urinary Elimination. Care planning will then flow from the specified nursing diagnosis.

Functional Incontinence

The obvious focus of care for patients with Functional Incontinence is to eliminate or compensate for the causative factors. The expected outcome for the patient is continence or a reduction in episodes of incontinence. In most cases this is a realistic outcome because the incontinence is functional in nature.

III

The approaches taken will vary greatly, depending on the identified related factors. The voiding or incontinence record should be the basis of the plan because that will show where, when, and under what conditions incontinent episodes occur. For instance, it may be that incontinence occurs only at night because the patient may be unable to get out of bed or may have poor night vision. Another patient with nighttime incontinence may drink more fluids in the evening before going to bed.

If the environment can be adapted to a patient's needs, that strategy should be tried first. Environmental changes are usually easiest to implement and the least disruptive to the patient. The following are some environmental adaptations that have been successful; (1) leave side rails down if safety factors allow, (2) place phosphorescent tape on the floor from the bed to the bathroom, (3) leave the bathroom door ajar with the light on, (4) move all unnecessary items away from the path to the bathroom, and (5) install support bars by the toilet. If clothing requires much effort to remove, applying velcro closures will ease removal. Bedpans, urinals, and call lights should be placed with easy reach. Nurses themselves may be part of the environmental problems. If call lights are not being answered promptly, staffing changes should be made so that this problem is eliminated.

When the environment is as conducive to normal voiding as possible, other strategies are directed toward the patient. If the secondary problem causing the incontinence can be eliminated, that should be done first. Further strategies may be unnecessary if the secondary problem is eliminated. If there is a stool impaction, a bowel evacuation plan is needed, and a program to prevent future impaction should be started.

If the patient has a mobility problem that can be treated, that should be addressed. For example, if the person has morning stiffness from arthritis that makes movement difficult, pain medications may need to be given more frequently or earlier in the morning. Adaptive devices, such as a trapeze on the bed, may assist with mobility. If drug use is affecting urinary elimination, the nurse should collaborate with the physician to consider if alternate drugs can be given or if schedules may be changed so that the drug's peak action time coincides with the optimal toileting time.

Habit training, bladder training, or timed voiding are frequently used behavioral interventions.[1] The rationale for these interventions is that old

---

◢ **NURSING CARE GUIDELINES**
Nursing Diagnosis: Functional Incontinence

Expected Outcome: The patient will be continent at all times or at a specified percentage of times (indicate realistic percentage).

- Identify incontinence pattern. *The pattern will show where, when, and under what conditions incontinent episodes occur and will direct all other interventions.*
- Remove environmental obstacles. *These are usually easiest to implement and least disruptive to the patient.*
- ▲ Remove or control secondary patient problems. Begin bowel management program. Maximize mobility. Assess drug use to identify any incontinence-related side effects. Change drug regimens if possible. *Further interventions may be unnecessary if underlying problems are removed.*
- Institute bladder training, habit retraining, timed voiding, or prompted voiding regimen, based on patient characteristics; provide reinforcement for continence. *Habits can be changed through behavior modification and reinforcement.*
- Adjust time of fluid intake to coincide with optimal voiding times. *Frequency of voiding is related to amount of fluid intake.*
- Maintain voiding record. *Success, reinforcement, and need for changes in plan will be seen more easily with a consistent recording of patterns.*

■ = nursing intervention; ▲ = collaborative intervention.

habits can be changed through behavior modification and reinforcement. Bladder training encourages the patient to suppress the voiding urge while intervals between voidings are gradually increased to 3 or 4 hours. Habit retraining encourages suppression of voiding while intervals between voiding are adapted to the person's voiding pattern. Timed voiding involves a fixed schedule of voiding, such as every 2 hours. Prompted voiding depends on asking patients at regular intervals if they need to void and assisting them if the answer is yes. A study by Schnelle and others[37] showed that prompted voiding is effective in reducing Functional Incontinence. The choice of one of these interventions largely depends on the pattern of incontinence found on the voiding or incontinence record used for assessment and on the underlying related factors for the individual patient.

Those who have cognitive deficits might respond best to timed voiding or prompted voiding. Those with mobility or sensory deficits might respond better to habit retraining. Patients with psychological or emotional problems and some with neurological or cognitive problems may respond to other behavioral therapies. Also called contingency management, behavioral therapies use reinforcers to promote continence. Verbal or social rewards are given when the patient is continent in voiding. These interventions must be well coordinated so that all staff take a similar approach. Behavioral therapies are ineffective if consistency is not maintained.

The Nursing Care Guidelines for a patient with Functional Incontinence provide a general guide to interventions. It is general in nature because specific approaches depend very much on the identified related factors. The general guidelines must be individualized according to each unique situation.

Stress Incontinence

Some interventions for Stress Incontinence are within the realm of nursing, especially if the severity of the problem is minimal and if the related factor is poor tone of pelvic floor muscle. When the problem is more severe and related to structural defects or estrogen deficiency, medical or surgical interventions are needed. Medical interventions may be needed if the patient with mild Stress Incontinence also has cognitive deficits. In these cases the problem becomes a medical diagnosis. Sometimes the care is collaborative and is planned and implemented by a physician and a nurse.

With mild Stress Incontinence in an alert patient, a realistic patient outcome is the elimination or significant reduction of incontinent episodes over several weeks or months, with a progressive decrease in the number of episodes in that time period. During that time, patients can learn to minimize the discomfort and embarrassment of incontinent episodes with planning aimed at maintaining dryness.

These patient outcomes can be achieved with exercises to increase pelvic and abdominal muscle tone and with weight loss if needed. Kegel exercises are a time-honored and research-supported intervention for stress incontinence.* These exercises, first introduced in the late 1940s by Kegel,[19] focus on strengthening the pubococcygeal muscle, the main support for the pelvic floor surrounding the urethra, the vagina, and the rectum. Many women are unaware of these muscles and how to exercise them, so they must be taught. Wells[43] suggested using the description "pelvic muscle exercise" because some women thought "pelvic floor exercises" had to be done on the floor. One simple method of teaching is to have the patient sit with legs apart and urinate. Ask her to squeeze the muscles to stop the stream of urine. If this can be done, the pubococcygeal muscle has been contracted. Another method is for the nurse to place a finger at least three quarters of the way into the patient's vagina and ask the patient to squeeze the finger. The patient also can do this herself and feel the contracting muscle.

Some studies have shown that a greater reduction in incontinence is achieved when biofeedback is used with Kegel exercises.[5,40] Biofeedback is achieved with a device called a perineometer placed in the vagina that can register on a gauge the pressure exerted with the muscle so that the

III

patient can see how well she is doing with the exercises. If a perineometer is available, it should be used for optimal teaching and evaluation of exercises. After it is established that the patient can contract the pubococcygeal muscle, she should be instructed to tighten the muscle, hold it for the count of 10, relax it, and then repeat the procedure 100 times per day. Another method, quick Kegels, is to tighten and relax this muscle repeatedly as rapidly as possible. Whatever exercise is used, the patient should accept that these should be done for the rest of her life to maintain that muscle tone. It is also helpful to teach patients to strengthen abdominal muscles so that these muscles can help in supporting the bladder in its correct anatomical position. Some nurses teach "pull in, push out" exercises along with Kegel exercises. Patients are taught to pull up the pelvic floor as though trying to suck water into the vagina and then to push out as though trying to push water out.

◢ **NURSING CARE GUIDELINES**
Nursing Diagnosis: Stress Incontinence

Expected Outcome: The patient will achieve continence (or significantly decrease incontinent episodes) within 2 to 6 months.
- Have the patient identify pubococcygeal muscle, and instruct on how to contract muscle by successfully stopping a stream of urine during voiding while sitting with legs apart; squeezing vaginal muscles against examiner's finger; or observing a biofeedback instrument activated by squeezing a perineometer in vagina. *External feedback makes it easier to identify this muscle.*
- Describe how to do Kegel exercises: slow Kegels—squeeze muscle, hold to count of 10, relax, and repeat 100 times daily; quick Kegels—repeatedly contract and relax muscle as rapidly as possible. *Kegel exercises repeatedly have been shown to be effective in strengthening pubococcygeal muscles and decreasing Stress Incontinence.*
- Teach abdominal muscle exercises: "pull in, push out"—pull up pelvic floor as though trying to suck water into the vagina, then push out as though trying to push water out; then repeat exercise. *Strengthening abdominal muscles will increase bladder control.*
- Discuss a total body exercise program that is conducive to the patient's lifestyle. *Overall muscle tone will decrease Stress Incontinence.*
- If the patient is obese, plan weight-reduction and exercise programs. *There is a correlation between obesity and Stress Incontinence; a reduction in weight has been effective in reducing Stress Incontinence.*

Expected Outcome: The patient will maintain optimal dryness at all times.
- Encourage the patient to wear a pad, especially during strenuous activity or when there is an increased likelihood of coughing or sneezing. *Because the amount of urine expelled is usually small, a pad effectively protects clothing. Strenuous activity, coughing, or sneezing are often stimuli to an episode of Stress Incontinence.*
- Have the patient assess fluid intake, decrease intake of caffeine drinks, and schedule the least intake before periods of strenuous activity. *Bladder fullness or irritability will increase the likelihood of incontinent episodes.*
- Advocate that the patient carry an "incontinent episode bag" with a change of underwear and stockings. *Because of the unpredictability of Stress Incontinence, such preplanning could save the person unnecessary embarrassment and discomfort.*
- Encourage the patient to empty the bladder more often if overdistention is a problem. *An overdistended bladder is more prone to Stress Incontinence.*
- Advise obese or pregnant patients to avoid long periods of standing. *Standing for a long time increases bladder pressure, especially in obese or pregnant persons.*

■ = nursing intervention; ▲ = collaborative intervention.

If the patient has generalized poor body muscle tone, a complete exercise program to strengthen muscles should be planned. If the patient is obese, a diet and exercise plan should also be included in care.

Another focus of care is to assist the patient in managing the incontinent episodes until the incontinence is cured through nursing, medical, or surgical treatment. Although many patients develop such strategies themselves,[9] additional suggestions may be helpful. Instruct the patient to wear a menstrual pad, especially during strenuous exercise or when she has a cold and is coughing and sneezing. Encourage the patient to carry an "incontinence episode bag" (a bag containing an extra pair of underwear and stockings). The patient should also be taught to avoid caffeine drinks that are irritable to the bladder and to empty the bladder more frequently so that there is less pressure on the sphincter. Patients also may be able to change their schedule of fluid intake so that the bladder is not overdistended during periods of peak stress. Patients who are obese or pregnant should avoid long periods of standing, which increase intraabdominal pressure.

It is important that nurses understand the medical and surgical interventions available for more severe Stress Incontinence, although these are outside the realm of nursing. If the bladder has descended in the pelvis, a surgical bladder suspension can be done. This is often done after pelvic floor exercises have failed. For patients who have damaged sphincters, artificial urinary sphincters can be implanted. Vaginal pessaries have been used in the past, but because they are uncomfortable and impractical, they have limited use today. Medication treatments are effective for some patients. For estrogen deficiency with accompanying atrophic vaginitis, oral or intravaginal estrogen may be administered.[7] Alpha-adrenergic agonists, such as pseudoephedrine and phenylpropanolamine, are useful for increasing sphincter contractions. Imipramine, an antidepressant anticholinergic drug, has been used to decrease bladder contractility and increase the sphincter resistance.[12] Interestingly, although acknowledging the

need for further study, Wells and others[44] found that pelvic exercises were as effective as phenylpropanolamine.

Reflex Incontinence

Because of the nature of the diseases that cause Reflex Incontinence, it usually is not possible to cure this problem. It is, however, possible to control the voiding so that the patient can remain dry most of the time and can use a voiding stimulus to urinate into a receptacle at appropriate intervals.

Because of the risk of autonomic dysreflexia, another important patient outcome is the avoidance of an overdistended bladder. To achieve that outcome the patient needs to coordinate voiding times with fluid intake. It also is important for the patient to empty the bladder enough so that residual urine volume is low. Limits for acceptable residual volume range from 50 to 150 ml. This outcome often is set collaboratively by the nurse and physician or is set by protocol guidelines. Residual urine increases the risk of infection, stone formation, and overdistention. Patients need to be able to recognize signs of overdistention and infection so that cures can be sought. Patients also need to have a plan of action for unscheduled voiding or incontinent episodes because reflex voiding can be triggered at unpredictable times.

To achieve these outcomes nursing interventions must be tailored to the patient's unique characteristics. Many patients with Reflex Incontinence have gone through an acute state of illness when an indwelling catheter was in place. Long-term indwelling catheters are now used as a treatment of last resort because of the associated dangers of infection. After the catheter is out, patients can begin to explore triggering mechanisms that will initiate reflex voiding. The rationale for such interventions is that stimulated sacrolumbar dermatomes may activate the micturition reflex. Different mechanisms work for different people. Some possibilities are stroking the inner thigh, pulling lightly on pubic hairs, tapping or jabbing over the bladder area, digital stimulation of anal sphincter, stroking the glans penis or vulva, or even flexing the toes. Any or all of these can be ex-

III

plored. While trying these mechanisms, the patient should be sitting on a commode or toilet so that the normal voiding position is promoted. If the patient has functioning abdominal muscles and no medical contraindication, Valsalva's maneuver should be used during voiding to increase emptying. After the patient has voided, a straight catheter or a bladder ultrasound scanner should be used to check for residual urine in the bladder. If the residual volume is consistently lower than the limit set, this type of patient-stimulated reflex voiding may be adequate. If the residual volume is too high, other interventions may be necessary.

Intermittent catheterization is used widely today. The patient or a significant other may do this, usually after being taught by the nurse. A catheter is inserted through the meatus into the bladder, the bladder is emptied, and the catheter is removed. This procedure may be done as a sterile or as a clean technique.[25,26,33] A sterile procedure is sometimes performed in the hospital in which a new catheter is used for each catheterization. Patients at home usually use a clean technique in which they clean the catheter after each use and reuse it. The Nursing Care Guidelines for the patient with Reflex Incontinence include the steps for teaching intermittent self-catheterization.

For a trigger-stimulated voiding or an intermittent catheterization, a schedule for voiding is imperative. This schedule is initiated by setting the times at fixed intervals, then recording the amounts voided or released by the catheter. The object is to keep the bladder from filling beyond a limit of 300 to 400 ml. Times between voidings or catheterizations are adapted until this goal is reached. At the same time, a fluid intake schedule is set up, and the patient is urged to maintain this schedule so that a regular pattern of intake and output can be established. Overdistention of the bladder is thought to contribute to urinary tract infection.[25] To avoid the risk of autonomic dysreflexia as a result of an overdistended bladder, the patient must be taught to recognize any signs of this problem and to empty the bladder immediately if signs appear. It also is important that the patient know to shorten the interval between voidings or catheterizations if there has been an increase in fluid consumption. Patients who can void successfully using a trigger mechanism also need to know how to catheterize themselves in case of overdistention. They should carry a catheter with them at all times.

Because of the increased risk of urinary tract infections from residual urine, overdistention of the bladder, and intermittent catheterization, patients must be taught to observe and smell the

---

■ **NURSING CARE GUIDELINES**
Nursing Diagnosis: Reflex Incontinence

Expected Outcome: The patient will participate in a planned voiding schedule, using a voiding stimulus or intermittent catheterization, until a regular pattern of bladder emptying is achieved.

- Explain mechanics of bladder reflex to the patient. *The greater the understanding, the better the patient will accept this new task.*
- Explore various triggering mechanisms (stimuli) to initiate voiding, such as stroking inner thigh, pulling lightly on the pubic hairs, tapping or jabbing lower abdomen, digital stimulation of anal sphincter, stroking glans penis or vulva, and flexing toes. *These mechanisms trigger the neurological reflex in some persons.*
- Have the patient practice these mechanisms in optimal voiding positions, using Valsalva's maneuver during voiding if possible. *Using usual voiding patterns will increase the likelihood of reflex voiding. Valsalva's maneuver will allow abdominal muscles to squeeze the bladder and help it empty. Caution: this maneuver may be contraindicated in some patients. The nurse should check with the physician before teaching this.*

■ = nursing intervention; ▲ = collaborative intervention.

▲ If the triggering mechanism is effective, catheterize the patient after voiding to check for residual urine. Continue checking postvoiding residual urine volume until the volume is less than 75 ml. *Some triggered reflex voiding is ineffective in emptying the bladder completely.*

▪ If the triggering mechanism is ineffective or if postvoiding residual volumes are too high, teach the intermittent self-catheterization technique to the patient (or significant other, if the patient is unable to do it). Instruct the patient to use the following regimen: (1) gather equipment; (2) wash hands; (3) get in a comfortable position—sitting up in bed or chair or standing; (4) lubricate 1 in. of catheter tip with water-soluble lubricant; (5) wash perineal area or penis; (6) for women (after practice viewing meatus with mirror and feeling it), spread labia with nondominant hand and insert catheter until urine flows; (7) for men, hold penis at about 60° angle from body and insert catheter until urine flows; (8) allow urine to flow until stream stops; (9) rotate catheter and check for further urine flow; (10) remove catheter slowly; (11) wash catheter inside and out; and (12) store catheter in clean, dry place. *Intermittent self-catheterizations allow the patient to be independent in bladder emptying. Principles of teaching should be applied individually, as with all patient teaching.*

Expected Outcome: The patient will coordinate voiding times with fluid intake schedule.

▪ Monitor fluid intake and urine output to determine optimal times for voiding or catheterization to keep urine volume lower than 300 ml. *A bladder volume above 300 ml may predispose the patient to infections.*

▪ Plan a schedule for amount and timing of fluid intake. *There is a direct relationship between amount and timing of fluid intake and urinary output.*

▪ Start timing of voiding or catheterization at 2- to 3-hour intervals, and extend time to 4- to 6-hour intervals until desired volume is reached. *Because there is wide variation in the amount of time for bladder filling, schedules must be individualized.*

Expected Outcome: The patient will identify the signs of autonomic dysreflexia.

▪ Discuss with the patient any signs of sympathetic nervous system response to a full bladder. *Patients have varied responses, so an individualized baseline is very important.*

▪ Teach the patient and significant others the signs of autonomic dysreflexia: throbbing headache, profuse perspiration, blurred vision, nausea, flushing of the skin, severe pilomotor spasms, hypertension, bradycardia, shortness of breath, and anxiety. Urge patient to empty bladder at any hint of these signs of autonomic dysreflexia. *Autonomic dysreflexia can be life-threatening. Because the patient's condition may render him incapable of action, significant others need to know these signs. Recognition of the signs and prompt action can save the patient's life.*

Expected Outcome: The patient will identify the signs of urinary tract infection.

▪ Teach the patient to recognize the signs of urinary tract infection: increased temperature; malodorous or cloudy urine; change in color, sediment, or blood in urine; or increasing bladder irritability. *Because infection is a high risk, the patient must be able to recognize the signs so that interventions can be sought in a timely manner.*

Expected Outcome: The patient will devise a plan for dealing with unexpected incontinent episodes.

▪ Discuss with the patient a plan for preventing and dealing with unexpected incontinent episodes that fits the patient's lifestyle. *The individuality of the patient must be considered at all times so that interventions will be relevant.*

▪ Urge the patient to carry a catheter at all times and extra clothing; to empty the bladder earlier if lack of opportunity to void on schedule is anticipated; and to empty the bladder before sexual activity. *Such anticipatory activities can prevent undue discomfort from accidents and prevent overdistention of the bladder.*

▪ Consider the need for incontinence underwear, depending on frequency of unexpected incontinence. *Many patients, in spite of diligent preplanning, will have accidental incontinent episodes.*

III

urine so that any abnormalities can be reported to their physician or nurse. Any cloudiness, blood, or sediment in the urine or a change in the color or odor of urine may indicate an infection. Sometimes an infection can increase bladder irritability, which can cause unexpected incontinent episodes or difficulty voiding.

One other area of intervention helps the patient be prepared for "accidents." A reflex bladder may be triggered at unscheduled times. It may be triggered by odd kinds of activities such as scratching a leg. Fondling or stroking, especially in the genital or leg area, may trigger voiding. Strict adherence to the set voiding schedule will minimize the number of accidents, but other actions can also help the patient and significant others cope with accidents. Patients should be encouraged to carry extra underwear and pants or skirts with them. If they are going to be some place where voiding will be difficult at their scheduled time, they should empty the bladder before the activity. Sexual activity should be planned if possible so that the patient can empty the bladder first. Those who have frequent accidents may choose to wear incontinence underpants.

Urge Incontinence

Depending on the related factors for Urge Incontinence, care may be focused on eliminating the problem or on managing the problem. Care may be within the realm of nursing or medicine or a combination of both. If the cause is a medical problem, medical treatment may lead to a cure of the incontinence when the medical problem is cured. However, many of the medical problems that cause Urge Incontinence cannot be cured. In that case, because the related factor cannot be eliminated, the incontinence must be managed through medical or nursing measures.

The expected patient outcome will be an elimination of incontinent episodes (cure) or a reduction in the number of incontinent episodes (management). The outcome chosen as a realistic goal of care will depend on the nature of the related factors. Other secondary expected patient outcomes will flow from one of these two primary outcomes.

Nursing care plans with elimination of incontinent episodes as a goal will likely apply to patients with the following types of related factors: (1) decreased bladder capacity; (2) previous use of an indwelling catheter; (3) increased bladder irritability from alcohol or caffeine intake and increased urine concentrations; and (4) overdistention of the bladder from increased fluid intake, decreased voiding frequency, and use of diuretics. Secondary patient outcomes will be to increase bladder capacity, to decrease bladder irritability, or to decrease bladder distention.

Nursing care plans aimed at reduction of the number of incontinent episodes will apply to patients with the following types of related factors: (1) increased bladder irritability from chronic cystitis and urethritis and (2) incurable neurological disorders such as cerebrovascular accident, Alzheimer's disease, Parkinson's disease, and spinal cord injuries. Secondary patient outcomes will relate to a reduction in bladder irritability or to participation in a voiding schedule that permits voiding before the bladder is full enough to stimulate the strong urge to void.

Nursing interventions aimed at eliminating incontinent episodes focus on eliminating causative factors. For example, decreased bladder capacity may be caused by the extended use of an indwelling catheter. A plan for progressively lengthening the intervals between voiding will cause a gradual increase in the threshold of the bladder stretch receptor. With data on the incontinence record, the initial interval for voiding can be set at a time before the incontinence usually happens. With careful recording, that interval should be increased gradually. The patient should be reminded to continue to void at these optimal intervals to avoid overdistention and to allow the bladder to reach full capacity.

Urge Incontinence, like Stress Incontinence, may be related to weakened pelvic muscles.[11] Interventions similar to those described under Stress Incontinence can be used with these patients.

If increased bladder irritability caused by alcohol or caffeine intake is the related factor, the patient should be educated about the effect of these irritants and about alternate fluids to consume. If increased urine concentration is causing bladder irritability, patients should be encouraged to increase fluid intake.

Patients with Urge Incontinence from other causes sometimes will decrease their fluid intake to decrease incontinent episodes; they should be taught that this makes the situation worse because the urine becomes more concentrated. Diabetic patients whose disease is not well controlled may have concentrated urine; if so, these patients should be assisted in adjusting their diet and fluid intake. If overdistention of the bladder is the related factor, patients should be encouraged and helped to void more frequently. Those taking diuretics should be taught to recognize peak action times so that they can plan to void more frequently at that time. If patients who need assistance with toileting are experiencing Urge Incontinence, they should be put on a voiding schedule so that help is available more frequently. Call lights should be answered promptly, and bedpans, urinals, and commodes should be made readily accessible to such patients.

It is vital that the nurse study the voiding or incontinence record before initiating these interventions. It would be counterproductive to use an intervention aimed at reducing overdistention with a patient who has reduced bladder capacity. Selecting the appropriate interventions therefore critically depends on accurate identification of the related factors for Urge Incontinence.

Nursing interventions directed toward managing incurable Urge Incontinence focus on helping the patient to reduce the number of incontinent episodes. Patients with increased bladder irritability from chronic cystitis or urethritis need interventions to decrease the irritability. Medication often helps. In addition, nurses should focus on keeping the urine dilute by helping the patient increase fluid intake. These patients also may respond to a toileting schedule aimed at emptying the bladder before it gets full enough to trigger incontinence. Choosing this approach depends on the individual's bladder capacity, and the decision should be made jointly by the patient's nurse and physician.

For patients with neurological disorders, bladder training and toileting regimens seem to be the most widely used and successful intervention.[20] Bladder training and habit retraining are discussed in more detail under the diagnosis Functional Incontinence. Generally the patient with Urge Incontinence is put on a schedule of fluid intake, and a voiding schedule is set up. After a schedule is established, the intervals between voidings are progressively increased. Merely toileting these patients more often is not recommended; with an overly frequent voiding schedule there is a risk of decreasing bladder capacity, which will only compound the Urge Incontinence problem.

Biofeedback may be another treatment option for patients with Urge Incontinence. A method of recording bladder pressure, abdominal pressure, and anal sphincter activity (with innervation identical to that of the urinary sphincter) is made visible to the patient. This allows the patient to try to control the sphincter, the detrusor, and the abdominal muscles. This type of intervention has produced improvement in incontinence in some patients, but biofeedback is not practical for patients with severe cognitive impairments.

Because medical interventions often are used along with nursing measures to eliminate or reduce Urge Incontinence, a short overview of these measures is important to the nurse's full understanding of care. Corrective surgery of the genitourinary system, bladder denervation (selected central or peripheral nerves are cut), and hydrostatic dilation (the bladder is distended while the patient is anesthetized) are some of the medical treatments used for Urge Incontinence.

Some medications can reduce detrusor instability or overactivity. Imipramine, oxybutynin, and propantheline are examples of drugs that are sometimes effective in the treatment of Urge Incontinence.[1,12] These drugs relax the bladder and expand its capacity, but they have potentially serious side effects, especially when used by elderly patients. Dry mouth, decreased sweating, constipation, and urinary retention are but a few of the noted side effects for which nurses must monitor patients.

III

For nurses and physicians Urge Incontinence continues to be a frequently encountered treatment challenge. Some new treatments, such as electrical stimulation of selected nerves, are being explored.[1,39] However, at present these are still under study. Cure or management care requires creativity and a controlled set of interventions tailored to each patient. As evident from the care plan, there are few interventions that work with all patients.

◢ NURSING CARE GUIDELINES
Nursing Diagnosis: Urge Incontinence

Expected Outcome: The patient will experience an elimination of incontinent episodes or a reduction in the number of incontinent episodes.
- Assess related factors to determine choice of realistic outcome and reasonable time frames for meeting outcomes. *The plan must be individually tailored to each patient. All future outcomes and actions will depend on the accurate identification of related factors.*
- ▲ Monitor patient for side effects of medications used to treat incontinence. *Medications that relax the bladder and expand its capacity have potentially serious side effects, including constipation and Urinary Retention.*
- Maintain a voiding record. *Patterns of voiding can be seen more clearly and changes in plan may become evident.*

Expected Outcome: Depending on related factors identified, the patient will have (1) increased bladder capacity (increased urine volume and lengthened voiding intervals), (2) decreased bladder irritability (lengthened voiding intervals), or (3) decreased bladder distention (shortened voiding intervals and decreased urine volume).
- To increase bladder capacity, plan the voiding schedule: start the voiding at intervals shorter than intervals between incontinent episodes; progressively increase time between voidings until incontinence is decreased or eliminated; teach the patient to maintain the schedule; and coordinate fluid intake with the voiding schedule. *Increasing the interval will gradually increase the bladder stretch receptor threshold.*
- To decrease bladder irritability, eliminate the patient's intake of irritants such as alcohol and caffeine, increase the patient's fluid intake to maintain dilute urine, and educate the patient on the irritating effects of concentrated urine and how to counteract this with increased fluid intake. *Concentrated urine is irritating to the bladder. Irritants make it more difficult for the bladder muscle to relax.*
- To decrease bladder overdistention, encourage and assist the patient to void more frequently; set up a voiding schedule that balances with fluid intake, but be careful not to decrease time between voidings so much that bladder capacity decreases; have call light, bedpan, urinal, and commode within easy reach; and for the patient taking diuretics, teach peak action times, and plan increased voiding at that time. *There is a direct relationship between fluid intake and urine output. Diuretics have peak action times during which urine output increases. Convenience of toileting prevents Functional Incontinence episodes.*

Expected Outcome: The patient will participate in a set voiding and treatment schedule.
- Help patient set up a schedule that accounts for individual needs and routines. *Maintaining a schedule will train the bladder to empty at regular intervals, decrease the likelihood of overdistention, and maintain stretch receptor stimulus for full bladder.*
- If equipment is available and if the patient is cognitively intact, attempt the use of biofeedback to assist in patient control of bladder and sphincter. *Biofeedback gives an active message to the patient, allowing for control of sphincter, detrusor, and abdominal muscles.*

■ = nursing intervention; ▲ = collaborative intervention.

Total Incontinence

Patients with Total Incontinence whose problem cannot be corrected medically or surgically are a nursing challenge. Often their care is planned for other nursing diagnoses that have been caused by the Total Incontinence. Risk for Infection and Impaired Skin Integrity or Risk for Impaired Skin Integrity related to Total Incontinence often become the priority nursing diagnoses. Planning and implementation of treatment for these problems should include nursing actions aimed at managing Total Incontinence.

When Total Incontinence can be corrected through medical or surgical procedures, nursing care shifts away from managing the incontinence. Fistulas, especially those caused by trauma or obstetrical injuries, often can be closed surgically or with electrodes. Congenital anomalies such as bladder exstrophy may be corrected surgically. Patients with sphincter damage can have artificial sphincters implanted. Artificial sphincters allow patients to deflate a cuff that, when inflated, acts to keep urine in the bladder. The bladder sometimes can be totally bypassed when an artificial bladder is made, into which the ureters are transplanted. An ileal conduit is a pouch of resected ileum with an opening to the abdominal wall. A ureterosigmoidostomy transplants the ureters into the sigmoid colon. A continent ureterostomy via a Koch pouch is an ileal conduit with two valves: one keeps urine in the pouch until released by the patient by catheterization, and one prevents reflux of urine into the kidneys. Patients who undergo these procedures need nursing care to help them adapt to these new methods of urinating. However, their problems would be identified by other diagnostic categories.

Unfortunately, many diseases that cause Total Incontinence cannot be corrected medically or surgically. In these cases a urine collection device is needed. For men this can be a condom catheter or an indwelling urethral catheter. For women indwelling catheters are used more often because external devices are difficult to apply and are not always successful. Such devices are still quite new and need further testing.[18,42] Most men can wear an external condom catheter attached to a collection bag. These should be changed on a regular schedule, and the penis should be checked for any skin breakdown or constriction. Bacteria can build up inside an external catheter, and if it is applied tightly, blood supply can be restricted. Therefore these catheters should be checked for twisting, which can restrict the flow of urine.

Indwelling Foley catheters generally are used only as a last resort; long-term catheter use has many risks, the greatest being life-threatening infections. Diligent nursing care often can prevent the need for indwelling catheters; patients without catheters need nursing care focused toward managing Total Incontinence. These patients need creative and time-consuming nursing care. Approaches that work for one patient often will not work for another, so care must be individualized.

Determining expected outcomes is therefore difficult. Often, maintaining optimal dryness is the only realistic outcome. For some patients it may be possible to reduce the number of incontinent episodes. Patients who have intact verbal or nonverbal communication skills may be able to identify their need for assistance in keeping dry. Those who have motor ability may be able to participate in an incontinence management regimen.

Nursing actions will depend on the expected outcome, so these too will be highly individualized. It is helpful to place these patients on a set schedule of fluid intake so that urine output is predictable. There is sometimes a temptation to restrict fluid. This should never be done because it increases the already present risk of urinary tract infection. A fluid intake of at least 2000 ml per day should be maintained.

Containment garments, such as incontinence underpants, usually are necessary. Sometimes large menstrual pads may be used. These can be changed on a regular schedule.

Disposable, waterproof pads on beds are often used to keep patients dry. Unfortunately they often wrinkle and stay wet. They also are very expensive. If used, they should be straightened and changed frequently so that they do not cause skin breakdown. Recently, however, alternatives to these

III

"blue pads" have become available. These include disposable diapers and pads and washable pants with removable pads.[3]

Whether containment garments or disposable pads are used, the nursing plan should have a set schedule for changing them. Strict adherence to a preset schedule, such as every 2 hours during the day and evening and every 3 hours at night, will minimize the risks of skin problems and infections. It also will ensure comfort for the patient and decrease undesirable odor.

It also is important that family members are aware of the plan for managing incontinence. They need to be educated about options for maintaining dryness so they understand that their family member is not being left wet for long periods of time because of lack of care. If patients are able to communicate their needs, they should be involved in the incontinence management schedule. Because patients may feel embarrassed about incontinence, they should be made to feel free to ask for clothing or for changes of bed linen. They may be able to indicate a linen-changing schedule that works best for them. Patients who are adequately mobile should have undergarments, linens, or incontinent pads for their own care. These should be available in sufficient quantities to allow for frequent changes.

Intermittent catheterization (discussed under Reflex Incontinence) is not appropriate for patients

---

◢ NURSING CARE GUIDELINES
Nursing Diagnosis: Total Incontinence

Expected Outcome: The patient will maintain optimal dryness.
- Use containment garment and change garment on regular schedule, such as every 1 to 2 hours during the day and every 2 to 3 hours at night. *Maintaining dry skin will prevent skin breakdown. Moisture in a closed system will promote bacterial growth.*
- Set up a schedule for linen and pad changes; use checklist to record times. *External reminders will promote staff adherence to a schedule.*

Expected Outcome: The patient will reduce the number of incontinent episodes (if realistic).
- Set up a fluid intake schedule so that at least 2000 ml is taken in per day at regular intervals; do not restrict fluids unless medically ordered. *Dilute urine is less irritating to the bladder and the skin.*
- For men, apply condom catheter and drainage bag, check penis regularly for constriction and excoriation, and check condom regularly for twisting. *Constriction of the penis can cause severe tissue damage.*
- Use waterproof pads or special bed sheets as needed, and check these frequently for wrinkles. *Wrinkles and wetness increase the risk for skin damage.*
- ▲ Perform intermittent catheterization if enough urine is stored in the bladder to make the procedure worthwhile. *Intermittent catheterization will decrease the amount of urine spilled on the skin.*

Expected Outcome: The patient will identify the need for assistance with keeping dry (if realistic).
- If the patient can communicate needs, set up message system for indication of wetness. *The patient is in the best position to determine when wetness is a problem.*
- Encourage the patient not to remain wet for long periods. *Moisture promotes bacterial growth.*

Expected Outcome: The patient and family will participate in an incontinence management regimen (if realistic).
- Discuss incontinence care with family members, and encourage their participation in changing garments and pads. *Incontinence is often embarrassing. Self-care will decrease the need to involve others in a private matter.*
- If the patient can move well enough, have supplies readily available for self-changing of garments, pads, and linens. *Self-sufficiency will promote a feeling of control.*

■ = nursing intervention; ▲ = collaborative intervention.

who have true Total Incontinence with constant leakage of urine. It may be helpful to patients who have some urine storage capabilities that reduce the quantity of leaked urine. The potential risks must be weighed against the benefits of intermittent catheterization for each patient. This decision is made collaboratively with the physician.

Ultimately some patients with Total Incontinence may need to be managed with indwelling catheters. Technically the maintenance of dryness for these patients is being treated medically by the catheter, and nursing care is supportive of the medical treatment. The patient's response to the use of the catheter must be assessed, and other diagnoses should be made. The reader should refer to diagnoses such as Risk for Infection and devise plans aimed at reducing the risk of infection in patients with indwelling catheters.

Urinary Retention

Realistic patient outcomes depend on the severity of Urinary Retention and the factors contributing to retention and whether the patient has difficulty starting a stream of urine. Several outcomes are possible but may not all apply to any one patient. The ideal general outcome is for the patient to be able to empty the bladder completely. This may be achieved through interventions aimed at aiding the patient to void or through an intermittent catheterization program. Therefore secondary outcomes may be for the patient to participate in an augmented voiding program or to perform intermittent catheterization. The usual criterion for determining adequate emptying of the bladder is if the patient has a postvoiding residual urine volume of 75 to 100 ml or another amount deemed safe by the patient's physician.

Interventions derive from whichever patient outcome is reasonably expected. If the patient has postoperative Urinary Retention, strategies oriented toward initiating a stream of urine are often effective. Getting the patient into as near a normal voiding position as possible helps initiate patterned responses. Many nurses use "tricks" that help trigger the micturition reflex, such as running water near the patient, putting the patient's hands in water, stroking the lower abdomen with ice, or pouring water over the perineal area. These maneuvers stimulate the micturition reflex. Many of these strategies also work for postpartum patients. In addition, if swelling of the perineal area is contributing to Urinary Retention, application of ice to the perineum will decrease swelling and remove this obstruction.

If fear of discomfort with voiding is a factor, giving pain medication before the initiation of voiding and providing calming communication and support can help. For postoperative or postpartum patients the nurse must assess fluid intake and fluid loss to determine the probable urine volume in the bladder. In addition, the bladder area should be palpated and percussed to check for distention. These data help determine how long a patient can safely go without voiding. If patients cannot void and the bladder is not overdistended, it helps to have them rest and then try again. If none of these strategies is effective, catheterization will be needed to empty the bladder. A patient should never be "threatened" with catheterization; this merely causes more tension.

A bladder obstruction causing incontinence should be removed if possible. Nurses can remove fecal impaction and start bowel regimens when constipation is causing Urinary Retention. Hemorrhoids causing obstructive pressure on the bladder outlet may be treated medically or may be reduced with sitz baths and bed rest. Sitz baths increase circulation to the hemorrhoid area, and bed rest decreases the downward pressure on the rectal area.

Other obstructive problems, such as prostatic hypertrophy, tumors, or urethral strictures, are treated medically or surgically. Prostate gland surgery or the insertion of a suprapubic catheter are common treatments for prostatic hypertrophy. Strictures are sometimes treated by dilating the urethra. In these cases nursing care is supportive to the medical treatment, and other nursing diagnoses may apply.

Patients with neuromuscular conditions causing Urinary Retention may respond to an augmented voiding regimen, but often patients need intermittent catheterization to empty the bladder completely. Augmented voiding regimens include setting a schedule for voiding that is correlated with

III

fluid intake; double voiding (having the patient void and then try to void again); using Valsalva's maneuver (bearing down on the bladder with abdominal muscles); Credé's method (pressing down on the bladder area); and using an optimal voiding position and receptacle. In addition, because the innervation of the anal and urinary sphincter muscles is identical, stretching the anal sphincter may cause the urinary sphincter to relax. Such procedures compensate for weak bladder muscles and maximize the natural voiding reflex patterns. These tactics should not be used when there is an obstruction; the extra pressure will not help open a blocked urethra and may cause reflux of urine into the kidneys. Valsalva's maneuver is contraindicated in patients with certain conditions such as myocardial infarction, aneurysms, eye surgery, and glaucoma.

When the patient uses augmented voiding regimens, the postvoiding residual urine volume should be monitored by catheterization or ultrasound scanner to determine if the bladder is being emptied adequately. If there is a high residual urine volume, intermittent catheterization may be indicated. (Intermittent catheterization is discussed under the Nursing Care Guidelines for Reflex Incontinence.)

Medications producing Urinary Retention should be changed if possible. Nursing interventions are usually limited to detection of medication side effects and notifying the patient's physician of the problem.

When environmental or psychosocial factors contribute to Urinary Retention, care should focus on alleviating those that inhibit sphincter relaxation. Maintaining complete privacy and setting up nearly normal voiding conditions will promote reflex voiding. If the patient is anxious or tense, contributing factors should be addressed and relaxation-promoting interventions implemented.

◾ NURSING CARE GUIDELINES
Nursing Diagnosis: Urinary Retention

Expected Outcome: The patient will achieve complete emptying of the bladder or will maintain a postvoiding residual urine volume of less than 75 ml (or another amount deemed safe by the patient's physician).

- Assure privacy for patient. *Privacy promotes total body relaxation.*
- Help patient into voiding position as near normal as possible. *Familiar patterns promote reflex voiding.*
- Encourage relaxation: deep breathing, loosening muscles, closing eyes. *Total body relaxation helps relax the bladder muscle.*
- Assist with initiating voiding reflex by trying techniques such as running water near patient, placing patient's hands in water, stroking the lower abdomen with ice, or pouring water over the perineum. *These techniques promote the micturition reflex.*
- ▲ Alleviate constrictions or obstructions: for perineal edema, apply ice; for fecal impaction, remove impaction or give an enema; for constipation, start bowel regimen; for hemorrhoids, give sitz baths and bed rest. *Constrictions interfere with the passage of urine through the bladder neck and urethra.*
- ▲ Reduce discomfort or fear of discomfort by giving pain medications before voiding attempts; use calming communication and support. *Discomfort adds to muscle tension.*
- ▲ Determine safe duration for patient to go without voiding by comparing intake and output and palpating for bladder distention. *Realistic expectations for urination are dependent on fluid intake.*
- If bladder is not overdistended, have patient rest, then try the above strategies again. *Promoting relaxation enhances muscle relaxation.*
- ▲ If the above strategies are ineffective and the bladder is overdistended, catheterize and then wait for bladder fullness; then repeat interventions. *Risks for infection and sympathetic neural response increase when the bladder is overly distended.*

◾ = nursing intervention; ▲ = collaborative intervention.

▲ Check postvoiding residual urine volume if voiding is accomplished. *Patients with urinary retention are less likely to empty the bladder fully. Residual urine increases the risk for infection.*

■ If voiding is repeatedly unsuccessful, go to the next part of plan. *Individualized planning is essential for success.*

Expected Outcome: The patient will participate in an augmented voiding regimen.

■ Set up a voiding schedule correlated with fluid intake. *Output is directly related to input.*

■ Position patient in optimal voiding position, preferably on toilet or commode. Women should sit, leaning slightly forward, with feet and legs apart. Men who usually stand to void should stand if possible. *Patterned responses will occur most easily when the circumstances surrounding the usual pattern of voiding are replicated.*

■ Teach the double-voiding technique. *More complete emptying of the bladder can be achieved when the voiding is initiated twice.*

▲ Encourage patient to use Valsalva's maneuver (check with physician first; this may be contraindicated in patients with some health problems). *Valsalva's maneuver optimizes the use of abdominal muscles to aid in emptying bladder.*

■ Use Crede's method over bladder area (use only if no obstruction). *Manual pressure will help complete emptying of the bladder.*

■ Teach patient and assist with anal sphincter stimulation while the patient bears down to void (insert finger into anus and pull slightly). *The innervation of the anal and urinary sphincter muscles is identical. Stimulating one can stimulate the other.*

■ If voiding is successful, check the postvoiding residual volume. *Residual urine will increase the risk for infection.*

■ If voiding is repeatedly unsuccessful, catheterize and go to the next part of plan. *Starting with the least invasive measures promotes natural voiding; however, complete emptying of the bladder is essential.*

Expected Outcome: The patient will perform (or participate in) intermittent catheterization.

■ Assess patient's or significant other's ability to learn technique. *Self-care allows independence. Teaching should be done when learners are ready and able to learn.*

■ Refer to Nursing Care Guidelines for Reflex Incontinence for intermittent self-catheterization procedure.

EVALUATION

Evaluating patterns of urinary elimination always focuses on an expected outcome of voiding that is as close to normal as possible for each individual patient. Accepting wetness from incontinence, incomplete bladder emptying, and long-term indwelling catheterization should be last resorts.

Functional Incontinence

Because the expected patient outcome is complete continence, or at least continence for a given percentage of times, the first step in evaluation is to compare the new voiding record with the one kept before treatment to determine if this goal was achieved. Depending on the severity of the related factors and the unique characteristics of the patient, complete continence or a reduction in incontinent episodes should occur. If not, the nurse must evaluate interventions to determine which were effective and which were not. If interventions are ineffective, alternate ones should be tried, and the related factors should be reevaluated. Often, as a plan is being implemented, additional related factors surface; these must then be addressed, and the care plan must be amended.

Stress Incontinence

Patients should be asked to keep a voiding record, noting incontinent episodes and precipi-

III

tating factors so that evaluation of the first outcome is possible. Comparing the posttreatment voiding record with the pretreatment voiding record will determine if the incontinent episodes have decreased. The time frame for achieving the outcome will vary from one patient to another. If the patient is not overweight and has mild incontinence, positive results should be achieved more quickly than if the patient is obese and needs time to lose weight.

The patient's ability to do the Kegel exercises correctly should be evaluated. If a perineometer is available, this is the most objective instrument to show if the pubococcygeal muscles are being contracted and if muscle tone is increasing. If such an instrument is unavailable, the nurse can check the muscle contractions by inserting a finger into the vagina and having the patient do the Kegel exercise. Deciding how often this should be evaluated will depend on how well the patient meets the first outcome. If the incontinent episodes are decreasing quickly, it is likely that the patient is doing the exercise correctly. If not, more frequent checks of the patient's ability to do the exercise will be needed.

The second outcome is an ongoing one. With each patient encounter, the nurse can check on what the patient is doing to maintain dryness.

Reflex Incontinence

A great deal of time and effort are needed to implement the plan of care for a patient with Reflex Incontinence. The time needed to achieve the stated outcomes will vary from patient to patient depending on manual dexterity, education level, age, and intake and output patterns.

The first outcome can be evaluated at intervals until it is fully achieved (e.g., when a regular pattern of bladder emptying is achieved); this may take several weeks. The patient will need constant encouragement and reteaching during this period of time. The postvoiding residual urine volume will determine whether to use a voiding triggering mechanism or to implement a plan for catheterization. If postvoiding residual volumes are greater than the set amount, the intermittent self-

catheterization plan must be initiated. The second outcome is evaluated along with the first one because a fluid intake schedule is critical to a successful voiding schedule. It may be easier to achieve a set fluid intake schedule for patients in the hospital than for those at home. Therefore the nurse can expect to adapt the schedule on discharge of the patient from the hospital. Follow-up by a home care nurse or at an outpatient clinic is critical to the continued achievement of the second outcome. The third and fourth outcomes are critical to the patient's safety while he or she manages bladder emptying. The nurse needs positive evidence that the patient understands the signs of infection and autonomic dysreflexia so that these problems can be corrected immediately.

The last outcome should be evaluated in the hospital and after the patient goes home. Each patient's individual lifestyle affects the frequency of unexpected incontinent episodes and dictates the best interventions.

Urge Incontinence

To determine if the expected patient outcomes have been met, the nurse, the patient, or both need to maintain a voiding record that notes the number of incontinent episodes, each interval between voidings, the amount of urine voided, and the nature of the urge to void. From such a record the nurse will know if the number of incontinent episodes has decreased. Data from this record also will indicate if changes in bladder capacity, irritability, and distention are occurring.

Evaluation of these patients must be part of a cycle of looking at results and adapting interventions to changes that occur. Some patients will show changes very quickly; others will need more time. Schedules for evaluation will need to be set for each patient.

Total Incontinence

The expected outcome, optimal dryness, must be defined for each patient. Each patient's tolerance for wet skin is different. What is critical for evaluation is that optimal dryness is defined from the patient's perspective and not from a staff's perspective of how often a patient's clothing, linen, or pads must be changed. Whereas nurses may feel they change clothing and linen only every 2 or 3 hours, this may not be sufficient to maintain adequate dryness for some patients.

The other expected outcomes in the plan should be stated only if they are truly realistic. If it seems possible to reduce the number of incontinent episodes, this can be measured with a voiding record. For patients who have constant leakage, with no ability to store urine in the bladder, it is unlikely that this outcome would apply. For communicative patients, the expectation that they will identify their needs may apply. Evaluation of this outcome may be possible through use of the voiding record or from direct interaction with the patient. The fourth outcome depends on the patient having some mobility. All patients should be urged to participate in care at any level possible. Evaluation of this outcome depends on the patient being involved in self-care.

Urinary Retention

The time needed for meeting expected outcomes will vary greatly, depending on the factors contributing to Urinary Retention. Some patients will meet the first outcome quickly after a few interventions and the problem will be resolved; others will need all of the interventions just to reach a level of control of Urinary Retention.

The three parts of the care plan can be implemented sequentially and evaluated accordingly. If the first outcome is unrealistic, the next one can be attempted. If augmented voiding is unsuccessful in maintaining a low postvoiding residual urine volume, then the final outcome, intermittent catheterization, is sought.

In evaluating this care it is important that all possible attempts are made to get the patient to void without the invasive catheter. Therefore it is vital that nurses continuously evaluate the outcomes and all attempted nursing interventions.

III

◤ CASE STUDY WITH PLAN OF CARE

Mrs. Jolynn F., a 78-year-old Hispanic woman, has been a resident of a nursing home for 6 years. She is 5'2" tall and weighs 192 pounds, which she says has been her usual weight all her life. She resides in a nursing home because she is wheelchair-bound as a result of severe osteoarthritis and degenerative joint disease, which have greatly decreased her hip and knee mobility. She also has mild congestive heart failure with dependent edema. She is a quiet woman, who spends much of the day sitting in her wheelchair in the main floor lounge, in the chapel, or in the crafts room working on a hooked rug. She likes to get out of bed early in the morning and stay downstairs until after lunch time. After lunch she returns to her unit until about 3 P.M., after which she returns to the main floor until supper time. Until a month ago, Mrs. F. was continent. She was able to stand and pivot onto the toilet with the help of two aides. Then her arthritis progressively worsened and she could not stand. So that she would not fall, three aides were needed to lift her onto the toilet. With each toileting Mrs. F. apologized for taking up so much of their time. The aides privately complained about how difficult it was to toilet her. Soon Mrs. F. was remaining off the unit

all day, returning only to get her 1 P.M. medication and after supper. Each evening her clothing and chair were very wet with urine. At night she was continent; she could get on and off a bedpan with the assistance of one person. Her medications were aspirin, two tablets at 9 A.M., 1 P.M., and 5 P.M.; Lasix, 40 mg at 9 A.M.; and digoxin, 0.125 mg at 9 A.M.

At first the nurses thought Mrs. F. had Stress Incontinence because she was obese and had delivered five children, including one set of twins. They considered that she might have Urge Incontinence because she couldn't hold urine long enough to get to the toilet. When questioned, Mrs. F. said she didn't necessarily void when she moved or coughed. She also said she could hold her urine for a while. She held it at night until help arrived to get her onto the bedpan. She admitted that she felt very bad about wetting herself, but she felt even worse having to take up the time of three people to help her to the toilet. Saying "I've never been such a bother to anyone in my whole life," she conceded that she would rather be wet than to be a bother. The nurse made the diagnosis of Functional Incontinence related to mobility deficits, avoidance behavior, and medication effects.

III

▶ **PLAN OF CARE FOR MRS. JOLYNN F.**
Nursing Diagnosis: Functional Incontinence Related to Mobility Deficits, Avoidance Behavior, and Medication Effects

---

Expected Outcome: Mrs. F. will be continent at all times within 2 weeks.
▲ Change time of Lasix administration to 6 A.M. (peak action 1 to 2 hours).
▪ Assist Mrs. F. to toilet before she leaves unit (by 8 A.M.).
▲ Consult with physician to consider an increase in pain medication.
▪ Provide Mrs. F. with positive reinforcement for continent behavior.
▲ Consult with nutritionist to plan a weight-loss program for Mrs. F.
▪ Maintain voiding record to evaluate plan.

Expected Outcome: Mrs. F. will participate in a set toileting regimen within 1 week.
▪ Contract with Mrs. F. for specific times, at least once in the morning and once in the afternoon, when she will return to the unit for toileting.
▪ Assure Mrs. F. that three staff members will be available at contracted times.
▪ Instruct Mrs. F. to increase her fluid consumption in the late afternoon and to decrease it early in the afternoon.

▪ = nursing intervention; ▲ = collaborative intervention.

■ **CRITICAL THINKING EXERCISES**

1. Develop a mnemonic device (a memory aid) that would help you remember the critical data to collect to differentiate Functional Incontinence from other types of incontinence.
2. What anatomy and physiology knowledge does a nurse need to diagnose Stress Incontinence and plan care for a patient who has this diagnosis?
3. What is the reasoning behind not having patients decrease their fluid intake to decrease the incidence of Urge Incontinence? Why is Urge Incontinence often misdiagnosed as Functional Incontinence?
4. If a patient with Total Incontinence is cognitively alert, how can that ability be used as a strength in planning care?
5. Some persons with Urinary Retention can void but cannot adequately empty their bladders. Given that these persons still void, how would a nurse know that urine was being retained?
6. Why is Urinary Retention often misdiagnosed as Urinary Incontinence? What assessment parameters are needed to differentiate these diagnoses?

REFERENCES

1. Agency for Health Care Policy and Research, *Urinary incontinence in adults: clinical practice guidelines,* AHCPR Pub No 92-0638, Rockville, Maryland, 1992, Public Health Service, U.S. Department of Health and Human Services.
2. Braddom RL and Rocco JF: Autonomic dysreflexia: a survey of current treatment, *Am J Phys Med Rehabil* 70:234–241, 1991.
3. Brink CA: Absorbent pads, garments, and management strategies, *J Am Geriatr Soc* 38:368–373, 1990.
4. Brink CA and others: A digital test for pelvic muscle strength in women with urinary incontinence, *Nurs Res* 43:352–356, 1994.
5. Burgio KL and Engel BT: Biofeedback-assisted behavioral training for elderly men and women, *J Am Geriatr Soc* 38:338–340, 1990.
6. Burns PA and others: Treatment of stress incontinence with pelvic floor exercises and biofeedback, *J Am Geriatr Soc* 38:341–344, 1990.
7. Cardozo L: Role of estrogen in the treatment of female urinary incontinence, *J Am Geriatr Soc* 38:326–328, 1990.

8. Diokno AC: Diagnostic categories of incontinence and the role of urodynamic testing, *J Am Geriatr Soc* 38:300–305, 1990.
9. Engberg SJ and others: Self-care behaviors of older women with urinary incontinence, *J Geront Nurs* 21(8):7–14, 1995.
10. Fantl IA, Wyman IF, Harkins SW, and Hadley EC: Bladder training in the management of lower urinary tract dysfunction in women, *J Am Geriatr Soc* 38:329–332, 1990.
11. Flynn L, Cell P, and Luisi E: Effectiveness of pelvic muscle exercises in reducing urge incontinence among community residing elders, *J Geront Nurs* 10(5):23–27, 1994.
12. Fowler EM, Ouslander JG, and Papen L: Managing incontinence in the nursing home population, *J Enterostom Ther* 17(2):77–86, 1990.
13. Goldstein M and others: Urinary incontinence: why people do not seek help, *J Geront Nurs* 18(4):15–20, 1992.
14. Gray M: Congenital causes of incontinence in childhood: presentation and treatment, *J Enterostom Ther* 17(2):4753, 1990.
15. Grosshans C, Passadori Y, and Peter B: Urinary retention in the elderly: a study of 100 hospitalized patients, *J Am Geriatr Soc* 41:633–638, 1993.
16. Herzog AR and Fultz NH: Prevalence and incidence of urinary incontinence in community-dwelling populations, *J Am Geriatr Soc* 38:273–281, 1990.
17. Hu TW: Impact of urinary incontinence on health care costs, *J Am Geriatr Soc* 38:292–295, 1990.
18. Johnson DE, Muncie HL, O'Reilly IL, and Warren IW: An external urine collection device for incontinent women, *J Am Geriatr Soc* 38:1016–1022, 1990.
19. Kegel AH: Progressive resistance exercises in the functional restoration of the perineal muscles, *Am J Obstet Gynecol* 56:238–248, 1948.
20. Lockhart-Pretti P: Urinary incontinence, *J Enterostom Ther* 17:112–119, 1990.
21. McCormick KA: From clinical trial to health policy—research on urinary incontinence in the adult, part I, *J Prof Nurs* 7:147, 1991.
22. McCormick KA: From clinical trial to health policy—research on urinary incontinence in the adult, part II, *J Prof Nurs* 7:202, 1991.
23. McCormick KA and Palmer MH: Urinary incontinence in older adults. In Fitzpatrick JJ, Taunton RL, and Jacox AK, editors: *Focus on current critical nursing problems: annual review of nursing research,* vol 10, New York, 1992, Springer.
24. Miller J: Assessing urinary incontinence, *J Geront Nurs* 16(3):15–19, 1990.
25. Moore KN: Intermittent catheterization: sterile or clean? *Rehab Nurs* 16(1):15–18, 33, 1991.
26. Moore KN, Kelm M, Sinclair O, and Cadrain G: Bacteriuria in intermittent catheterization users: the effect of sterile versus clean reused catheters, *Rehab Nurs* 18:306–309, 1993.
27. North American Nursing Diagnosis Association: *NANDA nursing diagnoses: definitions and classification, 1995–1996,* Philadelphia, 1994, The Association.
28. Ouslander JG: Urinary incontinence in nursing homes, *J Am Geriatr Soc* 38:289–291, 1990.
29. Ouslander JG and others: Use of a portable ultrasound device to measure post-void residual among incontinent nursing home residents, *J Am Geriatr Soc* 42:1189–1192, 1994.
30. Owen DC, Getz PA, and Bulla S: A comparison of characteristics of patients with completed stroke: those who achieve continence and those who do not, *Rehab Nurs* 20(4):197–203, 1995.
31. Palmer MH: A health-promotion perspective of urinary continence, *Nurs Outlook* 42:163–169, 1994.
32. Penn C and others: Assessment of urinary incontinence, *J Geront Nurs* 22(1):8–9, 1996.
33. Rainville NC: The current nursing procedure for intermittent urinary catheterization in rehabilitation facilities, *Rehab Nurs* 19:330–333, 1994.
34. Resnick B: A bladder scan trial in geriatric rehabilitation, *Rehab Nurs* 20:194–196, 1995.
35. Resnick B: Retraining the bladder after catheterization, *Am J Nurs* 93(11):46–50, 1993.
36. Resnick NM: Initial evaluation of the incontinent patient, *J Am Geriatr Soc* 38:311–316, 1990.
37. Schnelle IF and others: Assessment and quality control of incontinence care in long-term nursing facilities, *J Am Geriatr Soc* 39:165–171, 1991.
38. Skoner MM, Thompson WD, and Caron VA: Factors associated with risk of stress urinary incontinence in women, *Nurs Res* 43:301–306, 1994.
39. Tanagho EA: Electrical stimulation, *J Am Geriatr Soc* 38:352–355, 1990.
40. Tries I: Kegel exercises enhanced by biofeedback, *J Enterostom Ther* 17:67–76, 1990.
41. Warkentin R: Implementation of a urinary continence program, *J Geront Nurs* 18(1):31–36, 1992.
42. Warren IW: Urine-collection devices for use in adults with urinary incontinence, *J Am Geriatr Soc* 38:364–367, 1990.
43. Wells TI: Pelvic (floor) muscle exercise, *J Am Geriatr Soc* 38:333–337, 1990.
44. Wells TI and others: Pelvic muscle exercises for stress urinary incontinence in elderly women, *J Am Geriatr Soc* 39:785–791, 1991.
45. Williams ME and Gaylord SA: Role of functional assessment in the evaluation of urinary incontinence, *J Am Geriatr Soc* 38:296–299, 1990.
46. Williams MP, Walhagen M, and Dowline G: Urinary retention in hospitalized elderly women, *J Geront Nurs* 19(2):7–14, 1993.
47. Woodtli A: Stress incontinence: clinical identification and validation of defining characteristics, *Nurs Diagnosis* 6(3):115–122, 1995.
48. Woodtli A: Mixed incontinence: A new nursing diagnosis? *Nurs Diagnosis* 6(4):135–142, 1995.

III

Risk for Activity Intolerance

▶ ─────────────────────────────────

Activity Intolerance

▶ ─────────────────────────────────

Risk for Activity Intolerance *is the state in which an individual is at risk of experiencing insufficient physiological or psychological energy to endure or to complete required or desired daily activities.*[17]

Activity Intolerance *is the state in which an individual has insufficient physiological or psychological energy to endure or to complete required or desired daily activities.*[17]

OVERVIEW

Activity in which individuals engage reflects their physical capacity and their structural and functional abilities, interests, and desires. Activity is a basic human need that contributes to physical and emotional well-being. Activity is action; it requires intent and expenditure of energy. Activity is purposeful; it is required to maintain self-care, to accomplish occupational tasks, and to engage in physical exercise.

Unrestricted choice of activities contributes to one's sense of autonomy and independence. When an individual has no physiological or psychological constraints on choice of activities, that person feels a sense of control. But when limitations are imposed on an individual's usual activity pattern, this sense of control can be altered. White and associates,[21] in their discussion of the effects of the prolonged inactivity that was recommended for myocardial infarction patients in the 1950s, confirm this effect. They state, "The end of the ability

to engage in constructive, purposeful activity is, for most persons, a tragedy — it symbolizes the end of independence and purpose in life."

Yura and Walsh[22] define the human need for activity as "a behavior or action requiring an expenditure of energy by the person with volition and intent." The need is further described as one that contributes to a person's survival. The potential inability to tolerate activity can threaten a person's well-being. The consequences of inactivity, imposed or assumed, affect the individual's total well-being — physiological, psychological, social, cultural, and spiritual. Any alteration in an individual's activity pattern that occurs in response to a potential or actual health problem is of concern to professional nurses. When a potential or actual health problem interferes with the individual's ability to tolerate physical activity, the response is labeled Activity Intolerance; if the problem puts the individual at risk for becoming intolerant of activity, the response is labeled Risk for Activity Intolerance.

The diagnoses Activity Intolerance and Potential for Activity Intolerance were accepted for clinical testing in 1982 at the Fifth National Conference on the Classification of Nursing Diagnoses.[12] Although definitions for these diagnostic labels were not presented at the conference, Gordon[5] offered a similar diagnostic label (Activity Tolerance, Decreased) that implies a change (decrease) in the level of tolerance for activity. She defined Decreased Activity Tolerance as "insufficient energy to complete required or desired daily activities due to physiological or therapeutic limitations." The physiological and therapeutic limitations addressed by Gordon in this definition could be related to etiologies that are functional, structural, or situational in nature.

In 1985 Gordon[6] adopted the diagnostic labels Activity Intolerance and Potential for Activity Intolerance and provided definitions for the labels. Activity Intolerance was defined as "abnormal responses to energy-consuming body movements involved in required or desired activities"; Potential Activity Intolerance was defined as "presence of risk factors for abnormal responses to energy-consuming body movements." Gordon[7] continues to use these definitions but addresses "energy-consuming activities," and she has changed the label Potential for Activity Intolerance to reflect guidelines of the North American Nursing Diagnosis Association (NANDA) for labeling risk diagnoses.[17]

NANDA included definitions for the actual and potential activity intolerance diagnostic labels in the 1987 publication of the *Proceedings of the Seventh Conference.*[14] Activity Intolerance was defined as "a state in which an individual has insufficient physiological or psychological energy to endure or complete required or desired daily activities." The definition for Potential Activity Intolerance was the same as that for Activity Intolerance except for identifying that the individual was "at risk of experiencing" insufficient energy to endure or complete activities. (Potential Activity Intolerance was renamed Risk for Activity Intolerance.) These definitions, which continue to be considered appropriate,[17] imply that the diagnoses would be identified in patients who are experiencing a potential or actual disruption of the physiological and psychological resources necessary to carry out their daily activities.

Activity Intolerance, actual or Risk for, is a diagnosis frequently made in critical care[10] and acute care[11] settings as well as in long-term care,[4,18] home care,[20] and rehabilitation settings.[8,9] A comprehensive assessment will assist the nurse in determining a patient's status as it relates to Activity Intolerance.

ASSESSMENT

The initial nursing assessment provides the opportunity to collect data relevant to the patient's ability to engage in activity and that person's response to activity. Review of the patient's usual lifestyle and current physiological and psychological status is incorporated into a thorough health assessment with special attention to the patient's Activity-Exercise Pattern.[7,19] Patients with cardiovascular, respiratory, musculoskeletal, and neurological alterations are especially at risk for experiencing Activity Intolerance.[3,16] Treatments for a particular physical alteration may in themselves make a patient more vulnerable to Activity Intolerance (e.g., prolonged bed rest). Therefore ongoing assessment is critical and should focus on changes in a patient's level of activity as well as the patient's response to activity in terms of cardiovascular and respiratory changes and feelings of fatigue and weakness.[13]

The following parameters provide a general guide for gathering data relative to assessing a patient's tolerance for activity. The type, intensity, duration, and frequency of each activity in which an individual engages also must be considered when evaluating response to activity.

1. Activity pattern, past and present
   a. In the past, what activities (self-care, exercise, and leisure) did the patient engage in? How are these activities now tolerated?
   b. What activities are now engaged in? How are these activities tolerated?
2. Physical impediments
   a. Are there physical impediments that restrict participation in particular activities?
   b. Are there physical impediments that prevent active participation in activities?
3. Physiological status
   a. Is there a change in physiological status when the patient engages in activity?
   b. Cardiovascular response: Note heart rate and rhythm, pulse strength, and blood pressure.
   c. Respiratory response: Note rate, depth, and rhythm of respirations.

IV

d. Skin: Note color, temperature, and moistness.

e. Posture: Note signs of muscle fatigue.

f. Equilibrium: Note gait and fine and gross movements.

4. Emotional status

a. Is there a change in emotional status before or during activity?

b. Is the patient fearful of harming self?

In using this assessment guide, the nurse will collect data that may indicate the patient is at risk for or is experiencing Activity Intolerance. The nurse should seek additional data to determine whether the diagnosis of Risk for Activity Intolerance or Activity Intolerance should be made.

Risk for Activity Intolerance

The data from the health history and initial assessment should provide cues that indicate whether a patient may be at Risk for Activity Intolerance. The nurse should review specific assessment data to determine whether any of the risk factors for Activity Intolerance are present, and answers to specific questions should be sought. For example, does the patient have a history of intolerance to activity? If so, what type of intolerance did the patient experience? What was the reason for the intolerance? Was there a related medical condition?

During the review of data related to the patient's current physical condition, the following questions should be addressed:

- What is the current status of the patient's circulatory system? For example, does the patient experience bradycardia or tachycardia?
- Has the patient had a decrease in pulse strength, a decrease in systolic pressure, or an excessive increase in systolic or diastolic pressure?
- Does the patient have respiratory problems, such as dyspnea or an irregular respiratory rhythm?
- Does the patient have arthritis or any other condition that would lead to functional limitations?

The mental and emotional status of the patient also should be considered. The nurse should determine whether the patient has experienced emotional or mental stress that would lead to

refusal to participate in prescribed activities.

Finally, the overall condition of the patient should be evaluated. Does the patient have a sedentary lifestyle? Is the patient overweight? The presence of any or all risk factors listed below could lead to the diagnosis of Risk for Activity Intolerance.

■ Risk Factors

The presence of the following behaviors, conditions, or circumstances render the patient more vulnerable to Risk for Activity Intolerance:

- History of intolerance to activity
- Fatigue or weakness
- Sleep disorders
- Deconditioned status (e.g., prolonged bed rest or inactivity)
- Pain
- Chronic or progressive disease (e.g., chronic obstructive pulmonary disease, multiple sclerosis, coronary artery disease, arthritis, depression)
- Circulatory or respiratory problems
- Weight more than 15% over accepted standard
- Climate extremes affecting tolerance of activity
- Inexperience with activity
- Sedentary lifestyle
- Expressions of concern about ability to perform an activity
- Expressions of disinterest in an activity
- Refusal to participate in prescribed activities

Activity Intolerance

After completing the initial health assessment and assessing the patient's tolerance for engaging in activity, the nurse identifies the specific signs and symptoms (defining characteristics) that indicate that the patient may be experiencing Activity Intolerance. The defining characteristics may be vague, as in the patient making a single report of feeling exhausted after taking a shower, or obvious, as in the patient experiencing dysrhythmia, dyspnea, and profuse diaphoresis after walking up a flight of stairs.

The assessment data is analyzed further to determine a specified etiology or related factor that is limiting the patient's ability to tolerate activity. The limitations that can contribute to intolerance of activity can be classified as functional, structural, or situational.

Functional limitations include those factors reflecting altered or impaired physiological functioning. The energy required to perform the activity may be more than the patient has to expend. For a patient with cardiac disease the required myocardial oxygen consumption during various activities may exceed the amount of oxygen available. Pulmonary diseases are often characterized by alterations of the oxygen and carbon dioxide transport process, which compromise the supply of oxygen available to support the performance of activities.

Diseases causing endocrine disturbances (e.g., hypothyroidism), fluid-electrolyte imbalances (e.g., chronic renal disease), neurological alterations (e.g., multiple sclerosis and Guillain-Barré syndrome), hepatic dysfunction (e.g., hepatitis), and circulatory and hematological disorders (e.g., Raynaud's disease and anemia) also present functional limitations that can cause discomfort during activity. These disease-related functional limitations include generalized weakness, decreased mobility or immobility, and an imbalance between oxygen supply and demand.

Structural limitations that can lead to Activity Intolerance are associated with an impairment or alteration of the anatomical structure. A structural impairment is related to a congenital or acquired anatomical deficit that limits mobility (e.g., a patient whose right leg is shorter than the left leg). A structural alteration can be caused by a therapeutic intervention (e.g., a painful surgical incision or a cast applied to a leg that renders it immobile) or by the use of therapeutic equipment (e.g., a leg or back brace). The intervention or the use of equipment, although therapeutic in nature, can temporarily or permanently impose constraints that decrease a patient's willingness or ability to be mobile and active. The extent of the structural impairment or alteration influences the degree to which the patient's mobility is restricted and the consequent effect on the ability to tolerate activity.

Situational limitations that can alter a patient's tolerance for activity include factors relevant to the patient's cognitive and emotional status and environment. These limitations include lack of knowledge, lack of motivation, deconditioning, lack of support, and climate extremes (e.g., living at high altitude or in areas where inclement weather impedes activity). The patient may lack the knowledge necessary to engage in a particular activity in a manner that would provide for conservation of energy. An example of this is a patient with chronic obstructive pulmonary disease who avoids all activity to prevent shortness of breath. The patient becomes more and more deconditioned and experiences increasing resting oxygen consumption. Although the disease imposes functional constraints, the patient's avoidance of all activity because of a lack of knowledge imposes unnecessary restrictions on certain activities in which that person could participate comfortably and safely. With proper instruction the patient can be made aware of the importance of specific conditioning exercises tailored to meet individual physiological needs.

Even though a patient may be knowledgeable about the importance of a physical activity and how to engage in it to conserve energy, he or she may avoid activity because of depression. Consequently the patient lacks the motivation required to endure physical activity. Even when the cognitive and emotional status of the patient is such that participation in activity is encouraged, the environment can contribute to a reluctance to become involved. A sedentary lifestyle that promotes deconditioning also promotes intolerance of activity.

■ Defining Characteristics

The presence of the following defining characteristics indicates that the patient may be experiencing Activity Intolerance:

- Decrease in activity (self-care, exercise, or leisure)
- Avoidance of activity
- Verbal report of fatigue or weakness
- Cardiovascular response to activity: bradycardia, inappropriate tachycardia, dysrhythmia, decrease in pulse strength, or inappropriate increases or decreases in blood pressure

IV

- Respiratory response to activity: dyspnea, tachypnea, or irregular rhythm
- Skin response to activity: pallor, cyanosis, flushing, profuse diaphoresis, or dryness with strenuous activity
- Posture: drooping of shoulders or head or decrease in muscle tone and strength
- Altered equilibrium (e.g., ataxia, dizziness, vertigo, syncope)
- Emotional status: depression, lack of interest in activity, fear of activity or its consequences

■ Related Factors

The following related factors are associated with Activity Intolerance:

Functional limitations
- Generalized weakness
- Decreased mobility or immobility
- Imbalance between oxygen supply and demand
- Obesity
- Pain

Structural limitations
- Anatomical alteration that limits mobility or activity (e.g., amputation of leg)
- Therapeutic intervention that limits mobility or activity (e.g., leg cast, prescribed bed rest)

Situational limitations
- Lack of knowledge, motivation, or support
- Deconditioning (related to lifestyle)
- Climate extremes

DIAGNOSIS

■ Differential Nursing Diagnosis

Differentiating Risk for Activity Intolerance from Activity Intolerance depends on whether or not the patient is able to endure or complete required or desired daily activities. If the patient attempts to engage in but cannot complete an activity because of the presence of any of the defining characteristics, that person is experiencing Activity Intolerance. The patient who is at Risk for Activity Intolerance may complete the activity, but because of the presence of risk factors the patient is more vulnerable to Activity Intolerance.

There are nursing diagnoses that in themselves are risk factors and, once diagnosed, indicate that the patient may be at Risk for Activity Intolerance. Examples of these are Impaired Physical Mobility, Fatigue, and Sleep Pattern Disturbance. Conversely, the diagnosis of Activity Intolerance could indicate that the patient is at Risk for Disuse Syndrome. Other nursing diagnoses that imply an alteration in physiological status (e.g., Decreased Cardiac Output, Impaired Gas Exchange, Ineffective Breathing Pattern, or Pain) or psychological status (e.g., Social Isolation, Post-Trauma Response, Knowledge Deficit, or Ineffective Individual Coping) can be an indication that a patient is at risk for or is experiencing Activity Intolerance.

■ Medical and Psychiatric Diagnoses

Patients with medical diagnoses that imply alterations in physiological functioning, particularly of the cardiovascular, respiratory, nervous, and musculoskeletal systems, are at Risk for Activity Intolerance and often can experience Activity Intolerance. Examples of these medical diagnoses are cerebrovascular accident, congestive heart failure, hepatitis, multiple sclerosis, and rheumatoid arthritis. Psychiatric diagnoses resulting in a decrease in motivation or desire to engage in required activities include depression, degenerative dementia of the Alzheimer type, and bipolar depression. Ongoing assessment by members of the health care team of patients with these diagnoses should focus on early identification of the risk factors and defining characteristics of Activity Intolerance.

OUTCOME IDENTIFICATION, PLANNING, AND IMPLEMENTATION

The overall goal of treatment for the patient experiencing potential or actual Activity Intolerance is to have the patient maintain, regain, or develop an optimal level of activity that permits completion of required or desired daily activities.[15] To achieve this goal the involvement of the patient and significant others in planning interventions is very important. Outcomes and specific intervention strategies for Risk for Activity Intolerance and Activity Intolerance are discussed below.

Risk for Activity Intolerance

The person at Risk for Activity Intolerance requires support and guidance in choosing activities that promote optimal well-being. Most important, the nurse must consider the patient's physiological response to particular activities when developing an appropriate plan for the patient's participation in required or desired activities. The patient should be given information that will assist in identifying activities that are therapeutic, enjoyable, and within the patient's physiological capabilities.

It is important that the prescribed exercise program is of appropriate duration and frequency. The nurse should instruct the patient on the performance of unfamiliar activities and on alternative ways of performing familiar activities. The patient should be informed about factors that might interfere with the ability to tolerate activity so that appropriate changes that will promote activity tolerance can be made. Factors that may aggravate Activity Intolerance include inadequate sleep or diet, inappropriate use of medications, excessive alcohol intake, noncompliance with the treatment regimen, and stressful environmental conditions. These factors should be discussed with the patient.

The nurse should also consider the patient's psychological response to particular activities. The patient's values as they relate to engaging in health-promoting activities should be assessed. This can be accomplished by encouraging the patient to describe his or her feelings about engaging in an exercise program. If the patient lacks the motivation to participate in required or desired activities on a regular basis, the nurse should elicit support for the patient from significant others or through organized activities or programs. Finally, the patient should be encouraged to seek consultation with appropriate health professionals (e.g., a physician, physical therapist, or occupational therapist) to support the integration of appropriate activities into the daily routine.

Activity Intolerance

The expected outcomes for a patient with Activity Intolerance include (1) participation in activities that enhance physiological well-being, (2) development of an activity-rest pattern that supports increased tolerance of activity, and (3) development of a support network (family, friends, and health care providers) to assist in adjusting the activity-rest pattern to meet the need for activity.

Although the expected patient outcomes and interventions are presented in general terms, these should be adapted and expanded as needed for the patient. The activity-exercise prescription must be tailored to each patient's needs and abilities. Primary considerations in planning nursing care include the general physiological and emotional status of the individual and the optimal therapeutic level of activity that should be attained.

The data gathered in the assessment phase of the nursing process and the consequent development of the treatment goals should be validated with the patient. The nurse should review the patient's past and present activity pattern and physiological and emotional responses to participation in activity and exercise. Any change in the patient's physiological status when the patient engages in activity should be noted. For example, the cardiovascular response is assessed for changes in heart rate and rhythm, pulse strength, and blood pressure; the respiratory response is assessed for changes in rate, depth, and rhythm of respirations; and the color, temperature, and moistness of the skin, as well as signs of muscle fatigue and changes in gait and fine and gross movements are noted. The patient's emotional response when engaging in activity also is assessed.

The nurse should share information with the patient to assist in the identification of activities that will enhance the patient's physiological well-being. In the same manner, the patient should be assisted in identifying factors that reduce activity tolerance (e.g., inadequate sleep, medications, or stressful environmental conditions). While the patient's independence in the performance of activities is to be encouraged, assistance should be provided as needed. To ensure a patient's adher-

IV

◢ NURSING CARE GUIDELINES

Nursing Diagnosis: Risk for Activity Intolerance

Expected Outcome: The patient will participate in activities that promote optimal well-being (within 1 week), as evidenced by daily performance of recommended self-care, exercise, and leisure activities.

- Review with the patient and significant others the patient's present activity pattern and discuss desired and required activities that could be introduced into daily routine. The activities should be discussed in terms of type of activity and desired intensity, duration, and frequency.
- ▲ Assist the patient in selecting enjoyable activities that can be integrated into his or her lifestyle and that promote an increase in activity tolerance within therapeutic limits.
- ▲ Provide information about organized activities and programs in which the patient might participate.
- Discuss with the patient and significant others how to monitor activity in terms of physiological and psychological responses.
- Assist the patient in identifying (1) risk factors that interfere with the ability to tolerate activity and (2) those risk factors over which the patient may have some control (e.g., changing a sedentary lifestyle or dressing to acclimatize to extremes of weather).
  When the patient and significant others participate in care planning (i.e., identifying appropriate activities and monitoring response to activities), it is more likely that lifestyle changes will be introduced and maintained.
- ▲ Encourage significant others to support the patient and to participate in activities and programs with the patient when feasible.
- Arrange a consultation with physical therapist and occupational therapist as needed.
  Involving significant others and other members of the health care team provides the patient with a network of support.

Expected Outcome: The patient will appreciate the need to participate in required and desired activities (within 1 week), as evidenced by his or her describing the benefits of engaging in activity and identifying factors that could inhibit activity tolerance.

- Review benefits of regularly engaging in activities that promote physical and psychological well-being and of identifying factors that could inhibit activity tolerance.
- Assist the patient in developing a realistic plan that includes self-care, exercise, and leisure activities.
- Encourage the patient to plan activities with people who participate in activities that enhance well-being.
  Knowledge of and participation in desired and necessary activities, as well as participation with people who appreciate the need for activity, supports the development of a sense of appreciation for activity.

■ = nursing intervention; ▲ = collaborative intervention.

◢ NURSING CARE GUIDELINES

Nursing Diagnosis: Activity Intolerance

Expected Outcome: The patient will participate in activities that enhance his or her physical and psychosocial well-being (within 1 week), as evidenced by a balance between oxygen supply and demand, the absence of weakness and fatigue during and after engaging in activity, and a verbal report of activity tolerance.

- Assess patient's past and present activity pattern *to determine the type, intensity, duration, frequency, and toleration of former activities, as well as the potential for resuming former activities.*
- Assess physical impediments *to determine if they restrict or prevent active participation in relevant activities.*

■ = nursing intervention; ▲ = collaborative intervention.

- Assess physiological status before, during, and after engaging in activity *to determine if there is any change in cardiovascular and respiratory responses, skin (color, temperature, moistness), posture (muscle fatigue), and equilibrium (gait, fine and gross movements).*
- Assess psychosocial status before, during, and after engaging in activity *to determine if there are changes in emotional status or if the patient fears being harmed by the activity.*
- ▲ Provide the patient information about activities in which to participate.
- ▲ Assist the patient in interpreting the activity-exercise prescription.
- Assist the patient in identifying factors that reduce tolerance to activity (e.g., inadequate sleep, medications, treatments, and environmental conditions).
- ▲ Provide assistance to the patient as needed, encouraging independence in performing activities.
- ▲ Encourage the patient to engage in all self-care, exercise, and leisure activities that can be tolerated.
- ▲ Guide the patient in increasing activity within therapeutic limits.
  Providing the patient with information and guiding the patient in choosing the level and type of activities contributes to outcome achievement.

Expected Outcome: The patient will develop an activity-rest pattern supportive of increasing activity tolerance (within 2 weeks), as evidenced by adherence to a schedule that promotes increased activity without increasing weakness, fatigue, and untoward physiological responses to activity.
- Discuss with the patient usual activity-rest pattern; suggest ways to modify an ineffective pattern.
- Review with the patient the importance of increasing activity tolerance.
- Encourage the patient to participate in planning daily rest and activity periods.
- Encourage the patient to increase activity periods gradually to provide for required and desired self-care, exercise, and leisure activities.
- Encourage the patient to adhere to activity-rest schedule that best promotes an increase in activity tolerance.
  Planned rest periods will support the patient's attempts to increase activity gradually.
- ▲ Adjust the patient's medication and treatment schedule *to provide adequate periods of rest.*
- ▲ Teach the patient to monitor response to activity *so that the patient can stop activity when symptoms of anoxia or excessive fatigue are present.*

Expected Outcome: The patient will use the support of family, friends, and health care providers in adjusting the activity-rest pattern to increase activity tolerance (within 1 week).
- Provide the patient and significant others with information about the importance of establishing a therapeutic activity-rest pattern.
- Encourage the patient and significant others to participate in planning a mutually agreeable daily schedule of activity and rest periods.
- Encourage the patient and significant others to express any concerns about the proposed schedule.
- Encourage family and friends to support the patient in efforts to enhance tolerance to increased activity.
  When significant others are aware of the importance of establishing a therapeutic activity-rest pattern and are involved in planning the schedule, they are more likely to be available to assist and support the patient.
- ▲ Discuss with the patient and significant others support services available from other health care providers (e.g., an exercise physiologist or physical therapist) and agencies (e.g., outpatient rehabilitation services or home health care services) if continued support in refining or revising the activity-rest schedule is needed after discharge. *Knowledge of available services makes it more likely that the patient will seek necessary support in a timely manner.*

ence to a recommended Activity-Exercise Pattern, it is important that the pattern be integrated into the patient's lifestyle. The patient should be assisted in developing and implementing an activity-rest schedule that supports an increased tolerance of activity. The schedule should incorporate the patient's requirements for medications and treatments, as well as participation in self-care and leisure activities. The patient is also taught to monitor responses to activity and to adjust the activity-exercise schedule as needed.

The patient's lifestyle incorporates the lifestyles of family, friends, and significant others. Family members may be required to alter or revise their daily activities to support a therapeutic activity and rest schedule for the patient. The support of family and friends can be essential in assisting the patient to adhere to an activity-rest pattern that will promote optimal participation in therapeutic activities and exercise. The willingness of family members and friends to schedule meals, group activities, and time for personal activities around the patient's activity needs contributes to the patient's tolerance of and adherence to therapeutic activities. Encouragement and guidance from health care profes-

sionals can further enhance the patient's motivation and willingness to engage in activity.

EVALUATION

The effectiveness of the nursing interventions is determined by the patient's achievement of the expected outcomes. Each identified outcome reflects the elimination or reduction of a specific related factor, which enhances the patient's tolerance of activity. The effectiveness of the nursing interventions for Risk for Activity Intolerance and Activity Intolerance is evidenced by the following:

1. The patient demonstrates increased participation in self-care, exercise, and leisure activities.
2. The patient does not report fatigue or weakness after engaging in activity, and there is evidence of a balance between oxygen supply and demand.
3. The patient describes the benefits of engaging in activity and participates in the prescribed activity and exercise.
4. The patient seeks and uses the support of significant others and health care professionals to maintain a therapeutic activity schedule.

■ CASE STUDY WITH PLAN OF CARE

Mr. John R., an 82-year-old retired railroad engineer, has recently been accepted for home health care services. Six months ago Mr. R. fell and fractured his left hip; subsequently he had a total hip replacement. He walks with the aid of a walker ("So I can keep my balance and not fall again"). Mr. R. reports that before his fall and surgery he was very active. He drove his own car and was able to be involved in church and community activities on an almost daily basis. Over the past 6 months, he reports, he has experienced a gradual decrease in activity and a generalized lack of energy. He also has been

experiencing bradycardia and dysrhythmias and is being treated with digoxin and furosemide (Lasix). His appetite is poor and he is mildly depressed. Mr. R.'s only son lives about 2 hours away by car from him and tries to visit monthly. Immediate neighbors and members of his church provide him with a valuable support system. One of the nursing diagnoses for Mr. R. was Activity Intolerance related to functional limitations (i.e., generalized weakness, decreased mobility, and imbalance between oxygen supply and demand) and situational limitations (i.e., deconditioning related to lifestyle).

■ PLAN OF CARE FOR MR. JOHN R.
Nursing Diagnosis: Activity Intolerance Related to Functional and Situational Limitations

---

Expected Outcome: Mr. R. will participate in activities that enhance his physical and psychosocial well-being, as evidenced by a balance between oxygen supply and demand, the absence of weakness and fatigue during or after engaging in activity, and a verbal report of tolerating increased activity.

- Counsel Mr. R. on maintaining adequate nutritional intake, including sufficient protein and calcium.
- Monitor Mr. R.'s cardiovascular status; advise Mr. R. to take digoxin and Lasix as ordered.
- With Mr. R., review his activity-rest pattern and identify periods for rest before he engages in activities, particularly daily self-care activities.
- ▲ Refer Mr. R. to physical therapy for evaluation.
- ▲ Describe active range-of-motion exercises Mr. R. should be able to perform, and have Mr. R. demonstrate the exercises; evaluate his tolerance and revise exercises as necessary.
- Assess Mr. R.'s hobbies and interests; encourage participation in leisure and diversional activities as tolerated.
- Reassure Mr. R. that increasing tolerance for activity is a slow process, so that he does not become discouraged.
- ▲ Teach Mr. R. to monitor his response to activity and to alter the activity when signs and symptoms of fatigue and imbalance between oxygen supply and demand are present.
- Encourage Mr. R. to increase his participation in activities gradually.
- Discuss with Mr. R. how he might again become active in his church (e.g., identify neighbors and friends who can give him rides to church activities).
- ▲ Describe community activities and support services that could be helpful to Mr. R. (e.g., transportation services for senior citizens or Seniors' Day out at the local recreation center).

■ = nursing intervention; ▲ = collaborative intervention.

■ CRITICAL THINKING EXERCISES

1. What questions should be asked of Mr. R. to plan activity and rest periods for him throughout the day?
2. What issues and factors affecting Mr. R.'s level of activity tolerance should be included in a teaching plan for him?
3. Identify community activities and support services in your city that could be used by a patient such as Mr. R. Develop a list of these services, identifying the following: how to contact; contact person; description of activity or service provided; cost or fee for services.

REFERENCES

1. Carroll-Johnson RM, editor: *Classification of nursing diagnoses: proceedings of the Eighth Conference*, Philadelphia, 1989, JB Lippincott Co.
2. Carroll-Johnson RM, editor: *Classification of nursing diagnoses: proceedings of the Ninth Conference*, Philadelphia, 1991, JB Lippincott Co.
3. Chyun D, Ford CF, and Yursha-Johnston M: Silent myocardial ischemia, *Focus Crit Care* 18(4):295–302, 1991.
4. Glick OJ and Swanson EA: Motor performance correlates of functional dependence in long-term care residents, *Nurs Research* 44(1):4–8, 1995.
5. Gordon M: *Nursing diagnosis: process and application*, New York, 1982, McGraw-Hill.
6. Gordon M: *Manual of nursing diagnosis: 1984–1985*, New York, 1985, McGraw-Hill.
7. Gordon M: *Nursing diagnosis: process and application*, ed 3, St. Louis, 1994, Mosby–Year Book.
8. Gordon M: Report of an RNF study to determine which nursing diagnoses have high frequency and high treatment priority in rehabilitation nursing, part I, *Rehab Nurs Research* 4(1):3–10, 1995.
9. Gordon M: Report of an RNF study to determine which nursing diagnoses have high frequency and high treatment priority in rehabilitation nursing, part II, *Rehab Nurs Research* 4(2):33–46, 1995.

IV

10. Greenlee KK: The effects of implementation of an operational definition and guidelines for the formulation of nursing diagnoses in a critical care setting. In Carroll-Johnson RM, editor: *Classification of nursing diagnoses: proceedings of the Ninth Conference,* Philadelphia, 1991, JB Lippincott Co.

11. Hwu Y-J: The impact of chronic illness on patients, *Rehab Nurs* 20(4):221–225, 1995.

12. Kim MJ, McFarland GK, and McLane AM, editors: *Classification of nursing diagnoses: proceedings of the Fifth National Conference,* St. Louis, 1984, The CV Mosby Co.

13. Mason DJ and Redeker N: Measurement of activity, *Nurs Research* 42(2):87–92, 1993.

14. McLane AM, editor: *Classification of nursing diagnoses: proceedings of the Seventh Conference,* St. Louis, 1987, The CV Mosby Co.

15. National Institute of Nursing Research: *Long-term care for older adults: a report of the NINR priority expert panel on long-term care,* NIH Pub No 94-2418, Bethesda, Maryland, 1994, National Institutes of Health.

16. Neuberger GB and others: Determinants of exercise and aerobic fitness in outpatients with arthritis, *Nurs Research* 43(1):11–17, 1994.

17. North American Nursing Diagnosis Association: *NANDA nursing diagnoses: definitions and classification, 1995–1996,* Philadelphia, 1994, The Association.

18. Rantz M, Vinz-Miller T, and Matson S: Nursing diagnoses in long-term care: a longitudinal perspective for strategic planning, *Nurs Diagnosis* 6(2):57–63, 1995.

19. Rubenfeld MG and McFarlane EA: Health assessment. In Flynn JM and Heffron PB, editors: *Nursing from concept to practice,* ed 2, Norwalk, Connecticut, 1988, Appleton & Lange.

20. Tack BB and Gilliss CL: Nurse-monitored cardiac recovery: a description of the first 8 weeks, *Heart Lung* 19(5): 491–499, 1990.

21. White RD and others: *Rehabilitation of the cardiovascular patient,* New York, 1958, McGraw-Hill.

22. Yura H and Walsh MB: *The nursing process: assessing, planning, implementing, evaluating,* ed 5, Norwalk, Connecticut, 1988, Appleton & Lange.

Ineffective Airway Clearance

Ineffective Breathing Pattern

Impaired Gas Exchange

Ineffective Airway Clearance *is the state in which an individual is unable to clear secretions or obstructions from the respiratory tract to maintain airway patency.*[10]

Ineffective Breathing Pattern *is the state in which an individual's inhalation or exhalation pattern does not enable adequate pulmonary inflation or emptying.*[11]

Impaired Gas Exchange *is the state in which an individual experiences a decreased passage of oxygen or carbon dioxide between the alveoli of the lungs and the vascular system.*[11]

OVERVIEW

The overall purpose of respiration is the exchange of oxygen and carbon dioxide at the alveolar level to maintain homeostasis in the individual. Respiratory function can be divided into two major physiological activities: internal and external respiration. External respiration occurs as air is brought into the nose, the trachea, and the upper and lower airways. It includes the inspiratory effort of the muscles, the rib cage, and the diaphragm; the recoil response of the lung tissue in expiration; and the exchange of gases between alveolar cell walls and the blood.[7]

Internal respiration, in contrast, is the exchange of gases across the cell walls and the blood and the utilization of oxygen by the cells.[7] In normal gas exchange the following processes occur: (1) oxygen is delivered into the system so that adequate alveolar ventilation takes place (ventilation), (2) alveoli become adequately perfused with blood for the transport of oxygen and carbon dioxide (distribution), (3) the alveolar-capillary membrane diffuses the gases (diffusion), and (4) hemoglobin in the red blood cells picks up and delivers oxygen to the tissues (perfusion).[15] Therefore respiratory distress usually results from clinical disease states that alter these four processes.

Hemoglobin is essential to this process of gas exchange as the chemical carrier of oxygen and carbon dioxide. *Oxyhemoglobin* is oxygen combined with hemoglobin, and it gives arterial blood its bright red color. Oxyhemoglobin is a relatively unstable compound, and the body's cells have easy access to the oxygen contained in red blood cells.[8]

Carbon dioxide is carried by the blood in three different forms. It may be dissolved in the plasma as a bicarbonate ion or combined with hemoglobin to form a loosely bonded compound called carbaminohemoglobin. Carbon dioxide is easily released in tissues that are low in carbon dioxide (i.e., the alveoli) and thus eliminated through respira-

IV

tion. Oxygen from inspired air bonds with iron atoms in the blood, and carbon dioxide combines with the amino groups of the hemoglobin molecule. They do not compete for the same bonding sites, so the hemoglobin molecule can carry both gases at the same time.[8] The quality and amount of hemoglobin in the blood obviously has a direct influence on the effectiveness of gas transport throughout the body.

Hypoxia is most frequently caused by ventilation and perfusion (V/Q) imbalances.[15] The adequate matching of ventilation to perfusion results in an adequate oxygenation status. In the normal lung, ventilation to perfusion is unevenly distributed. The location of the pulmonary artery branches affects the amount of blood flow into the bases of the lung. Similarly, ventilation is unevenly distributed throughout the lung. The actions of the diaphragm and the rib cage during inspiration and the heavy concentration of blood cause the bases of the lung to receive more O_2 ventilation than the apices in the gravity-dependent areas of the lungs.[15] Certain pathological conditions, such as hypovolemic shock or emphysema, can cause the mismatching of ventilation to perfusion, resulting in symptoms of hypoxia.

The rate, rhythm, and depth of respiration are controlled neurologically. The breathing control center, located in the medulla of the brain stem, receives input from various subcenters in the body that interact to regulate breathing in a rhythmical pattern. The rate and depth of respiration are controlled by the amount of carbon dioxide, hydrogen ions, and oxygen present in the blood. The level of each of these chemicals is determined by structures called *chemoreceptors* located in carotid arteries and the aorta. Increased carbon dioxide concentration in the blood causes an alteration in pH level, thereby stimulating ventilation. Likewise, a drop in carbon dioxide concentration in the blood slows respiration. The activation of these homeostatic mechanisms normally results in regulation of carbon dioxide concentration and thus the rate and depth of respiration.

A secondary mechanism that helps control respiration includes chemoreceptors in the carotid arter-

ies that sense the presence of oxygen. These receptors stimulate respiration when oxygen levels fall below normal. Changes in level of oxygen have a greater effect on stimulating respiration than a constant low level. A low level of oxygen in the blood has less influence on changes in respiration than a high level of carbon dioxide and low blood pH.

Muscle strength and energy also affect respiratory function. The diaphragm is the main muscle involved in the ventilation process. In addition, the internal and external intrathoracic and abdominal muscles play important roles in the strength and depth of ventilatory air movement. These muscles are under neurological control primarily located in the respiratory centers in the brain. Respiration can also be voluntarily controlled to some degree, as exhibited by temporarily holding the breath or by voluntarily speeding up or slowing down the respiration rate or depth.

Many factors contribute to maintaining an open airway: warming, filtering, and humidifying inspired air; mucus and upward ciliary motion sweeping the airway clean; the macrophage clearance system; and the cough reflex. Likewise, the strength and enervation of the diaphragm contribute to the depth of inspiration, and the good muscle strength of associated muscles contributes to the effectiveness of the cough. All of these defense mechanisms can be affected by loss of body condition and strength through inactivity, cerebrovascular accident (CVA) or other neurological pathology, malnutrition, age, or other general systemic disease conditions.

Various preventive measures may help maintain or improve respiratory function. For example, deep breathing exercises before and after surgery will help clear the upper and lower airways and facilitate gas exchange in the alveoli. Patients should be counseled to avoid smoking cigarettes at any time, but especially during periods of acute respiratory infection and before and after surgery. Adequate fluid intake will help liquefy secretions and thus aid in their elimination from the respiratory tree through coughing.

Patients and their families should be taught basic principles of home care and infection control related to respiratory function. This includes hand washing, proper disposal of infected material such as tissues and sputum, and maintenance of adequate nutrition and fluid balance. Those whose immune systems are compromised should be taught to avoid crowded, inadequately ventilated areas and persons with obvious respiratory infections to reduce the risk of their spread.

Developmental factors, such as those associated with aging, may have an effect on maintaining airway clearance. In the elderly there is a general decline in the lung or host defense, which may lead to an increase in infections. Furthermore, the cough mechanism is impaired; ciliary function is less effective; there is a decrease in immunoglobulin A; and there is defective activity of alveolar macrophages. Also, the elderly may experience a reduction in exercise tolerance because the muscles of breathing weaken with age, thereby increasing the work of breathing.[1] Other changes with age include increased frequency of osteoporosis, chest wall changes that include increased calcification of the costal cartilage and vertebral collapse resulting in kyphosis, thus limiting lung expansion. There is also increased residual lung capacity with diminished vital capacity, maximum breathing capacity, and inspiratory reserve volume. These changes limit the ability to move air in and out of the lungs.[1,14] These factors have the greatest influence when the patient is exposed to tobacco smoke, is immobilized, or experiences a compromised immune system.[14] Infants with an anatomically small airway may be more susceptible to airborne infections because of the inability to warm and humidify the inspired air adequately, and their immature immune systems may not be able to fight off invading bacteria and viruses.[13]

ASSESSMENT

Ineffective Airway Clearance

Assessment related to this diagnosis involves the rate, depth, and sound of respiration; the use of accessory muscles; skin color; body temperature and hydration; and dyspnea.[11] Under normal circumstances the breathing pattern of an adult is quiet and smooth; the respiratory rate ranges from 12 to 20 breaths per minute; the skin appears well oxygenated, and quiet breathing is heard throughout all lung fields. The individual with a clear airway will be free from use of accessory muscles of the neck and shoulders and retraction of the sternum and intercostal spaces.[11]

Abnormal or adventitious breath sounds generally consist of rales (crackles) and rhonchi (sonorous wheezes) and indicate an alteration in normal function. Various definitions of rales and rhonchi can be found. In general, *rales* are described as crackles that occur mostly during inspiration as air passes through small, congested airways. The sounds are noncontinuous and usually are not cleared by coughing. Crackles may be heard in patients with congestive heart failure, pulmonary edema, consolidation, pulmonary fibrosis, atelectasis, and bronchitis.[17] *Rhonchi* are continuous sounds produced as air passes through narrowed airways. Wheezes are musical, squeaking noises that are known as rhonchi when they are low pitched and resemble loud snoring. Sonorous wheezes or rhonchi indicate the presence of secretions in the airway. The rhonchi usually clear by coughing or by suctioning. A narrowing of the airway results from secretions, tumors, foreign bodies, bronchial stenosis, bronchospasm, or a swelling of the mucosa.[17]

Changes in the rate or the depth of respiration, such as hyperpnea (an increase in the number of breaths), may indicate an obstruction of the airflow. The respiratory rate increases to maintain oxygenation and to increase airflow around a partially obstructed airway. Coughing is a normal defense mechanism of the airway, but a persistent cough can indicate abnormal function or underlying processes. Some causes of persistent cough are excessive mucus, foreign particles, irritation from erosive lesions, or airway hyperreactivity.[2,17] The presence of cough, with or without sputum production, is associated specifically with many diseases, such as acute sinusitis, bacterial pneumonia, aspiration, inhaled irritants, asthma, cystic fibrosis, lung abscess, bronchiectasis, bronchitis, and left ventricular failure.[18]

The color of the skin is often used as an indicator of body oxygenation. *Cyanosis* is a bluish discoloration of the skin and mucous membranes resulting from excessive concentration of reduced hemoglobin in the blood. Cyanosis may indicate hypoxemia (deficient oxygenation of the blood); however, it is a late indicator. At the same time, if cyanosis is located in the nail beds, it may only represent stagnant blood flow.[18] In cases where there are low levels of hemoglobin (anemia), the skin color may be pale or, in dark-skinned persons, gray. True cyanosis is more effectively assessed in highly vascular areas such as the lips, the nose, the ear helices, and the underside of the tongue.[17] When the amount of hemoglobin is low, the necessary level of unsaturated hemoglobin will not be achieved and the blue skin color of cyanosis will not be seen. When hemoglobin levels are adequate, but the hemoglobin is combined with carbon monoxide (carboxyhemoglobin), the individual will exhibit a cherry red skin coloration. Thus the alert nurse will avoid relying on skin color alone as a primary indicator of blood oxygenation and look for other data to validate this critical condition.

Dyspnea (breathing difficulty) is a subjective complaint of breathlessness and may be caused by several conditions that can increase ventilatory requirements, decrease ventilatory capacity, or increase resistance to breathing. Some examples are exercise, anemia, fever, weak respiratory muscles, pleural effusion, asthma, emphysema, and chronic bronchitis.[7] Dyspnea probably results from the work of breathing against an obstruction that inhibits adequate oxygenation.

Airway clearance is essential to maintaining adequate oxygenation. Decreased energy and fatigue may influence an individual's ability to cough effectively. Furthermore, the adequacy of food and fluid intake and an individual's mobility status will directly affect airway stability. Tracheobronchial factors such as infection and irritation cause the goblet cells to secrete large amounts of mucus, possibly leading to airway obstruction, especially when the cough reflex is weak or ineffective.[2] Normally, loose mucus can cause obstruction when it becomes thick because of dehydration. Individuals with perceptual or cognitive impairments are likely to develop airway obstruction resulting from noncompliance or resistance to therapy. For instance, these patients may refuse to use humidified oxygen or to follow coughing and deep-breathing exercises. Furthermore, neurologically impaired individuals may have a diminished cough, and patients affected by trauma or surgery may not be able to cough effectively because of injury, pain, or sedation.[3]

■ Defining Characteristics

The presence of the following defining characteristics indicates that the patient may be experiencing Ineffective Airway Clearance:

- Absent or adventitious breath sounds (e.g., rales or rhonchi)
- Dyspnea
- Changes in respiratory rate or depth
- Cough, effective or ineffective, with or without sputum
- Cyanosis
- Substernal, intercostal retraction
- Tachycardia
- Anxiety

■ Related Factors

The following related factors are associated with Ineffective Airway Clearance[11]:

- Decrease energy and fatigue
- Tracheobronchial infection, obstruction, or increased secretions
- Perceptual or cognitive impairment
- Trauma
- Aspiration of foreign matter

Ineffective Breathing Pattern

The assessment of Ineffective Breathing Pattern includes the rate, rhythm, and quality of respiration, and the presence of dyspnea, cough, nasal flaring, pursed-lip breathing, prolonged expiratory phase, use of accessory muscles, altered chest excursion, increased anteroposterior diameter, cyanosis, and anxiety.[3]

Several neuromuscular and musculoskeletal impairments can adversely affect an individual's breathing pattern. Generally, the problems result from the inability to innervate the proper muscles because of nerve damage, myelin degeneration, spinal cord and brain damage, and inconsistent impulses from the phrenic and intercostal nerves.[2,11] The location of the damage or degeneration and the extent of the disease usually determine the potential adverse effects on breathing patterns. For instance, spinal cord problems may interfere with the normal breathing pattern, depending on the site of damage and whether the phrenic nerve is involved. Specific diseases such as myasthenia gravis, muscular dystrophy, poliomyelitis, multiple sclerosis, and Guillain-Barré syndrome may cause altered breathing patterns resulting from the physiological destruction involved.[11] Furthermore, sedation and drug overdoses may depress the respiratory center and result in hypoventilation.

Conditions that decrease lung expansion will interfere with normal breathing patterns.[16] The presence of pain may limit lung expansion because of existing injuries to the chest or other body structures. Rib fractures will limit lung expansion and may produce paradoxical (uneven) breathing. Kyphoscoliosis, a disabling disease characterized by abnormal curvature of the spine, results in an uneven, limited breathing pattern because of the inability of the lungs to expand properly. Conditions that add pressure on the lungs, such as pneumothorax and hemothorax, will cause altered breathing patterns. Specific problems within the lungs themselves, which are associated with tracheobronchial obstruction and inflammation, may cause alterations in breathing patterns, especially in the individual who is already compromised. An example is the individual who suffers from asthma. The pathophysiology is as follows: the airway narrows from the constriction of the bronchial walls; the production of mucus increases; the bronchial walls may thicken; and airways narrow further from the presence of secretions. This course of events may lead to altered breathing patterns, depending on the extent of the symptoms.

Furthermore, conditions that affect the individual's ability to inhale adequately and consistently, such as decreased energy and fatigue, will result in altered breathing patterns stemming from alveolar hypoventilation. Effective muscle contraction and ventilation require energy and adequate nutrition. Emotional problems such as anxiety are primarily responsible for hyperventilatory breathing patterns.

Many of the defining characteristics of Ineffective Breathing Pattern generally are found in patients with chronic obstructive pulmonary diseases (COPD). COPD is a classifying term used for several respiratory diseases that manifest common characteristics.[4,8] Bronchial asthma, chronic bronchitis, and emphysema are diseases frequently encompassed by the COPD classification, although each disease has a distinct pathophysiological course.[11] The common clinical link among these obstructive pulmonary diseases is the pathological change in the airway or lungs that results in chronic airflow limitation (CAL).[11] The clinical manifestations of CAL and interventions used to treat CAL involve the pathophysiological processes of the trapping of air and the collapse of the airways on expiration.

To improve ventilation and force air out of the lungs, the accessory muscles of respiration are recruited involuntarily by patients with obstructive diseases. The scalene muscles, which elevate the first two ribs; the sternocleidomastoid muscles, which raise the sternum; and the trapezius muscles, which fix the shoulder,[15] are used and will often become pronounced and enlarge as a result of the excessive demands placed on them.

The affected individual often breathes through pursed lips to increased or to slow exhalation. This process helps create a back pressure that lessens the collapse of the airway and improves exhalation.[6] The three-point position—sitting forward, hands on knees, and shoulders elevated—is the position many patients with COPD choose because it allows for easier elevation of the diaphragm, leading to better airflow. The anteroposterior diameter of the chest will become enlarged over time because of the trapping and pulmonary overdistention of air. Diaphragmatic movement becomes greatly depressed or absent as the movement of the rib cage becomes taut as a result of changes in the chest wall. A chronic cough, with or without the expectoration of sputum, frequently accompanies

IV

an obstructive disease and will potentiate fatigue and inspiratory muscle weakness. Patients with obstructive diseases must undergo tests for abnormal pulmonary function such as a test for decreased forced expiratory volume (FEV1) in 1 second or a test for decreased forced vital capacity (FVC), which measures the maximum amount of air expired. Altered chest excursion refers to visual or palpable asymmetry of the chest cage.

The patient may appear to be short of breath or dyspneic as evidenced by pausing for breath after every seven or eight words when speaking. Dyspnea is a complex concept that describes the feeling that ventilatory requirements are not being met by the current ventilation pattern. Typically the respiratory rate increases to meet increased demands. Nasal flaring often shows distress and may be present during dyspnea. An intolerance for activity frequently accompanies dyspnea, especially in patients with CAL.[7]

■ Defining Characteristics

The presence of the following defining characteristics indicates that the patient may be experiencing Ineffective Breathing Pattern:

- Dyspnea
- Changes in pulse rate, quality, or rhythm
- Changes in respiratory rate, depth, or pattern
- Cyanosis
- Lips pursed when breathing
- Flaring of nostrils
- Prolonged expiratory phase
- Assumption of three-point position
- Use of accessory muscles
- Orthopnea
- Splinted or guarded respirations

■ Related Factors

The following related factors are associated with Ineffective Breathing Pattern:

- Neuromuscular impairment
- Musculoskeletal impairment
- Decreased energy or fatigue
- Inflammatory process
- Pain, fear, and anxiety
- Perception or cognitive impairment

Impaired Gas Exchange

Impaired Gas Exchange is a complicated diagnosis that obviously requires medical corroboration of clinical information for support. The arterial blood gas analysis is the most accurate indicator of oxygenation and gas exchange status.[12] However, other clinical signs such as mental status, agitation or restlessness, respiratory rate and rhythm, heart rate and rhythm, quality of the pulse, activity tolerance, breath sounds, tidal volume, body position, and skin color can indirectly measure gas exchange.[11,15] In general, the clinical characteristics of Impaired Gas Exchange result from the effects of hypoxia and hypercapnia on the individual. Hypoxia is a general deficiency of oxygen in body tissues. The signs and symptoms vary, depending on the extent and nature of the hypoxia. Mild hypoxia stimulates the peripheral chemoreceptors, increasing heart rate and respiratory rate to compensate for decreased oxygen. Other symptoms, such as confusion, somnolence, restlessness, and agitation, demonstrate altered mentation resulting from decreased delivery of oxygen to the tissues of the brain.[9,15] Hypercapnia is an abnormal increase of carbon dioxide in the blood that may be caused by many factors, including the presence of thick secretions that can cause airway obstruction and obstructive diseases such as chronic obstructive pulmonary diseases (COPD), which lead to chronic retention of carbon dioxide.

Arterial blood gas analysis will reveal oxygenation and ventilation status, as well as patient response to pulmonary interventions.[4] Arterial blood gas analysis will determine the efficiency of ventilation and gas exchange. The gas analysis measures the concentration of oxygen and carbon dioxide, the percentage of oxygen, and bicarbonate, and the pH of the arterial blood. The normal values for arterial blood gases at sea level are PO_2 90 ± 10 mm Hg; O_2 saturation, 96% ± 1%; PCO_2, 40 ± 3 mm Hg; pH, 7.4 ± 0.03; and bicarbonate, 22 to 26 mEq/L.[13,17]

Pulse oximetry can be used at the bedside to assess oxygenation through assessment of oxygen saturation (SaO_2). About 97% of oxygen in the blood binds with hemoglobin. <u>*Saturation* is a measure of the percentage of hemoglobin that is saturated by oxygen.</u> An SaO_2 of 90% to 100% is needed to replenish plasma adequately. Problems occur when SaO_2 goes below 85%, and a saturation below 70% is considered life threatening.[13,18] Pulse oximetry gives the practitioner a quick means to assess impending hypoxemia. It must be remembered that this test does not measure ventilation status.

Care should be used interpreting oxygen saturation determined by pulse oximetry alone. Patients with oxygen saturation well within normal levels (95% to 100%) who exhibit no symptoms of oxygen deficiency are at no risk. Others, who have identified low levels and symptoms (below 85%), will be under treatment. Those most at risk for misinterpretation are patients with pulse oximeter readings between 85% and 90% saturation. The pulse oximeter may have an error rate of 4%.[6] Patients with borderline readings may in fact be at 81% or 89% because of the possible error in measurement. Patients with factors that may interfere with pulse oximeter reliability include those persons exposed to tobacco smoke or suffering from smoke inhalation and those with thick digits, low blood pressure, vasoconstriction, or decreased temperature, which may result in poor perfusion.[7]

Other associated signs and symptoms must be included in the assessment to establish the actual oxygenation status. For example, respiratory rate is a very simple yet sensitive indicator of respiratory distress in all age groups, but it is nonspecific. Tachypnea is seen in cardiac, pulmonary, metabolic, and central nervous system disorders and infectious disease.[9] It needs to be investigated and explained.

The lungs function as a buffer system to maintain the close balance of pH in the blood by regulating the ratio of bicarbonate to carbon dioxide (CO_2). Alterations in blood gases, especially the pH, will result in changes in the respiratory pattern.[15,18] For instance, respiratory acidosis (a decrease in the pH and increase in CO_2), which results from alveolar hypoventilation, will cause hyperventilation in an individual with intact com-

pensatory mechanisms. This response decreases the concentration of CO_2 in the blood and restores balance.

The related factors of Impaired Gas Exchange are an altered oxygen supply, alveolar-capillary membrane changes, an altered blood flow, and the altered capacity of blood to carry oxygen.[11] An altered oxygen supply representing a low ventilation-to-perfusion (V/Q) ratio occurs when perfusion to the alveoli is adequate but ventilation is less than adequate. In this case, oxygen is not available to the cells, and carbon dioxide is not properly eliminated. Some clinical examples that can cause this are an airway obstruction, muscle weakness, central nervous system depression, chest trauma, emphysema, and high altitudes (low oxygen concentration).[3]

Changes in the alveolar capillary membrane may impair the diffusion of gases. Some examples include the reduction of the gas exchange area caused by lung resection; thickening of the alveolar membrane, which occurs with adult respiratory distress syndrome; and interference from the displacement of interstitial fluids, which occurs with pulmonary edema. Altered blood flow results in a high V/Q ratio; the alveoli are adequately ventilated but poorly perfused. Therefore ventilation is wasted, and hypoxia and hypercapnia result because blood is not available to pick up or remove the gases.[3] <u>Some causes of decreased perfusion are circulatory or hypovolemic shock, pulmonary embolism, cardiac dysrhythmia, myocardial depression, and the destruction of the capillary bed.</u>

Any alteration in hemoglobin, the blood's primary transporter of oxygen, results in an altered level of oxygen transported to the tissues. Some causes for this are (1) inadequate hemoglobin, as in anemia, (2) inadequate force to pump the blood, as with congestive heart failure, and (3) vessel patency that does not allow for the normal flow of blood, as in pulmonary embolism.[10,15]

Developmentally the elderly exhibit physiological changes that render them at risk for Impaired Gas Exchange. There is a reduction of alveolar surface area, so gas exchange and saturation are reduced. Furthermore, the signs of hypoxia that are manifested in the younger population, such as increased heart rate, increased blood pressure, and increased respiratory rate, are often blunted in the elderly. Sometimes the only early sign of hypoxia in the elderly is a change in mentation.[1,6]

■ Defining Characteristics

The presence of the following defining characteristics indicates that the patient may be experiencing Impaired Gas Exchange:

- Confusion
- Somnolence
- Restlessness
- Irritability
- Inability to move secretions
- Hypercapnia
- Hypoxia

■ Related Factors

The following related factors are associated with Impaired Gas Exchange:

- Ventilation perfusion imbalance
- Alveolar capillary membrane changes
- Altered blood flow
- Altered capacity of the blood to carry oxygen
- Altered oxygen supply

DIAGNOSIS

■ Differential Nursing Diagnosis

Ineffective Airway Clearance

Diagnosis of Ineffective Airway Clearance is made from the inability to clear rales or rhonchi from the lungs by effective coughing. Removal of the obstructing material by coughing or suctioning should result in clear lung sounds. Confounding diagnoses include Impaired Gas Exchange and Ineffective Breathing Pattern because of similarities in defining characteristics, such as increased respiratory and pulse rates and dyspnea. Cyanosis also may occur as a result of the inability to bring oxygen into the alveolar areas (Impaired Airway Clearance or Ineffective Breathing Pattern) or from the inability to exchange oxygen and carbon dioxide at the alveolar level (Impaired Gas Exchange).

Ineffective Breathing Pattern

Differential diagnosis in patients with Ineffective Breathing Pattern includes Ineffective Airway Clearance and Impaired Gas Exchange. With an Ineffective Breathing Pattern, the patient status is affected by the rate, rhythm, and depth of respiration, whereas in the patient with Ineffective Airway Clearance the ability to remove obstructing respiratory secretions is the principal focus. In Impaired Gas Exchange, the ability of the body to exchange gases at the alveolar level is impaired. Although certain conditions affect both gas exchange and breathing patterns (e.g., COPD), the focus of the diagnosis Ineffective Breathing Pattern is the movement of air in and out of the lung that is unobstructed by secretions.

Impaired Gas Exchange

Impaired Gas Exchange primarily focuses on the ability to transfer gases across the alveolar membranes. Ineffective Airway Clearance is frequently associated with increased mucus production and an ineffective cough. Ineffective Airway Clearance involves the ability to move oxygenated air in and carbon dioxide–laden air out of the lungs through clear airways. Ineffective Breathing Pattern, by contrast, describes the condition in which the lungs are unable to maintain movement of air, even though the airways remain open. This diagnosis is appropriate when adequate muscle strength or neurological control to maintain respiration is absent. Although the airway may be clear and adequate muscle strength and neurological control are intact, the body may still lack the ability to transfer oxygen and carbon dioxide across the lung cell walls (alveoli). In that case the diagnosis Impaired Gas Exchange is appropriate. Each process is separate and distinct, yet all are essential if adequate oxygen for body functions is to be maintained. Table 6 may help clarify the differential diagnosis involved in these three diagnoses.

TABLE 6 Comparison of Respiratory Related Diagnoses

Ineffective Airway Clearance	Ineffective Breathing Pattern	Impaired Gas Exchange
Increased pulse rate	Increased pulse rate	Increased pulse rate
Increased respiratory rate	Increased respiratory rate	Increased respiratory rate
Cyanosis	Cyanosis	Cyanosis
Weak, ineffective cough or absent cough reflex	Pursed-lip breathing	Dyspnea on exertion
Obstructive airway secretions	Three-point posture	Changes in blood gases
	Use of accessory muscles	$PO_2 < 90$ mm Hg
	Orthopnea	O_2 saturation $< 96\%$
	Splinted or guarded aspirations	$PCO_2 > 40$ mm Hg
	Increased anteroposterior diameter	pH < 7.4

IV

■ Medical and Psychiatric Diagnoses

Ineffective Airway Clearance

Ineffective Airway Clearance is associated with certain medical conditions such as asthma, chronic obstructive pulmonary disease (COPD), cerebrovascular accident (CVA), or coma. Asthma and COPD obstruct the airways with excessive mucus and are associated with bronchoconstriction. Lung sounds include wheezing, and there is a prolonged expiration phase in respiration. The trapped mucus prevents adequate oxygen and carbon dioxide exchange though the alveolar membrane. Chronic hyperinflation of the lungs results in an increased anteroposterior diameter. A cerebrovascular accident may result in Ineffective Airway Clearance because of diminished cough reflex, paralysis of the oropharyngeal muscles, diminished strength of the diaphragm and abdominal muscles, or Impaired Swallowing. Coma may result from several conditions, including (1) a neurological impairment such as head injury, (2) a disease such as meningitis, or (3) a drug overdose. In these cases relaxation of oropharyngeal structures or the pooling of secretions in this same location may result in obstruction of the airway.

Ineffective Breathing Pattern

Medical and psychiatric diagnoses related to the diagnosis Ineffective Breathing Pattern include any that affect energy or lung expansion. Because of the neurological control of breathing, cerebral injury may play an important role in the diagnosis of Ineffective Breathing Pattern. As previously discussed, centers in the brain control the rate, depth, and rhythm of breathing, and these can be disrupted if the brain suffers from trauma, resulting in edema or hemorrhage. Chest trauma, such as rib fracture or surgery, often causes pain with breathing, and the patient may voluntarily reduce the depth of respiration in an attempt to control the pain.[12] Medications such as narcotics, sedatives, and analgesics, an overdose of street drugs, or anesthesia reduces the body's response to the normal stimuli for breathing (increased CO_2), slowing the rate and depth of respiration. Oversedation also will reduce the cough reflex.[3]

Impaired Gas Exchange

The following are examples of related medical and psychiatric diagnoses for Impaired Gas Exchange: Anemia and leukemia are examples in which the body lacks adequate hemoglobin to transport oxygen. Atelectasis and pneumothorax both result in lack of exchange gases because the collapsed alveoli remain airless. Atelectasis may be prevented through effective preoperative teaching because the surgery patient is especially prone to this disorder. Pneumothorax affecting only a small area of a lung may resolve without intervention.

Large pneumothorax most often requires the placement of a chest tube with water seal drainage.

Pulmonary embolism is a serious and life-threatening condition in which a blood clot lodges in a pulmonary artery and prevents blood flow to the affected area. With inadequate blood flow to the lung tissue, oxygenation of the hemoglobin is prevented. Ventilation is adequate, but perfusion is prevented. The result is reduced oxygenation of the blood transported to body tissues. Emboli may travel from anywhere in the body, but the common origin is the lower extremities.

OUTCOME IDENTIFICATION, PLANNING, AND IMPLEMENTATION

Nursing care of patients with respiratory problems must focus first on the immediate oxygenation needs of the body. The ability to move air in and out of the lungs through clear airways and to exchange oxygen and carbon dioxide at the alveolar level is an essential body function. Brain, heart, and kidney tissue are especially susceptible to damage from hypoxia and cannot withstand prolonged periods of inadequate oxygen.

Ineffective Airway Clearance

Ineffective Airway Clearance is primarily diagnosed by the presence of abnormal breath sounds, changes in the rate and rhythm of respiration, an ineffective cough, and dyspnea. The ability to establish and maintain a patent airway early after patient admission is critical. This outcome is urgent and requires initial and repeated assessments of respiratory status. This assessment includes pulse and respiratory rate and rhythm, breath sounds, cough and sputum characteristics, and effectiveness in clearing secretions.

Effective response to pulmonary interventions will be demonstrated as the rate and depth of respirations improve and dyspnea is relieved. The cough will be effective in removing thin secretions from the respiratory tree. Teach the patient to cough effectively after taking several deep breaths. A high Fowler's position and splinting incisions (if applicable) will aid in the development of an effective cough. Patients who have limited muscle strength for an effective cough may need to be suctioned. Preoxygenate and hyperinflate the lungs before and after suctioning if the patient is intubated, and limit each suctioning period to no more than 15 seconds.[7]

After the airway has been opened, administer humidified oxygen and medications (e.g., bronchodilator, expectorants, steroids, and antibiotics) as ordered to help the patient maintain adequate ventilation and oxygenation status. Position the patient to facilitate respiration and lung expansion. The position of choice may be high Fowler's or it may be recumbent with the unaffected lung side down. Patient comfort and level of anxiety may also affect positioning. Provide adequate hydration to help liquefy secretions through oral or intravenous fluid as ordered. Provide chest physiotherapy as ordered.

Ineffective Breathing Pattern

The outcome for a patient with Ineffective Breathing Pattern is stated as follows: The patient will experience adequate airflow in and out of the lungs early in the admission process. Nursing Care Guidelines include the assessment of respiratory effectiveness upon which to develop appropriate interventions.[15] A complete health history should include questions about exposure to environmental irritants, present and past occupations, and the use of cigarettes. Assess the patient's current breathing pattern for rate, rhythm, and regularity. Document the patient's overall appearance, including skin color and body position. If the patient is breathing abnormally, document the pattern, the events preceding the alteration, and the patient's emotional state. Assess and document the presence of any defining characteristics, such as use of accessory muscles, chest expansion, dyspnea, pursed-lip breathing, and so on, to determine the etiology of the breathing alteration.

Instruct and position the patient to facilitate breathing and to maximize ventilation. This process is sometimes termed *breathing retraining* and involves (1) teaching and assisting the patient in breathing through pursed lips, (2) assisting the patient in assuming a position of maximum ventilation—often the three-point position, (3) teaching the patient diaphragmatic and abdominal breathing techniques, and (4) assisting the patient with progressive relaxation techniques and biofeedback. These interventions should increase the exhalation phase and reduce airway collapse.

Diaphragmatic breathing incorporates the abdominal muscle group for improved ventilation because these muscles are close to the diaphragm. To encourage full expansion of the diaphragm, patients are taught to relax abdominal muscles during inspiration and to tighten them slightly during expiration. Many positions can facilitate ventilation, including the forward-leaning position, the head-down position, and the supine position.[4,6,7] In general, patients usually assume the position of maximum ventilation and comfort without coaching.

Administer bronchodilator, anticholinergic, and antiinflammatory medications as ordered to improve airflow.[7] Evaluate the effectiveness of these medications. A comprehensive plan should be directed at (1) reducing the work of breathing, (2) minimizing the expenditure of energy by assisting the patient with daily activities as needed, (3) providing rest periods as necessary if Activity Intolerance is assessed, (4) maintaining adequate nutritional stores to support the respiratory muscles and supply the energy required for breathing, and (5) teaching the patient to avoid airway irritants such as cigarette smoke and to prevent respiratory infections.

Impaired Gas Exchange

The outcome for the individual with Impaired Gas Exchange is to experience adequate ventilation and oxygenation status throughout the admission process. The nurse helps the patient toward this outcome by assisting in the identification of the etiology designating Impaired Gas Exchange and by performing interventions to improve overall gas exchange. One must collaborate with the physician to assess gas exchange accurately through the analysis of arterial blood gas (ABG) levels.

Assess the patient's respiratory status to establish a baseline and to plan interventions. Document breath sounds, respiratory rate and rhythm, sputum production, skin color, body position, alterations in mental status, heart rate, and dysrhythmia. Also note the medical diagnoses. Assist the physician in obtaining the arterial blood gas sample, and report other laboratory values that affect oxygenation status, such as hemoglobin level. Monitor pulse oximetry to determine oxygen saturation.[5]

Perform nursing interventions that maximize and coordinate ventilation and perfusion. If partial airway obstruction is determined, instruct and assist the patient in coughing and expectorating secretions. Suction the patient's airway if the cough is ineffective. Provide supplemental oxygen if the patient is hypoxemic.

Depending on the specific lung pathology, place the patient in a position that facilitates ventilation and perfusion matching. Although clinical nursing research in this area is just developing, some support for therapeutic positioning is noted. The individual with unilateral lung disease exhibits the most noted effect. The lateral position with the "good" (unaffected) lung down (dependent) will improve oxygenation by increasing perfusion to the healthy tissue.[7,16] This research reveals evidence opposing the idea that patients should be repositioned frequently and arbitrarily and suggests the development of a more specific plan based on the patient's lung pathology. However, only future study can answer the many remaining questions about the effects of other positions on oxygenation and the frequency and duration of therapeutic position changes.

Facilitate gas exchange and adequate ventilation by providing maintenance and supportive treatment. Encourage and provide rest periods before and after physical activity to prevent exacerbation of hypoxia. Assist with activities of daily living to conserve patient energy and to reduce oxygen requirements. Administer medications as ordered and evaluate their effectiveness; these may include bronchodilators, expectorants, corticosteroids, antibiotics, and antihistamines to improve pulmonary function. Prevent the development of hypoxia by using measures to decrease oxygen consumption and demand.

Administration of blood, which requires a physician's order, may be the major response to anemias. Monitoring for untoward effects of the transfusion and ongoing assessment of respiratory function are major nursing responsibilities. Oxygen therapy is implemented in most conditions affecting respiration and circulation. Nursing responsibilities associated with this therapy include monitoring vital signs, mentation, skin color, hydration, and regulation of oxygen.

Chest drainage may be implemented in cases of pneumothorax or hemothorax. Nursing responsibilities beyond monitoring respiratory function include recording the quantity and quality of lung drainage, maintaining the patency of the water seal apparatus, and providing emotional support for the patient.

Prevention of venous stasis is a primary nursing responsibility for surgical patients and those confined to bed rest. Early ambulation, cough, deep breathing, turning, and the use of elastic stockings are the cornerstones of preventing pulmonary embolus. Once an embolus has lodged in the lungs, however, oxygen and anticoagulant therapy are often necessary.[10] This requires careful monitoring for evidence of bleeding and wound healing, as well as monitoring coagulation laboratory work (partial thromboplastin time [PTT]).

◢ NURSING CARE GUIDELINES
Nursing Diagnosis: Ineffective Airway Clearance

Expected Outcome: The patient will develop and maintain clear airways throughout admission.
- Assess respiratory status, documenting respiratory rate and rhythm, breath sounds, and cough and sputum characteristics.
- ▲ Monitor finger oximetry and ABG as ordered.
  A thorough assessment in performed to design and evaluate an appropriate plan.
- Assist the patient to a position most effective for lung expansion (e.g., high Fowler's or a recumbent position with affected lung side down).
- Teach the patient to breathe deeply.
- Teach the patient to cough effectively after deep breaths.
- Splint incisions if applicable.
- Suction the airway if necessary.
- Preoxygenate and hyperinflate the lungs before and after suctioning if patient is intubated.
- Limit each episode of suctioning to 15 seconds.
- ▲ Perform chest physiotherapy (e.g., percussion and postural drainage) as ordered.
  Removal of secretions facilitates ventilation.
- Reduce anxiety.
- Provide comfort measures through physical presence and reassurance as needed.
  Therapy is more effective in a relaxed patient.

Expected Outcome: The patient will maintain oxygenation status throughout admission.
- ▲ Administer humidified oxygen as ordered, especially if there is inadequate ventilation and patient has an artificial airway.
- ▲ Administer medications as ordered (e.g., bronchodilators, expectorants, steroids, and antibiotics).
- ▲ Provide the patient with adequate hydration—encourage intake of oral fluids and maintain IV fluids as ordered.

■ = nursing intervention; ▲ = collaborative intervention.

- Position the patient to maximize oxygenation (e.g., position patients with unilateral lung disease with the unaffected lung down as tolerated). Considerations during positioning include pathophysiology, comfort, medical problems, and related factors, such as obesity, fractures, and surgeries.
- Monitor respiratory status as above, as the patient responds to treatment.
  Medical management can increase airflow and maintain an adequate oxygenation status.

◢ NURSING CARE GUIDELINES
Nursing Diagnosis: Ineffective Breathing Pattern Related to Physiological Alterations

Expected Outcome: The patient will experience adequate airflow in and out of the lungs.
- Assess and document the patient's respiratory status, including a complete health history.
- Assess and document the patient's breathing pattern (rate, rhythm, chest expansion, breath sounds, use of accessory muscles, pursed-lip breathing, arterial blood gases, and skin color).
- Assess and document the patient's pulse rate, quality, and rhythm.
  A thorough assessment is performed to design and evaluate an appropriate plan.
- Administer medications as ordered to increase airflow, and evaluate their effectiveness (e.g., bronchodilators, anticholinergics, and antiinflammatory medication). *Available interventions may improve dyspnea and lead to effective breathing patterns.*
- Instruct and assist the patient in using the most effective respiratory position (e.g., the three-point position) if patient experiences pursed-lip breathing. *Positioning and other measures increase the exhalation phase and reduce airway collapse.*
- Assist the patient with activities of daily living. Assess the level of activity tolerance and provide adequate rest periods. *Conserve energy to enhance respiratory efforts.*
- Maintain adequate nutritional intake. *Supply the energy required for breathing.*
- Teach the patient to avoid airway irritants (e.g., cigarette smoke).
- Teach the patient to prevent respiratory infections.
  Prevention will preserve well-being and sense of control.

■ = nursing intervention; ▲ = collaborative intervention.

◢ NURSING CARE GUIDELINES
Nursing Diagnosis: Impaired Gas Exchange

Expected Outcome: The patient will experience adequate gas exchange as evidence by normal ABGs and the absence of hypoxia.
- Monitor for hypoxia: changes in mental status, tachycardia, irritability, and abnormal breath sounds.
- Monitor vital signs, arterial blood gas levels, ECG, and pulse oximetry every shift and PRN.
  A thorough assessment is performed to design and evaluate an appropriate plan.
- Position the patient to maximize ventilation and perfusion matching.
▲ Administer oxygen as ordered.
- Encourage coughing and deep breathing.
▲ Administer medications as indicated (e.g., bronchodilators, expectorants, inhalants, and antibiotics).
- Monitor mechanical ventilation and assist the patient as required. *Appropriate therapy enhances ventilation and perfusion relationship.*
- Encourage rest periods. *Conservation of energy enhances respiratory effort.*

■ = nursing intervention; ▲ = collaborative intervention.

EVALUATION

Evaluation of the diagnoses in this cluster focuses on adequate oxygenation of body tissues through respiration.

Ineffective Airway Clearance

Evaluation of effective nursing care includes the presence of clear breath sounds, a normal pulse rate, and a normal rate, depth, and rhythm of unlabored respirations. If a cough is present, it will be effective and produce loose, thin secretions. All of these results indicate that the nursing actions are effective. The patient will report that the symptom of dyspnea is relieved and that activity tolerance has increased.

Ineffective Breathing Pattern

Alleviation of the defining characteristics that support the diagnosis of Ineffective Breathing Pattern is evidence of improvement. The patient will demonstrate bilateral breath sounds, a less labored breathing pattern, normal blood gas levels, an increase in FEV1 and FVC, and a general decrease in symptoms.

Impaired Gas Exchange

Improvements in respiratory status are supported clinically by improvements in arterial blood gases, pulmonary function tests, and the patient's overall clinical picture, including a reduction in symptoms. Adequate oxygenation of tissues will be indicated by normal mental status, normal levels of blood gases, normal pulse rate and rhythm, natural skin color, lack of restlessness, and absence of cyanosis. The patient's ability to maintain adequate ventilation and oxygenation status can be determined by improved mental status and reduced anxiety.

If the above measures are ineffective in achieving the expected outcomes, intubation with ventilatory support should be considered. Otherwise, irreversible, serious brain and renal tissue damage will occur.

◤ CASE STUDY WITH PLAN OF CARE

Mr. Peter C. is a 75-year-old, widowed nursing home resident admitted to the medical unit with a diagnosis of chronic obstructive pulmonary disease (COPD) with spontaneous pneumothorax. Mr. C. has a lifelong smoking habit evaluated at 120 pack years. He has been on oxygen therapy at 2 L/min for the past 6 months. He suffered from an exacerbation of his COPD about 2 weeks ago with increased dyspnea, decreased activity tolerance, and a frequent cough that produced thick white mucus. He experienced a sudden episode of extreme dyspnea with chest pain, diagnosed on X ray as an upper left lobe pneumothorax. On admission, Mr. C. had a pulse rate of 94 beats/min, respiratory rate of 36/min, an increased anteroposterior diameter, three-point posture, and pursed-lip breathing. His skin was pale, with slight cyanosis of the lips and mild clubbing of his fingers. Further examination revealed absent lung sounds over the upper left lobe, limited respiratory excursion, and a Posat of 85%. The nursing diagnosis was Impaired Gas Exchange related to collapsed lung (pneumothorax).

◤ PLAN OF CARE FOR MR. PETER C.
Nursing Diagnosis: Impaired Gas Exchange Related to Collapsed Lung (Pneumothorax)

Expected Outcome: Mr. C. will experience adequate gas exchange as evidenced by normal levels of ABGs and normal mentation within 24 hours.
- Assess respiratory status for baseline: arterial blood gas level, ECG, and pulse oximetry every shift and PRN.
- Monitor mental status, breath sounds, and vital signs.

■ = nursing intervention; ▲ = collaborative intervention.

- ▲ Provide humidified O_2 at 2 L/min as ordered.
- ▲ Administer medications as indicated (e.g., bronchodilators, expectorants, and inhalants).
- ▪ High Fowler's position.
- ▪ Encourage coughing to remove secretions; suction the airway as needed.

Expected Outcome: Mr. C. will report increased comfort and relaxation.
- ▪ Alternate rest and activity to conserve energy.
- ▪ Offer reassurance to decrease the patient's fear and anxiety.
- ▪ Provide therapeutic interactions that require a minimum of verbalization by patient. Explain all procedures; anticipate needs. Allow patient to use yes or no responses to decrease communication effort.

IV

▒ CRITICAL THINKING EXERCISES

1. What should be included in the methods of history taking and interviewing to accommodate the dyspnea that Mr. C. is experiencing? Include pace, organization, and timing.

2. In assessing Mr. C.'s cough, what questions would be most helpful in determining the development and seriousness of the condition?

3. Given the fact that Mr. C. has had chronic obstructive pulmonary disease for a long period of time, how might the signs of chronic low-grade hypoxia be exhibited?

4. When Mr. C. is discharged, he will need continuous oxygen therapy. Discuss the various types of oxygen units used for home care, their cost, and the impact on patient mobility and energy cost in carrying them (portable systems).

5. Design a teaching plan for Mr. C.'s home care that includes diet, activity, and probable drugs (by classification).

REFERENCES

1. Bender P: Deceptive distress in the elderly, *AJN* 92(10):29–33, 1992.
2. Bolton PJ and Kline KA: Understanding modes of mechanical ventilation, *AJN* 94(6):36–43, 1994.
3. Calianno C, Clifford DW, and Titano K: Oxygen therapy giving your patient breathing room, *Nurs 95* 25(12):33–38, 1995.
4. Chang JT, Moran MB, Cugell DW, and Webster JR: COPD in the elderly, a reversible cause of functional impairment, *Chest* 108(3):736–739, 1995.
5. Clinical news: pitfalls of pulse oximetry, *AJN* 95(4):52, 1995.
6. Gift AG, Moore T, and Soeken K: Relaxation to reduce dyspnea and anxiety in COPD patients, *Nurs Res* 41(4):242–246, 1992.
7. Green E, editor: *Clinical practice guidelines for the adult patient,* St. Louis, 1995, Mosby–Year Book.
8. Hayden RA: What keeps oxygenation on track, *AJN* 92(12):32–42, 1992.
9. Jones M, Hoffman L, and Delgato E: ARDS revisited: new ways to fight an old enemy, *Nurs 94* 24(12):34–43, 1994.
10. Keep NB: Identifying pulmonary embolism, *AJN* 95(4):52, 1995.
11. Kim J, McFarland GK, and McLane AM: *Pocket guide to nursing diagnoses,* ed 4, St. Louis, 1991, The CV Mosby Co.
12. Laskowski-Jones L: Meeting the challenge of chest trauma, *AJN* 95(9):23–30, 1995.
13. Mays DA: Turn ABGs into child's play, *RN* 58(1):36–39, 1995.
14. Miller CA: *Nursing care of older adults,* Glenview, Illinois, 1990, Scott, Foresman.
15. Phipps WJ, Long BC, Woods NF, and Cassmyer VL: *Medical surgical nursing concepts and clinical practice,* ed 4, St. Louis, 1991, The CV Mosby Co.
16. Robichaud A: Alteration in gas exchange related to body position, *Crit Care Nurse* 10(1):56–59, 1990.
17. Stiesmeyer JK: A four-step approach to pulmonary assessment, *AJN* 93(8):22–28, 1993.
18. Strigfield YN: Back to basics: acidosis, alkalosis, and ABGs, *AJN* 93(11):23–30, 1995.

Decreased Cardiac Output

▶

Decreased Cardiac Output *is the state in which the blood pumped by the heart is sufficiently reduced so that it is inadequate to meet the needs of the body's tissues.*[16]

OVERVIEW

Since the 1970s, mortality from cardiovascular disease has declined as the result of the development of sophisticated emergency medical systems in coronary care units, advances in antidysrhythmic and fibrinolytic therapy, development of techniques for recanulization of coronary arteries via a percutaneous approach, and advances in cardiac surgery.[14] Because of the increasing level of acuity in today's long-term care population, interventions previously found in acute care only are not commonplace in the chronic care setting. These changes result from health care and reimbursement legislation, advances in medical technology, and the overall increased life expectancy of the population at large. As health care costs continue to escalate, policy makers, consumers, and insurers are questioning the value of the technologically intensive American health care system. They are demanding that providers demonstrate the effectiveness of their interventions. The need to evaluate, measure, and predict with some accuracy outcomes of care has emerged as the cultural issues of the 1990s.[22] Case management strategies incorporating clinical pathways are being implemented in various settings. Clinical pathways serve as tools to help organize care to achieve specific outcomes within designated time frames and resource parameters. This approach fosters shorter hospital stays and helps to conserve resources. Utilization of clin-

ical pathways provides a common language for clinical practice and business management. To meet these challenges, nursing leaders are making efforts to identify and anticipate patient care needs and to implement educational programs for staff to meet these needs.[25]

Decreased Cardiac Output is one of the most complex and most frequently encountered problems among patients. Often the patients experiencing this condition present life-threatening situations that require critical nursing judgments and immediate interventions.[4] It is important that nurses be knowledgeable and skilled in the diagnosis of this disorder.

Cardiac output is the volume of blood pumped by each heart beat (or stroke volume) times the number of beats per minute. Normal cardiac output averages about 5 L/min in an adult human being at rest.[8] The cardiac output of an individual may vary with activity, postural changes, and metabolic rate. If the heart rate and stroke volume decrease, cardiac output decreases. Homeostatic mechanisms regulating cardiac output involve factors controlling performance of the pump and also factors affecting the peripheral vascular system and resistance. Normally the heart can increase its output up to five or six times the resting level, depending on the age and physical condition of the patient. There are two basic methods by which the heart regulates cardiac output in response to stress or disease: (1) changes in heart rate and (2) changes in stroke volume.[7]

Numerous systemic and cardiac factors affect the ability of the heart to pump blood and thereby alter cardiac output.[3,11] Cardiac failure results from any condition that reduces the heart's ability to pump.[26] The most common cause of low cardiac output at rest is diminished myocardial function resulting from myocardial infarction with coronary artery disease.[6] The only peripheral factor that usually decreases cardiac output is decreased mean systemic pressure, most often caused by decreased blood volume. Rapid bleeding (25% to 30% of total blood volume) will reduce the cardiac output to zero, and slow bleeding (40% to 50% of total blood volume over a period of an hour) will do the same thing.[11] With deterioration of left ventricular function, left ventricular dilation may occur as a compensatory mechanism to maintain cardiac output.[8] When cardiac output is significantly diminished, heart failure can occur.

It is estimated that 3 million people in the United States have congestive heart failure and that this disorder affects nearly 15 million people worldwide. In 1985, hospital discharge records listed congestive heart failure as a secondary diagnosis for 1.7 million patients.[5] The incidence of congestive heart failure is escalating. Readmission rates as high as 57% within 90 days have been reported in patients over the age of 70, and many of these readmissions may be avoidable. Proper discharge planning is essential to prevent these unnecessary readmissions.[1] Congestive heart failure has been the objective of extensive research, yet it still remains the leading cause of death.[19] The Framingham Study[17] revealed a 5-year survival rate of 40%. The New York Heart Association has categorized heart failure into four classes based on cardiac reserve or functional capacity, as shown in Table 7. One-year mortality rates have been correlated with functional class and increased from 0% to 5% for class I, from 10% to 20% for class II, from 35% to 45% for class III, and from 85% to 95% for class IV.[15]

Decreased Cardiac Output resulting from heart failure may be caused by mechanical, electrical, or structural factors. Mechanical factors include alterations in preload, alterations in afterload, and alterations in inotropic changes of the heart. *Preload* is the pressure exerted by the blood volume and venous return to the heart.[2] Preload is related primarily to contractility; a reduction in contractility results in Decreased Cardiac Output. *Afterload* is the resistance against which the heart pumps, arterial pressure.[2] An increase in afterload decreases stroke volume. If stroke volume decreases, cardiac output decreases.

Noncardiac factors, as noted earlier, influence preload and afterload, resulting in Decreased Cardiac Output. Invasive hemodynamic monitoring, as performed with balloon-tipped pulmonary artery catheters, is the measurement of factors affecting preload and afterload and of the stimuli that affect the inotropic state of the heart. Inotropic changes occur in the normal heart during exercise. During exercise, catecholamines, tachycardia, and an increase in sympathetic nerve impulses augment myocardial contractility and

TABLE 7 New York Heart Association Functional Classification

Functional Class	Definition	Manifestation
I	Patients with cardiac disease, but without resulting limitations of physical activity	Ordinary physical activity does not cause undue fatigue, palpitations, dyspnea, or angina
II	Patients with cardiac disease resulting in slight limitation of physical activity, but comfortable at rest	Ordinary physical activity results in fatigue, palpitations, dyspnea, or angina
III	Patients with cardiac disease resulting in marked limitation of physical activity, but comfortable at rest	Less than ordinary physical activity causes fatigue, palpitations, dyspnea, or angina
IV	Patients with cardiac disease resulting in an inability to carry out any physical activity without discomfort	Symptoms of cardiac insufficiency or of angina may be present even at rest

From Wright SM: Pathophysiology of congestive heart failure, *J Cardiovasc Nurs* 4(3):12, 1990. Copyright © 1990 Aspen Publishers, Inc.

IV

stroke volume, resulting in an increase in cardiac output. In patients with heart failure the heart does not respond to exercise in the same way. The normal increase in cardiac output does not occur. The compromised myocardium is incapable of meeting the increased demands of exercise. As a result, cardiac output is decreased.

Electrical factors that decrease cardiac output include alterations in heart rate, rhythm, and conduction. Pacemaker therapy may be beneficial. Cardiac output may be optimized by increasing or decreasing the rate of the pacemaker.[13,20] Nursing responsibilities include (1) knowledge of the type and functional capabilities of the pacemaker, (2) early identification of changes in electrical factors affecting cardiac output, and (3) knowledge regarding appropriate interventions to correct electrical abnormalities (e.g., use of medications and reprogramming parameters).

Structural factors that decrease cardiac output include papillary muscle dysfunction and ventricular abnormalities. These structural problems interfere with normal functioning of the heart. Conditions such as papillary muscle dysfunction, ventricular aneurysm, rupture of the interventricular septum, and rupture of the ventricle can lead to a decline in cardiac output.

The patient with low-output failure shows clinical evidence of impaired peripheral circulation and peripheral vasoconstriction. The extremities are usually cold, pale, and cyanotic. In late stages the stroke volume decreases and the pulse pressure narrows. Low-output failure occurs in patients with congenital or rheumatic, valvular, coronary, hypertensive, and cardiomyopathic heart disease.[8] It is the responsibility of the nurse to (1) attempt to understand the cause underlying the symptoms of Decreased Cardiac Output, (2) initiate the appropriate nursing interventions, and (3) recognize the necessity for early medical intervention.

ASSESSMENT

The 11 Functional Health Patterns can provide conceptual direction for the initial assessment of the patient. Because of their apparent relevance to clinical practice, the Functional Health Patterns are useful in categorizing the NANDA nursing diagnoses.[10]

The defining characteristics of Decreased Cardiac Output are obtained from a complete biopsychosocial patient history. Subjective data from the history provide information about the disease process and the patient's lifestyle, family structure, and preexisting health problems. Health problems may include conditions such as heart enlargement, elevated cholesterol or triglyceride levels, diabetes, a heart murmur, a heart attack, rheumatic fever, or hypertension. In addition, the patient's family history may reveal pertinent information about certain familial diseases (e.g., hypertension, rheumatic fever, stroke, blood disease, asthma, glaucoma, or gout).

Objective data are obtained by assessing the patient's mental status, cardiovascular system, peripheral vascular system, respiratory system, and urinary output. The signs and symptoms of Decreased Cardiac Output may differ, depending on the etiology of the associated health problem. The four techniques of inspection, palpation, percussion, and auscultation are used to complete the assessment.[23]

The nurse begins the assessment by monitoring the patient's heart rate, blood pressure, and respirations. Low blood pressure may indicate low cardiac output. The nurse assesses respiratory status and notes any productive or nonproductive cough. The patient is observed for signs of fear or anxiety that may appear in Decreased Cardiac Output. Signs of dyspnea and orthopnea may be apparent in a patient with left ventricular failure. Distention of the external jugular veins may be seen in right-sided heart failure. Cyanosis of the lips and nail beds indicates venous distention and inadequate oxygenation of blood. Another characteristic of this diagnosis is pale, cool, diaphoretic skin. The patient may appear tired and weak because of sleep disturbances and poor perfusion of skeletal muscles caused by a decrease in cardiac output. Edema and ascites resulting from right ventricular failure may be noted. Dependent edema may be observed in the patient's ankles, feet, and hands.

The nurse inspects the patient for impression marks from socks, rings, and shoes. If the patient has been confined to bed, the nurse should observe the sacrum for dependent edema. Urine output is observed for signs of oliguria and anuria, which may indicate Decreased Cardiac Output and subsequent decreased renal blood flow.

The nurse auscultates the heart for rate and rhythm. Tachycardia and other dysrhythmias often reflect an attempt by the heart to compensate for Decreased Cardiac Output.[18] The nurse should document any noted dysrhythmias in the patient's medical record and report them to the physician for immediate treatment.

Alterations in hemodynamic parameters indicate early left ventricular failure, often preceding other signs and symptoms of failure; therefore noting such alterations is an essential part of nursing assessment.[18] It is important for the nurse to realize that even in hemodynamically stable patients, results may vary as a result of (1) errors in measurements or (2) physiological alterations occurring within the patient.[6,9,18]

The nurse should palpate the carotid, brachial, femoral, popliteal, dorsalis pedis, and posterior tibial pulses. These are evaluated for patency, rate, rhythm, and character.[2] Lungs are auscultated for rales and decreased breath sounds caused by excess fluid in lung fields. Percussion is an especially useful tool in assessing the pulmonary and abdominal systems.[23] Dull sounds are noted when abnormal fluid is present in the lungs or abdomen. The nurse should carefully record assessment data in the patient's medical record. A chest film will confirm pulmonary congestion. Evaluation of the results of the assessment will provide information from which the nurse can develop an effective plan of care.

Patients with symptoms of heart failure should undergo radionuclide ventriculography to measure left ventricular ejection fraction. The *ejection fraction* is the ratio of blood expelled from the ventricle in one contraction to the ventricle's total capacity. At rest the healthy heart has an ejection veracity of 60% to 70%. Most patients with signs and symptoms of heart failure are found to have ejection fractions below 40%.[1] If the radionuclide ventriculography is to be done only at rest, a single ejection fraction will be reported. If it is to be done during an exercise study, two ejection fractions will be reported: one at rest and one during exercise. If the resting ejection fraction is low or if the ejection fraction decreases with exercise, cardiac pumping has decreased and has compromised cardiac output. Patients with significant cardiovascular disease or other medical problems that limit their ability to exercise for a stress test may require a drug-induced stress test. Medications such as Adenosine, Persantine, or Dobutrex may be administered intravenously during exercise. The nurse should be aware of the ejection fraction reported in the summary of the radionuclide ventriculography study. The patient should know the test is quite accurate and involves little risk. The patient should be instructed regarding the preparations and protocol of the testing procedures. The nurse should emphasize that there is no danger of harmful radiation.[8]

Additional noninvasive testing may include an echocardiogram and a Holter monitor. An echocardiogram, at rest or during exercise, will provide information regarding chamber hypertrophy, wall motion, or stenosis. A Holter monitor will provide a 24-hour electrocardiographic tracing of the patient's heart.

Laboratory tests will reflect changes caused by impaired tissue perfusion, diuretic therapy, or renal insufficiency (e.g., elevated blood urea nitrogen or elevated serum potassium).

▪ Defining Characteristics

The presence of the following defining characteristics indicates that the patient may be experiencing Decreased Cardiac Output:

- Variations in hemodynamic readings
- Dysrhythmias, electrocardiographic changes
- Fatigue
- Rales, dullness percussed in lungs
- Dyspnea, orthopnea, nonproductive cough
- Cyanosis—pallor of skin and mucous membranes
- Altered arterial blood gases

- Hypotension
- Cold, clammy skin
- Edema, ascites
- Decreased urinary output
- Decreased peripheral pulses
- Jugular vein distention
- Anxiety
- Confusion
- Restlessness
- Oxygen saturation below 90% (not due to pulmonary disease)
- Weakness

■ Related Factors

The following related factors are associated with Decreased Cardiac Output:

Mechanical factors
- Alteration in preload
- Alteration in afterload
- Alteration in inotropic changes in the heart

Electrical factors
- Alterations in rate
- Alterations in rhythm
- Alterations in conduction

Structural factors
- Papillary muscle dysfunction
- Ventricular abnormalities[11]

DIAGNOSIS

■ Differential Nursing Diagnosis

Decreased Cardiac Output can be related to Altered Tissue Perfusion, Altered Urinary Elimination, Inability to Sustain Spontaneous Ventilation, Fatigue, and Fluid Volume Deficit. Decreased Cardiac Output can include all of these clinical diagnoses. The detection of rales, dysrhythmias, and electrocardiography changes may indicate cardiac failure. The identification of the defining characteristics promotes accuracy in assessing the potential global effect of Decreased Cardiac Output.

■ Medical and Psychiatric Diagnoses

The specific medical diagnoses often associated with Decreased Cardiac Output are cardiomyopathy, congestive heart failure, myocardial infarction, rheumatic heart disease, and valvular heart disease. Clinical pathways utilized in today's managed care environment focus on the underlying goal of maintaining an adequate cardiac output. Plans of care may vary to reflect the specificity of the diagnosis, although the underlying goal is the same.

OUTCOME IDENTIFICATION, PLANNING, AND IMPLEMENTATION

The expected outcomes for patients with Decreased Cardiac Output are based on measures to (1) improve cardiac pump performance, (2) reduce cardiac work load, and (3) control salt and water retention.[8] Independent nursing actions to achieve these measures are primarily monitoring functions and health teaching. Direct treatment of Decreased Cardiac Output requires collaboration of the nurse with the physician to institute appropriate interventions.

Nursing interventions to improve pump performance are based on the administration of medications and their subsequent actions. Independent nursing actions are primarily assessment and monitoring activities to denote impending signs of Decreased Cardiac Output. Collaborative actions are predominantly monitoring functions and include the evaluation of prescribed medications.

Nursing interventions to reduce the cardiac work is accomplished with the administration of vasodilators in conjunction with physical and emotional rest. These actions are primarily individual interventions for nurses in various care settings.

Nursing interventions to help and maintain normal fluid and electrolyte balance include independent and collaborative measures to monitor lab values, assess for the effectiveness of prescribed medications, and patient education in regard to food and fluid intake.

IV

◢ NURSING CARE GUIDELINES
Nursing Diagnosis: Decreased Cardiac Output

Expected Outcome: The patient will have improved cardiac pump performance.
- Monitor blood pressure.
- Note respiratory rate and pattern.
- Auscultate and monitor heart rate and rhythm.
- Auscultate the lungs.
▲ Monitor hemodynamic status; consult physician if values exceed normal ranges.
- Assess jugular veins for distention.
- Assess skin temperature and color.
- Observe for peripheral edema, and report daily weight gain to physician.
- Maintain accurate intake and output records.
▲ Assess effects of prescribed medications.

Digitalis and inotropic agents are commonly prescribed. Digitalis is given to patients with heart failure to improve the depressed myocardial contractility, increase cardiac output, and promote diuresis.[18,21] *Inotropic agents are given to augment heart rate, stroke volume, and myocardial contractility. Nursing intervention involves observation for side effects of the drugs, especially dysrhythmias. Any abnormality in cardiac rate and rhythm can result in a decrease in cardiac output. Patients who experience severe bradycardia or atrial or ventricular dysrhythmias may require a temporary pacemaker to restore heart rate to normal. Because drug therapy plays a major role in the management of heart failure, patient and family education is imperative to promote compliance with the overall plan of care.*

Expected Outcome: The patient will have a reduction in cardiac work load.
- Instruct the patient in ways to reduce energy expenditure, such as bed rest with bedside commode (as indicated); semi-Fowler's or high Fowler's position; frequent rest periods; possible need to restrict fluids as directed; need to take prescribed medication; and need to reduce salt intake as directed.
- Promote calm environment.

Restrictions in activity depend on the degree and severity of heart failure. Nursing interventions focus on observations for possible side effects, such as hypotension, bradycardia, headaches, and drug interactions. If needed, circulation may be assisted by the use of intraaortic balloon counterpulsation or ventricular assist devices. With cardiac output assistance, blood can be circulated through the body at a physiologically acceptable rate, relieving cardiac work and increasing oxygen supply to the failing ventricle, yet augmenting cardiac output and systemic coronary perfusion.[24] *The nurse should encourage obese patients to participate in a weight reduction program with dietary supervision.*

Expected Outcome: The patient will maintain a normal fluid and electrolyte balance.
- Weigh the patient daily (same clothes, same scales, same time each day).
▲ Monitor electrolyte values; consult physician if values are not within normal range.
- Monitor changes in vital signs (compare with baseline signs).
- Encourage the patient to adhere to fluid restrictions as ordered.
- Assess for effectiveness of prescribed medication.
- Maintain accurate intake records.
- Encourage the patient to adhere to low-sodium diet.

Sodium restriction should be managed through dietary supervision. Diuretics are administered to correct fluid volume overload. Accurate daily weights will reflect changes in fluid status. A gain or loss of 1 kg (2.2 lb) of body weight approximates the gain or loss of 1 L of fluid.[18] *The nurse should maintain accurate intake and output records because they are essential to assess the effectiveness of treatment with diuretics. Monitoring electrolyte levels daily is essential. The nurse should report and document any change in the patient's heart rate, heart rhythm, respirations, blood pressure, skin temperature, skin color, mental status, or urine output. Any change in these may indicate electrical factors corresponding to Decreased Cardiac Output. Nursing interventions should initiate actions to correct abnormalities.*

■ = nursing intervention; ▲ = collaborative intervention.

IV

EVALUATION

Throughout the process of evaluation, patients should be informed about their diagnosis, including the prognosis, symptoms, and what to do if these symptoms occur. It is important for patients to understand their disease and to be involved in developing the plan for their care. Family members and caregivers should be included in counseling and decision-making sessions.[1]

Improved cardiac pump performance will be evaluated by the following criteria: normal blood pressure; normal pulse; normal sinus rhythm; normal breath sounds without rales or wheezes; warm and dry skin without cyanosis; normal urine output; no cough, dyspnea, or orthopnea; no diaphoresis; no jugular vein distention; no peripheral or sacral edema; no ascites; normal hemodynamic status (cardiac output resting range, 4 to 8 L/min); cardiac index, 2.5 to 4 L/min/m^2; pulmonary artery wedge pressure, <13 mm Hg; and mean right atrial pressure, 4 ± 2 mm Hg central venous pressure, 4

to 15 cm H_2O or 3 to 11 mm Hg. A reduction in cardiac work will be evaluated by the criteria cited above under improved pump performance.

A normal fluid and electrolyte balance will be evaluated by the following criteria: intake equals output; normal electrolyte values (Na, 135 to 145 mEq/L; K, 3.5 to 5.5 mEq/L; Ca, 4 to 5 mEq/L or 8.6 to 10.5 mg/dl); no weight gain; no peripheral edema; no peripheral venous distention; no orthopnea or paroxysmal nocturnal dyspnea; no cough; no frothy sputum; normal hemodynamic readings (as noted); and no tachypnea.

If the outcomes are not achieved, collaboration must occur to attempt to resolve any variations in cardiovascular homeostasis that may increase the potential for Decreased Cardiac Output. Careful consideration should be given to any social or cultural factors that may influence the patient's adherence to the proposed interventions such as diet and activity. The nurse should assist the patient in setting realistic goals to help achieve the proposed outcomes in various care settings.

▶ CASE STUDY WITH PLAN OF CARE

Mr. Charles V., age 75, is a widowed, retired factory worker. He lives alone in a senior citizen housing development. He is 5'7" tall and weighs 185 pounds. He has two children who live in another city several miles away. He prepares his own meals and admits to opening "cans of food, not really cooking like my wife did when she was with me." He smoked for 23 years but quit 3 years ago after having a myocardial infarction. His daily activities consist of walking in his yard "when the weather is good and I feel like getting out." He watches television 4 to 5 hours a day. His reading is limited to the daily newspaper since his cataract surgery 6 months ago.

Over a 2-week period, Mr. V. noticed swelling in his hands and feet progressively increasing. His weight rose to 195 pounds. His belts felt snug. He developed a nonproductive cough. At night he required two pillows to breathe comfortably. He resorted to sleeping in a chair. He became increasingly anxious and fatigued for lack of

sleep. His shortness of breath worsened. A neighbor became concerned about Mr. V. after not seeing him for 3 days. After checking on Mr. V. he encouraged him to go to the emergency room. Because of the lack of transportation the neighbor called a cab to transport Mr. V. to the hospital. Physical findings were as follows: Mr. V. was anxious and short of breath. His lips and nail beds appeared dusky. His skin was cool and clammy. Bilateral jugular vein distention was present. Blood pressure was 102/60 mm Hg; heart rate was 118 beats/min with frequent irregularities; and respirations were 29/min and labored. Bilateral rales were present. A chest X ray revealed marked pulmonary congestion. The abdomen was distended. Edema of the hands was noted with pressure marks from his rings. Edema of both feet was observed with indentations from his socks. Pedal pulses were difficult to palpate.

■ **PLAN OF CARE FOR MR. CHARLES V.**
Nursing Diagnosis: Decreased Cardiac Output Related to Electrical, Mechanical, or Structural Factors

Expected Outcome: Mr. V. will have normal breath sounds without rales or wheezes and no cough.
- Note respiratory rate and pattern.
- Auscultate the lungs.
- Administer oxygen as ordered.
- Administer medications as ordered (e.g., diuretics).
- Reduce Mr. V.'s fluid intake if ordered.

Expected Outcome: Mr. V. will express no complaints of dyspnea, orthopnea, or paroxysmal nocturnal dyspnea.
- Instruct Mr. V. regarding the need for lung assessment, fluid restriction, and pacemaker therapy (when applicable).

Expected Outcome: Mr. V. will maintain normal blood pressure, pulse, and sinus rhythm.
- Monitor blood pressure.
- Auscultate and monitor heart rate and rhythm.

Expected Outcome: Mr. V. will have no jugular vein distention.
- Assess jugular veins for distention.

Expected Outcome: Mr. V.'s urine output will be normal.
- Maintain accurate intake and output records.
- Observe for peripheral edema; examine sacrum for dependent edema.
- Note ascites.

- Weigh Mr. V. daily, and instruct him on the need to weigh daily (same time of day, same clothes) after voiding and to report weight gain.
- Teach Mr. V. to observe for and report edema.

Expected Outcome: Mr. V. will experience reduced anxiety and fear.
- Teach Mr. V. about the disease process, including the following: medications—actions and potential side effects; correct way to take pulse; purpose of cardiac monitoring; and purpose of cardiac testing.

Expected Outcome: Mr. V. will maintain normal hemodynamic status as evidence by mean right atrial pressure of 4 ± 2 mm Hg; cardiac output resting rate of 4 to 8 L/min; cardiac index of 2.5 to 4 L/min/m^2; mean pulmonary artery pressure less than 13 mm Hg; and central venous pressure of 4 to 15 cm H$_2$O or 3 to 11 mm Hg.
- Monitor hemodynamic status; consult physician if values exceed normal ranges.
- Instruct Mr. V. in need and procedure for hemodynamic monitoring.
- Assess skin color and temperature: skin should be pink, warm, and dry; no cyanosis, decrease in temperature, or diaphoresis.
- Arrange for home health care follow-up after discharge for patient assessment, proper adherence to medication regimen, and continued patient evaluation.
- Arrange for homemaker services after discharge to assist Mr. V. with housekeeping during his recovery.

Expected Outcome: Mr. V. will demonstrate a reduction in cardiac work load: he maintains bed rest with bedside commode; uses semi-Fowler's or Fowler's position; takes rest periods; demonstrates no anxiety or fear; has no daily weight gain; adheres to fluid restriction if indicated; has positive reaction to medications, without side effects; and is normothermic.

■ = nursing intervention; ▲ = collaborative intervention.   *Continued*

IV

◧ **PLAN OF CARE FOR MR. CHARLES V.— CONT'D**

- Encourage bed rest with bedside commode.
- Encourage frequent rest periods.
- Instruct Mr. V. in the need to reduce fluid intake; take prescribed medications (instruct regarding action and potential side effects); monitor temperature; and use stress-management techniques.

Expected Outcome: Mr. V. will maintain normal fluid balance as evidenced by the following: normal electrolyte values; Na, 135 to 145 mEq/L; K, 3.5 to 5.5 mEq/L; Ca, 4 to 5 mEq/L or 8.6 to 10.5 mg/dl; no rapid weight gain; no peripheral edema; adherence to sodium-restricted diet as indicated; adherence to fluid restriction as indicated; and no side effects from prescribed medications.

- Instruct Mr. V. in the importance of maintaining accurate daily weight; monitor electrolyte levels (consult physician if levels are not within normal range); monitor sodium intake as directed; encourage cardiac rehabilitation exercise (with appropriate prescription note for limitations and potential complications); and assess for effectiveness of prescribed medications and potential side effects.
- Arrange for a dietary assistance program after discharge that adheres to prescribed diet.

◧ **CRITICAL THINKING EXERCISES**

1. Which physical findings indicated that Mr. V. may be experiencing low cardiac output related to the mechanical factor of poor cardiac pump performance resulting in congestive heart failure?
2. Which aspects of Mr. V.'s activities of daily living place him at risk for complications resulting from low cardiac output?
3. What would be the initial priority in regard to nursing interventions when Mr. V. is evaluated?
4. What should the nurse consider regarding discharge planning for Mr. V.?
5. What are the topics to be addressed in regard to patient education for Mr. V. in the hospital and on discharge?

REFERENCES

1. Agency for Health Care Policy and Research: *Heart failure: management of patients with left-ventricular systolic dysfunction*, AHCPR Pub No 94-0613, Rockville, Maryland, 1994, U.S. Department of Health and Human Services.
2. Andreoli KG and others: *Comprehensive cardiac care*, ed 6, St. Louis, 1987, The CV Mosby Co.
3. Berne RM and Levy MN: *Physiology*, ed 2, St. Louis, 1987, The CV Mosby Co.
4. Bumann R and Speltz M: Decreased cardiac output: a nursing diagnosis, *Dimen Crit Care Nurs* 8(1):6–15, 1989.
5. Chesebro J: Cardiac failure. In Brandeburg RO, Fuster V, Giuliani ER, and McDoon DC, editors: *Cardiology: fundamentals and practice*, Chicago, 1987, Year Book.
6. Daily EK and Mersch J: Thermodilution cardiac outputs using room and ice temperature injectate: comparison with the Fick method, *Heart Lung* 16:294, 1987.
7. Daily EK and Schroeder JS: *Techniques in bedside hemodynamic monitoring*, ed 4, St. Louis, 1989, The CV Mosby Co.
8. Dossey BM, Guzzetta CE, and Kenner CV: *Essentials of critical care nursing*, Philadelphia, 1990, JB Lippincott Co.
9. Gardner PE, Monat LA, and Woods SL: Accuracy of the injectate delivery system in measuring thermodilution cardiac output, *Heart Lung* 16:552, 1987.
10. Gordon M: *Nursing diagnosis: process and application*, New York, 1987, McGraw-Hill.
11. Guyton AC: *Textbook of medical physiology*, ed 8, Philadelphia, 1990, WB Saunders Co.
12. Guzzetta CE and Dossey BM: *Cardiovascular nursing: body-mind tapestry*, St. Louis, 1984, The CV Mosby Co.
13. Iskandrian AS and Mintz GS: Pacemaker therapy in congestive heart failure: a new concept based on excessive utilization of Frank-Starling mechanism, *Am Heart J* 112:867, 1986.
14. Jaffe A, Albarran-Sotelo R, and Athins J: *Textbook of advanced cardiac life support*, ed 2, Dallas, 1987, American Heart Association.
15. Killip T: Epidemiology of congestive heart failure, *Am J Cardiol* 56:2A–7A, 1985.
16. Kim MJ, McFarland GK, and McLane AM: *Pocket guide to nursing diagnoses*, ed 6, St. Louis, 1995, Mosby–Year Book.

17. McKee P and Castell W: The natural history of congestive heart failure: the Framingham study, *N Eng J Med* 285: 1441–1446, 1971.
18. Metheny NM: *Fluid and electrolyte balance: nursing considerations,* Philadelphia, 1987, JB Lippincott Co.
19. Michaelson C: *Congestive heart failure,* St. Louis, 1983, The CV Mosby Co.
20. Miura DS: Indications and guidelines for cardiac pacing in the 1980s, *Cardiovasc Rev Rep* 8:51, 1987.
21. Packer M: Prolonging life in patients with congestive heart failure: the next frontier, *Circulation* 75(supplement IV):1, 1987.
22. Reiley P and Howard E: Predicting hospital length of stay in elderly patients with congestive heart failure, *Nurs Econ* 13(4):210–216, 1995.
23. Reuther MA and Hansen CB: *Cardiovascular nursing,* New York, 1985, Medical Examination Publishing.
24. Teplitz L: An algorithm for ventricular assist devices, *Dimen Crit Care Nurs* 9(5):256–265, 1990.
25. Wengate S: Nursing grand rounds, *J Cardiovasc Nurs* 4(3):71, 1990.
26. Wright S: Pathophysiology of congestive heart failure, *J Cardiovasc Nurs* 4(13):1–15, 1990.

IV

Risk for Disuse Syndrome

▶

Risk for Disuse Syndrome *is the state in which an individual is at risk for deterioration of body systems as the result of prescribed or unavoidable musculoskeletal inactivity.*[16]

OVERVIEW

Disuse syndrome is a term used to describe the multisystem deterioration that occurs with inactivity.[8] Disuse syndrome is often referred to as *deconditioning* and is related to the complications of immobility, bedrest, or inactivity.[11,13,17] Inactivity is associated with many conditions and can have deleterious effects on every body system.[9,13,17] The hazards of inactivity as it relates to disuse syndrome are omnipresent for all patients regardless of age, medical diagnosis, or health care setting. Nursing interventions directed toward the prevention of disuse syndrome are critical to averting temporary or permanent disability. Risk for Disuse Syndrome can be best understood through a review of assessment parameters, particularly in relation to the status of the body systems and the psychosocial status of the patient with this diagnosis.

ASSESSMENT

Nurses are responsible for recognizing an inactive patient's predisposition for developing disuse syndrome as a consequence of disease, injury, or prescribed therapy.[4] This recognition is based on a thorough and systematic assessment of the potential and actual effects of a patient's inactivity. The patient's previous health history, current health problems, and prescribed medical regimen are taken into consideration. Because of the multiple and complex human responses to inactivity, the nurse uses a head-to-toe technique based on body systems.[6] This method ensures that important assessment data are not missed, and risk factors for Risk for Disuse Syndrome are identified.[12,16]

Cardiovascular Status

Cardiovascular effects associated with inactivity are (1) decreased venous return, (2) decreased orthostatic capacity, and (3) decreased work capacity.[14] Increased risk of thrombus formation is due to the absence of the skeletal muscle pump (muscle contraction with exercise), subsequent venous pooling in the extremities, and external pressure on the blood vessels by pillows and use of the knee gatch.[14,17] A combination of fluid and electrolyte shifts, shifts in blood volume, and an altered neurovascular response to upright position changes results in orthostatic hypotension.[14,15,18] The patient should be observed for dizziness, lightheadedness, giddiness, pallor, hypotension, and fainting. A patient's response to physical activity may indicate that the heart has a decreased work capacity. Tachycardia, fatigue, and weakness in response to changing positions in bed or performing active range-of-motion exercises indicate deconditioning of the cardiovascular system.[17]

Cardiovascular assessment involves monitoring blood pressure for postural changes; heart rate and rhythm before, during, and after activity or movement in bed; and signs indicating that the patient may be experiencing Activity Intolerance. The lower extremities are checked for the signs indicative of a thrombus or phlebitis: color (erythema), size, edema, warmth, presence of palpable masses, and Homan's sign (dorsiflexion of the foot resulting in pain in the calf).

Respiratory Status

The main physiological effects of inactivity on the respiratory system are decreased respiratory movement, stasis of secretions, and altered oxygen–carbon dioxide balance.[17] Assumption of the supine position affects respiratory function by decreasing all lung volumes except tidal volume and by impairing gas exchange.[19] This makes the recumbent patient susceptible to arterial oxygen desaturation, atelectasis, and pneumonia.[11] Pulmonary embolism, with sudden onset of dyspnea, tachycardia, and tachypnea, is a life-threatening problem that may result from a dislodged thrombus in the legs.[5] Respiratory assessment would include frequent monitoring of respirations (rate, rhythm, and depth), breath sounds, and arterial blood gases to detect complications.

Musculoskeletal Status

Musculoskeletal system alterations involve muscle atrophy, decreased muscle strength, decreased endurance, decreased range of joint movement, and contractures. The loss of weight-bearing forces on joints results in osteoporosis (decreased bone density) because of increased bone resorption with resultant risk for fractures. The mobilization of calcium from the bones also predisposes the patient to hypercalcemia and renal calculi formation.[17,18] A musculoskeletal assessment involves a comprehensive assessment of the patient's muscle strength, range of joint motion, ability to move in bed, and ability to perform activities of daily living (e.g., eating, bathing, dressing, and toileting).[20]

Gastrointestinal Status

Results of inactivity on the gastrointestinal system include constipation, impaction, negative nitrogen balance, and decreased appetite. Generalized muscular weakness and longer transit time of food through the gastrointestinal tract can interfere with the complete evacuation of the bowel.[11,17] Personal factors, such as the inability to toilet independently and use a bedpan in the supine position or the lack of prompt assistance when needed, may predispose the inactive patient to constipation.[11] Gastrointestinal assessment includes gathering data about the patient's dietary likes and dislikes, dietary intake of nutrients and vitamins (especially protein and vitamin C for wound healing), fluid intake, previous bowel elimination pattern, and the use of pharmacological agents that affect bowel function. A patient with a history of hiatal hernia may experience reflux of stomach contents in the supine position.[18]

Renal Status

Assessment of the renal system is directed toward the detection of evidence indicating Urinary Retention, incontinence, urinary tract infections, and renal calculi. The supine position alters the normal mechanism of micturition by interfering with the relaxation of perineal muscles and the external sphincter, thereby contributing to Urinary Retention.[17] Urinary stasis in the supine position and hypercalcemia both contribute to the formation of renal calculi. Assess the patient for abdominal distention; the presence of frequency, urgency, or burning on urination; fever; flank pain; and renal colic (e.g., waves of severe pain). The patient's intake and output and the characteristics of the urine (e.g., color, clarity, and presence of hematuria) should be noted.

Status of the Integument

Immobility is the most significant risk factor for pressure ulcer development.[3] Large body surfaces, including bony prominences, may be exposed to prolonged pressure in a recumbent position.[18] The most common sites for pressure ulcers include the occiput (posterior head), ears, scapula, elbows, hips, sacrum, knees, ankles, and heels. When performing a complete skin assessment, the nurse also considers the patient's mobility status in bed, bowel and bladder incontinence, mental status, nutritional intake, previous history of pressure ulcers, and laboratory values (e.g., albumin and total protein).[3] The skin should be assessed every time the patient is turned and repositioned. Risk factors, such as shearing forces and friction, can be eliminated with the use of a turn/lift sheet or trapeze.

IV

Psychosocial Status

Inactivity or immobility may affect the patient's personality by altering ability to concentrate, motivational level, emotional expression, sensory perception, time estimation, and social role activities.[17] External immobilization (e.g., casting) and internal immobilization (e.g., paralysis) result in confinement and decreased sensory stimulation, which can result in a change in intellectual, emotional, or social reactions.[10] Common reactions include anger, hostility, altered body image, frustration, anxiety, regression, withdrawal, apathy, loss of personal worth, and fear.[10,15] Intellectual reactions may be reflected in changes in learning capacity such as decreased problem-solving ability. The way an individual reacts intellectually and emotionally to immobility can affect social interactions (e.g., the patient may lose interest in maintaining social contacts).[10]

■ Risk Factors

The presence of the following behaviors, conditions, or circumstances[12,16] renders the patient more vulnerable to Risk for Disuse Syndrome:

Physiological response risk factors
- Paralysis (from disease or trauma)
- Pain (acute or chronic)
- Altered level of consciousness
- Coma
- Contractures
- Cachexia or debilitated state
- Shock
- Impaired muscular strength
- Ischemia
- Fatigue
- Obesity
- Malnutrition
- Altered sensation

Treatment-related risk factors
- Major surgery
- Confining treatment modalities
- Mechanical immobilization (e.g., traction and physical restraints)
- Prescribed immobilization (e.g., bed rest)

- Mechanical ventilation
- Neuromuscular blocking agents

Disease and trauma-related risk factors
- Major or multiple trauma
- Burns
- Terminal or end stage of a disease
- Guillain-Barré syndrome
- Cerebrovascular accident
- Progressive debilitating diseases (e.g., Parkinson's disease)
- Diseases or injuries of the musculoskeletal system (e.g., muscular dystrophy, multiple sclerosis, rheumatoid arthritis, and fractures)
- Head trauma or head injury
- Brain tumors
- Cardiovascular and respiratory diseases causing hypoxia or hypoxemia

Psychosocial risk factors
- Major or severe depression
- Catatonic state
- Severe dementia
- Senile dementia, Alzheimer's type
- Lack of knowledge of pain control measures
- Hopelessness
- Altered cognitive functioning

DIAGNOSIS

■ Differential Nursing Diagnosis

Risk for Disuse Syndrome incorporates a number of risk and actual nursing diagnoses. Examples of these include Risk for Infection, Risk for Injury, Risk for Impaired Skin Integrity, Risk for Activity Intolerance, Risk for Loneliness, Constipation, Body Image Disturbance, Powerlessness, Impaired Physical Mobility, Sensory/Perceptual Alterations, and Altered Tissue Perfusion. Treatment of Risk for Disuse Syndrome incorporates interventions that should prevent the patient's development of Impaired Gas Exchange, Ineffective Airway Clearance, and Ineffective Breathing Pattern. The desired outcomes and interventions for Risk for Disuse Syndrome direct the focus of nursing care to the prevention of complex multisystem deterioration that may occur with inactivity.

IV

■ **Medical and Psychiatric Diagnoses**

Risk for Disuse Syndrome is commonly related to several medical diagnoses, including cerebrovascular accident, neuromuscular disorders, diseases of the central nervous system, major or multiple trauma, and major burns. Catatonia and major or severe depression are two psychiatric diagnoses that are frequently related to Risk for Disuse Syndrome.

OUTCOME IDENTIFICATION, PLANNING, AND IMPLEMENTATION

Nursing care planning is directed toward the prevention of deterioration of body systems and the maintenance of functional independence to the fullest extent possible.[7] The overall outcome that the patient should achieve is that he or she will not develop disuse syndrome during the period of prescribed or unavoidable inactivity. The nurse must be knowledgeable about and anticipate the possible deterioration that may occur. Preventive measures for the inactive patient must be implemented promptly. Through the implementation of outcome-specific interventions, optimal physical and psychosocial functioning is expected and desired.

The Nursing Care Guidelines present a detailed description of nursing interventions directed toward supporting achievement of seven outcomes. The outcomes are specific for preventing altered functions or maintaining normal function of the cardiovascular, respiratory, musculoskeletal, gastrointestinal, renal, and integumentary systems as well as the supporting psychosocial function. Interventions are grouped according to the potential effects on a particular body system and psychosocial functioning.

■┘ **NURSING CARE GUIDELINES**
Nursing Diagnosis: Risk for Disuse Syndrome

Expected Outcome: The patient will have no evidence of altered cardiovascular functioning.
- ■ Monitor apical heart rate and rhythm and blood pressure at least every 4 hours *to assess cardiovascular status and to monitor signs and symptoms of complications.* If dizziness or lightheadedness is present, monitor blood pressure in lying, sitting, and standing (if appropriate) positions *to detect the presence of orthostatic hypotension.*
- ■ Assess lower extremities for color, temperature, edema, peripheral pulses, and Homan's sign *to assist in the early detection of deep venous thrombosis or thrombophlebitis.*
- ▲ Apply antiembolism stockings as ordered. Teach the patient isometric and active foot and leg exercises (e.g., dorsiflexion and plantar flexion of the feet), if not contraindicated. *These measures increase venous return to the heart, decrease or prevent edema, and prevent thrombus formation.*
- ■ Change positions slowly. Gradually elevate head of bed from lying to sitting position *because the upright position may decrease orthostatic blood pressure changes.*[11] If standing or ambulation is allowed, dangle legs on side of bed beforehand and encourage active contraction of muscles of the lower extremities *to increase venous return and minimize orthostatic hypotension.*[14]
- ■ Encourage the patient to participate in activities of daily living as much as possible *because physical activity increases cardiac endurance.*
- ▲ Administer anticoagulants (e.g., Heparin or Coumadin) if ordered. Monitor blood clotting studies and observe for signs and symptoms of bleeding. *Anticoagulants, ordered to prevent deep vein thrombosis, alter blood clotting mechanisms and may cause hemorrhage.*

Expected Outcome: The patient will show no evidence of respiratory compromise.
- ■ Monitor respiratory rate, depth, rhythm, chest movement, and breath sounds at least every 4 hours *to detect signs and symptoms of respiratory complications (e.g., pneumonia, atelectasis, or pulmonary embolism).*

■ = nursing intervention; ▲ = collaborative intervention. *Continued*

◼ NURSING CARE GUIDELINES — CONT'D

- Position the patient in Fowler's position, if appropriate, *to facilitate chest expansion and promote ventilation.*
- Assist and teach deep breathing, coughing, and use of incentive spirometry *to foster lung expansion, to clear major airways, and to prevent pooling and stasis of secretions.*
- Suction the airway, *to stimulate the cough reflex and to maintain a patent airway.* Monitor characteristics of sputum and secretions (e.g., color, odor, and consistency) and sputum culture results *for evidence of respiratory tract infection.*

Expected Outcome: The patient will be free of musculoskeletal complications.

- Identify the patient's functional level. Assess and document muscle size, tone, strength, and joint range of motion (ROM). *Documentation of functional level provides a baseline for future comparisons and guides nursing interventions.*
- Perform active range-of-motion or passive range-of-motion exercises at least once per shift *to prevent joint contractures and to maintain muscle size and strength.*
- Encourage the patient to participate in activities of daily living (ADL) (e.g., bathing, dressing, and toileting). Provide help with ADL as needed. *Participation in ADL maintains functional level, improves the patient's self-esteem, and prevents other complications of immobility.*

Expected Outcome: The patient will maintain normal bowel function.

- Identify previous bowel elimination pattern *for future comparison of bowel function.*
- ▲ Provide adequate fluid intake. Confer with dietitian about increase in dietary fiber content, if not contraindicated. Record intake and output. *These actions monitor hydration status and assist bowel elimination.*
- ▲ Administer stool softeners, laxatives, or suppositories as ordered. Note the effectiveness of these drugs. *These pharmacological agents alter bowel function and assist in bowel elimination.*
- ▲ Administer antacids and histamine blockers, as ordered, *to reduce the symptoms of ulcer disease, hiatal hernia, and esophageal reflux disease.*

Expected Outcome: The patient will be free of signs and symptoms of Urinary Retention, urinary tract infection, or renal calculi.

- Assess urine output for color, clarity, odor, and amount *to detect urinary tract infections.* Record intake and output *to monitor hydration status.* Note urinary frequency. Question the patient about subjective symptoms such as urgency, burning, painful urination, or flank pain *to detect urinary tract complications early.*
- Encourage a minimum of 2 L of fluid per day, if not contraindicated, *to maintain urinary output and to prevent urinary calculi formation.*
- Ensure proper positioning and privacy *to facilitate urination.*
- ▲ Monitor blood studies (e.g., blood urea nitrogen, creatinine, and electrolytes) *to assess renal function.*

Expected Outcome: The patient will maintain skin integrity.

- Inspect skin with every position change *to detect skin breakdown at the earliest point.* Apply protective skin creams *to preserve intact skin and to protect susceptible areas from irritation.*
- Turn and reposition the patient as often as necessary based on nursing assessment data and the patient's Risk for Impaired Skin Integrity *to prevent pressure ulcers.*[2]
- Use positioning devices (e.g., pillows or wedges) to elevate the patient's heels off the bed and to prevent contact between bony prominences *to remove pressure and to foster soft tissue viability.*[2]
- If the patient is immobile, avoid positioning directly on trochanters when in the side-lying position *to reduce the adverse effects of pressure in this area and to prevent pressure ulcer formation.*[1,2]
- Keep the skin clean and dry. Keep bed linens wrinkle-free. *Moisture and creased linen can contribute to skin breakdown.*

Continued

- Use a turn/lift sheet or trapeze to move the patient in bed. *These measures reduce friction and shearing forces that contribute to skin breakdown.*[1]
- Provide ongoing education for the patient and family regarding pressure ulcer prevention *because education is an important factor in reducing the incidence of pressure ulcers.*[1]

Expected Outcome: The patient will express feelings about inactivity, treatment, and recovery.
- Encourage the patient to express feelings regarding inactivity and treatment. *Expression of feelings helps the patient cope with the illness and inactivity. It also helps reduce anxiety, decreases fear, and allows the patient to ventilate frustrations.*
- Provide privacy (e.g., pull curtains) or move the patient to a quiet or secluded area *to ease the expression of confidential feelings and concerns.*
- Help the patient identify coping strategies, their effectiveness, and new strategies, if needed, *to assist the patient in dealing with the prescribed or unavoidable musculoskeletal inactivity.*
- Teach the patient the rationale for the medical and nursing regimen. *Information assists the patient to cope with inactivity.*
- Encourage the patient's participation in activities that are meaningful and mentally stimulating *as a means of diversion. Group activities may increase socialization and sensory input from others.*
- Encourage participation of family members in the plan of care. *Collaboration with family members promotes continuity of care and achievement of desired outcomes.*
- Provide sensory stimulation (e.g., preferred music via headphones) *to assist in preventing the sensory and behavioral changes associated with inactivity.* Family members may provide sensory stimulation such as gently touching the patient's arm or face or verbally conversing with the patient *to prevent sensory deprivation.*
- Help the patient and family identify community resources *to assist in planning for patient care after discharge.*
- Refer patient and family members to appropriate individual counseling or support groups *to assist in coping with medical diagnosis, prescribed or unavoidable inactivity, treatment modalities, or recovery.*

EVALUATION

Overall, evaluation of the expected outcomes for the patient with the nursing diagnosis Risk for Disuse Syndrome involves a thorough and systematic assessment, including physical and psychosocial assessment as well as laboratory data. This data is compared to the baseline data or previous nursing assessment data to determine if the patient's functioning has been maintained or has deteriorated. Through the implementation of the nursing interventions described in the Nursing Care Guidelines, optimal physical and psychosocial functioning should be maintained.

Depending on the type and number of risk factors and each patient's unique physical and psychosocial characteristics, the signs and symptoms of disuse may be totally absent, or multisystem deterioration may be present. The nurse must evaluate how effective the nursing interventions were in achieving the overall goal of prevention of disuse syndrome and in maintaining the function of specific body systems. Nursing interventions must be evaluated to determine if they were effective or ineffective.

If a specific outcome was not achieved or only partially achieved, alternative interventions should be planned and implemented. New nursing diagnoses may need to be added to the plan of care. For example, the evaluation of a patient with the nursing diagnosis Risk for Disuse Syndrome may reveal evidence of the defining characteristics of the nursing diagnosis Ineffective Individual Coping (e.g., verbalization of the inability to cope with inactivity or a change in the usual communication pattern). This nursing diagnosis would be added to the plan of care and appropriate interventions carried out. The nursing diagnosis Risk for Disuse Syndrome would remain on the plan of care so that the potential deterioration of other body systems would be prevented.

The patient may experience prescribed or unavoidable inactivity for several weeks or months. Therefore the time frame for the achievement of the outcomes will reflect these longer time periods. The time frame will vary from one patient to another. For example, a pediatric patient in a body cast may be inactive for a few months, whereas a patient with quadriplegia may be inactive and wheelchair bound for several years. When the patient is discharged from an acute care setting to the home, continued evaluation of achievement of outcomes is necessary and should be done periodically.

Case Study with Plan of Care

Mr. James S. is a 22-year-old male who sustained a gunshot wound to the thoracic spine at the level of T6 1 year ago. His injury resulted in a complete loss of motor and sensory function below the level of the lesion. He is attending the outpatient follow-up clinic at a major medical center. He has normal upper body strength and sensation and is able to self-propel his wheelchair. He performs clean, intermittent urinary catheterization every 6 hours. He has a history of urinary tract infections, pressure ulcers, and constipation. Mr. S. lives with his mother in a handicap-accessible apartment building. When not attending vocational rehabilitation, Mr. S. plays wheelchair basketball on a local team.

Plan of Care for Mr. S.

Nursing Diagnosis: Risk for Disuse Syndrome Related to Paralysis Secondary to Spinal Cord Injury at T6 Level

Expected Outcome: Mr. S. will maintain optimal cardiovascular functioning.

- ▪ Discuss with Mr. S. the importance of wearing antiembolism stockings.
- ▪ Evaluate Mr. S.'s knowledge of proper positioning, including the need to avoid extreme hip and leg flexion for long periods of time.
- ▪ Teach Mr. S. the importance of avoiding crossing the legs and excessive pressure from tight stockings or clothing.
- ▪ Review the signs and symptoms of deep vein thrombosis, including how to assess lower extremities for thrombophlebitis and deep venous thrombosis. Stress the need to seek prompt medical treatment if any signs or symptoms are present.
- ▪ Provide positive reinforcement regarding Mr. S.'s active lifestyle, including incorporation of aerobic exercise.

Expected Outcome: Mr. S. will show no evidence of atelectasis, pneumonia, or pulmonary embolism.

- ▪ Encourage Mr. S. to cough and to deep breathe frequently and to maintain an upright position as much as possible.
- ▪ Review the signs and symptoms of respiratory tract infections and pulmonary embolism. Emphasize the need for recognition of early signs and symptoms and prompt medical intervention, if necessary.
- ▪ Encourage and support physical activities that maximize lung function.

Expected Outcome: Mr. S. will be free of musculoskeletal complications.

- ▪ Assess and evaluate current functional level and compare with previous documentation on medical record.

▪ = nursing intervention; ▲ = collaborative intervention.

▲ Assess proper wheelchair fit. Refer to physical therapist, if needed.

▲ Have Mr. S. give demonstration of his prescribed exercise program, including passive range-of-motion exercises of the lower extremities. Refer to physical therapist for changes, if needed.

▲ Promote and encourage exercises that maximize upper torso functioning and that maintain strength and endurance, including weight lifting, wheelchair sports, pushing or lifting the body in wheelchair, and daily living activities.

▪ Support and encourage Mr. S.'s physical activities with the wheelchair basketball team.

Expected Outcome: Mr. S. will maintain normal bowel function at least every 3 days.

▪ Review Mr. S.'s bowel elimination pattern and prescribed bowel program for effectiveness. Review the importance of regular bowel elimination because bowel distention from constipation may trigger autonomic dysreflexia. Consult with physician for changes in prescribed bowel program, if necessary.

▲ Instruct patient to take stool softeners as ordered.

▲ Teach Mr. S. to use rectal suppository every night after dinner to stimulate bowel movement. Reinforce the need to allow 15 to 60 minutes for results.

▲ Encourage adequate dietary fiber intake of 30 g of fiber per day, if not contraindicated.[21] Assess for any needed dietary changes, and refer him to dietitian.

▪ Instruct Mr. S. to avoid Fleet enemas as a means of bowel elimination because enemas cause significant rectal stretch, act as irritants, and may interfere with reflex emptying of the bowel.[21]

Expected Outcome: Mr. S. will maintain his normal urinary elimination pattern.

▪ Review Mr. S.'s urinary elimination pattern, including frequency of catheterization and bladder volumes obtained.

▪ Assess Mr. S.'s ability to perform clean, intermittent catheterization technique. Teach modification of technique, if needed.

▪ Stress the importance of maintaining a minimum fluid intake of 2 L per day.

▪ Review the signs and symptoms of urinary tract infections and renal calculi with Mr. S. Underscore the necessity of obtaining prompt medical treatment, if necessary.

▪ Review the signs and symptoms of autonomic dysreflexia and possible causative factors (e.g., bladder distention). Urinary catheterization may need to be performed more frequently or fluid intake decreased to prevent large bladder volumes and bladder distention that may trigger autonomic dysreflexia.

Expected Outcome: Mr. S. will be free of pressure ulcers.

▪ Assess condition of skin surface, especially previous area of breakdown on the ischium.

▪ Teach Mr. S. to use a mirror to monitor entire skin surface at least daily, with special attention paid to the sacrum, the hips, the ischium, and the heels.

▪ Stress importance of changing positions every 15 minutes by performing wheelchair lifts or by changing positions.[2]

▲ Monitor condition of pressure relief pad for wheelchair. Refer Mr. S. to physical therapy for evaluation, if needed.

▪ Reinforce importance of eating a balanced diet and drinking at least 2 L of fluid each day.

▪ Encourage Mr. S. to sleep in the prone position at night to keep pressure off ischium.

Expected Outcome: Mr. S. will express feelings about inactivity, treatment, and recovery.

▪ Assess with Mr. S. his coping strategies, evaluate their effectiveness, and identify new strategies, if necessary.

▪ Give Mr. S. positive reinforcement regarding his attendance at vocational rehabilitation training.

▪ Encourage and support attendance at spinal cord injury peer or support group meeting at outpatient clinic.

IV

■ CRITICAL THINKING EXERCISES

1. What are the specific physiological and psychosocial effects of a spinal cord injury that put Mr. S. at Risk for Disuse Syndrome?

2. In what ways would a patient's cultural or ethnic background affect the plan of care for a patient at Risk for Disuse Syndrome? Specify how you would tailor specific nursing interventions for patients of different backgrounds.

3. Consider the involvement of family members and significant others in the plan of care for the patient at Risk for Disuse Syndrome. How can Mr. S.'s mother participate in and augment Mr. S.'s plan of care? What specific organizations that could provide assistance to a patient such as Mr. S. are available in your city?

REFERENCES

1. Agency for Health Care Policy and Research: *Pressure ulcers in adults: prediction and prevention. Clinical practice guideline number 3,* AHCPR Pub No 92-0047, Rockville, Maryland, 1992, U.S. Department of Health and Human Services.

2. Agency for Health Care Policy and Research: *Treatment of pressure ulcers. Clinical practice guideline number 15,* AHCPR Pub No 95-0652, Rockville, Maryland, 1994, U.S. Department of Health and Human Services.

3. Alvarez OM, and Childs EJ: Pressure ulcers: physical, supportive, and local aspects of management, *Clin Podiatr Med* 8:869–890, 1991.

4. American Nurses' Association: *Nursing's social policy statement,* Washington D.C., 1995, The Association.

5. Andrews L: Medical management of pulmonary emboli, *Med Surg Nurs* 3(1):31–35, 1994.

6. Bates B: *A guide to physical examination and history taking,* ed 5, Philadelphia, 1995, JB Lippincott Co.

7. Blocker WP: Maintaining functional independence by mobilizing the aged, *Geriatrics* 47(1):42–56, 1992.

8. Bortz WM: The disuse syndrome, *Western J Med* 141:691–694, 1984.

9. Corcoran PJ: Use it or lose it—the hazards of bed rest and inactivity, *Western J Med* 154:536–538, 1991.

10. Hammer RL and Kenan EH: The psychological aspects of immobilization. In Steinberg FU, editor: *The immobilized patient: functional pathology and management,* New York, 1980, Plenum Publishing Co.

11. Harper CM and Lyles YM: Physiology and complications of bed rest, *J Am Geriatr Soc* 36:1047–1054, 1988.

12. Hayes KV: *Diagnostic content validation and operational definitions of risk factors for the nursing diagnosis high risk for disuse syndrome,* doctoral dissertation, The Catholic University of America, Ann Arbor, Michigan, 1994, University Microfilms.

13. Hoenig HM and Rubenstein LZ: Hospital-associated deconditioning and dysfunction, *J Am Geriatr Soc* 39:220–222, 1991.

14. Lentz M: Selected aspects of deconditioning secondary to immobilization, *Nurs Clin No Am* 16:729–737, 1981.

15. Mobily PR and Kelley LS: Iatrogenesis in the elderly: factors of immobility, *J Geront Nurs* 17(9):5–11, 1991.

16. North American Nursing Diagnosis Association: *NANDA nursing diagnoses: definitions and classification, 1995–1996,* Philadelphia, 1994, The Association.

17. Olson EV: The hazards of immobility, *Am J Nurs* 67:779–797, 1967.

18. Rubin M: The physiology of bed rest, *Am J Nurs* 88:50–56, 1988.

19 Tyler ML: The respiratory effects of body positioning and immobilization, *Respiratory Care* 29:472–481, 1984.

20. Vorhies D and Riley BE: Deconditioning, *Clin Geriatr Med* 9:745–763, 1993.

21. Weingarden SI: The gastrointestinal system and spinal cord injury, *Physical Med Rehab Clin No Am* 3:765–781, 1992.

Diversional Activity Deficit

▶

Diversional Activity Deficit *is the state in which an individual experiences decreased stimulation from or interest or engagement in recreational or leisure activities.*[12] *It involves "a personally defined dissatisfaction with a lack of sufficient leisure-time recreational activities."*[17]

OVERVIEW

Thoughts of diversional activities conjure up images of children at play, skiing on weekends, going to movies or parties, painting, or lounging in a bathrobe doing crossword puzzles. These images are highly personal, and many favorite activities could be added to the list. The significance of these activities has not yet been studied fully, but some themes about leisure and recreation are emerging. It has been suggested that leisure activities should be studied qualitatively to determine their personal meaning.[10] For example, ethnic issues relative to leisure have been studied qualitatively by nurse researchers.[7]

Leisure has been linked to health-related self-care activities, meaning and quality of life, and life satisfaction.[4,7,13] Diversional activities for elderly persons are increasingly acknowledged as important.[15] In early life, boredom or aimlessness is usually transitory, but time can drag on for elders, who have been poorly prepared by society for meaningful leisure time. Residents in long-term care facilities value recreational activities and keeping active. Activities such as watching TV, reading, partying, listening to music programs, and taking classes have been listed as very important.[1,6] Indeed, "working hard and staying active" have been cited as important to successful aging.[11]

General diversional activity does not suit all people, however. Vogel and Mercier[19] emphasize the need in nursing homes for diversional activities that are tailored to individual interests. Similarly, Ross[16] finds that elderly persons are more satisfied with individualized recreation. Group interests, the usual focus of standard recreational programs, although important, do not necessarily fill the participants' individual needs for diversional activity.

Further support for the need to individualize diversional activities is given by Ragsdale and colleagues, who studied the quality of life of hospitalized patients with AIDS.[14] One "management style" found in this population was that of "timekeeper." These patients often report being bored while waiting for things to happen. Although the timekeepers would benefit from diversional activities, persons using other management styles had less need for such distractions to cope with hospitalization.

At the other end of the continuum from patients who have too much time and too few diversional activities are those who have too many demands on their time to fit in their usual diversional activities. Recent research with people who care for ill family members at home reveals a recurrent theme of Diversional Activity Deficit.[2,3,9,18] Caregivers find their social lives restricted because responsibilities interfere with leisure activities. Frustration and self-sacrifice are feelings associated with Diversional Activity Deficit.

From studies such as these it can be seen that, although Diversional Activity Deficit as a nursing diagnosis has received little empirical study, there is support for the importance of diversional activities in relation to the quality of life. There is also ample evidence of the importance of defining unique diversional activities for each individual.

Diversional activities are determined by individuals' use of time, their environmental opportunities, and their functional abilities. Innate in all of these factors are a person's individual perceptions and interests. Individuals define for themselves what they can or want to do with their available time and opportunities for diversion.

Use of time combines work, rest, self-care, and leisure. Leisure is time free of obligations. However, the spectrum of available leisure time is highly variable. Many persons have little leisure time, either by choice or by circumstance. Others have too much. At both ends of this continuum are patients likely to have deficits.

The environment dictates cultural patterns, available space, resources, and social opportunities for leisure activities. For example, persons with limited finances are unlikely to pursue expensive hobbies. Those who live in northern climates are more likely to be skiers than their southern counterparts. People who live in one room are unlikely to collect large objects.

Functional ability defines what one is capable of doing and the energy available for diversional activities. Someone with a mobility deficit is unlikely to be a jogger. A person with a physically demanding occupation is more likely to have a sedentary, energy-conserving hobby.

Perhaps the most important aspect of diversional activities, however, is individual interest. There is a freedom in choosing leisure activities that is not always available in work, rest, or self-care. The overriding purpose of diversional activities is personal satisfaction. A satisfying balance of time, environmental factors, and personal abilities and interests varies greatly from person to person.

When there is a lack of diversional activities, part of the very essence of a person's self-concept and feeling of self-fulfillment is affected. From a review of the above components of diversional activities, we can see that a deficit may exist when there is an excess or a lack of unobligated time. A deficit can also occur when the environment is

changed so that usual activities or resources are unavailable. Similarly, a deficit can occur when functional ability changes. Any one factor—or a combination of factors—can lead to a situation in which a patient cannot achieve the personal satisfaction of chosen diversional pursuits.

Nurses in almost any work setting come in contact with patients of all ages who have Diversional Activity Deficit. Patients with too little leisure time may be seen with stress-related illnesses in clinics, homes, or treatment centers. Patients with too much leisure time may be seen in those settings also. For example, patients receiving lengthy, passive treatments, such as dialysis, may get bored without diversional activities. Being hospitalized, except with acute illness, can leave a patient with excess unobligated time but with no diversional activity.

ASSESSMENT

Because diversional activities have meaning, purpose, and value for the patient, the nurse must be persistent in focusing assessment on the patient's perception of the situation as well as on objective data. It is important to ascertain the patient's usual pattern of diversional activities before illness or whatever change brought him or her to the health care system. This assessment data may be categorized as (1) the amount of leisure time, (2) environmental factors related to activities, (3) personal functional abilities, (4) a description of usual activities, and (5) the patient's satisfaction with those activities.

The baseline assessment in some instances can predict the severity of the patient's Diversional Activity Deficit. Jongbloed and Morgan,[8] in studying patients' leisure activities after having a stroke, find that persons with multiple interests before an illness are better able to continue an activity after the illness than those who had limited activities before an illness.

The baseline assessment can be contrasted with data from the present situation. The following questions related to available time, the environment, functional abilities, and patient interest in activities can help focus data gathering: How much unobligated time does the patient have? Does this time seem to pass slowly or fast? What are the environmental constraints in terms of space or resources? What are the patient's functional abilities or constraints, actual and perceived? What activities has the patient attempted? Have these been successful? Can the patient undertake the same activities enjoyed before the illness or change in circumstances? What would the patient like to do?

Finally, answers to these questions should be combined with an objective assessment of the patient's behavior. Look for signs of boredom, such as flat affect, frequent yawning, daytime napping, or inattentiveness. Pay attention to seemingly unwarranted hostility or restlessness. To test time perception, ask the patient to let you know when a specific amount of time (e.g., 15 minutes) has elapsed without checking a clock. Those who feel that time drags will usually indicate that the time has elapsed more quickly than actual clock time; those with very busy schedules often feel that time goes by too fast, so they will tend to indicate that the time has elapsed more slowly than actual clock time.

Related factors contributing to Diversional Activity Deficits can also be assessed in terms of available time, the environment, functional abilities, and patient interest in activities. In regard to time, there may be too little or too much leisure time. Patients with too little time may have a problem with time management or an excess of obligations on their time. Those with too much time may have recently undergone a major change, such as retirement, grown children moving out of their home, or an illness that curtailed their usual obligations and increased free time.

Environmental factors tend to be different for home-based patients than for patients in treatment centers (e.g., hospitals, long-term care settings, dialysis centers, and clinics). Home environmental factors that contribute to Diversional Activity Deficit may be limited finances, lack of transportation, social isolation, or fear of crime. A thorough assessment of a patient's living conditions will reveal these types of factors. A treatment center environment may have space and resource constraints that are actual or perceived by the patient. Very often patients assume that they cannot do certain things in a hospital when in reality they may be able to. In addition, patients may be unfamiliar with routines or what is expected of them, so that they are unsure when or how they might engage in some self-chosen diversional activity.

Assessing functional abilities will reveal personal obstacles that may be preventing patients from pursuing their usual activities or starting new ones. Some of these deficits are impaired mobility and sensory or cardiopulmonary malfunctions. If the patient is fatigued, leisure time becomes needed rest time. Depression affects time perception and adversely influences diversional activities. A patient with many problems may become apathetic about diversional activities.

Finally, assessing interest in activities may show that some patients have Diversional Activity Deficit because something is interfering with their desire or interest in diversional activities. Some patients lack exposure to or an orientation toward diversional activities. They have a strong work orientation and think that leisure activities are not desirable, and they may have difficulty defining what to do with leisure time. Others lack knowledge of their options and therefore have no interest in those things.

▪ Defining Characteristics

The presence of the following defining characteristics indicates that the patient may be experiencing Diversional Activity Deficit:

- Frequent yawning
- Flat affect
- Overeating or eating too little
- Inattentiveness
- Restlessness
- Daytime napping (seemingly unwarranted)

IV

- Hostility or irritation
- Perception of time passing slowly
- Perception of time passing too quickly
- Statement of boredom
- Statement of missing recreational activity
- Statement of frustration
- Little or no unobligated time
- Increase in unobligated time
- No pattern of leisure activities
- Previous leisure activities impossible after illness or life change
- No substitute activities defined after illness or life change
- Statement of desire for something to do
- Unavailability (actual or perceived) of resources for desired activity
- Confined space
- Disinterest in television
- Refusal to attend planned recreational programs
- Selective attendance at planned recreational programs

■ Related Factors

The following related factors are associated with Diversional Activity Deficit:

Time factors
- Problematic time management
- Excess obligations on time
- Decrease in obligated time/increase in available unobligated time
- Major life change such as retirement, children leaving home, or long-term illness

Environmental factors
- Home-based patients: limited finances, lack of transportation, social isolation, and fear of crime
- Treatment-center-based patients: space constraints, lack of resources, and unfamiliarity with routines or expectations

Functional abilities
- Impaired mobility
- Activity intolerance
- Impaired senses or pain
- Impaired cardiopulmonary functions

- Fatigue
- Depression or lack of motivation
- Apathy
- Loneliness
- Maturational factors (e.g., a child who has no toys)

Interest in activities
- Lack of exposure or orientation to diversional activities
- Lack of knowledge of options
- Personal preferences at odds with available options

DIAGNOSIS

■ Differential Nursing Diagnosis

Many of the nursing diagnoses in the NANDA taxonomy "Relating" pattern can be likely conclusions for persons who have Diversional Activity Deficit. Social Isolation, for example, can contribute to a deficit in diversional activity. Caregiver Role Strain might manifest itself as Diversional Activity Deficit. The nurse needs to decide which is the primary diagnosis in these situations. One diagnosis might well be a related factor for the other. Similarly, several diagnoses in the "Choosing" pattern closely resemble Diversional Activity Deficit. Impaired Adjustment or Ineffective Individual Coping might be seen in patients whose lives have changed so that usual recreational activities are curtailed. Decisional Conflict might be found in patients who cannot decide if they should focus on the seemingly selfish need for diversion or on altruistic tasks such as caring for others.

■ Medical and Psychiatric Diagnoses

Any illness that curtails usual patterns of personally relevant diversional activities can contribute to deficits in this response. Diseases affecting the senses, such as blindness, could leave a patient incapable of engaging in usual activities. Diseases that restrict mobility, such as multiple sclerosis, spinal cord injuries, chronic obstructive pulmonary diseases, congestive heart failure, or arthritis, will curtail usual activities. Psychological illnesses, such as depression, might make a patient disinterested in usual activities. Illnesses requiring patient confinement for long periods of time for treatment, such as renal failure or cancer, can cause boredom.

OUTCOME IDENTIFICATION, PLANNING, AND IMPLEMENTATION

The essential principle of care for the patient with Diversional Activity Deficit is that interventions to correct the deficit must be personally meaningful. The patient's perception of the deficit in relation to usual patterns of activity must provide the groundwork for planning a new or adapted activity. Turning on a television for a patient who is bored is not enough. Telling the patient with the busy schedule to relax more is not enough. An expected outcome for the patient is exploring the personal meaning of usual or desirable diversional activities. The nurse can help the patient break down usual activities into meaningful components by prompting. The patient can be asked, "What is it about (the activity) that you like?" For the skier, is it movement, the speed, the outdoors, the solitary challenge, or the hot chocolate afterwards? For the antique collector, is it the history, the hunt, or the contemplation of the object itself? Such analysis will help broaden the patient's options in choosing a new or adapted activity because it focuses on the components that are gratifying to the patient more than on the activity itself. Similar or related activities may then be chosen and still be personally meaningful.

Another expected outcome is that the patient is able to choose a desired diversional activity that can be engaged in now. To meet this outcome the nurse should focus on the positive, or what the patient is able to do. Patients may tend to focus on what they cannot do, especially if an illness has radically changed their functional abilities. The nurse can prompt thinking along these positive lines without actually making a choice for the patient. This can be accomplished by asking questions such as, "What other activities might meet the need that you met with your usual activity?" Further prompting may be needed. The nurse can avoid suggesting an actual activity by listing possible categories of activities, such as music, games, arts, and crafts. Whenever possible, it is best if the patient can choose an activity related to one enjoyed in the past.

All too often, especially in hospitals, patients think they cannot engage in chosen activities because they have little say in the daily routine. It is imperative that nurses orient patients to routines and let them know what is within their control and what aspects of the environment can be adapted for their use. Allowing patients to control the environment means that nurses must be willing to be flexible and to acknowledge the value of diversional activities. Nurses must be willing to allow patients to choose to do unusual things, such as painting a watercolor during the morning, when the light is best in the room but a bath is scheduled, even if this means that the bath must be rescheduled for the afternoon. Or the nurse may allow the patient to set up Tibetan bells in a private area and to have an hour of uninterrupted time to chant daily.

After the patient chooses an activity, the nurse may help obtain resources or adapt the environment to the activity. Again, to promote personally meaningful activities, the nurse should encourage the patient to identify needed resources and, if possible, ways to obtain them. Getting resources may be simple or complex. If a patient has little leisure time but would like to have a quiet half hour each day for listening to music, counseling the patient about time management may be needed to set aside that half hour.

Finally, the nurse must not assume the problem is resolved once the patient is busy with a project. The patient must be allowed to have a change of mind if other or additional activities are desired. Remembering the principle that diversional activities must be personally meaningful, the nurse must allow for the patient's evaluation of the success of the activity.

IV

◢ **NURSING CARE GUIDELINES**
Nursing Diagnosis: Diversional Activity Deficit

Expected Outcome: The patient will identify the personal meaning of diversional activities.
- Encourage the patient to discuss usual or desired diversional activities. *Diversional activities are personally meaningful to each individual.*
- Prompt the patient to analyze usual activities in terms of components that are meaningful (e.g., ask, "What is it about this activity that you like?"). *A focus on the meaning rather than the activity itself will allow the patient to consider related activities that could provide similar satisfaction when usual activities are curtailed.*

Expected Outcome: The patient will choose a desired diversional activity in which he or she can engage.
- Focus on the positive more than the negative (e.g., say, "You can do this" rather than "You can't do that"). *Patients dealing with illness and change may initially see the negative aspects more than the positive possibilities.*
- Encourage the patient to choose an activity related to usual activities whenever possible. *Personal meaning is found in usual diversional activities.*
- Use prompting rather than actually suggesting a specific activity (e.g., ask, "What other activities might meet the need that you met with your usual activity?"). *Activities will be more personally meaningful if the patient identifies them rather than the nurse.*
- If necessary, prompt the patient's imagination by suggesting activities such as music, games, arts, crafts, physical exercise, toys, reading, writing, change of scene or routine, companionship, video or audio programs, talking, and productive chores (e.g., sorting and cleaning). *Sometimes patients cannot think of any possibilities because they are overwhelmed by their present restrictions.*
- For overstressed patients with little leisure time, assist them in setting activity priorities. *Some people need "permission" to engage in diversional activities because they may perceive such activities as selfish and less important than other demands on their time.*
- Orient patients to routines of care and describe areas that are within their control and routines that can be adapted for their use. *A full range of possible activities will be more evident if patients know the routines and what is expected of them in their present situation.*

Expected Outcome: The patient will satisfactorily engage in chosen diversional activities.
- Have the patient identify needed resources and assist in obtaining those resources. *Provide for the patient's control of the situation as much as possible to promote personal meaning.*
- Adapt the environment as necessary. *This will show the patient that the activity is a valued part of care.*
- If needed, teach time-management or stress-management strategies to optimize the opportunity for diversional activities for those with little leisure time. *Diversional activities may be seen as luxuries and as low priorities by patients with excessive demands on their time. The value of diversional activities, when communicated by the nurse, will give the patient "permission" to include them in daily life.*
- Allow for change of plans if an activity is unsatisfactory. *Personal satisfaction is vital; because the activity may be adapted from usual activities, the modified activity may not always work to the patient's satisfaction.*

■ = nursing intervention; ▲ = collaborative intervention.

EVALUATION

Evaluation of the effectiveness of the interventions centers on three patient outcomes: (1) Has the patient been able to identify the personal meaning of diversional activities? (2) Has an activity been chosen? (3) Was it successfully implemented by the patient?

More than the actual pursuit of an activity, the personal meaning of the pursued activity is the key to successful interventions. The patient who was bored but is now watching television may still be bored because television is not a personally meaningful diversion. However, the patient who identifies carpentry as a usual leisure activity and is watching a television program on renovating old houses may be experiencing a meaningful diversion. That same person, even in a hospital bed, may try small-scale wood carving to round out a set of activities, all of which relate to the usual meaningful activity of carpentry.

The important component of evaluation is asking the patient about satisfaction with the diversional activity and not merely focusing on the fact that the patient is doing something. If the patient is not satisfied, planning for other diversional activities is needed.

▶ CASE STUDY WITH PLAN OF CARE

Mr. Frank F. is a 46-year-old African-American construction foreman who recently started outpatient hemodialysis treatments three times a week because of chronic renal failure secondary to diabetic nephropathy. An internal arteriovenous fistula in his left arm is used as access for dialysis. Physically he has been tolerating the dialysis treatments well, with only mild dizziness at the end of each session. The nurses noted, however, that increasingly Mr. F. gets irritated about an hour into the treatment. He calls to the nurses often to check the machine or his blood pressure, both of which are normal. He frequently turns the channel selector on his TV set but doesn't seem to watch anything for long. Because he doesn't feel well enough to drive after dialysis, Mr. F.'s wife brings him to the dialysis center during her lunch hour at noon on Monday, Wednesday, and Friday; she returns after work to pick him up at 6:00 P.M. His treatment is scheduled from 1:00 to 6:00 P.M.

When asked about his usual routines, Mr. F. reports that his greatest joy is fishing with his 13-year-old son. Because his job is stressful (he still works 30 hours per week), he likes the quiet of this sport. Between fishing trips he designs and ties flies. He doesn't watch much television except for old movies at night, and he doesn't read much except for sporting magazines. When asked how he feels about the dialysis treatments, he replies, "It's better than dying, so I'm adjusting. It's just that these 5 hours seem to drag on and on. I can't read magazines and watch TV that long."

▶ PLAN OF CARE FOR MR. FRANK F.
Nursing Diagnosis: Diversional Activity Deficit Related to Long Hours of Treatment and Relative Immobility During Treatment

Expected Outcome: Mr. F. will identify the personal meaning of his usual diversional activities, fishing and tieing flies.
- Encourage Mr. F. to discuss fishing and fly tieing in detail.
- Ask Mr. F. to list what parts of these activities are most meaningful to him.
- Prompt Mr. F.'s thinking if necessary, using reminders of fishing (e.g., the solitude, nature watching, the fish, the beauty of the surroundings, the timing of the catch, the testing of various flies, and the creativity of the flies).

Expected Outcome: Mr. F. will choose a desired diversional activity in which he can engage.
- Focus on what Mr. F. can do with one hand and his senses while sitting for 5 hours rather than on what he cannot do.
- Encourage Mr. F. to analyze the meaningful aspects of fishing and fly tieing and to identify other activities that have similar meaning.

■ = nursing intervention; ▲ = collaborative intervention.   *Continued*

IV

▶ PLAN OF CARE FOR MR. FRANK F. — CONT'D

- If necessary, prompt Mr. F. with ideas related to his analysis, such as listening to a tape of water sounds, playing a magnetic fishing game, drawing plans for flies with colored pencils, tying flies with the assistance of a clamp on a table, writing fishing stories, or watching fish in a tank. (Use specific suggestions sparingly until he begins to list possibilities.)
- Let Mr. F. know what areas of the environment could be adapted for his use (e.g., moving a larger table close by, allowing him time to set up before hooking up the machine, and providing periods of uninterrupted time).

Expected Outcome: Mr. F. will satisfactorily engage in a chosen diversional activity.
- Have Mr. F. identify needed resources and plan with him how to obtain them.
- Adapt the environment as needed for the chosen activity.
- Observe Mr. F. for initial frustrations with attempts to adapt the environment, and assist him as much as possible. If frustrations are noted, discuss these with him.
- Let Mr. F. know that making changes in plans for diversional activities or adding new activities is possible.

▦ CRITICAL THINKING EXERCISES

1. Describe resources available in the community that could be used to support Mr. F.'s choice of diversional activities. Be specific in specifying personal and material resources.
2. Why is Diversional Activity Deficit often overlooked as a nursing diagnosis?
3. Spend more time thinking about your personal diversional activities. What is the personal meaning of them? If you could not engage in these activities, how would you feel? Could you adapt them to something you could do if you were confined to a wheelchair?

REFERENCES

1. Aller LJ and Van Ess Coeling H: Quality of life: its meaning to the long-term care resident, *J Geront Nurs* 21(2):20–25, 1995.
2. Beach DL: Gerontological caregiving analysis of family experience, *J Geront Nurs* 19(12):35–41, 1993.
3. Boykin A and Winland-Brown J: The dark side of caring: challenges of caregiving, *J Geront Nurs* 21(5):13–18, 1995.
4. Burbank PM: an exploratory study: assessing the meaning in life among older adult clients, *J Geront Nurs* 18(9):19–28, 1992.
5. Chin-Sang V and Allen KR: Leisure and the older black woman, *J Geront Nurs* 17(1):30–34, 1991.
6. Daley OE: Women's strategies for living in a nursing home, *J Geront Nurs* 19(9):5–9, 1993.
7. Hartweg DL: Self-care actions of healthy middle-aged women to promote well-being, *Nurs Res* 42:221–227, 1993.
8. Jongbloed L and Morgan D: An investigation of involvement in leisure activities after a stroke, *Am J Occup Ther* 45:420–427, 1991.
9. Krach P and Brooks JA: Identifying the responsibilities and needs of working adults who are primary caregivers, *J Geront Nurs* 21(10):41–45, 1995.
10. Krefting L and Krefting D: Leisure activities after a stroke: an ethnographic approach, *Am J Occup Ther* 45:429–436, 1991.
11. Laferriere RH and Hamel-Bissell BP: Successful aging of oldest old women in the northeast kingdom of Vermont, *Image* 26:319–321, 1994.
12. North American Nursing Diagnosis Association: *NANDA nursing diagnoses: definitions and classification, 1995–1996*, Philadelphia, 1994, The Association.
13. Porter EJ: Older widows' experience of living alone at home, *Image* 26:19–24, 1994.
14. Ragsdale D, Kotarba JA, and Morrow JR: Quality of life of hospitalized persons with AIDS, *Image* 24:259–265, 1992.
15. Rantz M: Diversional activity deficit. In Maas M, Buckwalter UC, and Hardy M, editors: *Nursing diagnoses and interventions for the elderly*, Redwood City, California, 1991, Addison-Wesley Nursing.
16. Ross M: Time-use in later life, *J Adv Nurs* 15:394–399, 1990.
17. Rubenfeld MG: Diversional activity deficit. In Thompson J and others, editors: *Mosby's clinical nursing*, ed 3, St. Louis, 1993, Mosby–Year Book.
18. Sayles-Cross S: Perceptions of familial caregivers of elder adults, *Image* 25:88–92, 1993.
19. Vogel CH and Mercier J: The effect of institutionalization on nursing home populations, *J Geront Nurs* 17(3):30–34, 1991.

Dysreflexia

▶

Dysreflexia is the state in which an individual with a spinal cord injury at the seventh thoracic vertebra (T7) or above experiences a life-threatening, uninhibited sympathetic response of the nervous system to a noxious stimulus.[6]

OVERVIEW

To understand Dysreflexia one must understand the basic mechanisms of the normal autonomic nervous system and its two divisions, the sympathetic and the parasympathetic. The sympathetic division reacts to noxious stimuli by accelerating the "fight or flight" reflex of the human system. The parasympathetic division assists the body by counteracting the sympathetic response and returning the body to homeostasis.[2]

The sympathetic nervous system controls chemical neurotransmitters to accelerate the heart rate, constrict blood vessels, increase blood pressure and muscle blood volume, shunt blood from nonvital areas, increase energy by liver glycolysis, and increase mental activity. The parasympathetic nervous system helps the body relax by slowing the heart rate, increasing intestinal peristalsis and glandular activity, and relaxing sphincter control.

In individuals with spinal cord injury (SCI) at the seventh thoracic vertebra (T7) or higher, this mechanism is no longer intact. Basically the spinal cord lesion obstructs neurotransmission from below T7 up to the vasomotor centers of the nervous system. The parasympathetic neurons located in the gray matter of the sacral cord and in the brain stem are above and below the level of injury, whereas the neurons of the sympathetic system are located only below the level of injury.[2]

A major concept in Dysreflexia is that the sympathetic system information goes virtually undetected in an individual with SCI, but the parasympathetic system response provides observable and detectable signs and symptoms. Therefore the human system works without its normal protective checks and balances for maintaining homeostasis.

This is particularly crucial in regard to the autonomic reflexes. These reflexes are homeostatic and involuntary neurological processes. Such sympathetic reflexes regulate the body's cardiovascular, gastrointestinal, and bladder systems. These visceral functions are also the major concerns in Dysreflexia. If problems arise in any of the reflex areas, the normal sympathetic reflex occurs along with its parasympathetic counterpart. The result is the symptoms and problems of autonomic Dysreflexia in patients with SCI.[4]

ASSESSMENT

The nurse's role in the assessment process is to determine which patients will experience Dysreflexia. In 85% of the cases, individuals with SCI at T7 or above are likely to be affected.[1] Therefore it is essential that patients receive instruction in symptom recognition, causative factors, and treatment.

The nurse needs to know if the patient has a history of Dysreflexia. If so, the patient will be aware of his or her own unique set of symptoms and causative factors and the plan for their prevention and treatment. Patients with a new injury or experiencing a first episode of Dysreflexia will need the nurse to explain the relevance of the signs and symptoms they might experience and to help iden-

IV

tify the cause. These symptoms, if prolonged, can lead to seizures, cerebral hemorrhage, myocardial infarction, and death.[2] Therefore it is crucial that, while the nurse assesses the patient, intervention occurs simultaneously. The assessment must include the identification of the causative factors of Dysreflexia. Dysreflexia should be diagnosed by assessing for the presence of defining characteristics and related factors, alleviating the cause, and returning the patient to the baseline condition.

■ Defining Characteristics

The presence of the following defining characteristics indicates that the patient may be experiencing Dysreflexia:

- Spinal cord injury at T7 or above
- Paroxysmal hypertension (i.e., sudden, periodic elevated blood pressure where systolic pressure is over 140 mm Hg and diastolic is above 90 mm Hg)
- Bradycardia or tachycardia (i.e., pulse rate of less than 60 or more than 100 beats per minute)
- Diaphoresis (above the injury)
- Red splotches on skin (above the injury)
- Pallor (below the injury)
- Headache (i.e., a diffuse pain in different portions of the head and not confined to any nerve distribution area)

■ Related Factors

The following related factors are associated with Dysreflexia:

- Bladder distention
- Bowel distention
- Skin irritation
- Lack of knowledge by patient and caregiver

DIAGNOSIS

■ Differential Nursing Diagnosis

Dysreflexia is its own unique diagnosis and should not be confused with medical conditions such as hypertensive crisis or cardiac arrhythmias such as tachycardia or bradycardia. The major difference is that Dysreflexia can be resolved by elim-

inating the causative factor or noxious stimulus. After the cause is eliminated, the patient's blood pressure and heart rate will return to the baseline level.

■ Medical and Psychiatric Diagnoses

The related medical diagnosis for Dysreflexia is spinal cord injury at the seventh thoracic vertebra (T7) or above. Patients with this diagnosis must be assessed for factors related to the cause of Dysreflexia.

OUTCOME IDENTIFICATION, PLANNING, AND IMPLEMENTATION

Nursing interventions for Dysreflexia include assessment of symptoms and related factors, diagnosis, relief intervention, medication administration, education, precautions for prevention, and wellness planning. The nurse may assist the physician in the management of dysreflexic crisis and in addressing related factors such as bladder and bowel programs.

Dysreflexia creates a hypertensive crisis that can produce seizures, cerebral hemorrhage, and possibly death. The patient must not reach this climactic point. When Dysreflexia presents, the nurse's first action is to support the reversal of the hypertensive state and to lower cerebral pressures by elevating the patient's head at last 45° or, if possible, by placing the patient in an upright sitting position. The patient's vital signs are monitored at least every 5 minutes until the cause is determined and alleviated and the vital signs return to baseline levels. The nurse notifies the physician of the hypertensive emergency, administers ordered medications, and assists with the prevention of complications. After the patient's safety has been assured, interventions are directed toward identifying and resolving the causative factor of Dysreflexia.[4]

Visceral stimuli that may prompt occurrences of Dysreflexia are classified and prioritized according to the most common causes: (1) bladder distention, (2) bowel distention, and (3) skin irritation. All patient outcomes focus on freeing the patient of all related factors.

Bladder distention is typically the most common cause of Dysreflexia and is the easiest to resolve; all nursing interventions are focused on emptying the bladder. Patients with SCI, because of their impaired ability to void, are on bladder treatment plans.

The nurse must verify the patency of any urinary adjunctive equipment. The patient's bladder treatment plan may include a Foley or suprapubic catheter, a condom catheter, or an intermittent catheterization program. All tubing must be checked for twisting, kinks, or other obstructions to urinary flow.[3] Catheter irrigation can validate the tube's patency. If the catheter is obstructed, it is removed and replaced immediately and the bladder emptied. Although irrigation of an obstructed catheter may facilitate urine flow and bladder emptying, the catheter should be replaced with a new one to prevent recurrence of an obstruction and Dysreflexia.[7]

For a patient on an intermittent catheterization program, catheterization needs to be performed to determine the patient's bladder volume. A large bladder volume may necessitate a modification in the patient's catheterization program. The frequency of catheterization may need to be increased and schedules changed (e.g., from every 6 hours to every 4), or the patient may require fluid restriction to prevent excess urinary volume and potential bladder distention.

The patient must not experience any additional bladder stimulation during bladder catheterization and interventions. To prevent this, the nurse applies lidocaine jelly 2% as a lubricant for the tube insertion; the jelly will act to anesthetize the urethra and reduce stimulation caused by manipulation.

If the bladder assessment and interventions do not resolve the Dysreflexia symptoms, the next potential source of visceral stimuli must be assessed (i.e., the bowel). The patient is assessed for constipation or hard stools. It is essential that patients with SCI have a regulated scheme for bowel care because this is a limitation of the disability. The patient's bowel should be empty and not distended with stool.

The nurse can physically assess the bowel by digital examination of the rectum and lower colon.

Nupercainal ointment should be ordered, placed around the rectum, and used as a lubricant for the examining finger. Nupercainal ointment acts as an anesthetic and reduces any further stimulation of the bowel during the examination. If the bowel is distended and stool is present, the nurse digitally removes any impaction. If the patient's vital signs are stable, digital rectal stimulation and cleansing enemas may facilitate bowel emptying. The bowel program then needs modification in relation to frequency of defecation, oral administration of stool softeners, and diet control.

If the bladder and bowel are not the cause of Dysreflexia, the nurse then seeks to rule out skin stimulation as the related factor. Skin stimulation can result from constrictive clothing, the lack of relief from pressure caused by infrequent changes of position, the presence of skin insults such as decubitus ulcers, and thermal exposures. The skin should be free of any adverse stimulation.[2]

The nurse should observe for any skin redness or indentations, sores, burns, or early signs of skin breakdown. The nurse should assess the fit of any straps, splints, casts, or any item that can result in pain or skin insult.[2] The nurse's role in intervention is treatment and the prevention of further painful stimuli to the skin. Wounds are kept clean, dry, and free of infection. Analgesics should be administered to prevent pain and potential visceral stimulation. Because thermoregulation is altered in a patient with SCI, the patient will be sensitive to extremes of heat and cold. Such exposure can result in visceral stimulation caused by shivering or by the body's response to any sudden temperature change.

Emergency episodes of Dysreflexia are managed by physicians. Pharmacological agents may be ordered on a single-episode basis or for permanent prophylaxis. Hydralazine hydrochloride (Apresoline) may be injected for life-threatening hypertension. Nifedipine (Procardia) may be given sublingually in urgent hypertension or orally to prevent further occurrences. Mecamylamine hydrochloride (Inversine) is another preferred oral agent.[5]

The nurse's major role in Dysreflexia is to prevent its recurrence. It is essential that the patient

IV

and family be taught how to solve problems independently for any aspect of the care and prevention of Dysreflexia. Teaching should include the signs, symptoms, and treatment of Dysreflexia as well as bladder, bowel, and skin care techniques. Teaching needs to be specific yet flexible to match lifestyles and to allow self-maintenance and self-control.

◢ **NURSING CARE GUIDELINES**
Nursing Diagnosis: Dysreflexia

Expected Outcome: The patient's blood pressure will be stabilized within 20 minutes.
- Elevate the head of the patient's bed at least 45° or, if possible, place patient in an upright sitting position. *This will decrease cerebral pressures and prevent cerebral hemorrhage.*
- ▲ Notify physician of the patient's hypertensive emergency and administer prescribed medications. *The blood pressure must be returned to the baseline level to prevent cerebral hemorrhage.*
- Institute seizure precautions. *This is done to prevent injury.*
- Monitor patient's vital signs until the cause of the Dysreflexia has been determined and alleviated and the patient's vital signs have returned to baseline levels. *Continued elevation of vital signs may require aggressive medication orders by the physician.*
- Assess the patient for presence of visceral stimulation and institute interventions directed toward relieving such stimulation. *The related factor and stimulus for Dysreflexia must be eliminated to prevent seizures, strokes, and possibly cardiopulmonary arrest.*

Expected Outcome: The patient's bladder distention will be eliminated within 20 minutes.
- Assess for bladder fullness *to determine this as a factor.*
- Assess patency of the urinary equipment; correct any problem that may be interfering with bladder emptying and free urinary flow.
- If the patient does not have an indwelling catheter and if bladder is distended, the patient should be catheterized. *The bladder needs to be emptied as quickly as possible to prevent complications.*
- After the acute episode, monitor fluid intake and output, modify or develop an individualized bladder program; frequently assess and evaluate program effectiveness.

Expected Outcome: The patient's bowel distention will be eliminated within 25 minutes.
- Review patient's bowel history and assess for bowel distention or presence of impaction.
- If the patient is impacted, remove stool. *This is done to eliminate the visceral stimuli and the cause of Dysreflexia.*
- ▲ An ointment such as Nupercainal should be ordered and used when examining the rectum or removing the impaction. *This medication anesthetizes the rectum, preventing further noxious stimulation.*
- ▲ Assess the need for diet change and discuss possible changes with the patient and the dietitian *to maximize bowel motility.*
- ▲ Assess the need for a cleansing enema and, if needed, obtain an order and administer the enema *to expedite stool removal.*
- ▲ Assess the need for stool softeners. *If the stool is too hard it may be too difficult for the patient to pass.* If necessary, obtain order for softeners and administer.

Expected Outcome: The patient's skin will be free of pressure and irritation within 30 minutes.
- Inspect the patient's skin and fit of clothing. Remove any restrictive clothing or appliances. *Tight clothing can be a noxious stimulus, producing Dysreflexia.*
- Control the patient's exposure to temperature extremes indoors.
- After the acute episode, keep wounds dry and clean, assess skin for any breakdown and infection, and teach patient to monitor fit of clothing and appliances.

■ = nursing intervention; ▲ = collaborative intervention.

EVALUATION

The clinical evaluation of Dysreflexia is based on the resolution of the crisis episode and the prevention of its recurrence. The key evaluation criterion is the patient's performance in recognizing and independently resolving any acute events and in preventing future episodes. The long-term goal is for the patient to maintain wellness and to achieve it independently.

Short-term evaluation is based on the effectiveness of the teaching plan and the achievement of its goals. Patients should be able to demonstrate an understanding of the identifying characteristics of Dysreflexia, the steps to resolve and prevent episodes, bowel and bladder programs, fluid restriction, catheterization and defecation techniques, and complications.

Dysreflexia is a lifelong concern for the individual with SCI. It is a complex health issue. The nurse plays a major role in assisting these individuals in maintaining wellness and independence in a disabled state.

IV

▶ CASE STUDY WITH PLAN OF CARE

Mr. Virgil W. is admitted to the rehabilitation center for independent living skill training. He is 41 years old. He works as a computer operator but has not been employed since his car accident 4 months ago. He owns an inaccessible two-story dwelling, where he lives alone. His medical history includes an injury at the T3 level of the spinal column; otherwise his history is unremarkable. Physical examination reveals a flushed face and warm skin. The patient complains of a throbbing headache. An indwelling Foley catheter leads to a leg bag. The bag is empty of urine. His blood pressure is 200/100 mm Hg; pulse is 60 beats per minute and regular; respirations are 14 per min; and oral temperature is 98.6°F. The patient has daily bowel movements.

▶ PLAN OF CARE FOR MR. VIRGIL W.
Nursing Diagnosis: Dysreflexia Related to Inability to Empty Bladder

---

Expected Outcome: Mr. W.'s blood pressure will be within normal limits within 20 minutes.
- Place Mr. W. in upright sitting position.
- Assess and monitor vital signs every 5 minutes until episode resolves.
- ▲ Notify physician of assessment findings.
- ▲ Administer medications as ordered.

Expected Outcome: Mr. W.'s bladder will be empty and his urinary equipment will be functional within 20 minutes.
- Assess Mr. W.'s catheter and tubing for patency.
- Have Mr. W. empty his bladder; if he is unable to do so, catheterize patient.
- Reassess Mr. W. for status of symptoms, if symptoms continue.

Expected Outcome: Mr. W. will experience a decrease in frequency of episodes of Dysreflexia within 2 days.
- Assist Mr. W. in developing a bladder treatment program that eliminates bladder distention.
- Working with Mr. W., monitor his progress related to program adherence and make revisions to the program as needed.

■ = nursing intervention; ▲ = collaborative intervention.   *Continued*

IV

▶ PLAN OF CARE FOR MR. VIRGIL W. — CONT'D

Expected Outcome: Mr. W. will describe the symptoms of Dysreflexia and its treatment within 3 days.
- Teach Mr. W. signs and treatment measures of Dysreflexia.
- Encourage Mr. W. to ask questions.
- Provide written material supporting the verbal information given to Mr. W.
- Ask Mr. W. to describe the signs and symptoms of Dysreflexia.
- Have Mr. W. demonstrate interventions he may use to prevent or control an episode of Dysreflexia.

▦ CRITICAL THINKING EXERCISES

1. What other factors in the case study need to be addressed for Mr. W. to continue living independently in his home?
2. Knowing that Mr. W. is going home alone, what equipment does he need at home to resolve an episode of Dysreflexia independently?
3. What prescription medications will Mr. W. need at home to manage an episode of Dysreflexia?
4. What guidance would you give Mr. W. about reporting Dysreflexia events to his physician?
5. What recommendations would you make about diet control for preventing Dysreflexia?

REFERENCES

1. Ceron G and Rakowski-Reinhart A: Action stat! Autonomic dysreflexia, *Nursing* 21:33, 1991.
2. Chancellor MB and others: Prospective evaluation of terazosin for the treatment of autonomic dysreflexia, *J Urol* 151:111–113, January 1994.
3. Chang C, Chen M, and Chang L: Autonomic hyperreflexia in spinal cord injury patient during percutaneous nephrolithotomy for renal stone: a case report, *J Urol* 146:1601–1602, December 1991.
4. Finocchiaro DN and Herzfeld ST: Understanding autonomic dysreflexia, *Am J Nurs* 90:56–59, September 1990.
5. Kabalin JN and others: Incidence and management of autonomic dysreflexia and other intraoperative problems encountered in spinal cord injury patients undergoing extracorporeal shock wave lithotripsy without anesthesia on a second generation lithotriptor, *J Urol* 149:1064–1067, May 1993.
6. North American Nursing Diagnosis Association: *NANDA nursing diagnoses: definitions and classification, 1995–1996,* Philadelphia, 1994, The Association.
7. Trop CS and Bennett CJ: Autonomic dysreflexia and its urological implications: a review, *J Urol* 146:1461–1469, December 1991.

Fatigue

▶─────────────────────────────────

Fatigue *is the overwhelming, sustained sense of exhaustion and decreased capacity for physical and mental work.*[12]

OVERVIEW

Fatigue is a universal complaint that occurs with almost every illness, mental or physical.[5] Until recently, however, scant literature contributed to understanding its nature. It has been estimated that the rate of unexplained Fatigue in primary care patients may be as high as 20%.[14]

Historical accounts of fatigue were seldom reported before the second half of the nineteenth century. At that time an epidemic of Fatigue spread mainly among women of the middle and upper classes, rendering countless of them bedridden with complaints of Fatigue and weakness. Reports of debilitating Fatigue multiplied greatly from 1870 to 1900; the epidemic spread to virtually every country in Western society. Curiously, the wave of chronic Fatigue ebbed around the time of the First World War.[13]

In the 1980s chronic mononucleosis, or chronic Epstein-Barr virus (EBV) infection, drew media attention. Patients who suffered unexplained Fatigue and a prolonged attack of acute mononucleosis often received the diagnosis of chronic EBV infection or Epstein-Barr virus syndrome. However, EB viral serological tests were shown to be of little diagnostic value because of (a) poor reproducibility within and among laboratories and the serological associations between the syndrome and (b) other viruses such as cytomegalovirus and *Herpes simplex*.[6]

Chronic fatigue syndrome (CFS) was formally defined in the literature in 1988 to describe a syndrome of disabling Fatigue lasting longer than 6 months and associated with a variable number of physical and psychological symptoms. The syndrome usually occurs sporadically, but occasionally manifests in outbreaks. Females comprise the majority of cases; age at presentation is between 20 and 50 years, with a median of 36 years.[1] The cause of CFS is still poorly understood, although an infectious etiology is still a possibility. Many studies point to immune function defects, although in most cases few findings have been reproducible.[9] Attempts at treatment have included such pharmacological agents as antidepressants, antivirals, immune modifiers, immunosuppressants, vitamins, and minerals.

Fatigue is also a central feature in fibromyalgia, a rheumatological condition gaining increasing notoriety in the literature. It is estimated that 6% to 11% of patients in medical clinics exhibit presenting symptoms of fibromyalgia; the rate of hospitalizations for these patients is higher than that for rheumatoid arthritis.[7] This chronic rheumatic disorder affects middle-aged women, who typically complain of generalized musculoskeletal pain and widespread but localized tender points. Fatigue is a very prominent feature seen in 75% of fibromyalgia patients along with the problem of unrefreshed sleep.[11]

The inexplicable Fatigue in both CFS and fibromyalgia has been studied in relation to altered sleep patterns. A sleep study comparing 14 fibromyalgia patients with control subjects demonstrated increased wakefulness, reduced sleep efficiency, and a decreased percentage of slow wave and REM sleep among fibromyalgia patients.[2] Similarly, sleep study data from 14 CFS patients revealed a prominent, alpha-wave, non-REM sleep disturbance not unlike that reported in fibromyalgia patients.[4]

Moderate to severe Fatigue has been recognized as a major problem in most patients with systemic lupus erythematosus (SLE).[10] According to many SLE patients, Fatigue seems to be directly related to disease activity. This finding was borne out in a study in which Fatigue in SLE patients was found to be significantly associated with depression and disease activity and also with the patient's perception of disease. That is, patients who perceived their disease to be more active also felt more Fatigue.[8]

The economic and personal effects related to Fatigue in these and other conditions are great. The economic impact of Fatigue was calculated in Australia, where the health care system facilitates estimates of the financial impact of illness. Fatigue cost the country $59 million per year, or approximately $9429 per afflicted individual.[3] The personal impact of Fatigue on the patient is also striking. Because Fatigue is subjective and difficult to measure, some still regard it to be a psychological problem. Studies of Fatigue almost always include a tool to assess the presence of depression. Fatigue versus depression remains as controversial as the chicken and the egg metaphor.

Fatigue can have a profound effect on patients' lives. In one study, Fatigue adversely affected the ability of one group of chronically ill patients to maintain full-time employment and perform acceptably on the job. Fatigue also can affect family relationships, because Fatigue can make it virtually impossible to fulfill the many roles society places on individuals. Moreover, the number and types of social activities and commitments dwindle greatly because of Fatigue. One patient stated, "Limiting activities is an effective mechanism against Fatigue, but it can also be a defense mechanism, resulting in reclusiveness. I have not developed many friendships, so I am not asked out and don't have to say no."[8]

Fatigue can accompany acute and chronic illnesses. In acute illness, Fatigue is usually self-limiting and will abate when the acute phases of illness pass. In chronic illness, however, Fatigue may be ubiquitous and distress the patient as much as the chronic illness itself.

ASSESSMENT

The diagnosis Fatigue usually cannot be attributed to one single cause; rather, it involves a constellation of related factors. Because Fatigue is subjective, its identification, extent, and effect must come from the patient. The nurse should seek information about the related factors associated with Fatigue during assessment. Data related to current or recent illnesses, emotional stress, medication regimen, anemia, sleep disorders, and altered nutritional status are especially important.

The relationship between Fatigue and illness must be determined during assessment. Whether to encourage rest or physical activity will depend on the nature and extent of illness. The nurse can determine this by considering the following questions: Is the illness acute or chronic? Is it inflammatory or degenerative, or is it a viral infection? In the patient's view, how does the Fatigue that has been experienced relate to the illness? Is Fatigue experienced all the time, or does it wax and wane?

The nurse must also assess for the presence of emotional stressors and depression, because the diagnosis of a chronic illness can be physically and emotionally traumatic. In many cases, trying to cope with an illness that can disrupt virtually all aspects of one's life can cause situational depression. Allowing the patient to explain the meaning that this illness has for him or her may provide some insight into emotional stress or depression.

Various medications have been known to cause Fatigue. Antihypertensives, including beta blockers and calcium channel blockers, may be suspect. Tranquilizers, alcohol, muscle relaxants, and soporifics should be considered potential contributors. Corticosteroids taken in high doses over prolonged periods of time can cause myopathy and muscle wasting, making physical activity more difficult.

Iron deficiency anemia, deficiencies of certain vitamins such as folate and B_{12}, and anemia related to chronic disease will readily cause Fatigue. Assess the laboratory data to determine if an anemia is present. The nurse should also ask about the patient's sleep patterns, keeping in mind that people generally evaluate the quality of their sleep based on (1) how long it takes to fall asleep, (2) subjective feelings of how soundly or deeply they sleep, and (3) how rested they feel on awakening.

A nutritional assessment also must be done because symptoms such as lethargy, irritability, insomnia, and difficulty concentrating may reflect an underlying nutritional deficiency. The nurse should also evaluate the patient's energy requirements and demands. The patient may state that daily tasks seem to require more energy; therefore it is important to assess any changes in psychological, social, and role demands. Inquire whether new or expanded demands have been placed on the patient. If so, the nurse should determine the patient's ability to cope with these demands.

■ Defining Characteristics

The presence of the following defining characteristics indicates that the patient may be experiencing Fatigue:

- Verbalization of unremitting and overwhelming lack of energy
- Inability to maintain usual routine
- Increase in rest requirements
- Inability to restore energy, even after sleeping
- Decreased performance
- Lethargy or listlessness
- Disinterest in surroundings
- Impaired ability to concentrate
- Noninvolvement in social activities
- Decreased libido
- Perceived need for additional energy to finish required tasks
- Feelings of guilt for not keeping up with responsibilities

■ Related Factors

The following related factors are associated with Fatigue:

- Acute or chronic illness
- Anemia
- Nutritional deficiencies
- Radiation therapy
- Chemotherapy
- Certain medications
- Increased energy requirements
- Depression
- Overwhelming psychological, social, or role demands

DIAGNOSIS

■ Differential Nursing Diagnosis

Fatigue is subjective and variable, making it difficult to evaluate its presence and magnitude without obtaining patient input and considering multiple factors. Assessment data must be sought that assists the nurse in distinguishing Fatigue from other nursing diagnoses, such as Activity Intolerance, Sleep Pattern Disturbance, Altered Role Performance, and Altered Nutrition.

■ Medical and Psychiatric Diagnoses

Fatigue and Depression are closely related and often difficult to diagnose based on the patient's affect alone. A diagnosis must be based on discussion with the patient and evaluation of multiple factors relevant to the situation. Certain physical illnesses (e.g., congestive heart failure or chronic obstructive pulmonary disease) cause inherent Fatigue. Emotional stress and despair over the death of a loved one, loss of employment, or financial burdens can be responsible for an overwhelming sense of Fatigue.

OUTCOME IDENTIFICATION, PLANNING, AND IMPLEMENTATION

The nursing care outcomes are intended to assist patients diagnosed with Fatigue to live their lives as normally as possible. It is important for patients to identify what activities they see as important to maintaining an independent lifestyle and for the nurse to help them conserve energy to achieve them.

IV

It is expected that the patient will be able to identify and to use appropriate energy conservation techniques. To accomplish this, the nurse should explain the underlying principles of energy conservation. Discuss a typical day with the patient to determine what activities could be curtailed or combined. Determine who else in the household or social network can be available to assume or assist with chores, shopping, and so on.

It is also important that the patient understand the need to incorporate rest periods into daily activities. The nurse should ascertain the types of rest or respite that benefit the patient the most.

For some patients, a short nap in the afternoon may alleviate Fatigue. If that isn't practical, perhaps an earlier bedtime may be in order. The type of rest and the hour of bedtime will need to be individualized for the patient.

The patient must learn to ask for help and to delegate tasks when necessary. Some people find it difficult to ask for help. Discussions with the patient's family may provide some insight into who can and will assist with certain tasks and responsibilities. Such discussions can also provide the family with an understanding of why the patient is feeling fatigued and how they can help.

◢ **NURSING CARE GUIDELINES**
Nursing Diagnosis: Fatigue

Expected Outcome: The patient will incorporate at least one energy conservation technique into his or her daily routine within 48 hours.
- Teach the patient the principle of energy conservation; provide two or more sessions to teach and determine patient's understanding. *Patients are more inclined to comply with a regimen when they understand the basis or rationale for it.*
- Discuss with the patient realistic and practical ways to combine or curtail activities. Assessment of the patient's typical routine can be accomplished at the time the nurse is teaching about energy conservation. *Compliance is more likely when it is possible to modify activities in which the patient engages.*
- With the patient, monitor the effectiveness of the energy conservation technique. *The situation may change or additional strategies may need to be considered.*
- Encourage patience in regard to the effectiveness of the employed technique(s). *It can take several weeks to determine if the conservation techniques are working and feelings of fatigue are reduced.*

Expected Outcome: The patient will incorporate a rest period into the daily routine within 48 hours.
- Review the patient's daily routine. *There may be obvious reasons for the patient's Fatigue that could be eliminated.*
- Assist the patient in assigning priority to activities deemed essential. *Activities of lesser importance to the patient can be delegated to someone else.*
- Discuss with the patient any arrangements that will accommodate rest periods. *Individualized and practical rest periods are more likely to be incorporated into the daily routine.*

Expected Outcome: The patient will seek help and delegate tasks when necessary within 1 week (continue to monitor weekly).
- Assess the understanding of family and friends about the reasons the patient experiences Fatigue. *The better informed the family and friends are about the nature and extent of the patient's Fatigue, the more willing they will be to assist the patient.*
- Assist the patient in identifying specific tasks that family and friends can perform; encourage the patient to discuss these tasks with specific family members and friends and to seek their acceptance of helping with specific tasks. *When expectations are made very clear, a family member or friend is more likely to maintain a commitment to assist the patient.*

■ = nursing intervention; ▲ = collaborative intervention.

EVALUATION

Evaluation of the outcomes initially should be monitored on a daily basis and then weekly. Where behavior changes are involved, more time may be required to implement and maintain new strate-gies to reduce Fatigue. The exact time frame for evaluating the outcome achievement will depend on the specific patient, family, and unique set of circumstances. The patient should be guided in evaluating outcome achievement.

⚑ CASE STUDY WITH PLAN OF CARE

Mrs. Alice Z. is a 35-year-old woman with a 7-year history of systemic lupus erythematosus. She is married and has an 8-year-old daughter. She works full-time as a secretary at a publishing firm, where her main duties include typing manuscripts and updating files. During the assessment of Mrs. Z. in the outpatient clinic, she stated that her Fatigue has become constant throughout the day and that she's unable to keep up with her house or her child.

Mrs. Z.'s medical history shows that flares of her disease have been predominantly manifested by rash, alopecia, and migratory joint pains. She is currently taking 15 mg of prednisone every other day, indomethacin 25 mg three times a day, and hydrochlorothiazide 50 mg every day for mild hypertension.

Her parents live in a midwestern city about 800 miles away. Her maternal grandmother had rheumatoid arthritis and died when Mrs. Z. was 8 years old. She has no relatives living in the area. Her husband works as a plumber's apprentice and, according to Mrs. Z., "doesn't understand my disease." A physical exam reveals a blood pressure of 140/90 mm Hg, pulse of 86 beats per min, respirations of 20/min, temperature of 98.4°F, height 5'4", and weight of 128 pounds. Mrs. Z. is also slightly cushingoid, with an erythematous malar rash. When asked about her support system, Mrs. Z. identifies members of her church and neighbors as people she can count on to help when her disease flares up and she is unable to do much. Her daughter, although she is only 8 years old, is a tremendous help to her mother around the house. Mrs. Z. feels guilty for having to rely so heavily on her daughter.

⚑ PLAN OF CARE FOR MRS. ALICE Z.
Nursing Diagnosis: Fatigue Related to Chronic Illness

Expected Outcome: Mrs. Z. will assign priority to tasks and arrange for their completion.
- Review with Mrs. Z. those tasks she feels are essential.
- Guide her in prioritizing the tasks.
- Assist in identifying energy conservation principles appropriate for those tasks she will perform herself.
- Discuss with Mrs. Z. those tasks with which family members and friends can and are willing to assist.

Expected Outcome: Mrs. Z. will ask for help and delegate tasks necessary.
- If Mrs. Z. desires, be available to discuss with Mrs. Z.'s family members and friends how her illness relates to the Fatigue she experiences.
- With Mrs. Z., evaluate the willingness and availability of family members and friends to assume selected tasks or chores.
- Encourage Mrs. Z. to meet with selected family members and friends to determine whether they will help perform chores, and to make a schedule for persons who will help.

Expected Outcome: Mrs. Z. will establish regular rest periods each day.
- Review a typical day's activities with Mrs. Z.
- Assist Mrs. Z. in developing a daily schedule that incorporates daily rest periods.

■ = nursing intervention; ▲ = collaborative intervention.   *Continued*

IV

▶ PLAN OF CARE FOR MRS. ALICE Z. — CONT'D

Expected Outcome: Mrs. Z. will participate in social activities.
- Discuss with Mrs. Z. the importance of remaining active socially.
- Assist Mrs. Z. in identifying activities in which she would like to participate.
- Encourage Mrs. Z. to schedule a rest period before participating in a social activity.

Expected Outcome: Mrs. Z. will verbalize increased energy and improved well-being.
- Provide Mrs. Z. and her family information about energy conservation techniques and how they can be incorporated into Mrs. Z.'s daily routine.
- Review the activity-rest schedule and discuss with Mrs. Z. the options available to her to balance activity and rest periods.

■ CRITICAL THINKING EXERCISES

1. Considering the history of Fatigue, its recent resurgence, and its prevalence in young to middle-aged females, what factors may explain its causes?
2. How would you explain the principles of energy conservation to Mrs. Z., and what specific conservation techniques would you recommend to her?
3. What aspects of Mrs. Z.'s disease are important to convey to her husband and her daughter? Why are these important, and how would you convey them to the family members?

REFERENCES

1. Blondell-Hill E and Shafran SD: The treatment of chronic fatigue syndrome, *Drugs* 46(4):639–651, 1993.
2. Branco J, Atalia A, and Paiva T: Sleep cycles and alpha-delta sleep in fibromyalgia syndrome, *J Rheumatol* 6:223–233, 1994.
3. Buchwald D and Garrity D: Comparison of patients with chronic fatigue syndrome, fibromyalgia, and multiple chemical sensitivities, *Arch Int Med* 154:2049–2053, 1994.
4. Goldenberg DL: Fibromyalgia, chronic fatigue syndrome, and myofacial pain syndrome, *Curr Opinion Rheumatol* 6: 223–233, 1994.
5. Hart LK: Fatigue in patients with multiple sclerosis, *Res Nurs Health* 1(4):147–157, 1978.
6. Holmes GP, Kaplan JE, and Nelson M: Chronic fatigue syndrome: a working case definition, *Ann Int Med* 108:387–398, 1988.
7. Keller R: Psychosomatic syndromes, somatization, and somatoform disorders, *Psychotherapy Psychosomatics* 61: 4–24.
8. Knippen MA: The relationship among selected variables associated with fatigue in women with systemic lupus erythematosus, doctoral dissertation, 1988, The Catholic University of America, Washington, D.C. (University Microfilms International Dissertation Information Service, Order No 8919391.)
9. Krupp LB, Mendelson WB, and Friedman R: An overview of chronic fatigue, *J Clin Psychiatry* 52:403–410, 1991.
10. Moldofsky H: Fibromyalgia, sleep disorder, and chronic fatigue syndrome, *Ciba Foundation Symposium* 173:262-279, 1993.
11. Ng SC: The fibromyalgia syndrome, *Singapore Med J* 33:294–295, 1992.
12. North American Nursing Diagnosis Association: *NANDA nursing diagnoses: definitions and classification, 1995–1996*, Philadelphia, 1994, The Association.
13. Shorter E: Chronic fatigue in historical perspective, *Ciba Foundation Symposium* 173:6–16, 1993.
14. Wilson MMBS and others: The treatment of chronic fatigue syndrome: science and speculation, *Am J Med* 96(6): 544–550, 1994.

Altered Growth and Development

▶

Altered Growth and Development *is the state in which an individual demonstrates deviations from the norms of his or her age group.*

OVERVIEW

The developmental process in humans is continuous and dynamic throughout the entire life span. The study of that process encompasses the physical, cognitive, interpersonal, emotional, sexual, and spiritual aspects of a person. The result of growth and development is change. Change occurs in the external dimensions of the body, in the form and function of internal organs, and in the personality. All of these changes are interconnected and interdependent.

Whereas the medical or physiological model of development focuses on the changes that occur in the nervous, endocrine, cardiovascular, musculoskeletal, gastrointestinal, and other systems during the major period of growth through the first 18 years of life, developmental theorists have focused on other aspects of growth and development.[7,21] Maturational theorists such as Gesell view development as a continuum of unfolding, predictable, behavioral sequences determined by genetic endowment. The child's environment is seen as contributing to but not determining behavior. The maturationists' early observations of children led to the elaboration of norms for the developmental process. Freud's psychoanalytic theory emphasizes affective and emotional development. The focus of psychoanalytic theory is the development of one's self-concept, which is said to arise when the child's inner sexual and aggressive

needs, or drives, meet the conflicting demands of the external environment. Personality development in this theory is mainly determined by one's childhood experience with the parents. Erikson expanded on the psychoanalytic framework, moving beyond the influence of the immediate family and incorporating one's interaction with society as the important factor in personality development. As conceptualized by Erikson, the process of personality development continues through the entire life cycle. As in Freud's theory, successfully negotiated conflicts at each life stage facilitate the growth process. The learning theorists, such as Skinner and Pavlov, view development as a continuum of increasingly complex behaviors and associations that, for the most part, are learned. The environment is viewed as the source of the reinforcements or rewards that shape behavior. A theory of cognitive development and the development of logical thought was proposed by Piaget. In this framework the child progresses through a series of stages using evolving sensory-motor and neurological competence to interact with and understand the environment. There is no single theory of development that is comprehensive in that it encompasses all of the various aspects of development; therefore it is useful to look at a variety of theoretical frameworks in attempting to understand the significance of deviations from the normal developmental process in terms of eventual outcome.

Individuals with Altered Growth and Development generally have an irregularity in physical growth or an irregularity in structure or function that interferes with the evolution of motor, com-

IV

munication, adaptive, or social skills, causing them to progress at a significantly slower rate than others in their peer group and limiting their ability to fulfill role expectations. Children with the diagnosis Altered Growth and Development might be developmentally delayed, meaning that they have failed to meet certain developmental milestones, or they may have been diagnosed with a developmental disability. Developmental disabilities, defined by the Rehabilitation, Comprehensive Services and Developmental Disabilities Amendments of 1978 (P.L. 95-602), are severe, lifelong, disabling conditions that interfere with a person's ability to function in society and complete personal developmental tasks. These conditions are acquired before a person reaches the age of 22 and are the result of a mental and/or physical impairment.[44] Children with special health care needs or those who are medically fragile, chronically ill, or technology dependent, may also have the diagnosis Altered Growth and Development.[35,45]

Causative factors of Altered Growth and Development fall into four broad categories: heredity, which includes genetic and metabolic abnormalities; problems that occur during pregnancy or in the perinatal period; acquired diseases; and environmental and behavioral problems.[6,9,19,20] The dysfunction that causes Altered Growth and Development can occur before a child's birth, during delivery, after birth, or later. For instance, an infant who is normal at birth can later develop a dysfunction as a result of maladaptive family relationships or other harmful environmental conditions. During adolescence, a person can experience an injury or acquire a chronic illness that can adversely affect development.

The terms *growth* and *development,* used concurrently, refer to "the process by which the fertilized ovum becomes an adult person." *Growth* is defined as "changes in [the] size of the body as a whole or of its individual parts."[7] Development involves change and an increase in complexity of structure and function.[7] Development begins as a general response to the environment and progresses to a more specific, refined, and skilled

response. As development progresses, skills and behaviors become integrated, and new skills and behaviors are built on previously acquired ones.

Several general principles relate to the study of growth and development.[35,45] Although the timetable is unique for each person, normal growth and development follow a predictable pattern that progresses in a continuous, orderly fashion. Growth and development occur in a head-to-toe, or cephalocaudal, pattern. These processes are linked to central nervous system maturation; therefore, the most rapid period of development occurs during the early years of life when the most rapid brain growth occurs. Within the predictable sequence of growth and development there can be great variation in the age at which developmental milestones are achieved. Failure to attain anticipated milestones results in Altered Growth and Development.

As growth and development proceed, they are influenced by a wide variety of factors. There are "critical periods" of development when a person is particularly receptive to and requires certain environmental stimulation for optimal development to occur.[42] If a person is unable to utilize this stimulation or if the stimulation is not present in the environment, Altered Growth and Development may occur. For instance, a young child with a hearing loss secondary to repeated middle ear infections would be unable to receive the necessary verbal stimulation from the environment that is required for normal speech development. There are also "sensitive periods" or "vulnerable periods" of development during which certain organs or tissues may be particularly susceptible to the harmful effects of environmental conditions. This increased vulnerability coincides with the period of rapid brain development from pregnancy through early childhood.[42] For example, it is thought that the developing fetus is especially sensitive to the effects of alcohol during the very earliest weeks of pregnancy.[14]

The processes involved in growth and development are driven by genetic endowment, biological conditions, and environmental influence. The extent to which each person realizes the potential for growth and development is determined by the interaction of certain biological and/or environmental conditions and heredity. There is, at a minimum, an additive effect when detrimental biological and environmental conditions are simultaneously operative.[2] The presence in an infant of a biological condition, such as intracranial hemorrhage, sepsis, or bronchopulmonary dysplasia, increases the chance of future developmental deficits. The existence of more than one such condition creates "much greater risk of disability."[2] Environmental factors can prevent full expression of genetic traits or can distort potentially normal development, as in the case of encephalopathy caused by exposure to high doses of lead. In other cases, factors in the environment may serve to limit the deleterious effects of a genetic abnormality. For example, the injurious effects of the abnormal genes in phenylketonuria may be halted if the newborn's diet restricts phenylalanine intake.

The presence of trauma, prenatally or postnatally, compromises the genetic potential for growth and development. This may include chemical trauma, such as the effects of teratogenic drugs; physical trauma, such as birth injury or child abuse; the effects of an infection; exposure to radiation; or reaction to an immunological agent, such as pertussis vaccine.

Good prenatal and postnatal nutrition is basic to optimal growth and development. Nutritional status can be affected by the presence of a medical condition that precludes sufficient caloric intake or by psychosocial or socioeconomic factors that determine the extent to which adequate health care, education, and housing are available to the child. Psychosocial and socioeconomic factors modify developmental potential by influencing the child-rearing environment and the interaction between parents and the child. These factors shape the parents' personal needs and concerns and their ability to nurture effectively, thereby having a profound effect on the child's ability to achieve self-realization. Diverse issues, such as birth order, maternal age, and maternal health status, also influences a child's ability to achieve optimal development. Finally, cultural factors establish norms and expectations against which the acquisition of developmental milestones is measured.

ASSESSMENT

To assess growth and development, comparisons can be made with age- and gender-matched groups by utilizing standardized screening and assessment tools. Using representative groups, norms and standards have been established for physical measurements and developmental milestones.[7,45] Accurately determined anthropometric measurements are one of the best indicators of growth in children.[45] The usefulness of a single measurement is limited, but serial measurements are valuable in assessing body composition changes or growth over time.[7,24] Height (or length in the case of children less than 2 years old or not able to stand), weight, and head circumference (when children are less than 3 years old) are measured and compared with standard National Center for Health Statistics (NCHS) growth charts.[12,45] Special growth charts are available for premature infants and for those with Down, Turner, and Klinefelter syndromes and achondroplasia.[7] Altered growth patterns are not uncommon in children with chronic illnesses and developmental disabilities.[12]

Assessment will lead to a nursing diagnosis of Altered Growth and Development when there is a deviation from accepted norms in the quality and the quantity of maturational changes. This diagnosis can be assigned to an individual who has failed to progress at a normal rate in physical growth or in acquiring certain developmental skills in the areas of motor, adaptive, communication, and social functioning. Altered development of motor skills includes abnormal body movement (e.g., spasticity and athetoid movement), and the lack of coordination and balance necessary for such developmental milestones as rolling over, standing up, walking, and running. This also includes the inappropriate presence or absence of primitive reflexes. Altered development of adaptive skills encompasses deficits in problem-solving abilities

IV

and in hand control necessary for self-sufficiency and effective interaction with the environment, such as feeding, dressing, and toileting. Altered development of communication skills involves some degree of inability to understand or express oneself verbally and nonverbally. This includes the entire range of communication, from expressing oneself only by gesture to being unable to construct a complex sentence. Deficits in comprehension are exhibited by the inability to follow simple or complex instructions. An alteration in the acquisition of social skills involves a delay in the development of or a deficit in those abilities that a person needs to interact with others, such as social smiling and the ability to engage in appropriate peer relations.

Assessment of developmental progress can confirm normal development or identify developmental delays. A nurse is frequently the first professional to identify a child as having abnormal development in one or more areas. Dworkin advocates utilization of developmental surveillance—a continuous, skillful observation of children during any child health encounter—and soliciting input from parents, teachers, and others who have contact with the child. He suggests that screening tools can be used to confirm suspicions of delay.[23]

An individual with the nursing diagnosis Altered Growth and Development often undergoes a comprehensive developmental evaluation by a multidisciplinary team that includes a nurse. Gross and fine motor, cognitive, language, and social development as well as health, physical growth, family dynamics, parent-child interaction, and environmental factors are assessed.[15] The home is evaluated for safety and accessibility. Also evaluated are the family's knowledge about their child's condition and its management as well as family strengths, needs, resources, and coping skills. Family assessment is done *with*, not *to*, the family and should be nonintrusive and geared toward the family's practical needs and concerns.[9] The resulting information is used by the team in partnership with the family to set goals and priorities, to plan care, to mobilize resources, and to evaluate outcomes. Nursing assessment for Altered Growth and Development involves the use of an array of

screening methods and assessment tools, some of which are described in Table 8.

■ **Defining Characteristics**

The presence of the following defining characteristics[6,34,44] indicates that the patient may be experiencing Altered Growth and Development:

- Impaired physical growth
- Cognitive development inappropriate for age
- Impaired sensory function
- Delayed, altered, or compromised development of motor skills
- Abnormal movement patterns
- Abnormal neurological function
- Abnormal muscle tone
- Decreased coordination
- Decreased balance
- Unable to perform appropriately for age in activities of daily living
- Delayed, altered, or compromised development of receptive and/or expressive communication skills
- Deficient in following instructions
- Delayed, altered, or compromised development of social skills
- Impaired ability to interact with others
- Deficient in modulating behavior
- Limited ability for self-direction
- Limited capacity for independent living
- Limited capacity for economic self-sufficiency

■ **Related Factors**

The following related factors* are associated with Altered Growth and Development:

- Prenatal, maternal, chronic, or acute disease
- Inadequate prenatal care
- Maternal age
- Exposure to teratogens
- Fetal distress
- Prolonged or precipitous labor
- Interruption of oxygen intrapartally
- Prematurity
- Low birth weight

*References 2, 6, 18, 24, 38, 43.

TABLE 8 Screening and Assessment Tools for Nursing Diagnosis Altered Growth and Development

Tool	Applicable Age	Areas Assessed	Procedure	Additional Information	Source
Brazelton Neonatal Behavioral Assessment Scale	3 days to 4 weeks	Motor, social, and neurological functioning	Direct observation	Special training required, valuable for demonstration to parents to increase awareness of infant cues	Cambridge University Press, 110 Midland Ave., Port Chester, NY 10573, (800) 872-7423
Alpern-Boll Developmental Profile II (DPII)	Birth to 9½ years functional age	Physical development and self-help; social, academic, and communication skills	Direct observation and interview	Self-instructional manual available; developmental screening tool	Western Psychological Services, 12031 Wilshire Blvd., Los Angeles, CA 90025, (800) 648-8857
McCarthy Scales of Children's Abilities	2½ to 8½ years	Verbal, perceptual-performance, quantitative, general cognitive, memory, and motor	Direct observation	Self-instructional manual available; developmental assessment tool with manipulative items, gross motor tests, and verbal response items	McCarthy Scales of Children's Abilities, The Psychological Corp., 555 Academic Court, San Antonio, TX 78204-2498, (800) 228-0752
Infant-Toddler Developmental Assessment (IDA)	Birth to 3 years	Six phases of framework include: health review, parent interview, and developmental observation and assessment of eight domains: gross motor, fine motor, cognitive, language, self-help, relationship to persons, emotions and feeling states, coping	Direct observation and interview	Team-based, family-centered approach to developmental assessment; training manuals, recording forms, and manipulatives kit available	Riverside Publishing Company, 8420 Bryn Mawr Ave., Chicago, IL 60631, (800) 767-8378
Nursing Child Assessment Satellite Training (NCAST) Tools		Parent or caregiver behaviors (sensitivity to cues, response to distress, social-emotional growth fostering, cognitive growth fostering) and child behaviors (clarity of cues, responsiveness to parent or caregiver)	Observation	Used to assess parent-child interaction; extensive training is required, manual available to trained individuals; for more information contact NCAST Programs	NCAST Programs: University of Washington, School of Nursing, Campus Box 357920, Seattle, WA 98195-7920, phone: (205) 543-8528, fax: (206) 685-3284
Nursing Child Assessment Feeding Scale (NCAFS)	NCAFS: Birth to 1 year				
Nursing Child Assessment Teaching Scale (NCATS)	NCATS: Birth to 3 years				

Continued

IV

TABLE 8 Screening and Assessment Tools for Nursing Diagnosis Altered Growth and Development—cont'd

Tool	Applicable Age	Areas Assessed	Procedure	Additional Information	Source
Denver II	1 month to 6 years	Personal-social, fine motor-adaptive, language, and gross motor skills	Observation and parent report	Instructional manual, kit, and proficiency test available; updated version of Denver Developmental Screening Test (DDST)	Denver Developmental Material, Inc., P. O. Box 6919, Denver, CO 80206-0919, (303) 355-4729
Milani-Comparetti Motor Development Screening Test	Birth to 24 months	Motor development, primitive reflexes, mature patterns of movement and postural control	Direct observation	Manual and film available for instruction in administration and scoring; provides a framework for neuromotor assessment; does not yield a standardized score	Media Dept., Meyer Rehabilitation Institute, University of Nebraska Medical Center, 600 S. 42nd St., Omaha, NE 68198-5450, phone: (402) 559-7467, fax: (402) 559-5737
Adaptive Behavior Scale	3 to 69+ years	Adaptive behavior in the following domains: independent functioning, physical development, economic activity, language development, numbers and time, domestic and vocational activity, self-direction, responsibility, and socialization	Direct observation, parent or caretaker interview	Administration manual available; training not required; evaluates and describes effectiveness of coping with demands of environment; also includes maladaptive behavior scale	Pro-Ed, 8700 Shoal Creek Blvd., Austin, TX 78758, (512) 451-3246
Home Observation and Measurement of the Environment (HOME)	Birth to 3 years, 3 to 6 years, 6 to 10 years	Home environment and support for emotional, social, and cognitive development	Parent interview and structured observation	Administration manual available; training desirable; can be used to plan interventions	HOME Inventory Limited Liability Co., 13 Saxony Circle, Little Rock, AR 72209, (501) 569-3423
Adapted HOME for children with moderate handicaps	Infant Preschool Elementary	Home environment and support for emotional, social, and cognitive development	Parent interview and structured observation	Administration manual available; training desirable; modified for mental retardation, orthopedic, hearing, and vision impairment	Same as above
Extended HOME for children with severe handicaps	Same as above	Same as above	Same as above	Same as above	Same as above

Instrument	Age/Respondent	Content	Type	Comments	Source
Early Language Milestone Scale (ELM Scale 2)	0 to 36 months	Expressive and receptive language functioning	Interactive test and parent interview	Manual and test kit available; training not required; screening tool	Pro-Ed, 8700 Shoal Creek Blvd., Austin, TX 78758, (512) 451-3246
Family Needs Survey (Revised)	Parents	Perceived needs and extent of each need grouped into six subscales: needs for information, needs for support, explaining to others, community services, financial needs, and family functioning	Questionnaire	Helps family become aware of available services; designed to document family needs for early intervention program planning	D. B. Bailey, Jr., PhD, Director, Frank Porter Graham Child Development Center, CB #8180, University of North Carolina, Chapel Hill, NC 27599, (919) 966-4250
Parent Perception Inventory (PPI)	Parents	Demographics, concerns, beliefs, feelings, coping; separate instruments for siblings and for spouse	Questionnaire	Modification of Chronicity Impact and Coping Instrument: Parent Questionnaire (CICI:PQ); training not required; entire inventory or individual scales can be used; for use with families of individuals with long-term disabilities or chronic illness; packet of 6 instruments available for $20.00	D. P. Hymovich, PhD, Department of Family Nursing, College of Nursing, University of North Carolina at Charlotte, 9201 University City Blvd., Charlotte, NC 28223-0001, (704) 547-4684

References for table: 3, 4, 10, 11, 13, 15, 17, 25, 26, 28, 29, 32, 33, 34, 41.

- Asphyxia in neonatal period
- Low Apgar score
- Birth injury
- Significant blood loss
- Kernicterus
- Congenital defect(s)
- Genetic abnormality
- Metabolic disorder
- Familial history of mental retardation or genetic disorders
- Unknown mechanism
- Neonatal disease
- Neonatal infection
- Chronic illness or infectious illness
- Critical illness
- Malnutrition of mother or infant
- Trauma: physical, chemical, infection, radiation, immunological, psychological, or emotional
- Difficult infant temperament
- Inadequate caretaking
- Poor support system
- Disadvantaged social environment: poverty or homelessness
- Suboptimal infant-parent attachment
- Separation from significant others
- Lack of stimulation in the environment
- Overstimulation from the environment
- Substance abuse

DIAGNOSIS

■ Differential Nursing Diagnosis

Altered Growth and Development is unique among nursing diagnoses. The focus of this diagnosis is the deviation from peer-referenced norms caused by abnormal physical growth, structure, and function. These abnormalities may be physiological, anatomical, or psychological in nature and may interfere with the development of capabilities in the areas of motor, communication, adaptive, or social functioning. Other nursing diagnoses address the same issues (e.g., Self-Care Deficit, Impaired Verbal Communication, and Impaired Physical Mobility) and address many of the same family-related concerns (e.g., Family Coping: Potential for Growth and Altered Family Processes). These

and other nursing diagnoses may be used in conjunction with the diagnosis Altered Growth and Development. Selection of the diagnosis Altered Growth and Development implies that the problem is rooted in a deviation in the processes of growth and development, that it develops early in life (before age 22), that it will have profound effects on the entire family, and that it is likely to be a lifelong problem that affects the patient's ability to develop fully and to function independently.[44]

■ Medical and Psychiatric Diagnoses

The nursing diagnosis Altered Growth and Development can be applied to patients who have a broad spectrum of medical diagnoses and conditions. Medical diagnoses related to the nursing diagnosis Altered Growth and Development include deficits in cardiac formation and structure, such as tetrology of Fallot; metabolic dysfunction that affects the chemical processes in the body, such as galactosemia, or that causes abnormal growth patterns, such as hypothyroidism. Also included are congenital malformations of the nervous system, such as spina bifida; chromosomal abnormalities, such as Down syndrome; chronic diseases, such as acquired immunodeficiency syndrome (AIDS); and an array of systemic disorders affecting the child's physical development, such as cystic fibrosis and diabetes. Prematurity is frequently associated with Altered Growth and Development, although it is not the early delivery itself "but rather the causes or complications of prematurity" that cause developmental problems.[2] In addition, a group of conditions relates to the abnormal structure, maturation, and function of the brain that cause a child to fail to progress or to progress at a delayed rate. These developmental disorders include mental retardation, language delay, learning disabilities, microcephaly, autism, cerebral palsy, sensory deficits, and seizure disorders. Though developmental disorders have great variation in their cause and how they symptomatically appear in each individual, the common thread in these disorders is abnormal brain development.[8] Current policy and legislation reflect the fact that most if not all of these diagnoses have many issues and service requirements in common and that a "generic" approach to the care of individuals with these conditions is currently recommended.[30]

OUTCOME IDENTIFICATION, PLANNING, AND IMPLEMENTATION

Nursing interventions for patients with Altered Growth and Development and their families may occur at any point throughout the life span. Certain principles underlie the provision of all care to individuals with Altered Growth and Development and their families. All interventions should be family centered, recognizing the family's ultimate responsibility for making decisions about care and supporting the family's role as the primary and constant caregiver, educator, and advocate.[1,9,39] Nursing interventions should be part of a system of supports that is driven by family-identified needs and that is well coordinated, flexible, and accessible within the family's community.[39] The privacy and confidentiality of the family must always be respected.[22] It is important to be aware of the unique significance to the family of racial, cultural, ethnic, spiritual, and socioeconomic variables, respecting the diversity of families and not making assumptions about how a family will behave based on stereotypes.[31,39] Working collaboratively with the family and acknowledging their expertise, the nurse acts as a consultant to the family in assessing needs, setting goals and priorities, planning care, identifying and mobilizing resources, and evaluating outcomes. Dunst, Trivette, and Deal suggest that the focus of family-centered assessment and intervention efforts is to "help families use existing capabilities as well as learn new skills (these are referred to as "enabling experiences") in order to mobilize needed resources." Families are "empowered" by enhancing their competencies "in ways that support and strengthen family functioning."[22]

Regular monitoring of growth and development facilitates early recognition of developmental delay or dysfunction and enables referral for further testing, treatment of disabling conditions, and possible avoidance of secondary disabilities. The long-term goal of treatment for the individual with Altered Growth and Development is to maximize their developmental potential.[36] Developmental surveillance and screening for developmental disabilities can occur in many settings: in schools, as a part of well-child visits, or during hospital admissions or home care visits. Screening tools are used to distinguish "between children at high and low risk for developmental problems."[23] They are not diagnostic. In addition to screening tools, the nurse also uses assessment tools to discern functional levels across multiple developmental domains and to facilitate anticipatory guidance that enhances the parents' ability to encourage and to participate in the evolving process of development.[35]

The planning and implementation of a comprehensive educational and habilitative program for the patient with Altered Growth and Development frequently requires coordination of services involving multiple disciplines. The patient with Altered Growth and Development is often seen by many specialists, who may not always communicate effectively with each other, causing confusion for the family and resulting in gaps in the child's health care. The nurse can facilitate communication among the family, physicians, and other professionals and can clarify information for the family. Improved communication and collaboration will help ensure that the family has access to all necessary equipment and professional services, such as physical, occupational, and speech therapy; nutrition counseling; social work intervention; legal advice; and financial resources. Coordination of professional services is frequently required after a hospitalization to ensure a smooth transition from hospital to home. Interaction with school personnel is another aspect of providing care for the individual with Altered Growth and Development. Often this involves interpretation of health needs as they relate to the educational or vocational program. Because of improved medical care in recent years, developmentally disabled individuals are able to live longer. Collaboration is necessary to prevent discontinuity as an individual makes the shift between service delivery systems that are

IV

geared to certain age groups, especially during the major transition from pediatric to adult services.[5]

The nurse must also address the behaviors known collectively as activities of daily living. Teaching the family to deal with difficulties in feeding, sleeping, bathing, dressing, and toileting and to deal with difficult or inappropriate behavior is critical, and it requires much insight into the family's coping strategies, the family's personal and group goals, and the practical limitations and realities of the situation. These activities of daily living evolve as the patient grows in size and attains or does not attain new levels of functioning. The family dynamics and the family's ability to cope are not static, and the nurse must be sensitive to the family's needs at different stages of development. The patient should attain the highest possible degree of independence in activities of daily living.

The nurse has an ongoing responsibility to assist the family in anticipating, understanding, and cop-

---

◢ NURSING CARE GUIDELINES
Nursing Diagnosis: Altered Growth and Development

Expected Outcome: The patient will have growth and development monitored during all child health encounters.
- ■ Assess anthropometrics. *Accurately determined serial anthropometric measurements are one of the best indicators of growth in children.*[7,24,45]
- ▲ Initiate developmental surveillance at initial encounter, and continue it as an ongoing process.
- ■ Utilize screening tools to confirm suspicious of developmental delay.
- ▲ Rescreen or refer patient for further testing and treatment.
  Early detection of developmental delays facilities initiation of interventions to maximize potential for development and to minimize secondary problems.

Expected Outcome: The patient will engage in comprehensive, developmentally appropriate educational and habilative interventions.
- ▲ Work collaboratively with the family and the interdisciplinary team to identify and meet health, psychological, social, educational, and emotional needs.
- ▲ Identify community resources.
- ▲ Assist the family in gaining access to needed professional services, equipment, and financial resources.[46] *Individuals with Altered Growth and Development often have a variety of needs that change over time and that require services from multiple professionals and service providers. Coordination of services can help prevent fragmentation and gaps in care. Resources provided must meet the needs identified by the family.*[22,39]

Expected Outcome: The family will demonstrate successful management of difficulties relating to activities of daily living.
- ▲ Assist the family in dealing with difficulties in behavior, feeding, sleeping, bathing, dressing, and toileting.
- ▲ Within the limits of the child's capabilities, teach the skills necessary for self-care in activities of daily living. *Children with disabilities should learn skills associated with activities of daily living when they have reached the developmental stage at which they would normally be learned.*[45]

Expected Outcome: The family will successfully adapt to the changing needs of the individual with Altered Growth and Development throughout his or her life span.[37,40]
- ■ Provide anticipatory guidance in recognizing changing needs as the patient ages.
- ▲ Assist the family in dealing with transition issues.
  Parents may revisit feelings of disappointment and grief as they experience life cycle transitions and again mourn for the loss of their "ideal" child.[16]

■ = nursing intervention; ▲ = collaborative intervention.

ing with the unique and changing needs of their family member at various stages of development.[37,40] Feelings of grief and disappointment first experienced at the time of diagnosis may resurface periodically, especially at important transitions, such as the start of formal education, the development of the physical changes associated with puberty, emerging sexuality in an adolescent, and the time when parents face their own aging and deal with issues of guardianship and lifelong care.[16] Nonjudgmental listening helps to clarify concerns and lets the family know that their ideas and concerns are valid. To help avoid a crisis at these times of transition the nurse can provide anticipatory guidance and can recommend appropriate literature, community resources, and support groups for parents, siblings, and in some cases the individual with Altered Growth and Development. The nurse supports the parents' decision making as alternatives in care or residential placement are identified and examined and goals are reevaluated and clarified.

EVALUATION

Continual reassessment and evaluation of progress toward goal attainment are an integral part of the nursing process for patients with Altered Growth and Development. Evaluating progress toward meeting the needs that the family has identified can be done informally and should be done at every encounter with the family.[22]

Evidence that the patient has regular surveillance of growth and development is seen in the early detection of irregularities and the initiation of interventions aimed at maximizing the potential for development and preventing secondary complications.

The patient and family indicate that they are successfully managing activities of daily living by resolving problems associated with these activities in a manner that meets the needs of the patient and family and by the patient eventually becoming independent as much as possible in age-appropriate skills associated with feeding, sleeping, dressing, toileting, and bathing.

Evidence that the patient is involved in and is deriving benefit from appropriate educational and habilitative programs is seen in goals that are met in physical, occupational, and speech therapy and in the use of prescribed adaptive equipment and prosthetic or orthotic devices. Evaluation of the plan of care should determine to what extent the family successfully uses health care resources, educational and habilitative services, and social and emotional support systems.

Evidence of the family's ability to adapt to the changing needs of the individual with Altered Growth and Development throughout the life span is seen in the family's ability to anticipate and cope with life cycle transitions.

It is difficult if not impossible to attach a time frame to any of these outcomes because of the nature of this nursing diagnosis. This is a diagnosis that spans the entire life cycle. As a patient with Altered Growth and Development grows and changes, the needs of the patient and the family change. Adjustments that were successfully made may need to be made again; feelings that were resolved may resurface and need to be explored again; and problems that were solved may appear in a different form at a later stage in life. Families resolve issues and find ways to meet their needs in their own unique manner and in their own unique time. It is the job of the nurse and other professionals working in collaboration with the family to make it possible to meet the needs that the family has identified in the most expeditious way and to support the family as they work to achieve their goals.

IV

IV

◤ CASE STUDY WITH PLAN OF CARE

Sam is a 4-month-old diagnosed with Down syndrome shortly after birth. He was born with congenital heart disease and will need surgery to repair an atrioventricular (AV) canal. He has had frequent occurrences of respiratory infections and otitis media and has just been discharged after a hospitalization to treat respiratory syncytial virus (RSV). Sam has had feeding problems and slow weight gain. He is currently at the 25th percentile for weight (9.25 lb) and between the 10th and 25th percentile for height (22″) when plotted on the Down syndrome growth chart. Sam is hypotonic and is delayed in his development. He is the youngest of six children, who range in age from 10 to 20 years. The two eldest children do not live at home. Sam's parents had a difficult time accepting his diagnosis and have many concerns about prognosis. Many relatives live in the area, but they have been distant since Sam's birth, rarely calling, and the family has been reluctant to initiate contact.

◤ PLAN OF CARE FOR SAM AND HIS FAMILY
Nursing Diagnosis: Altered Growth and Development Related to Congenital Heart Disease and Down Syndrome

Expected Outcome: Sam will have adequate growth.
- Assess anthropometrics regularly.
▲ Consult with nutritionist; determine appropriate caloric intake for sufficient weight gain; discuss need for increased calorie formula.

Expected Outcome: Sam's parents will demonstrate successful management of feeding difficulties.
- If increased calorie formula is used, ascertain correct preparation.
▲ Instruct parents regarding physical anomalies that make feeding problems common in children with Down syndrome; refer them to occupational therapist for ongoing feeding problems.

Expected Outcome: Sam's parents will have an awareness of Sam's current abilities and needs to promote his development.
- Assess Sam's development periodically, and involve his parents.
- Assess parental concerns, perceptions, expectations, and knowledge about their child's development.
- Teach parents that difficulty in holding Sam is related to physical characteristic of Down syndrome and is not an indication of rejection by Sam; model appropriate handling for a hypotonic infant.
- Teach Sam's parents to encourage emerging skills (e.g., allow time each day for Sam to play in the prone position to develop upper body muscle tone).

Expected Outcome: Sam will participate in an early intervention program with a strong family-support component.
▲ Assist family in identifying community resources for early intervention and in completing the application process.
▲ Encourage parent involvement in parent-to-parent support to help deal with issues of accepting the diagnosis and of communicating with family members about the diagnosis.

■ = nursing intervention; ▲ = collaborative intervention.

■ CRITICAL THINKING EXERCISES

1. Although positive parent-child interaction is necessary for optimal growth and development, physical and behavioral characteristics of infants with Down syndrome (such as lack of cuddliness, feeding problems, delays in reaching motor milestones, and slow weight gain) in combination with parental characteristics related to the response to the birth of a child with a congenital disorder cause an increased risk for poor parent-infant interaction. What are some of the nursing interventions that would be helpful in promoting positive, nurturing parent-infant interactions?

2. Families with an infant who has Down syndrome or other alterations in the normal patterns of growth and development are often in need of the services of many professionals. The nurse must understand the role of all professionals who provide services to children with Altered Growth and Development and must have knowledge of the variety of informal and formal supports that are available to the family. What are some of the programs and professional services that Sam and his family will need? How can the nurse work with Sam's family to help them meet their needs?

3. Sam's family was informed of his diagnosis shortly after his birth. Why is it important for the nurse to assess his development periodically even though it has already been established that Sam has a developmental problem?

REFERENCES

1. Ahmann E: Family centered care: shifting orientation, *Pediatr Nurs* 20:113–117, 1994.
2. Allen MC: The high-risk infant, *Pediatr Clin North Am* 40:479–490, 1993.
3. Alpern G, Boll T, and Shearer M: *Developmental profile II manual*, Los Angeles, 1986, Western Psychological Services.
4. Bailey DB: Issues and perspectives on family assessment, *Infants Young Children* 4:26–34, 1991.
5. Batshaw ML: Mental retardation, *Pediatr Clin North Am* 40:507–521, 1993.
6. Batshaw ML and Perret YM: *Children with disabilities: a medical primer*, ed 3, Baltimore, 1992, Paul H. Brookes Publishing Co.
7. Behrman RE, editor: *Nelson textbook of pediatrics*, ed 14, Philadelphia, 1992, WB Saunders Co.
8. Blondis TA and others: Developmental disabilities: a continuum, *Clin Pediatr* 32:492–498, 1993.
9. Bond N, Phillips P, and Rollins JA: Family-centered care at home for families with children who are technology dependent, *Pediatr Nurs* 20:123–130, 1994.
10. Bradley RH and others: *Addendum to HOME manual: use of the HOME inventory with children with handicaps*, Little Rock, Arkansas, 1987, University of Arkansas at Little Rock.
11. Brazelton TB: *Neonatal behavioral assessment*, ed 3, New York, 1995, Cambridge University Press.
12. Brizee LS, Sophos CM, and McLaughlin JF: Nutrition issues in developmental disabilities, *Infants Young Children* 2:10–21, 1990.
13. Caldwell B and Bradley RH: *Manual of home observation for measurement of the environment*, rev ed, Little Rock, Arkansas, 1984, University of Arkansas at Little Rock.
14. Caruso K and ten Bensel R: Fetal alcohol syndrome and fetal alcohol effects: the University of Minnesota experience, *Minnesota Med* 76:25–29, 1993.
15. Clark R, Paulson A, and Conlin S: Assessment of developmental status and parent-infant relationships: the therapeutic process of evaluation. In Zeanah CH: *Handbook of infant mental health*, New York, 1993, Guilford Press.
16. Clubb RL: Chronic sorrow: adaptation patterns of parents with chronically ill children, *Pediatr Nurs* 17:461–466, 1991.
17. Coplan, J: *Early language milestone scale*, ed 2, Austin, Texas, 1993, Pro-Ed.
18. Crocker AC and Nelson RP: Mental retardation. In Levine MD, Carey WB, and Crocker AC, editors: *Developmental behavioral pediatrics*, Philadelphia, 1992, WB Saunders Co.
19. Curry DM and Duby JC: Developmental surveillance by pediatric nurses, *Pediatr Nurs* 20:40–44, 1994.
20. Danielson CB, Hamel-Bissell B, and Winstead-Fry P: *Families, health, and illness: perspectives on coping and intervention*, St. Louis, 1993, Mosby–Year Book.
21. Dixon SD: Setting the stage: theories and concepts of child development. In Dixon SD and Stein MT: *Encounters with children: pediatric behavior and development*, ed 2, St. Louis, 1992, Mosby–Year Book.
22. Dunst CJ, Trivette CM, and Deal AG, editors: *Supporting and strengthening families, vol 1: methods, strategies, and practices*, Cambridge, Massachusetts, 1994, Brookline Books.
23. Dworkin PH: British-American recommendations for developmental monitoring: the role of surveillance, *Pediatrics* 84:1000–1009, 1989.

IV

IV

24. Foye HR and Sulkes SB: Developmental and behavioral pediatrics. In Berhman RE and Kliegman RM, editors: *Nelson essentials of pediatrics,* ed 2, Philadelphia, 1994, WB Saunders Co.

25. Frankenburg WK and Dodds JB: *Denver II,* Denver, 1990, Denver Developmental Materials.

26. Glascoe FP: Developmental screening: rationale, methods, and application, *Infants Young Children* 4:1–10, 1991.

27. Hayes A and Batshaw M: Down syndrome, *Pediatr Clin North Am* 40:523–535, 1993.

28. Huber C: Documenting quality of parent-child interaction: use of the NCAST scales, *Infants Young Children* 4:63–75, 1991.

29. Hymovich DP: Measuring parental coping when a child is chronically ill. In Strickland OL and Waltz CF, editors: *Measurement of nursing outcome, vol IV: measuring client self-care and coping skills,* New York, 1990, Springer.

30. Ireys HT: New federal policy for children with special health care needs: implications for pediatricians, *Pediatrics* 90:321–327, 1992.

31. Konstantareas MM and Homatidis S: Effects of developmental disorder on parents: theoretical and applied considerations, *Psychiatr Clin North Am* 14:183–198, 1991.

32. Lambert N, Leland H, and Nihira K: *Adaptive behavior scale,* ed 2, Austin, Texas, 1993, Pro-Ed.

33. McCarthy D: *Manual: McCarthy scales of children's abilities,* New York, 1972, The Psychological Corporation.

34. Milani-Comparetti A and Gidoni EA: *Milani-Comparetti developmental scale,* Omaha, 1973, University of Nebraska Medical Center.

35. Morse JS: An overview of developmental disabilities nursing. In Roth SP and Morse JS: *A life-span approach to nursing care for individuals with developmental disabilities,* Baltimore, 1994, Paul H. Brookes Publishing Co.

36. Nehring W: The nurse whose specialty is developmental disabilities, *Pediatr Nurs* 20:78–82, 1994.

37. O'Brien DR: Health maintenance and promotion in adults. In Roth SP and Morse JS: *A life-span approach to nursing care for individuals with developmental disabilities,* Baltimore, 1994, Paul H. Brookes Publishing Co.

38. Russell FF and Free TA: The nurse's role in habilitation. In Roth SP and Morse JS: *A life-span approach to nursing care for individuals with developmental disabilities,* Baltimore, 1994, Paul H. Brookes Publishing Co.

39. Shelton TL and Stepanek JS: *Family-centered care for children needing specialized health and developmental services,* Bethesda, Maryland, 1994, Association for the Care of Children's Health.

40. Steadham CI: Health maintenance and promotion: infancy through adolescence. In Roth SP and Morse JS: *A life-span approach to nursing care for individuals with developmental disabilities,* Baltimore, 1994, Paul H. Brookes Publishing Co.

41. Stuberg W: *Milani-Comparetti motor development screening tool test manual,* ed 3, Omaha, 1992, Meyer Rehabilitation Institute.

42. Touwen BCL: Perspective: critical periods of brain development, *Infants Young Children* 1:vii–x, 1989.

43. Uauy R, Mena P, and Warshaw JB: Growth and metabolic adaptation of the fetus and newborn. In Oski FA and others, editors: *Principles and practice of pediatrics,* ed 2, Philadelphia, 1994, JB Lippincott Co.

44. U.S. Department of Education: *Summary of existing legislation affecting people with disabilities,* Washington, D.C., 1992, U.S. Government Printing Office.

45. Wong DL: *Whaley and Wong's nursing care of infants and children,* ed 5, Philadelphia, 1995, Mosby–Year Book.

46. Youngblut JM, Brennan PF, and Stewart LA: Families with medically fragile children: an exploratory study, *Pediatr Nurs* 20:463–468, 1994.

Impaired Home Maintenance Management

Impaired Home Maintenance Management *is the state in which an individual or family is unable to maintain independently a safe, hygienic growth-promoting environment.*

OVERVIEW

Home is a special place for Americans. Personal privacy and personal property are valued so much that they are protected by the Constitution. Living in a private home is believed to provide a higher quality of life than institutional care because it supports independence and individuality. Private home life facilitates self-care, which is associated with self-esteem.[19] The current trend to support community-based living for high-risk populations and to discharge stable, acutely ill patients has led to a dramatic increase in home health care services.

These trends are an outgrowth of three separate social movements that have occurred since the 1960s. The first is the deprofessionalization of health care. In the 1950s Americans had come to expect the physician and other health care providers to cure their health problems through accurate diagnosis and intervention, which included pharmacological agents and high technology. Americans viewed the hospital as a place to go to be cured. By 1960 health professionals realized that America's major health problems were long-term and required active participation by the public for prevention and treatment. Disease was multicausal and related to lifestyle patterns. The patient and family were recognized as important members of the health team.

Until the 1960s home health care had been done by the family, the physician, and the nurse. Then home health care agencies began to employ professionals from other disciplines, such as social workers, physical therapists, speech therapists, and nutritionists, as well as paraprofessional aides and trained homemakers, to broaden the scope of home care. Home care then involved a multidisciplinary team with various levels of preparation that included family caregivers and the patient.[10]

The second social movement was the medical self-care or consumer movement. It is related to the deprofessionalization of health care. As Americans became more aware that they had a role in health care, they also sought a more active role in planning, evaluating, and controlling care decisions. Health care knowledge no longer belonged exclusively to professionals such as physicians and nurses. New courses were developed in schools and the community in response to the public's interest in health promotion and the evaluation of professional health care.

The third social movement was cost containment. With the advent of the Social Security Act of 1963, Medicare paid for acute skilled nursing care in the home but not custodial care.[15] Each year health care costs have escalated at a higher rate than the consumer price index. This has resulted in several attempts by the federal government to control costs. One significant attempt was to change payment for hospital services from retrospective payment for services rendered to a prospective payment system (PPS) by medical diagnosis (DRG). The most recent attempt has been the expansion of integrated health systems to charge annual capitated payments (with patient co-pay charges for encounters) over the entire continuum of care.

IV

One outcome of these changes has been shorter hospitalizations, resulting in a growth of home-based health care. Also associated with cost containment has been the increase in ambulatory surgical treatment and the decrease in long-term institutionalization of the infirm, mentally ill, mentally retarded, and other high-risk, disabled populations. State and federal funding has been structured to provide incentives for the development of community-based treatment programs.[15] One example is case management for high-risk groups, such as the frail elderly, AIDS patients, and the chronically mentally ill.

Today the community health nurse provides home-based care for the patient by working with the family unit to provide skilled nursing care; to coordinate care provided by the family, paraprofessionals, social agencies, and other health care professionals; and to assist them to increase their level of self-care and home maintenance management.[1] Home health care nursing is now recognized as a specialized field of community health nursing, with separate standards of practice established by the American Nurses' Association.[2]

In providing care the nurse, in cooperation with the patient, must assess the health care demands of the patient and family and also the home and community environment. The nurse's documentation of services must include these activities. Mundinger[15] found that community health nurses routinely provide health promotion and maintenance services to the entire family unit. She also found that nurses assessed and intervened at the environmental level but only recorded direct care given to the patient. Documentation must reflect all nursing activities performed to ensure demonstration of the scope of nursing practice and justification of adequate compensation.

ASSESSMENT

Impaired Home Maintenance Management is rarely the reason that a patient seeks nursing care. However, in the nursing assessment the nurse may identify current home maintenance management

as a barrier to healthful living or to providing nursing care. Necessary adaptations of the structure or furnishings for home care may be missing. Aids that could increase the patient's independence may be missing. Knowledge of how to obtain necessary durable medical equipment for treatment or how to operate it safely may be needed. Intervention for this diagnosis may take precedence over others to create a workplace for safe care or to prevent injury to the patient and family. The home maintenance practices and facilities may be adequate for a family with healthy members but hazardous for a patient.

A number of excellent tools developed for the assessment of the family and the home environment are printed in the community health literature. A home assessment tool for use with all families is illustrated in the box on pages 377–378. It demonstrates the importance of assessing a home from room to room for safety and hygiene. When conducting a home assessment, the nurse may find that personal standards or values of cleanliness are different from the patient's. For example, the home might seem dirty to the nurse but not necessarily affect the resident's health.[13] Impaired Home Maintenance Management applies only when the home environment presents an actual or potential risk to the resident's health.[4]

Two high-risk populations needing specific home assessments are children and the elderly. Several tools are available to assess the home environment in regard to safety and developmental stimulation of children at several stages.[5]

When planning home health care for the elderly, the nurse needs to include a safety assessment that is sensitive to their special needs. One tool written for use by professionals or by the elderly patient or family is the *Home Safety Checklist* published by the U.S. Consumer Product Safety Commission.[20] If the elderly person depends on a caregiver, the nurse needs to assess both the burden of care and the environment.[7] Greif[9] has developed a caregiver assessment guide.

When assessing for the nursing diagnosis Impaired Home Maintenance Management, the

HOME ASSESSMENT CHECKLIST

TYPE OF DWELLING

Apt. _____ Rowhouse _____ House _____ Owned _____ Rented _____
No. of rooms in dwelling _____ No. of persons in the home _____
Water: Public _____ Well _____ Sewer: Public _____ Septic _____
Plumbing: Indoor _____ Outdoor _____

HOME EXTERIOR AND ENVIRONMENT	YES	NO	COMMENTS
Are there any pollutants in the external environment?			
Are sidewalks and steps in good condition?			
Do steps have railings?			
Are handrails adequately fastened?			
Are there barriers to accessing this home for any household members (e.g., need ramp)?			
Is entrance adequately lighted?			
Has the home been tested for radon?			

HOME INTERIOR: GENERAL

	YES	NO
Are emergency numbers posted by the phone?		
Are smoke detectors available and working?		
Is there an emergency exit plan?		
Are electrical cords in good condition?		
Are there pests (e.g., vermin or roaches)?		
Are rooms uncluttered to permit easy mobility?		
Are doorways wide enough to permit assistive devices?		
Are carpets, rugs, and flooring in good condition?		
Are scatter rugs secured by two-way tape or a rubber backing?		
Is the water heater thermostat set at 110°F or lower?		
Is lighting adequate?		
Is the temperature kept within healthful range (68° to 75°F)?		
Are medications stored safely and properly?		
Are chemicals stored safely and properly?		

STAIRS AND HALLS

	YES	NO
Are stairways and halls well illuminated, with light switches at top and bottom of stairs?		
Are steps in good condition and free of objects?		
Do steps have nonskid strips or securely fastened carpet?		
Are handrails sturdy and securely fastened?		

KITCHEN

	YES	NO
Is there adequate light around the stove and the sink?		
Is a gas stove pilot light equipped with automatic cutoff if flame fails?		
Are small appliances unplugged when not in use?		
When working in the kitchen, does worker		
Turn pan handles away from edge of stove?		
Avoid wearing garments with loose, long sleeves?		

Continued

IV

HOME ASSESSMENT CHECKLIST—cont'd
TYPE OF DWELLING

BATHROOM
Are there skidproof strips or a mat in the tub or shower?   _____ _____
Are there grab bars on the tub, the shower, and the toilet?   _____ _____
Is the medication cabinet well illuminated?   _____ _____
Is medication safely stored?   _____ _____

BEDROOM
Are bed and chairs adequate height to allow getting on and off   _____ _____
    easily (e.g., elderly)?
Are night-lights available?   _____ _____
Is there a flashlight or lamp within easy reach of the bed?   _____ _____
Other comments and observations   _____ _____

nurse must consider the individual, the family, the dwelling, and the community. The key observation is of the dwelling and its organization, cleanliness, and safety for both daily living and patient care. Observation for signs of provision for personal growth and individuality of family members is also necessary.

■ Defining Characteristics

The presence of the following defining characteristics[4,6,8,10,11] indicates that the patient may be experiencing Impaired Home Maintenance Management:

- Presence of disease or disability necessitating adaptation of home maintenance
- Repeated hygienic disorder, infestations, or infections
- Knowledge of home maintenance inconsistent with current environment (e.g., family moving from one country or culture to another may not know how to maintain a home in the new environment)
- Expresses ignorance in providing environment conducive to patient care
- Appears too exhausted or anxious to maintain the home
- Expresses need for assistance in home maintenance management
- Accumulation of dirt, food waste, or hygienic waste
- Inadequate or contaminated water supply
- Inadequate lighting
- Inappropriate household temperature or ventilation
- Presence of vermin or rodents
- Offensive odors
- Presence of indoor pets that are not housebroken
- Disorderly surroundings
- Overcrowding of available space
- Presence of structural barriers (e.g., doorways too narrow for wheelchair)
- Home structure needs adaptation to facilitate safe use of equipment (e.g., wiring outlets)
- Unrepaired defects in structure or utilities
- Insufficient supply of or unwashed cooking utensils, linens, or clothes
- Lack of necessary equipment or aids
- Lack of durable medical equipment
- Home lacks personal items and decorations
- Lack of support for personal growth of family members

- Overtaxed family members (e.g., exhausted or anxious)
- Lack of knowledge of caregiver
- Lack of knowledge regarding community resources
- Inadequate support system
- Apparent lack of economic resources (e.g., for services, purchases of equipment, supplies, repairs, or fuel)
- Characteristics of neighborhood make effective home maintenance difficult
- Characteristics of neighborhood make home visiting unsafe or unavailable
- Community resources insufficient to provide needed equipment, aids, repairs, or support
- Inability to maintain home consistent with spiritual beliefs and practices

■ Related Factors

The following related factors are associated with Impaired Home Maintenance Management:

- Disabled by acute illness, injury, or congenital anomaly
- Disabled by chronic, debilitating disease or impaired sensory functioning
- Disabled by impaired cognitive or emotional functioning
- Lack of sufficient knowledge about home maintenance, adaptation of home maintenance, use of durable equipment, or neighborhood health plan, or governmental resources
- Lack of socialization (role model for socialization)
- Insufficient family organization or planning
- Inadequate amount or quality of social support
- Insufficient finances or insurances
- Insufficient dwelling or furnishings (e.g., structural defects or lack of equipment or aids)
- Insufficient community environmental sanitation or control of environmental contaminants or pollutants
- Lack of needed professional or paraprofessional home care or support services in community
- Neighborhood too dangerous for safety of professional or paraprofessional care or support services to visit

DIAGNOSIS

■ Differential Nursing Diagnosis

Impaired Home Maintenance Management may appear as a secondary nursing diagnosis associated with a primary medical-psychiatric diagnosis (e.g., major depression) or nursing diagnosis (e.g., Urinary Incontinence) that renders a patient unable to maintain the home. The extent to which the primary diagnosis affects the patient's ability to maintain the home determines whether the nursing diagnosis would be Impaired Home Maintenance Management or Ineffective Coping. The presence of environmental hazards or structural barriers in the home or the surrounding community are the defining characteristics that indicate this diagnosis instead of Risk for Injury or Risk for Trauma. When environmental factors in the home or neighborhood are the primary cause of lack of adherence to a therapeutic regimen, this diagnosis is preferred over Ineffective Management of Therapeutic Regimen: Individuals, Families, or Communities. For example, lack of finances to pay for the electric bill may be the primary cause of nonadherence to the use of an oxygen concentrator as part of the medical regimen for chronic obstructive pulmonary disease (COPD).

■ Medical and Psychiatric Diagnoses

Conditions or disorders that cause physical, emotional, or cognitive disability of patients such as chronic diseases (including COPD, cardiovascular accident, and multiple sclerosis), congenital anomalies or traumatic injuries (including quadriplegia), and psychiatric diseases or disorders (including substance abuse, major depression, and Alzheimer's disease) may necessitate adaptation of the home itself or patterns of caring for the home to ensure safety, provide effective care, and facilitate personal growth of residents. In cases where the level of home maintenance deteriorates or is at high risk of threatening the health or safety of the patient or family, Impaired Home Maintenance Management is an appropriate diagnosis. The level of danger to the patient's well-being will dictate if this diagnosis is primary or secondary. This diagnosis illustrates the importance of collabora-

IV

IV

tion by the episodic care nurse with home care nurses, case managers, social workers, and family members who will assist in the environmental assessment for discharge planning.

OUTCOME IDENTIFICATION, PLANNING, AND IMPLEMENTATION

Case management over the continuum of care[3] is becoming more important in this era of increasingly complex ambulatory care, limited hospice care,[12] and home care, and of hospitalizations being limited to periods when the patient is medically unstable. Whether the patient is chronically ill, newly disabled, terminally ill, or recovering from an acute illness or trauma, the family will be the principal caregiver.[14] The multidisciplinary team needs to include the family for information on the home and the feasibility of adapting their lifestyles and committing resources to include caregiving activities.[17] The desired outcome is to maintain the patient at home with maximum independence as long as possible and desired. Other intermediate outcomes associated with specific defining characteristics and the process of assessment and intervention need to be identified for specific individuals.

As part of the planning process, the nurse assists the patient to assess the safety of the home and need for adaptation. Structural changes, equipment, aids, and supplies needed and financing for acquisition must be planned. Discussion of the need for and meaning of lifestyle adaptation of the patient, caregivers, and family supports effective planning. During this time, patients, caregivers, and families need to explore and identify potential supportive resources available from friendship networks, work associations, health plans, the neighborhood, the extended family, governmental programs, and community-based professional and paraprofessional services to augment personal resources and to provide respite services. Environmental assessment should include identification of constraints such as neighborhood safety, the depth and variety of community resources, environmental pollution, and the condition of the home.[18] These activities will help achieve the first intermediate desired outcome for all patients: development of a realistic, feasible, and satisfactory plan for home adaptation and maintenance.

Once a plan is in place, activities focus on structural adaptation and repair; training in the use of equipment and aids for care and home maintenance; training in safety measures,[16] contact of appropriate supports and services; and arrangements for scheduling, payment, and other essential steps to assure participation. Collaboration between patients, case managers, nurses, other health professionals and paraprofessionals, social workers, caregivers, and family members is essential to coordinate activities and plan for a smooth discharge or adaptation to a new level of dependency. These activities help achieve the second and third intermediate desired outcomes for all patients: making needed changes and seeking appropriate resources. Patients should participate in activities of daily living as much as possible within a home environment that is safe and promotes the health of all family members.

The maintenance of such an environment requires the persistence of new behaviors and the efficient coordination of services and supports over time. The nurse promotes maintenance through recognizing change, periodically evaluating safety and health promotion levels, and praising the patient and family for sustaining a clean, safe, growth-promoting environment (the fourth intermediate desired outcome for all patients).

■◢ Nursing Care Guidelines
Nursing Diagnosis: Impaired Home Maintenance Management

Expected Outcome: The patient will participate with the family and the nurse in the development of a feasible home maintenance and adaptation plan as evidenced by a realistic plan that is satisfactory to all parties by the end of the first visit.
- Have members state what factors in their home environment affect their health and how.
- Patient, family, and nurse collaboratively and systematically identify factors that impede meeting the household standard.
- Compare the patient's perceptions with the observations; share the nurse's observations.
- Assist family in completing a home safety assessment; follow up on identified deficits.
- Identify factors in the community that adversely affect the family's ability to maintain their home.
- Identify local resources that work to promote changes,
- ▲ Make appropriate referrals, utilizing the multidisciplinary team.
- Order necessary durable medical equipment for home treatment.
- Establish necessary adaptations to the home to facilitate use of durable medical equipment.
- ▲ Teach the patient and family as appropriate.

  Awareness of the relationship of health to the home environment is the antecedent to realistic planning. The nurse, along with the patient and the family, will systematically and collaboratively assess household standards of cleanliness and maintenance, the home safety level, the perceived need for structural changes and repairs, the need for equipment and aids, and necessary patient and family lifestyle changes to provide a base for planning change. Increasing patient and family awareness of available equipment, aids, community resources, and health plan and government program resources, and a review of the patient's social network and extended family assist in realistic planning.

Expected Outcome: The patient will be aware of his or her own capacity for daily home maintenance and adaptation and will provide for appropriate support as evidenced by making needed changes or acquiring appropriate supports by the end of the second visit.
- ▲ Identify members of current support system and assess their capabilities.
- ▲ Discuss what each member now does and how often; if necessary, discuss possible role changes.
- Listen (without judging) to the realities of the home situation,
- ▲ Mutually develop a plan of care to increase supports consistent with family values.
- Differentiate aesthetic hygienic factors from those that adversely affect health.
- ▲ Discuss community resources for daily home maintenance.
- Initiate referrals for supplementation of daily home maintenance.
- Have patient or caregivers demonstrate use of durable medical equipment.
- Investigate community resources for long-term maintenance.
- ▲ Review with support system members how to utilize nurse as continuing resource.

  Adaptation of the home environment, home maintenance patterns, and caregiving patterns and seeking appropriate support are necessary for home maintenance to be sufficient and adequate to support a safe, personal, growth-enhancing environment.

Expected Outcome: The patient will optimally participate in activities of daily living and personal health regimen with appropriate support. The caregiver will appropriately utilize equipment, supplement home maintenance as planned, and assist in coordination of services and purchases by the end of the third visit.
- ▲ Discuss specific lifestyle and home changes that will promote health.
- Discuss relationship of deficits to health.
- Discuss possible disease caused by defects.
- ▲ Assist family to complete a home safety assessment and follow up on deficits found.
- Encourage removal of clutter that may endanger patient and caregiver safety.

■ = nursing intervention; ▲ = collaborative intervention.

Continued

IV

IV

- Teach universal precautions for infection control.
- Reinforce changes by discussing positive effect and praise attempts at adaptation.
▲ Review with family a plan to respond to emergencies.
  Patient participation at an optimum level in activities of daily living and home maintenance fosters independence, self-esteem, and personal growth.

Expected Outcome: Identify the degree to which the patient and the family have sustained the levels of improved safety, home maintenance, and healthy lifestyles indicated throughout the plan of care by the end of the fourth visit.
▲ Have caregiver and family establish a mutually agreeable standard of cleanliness and order that is safe.
- Determine equipment and supplies needed, identify sources, and obtain them.
- Teach appropriate use and maintenance of equipment.
- Teach caregiver to support maximum independence of patient.
- Review means of maintaining sufficient supplies.
- Investigate alternative ways to have repairs made within financial capabilities of family.
- Support attempts to obtain repairs.
- Arrange for additional support on a regular or periodic basis for caregiver respite.
- Observe for increased level of health secondary to cleaner home environment, and when observed, compliment on changes.
  The sustaining of behavioral change and a safe, personal-growth-enhancing environment over time is necessary to promote health and prevent increased disability.

EVALUATION

The next step in the nursing process is to evaluate whether the desired patient outcomes have occurred. For the nursing diagnosis Impaired Home Maintenance Management, outcomes focus on maintaining the patient at home with maximum independence as long as possible and desired.[8] At the first visit the nurse should guide the patient, the caregiver, and the family in a comprehensive safety and home adequacy assessment; in a discussion of standards of home maintenance and associated activities as perceived by each person present; and in the interpretation of the meaning of lifestyle changes and learning needs for each person. A specific plan will be developed by the end of this visit. If the plan is incomplete the nurse will contact the family in 1 week to assess progress and encourage completion. The location of the visit will depend on the patient's location: in the hospital, at a health center planning for a major surgical procedure, or at home experiencing changes in dependency level. If major changes are needed or if the family

appears unable to complete the plan efficiently, the nurse should contact the case manager and consider referring the patient to a social worker.

At the second visit the nurse discusses progress in achieving the plan and acts as a consultant in solving problems with emerging barriers and in supporting the implementation of the plan. Evidence of achievement includes changes in the cleanliness and orderliness of the home, the acquisition of needed equipment, aids, repairs, and required structural changes, and the scheduling of professional and paraprofessional services, support, and respite services. If progress appears unsteady the nurse will reassess the feasibility of the initial plan and make indicated changes. By the third visit the patient and family should be exhibiting behavior that includes the patient participating in activities of daily living and personal health regimen as much as possible; the caregiver should be proficient in the use of supplies and equipment, and the patient should participate in the scheduling of appropriate support activities for caregiver respite and the personal growth of all family members. If this is not achieved, the nurse should consider a referral for additional support, education, or other services as needed.

The final, fourth visit is to evaluate the degree to which the patient and the family have sustained the levels of improved safety, home maintenance, and healthy lifestyles indicated throughout the plan of care. Evidence of positive outcomes will emerge from a comparison of the evidence noted for the third visit with evidence noted in the fourth visit. If a substantial decline is observed, the nurse should review the original plan and barriers to achievement with the family, act as a problem-solving consultant, and make appropriate referrals.

▪ CASE STUDY WITH PLAN OF CARE

Mrs. Sarah S. is a 72-year-old widow who lives alone in a three-bedroom house in which she has resided for the last 35 years. Mrs. S. was discharged from the community hospital yesterday after hospitalization because of a cerebrovascular accident with right-side hemiplegia. She has been referred to the home health agency, and a home health nurse will make the initial home visit. The referral indicates that Mrs. S. was discharged with medications, a splint for her right arm, a quad cane, wheelchair, and orders and supplies for dressing change of a decubitus on her coccyx. Physical therapy, a registered nurse, and home health services were requested. On the nurse's first visit Mrs. S. is alert, oriented, and adamant about staying in her home. She says, "I'm going to do everything I can to stay here. I don't know how, but I'll manage!" Her daughter is visiting from out of state and plans to stay "until I can get Mom situated." She says. "I feel so helpless. I don't know what to do or who to call. I was so relieved when the social worker at the hospital told me a nurse would come to visit." The nurse observes that (1) Mrs. S. has decubitus on her coccyx, which neither she nor her daughter knows how to care for; (2) she needs assistance with personal care; (3) she can transfer by pivoting from bed to wheelchair with minimal assistance; (4) the wheelchair cannot fit through the narrow doorway to the bathroom; (5) the bathroom has no assistive device such as railings on the tub or the commode; and (6) Mrs. S. can ambulate with a quad cane with a great deal of assistance.

▪ PLAN OF CARE FOR MRS. SARAH S.
Nursing Diagnosis: Impaired Home Maintenance Management Related to Restricted Mobility[7]

Expected Outcome: Mrs. S. and her daughter will make an accurate assessment of factors associated with home maintenance as evidenced by Mrs. S. and her daughter stating personal home maintenance standard and identifying factors that maintain or impede this standard by end of first visit.[1]
- Observe limitations on mobility.
- Make a home assessment, using a tool as a guide.
- Have Mrs. S. and her daughter state home factors that adversely affect recovery.

Expected Outcome: Mrs. S. will utilize community resources as evidenced by remaining in own home as long as desirable and feasible by fourth visit.[4]
- Discuss need for home health aide and daughter to assist with cleaning, shopping, and laundry, and the method of payment.
- Devise and review plans for handling emergencies.
- Refer Mrs. S. to appropriate resources.

Expected Outcome: Mrs. S. will adapt her home and lifestyle to accommodate restrictions as evidenced by remaining in her own home as long as desirable and feasible by fourth visit.[4]
- Discuss need for and ways to obtain safety aids for bathroom, bedroom, and kitchen.
- Asses the likelihood of Mrs. S. resuming social activities engaged in before her cerebrovascular accident.

▪ = nursing intervention; ▲ = collaborative intervention.

Continued

IV

▶ PLAN OF CARE FOR MRS. SARAH S.— CONT'D

Expected Outcome: Mrs. S. will arrange to have structural defects of her home repaired as evidenced by observation of repaired defects by second visit.[2]
- Make plans for repairs identified in home assessment.
- Refer to available resources.

Expected Outcome: Mrs. S. will demonstrate increased awareness of effect of neighborhood on home maintenance as evidenced by identifying neighborhood improvement resources by second visit.[2]
- Discuss with Mrs. S. how she arranged for home maintenance in the past and whether she can continue.
- Refer Mrs. S. to community programs to assist with utility bills, if appropriate.
- Observe immediate neighborhood for level of danger for an immobilized resident.

▦ CRITICAL THINKING EXERCISES

1. What community resources are appropriate for the case of Mrs. Sarah S?

2. What tool would you use to assess the home for this specific case?

3. Identify two specific, intermediate, desired patient outcomes, based on the defining characteristics for this case.

4. Discuss how the patient's health plans (e.g., Medicare or HMO Medigap insurance) in this case affect Mrs. S.'s access and quality of care (consider regulations and policy requirements for access to medical equipment, home care nursing, home health aids, etc.)

REFERENCES

1. American Nurses' Association: *A conceptual model of community health nursing,* Washington, D.C., 1986, The Association.
2. American Nurses' Association: *Standards of home health nursing practice,* Washington, D.C., 1986, The Association.
3. Bower K: *Case management by nurses,* Washington, D.C., 1992, American Nurses Publishing.
4. Carpentino L: *Nursing diagnosis: application to clinical practice,* ed 6, Philadelphia, 1995, JB Lippincott Co.
5. Clemen-Stone S, Eigsti D, and McGuire S: *Comprehensive community health nursing: family, aggregate, and community practice,* ed 4, St. Louis, 1995, Mosby–Year Book.
6. Dienemann J and Trotter JO: Home maintenance management, impaired. In Thompson J and others, editors: *Clinical nursing,* ed 4, St. Louis, 1996, Mosby–Year Book.
7. Ebersole P and Hess P: *Toward healthy aging: human needs and nursing response,* St. Louis, 1994, Mosby–Year Book.
8. Gordon M: *Nursing diagnosis,* ed 3, St. Louis, 1991, Mosby–Year Book.
9. Greif J and Golden B: *AIDS care at home: a guide for caregivers, loved ones and people with AIDS,* New York, 1994, John Wiley & Sons.
10. Jaffe M and Skidmore-Roth L: *Home health nursing care plans,* St. Louis, 1993, Mosby–Year Book.
11. Kim M, McFarland GK, and McLane A: *Pocket guide to nursing diagnoses,* ed 6, St. Louis, 1995, Mosby–Year Book.
12. Laferriere RH: Orem's theory in practice: hospice nursing care, *Home Healthcare Nurse* 13 (5):50–54, 1995.
13. Lentz J and Meyer E: The dirty house, *Nurs Outlook* 27(9): 590–592, 1979.
14. Marrelli TM and Hillard LS: *Home care and clinical paths: effective care planning across the continuum,* St. Louis, 1996, Mosby–Year Book.
15. Mundinger M: *Home care controversy,* Rockville, Maryland, 1983, Aspen Systems Publishing.
16. Rankin SH and Stallings KD: *Patient education: issues, education, practice,* Philadelphia, 1995, JB Lippincott Co.
17. Smith CM and Maurer F: *Community health nursing: theory and practice,* Philadelphia, 1995, WB Saunders Co.
18. Stanhope M and Knollmueller R: *Handbook of community and home health nursing: tools for assessment, intervention, and education,* ed 2, St. Louis, 1996, Mosby–Year Book.
19. Stuart G and Sundeen S: *Principles and practice of psychiatric nursing,* ed 5, St. Louis, 1994, Mosby–Year Book.
20. U.S. Consumer Product Safety Commission: *Home safety checklist,* Pub No 1985-475981: 32202, Washington, D.C., 1985, U.S. Government Printing Office.

Risk for Disorganized Infant Behavior

Disorganized Infant Behavior

Potential for Enhanced Organized Infant Behavior

Risk for Disorganized Infant Behavior *is a state in which the infant is at risk for developing an alteration in integration and modulation of the physiological and behavioral systems of functioning (i.e., autonomic, motor, state organizational, attentional-interactional, and self-regulatory systems).*[10]

Disorganized Infant Behavior *is an alteration in integration and modulation of the infant's physiological and behavioral systems of functioning (i.e., autonomic, motor, state organizational, attentional-interactional, and self-regulatory systems).*[10]

Potential for Enhanced Organized Infant Behavior *is that pattern of modulation of the infant's physiological and behavioral systems of functioning (i.e., autonomic, motor, state organizational, attentional-interactional, and self-regulatory systems) that is satisfactory but could be improved, resulting in higher levels of integration in response to environmental stimuli.*[10]

OVERVIEW

The care of preterm infants in this century has evolved from merely keeping babies warm in incubators to the high-tech specialty of neonatology. Infants born as early as the twenty-third or twenty-fourth week of gestation now survive; but most require long hospitalizations and may display sequelae related to body system immaturity and the stress of a prolonged hospitalization.

Interaction with their environment is the primary source of stimuli for infants. A mother's touch, the sound of a parent's voice, and the sight of a mother's face are sensory images that serve as stimuli for the infant. The infant responds in certain ways to those stimuli; these responses develop into an interactional pattern. Full-term infants are able to adapt to a complex and changing environment because of the maturity and integration of their physiological and behavioral systems. The third trimester is a time of brain growth and neuronal maturation for the fetus.[12] Preterm infants lack that brain development and maturity and are unable to integrate or "organize" their physiological and behavioral functions to respond to the stimuli generated from the environment. This "disorganization," if not recognized and corrected, can lead to long-term sequelae for the infant.[6]

In the early years of neonatal care, it was felt that preterm infants hospitalized for long periods of time experienced sensory deprivation.[7] Thus programs were developed to stimulate infants continually to enhance their growth and development.

Subsequent research demonstrated that infants are oversensitive and overresponsive to stimuli and are unable to buffer and differentiate the stimuli.[13] This necessitated a shift in the focus of care to a modulation of the stimuli presented, relative to the infant's responses.

In her hallmark work, Als describes the Synactive Theory of Neurobehavioral Organization as the interaction of subsystems within an individual—in this case, a preterm infant—for the development and maintenance of self-regulation in response to stimuli.[1] There are five subsystems: (1) the autonomic subsystem, which regulates physiological functions such as cardiorespiratory function, temperature control, and visceral functions (e.g., digestion); (2) the motor subsystem, which regulates movement, muscle tone, and posture; (3) the state subsystem (sometimes referred to as state organizational subsystem), which regulates levels of alertness, from deep sleep to fussiness, and the quality of the transitions from one state to another; (4) the attentional subsystem, which refers to the infant's ability to interact with the environment and those in it and to respond to the stimuli received; and (5) the self-regulation subsystem, which refers to the infant's ability to maintain a balance within and modulate between the subsystem in response to stimuli or when disruptions occur.

The subsystems are interdependent and develop in a hierarchical pattern; the autonomic system is the first subsystem to mature and provides the basis for the maturation of the others. When development progresses smoothly, these susbsystems are mutually supportive and behavior is classified as organized. If development does not progress smoothly, as in preterm infants, development and behaviors become disorganized.[13] The goal is for the infant successfully to regulate responses to stimuli without intervention from caregivers. This is demonstrated by self-quieting behaviors. Once competence (i.e., self-regulation and the modulation of behaviors) is demonstrated in one subsystem, maturation begins in the next.[8]

This theory suggests that successful integration and regulation of the subsystem functions indicate the infant's level of maturation or development. D'Apolito describes organization as the integrated

functioning of the infant's physiological and behavioral systems.[6] The ability of infants to interact with the environment in an organized, smooth fashion, indicates neurobehavioral maturation. If a disruption occurs, the infant may regress and display instabilities within a previously competent subsystem. These instabilities are described as disorganization.

To illustrate this point, when a premature infant is born, one of the initial responses to a stimulus or stressor (e.g., the light and noise of the neonatal intensive care unit) is an increase in the heart rate and/or blood pressure. When a quiet environment is provided, the heart rate and blood pressure normalize. As the infant matures, fewer fluctuations in vital signs occur in response to stimuli, indicating competence and maturation of the autonomic subsystem. This same infant 1 month later displays quiet, alert states before feedings, indicating competence in the state organizational subsystem. This competence in state organization is related to maturation of other subsystems. When there is a disruption in the autonomic or physiological subsystem, as in sepsis, the infant regresses and is unable to achieve a quiet, alert state and experiences an intolerance of handling, indicating a deterioration in maturation.

Practitioners must assess the ability of infants to adapt to their illness and environment and modify the environment of care to enhance the infant's self-regulatory ability and ultimately to maximize the potential for growth and development.

The current standard in neonatal intensive care is a developmentally supportive approach to care, in which the infant's developmental stage and responsiveness are incorporated into the plan of care for that infant.[4,5] The Synactive Theory is an important framework to use in delivering that care. Knowledge about neurobehavioral organization enables health care providers to evaluate the infant's responses to the environment or to caregiving activities. Rather than nursery routines, the care is individualized, based on each preterm infant's strengths. This is a shift from protocol-dependent care to care based on strategic or critical thinking.[3] If an infant is easily "stressed out" or becomes disorganized by handling or procedures, the nurse can cluster activities to maximize rest periods or to allow the infant "time out" between procedures so the infant can recover from the stress.

In an experimental study of 43 preterm infants, Als and colleagues[3] developed a training program for nurses about the provision of developmentally supportive nursing care and an observation system to assess those infants. They found that the infants in the experimental group had less intraventricular hemorrhage, less severe lung disease, and a shorter length of stay. Most importantly, these infants demonstrated better modulation and maturation in autonomic and motor system regulation and self-regulation at 42 weeks after conception.

Becker and colleagues[4] studied 52 infants and provided a developmentally supportive approach to neonatal intensive care. A developmentally supportive environment is described as one that can be altered to meet the variable needs of an infant, to decrease the exposure to stressors, to support the infant's self-regulatory behaviors, and to enhance interaction. The infants in the control group (receiving no intervention) displayed more disorganized behavior, and the experimental group (receiving intervention) exhibited more organized behavior.

ASSESSMENT

The most important tool in the assessment of an infant's behavior, whether it is an actual or a potential problem, is observation. There are certain behaviors exhibited by infants in response to stimuli (e.g., environmental stress or caregiving activities) thought to indicate stress as well as self-regulatory efforts and maintenance.[2] These behaviors can be classified to five subsystems; the presence or absence of these behaviors suggests competence within that subsystem. When the nurse is assessing the infant, the disorganized behaviors should be noted as well as those behaviors that indicate neurobehavioral maturity.

These behaviors have been described and organized in a behavioral assessment tool referred to as APIB (Assessment of Preterm Infant's Behavior.).[3] This system provides for structured assessment

and is often used by nurses. Als and colleagues have developed a program of instruction on the use of APIB; the program is called the Neonatal Individualized Developmental Care Assessment Program (NIDCAP).[3]

Risk for Disorganized Infant Behavior

Risk for Disorganized Infant Behavior reflects those influences that predispose an infant to develop disorganized behavior. Preterm infants are especially susceptible to external influences, such as environmental stressors, altered parent-infant interaction, and handling during caregiving activities. This is related to their immaturity and their inability to buffer stimuli from the environment. Full-term infants experiencing alterations in physiological function or illnesses can develop disorganized behavior related to deterioration in their neurobehavioral system. After the alteration or illness is resolved, the full-term infant's competence in self-regulation returns.

■ Risk Factors

The presence of the following conditions renders the infant at Risk for Disorganized Infant Behavior:

- Immaturity of body systems related to prematurity
- Physiological illness in full-term infants
- Environmental stress (e.g., excessive noise, lights, or invasive procedures)
- Neurological deficits
- Lack of environmental support (e.g., sleep cycle interruption or poor positioning)
- Altered sensory abilities (e.g., visual impairment or hearing loss)
- Pain
- Intrauterine exposure to toxic substances or infections

Disorganized Infant Behavior

The diagnosis Disorganized Infant Behavior refers to infant behavior that reflects an alteration in the stability of the neurobehavioral system. This is related to the stress of interaction with the environment. Immaturity and other risk factors affect

IV

the stability of an infant's behavioral system and subsequently the ability to interact and respond to the environment appropriately. The persistence of characteristics reflecting disorganized behavior may be decreased through ongoing assessment and supportive intervention by caregivers. The nurse assesses each of the five subsystems for the purpose of identifying subsystem behaviors characteristic of Disorganized Infant Behavior.

■ Defining Characteristics

The presence of the following defining characteristics indicates that the infant may have Disorganized Infant Behavior:

Autonomic subsystem

- Irregular respirations or heart rate
- Apnea
- Color changes: cyanosis, pallor, ruddiness, or mottling
- Visceral reactions: gagging, spitting up, or hiccoughs
- Yawning or sighing

Motor subsystem

- Motor activity: twitching, tremors, clonus, jitteriness, or finger splaying
- Muscle tone: flaccidity, hypertonicity, extension of extremities, or back arching
- Facial expressions: grimacing, gaping face, furrowed brow, mixed muscle tone, or yawning
- Frantic, diffuse activity

State subsystem

- Inability to breastfeed or bottle feed without physiological decompensation
- Irritability
- Inconsolable, unrelieved fussiness

Attentional subsystem

- Gaze aversion
- Inability to attend to objects or faces
- "Tuning out" (a halting of interaction) when faced with one or more stimuli
- Fixed staring

Self-regulatory subsystem

- Spontaneous oxygen desaturation associated with activity and handling

■ Related Factors

The following related factors are associated with Disorganized Infant Behavior:

- Prematurity or immaturity
- Motor problems
- Oral problems
- Pain
- Invasive procedures
- Environmental overstimulation (e.g., noisy, bright environment)
- Lack of containment or boundaries

Potential for Enhanced Organized Infant Behavior

Infants with the diagnosis Potential for Enhanced Organized Infant Behavior display adequate self-regulation and can interact with their environment without decompensation within their neurobehavioral systems. Although the infant's physiological and behavioral systems function satisfactorily, such functioning can be optimized. The nursing assessment focuses on evaluating the functioning of the five subsystems to determine if the infant is capable of higher levels of integration in response to environmental stimuli.

The infant with this diagnosis would be expected to display maturation and competence related to the more primitive autonomic and motor subsystems. The nurse might observe self-quieting behaviors, flexed positioning, and good hand-to-mouth activities. The diagnosis implies that maturation and competence is not as well developed in the attentional, state, and self-regulatory subsystems. The nurse might observe that the preterm infant or the infant in pain has difficulty attending to more than one stimulus at a time or is not consistent in modulating between sleep and quiet alertness. Assessment of the following characteristics can be an indication that the infant's behavior, although adequate, can be optimized through environmental and interactional support.

■ Defining Characteristics

The presence of the following defining characteristics indicates that the infant may have Potential for Enhanced Organized Infant Behavior:

Autonomic subsystem

- Regular respirations and heart rate
- Absence of signs of autonomic stress
- Pink color without variations during activity

Motor subsystem

- Grasping
- Hand to mouth or on the face
- Nonnutritive sucking on a pacifier or own hand
- Fisting
- Rooting or mouthing
- Bringing hands to the midline
- Hand clasping
- Flexed or tucked extremities
- Smooth movements
- Relaxed tone and posture

State subsystem

- Environmental and interactional support can promote and enhance:
    - Modulation of states between sleep, quiet, and alert
    - Focused expressions such as lip pursing, "ooh face," and smiling

Attentional subsystem

- Environmental and interactional support can promote and enhance:
    - Purposeful attention to stimuli
    - Seeks out interaction with stimuli and can modulate interest between two stimuli

Self-regulatory subsystem

- Environmental and interactional support can promote and enhance:
    - Tolerance of handling and caregiving activities
    - Tolerance of stimuli

■ Related Factors

The following related factors are associated with Potential for Enhanced Infant Behavior:

- Prematurity
- Pain

DIAGNOSIS

■ Differential Nursing Diagnosis

This cluster of diagnoses describes infant behavior on a continuum. At the wellness end of the continuum is Organized Infant Behavior, followed by Potential for Enhanced Organized Infant Behavior. The infant behaviors observed at this end of the continuum indicate behavioral competence, maturation, and self-regulation. Farther along the continuum, toward the illness end, is Risk for Disorganized Infant Behavior, which, if not diagnosed and treated, will increase the likelihood of an infant developing Disorganized Infant Behavior. This diagnosis reflects an alteration in functioning that is accompanied by discrete signs and symptoms.

■ Medical and Psychiatric Diagnoses

Examples of specific medical diagnoses related to Disorganized Infant Behavior and Risk for Disorganized Infant Behavior include respiratory distress syndrome; intracranial hemorrhage, bronchopulmonary displasia, and retinopathy of prematurity. Preterm infants with medical diagnoses that are accompanied by pain, feeding intolerance, and oral and motor problems should be considered at Risk for Disorganized Infant Behavior.

OUTCOME IDENTIFICATION, PLANNING, AND IMPLEMENTATION

A goal of nursing care for all infants is to foster their growth and development and to teach families to recognize the infant's cues to enhance development.[9] The expected outcomes for the diagnoses related to organized or disorganized infant behavior focus on the development, promotion, and enhancement of infant self-regulation. Self-regulation is evidenced by the presence of those infant behaviors that indicate competence (e.g., self-comforting behaviors and smooth transitions between sleep and wakefulness). The nursing interventions focus on providing support for the infant during interactions or care activities to reduce the incidence or prevent the development of Disorganized Behavior.

Risk for Disorganized Infant Behavior

All preterm infants are at Risk for Disorganized Infant Behavior related to their immaturity. The

IV

IV

physiological and sociological alterations, such as sensory deficits and altered parent-infant attachment, take time to correct; yet the effects of these alterations can be controlled and limited. For the infant at Risk for Disorganized Behavior, the goal of care is to maintain the infant's current level of functioning in terms of self-regulation abilities.

Developmental care and environmental modifications (e.g., modulating light or clustering caregiving activities) are described in the Nursing Care Guidelines. These have been identified as appropriate interventions to stimulate the self-regulation activities of preterm infants.[2–5,11] For infants with pathophysiological conditions, whether preterm or full-term, the treatment of the condition can itself decrease the Risk for Disorganized Behavior; however, nursing interventions (i.e., developmental care and environmental modifications) are important in supporting the infant's maintenance of self-regulation abilities throughout the course of the treatment.

Disorganized Infant Behavior

The desired outcome for the infant at Risk for Disorganized Infant Behavior is for the infant to demonstrate self-regulation as evidenced by the presence of organized behavior and a decrease in the number of characteristics reflecting disorganized behavior. Although many of the factors promoting disorganized behavior (e.g., motor problems and prematurity) may be resolved with the passage of time, immediate nursing interventions can be implemented that will support self-regulation activities. These interventions can decrease or mitigate the risks that the disorganized behavior factors pose for the infant. Specifically, a program of individualized intervention based on an assessment of behavioral cues should be implemented; such a program should modify the environment to support the infant's needs.[7]

Environmental modifications and activities to structure the interaction between the infant and caregivers should be introduced. These modifications and activities are designed to promote the infant's self-regulation, thereby decreasing the incidence of the disorganized behaviors. Cluster-

ing caregiving activities to maximize rest periods will give the infant time to recover from stressful activity, if any. It is important to reassess the infant to determine if this strategy is successful, taking care to ensure that there are not too many activities occurring at one time, and that the rest periods are long enough. Environmental modifications such as decreased or cycled light, less noise, and the use of positioning aids are less intrusive; the infant can then use his or her energies for interaction rather than filtering out external stimuli.[7,11] Minimal and gentle handling increases the infant's ability for self-regulation, easing the transition from deep sleep to alertness.

Using the infant's cues to regulate nursing activities individualizes the infant's care. The nurse can place his or her hands on the infant's torso and extremities and place rolls around the infant for supportive positioning. These interventions provide containment, encourage flexion of the extremities, and decrease the hypertonicity resulting from extension of extremities and back arching. Small hand rolls provide an opportunity for the infant to develop the self-consoling activity of grasping or holding on to things. Swaddling with blankets encourages proper positioning and posture and assist the infant in bringing the hands to the midline. Hands-to-midline activity is the infant's first step toward hand-to-mouth activities and keeps the extremities in flexion.

Support the infant while feeding through positioning (i.e., a tucked position), which provides oral support and decreases environmental stimulation. These interventions serve to encourage the infant's ability to breastfeed. Skin-to-skin contact between the infant and parents, such as placing the infant on the parent's chest, not only enhances parent-infant interaction but also has been shown to enhance quiet sleep and more regular respirations and heart rate.[7]

Potential for Enhanced Infant Behavior

As previously described, the assessment of the infant with the Potential for Enhanced Behavior identifies those behaviors that indicate the integration of all the subsystems in the neurobehavioral system. Infants who display organized behavior, without environmental modification and caregiver support, can display enhanced behavior when modifications and support are provided. The desired outcome is to optimize the infant's self-regulation abilities.

A developmental plan of care for such infants should take into consideration the competent behaviors displayed by the infant and the "time out cues" (disorganized behaviors) that the infant displays when overstressed. The "time out cues" indicate that environmental and interactional support is needed to optimize the attentional, state, and self-regulatory subsystems. Interventions to support outcome achievement relate to introducing environmental controls (e.g., dimming the lights and reducing noise) and caregiver interactions (e.g., the use of blanket wraps or modulating physical caregiving and verbal interaction).

IV

■ **NURSING CARE GUIDELINES**
Nursing Diagnosis: Risk for Disorganized Infant Behavior

Expected Outcome: The infant will maintain self-regulation as evidenced by organized behavior.
- ■ Monitor infant's responses to interactions *to determine the presence or absence of disorganized behavior*.
- ▲ Modulate the light around the infant (no bright lights, only dim lights when interacting with the infant) *to decrease environmental stress*.
- ▲ Cluster caregiving activities according to the infant's "time out cues" *to offer the infant rest periods in which to recover from stressful interactions*.
- ▲ Place blanket rolls, and position the infant prone and tucked in the crib *to provide physical support for the infant at rest*.
- ▲ Support the infant with blanket wraps, wrap the infant bringing the hands to the midline, and use upright positioning as appropriate (e.g., a mattress tilt) *to assist the infant in self-comforting activities*.
- ▲ Instruct the family about the infant's "time out cues" *to enhance their parent-infant interaction*.

■ = nursing intervention; ▲ = collaborative intervention.

■ **NURSING CARE GUIDELINES**
Nursing Diagnosis: Disorganized Infant Behavior

Expected Outcome: The infant will demonstrate self-regulation as evidenced by a decrease in the presence of disorganized behaviors.
- ■ Assess autonomic and motor system functions before and during interaction *to determine the infant's abilities and instabilities ("time out cues")*.
- ■ Monitor infant responses to interactions *to determine the presence or absence of disorganized behavior*.
- ▲ Discontinue interaction in response to the infant's decompensation *to prevent the development of disorganized behaviors*.
- ▲ Modulate the light around the infant (no bright lights, only dim light when interacting with the infant) *to decrease environmental stress*.
- ▲ Cluster caregiving activities according to the infant's "time out cues" *to offer the infant rest periods in which to recover from activity*.
- ▲ Place blanket rolls, and position the infant prone and tucked in the crib *to provide physical support for the infant while at rest*.

■ = nursing intervention; ▲ = collaborative intervention.

Continued

IV

◀◼ **NURSING CARE GUIDELINES — CONT'D**

▲ During interactions, support the infant with blanket wraps and hold the infant in an upright position, bringing the hands to the midline *to assist the infant in self-comforting activities, to promote flexion of the extremities, and to decrease extension and back arching.*

▲ Present one interaction (physical or verbal) to the infant at a time *to modulate the stimuli from the environment.*

▲ Instruct the family about the infant's "time out cues" *to enhance their parent-infant interaction and to support the infant's organized behaviors.*

◀◼ **NURSING CARE GUIDELINES**
Nursing Diagnosis: Potential for Enhanced Infant Behavior

Expected Outcome: The infant's self-regulation abilities will be optimized through environmental and interactional support as evidenced by the persistence of self-regulating behaviors.

▪ Identify those behaviors and activities that comfort the infant *so they can be used in caring for the infant.*

▲ Care for the infant using blanket wraps; wrap the infant, bringing the hands to the midline; and use upright positioning as appropriate (e.g., mattress tilt) *to support the infant in self-comforting activities, to promote flexion of the extremities, and to prevent extension and back arching.*

▲ Modulate physical caregiving and verbal interaction for the infant *to prevent the stress of introducing two stimuli simultaneously.*

▲ Utilize the infant's self-comforting behaviors (e.g., pacifier) when anticipating a stressful situation *to prevent decompensation in self-regulation.*

▪ = nursing intervention; ▲ = collaborative intervention.

EVALUATION

When evaluating the nursing care delivered to infants, whether preterm or full-term, the nurse takes into account that the infant's response is related to a complex combination of many variables. Not only does the nurse evaluate the effectiveness of the intervention itself but also the infant's response to the caregiving activities, the effect of the environment, and the infant's behavioral cues.

Risk for Disorganized Behavior

The effectiveness of nursing care for the infant at Risk for Disorganized Behavior is determined through ongoing evaluation of the infant's status as it relates to maintaining organized behavior. If the infant's behavior continues to be organized, the interventions are considered effective and should continue. If the defining characteristics of Disorganized Behavior are observed, further assessment and evaluation are necessary to confirm a change in diagnosis from Risk for Disorganized Behavior to Disorganized Behavior.

Disorganized Behavior

Evaluation of the effectiveness of the nursing care for the infant with Disorganized Behavior focuses on determining whether or not the infant is demonstrating self-regulation abilities. Through the initial assessment, specific characteristics reflecting the infant's Disorganized Behavior and the situations in which the infant is unable to maintain self-regulation should have been noted. During the ongoing evaluation of the infant, the nurse directs attention to the alleviation of the characteristics and infant's response to the noted situations. This is done to determine whether those nursing interventions identified in the plan of care have supported the infant's integration of organized behaviors.

The addition of new competencies into the infant's repertoire of behaviors that reflect organized behavior indicates that interventions have been supportive. If the infant displays new disorganized behaviors, or behaviors not previously assessed, this indicates a possible deterioration in self-regulation. The nurse then reevaluates the infant for causes of the deterioration and revises the plan of care.

Potential for Enhanced Organized Infant Behavior

The nursing interventions for the infant diagnosed with Potential for Enhanced Organized Infant Behavior should support the infant in optimizing self-regulation abilities. Such infants demonstrate self-regulation and competence in behavior (e.g., self-quieting behaviors, flexed positioning, and good hand-to-mouth activities). The interventions are effective if they elicit and promote further self-regulatory abilities (e.g., purposeful attention

IV

▐ CASE STUDY WITH PLAN OF CARE

Baby girl S. is 30 days old. She was born at 28 weeks gestation with Respiratory Distress Syndrome. Currently she weighs 1600 g and is taking 30 cc of 24-calorie premature formula (150 cc/120 kcal/kg) every 3 hours. She has recently weaned to room air, is cared for in an incubator, and is on a cardiorespiratory and an oxygen saturation monitor. She is beginning to bottle feed and likes to sleep on her stomach and suck on a pacifier. Her mother is 16 years of age and visits infrequently. The nurses have observed her to experience oxygen denaturation, extension of the extremities, and arching when vital signs are measured and feedings are given. She frequently spits up and gets hiccoughs after feedings. When her mother visits, Baby girl S. comes out of the incubator and is held, but she does not open her eyes.

▐ PLAN OF CARE FOR BABY GIRL S.
Nursing Diagnosis: Disorganized Infant Behavior Related to Prematurity or Immaturity

Expected Outcome: Baby girl S. will display self-regulation as evidenced by a decrease in the presence of disorganized behaviors.
- Assess Baby S.'s vital signs before nursing care activities and again during activities.
- Place a blanket roll around Baby S. in the incubator, as well as a hip roll when positioned prone.
- Offer Baby S. a pacifier during her feedings to console her and to assess her feeding readiness.
- Cover Baby S.'s incubator with an incubator quilt and turn down the light when her mother visits.
- Demonstrate to her mother how to wrap Baby S. (i.e., maintaining Baby S.'s hands at the midline when her mother holds her).
- Suggest to Baby S.'s mother that she hold Baby S. quietly, without talking, until Baby S. begins to open her eyes.
- Once Baby S. opens her eyes while being held, demonstrate to the mother how to hold Baby S. (i.e., 6 to 8 inches away from her face) so Baby S. can begin to focus.
▲ Consult with the physicians about using an oxygen cannula for feedings and when Baby S. is held to prevent hypoxia.
▲ Develop a developmental care plan for Baby S. as a reference for the care provider to refer to when they care for Baby S.

▪ = nursing intervention; ▲ = collaborative intervention.

IV

to a stimulus, attending to more than one stimuli [such as voices and faces], and modulating between different states such as sleep and quiet alertness). These behaviors reflect interaction of the attentional, state, and self-regulation subsystems.

■ CRITICAL THINKING EXERCISES

1. Specify and describe the self-regulating behaviors that Baby girl S. would display if nursing interventions were effective in treating her Disorganized Infant Behavior.

2. If you involve Baby S.'s mother in the development of a plan of care for Baby S. that incorporates increased mother-baby interactions, what mother-related and baby-related factors should be considered to assure implementation of the plan? Describe how these factors would influence how you would individualize Baby S.'s plan of care to her and her mother.

3. Baby girl S. is to be discharged after being hospitalized for 3½ months. What information about Baby S.'s mother and significant others would assist you in preparing a realistic discharge plan? What support services should be contacted before discharge? If Baby S. and her mother lived in your city, what specific services would you contact for them?

REFERENCES

1. Als H: Toward a synactive theory of development. A promise for the assessment and support of infant individuality, *Infant Mental Health J* 3:229–243, 1982.
2. Als H and others: Individualized behavioral and environmental care for the very low birthweight preterm infant at high risk for bronchopulmonary dysplasia: neonatal intensive care unit and developmental outcome, *Pediatrics* 78: 1123–1132, 1986.
3. Als H and others: Individualized developmental care for the very low-birth-weight preterm infant, *JAMA* 272: 853–858, 1994.
4. Becker PT and others: Effects of developmental care on behavioral organization of very low birthweight infants, *Nurs Res* 42:214–220, 1993.
5. Burns K and others: Infant stimulation: Modification of an intervention based on physiologic and behavioral cues, *JOGNN* 23:581–589, 1994.
6. D'Apolito K: What is an organized infant? *Neonatal Network* 10(1):23–31, 1991.
7. Klaus MH and Kennell JH: *Maternal-infant bonding*, St. Louis, 1976, The CV Mosby Co.
8. Mouradian LE and Als H: *The influence of neonatal intensive caregiving practices on motor functioning of preterm infants*, Am J Occup Ther 48:527–533, 1994.
9. National Association of Neonatal Nurses: *Infant developmental care guidelines*, ed 2, Petaluma, California, 1995, The Association.
10. North American Nursing Diagnosis Association: *NANDA nursing diagnoses: definitions and classification, 1995–1996*, Philadelphia, 1994, The Association.
11. Vandenberg KA: Revising the traditional model: an individualized approach to developmental interventions in the intensive care nursery, *Neonatal Network* 4(1):32–38, 1985.
12. Volpe JJ: *Neurology of the newborn*, ed 2, Philadelphia, 1987, WB Saunders Co.
13. Yecco GJ: Environmental stress and premature infants, *J Perin Neonat Nurs* 7:56–65, 1993.

Impaired Physical Mobility

▶

Impaired Physical Mobility *is a state in which the individual experiences a limitation of ability for independent movement.*[12]

OVERVIEW

The nursing diagnosis Impaired Physical Mobility is one of the most frequent and most important that nurses encounter in their practice. Impaired Physical Mobility is found in conjunction with numerous medical-surgical conditions. In addition, this nursing diagnosis can occur as a result of prescribed medical-surgical treatments. Impaired Physical Mobility can affect persons across the life span in all settings.[1,5,10,14,15,16]

The three elements necessary for mobility include the ability to move, the motivation to move, and an unrestrictive environment in which to move.[3] Much of the theoretical and research literature basic to an understanding of the nursing diagnosis Impaired Physical Mobility is found in such areas of subspecialty as neuroscience nursing, orthopedic nursing, rehabilitation nursing, and geriatric nursing.

ASSESSMENT

Thorough assessment of Impaired Physical Mobility begins with data collection and culminates in the identification of specific nursing diagnoses. The following assessment parameters should be included: gait, balance, symmetry and strength of muscle movements, presence of involuntary muscle movements, ability to perform activities of daily living, presence of structural deformities, range of motion in joints, muscle strength, and overall phys-

ical fitness. In addition, the need for equipment and prostheses for activity and ambulation is an important assessment factor.[3] The following functional levels have been described relative to Impaired Physical Mobility[12]:

Level   0: Completely independent
Level   I: Requires use of equipment or device
Level II: Requires help from another person for assistance, supervision, or teaching
Level III: Requires help from another person and use of equipment or device
Level IV: Dependent, does not participate in activity

■ Defining Characteristics

The presence of the following defining characteristics indicates that the patient may be experiencing Impaired Physical Mobility[2,7,9,12,13]:

- Inability to move purposefully within the physical environment, including bed mobility, transfer, and ambulation
- Decreased muscle strength, control, or mass
- Impaired coordination
- Imposed restrictions of movement, including mechanical or medical protocol restrictions
- Range-of-motion limitations
- Reluctance to attempt movement

■ Related Factors

The following related factors are associated with Impaired Physical Mobility[2,7,9,12,13]:

- Intolerance to activity
- Decreased strength or endurance
- Pain or discomfort
- Neuromuscular impairment

- Musculoskeletal impairment
- External devices such as casts, splints, braces, or intravenous tubing
- Advanced age
- Trauma
- Surgical procedures such as amputation
- Nonfunctioning or missing limbs
- Perceptual or cognitive impairment
- Depressive disorders
- Anxiety disorders

DIAGNOSIS

■ Differential Nursing Diagnosis

Impaired Physical Mobility should not be used to describe complete immobility. Instead, Risk of Disuse Syndrome is the appropriate diagnosis to select when there is complete immobility.

■ Medical and Psychiatric Diagnoses

Medical diagnoses most frequently related to Impaired Physical Mobility include disorders of the musculoskeletal system, the neurological system, and connective tissue. Specifically, musculoskeletal system diseases, such as muscular dystrophy, and trauma, such as fractures, are often related to Impaired Physical Mobility. In addition, neurological system diseases, such as Parkinson's disease, and trauma, such as spinal cord injury, are often related to Impaired Physical Mobility. Finally, disorders of the connective tissue, such as rheumatoid arthritis, are often related to Impaired Physical Mobility.

OUTCOME IDENTIFICATION, PLANNING, AND IMPLEMENTATION[4,6,8,11]

The identification of outcomes from which planning and implementation proceed is based on an understanding of the underlying principles of care for patients with Impaired Physical Mobility. Each of the six expected patient outcomes is briefly addressed.

The expected patient outcome relating to increasing mobility is based on the principle of restoring function. Specifically, planning and implementation are directed toward the restoration of the highest possible level of functioning.

The expected patient outcome relating to demonstrating maximum range of motion in all joints is based on the principle of preventing deterioration. Specifically, planning and implementation are directed toward maintaining strength in the unaffected limbs and maintaining joint mobility in the affected limbs.

The expected patient outcome relating to the use of adaptive devices is based on the principle of promoting independent functioning. Specifically, planning and implementation are directed toward instruction of patients in the appropriate use of adaptive devices to compensate for loss in mobility, either temporary or permanent.

The expected patient outcome relating to the utilization of safety measures is based on the principle of promoting physical safety. Specifically, planning and implementation are directed toward instructing patients in appropriate safety precautions that they or their caregivers need to follow.

The expected patient outcome relating to participating in a plan for integrating the mobility impairment into established lifestyle patterns is based on the principle of promoting psychosocial adaptation. Specifically, planning and implementation are directed toward counseling patients to accept and integrate their specific mobility impairments.

The expected patient outcome relating to identifying and using institutional or community resources to manage impaired mobility is based on the principle of promoting independent functioning. Specifically, planning and implementation are directed toward instructing patients regarding appropriate resources and services.

Providing time estimates for the attainment of these six expected patient outcomes is complex and difficult because of the extreme diversity covered in the diagnostic label Impaired Physical Mobility. One guideline that can be provided in terms of time estimates is that these outcomes will be attained not within hours or days but within weeks or even months. A second guideline is that these outcomes need to be attained on an ongoing basis. For example, the expected patient outcome

Continued on p. 398

◀ **NURSING CARE GUIDELINES**

Nursing Diagnosis: Impaired Physical Mobility°

Expected Outcome: The patient will demonstrate measures to increase mobility as evidenced by the performance of progressive mobilization and functional activities.

▲ Provide for progressive mobilization.

▲ Assist the patient to progress from active range-of-motion exercises to functional activities, as indicated.

■ Teach transfer techniques.

The use of such approaches will improve the functional abilities of the patient.

Expected Outcome: The patient will demonstrate maximum range of motion in all joints as evidenced by maintenance of strength in the unaffected limbs and maintenance of joint mobility in the affected limbs.

■ Teach patient to perform active range-of-motion exercises on unaffected limbs at least four times a day.

■ Perform passive range-of-motion exercises on affected limbs at least four times a day.

Active range-of-motion exercises increase muscle mass, tone, and strength, whereas passive range-of-motion exercises maintain joint mobility.

Expected Outcome: The patient will demonstrate the use of adaptive devices to increase mobility.

▲ Teach and observe proper use of appropriate devices: crutches, walkers, wheelchairs, prostheses, and slings.

▲ Teach and observe use of appropriate adaptive equipment to enhance use of arms.

The use of adaptive devices can significantly improve mobility and independent functioning.

Expected Outcome: The patient will utilize safety measures to minimize potential for injury.

■ Teach and observe safety precautions, such as protecting areas of decreased sensation from extremes of heat and cold, instructing patients confined to wheelchairs to shift position and lift up the buttocks every 15 minutes, and instructing patients with decreased perception of the lower extremities to check where limbs are placed when changing positions.

The use of such approaches will decrease the possibility of physical injury.

Expected Outcome: The patient will participate in a plan for integrating the mobility impairment into established lifestyle patterns.

■ Explore patient perceptions of mobility impairment in terms of previous lifestyle patterns, chance to resume prior patterns, and willingness to accept limitations.

■ Discuss alternatives (i.e., substitutions or modifications) for activities that are unachievable (temporarily or permanently).

■ Identify resources, special equipment, devices, and environmental modifications necessary to permit functioning, despite physical limitations.

These approaches will enhance the patient's sense of control and actual control.

Expected Outcome: The patient will identify and use institutional or community resources to manage impaired mobility.

■ Provide patient with information about available resources.

■ Facilitate access to available resources by means of printed materials, computer bulletin boards, telephone contacts, introductions, or written referrals.

■ Mobilize resources existing within the patient's support network.

■ Refer patient to support services according to need: physical therapy, occupational therapy, or social services.

The use of such approaches will assist the patient to achieve the highest level of independence possible.

■ = nursing intervention; ▲ = collaborative intervention.

°References 4, 6, 8, 11.

IV

relating to the utilization of safety measures is an outcome that needs to be attained on a daily basis. It is not an outcome that is attained once and then neglected.

EVALUATION

Evaluation[4,6,8,11] is the process of comparing actual patient status with expected patient outcomes. The outcome of demonstrating measures to increase mobility can be measured by the performance of progressive mobilization, the performance of functional activities, and the use of appropriate transfer techniques by the patient. The outcome of demonstrating maximum range of motion in all joints can be measured by the maintenance of range of motion, muscle mass, and strength in unaffected limbs at the patient's usual level. Measurement of the outcome for affected limbs is based on the maintenance of joint mobility. The outcome of demonstrating the use of adaptive devices to increase mobility can be measured by the proper use by the patient of whatever adaptive devices are appropriate for use in the particular situation.

The outcome of utilizing safety measures to minimize potential for injury can be measured by observing the patient's compliance with whatever safety precautions are appropriate for use in the particular situation. The outcome of participating in a plan for integrating the mobility impairment into established lifestyle patterns can be measured by the patient's active participation in discussions about and positive responses to possible alternatives and modifications necessary in his or her lifestyle patterns. The outcome of identifying and utilizing institutional or community resources to manage impaired mobility can be measured by the patient's acceptance of and use of whatever support services are appropriate in the particular situation.

If expected patient outcomes are not achieved, this could be due to several factors. One factor could be an incomplete or inaccurate data base leading to inappropriate expected patients outcomes. Another factor could be inappropriate nursing interventions. Often a reassessment of the patient's situation leads to the establishment of more realistic outcomes. Also, improved clarity about the patient's situation can lead to more individualized nursing interventions, with a higher probability of bringing about the expected patient outcomes.

▶ CASE STUDY WITH PLAN OF CARE

Mrs. Florence C. is 76 years old. Mrs. C. has lived alone since the death of her husband 7 years ago. She has two daughters, one of whom lives in the same small town. Three weeks ago, Mrs. C. sustained a vertebral compression fracture of the L1 vertebra secondary to spinal osteoporosis. She was hospitalized for 1 week on bed rest, then spent 2 weeks at the home of her daughter. Now she is returning to her own home. She is still experiencing pain caused by the fracture and associated muscle spasms. She has a prescription for a mild analgesic and is permitted to have activity as tolerated.

▶ PLAN OF CARE FOR MRS. FLORENCE C.
Nursing Diagnosis: Impaired Physical Mobility Related to Back Pain Resulting from Vertebral Compression Fracture and Muscle Spasms

---

Expected Outcome: Mrs. C. will demonstrate increasing mobility as evidenced by a return to her previous level of functional activities within 1 month.
- Negotiate with Mrs. C. a plan of care that allows a gradual return to previous level of activities, including, for example, increasing number of hours out of bed; increasing amounts of walking, standing, and sitting;

■ = nursing intervention; ▲ = collaborative intervention.

increasing independence in personal care; and increasing independence in home maintenance activities.
▲ Facilitate pain management (analgesic use, as ordered, and periodic rest periods).

Expected Outcome: Mrs. C. will utilize safety measures to minimize potential for injury as evidenced by adherence to specified precautions.
■ Teach Mrs. C. to avoid jarring movements and to avoid heavy lifting to help prevent another vertebral fracture.

Expected Outcome: Mrs. C. will identify and utilize resources to manage impaired mobility as evidenced by the use of existing support networks.
■ Negotiate with Mrs. C. a plan that allows for input from all available and willing members of her support network. Tasks to be shared include items such as food preparation, house cleaning, laundry, shopping, errands, and companionship until Mrs. C. is fully functional.

IV

■ CRITICAL THINKING EXERCISES

1. Mrs. C. hesitates to use her prescribed analgesic because she claims that she "has never liked taking pills." How would you advise her?
2. Mrs. C. has always been an independent person and is resistant to the idea of accepting assistance from others. How would you advise her?
3. Mrs. C. expresses fear of another vertebral fracture and reasons that the more she limits her activity, the less chance she has of another fracture. What points would you include in your patient teaching to address this issue?

REFERENCES

1. Creason NS: Mobility: current bases for practice. In Funk SG and others, editors: *Key aspects of recovery: improving nutrition, rest, and mobility,* New York, 1990, Springer Publishing Co.
2. Creason NS: Toward a model of clinical validation of nursing diagnoses: developing conceptual and operational definitions of impaired physical mobility. In Carroll-Johnson RM, editor: *Classification of nursing diagnoses: proceedings of the Ninth Conference,* Philadelphia, 1991, JB Lippincott Co.
3. Edlund BJ: Activity-sleep assessment. In Bellack JP and Edlund BJ, editors: *Nursing diagnosis and assessment,* ed 2, Boston, 1992, Jones & Bartlett Publishers.
4. Engelking CH and Lestz PW: Impaired physical mobility. In Daeffler RJ and Petrosino BM, editors: *Manual of oncology nursing practice: nursing diagnoses and care,* Rockville, Maryland, 1990, Aspen Publishers.
5. Gordon M: Report of an RNF study to determine which nursing diagnoses have high frequency and high treatment priority in rehabilitation nursing, part 1, *Rehab Nurs Res* 4(1):3–10, 1995.
6. Halar EM and Bell KR: Rehabilitation's relationship to inactivity. In Kottke FJ and Lehmann JF, editors: *Krusen's handbook of physical medicine and rehabilitation,* ed 4, Philadelphia, 1990, WB Saunders Co.
7. Johnson PA and others: Applying nursing diagnosis and nursing process to activities of daily living and mobility, *Geriatr Nurs* 13(1):25–27, 1992.
8. Loeper JM: Positioning. In Bulechek GM and McCloskey JC, editors: *Nursing interventions: essential nursing treatments,* ed 2, Philadelphia, 1992, WB Saunders Co.
9. Mehmert PA and Delaney CW: Validating impaired physical mobility, *Nurs Diagnosis* 2(4):143–154, 1991.
10. Mobily PR and Kelley LS: Iatrogenesis in the elderly: factors of immobility, *J Geront Nurs* 17(9):5–10, 1991.
11. Neal MC, Paquette M, and Mirch M: *Nursing diagnosis care plans for diagnosis-related groups,* Boston, 1990, Jones & Bartlett Publishers.
12. North American Nursing Diagnosis Association: *NANDA nursing diagnoses: definitions and classification, 1995-1996,* Philadelphia, 1994, The Association.
13. Ouellet LL and Rush KL: A synthesis of selected literature on mobility: a basis for studying impaired mobility, *Nurs Diagnosis* 3(2):72–80, 1992.
14. Pierce L and others: Frequently selected nursing diagnoses for the rehabilitation client with stroke, *Rehab Nurs* 20(3):138–143, 1995.
15. Rantz M, Vinz-Miller T, and Matson S: Nursing diagnoses in long-term care: a longitudinal perspective for strategic planning, *Nurs Diagnosis* 6(2):57–63, 1995.
16. Sawin KJ and Heard L: Nursing diagnoses used most frequently in rehabilitation nursing practice, *Rehab Nurs* 17(5): 256–262, 1992.

Risk for Peripheral Neurovascular Dysfunction

▶

Risk for Peripheral Neurovascular Dysfunction *is a state in which an individual is at risk of experiencing a disruption in circulation, sensation, or motion of an extremity.*[9]

OVERVIEW

The nursing diagnosis Risk for Peripheral Neurovascular Dysfunction was developed out of the need to describe accurately phenomena that were of specific concern to orthopedic nurses.[15] However, this diagnosis is also useful in numerous conditions where the patient is in jeopardy of any circulatory or neurological compromise.

Individuals across the life span are at Risk for Peripheral Neurovascular Dysfunction. Poor nutrition in any age group may predispose an individual to peripheral neurovascular dysfunction from a B vitamin deficiency.[14] Ingestion of tri-*o*-cresyl phosphate found in cooking oil in Morocco, Ginger Jake found in patent medicine in the United States, and large quantities of the cassava root found in Cuba, Jamaica, Mozambique, Nigeria, and Zaire may result in peripheral neurovascular dysfunction.[8,14] Chronic intake of high levels of alcohol can cause peripheral neuropathy from thiamine deficiency and the direct effects of ethanol or acetaldehyde. Prolonged cigarette smoking is a risk factor for peripheral neurovascular dysfunction because nicotine stimulates the sympathetic nervous system, causes arterial constriction, and increases platelet aggregation. Children at risk for lead poisoning and those who engage in glue sniffing activities are also risk for the development of peripheral neurovascular dysfunction.[8]

Individuals, regardless of age, who engage in athletic activities are at risk for the development of peripheral neurovascular dysfunction secondary to nerve entrapment syndromes or vascular syndromes in the chest, back, shoulders, elbows, hands, wrists, hips, knees, ankles, and feet. Cyclists, baseball players, and those who play racquet sports are at risk for compression injuries involving the median nerves (carpal tunnel syndrome) and ulnar nerves (Guyon's canal syndrome). Bowlers are at risk for injury to the digital nerve in the hand and may develop a syndrome known as Bowler's thumb. A single, traumatic event to the hand from sports such as judo, karate, lacrosse, or hockey, may result in vascular injury to the hand and the development of hypothenar hammer syndrome. Repetitive trauma from sports such as handball and baseball (catching and pitching) may cause vascular damage to the hand and digitial ischemia.[11] Athletic sports that involve throwing activities, such as football and baseball, can cause neurovascular injuries to the shoulder. The most commonly recognized neurovascular shoulder compression syndromes are axillary artery occlusion, effort thrombosis, quadrilateral space syndrome, and thoracic outlet syndrome.[1] Overtraining in sports such as cross country, basketball, and volleyball may result in popliteal artery entrapment.[13]

Musicians may be at risk for peripheral neurovascular disease from playing their instruments. Palmer and others[10] reported a case of intermittent compression of the right subclavian artery in a cellist. After approximately 30 minutes of cello playing, the cellist began to experience symptoms of neurovascular dysfunction in the right (bow) arm. Symptoms included numbness in the right little finger; aching and a sensation of coldness in the right elbow, forearm, arm, and shoulder; and pain in the region of the right rhomboid muscles. Musicians who play the violin, viola, cello, or bass violin are also at risk for peripheral neurovascular dysfunction from repetitive trauma to their wrists from bowing.

Certain occupations place individuals at Risk for Peripheral Neurovascular Dysfunction. Jobs requiring repetitive use of the wrist and hand— for example, word processing, assembly-line work, and construction work—may cause damage to the median and ulnar nerves. Individuals who have occupations that place them at risk for severe, extensive burns, such as firemen, those who work with electricity, and individuals who are exposed to toxins such as organophosphorus pesticides, mercury, some chlorinated hydrocarbons, arsenic, lead, and glue, are at risk for peripheral neurovascular dysfunction.[8]

Age-related changes in the peripheral nervous system that place the elderly at Risk for Peripheral Neurovascular Dysfunction include a gradual decline in nerve conduction velocity and amplitude, loss of vibration sense, and absence of ankle reflexes.[2] Prolonged immobility, frequently seen in the elderly, is also a risk factor for peripheral neurovascular dysfunction.

Many medical conditions place an individual at Risk for Peripheral Neurovascular Dysfunction. Some of these include diabetes mellitus, renal failure, late-stage AIDS, fractures, spinal stenosis, lumbar disc syndromes, sciatic nerve syndromes, Raynaud's disease, Buerger's disease, conversion disorder, vascular obstruction, thrombophlebitis, deep venous thrombosis, and arterial insufficiency. Ingestion of medications, such as cancer chemotherapeutic agents, isoniazid, and overdosage of vitamin B_6 may cause peripheral neurovascular dysfunction. Surgical patients who are improperly positioned during procedures or those who are maintained in a position for several hours are at Risk for Peripheral Neurovascular Dysfunction.[5] Circumstances that may cause an increase in pressure within a muscle compartment may place an individual at Risk for Peripheral Neurovascular Dysfunction. Pressure within a muscle compartment may increase because of (1) a decrease in the size or volume of the compartment, such as from premature closure of fascial defects before edema has subsided, (2) an increase in compartment contents, such as from edema or hemorrhage, or (3) application of external pressure from tight casts, dressings, air splints, or pressurized antishock garments.[12] Use of the intermittent pneumatic compression device for the prevention of deep venous thrombosis has been shown to cause perineal nerve palsy, pressure necrosis, and compartment syndrome.[7] Therefore patients are at Risk for Peripheral Neurovascular Dysfunction whenever this device is used. Patients who undergo invasive radiological procedures, such as cardiac catheterization and cerebral arteriography, are at Risk for Peripheral Neurovascular Dysfunction secondary to bleeding, pseudoaneuyrsm formation, or nerve irritation.[6]

ASSESSMENT

Identification and observation of the patient at Risk for Peripheral Neurovascular Dysfunction may prevent its occurrence. Assessment of a patient at Risk for Peripheral Neurovascular Dysfunction should center on the examination of subjective and objective data. In gathering subjective data, the nurse should focus on whether the patient has a history of peripheral vascular disease or any condition that may predispose him or her to peripheral neurovascular disease. The nurse should obtain a diet history, tobacco and alcohol history, an occupational history, a recreational history, a travel history, a list of the patient's routine daily activities, and a list of the patient's current medications. The nurse should ascertain if the patient experiences any pain. An affirmative answer should prompt further inquiry as to its location, severity, onset, characteristics, radiation, aggravating factors, and relieving factors.

Changes in circulation, sensory function, or motor function may be indicative of neurovascular dysfunction. Therefore, in obtaining objective data, the nurse must assess circulation, motor function, and sensory function. Circulation assessment should include evaluation of arterial pulses, skin temperature, and skin color. Sensory function assessment should include evaluation of pain, temperature, light touch, position, vibration, two-point discrimination, point localization, and extinction. Motor function should be assessed using tests to evaluate muscle tone, muscle strength, reflexes, range of motion, flexion, extension, abduction, and adduction.[3,4] Special techniques may need to be employed to evaluate for specific vascular or nerve problems. Examples include the Allen's test for evaluation of arterial insufficiency in the arm or hand and the Phalen's test and the Tinel's sign for evaluation of injury to the median and ulnar nerves.

■ Risk Factors

The presence of the following behaviors, conditions, or circumstances renders the patient more vulnerable to Risk for Peripheral Neurovascular Dysfunction:

- Fractures
- Mechanical compression
- Orthopedic surgery
- Trauma
- Peripheral revascularization
- Hematoma
- Snake or spider bites
- Postischemic swelling
- Crush injuries
- Electrical injuries
- Prolonged use of tourniquet
- Diabetes mellitus
- Renal failure
- Vascular injuries
- Arterial insufficiency
- Venous insufficiency
- Thermal injuries
- Poor nutrition
- Tobacco use
- Alcohol use
- Sports activities
- Occupational hazards
- Hyperventilation

DIAGNOSIS

■ Differential Nursing Diagnosis

The nursing diagnosis Risk for Peripheral Neurovascular Dysfunction is used to identify individuals in jeopardy of experiencing a disruption in circulation, sensation, or motion of an extremity. Patients with Altered Tissue Perfusion are at Risk for Peripheral Neurovascular Dysfunction; however, the nursing diagnosis Altered Tissue Perfusion is used specifically to address the needs of those individuals who experience symptoms as a result of diminished capillary blood flow. Nursing interventions for the diagnosis Risk for Peripheral Neurovascular Dysfunction are directed toward preventing neurovascular dysfunction in healthy and ill individuals in a variety of settings across the life span. Nursing interventions for the diagnosis Altered Tissue Perfusion are primarily directed toward maintaining adequate tissue perfusion.

■ Medical and Psychiatric Diagnoses

The diagnosis Risk for Peripheral Neurovascular Dysfunction is unique to nursing. Prevention of peripheral neurovascular dysfunction is a collaborative effort between nurses and other health care providers. Nurses collaborate with dietitians to provide optimal nutrition to prevent B vitamin deficiencies and subsequent peripheral neurovascular dysfunction. Occupational health nurses and physicians work together to identify individuals at Risk for Peripheral Neurovascular Dysfunction in the work place and to institute measures to prevent its occurrence. Nurses and physicians collaborate to prevent athletic injuries in the school setting as well as across the life span. Nurses and physicians in the hospital setting work together to prevent peripheral neurovascular dysfunction in the surgical, orthopedic, trauma, and burn patient as well as in those patients who require deep venous thrombosis prophylaxis using compression devices. This is done through proper positioning and early identification and treatment of neurovascular compromise. Nurses collaborate with organizations that assist patients to cease their smoking and alcohol habits.

OUTCOME IDENTIFICATION, PLANNING, AND IMPLEMENTATION

The expected outcomes for the patient with a diagnosis of Risk for Peripheral Neurovascular Dysfunction are that the patient will have intact and maximal circulation, sensation, and motor function. Nursing interventions for patients who are at Risk for Peripheral Neurovascular Dysfunction should be directed toward (1) maximizing vascular integrity by maintaining sufficient blood flow and (2) maximizing sensory and motor integrity by preventing nerve irritation or compression.

Following trauma, surgery, or a vascular insult, adequate hydration is essential to sustain the patient's cardiac output and peripheral blood flow. Systolic blood pressure should be kept in the high normal range to increase blood flow to the affected extremity.

Education should be provided regarding the avoidance of circular garters, constricting garments, constricting devices, crossing the legs, prolonged standing, extremes in temperature, and trauma to the extremities. When casts are applied or when antishock garments or intermittent, pneumatic, compression devices are used, frequent neurovascular assessment should be performed to ascertain circulatory status and neurovascular function. Individuals who engage in sports activities and those who play musical instruments should be instructed in positions and activities that will prevent peripheral neurovascular dysfunction.

Lifestyle recommendations focus on adequate nutrition, smoking cessation, avoidance of excessive alcohol intake, the maintenance of ideal body weight, and exercise, particularly walking. Occupational hazards should be noted, and precautions should be developed and enforced to prevent peripheral neurovascular dysfunction in the workplace.

IV

◢ NURSING CARE GUIDELINES

Nursing Diagnosis: Risk for Peripheral Neurovascular Dysfunction

---

Expected Outcome: The patient will have intact or maximum peripheral circulation.

- Assess extremities for pulse, color, temperature, capillary refill, and the presence and degree of edema. Compare with the contralateral extremity. *After trauma, surgery, or invasive procedures, circulation may be compromised secondary to edema, thrombus, embolus, bleeding, or pressure.*
- Maintain adequate hydration. *Adequate hydration is necessary to maintain an adequate cardiac output and peripheral blood flow.*
- Maintain systolic blood pressure in the high normal range without compromising cardiac function. *A systolic blood pressure in the high normal range will help to increase peripheral blood flow.*
- Position the extremity for maximum perfusion.
- Educate the patient to activate venous pumps (i.e., dorsiflex and plantar flex [in the foot]). *Activation of venous pumps facilitates venous return to the heart and aids in preventing clot formation.*
- ▲ Monitor any pharmacological agents that may have an effect on the peripheral vascular system, and educate the patient regarding these effects.
- If the patient smokes cigarettes, advise the patient to discontinue the habit. *Nicotine stimulates the sympathetic nervous system, causes arterial constriction, and increases platelet aggregation.*
- ▲ Advise the patient to follow a low-cholesterol, low-fat diet. *A low-cholesterol, low-fat diet will help prevent vascular insufficiency and/or decrease the progression of the disease.*
- Encourage walking. *Walking helps increase collateral circulation.*
- If the patient has diabetes mellitus, advise him or her to adhere to his or her prescribed diet, exercise, and medication regimen. *Maintaining blood glucose in the normal range will help decrease complications of diabetes mellitus, particularly progression of arterial insufficiency.*

■ = nursing intervention; ▲ = collaborative intervention.

Continued

■ NURSING CARE GUIDELINES — CONT'D

- Avoid wearing tight or constrictive clothing. *Constrictive clothing can obstruct blood flow.*
- Avoid prolonged standing, sitting, or crossing of the legs. *Prolonged standing, sitting, or crossing of the legs can interfere with venous return to the heart.*

Expected Outcome: The patient will have intact or maximum peripheral sensation.
- Assess the extremity for sensation to pain, temperature, light touch, position, vibration, two-point discrimination, point localization, and extinction. Compare with the contralateral extremity. *After trauma, surgery, or invasive procedures, sensation may be compromised secondary to nerve irritation or injury from pressure on a nerve or damage to a nerve.*
- Instruct the patient to report loss of sensation or sensations such as feelings of "pins and needles." *These are early signs of impaired neurovascular dysfunction.*
- Avoid use of ice, hot-water bottles, and heating pads. *Patients who are at Risk for Peripheral Neurovascular Dysfunction may have impaired sensation to thermal stimuli.*
- Avoid use of constricting garments or devices. *Constricting garments or devices compress nerves and can create neurovascular dysfunction.*
- ▲ Provide adequate nutrition, and instruct the patient about the benefits of a diet consisting of foods from the basic four food groups. *Adequate nutrition will help to prevent B vitamin deficiency and subsequent peripheral neuropathy.*
- ▲ Advise patients with diabetes mellitus and renal failure to adhere to their dietary restrictions, and educate them about the prescribed diet. *Adherence to a diet prescribed for the patient with diabetes or renal failure will help prevent the development of peripheral neurovascular dysfunction or slow its progression in these patients.*
- Advise patients to avoid or limit their intake of alcoholic beverages. *Excessive alcohol intake may result in peripheral neuropathy.*

Expected Outcome: The patient will have intact or maximum motor function.
- Assess muscle tone, muscle strength, reflexes, range of motion, adduction, abduction, flexion, and extension. Compare with contralateral extremity. *After trauma, surgery, or invasive procedures, motor function may be compromised secondary to nerve irritation or injury secondary to pressure on a nerve or damage to a nerve.*

Expected Outcome: The patient will verbalize knowledge of risk factors and demonstrate safety measures and preventive actions.
- Assess the patient's level of knowledge regarding his or her condition and activities to place him or her at Risk for Peripheral Neurovascular Dysfunction.
- ▲ Educate the patient regarding risk factors (i.e., B vitamin deficiencies, nicotine use, alcohol use, uncontrolled blood glucose if diabetic, exposure to extremes of temperature, use of constrictive garments or devices, crossing the legs, prolonged standing, occupational hazards, sports activities).
- Encourage health-promoting behaviors such as adequate nutrition, avoidance of cigarette smoking and alcohol use, and walking as an exercise.

EVALUATION

Neurovascular dysfunction can occur across the life span in a variety of clinical and nonclinical settings. Its onset may be insidious; therefore the nurse must have a high degree of suspicion in patients who are at risk. Nursing interventions are successful when the patient's circulation, sensory function, and motor function are intact. The absence of pain, pallor, paresthesia, pulselessness, paralysis, and coolness of a limb indicates adequate neurovascular function.[3,4]

◤ CASE STUDY WITH PLAN OF CARE

Mr. Nick C. is a 55-year-old government executive who visited the employee health unit for blood pressure monitoring and help with his diet. His physician had advised him to have his blood pressure monitored because at his last visit it was "borderline." Mr. C.'s past medical history is remarkable for hyperlipidemia for the past 10 years and non-insulin-dependent diabetes mellitus. His hyperlipidemia is currently being treated with medications because diet modification initially failed. His non-insulin-dependent diabetes mellitus is being treated with an oral hypoglycemic agent. He has been trying to make changes in his lifestyle to decrease his health risks despite having a very stressful job requiring long hours, frequent word processing activities, and frequent business travel. He stopped smoking 2 years ago and subsequently gained approximately 15 pounds. He drinks at least one alcoholic beverage every evening after work and beer or wine socially on weekends. He has occasional problems with insomnia. He exercises sporadically. He attempts to modify his diet by decreasing his intake of fats and sugars and increasing his intake of foods high in fiber. He also tries to eat three regular meals daily instead of skipping meals. He is intermittently successful with this diet because of job demands and business travel.

Physical examination revealed a well-groomed, slightly overweight male who appears fit. Pulse was 72 and regular; blood pressure (while sitting) was 142/90 mm Hg in the right arm and 138/92 mm Hg in the left arm. No significant postural changes were noted in his blood pressure. Heart sounds were normal, and the lung fields were clear to auscultation. His abdomen was benign. His neurovascular examination was normal except for complaints of paresthesias in both feet. He stated that his lower extremities have felt "cool" for several years. He has also noted intermittent numbness in his right hand over the palmar surface of the thumb, the index and middle fingers and part of the ring finger, and in his feet, especially at night, for the past 3 months. He attributes the numbness in his right hand to his word processing activities and in his feet to his diabetes. Pedal pulses were weak but equal bilaterally. Both feet demonstrated decreased sensitivity to sharp touch and dull touch. The skin of the feet was dry and cool, with anhydrosis. Dependent rubor was noted bilaterally in the lower legs and feet. He stated edema was occasionally present at the end of the day.

A plan of care was developed for Mr. C. that focused on patient education and prevention of peripheral neurovascular complications of hyperlipidemia and diabetes mellitus.

◤ PLAN OF CARE FOR MR. NICK C.

Nursing Diagnosis: Risk for Peripheral Neurovascular Dysfunction Secondary to Word Processing Activities and Complications of Diabetes Mellitus and Arterial Insufficiency

Expected Outcome: Mr. C. will have maximum peripheral circulation, sensation, and motor function in his hands.
- Assess the hands for pulse, color, capillary refill, and edema.
- Assess the hands for pain, temperature, light touch, position, vibration, two-point discrimination, point localization, and extinction.
- Assess the hands for muscle tone, muscle strength, range of motion, adduction, abduction, flexion, and extension.
- Assess for compression of the median nerve by performing the Phalen's test and assessing for a positive Tinel's sign.
- Assess word processing station for proper ergonomics.
- Correct any defects in word processing station to provide for proper ergonomics.

Expected Outcome: Mr. C. will have maximum peripheral circulation and sensation in his legs and feet.
- Assess legs and feet for pulse, color, capillary refill, and edema.
- Assess legs and feet for pain, temperature, light touch, position, vibration, two-point discrimination, point localization, and extinction.

■ = nursing intervention; ▲ = collaborative intervention.   *Continued*

IV

IV

◤ PLAN OF CARE FOR MRS. LOIS S. — CONT'D

- Encourage Mr. C. to continue his exercise program and to walk daily on his lunch hour to stimulate circulation and the venous pump.

Expected Outcome: Mr. C. will verbalize the significance of dietary modification to his current health problems.
- ▲ Collaborate with a registered dietitian to educate Mr. C. regarding the role of dietary fat in the development of atherosclerosis and its subsequent impairment of circulation.
- ▲ Collaborate with a registered dietitian to encourage Mr. C. to continue to eat regular meals that are high in fiber and complex carbohydrates.
- ▲ Advise Mr. C. to decrease his alcohol intake. Refer him to Alcoholics Anonymous or other alcoholic intervention programs.
- ▲ Instruct Mr. C. in the use of a blood glucose monitoring device and refer him to a diabetic nurse educator or diabetic support group for further instructions and support.

Expected Outcome: Mr. C. will comply with safety precautions to minimize risks for neurovascular complications.
- Advise Mr. C. to avoid activities that require prolonged sitting or standing.
- Advise Mr. C. to avoid exposure to extremes of temperature.
- Advise Mr. C. to avoid wearing tight-fitting clothing.
- Arrange Mr. C.'s workstation so that it is ergonomically correct.
- Advise Mr. C. to use the principles of proper ergonomics at his word processing station.

▥ CRITICAL THINKING EXERCISES

1. Mr. C.'s diminished pedal pulses, paresthesias, cool lower extremities, and 10-year documented history of hyperlipidemia reflect an increased process of atherosclerosis. What other organs or systems are also affected, and what signs and symptoms might one look for? Are further assessment data warranted?

2. Based on history and assessment data, what measure of compliance is usual for Mr. C.? As he ages and his disease progresses, is this sufficient? What measures can the nurse take to help the patient increase compliance?

3. Mr. C. consumes alcohol on a daily basis. Would it be appropriate to assess him further, using the CAGE questionnaire or other instruments to determine if referral or another intervention would help him decrease the risk?

4. What referrals to other health care providers would you consider discussing with Mr. C. to help him change his lifestyle and prevent further disease and Risk for Peripheral Neurovascular Dysfunction?

REFERENCES

1. Baker CL and Liu SH: Neurovascular injuries to the shoulder, *J Orthop Sports Phys Ther* 18(1):360–364, 1993.
2. Bouche P and others: Clinical and electrophysiological study of the peripheral nervous system in the elderly, *J Neurol* 240(5):263–268, 1993.
3. Dykes PC: Minding the five Ps of neurovascular assessment, *Am J Nurs* 93(6):38–39, 1993.
4. Eden-Kilgour S and Miller B: Understanding neurovascular assessment, *Nursing 93* 23(8):56–58, 1993.
5. Fowl RJ, Akers DL, and Kempczinski RF: Neurovascular lower extremity complications of the lithotomy position, *Ann Vasc Surg* 6(4):357–361, 1992.

6. Jones C, Holcomb E, and Rohrer T: Femoral artery pseudoaneurysm after invasive procedures, *Crit Care Nurse* 15(4):47–51, 1995.

7. Lachmann EA and others: Complications associated with intermittent pneumatic compression, *Arch Phys Med Rehabil* 73(5):482–485, 1992.

8. Landrigan RJ, Graham DG, and Thomas RD: Strategies for the prevention of environmental neurotoxic illness, *Environ Res* 61(1):157–163, 1993.

9. North American Nursing Diagnosis Association: *NANDA nursing diagnoses: definitions and classification, 1995–1996,* Philadelphia, 1994, The Association.

10. Palmer JB and others: A cellist with arm pain: thermal asymmetry in scalenus anticus syndrome, *Arch Phys Med Rehabil* 72(3):237–242, 1991.

11. Rettig AC: Neurovascular injuries in the wrists and hands of athletes, *Clin Sports Med* 9(2):389–417, 1990.

12. Ross D: Acute compartment syndrome, *Orthop Nurs* 10(2):33–38, 1991.

13. Turnipseed WD and Pozniak M: Popliteal entrapment as a result of neurovascular compression by the soleus and plantaris muscles, *J Vasc Surg* 15(2):285–294, 1992.

14. Tucker K and Hedges TR: Food shortages and an epidemic of optic and peripheral neuropathy in Cuba, *Nutr Rev* 51(12):349–357, 1993.

15. Weidman JR: Use of nursing diagnoses by the National Association of Orthopeadic Nurses. In Carroll-Johnson RM and Paquette M, editors: *Classification of nursing diagnoses: proceedings of the Tenth Conference,* Philadelphia, 1994, JB Lippincott Co.

IV

Self-Care Deficit: Feeding

▶
___

Self-Care Deficit: Bathing/Hygiene

▶
___

Self-Care Deficit: Dressing/Grooming

▶
___

Self-Care Deficit: Toileting

▶
___

Self-Care Deficit: Feeding *is a state in which the individual experiences an impaired ability to perform or complete feeding activities for him- or herself.*[15]

Self-Care Deficit: Bathing/Hygiene *is a state in which the individual experiences an impaired ability to perform or complete bathing and hygiene activities for him- or herself.*[15]

Self-Care Deficit: Dressing/Grooming *is a state in which the individual experiences an impaired ability to perform or complete dressing and grooming activities for him- or herself.*[15]

Self-Care Deficit: Toileting *is a state in which the individual experiences an impaired ability to perform or complete toileting activities for him- or herself.*[15]

OVERVIEW

Self-Care

Self-care, a concept fundamental to nursing, has received renewed interest in the health care arena. Its resurgence has been influenced by various political, social, economic, and environmental factors. Society's present focus on health promotion

and disease prevention and detection behaviors is a major factor in the self-care movement. From a heavy reliance on the health system and providers the responsibility for health is being transferred to the individual, with a greater focus on self-responsibility and independence.

The concept of self-care has numerous meanings, given the diverse perspectives from which it is viewed. It is typically conceptualized in terms of the degree of dependence on or interdependence with the health care system. Views on the meaning of self-care range from self-diagnosis and self-treatment to collaboration and partnership. Although self-care has a wide range of meanings, an underlying premise is that individuals have the ability to influence and participate in their own health.

Nurses frequently use Orem's definition of self-care[16]: "the practice of activities that individuals personally initiate and perform on their own behalf in maintaining life, health, and well-being." Orem clearly emphasizes the role of the nurse in meeting self-care demands for the patient when actual or potential deficits are present. Self-care is typically viewed in relation to the degree of assistance an individual needs to complete an activity or task. The degree of assistance can be depicted along a continuum ranging from total dependence on another to varying degrees of interdependence.

Self-care implies self-reliance, self-responsibility, independence, interdependence, and partnership. A self-care approach to health empowers people to meet their own needs, the needs of their families, and their communities. And it is nursing that enables and empowers people toward greater self-care.

Activities of Daily Living

Self-care activities that are commonly performed on a daily basis are termed *activities of daily living (ADLs)*. Nursing has traditionally identified them as feeding, bathing/hygiene, dressing/grooming, and toileting. ADLs are acquired or learned, mature over time, become sequential, and develop into lifelong habits. Children begin to learn ADLs at a young age, usually from immediate family members, and are expected to assume responsibility for them as soon as they become developmentally mature.

A number of factors influence the way in which an individual approaches ADLs (e.g., environmental and socioeconomic conditions such as the availability of plumbing and toilets and the size of the family). An individual's physical and cognitive abilities can greatly affect how an activity is performed. The cultural setting in which an individual is raised is particularly influential; spiritual factors are also influential. Because ADLs are habitual activities they have value not only with respect to what is done but how, when, where, and with whom it is done.[9]

When an individual lacks the physical and cognitive capacity to participate in any or multiple ADLs, a self-care deficit results. The ability to perform ADLs may be compromised by physiological aging, accidents, and acute and chronic illnesses. A physiological or cognitive insult may result in temporary or permanent self-care limitations, resulting in a need for assistance in performing or increasing self-care capacity. A period of rehabilitation is often necessary to relearn ADLs or to learn new ways of accomplishing those previously learned. The roles of the nurse, family members,

physical and occupational therapists, the chaplain, and other team member are important in assisting the patient to reach the optimal level of independence in performing self-care activities.

Performing ADLs is a personal matter and is intimately linked to an individual's self-concept. A threat to or actual loss of the ability to initiate or perform self-care can provoke a serious threat to self-perception and self-esteem, fostering feelings of fear and anxiety. Losing control over one's ability to perform a basic self-care activity is frequently not a negotiable option for many individuals. The thought of losing such control is frequently accompanied by statements such as "I would rather die than not be able to care for myself." Having the ability to perform personal self-care activities independently is valued by all, achieved by most, yet completely and permanently retained by few.

ADLs are affected by chronic illnesses and aging. In 1992 nearly 15% of noninstitutionalized persons of all ages reported some limitation in activity due to chronic conditions.[14] Of these, 45% of persons 75 years of age and over reported some limitation, of which 11% were unable to carry out a major activity. Wiener and others[20] reported that 5% to 8% of noninstitutionalized elders received help with one or more self-care activities: bathing, dressing, toileting, eating, and moving out of a bed, chairs, or both. These studies emphasize the impact that aging and chronic illness have on activity and self-care ability.

Deficits in self-care have been identified as a nursing problem commonly occurring in acute, rehabilitation, and long-term settings. Gordon[6] conducted a national survey of experts in rehabilitation nursing and found Self-Care Deficit to be a high-frequency and high-treatment priority. Rantz and others found over a 10-year period that Self-Care Deficit was the most frequently utilized diagnosis in a nursing facility. A study by Sheppard[18] identified the diagnosis Self-Care Deficit: Bathing/Hygiene as a significant predictor of home referral for patients in an acute setting with lung cancer diagnoses. The findings suggest that the nursing diagnosis describes the discharge planning needed and predicts the type of agency referral. As a fre-

IV

quently occurring nursing diagnosis, Self-Care Deficit challenges nursing to promote quality by finding innovative ways to assist patients to gain optimal independence in personal care activities or ADLs.

ASSESSMENT

The assessment phase of the nursing process involves a systematic and deliberate collection of data from which an individual's abilities, limitation, concerns, and problems can be identified. An assessment format or guide aids the nurse in gathering pertinent data in an efficient manner. There are various assessment formats that the nurse can utilize. Theory-based assessment guides are extremely beneficial in organizing data collection. Theoretical frameworks frequently utilized in assessment guides include Gordon's Functional Health Patterns and Orem's Self-Care Model. Each framework utilizes its specific approach to data collection.

Gordon's Functional Health Patterns framework[7] can be used for collecting and organizing data pertinent to the individual with self-care needs. Each of Gordon's 11 Functional Health Patterns provides a standard assessment format for a basic data base, regardless of a patient's age or level of care. The assessment specific to self-care activities would be found in the Activity-Exercise Pattern. Other assessment areas pertinent to Self-Care Deficit can be found in the Cognitive-Perceptual, Self-Perception—Self-Concept, Role-Relationship, Coping—Stress-Tolerance, and Value-Belief Patterns.

General assessment parameters for the individual with any Self-Care Deficit in ADLs include the individual's ability to carry out ADLs, the functional ADL status or degree to which an activity can be performed, and an assessment of underlying causes. As with any assessment, the nurse needs to consider the individual's age and developmental and mental status throughout the examination.

The assessment begins with an initial interview. A health history is obtained to identify the underlying injury or disease contributing to or causing the deficit. Data regarding its onset, duration, and

management, if applicable, are obtained. In addition, the nurse elicits as much information as possible from the patient regarding his or her ability to perform or complete feeding, bathing, dressing, and toileting activities. If the patient is unable to provide information, it should be sought from others, such as a family member or a friend. Other information gathered during this time, if appropriate, includes the use of assistive aids and devices. During this initial phase of the assessment, the nurse is especially alert for patient cues that support the defining characteristics of each Self-Care Deficit diagnosis. If evidence of a deficit is present, a further focused assessment is performed to confirm the presence of defining characteristics and the extent of the deficit and to appraise the underlying cause or related factor.

The nurse validates the patient's perceived ability to perform ADLs by observing the performance of an activity. The presence of defining characteristics indicates that one or more Self-Care Deficits may be present.[4,12,15] After validating the presence of a Self-Care Deficit, the nurse assesses the patient's ability to perform the activity (i.e., functional ADL status). This is most often accomplished when assessing the presence of defining characteristics. The ability of an individual with a Self-Care Deficit to perform ADLs can range from minimal independence to complete dependence on another. It is recommended that a standardized, physical, functional status index, which measures ADLs, be utilized. There are various functional status indices available to measure self-care abilities (e.g., the Barthel Index or the Katz ADL Index). A basic 0–4 scale can be used for determining the level of independence and need for assistance. The following 0–4 scale for classifying functional level is typical for the nursing diagnosis Self-Care Deficit: Feeding, Bathing/Hygiene, Dressing/Grooming, Toileting: 0 = completely independent; 1 = requires use of equipment or device; 2 = requires help from another person for assistance, supervision, or teaching; 3 = requires help from another person plus use of equipment or device; 4 = dependent, does not participate in activity. A patient's functional ADL status is evaluated on a regular basis to determine progress and the possible need for nursing plan modifications.

Related factors that contribute to the existence of the person's Self-Care Deficit are also assessed. Related factors associated with this diagnosis are primarily the result of long-time pathological disorders that impinge on cognitive-perceptual, musculoskeletal, neuromuscular, and sensory functions.

Cognition is an internal element that can affect a person's ability to perform any self-care activities. It is an important factor because abilities such as sequencing, selection, and judgment are necessary to perform ADLs. This is especially critical when relearning an activity previously performed or learning a new way of performing an old skill. Assessment of cognitive function includes ability with language, memory, decision making, orientation, and attention span.[7] Another related factor, intolerance to activity, occurs when an individual experiences insufficient energy to complete ADLs; this can significantly affect motor function necessary to perform ADLs. It is often a significant factor with individuals who have cardiovascular, respiratory, and musculoskeletal-related conditions, and it is also a factor in the physiological aging process.

Although the functional ADL status parameters are the same for all deficits, appraisal of defining characteristics is unique to each deficit. Additionally, assessment of motor and sensory function, although similar, are typically deficit-specific. Therefore assessment of defining characteristics and related factors for each deficit are addressed.

Self-Care Deficit: Feeding

A critical characteristic of Self-Care: Feeding is the inability to bring food from a receptacle to the mouth.[15] Other characteristics that have been identified, although not approved by NANDA, include the inability to select food and the inability to chew and swallow.[2,10] Functional ADL status is also assessed.

As the nurse observes self-feeding, he or she notes the patient's mobility, balance, coordination, range of motion, strength, stamina, and gross and fine motor movements.[5] Special attention is given to any evidence of involuntary movement, such as tremors and spasms that interfere with coordination. The nurse examines the upper extremities for muscle mass, size, and arm strength. The range of motion of the head, neck, shoulders, arms, wrists, and fingers is examined. Joints are examined for tenderness, swelling, and stability. Assessing proprioception, such as point-to-point localization, will assess the patient's ability to bring a feeding utensil to the mouth. An extremely important motor ability, necessary for all four ADLs, is opposition of the thumb and fingers to pitch and grasp objects (i.e., finger coordination). This can be assessed by asking the patient to pick up a small object, such as a pencil. The bilateral gag reflex is tested to determine swallowing ability, which, if impaired, results in aspiration. The patient is appraised for sensory (vision) function, including evidence of cataracts, ocular drift, and ptosis of the eyelid(s), which would limit or impair vision. The visual fields of both eyes are examined for hemianopia and diplopia.

Self-Care Deficit: Bathing/Hygiene

Assessment parameters for Self-Care Deficit: Bathing/Hygiene begin with appraising for the presence of the defining characteristics. The nurse observes for evidence of the critical defining characteristic: ability to wash the body or body parts.[15] Other attributes include the inability to obtain or get to the water source and the inability to regulate temperature control.[15] Functional ADL status is also assessed.

The process of bathing and hygiene requires the same basic motor, sensory, and proprioceptive abilities as feeding. However, attention needs to be given to sensory status because of its impact on safety issues. Assessment begins by observing the patient performing bathing and hygiene activities, noting mobility, coordination, range of motion, strength, and gross and fine motor movements.[5] If the patient has the ability to walk to the bathroom or shower, gait, posture, balance, and coordination should be assessed. Observations are made regarding safety precautions taken by the patient during bathing, especially if using the shower or bathtub. The assessment includes testing the sensory mode for touch, pain, temperature, vibratory sensation,

IV

and texture discrimination. Attention is given to sensation for evidence of anesthesia, hyperesthesia, hypoesthesia, and paresthesia, which, if present, could result in injuries such as water burns and fractured digits.

Self-Care Deficit: Dressing/Grooming

The critical defining characteristic for Self-Care Deficit: Dressing/Grooming is the inability to put on or take off necessary clothing.[15] If this attribute is present, the diagnosis is appropriate and accurate. Other assessment observations, although not critical, may include impaired ability to obtain or replace articles of clothing, impaired ability to fasten clothing, and inability to maintain appearance at a satisfactory level.[15] Functional ADL status is also assessed.

Dressing and grooming activities require the same motor and sensory functions as feeding and bathing/grooming; subsequently the assessment format is similar. Assessments of mobility, coordination, range of motion, finger dexterity, sitting balance, extremity strength, and stamina are performed. Special attention should be given to range of motion and finger dexterity because good range of motion is needed for applying and removing clothing and finger dexterity is needed for fastening clothing and applying makeup.

Self-Care Deficit: Toileting

Critical defining characteristics of Self-Care Deficit: Toileting include the inability to get to the toilet or commode, the inability to sit on or rise from the toilet or commode, the inability to manipulate clothing for toileting, and the inability to carry out toilet hygiene.[15] The inability to flush the toilet or commode may also be a presenting attribute. Functional ADL status is also assessed.

Toileting activities require the motor and sensory abilities required for feeding, bathing/hygiene, and dressing/grooming; thus assessment parameters are similar. Additionally, attention is given to gait, balance, coordination, endurance, and use of assistive walking devices, such as special adaptive shoes, a cane, and a walkerette. If the patient is not able to walk independently, the nurse assesses the mode of locomotion, such as manual or electric wheelchair, and maneuvering ability. If toileting requires transferring to get on and off a toilet, the patient's degree of independence is assessed. Whether walking is completely independent or modified, safety performance is assessed.

■ Defining Characteristics

The presence of the following characteristics indicates that the patient may be experiencing the following Self-Care Deficits: Feeding, Bathing/Hygiene, Dressing/Grooming, or Toileting[15]:

Feeding
- Inability to bring food from a receptacle to mouth

Bathing/Hygiene
- Inability to wash body or body parts
- Inability to obtain or get to water source
- Inability to regulate water temperature or flow

Dressing/Grooming
- Impaired ability to put on or take off necessary items of clothing
- Impaired ability to obtain or replace articles of clothing
- Impaired ability to fasten clothing
- Inability to maintain appearance at satisfactory level

Toileting
- Unable to get to toilet or commode
- Unable to sit on or rise from toilet or commode
- Unable to manipulate clothing for toileting
- Unable to carry out proper toileting hygiene
- Unable to flush toilet or commode

■ Related Factors

The following related factors are associated with Self-Care Deficit: Feeding, Bathing/Hygiene, Dressing/Grooming, or Toileting[15]:

Feeding, Bathing/Hygiene, and Dressing/Grooming
- Intolerance to activity
- Decreased strength and endurance
- Pain or discomfort
- Perceptual or cognitive impairment

- Neuromuscular impairment
- Musculoskeletal impairment
- Depression
- Severe anxiety

Toileting
- Impaired transfer ability
- Impaired mobility status
- Intolerance to activity
- Decreased strength and endurance
- Pain or discomfort
- Perceptual or cognitive impairment
- Neuromuscular impairment
- Musculoskeletal impairment
- Depression
- Severe anxiety

DIAGNOSIS

■ Differential Nursing Diagnosis

Self-Care Deficit has been closely associated with the diagnosis Impaired Physical Mobility. Although mutually exclusive, there is a conceptual tendency to perceive self-care and immobility as overlapping concepts.[3] Research is needed to address such conceptually based issues. To differentiate between the diagnoses Self-Care Deficit and Impaired Physical Mobility, a clear understanding of each definition and the defining characteristics is vital. Self-Care Deficit focuses on a limitation related to performance of a specific self-care task, whereas Impaired Physical Mobility focuses on limited ability for independent physical movement. Defining characteristics are also significantly different. Self-Care Deficits are characterized by performance problems related to specific activities—ADLs. However, Impaired Physical Mobility is characterized by the inability to maintain full movement.[15] The related factors for Self-Care Deficit that are diagnoses in their own right (i.e., Activity Intolerance, Anxiety, and Pain) can also cause confusion. The dilemma as to whether it is a diagnosis or a related factor can be addressed by determining whether or not the problem can be dealt with directly.[11] If the problem (i.e., Pain, Activity Intolerance, or Anxiety) can be dealt with directly, it should be the diagnosis of choice. How-

ever, if the problem cannot be resolved, attention needs to be directed to the diagnosis and treatment of Self-Care Deficit.

■ Medical and Psychiatric Diagnoses

A number of medical and psychiatric conditions can challenge an individual's self-care abilities. Pathophysiological conditions that can impair self-care abilities include multiple sclerosis, Parkinson's disease, arthritis, osteoporosis, Alzheimer's disease, central nervous system tumors, and cerebrovascular accidents. Chronic obstructive pulmonary disease, congestive heart failure, and coronary artery disease can alter the patient's activity tolerance and interfere with self-care activities. Injuries resulting in bone fractures can also lead to a deficit in self-care. Self-Care Deficit often accompanies sensory disorders that may be chronic or acute in nature (e.g., cataracts, macular degeneration, and retinal detachment). Mental health disorders, such as substance abuse, personality disorders, schizophrenia, depression, and severe anxiety, can also affect self-care abilities.

OUTCOME IDENTIFICATION, PLANNING, AND IMPLEMENTATION

After the nursing diagnosis Self-Care Deficit: Feeding, Bathing/Hygiene, Dressing/Grooming, or Toileting is made, expected outcomes and interventions are established. When planning care for the individual with this diagnosis, the specific deficit, functional ADL status, and related factors must be addressed.[9] The formulation of self-care outcomes is influenced by the patient's physical and cognitive abilities, whether the deficit is permanent or temporary in nature, and whether the underlying cause is subject to an acute or chronic trajectory. Expected outcomes must be realistic and attainable. For instance, if a deficit is severe and extensive, any degree of self-care independence may be an unrealistic outcome. In such a situation, the person may require the assistance of a nurse or personal attendant to perform all self-care activities. Outcomes must also be measurable and

IV

IV

observable. Short-term outcomes can be especially motivational when a self-care goal takes a great deal of time and effort to reach. Outcomes must also have a time designation. For the individual with a Self-Care Deficit, outcome target dates are relative to the extent of the deficit and the patient's abilities. If at all possible, expected outcomes should be mutually decided upon by the patient and family member(s), nurse, and other interdisciplinary team members (e.g., occupational and physical therapists, dietitian, and chaplain).

Patient outcomes and nursing interventions in the treatment of any of the four self-care deficits can be classified into three major areas: satisfactory completion of the self-care activity so that basic human needs are met; retention (by the patient) of as much situational control as possible; and avoidance or minimization of potential complications.[9]

Satisfactory completion of ADLs is the primary desired outcome for Self-Care Deficit. This outcome involves performing ADLs to an optimal level, with or without the use of assistive devices. If assistive devices are required, evaluation of use is documented on a regular basis. Satisfactory performance of basic ADLs is evidenced by adequate nutrition, cleanliness, neat appearance, comfort, adequate elimination, satisfaction with oneself, and, if applicable, effective use of adaptive devices. In addressing issues pertinent to satisfactory performance of ADLs, the nurse must determine each patient's functional ADL level and establish mutually attainable goals. Interventions are directed toward maximizing the patient's success in performing ADLs.

Being dependent on others for the most basic self-care activities signifies loss of control,[9] and with this loss there is likely to be a significant effect on self-concept and its components, self-esteem and self-image. A perceived lack of control of ADLs could result in a diagnosis of Powerlessness. The preservation of situational control involves allowing the patient to control an event directly (behavior control), providing the patient with necessary information (cognitive control), and allowing the patient to select among options (behavior control).[13] Providing the patient with options, facilitating discussion regarding therapy and treatment, and instituting referrals to assess the home environment for barriers to self-care can foster a sense of situational control.

Finally, complications should be avoided or minimized. Possible complications related to feeding include aspiration and nutritional deficit. Other possible complications as a result of limitations in ADLs include hot water burns and injuries associated with falls and the improper use of assistive devices. Problems related to toileting include skin breakdown due to inadequate cleansing and incontinence. Activity intolerance needs to be monitored to decrease fatigue and frustration. Loss of control or powerlessness should be avoided or minimized.[9] Interventions directed toward eliminating potential complications require a proactive approach that emphasizes prevention and early detection of problems.

The first set of Nursing Care Guidelines presents outcomes and interventions appropriate for a patient diagnosed with Self-Care Deficit, whether it be a deficit in feeding, bathing/hygiene, dressing/grooming, or toileting. The subsequent sets of guidelines address outcomes and interventions specific to Self-Care Deficit: Feeding, Self-Care Deficit: Bathing/Hygiene, Self-Care Deficit: Dressing/Grooming, and Self-Care Deficit: Toileting.

◢ NURSING CARE GUIDELINES
Nursing Diagnosis: Self-Care Deficit: Feeding, Bathing/Hygiene, Dressing/Grooming, Toileting*

Expected Outcome: The patient will demonstrate satisfactory self-care activities to the optimal extent possible, independently or with assistive devices, as evidenced by satisfactory fulfillment of basic human needs for nutrition, cleanliness, grooming, and elimination; expressions of comfort; effective use of assistive devices (if appropriate); and satisfaction with performance of activities.

- Carry out nursing and prescribed medical treatments for underlying disease conditions or disruptive symptoms, such as pain and discomfort, as necessary. *Pain and discomfort decrease movement and the ability to perform self-care activities to a satisfactory level.*
- Encourage the patient to do as much as possible for him- or herself as soon as possible. *Successful accomplishments early in recovery provide impetus to accomplish future tasks.*
- Encourage exercise to strengthen muscle groups on a regular basis. *Achieving maximum capacity to perform self-care activities requires optimal muscle and joint movement.*
- Provide guidance, support, and teaching regarding the use of assistive devices and ADL methods, as necessary. *Instructions and assistance facilitate the learning process. Assistive devices enhance the patient's ability to perform self-care tasks independently to a maximum capacity.*
- Provide positive feedback related to the patient's efforts and accomplishments. *Positive feedback promotes independence and encourages continued performance.*
- Plan activities to prevent fatigue during ADLs. *Fatigue magnifies stress and decreases concentration.*
- ▲ Request referrals to appropriate health care team members, such as occupational and physical therapists, speech therapist, dietitian, chaplain, or social worker. *Collaboration with interdisciplinary team members increases the patient's successful mastery of self-care tasks.*[1]
- Make changes in the environment, as needed, to provide easy access and foster safety (e.g., placing objects within reach and moving furniture). *Optimal satisfaction in performing self-care activities can be hindered by environmental barriers.*
- Initiate discharge planning upon admission; assess home and work environments for barriers that hinder self-care activities. *For maximum and long-term independence, self-care skills must be transferable to familiar settings (home or work).*

Expected Outcome: The patient will achieve or maintain as much situational control as possible as evidenced by stating a realistic appraisal of personal abilities, actively collaborating in the plan of care, and establishing reasonable goals.

- Assess the functional status of the patient on a regular basis, and discuss with the patient self-care behaviors that he or she can perform. *Accentuating the abilities enhances and fosters a positive self-image.*
- Consult with the patient in making choices regarding treatment or a restorative regime; allow the patient to take an active role in establishing and evaluating the plan of care; and encourage the patient to voice preferences. *Optimum decision making by the patient promotes feelings of control and enhances self-worth and self-esteem.*
- Discuss actual and anticipated therapy or treatment changes and their possible effects with the patient. *Advance knowledge of an event empowers an individual with a sense of control over the situation rather than being controlled by the situation.*
- Assist the patient in relating concerns to physician, therapists, and other pertinent team members. *Communicating concerns to appropriate individuals fosters self-responsibility and self-reliance and can improve self-care options.*

■ = nursing intervention; ▲ = collaborative intervention.   *Continued*
*References 1, 2, 8, 9, 10, 19.

IV

◢ **Nursing Care Guidelines — cont'd**

Expected Outcome: The patient will experience absence of complications or minimal complications as evidenced by freedom from physically limiting injuries; minimal signs and symptoms of powerlessness (i.e., perceived lack of situational control with decreased self-esteem or a sense of worthlessness); and no decline of abilities.

- Monitor patient during self-care activities to determine energy expenditure and tolerance level. *Fatigue can decrease ability to perform self-care activities successfully.*
- Teach, supervise, and assist in safety methods and maintenance.
- Evaluate patient's execution of safety precautions: maintenance of assistive devices and proper use of assistive devices. *A safety maintenance approach will serve to minimize physical hazards associated with the use of assistive devices.*
- Evaluate success of nursing interventions designed to increase behavioral, cognitive, and decision control. *Situational control can enhance self-concept and self-esteem and minimize the potential for powerlessness.*

◢ **Nursing Care Guidelines**
Nursing Diagnosis: Self-Care Deficit: Feeding

Expected Outcome: The patient will demonstrate optimum ability to feed him- or herself independently or with assistive devices as evidenced by consuming adequate nutritional intake, maintaining acceptable weight, and verbalizing satisfaction with level of independence.

- Incorporate patient food preferences (i.e., likes and dislikes) and familiar mealtime rituals (e.g., prayer before and after meal or a time for reflection). *Nutritional consumption is influenced by sociocultural factors.*
- ▲ Request consultations with dietitian and occupational and physical therapists, as needed. *Collaboration with interdisciplinary team members increases the patient's mastery of self-care tasks.*[1]
- Monitor nutritional status: intake, output, calorie count, weight. *Recording nutritional consumption provides data for an effective evaluation process and ongoing planning.*
- Assist patient to feeding position, preferably high Fowler's, and have patient remain in sitting position for at least 30 minutes after feeding. *Gravity aids digestion and decreases the possibility of aspiration.*
- Provide and encourage use of assistive devices (e.g., universal ADL cuff for utensils, straw, food guard, and rocking knife) at every meal. *Maximum independence in self-care can be improved by use of assistive devices.*
- Provide the patient with an environment that is quiet, private, and free from toileting devices. *Attention to aesthetics of feeding increases feeding success.*[1]
- Supervise and/or assist patient in setting-up the meal (i.e., cutting meat into small pieces, opening cartons, and applying condiments).
- Request referral to social services to assess and plan for needs following discharge (e.g., Meals on Wheels, The Visiting Nursing Association). *Supportive resources reinforce self-care plan. Discharge planning begins upon admission.*
- If needed, keep suction machine next to bedside and in working order. *Impairments in swallowing can result in aspiration.*

■ = nursing intervention; ▲ = collaborative intervention.

◢ **NURSING CARE GUIDELINES**
Nursing Diagnosis: Self-Care Deficit: Bathing/Hygiene

Expected Outcome: The patient will demonstrate optimal ability to bathe self independently or with assistive devices, as appropriate, as evidenced by clean skin and nails, clean and combed hair, brushed teeth (or cleaned dentures); shaved face, if appropriate; free from offensive odors; and verbalization of a sense of satisfaction in self-care progress.

- Initially encourage patient to perform the minimum of washing face and rinsing out mouth. *Initial successes foster motivation to accomplish future tasks.*
- Establish a bathing schedule, through mutual agreement with patient, that allows for adequate time to complete activities. *Bathing can be time-consuming and often requires significant energy.*
- Encourage the use of shower stall or tube, depending on what is available in the home setting. *When skills are transferable, long-term success is more likely.*
- Provide assistive devices: universal ADL cuff for bathing/hygiene utensils, long-handled brush, nail brush with suction cup, automatic toothbrush/adaptive toothbrush, shaver with holder, shower stool, hand-held shower handles, nonslip shower/bathtub mat. *Maximum independence in self-care can be improved by use of assistive devices.*
- Maintain an uncluttered, neat environment; provide adequate space. *An organized working area fosters progress when outcomes are complex.*
- Provide privacy during bathing (announce presence before entering). *Measures that ensure privacy enhance patient self-esteem.*

■ = nursing intervention; ▲ = collaborative intervention.

◢ **NURSING CARE GUIDELINES**
Nursing Diagnosis: Self-Care Deficit: Dressing/Grooming

Expected Outcome: The patient will demonstrate optimal ability to dress and groom him- or herself independently or with assistive devices, as appropriate, as evidenced by a neat appearance; clothing that is properly fastened; and a sense of satisfaction in level of independence and appearance.

- Provide or suggest clothing that is loose fitting around neck, arms, waist, and legs and that fastens in the front.
- ▲ Request consults for occupational and physical therapists as needed. *Collaboration with interdisciplinary team members increases the patient's mastery of self-care tasks.*[1]
- Provide dressing aids: zipper pull, buttonhook, long-handled shoehorn, and dressing stick. *Maximum independence in self-care can be improved by use of assistive devices.*
- Plan activities to prevent fatigue during meals. *Fatigue decreases the ability to concentrate and the ability to perform.*
- Supervise or assist patient in dressing by providing items and in a systematic order; provide assistance only when the patient needs it; avoid "rushing" the patient in carrying out activities.

■ = nursing intervention; ▲ = collaborative intervention.

IV

IV

◢ NURSING CARE GUIDELINES
Nursing Diagnosis: Self-Care Deficit: Toileting

Expected Outcome: The patient will demonstrate optimal ability to toilet independently or with assistive devices, as appropriate, as evidenced by avoidance of incontinence and satisfaction with management of toileting.

- Monitor intake and output and frequency and time of incontinence and bowel movements. *Accurate recording of intake and output can determine patterns of elimination and identify possible imbalances.*
- Establish a day-and-night toileting schedule. *Toileting schedules can prevent incontinence.*
- Provide and encourage use of assistive devices: raised toilet seat, grab bars, support side rails, fracture pans, spill-proof urinals, and commode chair. *Maximum independence in self-care can be improved by use of assistive devices.*
- ▲ Request consults for occupational and physical therapists if patient requires transferring to commode or toilet. *Collaboration with team members increases the patient's mastery of self-care tasks.*[1]
- Assist patient with toileting hygiene: cleansing and rearranging clothing if necessary.
- Provide privacy when toileting. *Privacy avoids possible embarrassment and withholding the need to toilet.*

■ = nursing intervention; ▲ = collaborative intervention.

EVALUATION

In clinical practice evaluation occurs during every phase of the nursing process. Evaluation involves the judgment to decide whether the outcome criteria have been met as evidenced by the stated behavioral indicators. If the expected outcome is not met, the care plan needs to be modified. The outcome may not be met because the expected outcome is unrealistic and unattainable,

the nursing diagnosis does not reflect the assessment data, and intervention strategies were not clearly and precisely described. Evaluation of Self-Care Deficit outcomes takes place on a continuing basis, especially when functional ADL status or general patient status changes as a result of pathology. When the patient masters a self-care activity, the nurse must continue to monitor the patient's ability to maintain the activity.

▶ CASE STUDY WITH PLAN OF CARE

Mr. Buel D., a 54-year-old assembly line worker at an auto plant, had a right hemisphere thrombotic stroke 4 days ago. He has a 2-year history of hypertension, which had been successfully controlled by diet and medication. Ten days before admission he stopped taking his medication because he had not been feeling well. He was admitted to the hospital, via the Emergency Department, after developing blurred vision, headache, and numbness in the left side of his face and weakness in his left arm and hand. Mr. D. was immediately started on an antihypertensive regime. The neurological assessment (after the acute period) reveals weakness on the right side of the body with minimal to moderate fine finger movement, moderate hand strength, decreased sensation in left extremities, minimal dysphagia, and homonymous hemianopia. When questioned about his

ability to perform basic ADLs he stated, "I just can't get my left hand to do what I want it to do. I can take off my clothes, but it takes a long time. I can't get food on my fork and usually can't get it to my mouth. . . . This is very frustrating. I have some trouble seeing, but if I remember to take time to look in all directions, I can usually see what's in front of me. It takes me so long to dress, and I get so tired . . . I also need help to get to the bathroom." Mr. D.'s functional ADL status (on a 0–4 scale) reveals: feeding, 3; bathing/hygiene (out of bed), 3; dressing/grooming, 3; toileting (out of bed), 2. The nurse diagnosed Mr. D. as having Self-Care Deficits in Feeding, Bathing/Hygiene, Dressing/Grooming, and Toileting related to paralysis and vision impairment. The plan of care that follows addresses Mr. D.'s Self-Care Deficit: Feeding.

⯈ **PLAN OF CARE FOR MR. BUEL D.**
Nursing Diagnosis: Self-Care Deficit: Feeding Related to Sensory and Motor Paralysis and
Visual Impairment

Expected Outcome: Mr. D. will maintain a sense of control over feeding as evidenced by participation in
decision making and by using assistive devices.
- Involve Mr. D. in formulating or modifying the plan of care; validate conclusions with him when updating the plan of care.
- ▲ Offer Mr. D. choices of food during all feeding activities.
- Provide supervision, assistance, and teaching, as needed, regarding use of adaptive devices (i.e., universal cuff and food guard).
- Consult with social services regarding possible home needs, such as Meals on Wheels.

Expected Outcome: Mr. D. will feed himself to an optimal level as evidenced by his consuming 75% to
100% of his meals and maintaining fluid intake at a minimum of 480 cc/day.
- Request consultation with the dietitian, occupational and physical therapists, and the speech therapist (minor swallowing problems may be associated with aphasia).
- Remain with Mr. D. during self-feeding and assist as necessary.
- Provide assistive aids (universal cuff and food guard) at every meal.
- Ensure that Mr. D. has his dentures securely in place.
- Remind Mr. D. to scan visual field when eating.
- Supervise or assist in meal preparations; assist Mr. D. to high Fowler's position during meals and maintain position for at least 30 minutes following meal; assist with meal setup (opening cartons and packages, applying condiments, cutting meat, etc.); keep suction machine at bedside and in working order.

Expected Outcome: Mr. D. will utilize feeding assistive devices effectively as evidenced by functional
feeding status of 1 (on a 0–4 scale) and satisfactory performance of feeding activities.
- Supervise, assist, and teach in using assistive devices.
- Provide short and clear instructions, repeating directions slowly.
- Provide positive feedback for accomplishments and encouragement for attempts.

■ = nursing intervention; ▲ = collaborative intervention.

▦ CRITICAL THINKING EXERCISES

1. What factors influence the way in which Mr. D. assesses his ADLs? What factors could present barriers to his independence?
2. Discuss the role of defining characteristics in determining the diagnosis of Self-Care Deficit. How are the defining characteristics different from related factors?
3. Describe how you would perform an assessment of Mr. D.'s functional ADL status. How often would you evaluate his status? Why?
4. Identify the physical assessment parameters that need to be included when examining Mr. D. Why are these parameters important?

5. Formulate an expected outcome and identify nursing interventions for Mr. D.'s Self-Care Deficit: Toileting. What ensures that the outcome is appropriate for Mr. D.?

REFERENCES

1. Ackley BJ and Ladwig GB: *Nursing diagnosis handbook: a guide to planning care,* ed 2, St. Louis, 1995, Mosby–Year Book.
2. Carnevali LJ: *Nursing diagnosis: application to clinical practice,* ed 5, Philadelphia, 1993, JB Lippincott Co.
3. Chang BL: Validity of concepts for selected nursing diagnoses, *Clin Nurs Res* 3(3):183–208, 1994.
4. Chang BL and others: Self-care deficit with etiologies: reliability of measurement, *Nurs Diagnosis* 1(1):31–36, 1990.

IV

5. Dittmar SS: *Rehabilitation nursing: process and application*, St. Louis, 1989, The CV Mosby Co.

6. Gordon M: Report of an RNF study to determine which nursing diagnoses have high frequency and high treatment priority in rehabilitation nursing, part I, *Rehab Nurs Res* 4(1):148–155, 1995.

7. Gordon, M: *Nursing diagnosis: process and application*, ed 3, St. Louis, 1994, Mosby–Year Book.

8. Gulanick M and others: *Nursing care plans: nursing diagnosis and intervention,* St. Louis, 1990, The CV Mosby Co.

9. Hoskins L: Self-care deficit: feeding, bathing/hygiene, dressing/grooming, toileting. In McFarland GK and McFarlane EA, editors: *Nursing diagnosis and intervention: planning for patient care,* ed 2, St. Louis, 1993, Mosby–Year Book.

10. Liddel BM: Principles and practices of rehabilitation. In Smelter SC and Bare BG: *Brunner and Suddarth's textbook of medical-surgical nursing,* ed 7, Philadelphia, 1992, JB Lippincott Co.

11. Lyke EM: Assessing for nursing diagnosis: a human need approach, Philadelphia, 1992, JB Lippincott Co.

12. McKeighen RJ, Mehmert PA, and Dickel CA: Bathing/hygiene self-care deficit: defining characteristics and related factors across age groups and diagnosis-related groups in an acute care setting, *Nurs Diagnosis* 1(4):155–161, 1990.

13. Miller JM: *Coping with chronic illnesses: overcoming powerlessness,* ed 2, Philadelphia, 1991, FA Davis.

14. National Center for Health Statistics: *Health United States 1993,* Department of Health and Human Services Pub No PHS 94-1232, Washington, D.C., 1994, Government Printing Office.

15. North American Nursing Diagnosis Association: *NANDA nursing diagnoses: definitions and classification, 1995–1996,* Philadelphia, 1994, The Association.

16. Orem DE: *Nursing: concepts of practice,* ed 5, St. Louis, 1995, Mosby–Year Book.

17. Rantz M, Vinz-Miller T, and Matson S: Nursing diagnoses in long-term care: a longitudinal perspective for strategic planning, *Nurs Diagnosis* 6(20):57–63, 1995.

18. Sheppard KC: The relationships among nursing diagnoses in discharge planning for patients with lung cancer, *Nurs Diagnosis* 4(4):148–155, 1993.

19. Thompson J and others: *Clinical nursing,* ed 3, St. Louis, 1993, Mosby–Year Book.

20. Wiener JM and others: Measuring the activities of daily living: comparisons across national surveys, *J Gerontol* 45(6):229–237, 1990.

Altered Tissue Perfusion: Renal
▶ _____

Altered Tissue Perfusion: Cerebral
▶ _____

Altered Tissue Perfusion: Cardiopulmonary
▶ _____

Altered Tissue Perfusion: Gastrointestinal
▶ _____

Altered Tissue Perfusion: Peripheral
▶ _____

Altered Tissue Perfusion: Renal *is the state in which an individual experiences a decrease in nutrition and oxygenation at the cellular level of the kidney because of a deficit in capillary blood supply.*

Altered Tissue Perfusion: Cerebral *is the state in which an individual experiences a decrease in nutrition and oxygenation at the cellular level of the brain because of a deficit in capillary blood supply.*

Altered Tissue Perfusion: Cardiopulmonary *is the state in which an individual experiences a decrease in nutrition and oxygenation at the cellular level of the heart and/or lungs because of a deficit in capillary blood supply.*

Altered Tissue Perfusion: Gastrointestinal *is the state in which an individual experiences a decrease in nutrition and oxygenation at the cellular level of the gastrointestinal system because of a deficit in capillary blood supply.*

Altered Tissue Perfusion: Peripheral *is the state in which an individual experiences a decrease in nutrition and oxygenation at the cellular level of* the peripheral tissues because of a deficit in capillary blood supply.*

OVERVIEW

Adequate tissue perfusion is essential to the life and functioning of each body organ and tissue. It depends on a competent circulatory system that will continuously deliver oxygen and nutrients to the cells and remove metabolic waste products. Oxygen and nutrients must pass through several steps from the time they enter the body until they reach the cells.[8] These steps include ventilation of the lungs, transport of oxygen into the plasma, attachment of oxygen to hemoglobin, transport of the oxygen-rich blood from the pulmonary circulation to the tissues, and diffusion of oxygen into the interstitial fluid and then to cells.

Altered Tissue Perfusion will ensue if there is an interruption at any point during the circulatory process, causing a decrease in the delivery of oxygen and nutrients to the cells, and thus a decrease in cellular function, energy metabolism, and removal of waste products. A local reduction in tissue perfusion is referred to as *ischemia,* and a systemic reduction is referred to as *shock.*

Ischemia is the result of occlusion or restriction of a vessel, resulting in a decrease in blood supply to the tissues. Pathophysiological conditions that cause ischemia include atherosclerotic plaque formation, vasoconstriction, vessel stenosis, the formation of a thrombus or embolus, and/or vasospasm.[8]

Shock is the result of a decrease in cardiac output, usually related to volume loss or impaired contractility such as that seen in patients with congestive heart failure. A decrease in cardiac output will affect all tissues because the heart is unable to maintain an adequate flow of oxygenated blood throughout the body.

Clinical manifestations of an Altered Tissue Perfusion can appear in any or all of the following tissues: renal, cerebral, cardiopulmonary, gastrointestinal, and peripheral. The extent of the effects of the decrease in tissue perfusion depends on the duration of the deficit and on the metabolic needs of the tissues. Its cause can be related to an interruption of arterial flow, an interruption of venous flow, exchange problems, hypervolemia, or hypovolemia.

Altered Tissue Perfusion: Renal is initially manifested by a decrease in urine output and signs of excess fluid volume. If the alteration is prolonged, the result may be ischemia, tissue death, and renal failure. The etiologies include any condition that results in an interruption of circulatory flow to the kidneys as indicated above.

In children, a common cause of Altered Tissue Perfusion: Renal is blunt trauma to the kidney.[6] This may be more difficult to detect because the initial symptom of hematuria is not present in 40% of children.

When renal tissue ischemia is present, a reflex arterial and venous vasoconstriction occurs, resulting in an increase in sodium and water retention by the kidneys. This vasoconstriction may improve venous return to the heart but will further impair blood flow through the kidneys, denying them the oxygen and nutrients needed for metabolism. Prolonged ischemia will result in renal insufficiency and eventual renal failure.

Some of the specific clinical conditions that are associated with renal tissue ischemia include diabetic neuropathy, rhabdomyolysis, renal trauma, and human immunodeficiency virus (HIV) infection.[5,11,15,16]

Once permanent damage occurs, the patient requires an artificial means of dialysis to remove excess waste products and fluid volume and to sustain life.

Altered Tissue Perfusion: Cerebral is often manifested by a change in mental status or loss of consciousness, due to any etiology, which results in decreased flow to the cerebral vessels as indicated above. Most etiologies are due to physiological inadequacy of the cerebral vessels, compression of surrounding tissues, or infection. These interruptions in flow to the cerebral tissues can produce temporary or permanent alterations in brain functions as a result of the ischemia.

Some specific clinical conditions that can result in Altered Tissue Perfusion: Cerebral include cerebral vascular accident, transient ischemic attacks, cerebral vasospasm, atherosclerosis, arteritis, hypertensive arteriosclerosis, trauma, orthostatic hypotension, cerebral aneurysm, tumors, hydrocephalus, and head injuries. Other disease states that result in degenerative changes in the central or peripheral nervous systems, endocrine system, and vascular system can also result in Altered Tissue Perfusion: Cerebral. These conditions are often seen in the elderly population, and the consequence is orthostatic hypotension, resulting in syncope and falls.[7] It may be further complicated by chronic disease, medications, decreased mobility, and confusion.

In children, head injuries from trauma are the most common cause of Altered Tissue Perfusion: Cerebral.[13] In some cases they are more vulnerable because of their increased head size and immature neck muscles. Some children, especially infants, may fair better than adults with a head injury because of the open fontanels and the rapid growth state of a child's brain.

Altered Tissue Perfusion: Cardiopulmonary is often manifested as cardiac ischemia or problems with oxygen delivery to heart and/or lung tissues.

Any condition that predisposes a patient to a decrease in cardiac output or interferes with blood flow through the alveolar capillary membrane may cause Altered Tissue Perfusion. Several conditions that cause this deficit of blood supply include: atherosclerotic, heart disease, coronary spasm, cardiogenic shock, congestive heart failure, anemia, chronic obstructive lung disease, and pulmonary infarction or embolus. Other possible etiologies are pulmonary edema, shock, atelectasis, and pneumothorax.

Each of these conditions interferes with the flow of blood within the circulatory or pulmonary systems. If it is prolonged, there may be permanent damage to the other body systems and tissues that are so highly dependent on the supply of oxygen and nutrients. Therefore Altered Tissue Perfusion: Cardiopulmonary can lead to Altered Tissue Perfusion in many other areas of the body.

Altered Tissue Perfusion: Gastrointestinal (GI) can be manifested by problems in the stomach, the liver, the bowel, and the pancreas. Any decrease in blood flow to the GI system can interfere with the normal function of the GI system and can cause a decrease in peristalsis. Postoperative complications of abdominal surgery, atherosclerosis of the GI vasculature, and shock are three main conditions that reduce blood flow to the GI tract. The result may be tissue necrosis and death.

Complete occlusion of the arterial blood supply can create severe abdominal pain, nausea, and vomiting, caused by ischemia of the tissues. If the interruption of blood supply is prolonged and severe, infarction and necrosis of tissue can occur. This situation requires prompt surgical intervention.

As with other body systems, the GI tract is affected by the prolonged vasoconstriction associated with shock.[14] The resulting ischemia can lead to ulceration of the stomach and the intestines, and the invasion of bacteria into the circulation. Another potential complication is GI hemorrhage.

Bowel ischemia and obstruction also may occur after abdominal surgery. It is referred to as *paralytic ileus* and occurs when a lack of peristalsis occurs following abdominal surgery. Paralytic ileus

may last from hours to days, and it is treated with gastric suction to prevent nausea, vomiting, and the potential for aspiration.

A decrease in tissue perfusion to the liver and pancreas also will result in ischemia and an alteration in function. During acute stages of shock there may be ischemic damage to the liver because the decrease in circulation does not provide enough nutrients to support the liver's high metabolic rate. If the deterioration continues, liver function is depressed, and cellular metabolism and detoxification of material and drugs are reduced.

Altered Tissue Perfusion: Peripheral can occur as a result of decreased blood flow, caused by structural problems such as vascular disease, functional problems such as vasospasm, or induced by other conditions such as shock and hypothermia. The extremities frequently are cold, blue, or purple and may have cellulitis and diminished arterial pulses. The legs may have ulcers. The patient may experience pain in the lower extremities during activity.

Causes of structural problems include arteriosclerosis, atherosclerosis, inflammation, emboli, thrombophlebitis, or thromboangiitis obliterans, also called Buerger's disease. Functional problems, such as vasospasm, interfere with tissue perfusion. Raynaud's disease can be caused by cold and is characterized by intermittent episodes of constriction of the small arteries. Hypothermia, as occurs with frostbite, can cause permanent damage to the tissues if not corrected.

ASSESSMENT

Each of the five related factors listed on page 428 impairs the cells' ability to obtain oxygen and nutrients needed for proper functioning and for excreting metabolic waste products. All of the medical diagnoses previously indicated can be associated with at least one of these factors. Therefore, when one of these related factors is present, the nurse should be alerted to begin a thorough assessment of its effects on physiological body systems and Functional Health Patterns. Specific Functional Health Patterns that may be affected include the

IV

Nutritional-Metabolic, Elimination, Activity-Exercise, and Cognitive-Perceptual Patterns.

There are many defining characteristics for Altered Tissue Perfusion: Peripheral, but those related to other body systems, tissues, and organs are still in the process of being developed. They are sometimes difficult to identify because they may differ from patient to patient, depending on the underlying disease. Therefore, if Altered Tissue Perfusion is suspected, a thorough assessment of each system is vital.

Altered Tissue Perfusion: Renal

When assessing a patient with Altered Tissue Perfusion: Renal, the nurse can first acquire subjective data by evaluating the Activity-Exercise Pattern, the Nutritional-Metabolic Pattern, and the Elimination Pattern and by obtaining a health history. A patient with renal insufficiency or failure may exhibit thirst, anorexia, and fatigue.[12] The patient may also have excessive urine output followed by decreased urine output. Other important symptoms include nausea, vomiting, pruritis, and neurological changes.

Urine output should be monitored along with any changes in weight. Is the patient taking any medications that are nephrotoxic? What are the serum lab values for blood urea nitrogen (BUN), creatine, and electrolytes? Is the patient's mental status within the baseline parameters, or are there problems with lethargy? Has the dietary intake of protein, calories, and fluid changed? Is the patient as active as usual, or has there been a noticeable decrease in activity due to fatigue?

Objective data can be obtained through physical examination and blood values. Besides BUN, creatine, and electrolytes, monitoring serum pH and hemoglobin is important. Acidosis is commonly associated with renal failure because of the inability of the kidneys to excrete waste products. If severe, it may be treated with sodium bicarbonate taken orally as prescribed. Hyperkalemia can be a life-threatening complication because of its effect on the cardiovascular system. Serial electrocardiograms (ECGs) will assist the nurse in identifying changes related to hyperkalemia. These ECG changes include peaked T waves, prolonged P-R intervals, and depressed ST segments.[15]

Kidneys also are responsible for the production of erythropoietin. This substance stimulates the bone marrow to produce red blood cells. Because erythropoietin levels decrease in patients with renal failure, these patients have chronic anemia and therefore a reduced oxygen-carrying capacity. This affects the patient's ability to tolerate activity. The inability to compensate for increased oxygen demand with activity may be exhibited by increased shortness of breath, weakness, palpitations, and fatigue.

As Altered Tissue Perfusion: Renal becomes more severe and as renal failure progresses, salt and water retention gradually increases. The fluid will be intracellular and extracellular. Patients usually exhibit chronic edema in dependent areas. If the edema is excessive, these areas must be monitored closely for Altered Tissue Perfusion: Peripheral and Impaired Skin Integrity. The nurse must assess the patient's breath sounds for signs of fluid overload and congestive heart failure.

Increased jugular vein distention (JVD) is another indication of excessive fluid volume. Under normal circumstances jugular veins cannot be seen more than 3 cm above the sternal angle when the patient is at a 30° to 45° angle.[10]

Monitoring blood pressure also becomes important because, as the glomerular filtration rate of the kidney decreases, the release of renin increases. This in turn raises blood pressure in an attempt to increase perfusion to the kidney. Patients with renal failure often require antihypertensive medications to control this increase in blood pressure.

■ Defining Characteristics

The presence of any of the following defining characteristics indicates that the patient may be experiencing Altered Tissue Perfusion: Renal:

- Decrease in urine output
- Complaints of thirst, anorexia, or fatigue
- Elevated BUN and creatine levels

- Weight gain
- Peripheral edema
- Hypertension
- Pruritis
- Changes in mentation
- Anemia

Altered Tissue Perfusion: Cerebral

When a patient is assessed for Altered Tissue Perfusion: Cerebral, subjective data can be obtained by evaluating the Cognitive-Perceptual Pattern and the Activity-Exercise Pattern. A pertinent history may include headaches, dizziness, and difficulty concentrating. The nurse must assess for an alteration in mental status or loss of consciousness. Does the patient black out, have problems remembering things, have periods of confusion, or have fainting spells? Is the patient oriented to person, place, and time? Is he or she restless?

When evaluating the history, the nurse should specifically ask about cerebral vascular accidents, tumors, transient ischemic attacks, head injuries, orthostatic hypotension, and seizures. What medications are being taken? Can the medications cause alterations in blood pressure or alter thought processes? Does the patient become lightheaded when moving from a lying position to sitting and then to standing?

Objective data can be obtained through physical examination. The nurse must assess the patient's blood pressure and pulse in the lying, sitting, and standing positions. An increase in heart rate greater than 20 beats per minute when position is changed from supine to vertical is a significant sign of orthostatic hypotension.[7]

If the patient has orthostatic hypotension, the nurse should assist in determining if it is due to medications, cardiac dysrythmias, or hypovolemia, or if it is an idiopathic problem. Temperature is also an important assessment parameter because hypothermia will alter cerebral blood flow. Pupils should be assessed for equality, shape, size, and reaction to light. Motor strength should also be evaluated.

If any of the above alterations are found in the history or physical examination, it is a clue to the nurse that the patient may have an acute or chronic neurological problem that can interfere with cerebral function. The nursing assessment then becomes one of the most important indicators of a potential or actual interruption of cerebral blood flow. It should be performed at routine intervals to recognize any progressive neurological deficit resulting from increased intracranial pressure (ICP).

Many different symptoms, alone or in combination, could indicate a change in cerebral blood flow and ICP. The nurse should monitor for headaches, nausea, vomiting, restlessness, confusion, hemiplegia, visual deficits, conjugate deviation of the eyes, sensory loss, stiff neck, otorrhea, or rhinorrhea.[4] Accurate identification of these early signs of increased ICP will aid in preventing further increases in ICP and the interruption of blood flow. If not prevented, tissue ischemia will progress to tissue death and loss of function.

Late signs of progressive, increased ICP include deterioration in the level of consciousness, coma, decorticate and decerebrate posturing, aphasia, and seizures.[4] Pupils may be unequal in size and may react sluggishly to light. Fixed and dilated pupils indicate a medical emergency that must be reported immediately because severe and potentially irreversible damage to cerebral tissue has probably occurred. Wide fluctuations in temperature can also be attributed to progressive increases in ICP.

A slow, falling pulse accompanied by a rise in systolic blood pressure is also an abnormal finding associated with an increase in ICP. Along with assessing for changes in vital signs, the nurse should closely monitor the patient's pulmonary status. As ICP rises it will interfere with the normal functioning of the respiratory center in the brain stem, and respiratory rate will fall. The patient's breath sounds, chest expansion, gag and cough reflexes, and ability to clear secretions may be impaired. If ICP continues to rise, these functions will cease, and respirations will become irregular, with progressively longer periods of apnea resulting in irreversible tissue damage and death.

IV

IV

■ Defining Characteristics

The presence of any of the following defining characteristics indicates that the patient may be experiencing Altered Tissue Perfusion: Cerebral:

- Fainting spells
- Restlessness
- Alteration in mental status
- Alteration in cognitive function
- Alteration in level of consciousness
- Headache
- Dizziness
- Memory Loss
- Confusion
- Disorientation
- Motor problem

Altered Tissue Perfusion: Cardiopulmonary

When a patient is being assessed for Altered Tissue Perfusion: Cardiopulmonary, information about current health perceptions, symptomatology, and a health history will provide the nurse with valuable information. Has the patient had a myocardial infarction, congestive heart failure, or respiratory failure? Is the patient taking any medications that can affect either the cardiac or the pulmonary system? Is there a history of smoking, hypertension, hypercholesterolemia, obesity, or a high stress level? Is there a family history of cardiovascular disease?

Subjective information can be obtained by a careful evaluation of symptoms evaluated. Chest pain should be evaluated for location, severity, radiation, duration, precipitating factors, accompanying symptoms, and alleviating factors. Complaints of palpitations and/or syncope may indicate the presence of a compromising dysrhythmia. Weight changes and ankle swelling are associated with congestive heart failure and hypertension.

Fatigue and dsypnea are both important symptoms that can be present with a cardiac or a pulmonary problem. Assess the activity level of the patient for a day. Determine when the patient first began to feel short of breath and whether it is associated with activity. How much activity can the patient tolerate without feeling short of breath or fatigued? Does the patient have paroxysmal nocturnal dyspnea or two- or three-pillow orthopnea? Is the patient able to cough up secretions?

During your interview, observe the patient's behavior as well as that of any family members present. Anxiety is common in patients with respiratory and cardiac problems and their families.

Objective data can be obtained through physical examination, electrocardiography, and monitoring of laboratory values. Important baseline laboratory assessments should include levels of BUN, creatine, creatine kinase (CK) and lactate dehydrogenase (LDH) enzymes and isoenzymes, baseline cholesterol, hemoglobin, and hematocrit. Cardiac enzymes will help confirm the diagnosis of myocardial infarction (MI), along with ECG changes and the presence of angina. If cardiac output decreases, the nurse will find the BUN and creatine levels increasing as blood flow to the kidneys is impaired. The presence of anemia may predispose the patient to chest pain as the oxygen-carrying ability of the blood is reduced. Arterial blood gas measurements are also helpful in determining if the patient's oxygenation is adequate, especially in the presence of anemia.

When the nurse suspects Altered Tissue Perfusion: Cardiopulmonary, a thorough physical exam is conducted. Cardiac rate and rhythm should be documented because dysrhythmias decrease cardiac output, which will further affect tissue perfusion. Abnormal heart sounds can indicate altered cardiac function. Blood pressure should be checked because the presence of hypertension is an important risk factor for coronary heart disease. Jugular vein distention, hepatojugular reflux, and peripheral edema can indicate congestive heart failure.

Respirations should be monitored for rate, depth, and character. Breath sounds should be auscultated for normal sounds and for any adventitious sounds. Bronchospasm or tumors that cause narrowing of the airways can be heard as wheezing. Crackles may indicate increased fluid in the lung or pneumonia. Rhonchi may indicate an increase in fluid or mucus within the pulmonary system, which can impair ventilation. Peripheral edema and peripheral cyanosis are also signs of an alteration in cardiopulmonary function.

A history of pulmonary emboli, pneumonia, obstructive or restrictive lung disease, plueral effusions, or lung abscesses may interfere with the ability of the pulmonary system to exchange oxygen and carbon dioxide. These medical conditions can precipitate Altered Tissue Perfusion.

The use of accessory muscles, an elevated respiratory rate, and the presence of an abdominal paradox or a respiratory alternans breathing pattern can indicate respiratory muscle fatigue and impending respiratory arrest.

■ Defining Characteristics

The presence of any of the following defining characteristics indicates that the patient may be experiencing Altered Tissue Perfusion: Cardiopulmonary:

- Shortness of breath
- Tachycardia or palpitations
- Abnormal breath sounds
- Peripheral edema and cyanosis
- Slow capillary filling
- Chest pain
- Tachypnea
- Dysrhythmias
- Hypotension
- Cold, clammy skin

Altered Tissue Perfusion: Gastrointestinal

When assessing a patient for Altered Tissue Perfusion: Gastrointestinal, the nurse can obtain subjective data by performing a nursing assessment that focuses on changes in bowel habits and complaints of nausea and vomiting.[2,3] Is the patient complaining of constipation or diarrhea, or is there blood in the stool? Has the patient had a surgical procedure? Is the abdomen distended?

If there has been vomiting, the nurse should determine the consistency of emesis and the presence of blood. The patient should be questioned regarding the location and quality of abdominal pain and its association with meals. Does the patient have a medical history of ulcerative colitis or ulcer disease? Has there been a recent weight gain or loss? Is the patient taking any medications that could affect the normal functioning of the gastrointestinal tract?

Objective data can be obtained through a physical exam. Low blood pressure can predispose the patient to a reduced blood flow in the GI tract. The nurse should auscultate bowel sounds before palpating the abdomen because palpation can reduce peristalsis. Assess for the presence of distension, guarding, and pain. If the patient complains of increasing distension, measuring the abdominal girth daily can be an objective tool for assessing increased abdominal size. All stools and emesis should be tested for occult blood.

■ Defining Characteristics

The presence of any following defining characteristics indicates that the patient may be experiencing Altered Tissue Perfusion: Gastrointestinal:

- Nausea
- Vomiting
- Lack of bowel sounds
- Abdominal pain that increases after meals
- Constipation
- Diarrhea
- Abdominal distension

Altered Tissue Perfusion: Peripheral

Subjective complaints that can suggest Altered Tissue Perfusion: Peripheral include pain, numbness, coolness of the skin, cramping, tingling, burning, or loss of motor or sensory function.[2,3] The nurse should determine if any of these are associated with any particular activities or time of day or exposure to cold.

A medical history of arteriosclerosis, Raynaud's disease, diabetes, phlebitis, deep vein thrombosis, or peripheral vascular disease may contribute to Altered Tissue Perfusion: Peripheral. Peripheral edema, leg ulcers, gangrene, and intermittent claudication can indicate significant risk. Low levels of hematocrit and hemoglobin can reduce the amount of oxygen reaching peripheral tissues, placing them at risk for ischemia. Hypothermia, shock, and vasoconstricting medications can cause decreased blood flow.

Physical examination can be helpful in collecting objective data that may indicate Altered Tissue Perfusion: Peripheral. The nurse should assess the extremities for color, temperature, presence and quality of pulses, edema and ulcerations. Redness or swelling in the calf can indicate thrombophlebitis. A positive Homan's sign, elicited by bending the knee and simultaneously dorsiflexing the foot, can indicate thrombophlebitis. A positive finding is calf pain.

Assess skin turgor and texture, lack of hair, shiny skin, and dry, thick slow-growing nails, which can indicate Altered Tissue Perfusion. Pressure changes in the extremities or the presence of bruits can indicate interruptions in blood flow to the peripheral tissues. Does the patient have problems with paresthesia or trophic skin changes, such as calluses or fissures found on the toes, heels, or soles of the feet? All of these findings are important to assess and document because they are characteristics of Altered Tissue Perfusion: Peripheral.

■ Defining Characteristics

The presence of any of the following defining characteristics indicates that the patient may be experiencing Altered Tissue Perfusion: Peripheral:

- Decreased or absent arterial pulse
- Cyanosis of extremities in a dependent position
- Pale extremities on elevation; color does not return after lowering leg
- Slow-growing, dry, brittle, thick nails
- Blood pressure changes in extremities
- Numbness and tingling in extremities
- Loss of motor or sensory function
- Decrease in capillary filling rate
- Slow healing of lesions
- Intermittent claudication
- Cold extremities
- Gangrene
- Lack of lanugo
- Shiny skin

- Peripheral edema
- Bruits
- Round scars with atrophied skin

■ Related Factors

The following related factors are associated with Altered Tissue Perfusion: Renal, Cerebral, Cardiopulmonary, Gastrointestinal, Peripheral:

- Interruption of arterial flow
- Interruption of venous flow
- Exchange problems
- Hypervolemia
- Hypovolemia

DIAGNOSIS

■ Differential Nursing Diagnosis

When choosing a nursing diagnosis that best addresses the problem the patient is experiencing, the nurse must first assess and evaluate the patient to determine the underlying etiology of the current problem to prioritize nursing interventions. For example, a patient with shortness of breath could be experiencing Altered Tissue Perfusion: Renal or Cardiopulmonary or another nursing diagnosis, such as Activity Intolerance, Ineffective Airway Clearance, Ineffective Breathing Pattern, Fluid Volume Excess, and Decreased Cardiac Output. Although more than one of these diagnoses can be present, one is often the result of the other. For example, suppose the patient has cardiac ischemia, resulting in dysrhythmias and a decrease in cardiac output. The patient would then experience an excess fluid volume and, subsequently, shortness of breath. The nursing care plan should address treatment of the primary etiology, cardiac ischemia, and all other problems should subside. In comparison, if only Fluid Volume Excess was treated, the ischemia could worsen and result in a negative outcome.

■ Medical and Psychiatric Diagnoses

The symptomatology of patients experiencing Altered Tissue Perfusion is directly linked to the physiological changes that occur with many disease states affecting the kidneys, brain, gastrointestinal tract, heart, and lungs and with all types of shock. Some of those medical conditions are aneurysm, atherosclerosis, Buerger's disease, cerebrovascular accident, congestive heart failure, deep vein thrombosis, hypovolemic shock, myocardial infarction, paralytic ileus, pulmonary embolism, Raynaud's phenomenon, and renal failure.

OUTCOME IDENTIFICATION, PLANNING, AND IDENTIFICATION

When planning care for Altered Tissue Perfusion, the nurse must first determine if the problem is local, resulting in ischemia to one organ, or systemic, resulting in possible effects in many organs. If the problem is local, then the specific nursing goals and interventions will depend on the tissue or organ involved. If the problem is systemic, the goals and nursing interventions will be directed toward the treatment of shock.

In either situation, however, the desired patient outcomes will be the same. These outcomes can be grouped into three major areas:

1. There will be adequate blood flow in the affected vessels, and tissue perfusion and cellular oxygenation will be maximized; the result will be maintenance of the integrity of the tissue or organ.
2. The metabolic needs of the tissue or organ will be reduced or maintained.
3. The patient and family will understand the cause of the problem and will modify their lifestyle to minimize the causative factors or side effects to the decrease in tissue perfusion.

Altered Tissue Perfusion: Renal

When planning care for a patient with Altered Tissue Perfusion: Renal, the first concern is adequate blood flow and tissue perfusion within the renal system. Nursing goals should include monitoring and maintaining cardiac output and blood pressure. This includes evaluating urine output, specific gravity, electrolytes, BUN, and creatine.[14] As blood flow through the kidneys decreases, there will be decreased glomerular filtration, retention of metabolic waste products, and metabolic acidosis. In the case of permanent renal damage, the nurse will see a gradual decrease in the hematocrit, due to a reduction in erythropoietin production.

If renal insufficiency is noted at any time, it is important to note if any of the medications the patient is receiving have nephrotoxic effects. As urine output decreases, the nurse should also monitor intake and output, daily weights, and any other signs of increased fluid volume, such as peripheral edema, lung crackles, and dyspnea.

Patient care includes maintaining the metabolic needs of the tissues. This is accomplished by controlling hyperthermia and monitoring hemoglobin. Some physicians may elect to use low-dose intravenous dopamine in an attempt to increase renal blood flow because of dopaminergic effects of vasodilatation of the renal vessels.

Teaching plans for patients with an alternation in renal function related to a decrease in tissue perfusion should emphasize frequent periods of rest. Because their disease may be associated with nausea, vomiting, and anorexia, dietary teaching can be a challenge for the nurse. Patients must be taught the importance of eating foods that are low in protein and potassium because of their limited ability to excrete these waste products of protein metabolism. Sodium intake is based on weight.

If the outcome of the decrease in renal tissue perfusion is chronic renal failure, the patient and family will need support after the decision is made for the patient to receive hemodialysis or peritoneal dialysis. The nurse should also provide information regarding the procedure and the need to make further lifestyle modifications.

◣ NURSING CARE GUIDELINES

Nursing Diagnosis: Altered Tissue Perfusion: Renal

Expected Outcome: The patient will have adequate tissue perfusion and cellular oxygenation of the renal system as evidenced by a urine output ≥ 30 ml/hr; normal BUN, creatine, and glomerular filtration rate; and absence of excess fluid volume.

- Monitor and document vital signs; notify physician of any changes. *An elevated heart rate may be a compensatory mechanism triggered by a decrease in cardiac output. Prolonged hypotension will put the kidneys at risk because of the decrease in the delivery of oxygen and nutrients.*
- Monitor fluid balance and specific gravity every 1 to 2 hours. *When renal function is impaired, the patient may have a decrease in urine output and the specific gravity will remain low as the kidney loses the ability to concentrate or dilute urine.*
- Weigh the patient daily. *When renal function is impaired, the patient will being to retain fluid.*
- Assess for peripheral edema. *When a patient with renal impairment begins to retain fluid, the patient develops venous pooling and peripheral edema.*
- Assess breath sounds at least once a shift and with any complaints of dyspnea. *The increasing fluid volume that results from renal insufficiency or failure will eventually cause pulmonary congestion.*
- ▲ Monitor BUN, creatine, and electrolyte levels. *An alternation in electrolytes and an elevation in BUN and creatine may indicate an alteration in renal function.*
- ▲ Monitor glomerular filtration rate as assessed by urine output. *A decrease in blood flow through the kidney will result in a decrease in urine output and demonstrate a decreased glomerular filtration rate.*
- ▲ Monitor serum pH and hematocrit. *As renal failure worsens, there is retention of metabolic waste products, resulting in metabolic acidosis. There will also be a decrease in hematocrit because of the decrease in erythropoietin.*
- ▲ Identify any medications with nephrotoxic effects. *Some medications can cause damage to the kidney and impair its function. If some renal insufficiency is already present, and if medication is metabolized and excreted by the kidney, the patient may be more likely to experience side effects.*

Expected Outcome: The patient will maintain the metabolic needs of the kidney as evidenced by a normal temperature and a normal level of hemoglobin.

- Monitor for hyperthermia and institute measures to decrease an elevated temperature. *Hyperthermia will increase the rate of cellular metabolism and metabolic needs of the tissues.*
- ▲ Monitor hematocrit and hemoglobin. *Because hemoglobin carries most of the oxygen to tissues, there must be adequate circulating blood volume to deliver the oxygen needed to the tissues.*
- ▲ Administer low-dose dopamine, if ordered. *In doses of 2 to 5 mcg/kg/min dopamine acts on the dopaminergic receptors in the renal vessels to cause vasodilation and increase perfusion.*

Expected Outcome: The patient will modify lifestyle to minimize the causative factors and/or side effects of a decrease in renal tissue perfusion.

- Help the patient and family to understand the need to restrict protein intake and foods high in potassium. *With inadequate renal function the patient will be unable to excrete the end products of protein metabolism or potassium.*
- Provide teaching about diet so the patient will have adequate caloric intake despite anorexia and decreased oral intake. *If anorexia is severe, the patient may need to eat small meals more frequently to provide a calorie intake that will meet their daily needs.*
- Teach the patient to base sodium intake on weight. *This is to prevent hyponatremia and problems with fluid overload.*
- If antihypertensives are used, instruct the patient on indications and side effects. *Provide the patient with the knowledge needed to monitor personal progress.*

■ = nursing intervention; ▲ = collaborative intervention.

- Provide the patient and family with psychological support if the outcome is chronic renal failure. *Dialysis will require patient and family to make lifestyle modifications.*
- Teach the patient about dialysis, whether hemodialysis or peritoneal dialysis. *The patient will need to decide which type of dialysis they will use.*
- Instruct the patient on the need for balancing exercise and rest periods to increase tolerance to activity. *Patients will have chronic anemia because of the reduction in erythropoietin production, resulting in decrease in activity tolerance.*

Altered Tissue Perfusion: Cerebral

When caring for a patient with Altered Tissue Perfusion: Cerebral, the nurse's first concern is adequate blood flow to the cerebral system. Monitoring the patient's neurological status, especially the level of consciousness, will assist the nurse to detect changes in cerebral function. Changes in systolic blood pressure have a direct effect on perfusion in the brain. When the intracranial pressure (ICP) measurement is available, the nurse should calculate the cerebral perfusion pressure (CPP). The formula for calculating CPP is mean arterial pressure (MAP) minus the ICP. If the CPP is less than 50 mm Hg, a vasopressor may be used to maintain arterial blood pressure.

In patients whose problem is the result of orthostatic hypotension, positioning can have a direct effect on outcome. They should lie flat in bed and, unless contraindicated, should be taught to wear waist-high elastic stockings when out of bed to promote venous return. They should learn to move slowly from a recumbent position to a sitting position and to dangle their feet before standing.

Patients with an elevated ICP should have the head of their bed elevated to promote venous return. Prompt recognition of problems in these patients is vital to preserving cerebral function.

Other types of treatment that may be used in these patients include osmotic diuretics, hyperventilation via a mechanical ventilator, barbiturate-induced coma, steroids, neuromuscular blocking agents and invasive intracranial pressure monitoring with cerebral drains. In concert with these medical treatments, the nurse can space out activities, institute seizure precautions, and evaluate the patient's neurological status.

Temperature is extremely important to preserving cerebral function because shivering can increase ICP. In some cases treatment of these patients will include hypothermia to decrease further the metabolic needs and oxygen consumption of the tissues. The nurse, in collaboration with the physician, can accomplish this by using a cooling blanket and ice packs, instilling cool intravenous fluids, or lavaging body orifices with cool fluids.

Before discharge, patients and families should be instructed about the possibility of taking medications such as antihypertensives and diuretics, especially if they are prone to orthostatic hypotension. They should also be aware of other medications, such as sedatives, that can alter thought processes. All of these side effects could result in symptoms associated with Altered Tissue Perfusion: Cerebral.

IV

◢ **NURSING CARE GUIDELINES**
Nursing Diagnosis: Altered Tissue Perfusion: Cerebral

Expected Outcome: The patient will maintain adequate tissue perfusion and cellular oxygenation of the cerebral system as evidenced by a wakeful, alert state of consciousness, a systolic blood pressure greater than 100 mm Hg, a cerebral perfusion pressure (CPP) of 60 to 90 mm Hg, and ICP of 0 to 15 mm Hg.

- Monitor and document the patient's mental status and level of consciousness; establish a baseline and ongoing neurological assessment. *Increasing restlessness and confusion are an early sign of an increase in intracranial pressure in adults. In children the nurse may find that the child no longer cries or fights during painful procedures.*
- Monitor and document the patient's vital signs; promptly report changes in vital signs or neurological status to the physician. *As the blood pressure decreases, blood flow to the cerebral tissues will not be adequate to prevent ischemia.*
- Monitor for signs of increased ICP: a decrease in consciousness; headache, vomiting, seizures, and hypertension, bradycardia, papilledema, pupillary changes, loss of motor or sensory function, and irregular respirations (Cheyne-Stokes respirations). *An elevated ICP can result in further compression of brain tissue and ischemia.*
- Monitor orthostatic vital signs, and notify physician if the difference is greater than 10 mm Hg. *Patients with orthostatic hypotension must be evaluated for a fluid volume deficit and treated if present. They should be positioned flat and moved slowly to a sitting position and then to a standing position to prevent loss of consciousness.*
- ▲ Monitor arterial blood gases for a decrease in P_{O_2} and an increase in P_{CO_2}. *In patients with cerebral edema, this is indicative of respiratory insufficiency, which may be due to increased pressure on the brain stem.*
- ▲ Administer medications as ordered. *The patient may require anticoagulants if the cause is related to emboli.*
- ▲ Administer vasopressors, as ordered by the physician, to maintain blood pressure. *A drop in blood pressure may result in a cerebral perfusion pressure less than 50 mm Hg; then cerebral tissue will not receive adequate amounts of oxygen and nutrients.*
- For patients with an increase in ICP, elevate the head of the bed. *This position promotes venous return.*

Expected Outcome: The patient will maintain the metabolic needs of the cerebral tissue as evidenced by normal temperature and by arterial blood gases within normal range for patient.

- ▲ Monitor temperature and induce hypothermia if ordered. *Shivering will result in an increase in ICP. Induction of hypothermia will decrease the metabolic needs and oxygen consumption of tissues.*
- ▲ If increased ICP is present, the following may be included in the plan of care: elevate head of bed, maintain controlled hyperventilation with P_{CO_2} between 25 and 35 mm Hg, maintain fluid restriction, maintain a quiet environment, space nursing activities with rest periods, administer osmotic diuretics as ordered, institute seizure precautions, and maintain barbiturate coma if indicated. *Elevation of the head will promote venous return. The other interventions, instituted alone or in combination, will preserve cerebral function and decrease ICP.*
- ▲ Monitor arterial blood gases, and maintain adequate oxygenation through ventilory support, if needed. *Alteration in neurological function and elevated ICP can result in respiratory depression, requiring mechanical support.*

Expected Outcome: The patient will make lifestyle modifications to minimize causative factors or side effects of a decrease in cerebral tissue perfusion.

- ▲ Identify medications that may contribute to Altered Tissue Perfusion: Cerebral, such as antihypertensives, diuretics, barbiturates, and phenothiazines. *Medications that result in hypotension and fluid volume loss and that alter the level of consciousness can result in decreased cerebral perfusion.*
- Prepare the patient for surgery, and do preoperative teaching, if indicated. *There are several etiologies of decreased cerebral tissue perfusion that may require surgery to correct the problem. Some of these include cere-*

■ = nursing intervention; ▲ = collaborative intervention.

bral aneurysm, arteriovenous malformation, head injury, and any other condition resulting in increased ICP.

- Teach the patient to change position slowly when rising from a recumbent position. *Orthostatic hypotension can occur after 2 to 3 days of bed rest. It can also be related to an autonomic dysfunction, resulting in decreased muscle tone and incompetent vein valves.*
- Discuss necessary dietary changes. *Patients who experience a cerebral vascular accident related to arteriosclerosis can limit their risk factors by diet modification.*
- Teach the patient to use elastic stockings and to apply and remove them when supine. *Elastic stockings promote venous return.*

Altered Tissue Perfusion: Cardiopulmonary

Planning the care of a patient with an alteration in cardiopulmonary function includes thorough monitoring of the cardiac and pulmonary systems. All complaints of chest pain and shortness of breath should be investigated. Cardiac output and blood pressure fall during the early phases of shock. The compensatory response is stimulation of the sympathetic nervous system, causing vasoconstriction and a redistribution of blood to the heart and brain. This vasoconstriction increases venous return, which may improve cardiac output and normalize the blood pressure. It is important to recognize that a normal blood pressure does not guarantee homeostasis and adequate organ perfusion.[9] If the compensatory response fails to improve blood pressure, vasodepressors such as dopamine may be administered. If the patient has poor cardiac output, an inotropic agent such as dobutamine may also be added to the medical treatment.

Hemodynamic parameters, such as central venous pressure (CVP), pulmonary artery pressure (PAP), and pulmonary artery wedge pressure (PAWP), should be monitored for abnormalities. If the patient's measurements are elevated and the patient has signs of congestive heart failure, diuretic therapy may be instituted. Vasoactive drugs, such as nitroglycerin and sodium nitroprusside, are useful in reducing the workload of the heart.

An electrocardiogram should be monitored for alterations in rate and rhythm. These patients are placed on a cardiac monitor and assessed for rate, rhythm, and presence of any dysrhythmias. If the patient is receiving antiarrythmics, such as lido-

caine, the nurse should document the effect of the medication on controlling the dysrhythmia during activity.

Chest pain that is prolonged can put the patient at risk for ischemia, injury, and infarction. An ECG will document the site and area at risk for damage. Nitroglycerin and rest are the first treatments for chest pain caused by altered cardiac tissue perfusion. If the patient experiences chest pain during common daily activities such as taking a shower, they can be taught to use nitroglycerin prophylactically to prevent chest pain. The patient should be informed how to use all medications and about their side effects. Dietary changes, such as limiting cholesterol and sodium intake, are part of the nursing priorities.

The nurse should assess the quality of the ventilatory effort of each patient, including rate, rhythm, use of accessory muscles, air movement, and breath sounds. If respiratory function is inadequate, hypoxemia or hypercarbia develops, and the patient may require artificial ventilatory support to supply the tissues and organs with adequate oxygen. This frequently occurs in patients with chronic obstructive pulmonary disease (COPD).

To control the metabolic needs of cardiopulmonary tissue, the patient will need to begin stress-reducing activities and take frequent rest periods. All medications should be evaluated to determine if their benefit outweighs any side effects. As with other organs, temperature control will reduce the metabolic needs of the tissue. Indications for modifications may include changing the diet, decreasing activity, carrying medications such as nitroglycerin, stopping smoking, and losing weight.

IV

■ **NURSING CARE GUIDELINES**
Nursing Diagnosis: Altered Tissue Perfusion: Cardiopulmonary

Expected Outcome: The patient will have adequate tissue perfusion and cellular oxygenation of the cardiopulmonary system as evidenced by a cardiac output ≥ 4 L/min, a systolic blood pressure ≥ 90 mm Hg; hemodynamic parameters within normal range, absence of dysrhythmias, chest pain, and shortness of breath, and a PO_2 > 80 with a saturation > 90%.

- Monitor and document vital signs, cardiac rhythm, central venous pressure (CVP), pulmonary artery pressures, wedge pressures, and cardiac output. *These parameters are important indicators of tissue perfusion.*
- Assess heart sounds and notify the physician of any abnormality. *Heart murmurs, such as those due to mitral regurgitation and aortic stenosis, can result in lowered cardiac output and chest pain.*
- ▲ Assess a baseline electrocardiogram and those taken during episodes of chest pain. *Ischemia, injury, and infarction can be assessed on the ECG and prompt interventions begun to improve myocardial tissue perfusion.*
- Assess for the presence of chest pain, shortness of breath, and breath sounds. *Abnormal breath sounds may indicate a condition that will interfere with the diffusion of oxygen and carbon dioxide across the alveolar capillary membrane. This can predispose the patient to hypoxia, hypercarbia, chest pain, and Altered Tissue Perfusion.*
- ▲ Monitor lab results for abnormalities in levels of hematocrit, hemoglobin, CK, LDH, isoenzymes, and arterial blood gases. *Arterial blood gases give an indication of adequate oxygen supply, whereas hemoglobin and hematocrit will indicate if oxygen-carrying capacity is reduced. Enzyme elevation indicates myocardial damage.*
- ▲ Administer vasopressors, inotropic agents, nitrates, and antidysrhythmic agents to maintain normal vital signs and hemodynamic ranges. *When compensatory mechanisms fail to improve vital signs, medications can improve cardiac output, blood pressure, and oxygen delivery and reduce oxygen demand.*
- ▲ Administer oxygen as needed. *Supplemental oxygen can reduce the work of breathing and improve oxygen availability.*
- ▲ Optimize fluid volume status and administer volume or diuretics as indicated. *Fluid volume affects cardiac output and myocardial oxygen demand.*

Expected Outcome: The patient will have control of metabolic needs of the cardiopulmonary tissues.

- ▲ Assess the metabolic effects of any medications. *Medications with side effects of dysrhythmias, tachycardia, or positive inotrope may cause an increase in myocardial oxygen consumption and precipitate chest pain.*
- Teach the patient to eliminate activities that result in chest pain or shortness of breath and to balance rest with activity. *Patients can reduce myocardial oxygen demand by reducing activities that place too high a demand on the myocardium and by allowing adequate rest periods.*
- Help the patient identify stressful situations and behavior modification activities to reduce stress response. *Stress increases circulating catecholamines, which increase the demand on the cardiopulmonary system.*
- ▲ Monitor for hyperthermia and institute measures to reduce temperature. *Hyperthermia increases demand on the cardiopulmonary system and causes an increased metabolic rate.*

Expected Outcome: The patient will make lifestyle modifications to minimize the causative factors or side effects of Altered Tissue Perfusion: Cardiopulmonary.

- Teach the patient and family how to modify their risk factors for heart and lung disease, including smoking cessation and dietary restrictions (low-sodium, low-cholesterol diet). *Risk factor modification can reduce the progression of heart and lung disease.*
- Instruct the patient about indications and side effects of medications. *Compliance with self-administration of medications is increased if patients understand the rationale. Patients should be informed of all side effects so they can report them quickly to prevent further complications.*

■ = nursing intervention; ▲ = collaborative intervention.

- Teach the patient to increase activity slowly and to balance rest and activity. *This helps conserve energy and reduces the chance of ischemia to myocardial tissues.*
- Reinforce the use of nitroglycerin, especially before activities that usually cause chest pain. *Nitroglycerin, a potent vasodilator, can reduce the incidence of chest pain.*

Altered Tissue Perfusion: Gastrointestinal

Postoperative patients as well as patients with shock, vascular disease, and hypotension are at risk for a shutdown in gastrointestinal functioning. The nurse should maintain gastric decompression until bowel function is restored. Assess bowel sounds in all quadrants, and assess for the presence of abdominal pain, nausea, and vomiting. A bowel program that helps prevent constipation and diarrhea needs to be incorporated into the care plan.

Intake and output should be monitored and intravenous fluids administered as needed. Gastric secretions and stools should be assessed for the presence of blood. Medications that irritate the gastrointestinal system should be avoided.

Assess the adequacy of nutritional intake, and note any recent changes. If the intake does not meet the patient's caloric requirements, easily digested diet supplements should be added.

Abdominal angina can be reduced if the patient is encouraged to rest after eating meals. The nurse should space activities over the course of the day so that the patient does not become fatigued. Stress-reducing activities also may help patients relax, which will decrease their metabolic needs.

IV

◢ NURSING CARE GUIDELINES
Nursing Diagnosis: Altered Tissue Perfusion: Gastrointestinal

---

Expected Outcome: The patient will have adequate tissue perfusion and cellular oxygenation of the gastrointestinal system as evidenced by normal bowel sounds in all four quadrants and the absence of nausea and vomiting.

- Assess blood pressure. *Hypotension can lead to a reduction in blood flow to the GI tract.*
- Monitor bowel sounds and document any changes. Assess for nausea and vomiting. *A reduction in bowel sounds or the presence of nausea and vomiting may indicate Altered Tissue Perfusion: Gastrointestinal.*
- Monitor for changes in bowel patterns. *A decrease in GI tissue perfusion can manifest itself in changes in bowel habits such as constipation.*
- Maintain gastric decompression and check all excretions for occult blood. *Patients with Altered Tissue Perfusion: Gastrointestinal and patients after surgery usually have an NG tube in for decompression until bowel function is restored. A positive test for occult blood is reportable to the physician and may indicate bleeding in the GI tract that can further alter tissue perfusion.*
- Maintain intake and output. *Patients with Altered Tissue Perfusion: Gastrointestinal may develop large amounts of nasogastric drainage and be unable to consume liquids without vomiting. IV hydration may need to be started to replace losses and inadequate intake.*

Expected Outcome: The patient will have control of the metabolic needs of gastrointestinal tissue.

- Encourage rest periods after meals. *Rest periods allow the blood flow to leave skeletal muscle and be redirected to the stomach and intestines.*
- Provide small meals or, if tube feedings are used, provide an elemental product. *Small meals and elemental tube feedings are digested more easily and place a lower metabolic demand on the GI system.*
- ▲ Assess medications and try to minimize those that decrease peristalsis and GI function. *Medications that can irritate the GI mucus should be given with meals or milk, if they are not contraindicated. Other medication choices should be considered.*

■ = nursing intervention; ▲ = collaborative intervention.

IV

Altered Tissue Perfusion: Peripheral

Planning the care of a patient with Altered Tissue Perfusion: Peripheral includes frequent patient assessment of the extremities. Along with vital signs, the quality of arterial pulses helps indicate the adequacy of flow. Different systolic blood pressures in each arm are also a sign of arterial disease. If capillary refill is checked, a finding of less than 3 seconds is normal.

Arm-ankle index should be assessed on admission in any situation where a patient is at risk for arterial insufficiency. A Doppler flow systolic pressure is taken in the dorsalis pedis and the posterior tibial.[1] This number is divided by the higher of the two brachial systolic pressures, with the normal range being 1.0 to 1.2. Any value less than this indicates a vascular problem.

If the patient has Altered Tissue Perfusion: Peripheral, activities should not interfere with blood flow to the area.[2,3] Extremities that have reduced arterial flow should be positioned in a dependent position to facilitate blood flow.[1,2,4] If the problem lies in the venous system, the extremity should be elevated to enhance venous return. The extremity should be assessed carefully to be certain that the delivery of oxygen and nutrients is adequate to maintain the integrity of the skin and the function of the extremity.

Many over-the-counter medications such as antihistamines have vasoconstrictive properties and should be avoided by patients with vascular insufficiency.

Teaching patients about diet is an important nursing function and focuses on modifying the diet based on the organs affected. For example, patients with peripheral arterial occlusive disease may need to reduce their intake of cholesterol.

The benefits of exercise can be reinforced by teaching the patient the importance of balancing activities with rest periods. Exercise helps promote the development of collateral circulation and the enlargement of the involved vessels. Exercise includes active and passive range-of-motion exercises and early ambulation for the hospitalized patient. All exercise should be increased gradually over time, provided the patient does not have signs and symptoms of fatigue or ischemia.[2]

The patient can be taught several preventive measures that can help reduce the side effects associated with Altered Tissue Perfusion.[2,3] First, the patient should be taught to inspect the skin daily for breaks and pressure points. Frequent foot care includes washing and thoroughly drying the feet as well as massaging them and keeping them well lubricated. Clean, warm footwear that fits comfortably should be worn.

Second, the patient should be discouraged from sitting and standing for long periods of time and from crossing the legs.[2,3] The patient should be taught to avoid constrictive clothes but to wear warm clothes to prevent further damage from exposure to cold weather. Appliances such as sheepskins and water mattresses can decrease pressure on certain areas and prevent damage.

◢ **NURSING CARE GUIDELINES**
Nursing Diagnosis: Altered Tissue Perfusion: Peripheral

Expected Outcome: The patient will have adequate tissue perfusion and cellular oxygenation of the peripheral system as evidenced by palpable pulses; warm dry skin; an ankle-arm index of 1.0 to 1.2; and normal motor function and sensation and skin integrity in the extremities.

- Monitor and document vital signs. *Patients with a reduction in blood pressure are at risk for Altered Tissue Perfusion: Peripheral.*
- Assess the quality of arterial pulses, skin temperature, presence of edema, color, and texture of extremities. Document skin integrity and the presence of ulcers. *Inadequate arterial flow may cause changes in color, hair growth, and skin temperature. Ulcers may form as a result of decreased tissue perfusion.*

■ = nursing intervention; ▲ = collaborative intervention.

- Assess ankle-arm index and notify the physician of any change. *Index values less than 1.0 indicate vascular problems.*
- Assess capillary refill. *Capillary refill that takes more than 3 seconds to occur can indicate impaired tissue perfusion.*
- Encourage active and passive range of motion. *Exercise enlarges vessels and encourages the development of collateral circulation.*

Expected Outcome: The patient will have control of the metabolic needs of organs and tissues by reduction or by maintenance at current level.

- If there is an arterial flow problem, maintain extremities in a dependent position to facilitate flow. For venous flow problems, elevate the extremities. *Elevation promotes venous return, whereas dependent positions facilitate arterial flow.*
- Avoid long periods of pressure on extremities. *Prolonged pressure can cause redness, interrupt tissue perfusion, and cause skin breakdown and ulcer formation.*
- Balance rest and activities. Promote early ambulation. *Rest periods prevent ischemia of tissues affected by decreased flow. Early ambulation reduces the risk of deep vein thrombosis.*
- ▲ Assess medications for vasoconstrictive side effects and collaborate with physician on selecting new medications. *Medications with vasoconstrictive properties can further decrease blood flow.*

Expected Outcome: The patient will modify lifestyle to minimize the causative factors or side effects related to the decrease in peripheral tissue perfusion.

- Teach the patient and family about the importance of diet. *Cholesterol reduction may reduce plaque buildup in blood vessels, which can cause reduction in perfusion.*
- Instruct patient to avoid standing for long periods of time, to avoid crossing the legs, to avoid hot water bottles, and to avoid heating pads and tight clothing. *All of these actions can reduce perfusion to the extremities. Because the patient may have reduced sensation, heat on an extremity can burn the patient accidentally.*
- Instruct patient on the use of foot cradles, water mattresses, and other appliances that decrease pressure on extremities. *These devices reduce pressure and avoid damage to tissues.*
- Teach skin care and the rationale for it. *Inspecting the lower extremities for skin breakdown and keeping skin lubricated prevents complications.*

EVALUATION

The first indicator of the effectiveness of nursing interventions, and therefore the attainment of expected patient outcomes, is maintenance of adequate tissue perfusion and cellular oxygenation of the tissues and organs involved. This can be determined by the absence of the defining characteristics that first alerted the nurse that an abnormality was present. Cardiac output and blood pressure, coupled with effective ventilation, will be adequate to maintain tissue perfusion and cellular oxygenation. Body systems will receive adequate circulation to prevent ischemia of the tissues or organs. Extremities will be warm, with palpable pulses. The gastrointestinal and renal systems will function properly so that food is digested, energy is available to the cells, and waste products are excreted. Patients will not experience chest pain, dyspnea, or an alteration in mental status.

A second important indicator of the effectiveness of nursing interentions is that the metabolic needs of the tissues and organs are being met. Body temperature and oxygenation will be maintained within normal limits. The patient will alternate activity with frequent rest periods to minimize the metabolic rate of the tissues. The patient will protect the extremities from long periods of pressure to any involved area and from exposure to cold environments. The patient will become involved in stress-reducing activities and will avoid increased tissue metabolism brought on by the emotions of fear, worry, and anxiety.

A third indicator that patients have achieved expected outcomes is modification of their lifestyles, including a change in dietary habits, and verbalization of the cause of their problem. The patient and family explain the uses and side effects of medications and how to minimize potential complications and balance rest with activity. They perform specialized skin care correctly.

▶ CASE STUDY WITH PLAN OF CARE

Mr. James T. is a 70-year-old retired electrician who was admitted to the emergency room with complaints of fever, a superficial left leg ulcer of 2 weeks duration, pain when walking, and some decreased sensation in his legs. The patient stated, "I haven't been sick a day in my life, but about 10 or 15 years ago my doctor told me that I had high blood pressure and diabetes. Because I never had problems, I never went back."

Social history revealed that his wife died about 7 years ago, and he has since lived alone and cooked for himself. His three children are married and live some distance away, so he sees them mainly on the holidays. Since he retired about 5 years ago, he spends many afternoons playing cards with his friends and his evenings watching television in the recliner chair his children bought as a retirement present.

Mr. T. attributes his leg ulcer to a cut he sustained when he bumped into the card table. On questioning, it was determined that he frequently has calf pain that goes away with rest. This he felt was due to the increased use of his leg muscles because he recently started to walk a mile before playing cards with his friends.

Physical examination revealed a well-groomed man who was slightly overweight. His lungs were clear, and heart sounds were normal. His abdominal exam was benign. His neurological examination was normal except for a decrease in sensation in his lower extremities. Pulses were equal bilaterally but barely palpable in the feet. The ankle-arm index was 0.9. His vital signs were temperature, 101°F; blood pressure, 154/86 mm Hg; pulse, 110 beats/min and regular; and respiratory rate, 20/min. Electrolyte, BUN, creatine, hematocrit, and hemoglobin values were all within normal limits. His white blood cell count was 15,000/mm³, and his blood glucose level was 264 mg/dl. The lower extremities were without hair and cool to the touch. The skin color was somewhat dusky, and vascular filling poor. The ulcer was about the size of a quarter and superficial. It was located on the lower portion of the shin, and the area around it was slightly swollen and erythematous. The medical diagnosis is peripheral vascular disease, diabetes mellitus, and ulcer of the left leg.

▶ PLAN OF CARE FOR MR. T.
Nursing Diagnosis: Altered Tissue Perfusion: Peripheral Related to Peripheral Arterial Disease and Diabetes Mellitus

Expected Outcome: Mr. T.'s lower extremity tissue perfusion will be maximized as evidenced by palpable pulses, warm, dry skin, and an ankle-arm index ≥ 0.9 and by normal motor function, sensation, and evidence of wound healing.
- Assess quality of arterial pulses and the color and temperature of extremities.
- Place Mr. T.'s lower extremities in a dependent position.
- Monitor vital signs, and notify the physician if systolic blood pressure falls below normal.
- Monitor ankle-arm index at least once a shift, and notify the physician of any change.
- Encourage active and passive range-of-motion exercises.
- Instruct Mr. T. to maintain a warm environment and to avoid excessive exposure to cold and pressure.

■ = nursing intervention; ▲ = collaborative intervention.

Expected Outcome: Mr. T.'s metabolic needs will be minimized as evidenced by a normal temperature, denial of leg pain, and a normal blood glucose level.
- ▲ Monitor temperature; administer acetaminophen, as ordered, to decrease fever.
- ▲ Administer antibiotics, as ordered, to fight infection.
- ▪ Provide local skin care to aid healing.
- ▲ Follow medical regimen to maintain Mr. T.'s blood glucose level within normal limits.
- ▪ Encourage frequent rest periods.
- ▪ Mr. T. will verbalize understanding of the cause of the leg pain and take action to minimize it.
- ▪ Explain to Mr. T. that the pain occurs because the narrowed arteries cause inadequate blood flow to the vessels during exercise.
- ▪ Help Mr. T. to develop an exercise plan that increases activity slowly, based on his tolerance.
- ▪ Explain the importance of frequent rest periods alternating with activity to prevent ischemia to the tissues.
- ▪ Encourage Mr. T. to stop activity and rest at the first sign of leg pain.
- ▪ Teach Mr. T. to avoid activity in cold environments.

Expected Outcome: Mr. T. will perform good wound care, and the ulcer will show signs of healing.
- ▪ Assess and document changes in the appearance of the wound.
- ▲ Provide local cleansing and topical treatments to the wound, as ordered.
- ▪ Explain to Mr. T. the importance of keeping the skin clean and dry.
- ▪ Teach the importance of adequate hydration and of keeping the skin well lubricated on a continual basis.
- ▪ Ask Mr. T. to demonstrate wound care.

Expected Outcome: Mr. T. will verbalize the importance of any dietary modifications that must be made.
- ▪ Explain the relationship between a high-fat diet and vascular disease.
- ▪ Teach Mr. T. the importance of following a diabetic diet.
- ▪ Work with Mr. T. to develop a diet plan low in fat.

Expected Outcome: Mr. T. will verbalize the safety precautions that can be taken to minimize the potential injury to affected tissues.
- ▪ Teach Mr. T. the rationale to keep his legs below heart level when sitting in the recliner.
- ▪ Instruct Mr. T. to avoid standing or sitting for long periods of time and to avoid crossing his legs.
- ▪ Introduce Mr. T. to the following safety devices, which can help decrease pressure to the affected areas: foot cradle, water mattresses, sheepskins, and padding.
- ▪ Help Mr. T. avoid hot water bottles and heating pads.
- ▪ Reinforce the need to avoid long periods of exposure to cold environments and the importance of wearing warm clothes.

■■ CRITICAL THINKING EXERCISES

1. Upon physical examination of Mr. T., you notice absent dorsalis pedis and posterial tibial pulses on the right foot. What could be causing this loss of pulses? What are your nursing interventions?
2. You are caring for Mr. T. on the third day of his hospitalization and notice a respiratory rate of 40/min, poor skin turgor, and a 2-pound weight loss. His leg ulcer does not appear to be healing. What possible etiologies could be causing this condition, and what nursing interventions would you undertake?
3. Mr. T. develops slurred speech, left facial droop, and lethargy. What possible etiologies could be causing this change? What nursing and collaborative interventions would you anticipate?
4. When caring for Mr. T. for the first time, you

note a green exudate draining from the ulcer. What additional assessments would be critical to make, and how would you change your nursing care plan?

5. Mr. T. is found with a blood pressure of 80/56, normal temperature, and an irregular heart rate of 150/min. What are your nursing priorities? What impact will this current situation have on his leg healing?

REFERENCES

1. Baker JD: Assessment of peripheral arterial occlusive disease, *Crit Care Nurs Clin North Am* 3(3):493–498, 1991.
2. Carpenito LJ: *Nursing diagnosis: application to clinical practice,* ed 4, Philadelphia, 1992, JB Lippincott Co.
3. Doenges ME and Moorhouse MF: *Nurse's pocket guide: nursing diagnosis with interventions,* ed 3, Philadelphia, 1991, FA Davis.
4. Drummond BL: Preventing increased intracranial pressure, *Focus Crit Care* 17(2):116–122, 1990.
5. Harper J: Rhabdomyolysis and myoglobinuric renal failure, *Crit Care Nurse* 10(3):32–36, 1990.
6. Lebet RM: Abdominal and genitourinary trauma in children, *Crit Care Nurs Clin North Am* 3(3):433–443, 1991.
7. Memmer MK: Acute orthostatic hypotension, *Heart Lung* 17(2):134–141, 1988.
8. Misasi RS and Keyes JL: The pathophysiology of hypoxia, *Crit Care Nurse* 14(4):55–64, 1994.
9. Murphy TG and Bennett EJ: Low tech, high-touch perfusion assessment, *AJN* 92(5):36–40, 42, 44, 1992.
10. Nelson DP: Congestive heart failure. In *Cardiopulmonary nursing,* Springhouse, Pennsylvania, 1991, Springhouse.
11. Pearlstein G: Renal system complications in HIV infection, *Crit Care Nurs Clin North Am* 2(1):79–88, 1990.
12. Reilly E and Yucha C: Multiple organ failure syndrome, *Crit Care Nurse* 14(2):25–26, 28–31, 1994.
13. Reynolds EA: Controversies in caring for the child with a head injury, *MCN* 17(5):246–251, 1992.
14. Rice V: Shock, a clinical syndrome: an update. Part 4, nursing care of the shock patient, *Crit Care Nurse* 11(7):28–40, 1991.
15. Roberto PL: Diabetic nephropathy: causes, complications and considerations, *Crit Care Nurs Clin North Am* 2(1):55–66, 1990.
16. Smith MF: Renal trauma: adult and pediatric considerations, *Crit Care Nurs Clin North Am* 2(1):67–78, 1990.

IV

Inability to Sustain Spontaneous Ventilation

▶

Dysfunctional Ventilatory Weaning Response

▶

Inability to Sustain Spontaneous Ventilation *(ISSV) is a response pattern of decreased energy reserves in which a patient is unable to maintain adequate breathing to support life.*[26]

Dysfunctional Ventilatory Weaning Response *(DVWR) is the state in which a patient's inability to adjust to lowered levels of mechanical ventilatory support interrupts and prolongs the weaning process.*[15,26]

OVERVIEW

Spontaneous ventilation (breathing), the ability of an individual to perform the necessary ventilatory work to maintain adequate gas exchange, occurs as a result of interactions among the pulmonary, cardiovascular, renal, musculoskeletal, and neurological systems.[2] Deterioration of these systems results in the need for mechanical ventilation. Successful weaning and extubation from mechanical ventilation may occur promptly or it may become a prolonged and complicated process for the patient and the health care team.[4,9,22] Although much progress has been made with mechanical ventilation, disagreements, controversies, and challenges continue to exist regarding the best ways to wean patients from mechanical ventilation.* Early recognition of the need for mechanical breathing support and a systematic team approach are keys

---

*References 4, 7, 9, 15, 18, 29.

to successful, early weaning of complex ventilator patients.[8,10,11]

The process of weaning consists of three phases: preweaning, weaning, and extubation.[18,20] *Weaning readiness* is a state in which the patient has the necessary physical and emotional resources to engage in the work of weaning.[4,22,20] For example, the patient must have adequate respiratory muscle function to maintain a sufficient tidal volume, to be able to cough effectively, and to breath deeply.[16] The patient's lungs must be able to ventilate sufficiently to maintain baseline arterial blood gases.[10] Caloric intake must be sufficient and specific to the individual's requirements to ensure appropriate nutritional support to meet the patient's energy needs.[27,30,31] Psychological readiness is influenced by emotionally charged events that can cause feelings such as anxiety, fear, frustration, and hopelessness. Reactions to emotionally charged events can precipitate physiological responses that increase shortness of breath, exacerbate the emotional response, and create a cycle of increased inability to breathe.[8,10]

Inability to Sustain Spontaneous Ventilation (ISSV) occurs when patients with hypermetabolic energy needs or depletion of energy reserves are unable to sustain the work load of spontaneous breathing.[3,8,9] The diagnosis of ISSV is based on deterioration of arterial blood gases, increased work of breathing, and decreasing energy. Patients with ISSV may present with outward manifestations of increased restlessness, increased use of

441

accessory muscles, and a compromised ability to cooperate.[26] Interpretations of findings from monitoring equipment may reveal other indications of ISSV, such as cardiac arrhythmias and decreased SaO_2.[9,29] Mechanically ventilated patients recovering from surgery, cachectic patients with chronic obstructive pulmonary disease (COPD), and patients with head injuries may present with hypermetabolic energy requirements that impair their ability to sustain spontaneous ventilation.

Dysfunctional Ventilatory Weaning Response (DVWR) refers to a patient state or response to a health problem, ventilator dependency.[15] DVWR is a temporary state in which a patient is not ready to mobilize the required physical and emotional resources for adjusting to lowered levels of mechanical ventilatory support. This inability to adjust to lowered levels of mechanical ventilatory support interrupts and prolongs the weaning process.[4,21,22] DVWR encompasses any specific behaviors associated with failure to wean, such as dyspnea, anxiety, or increased muscle tension that increases metabolic energy expenditure and exacerbates respiratory muscle fatigue, and an overall perception by the patient of a loss of control.[15]

Jenny and Logan,[15] who conducted research on DVWR, found in their literature review that up to 20% of patients who are mechanically ventilated are unable to tolerate discontinuation. Patients with severe, complicated acute or chronic lung disease, patients with multisystem extra pulmonary disease or neuromuscular disease who are on mechanical ventilation, and patients who have been on the ventilator more than 30 days, often experience difficulties that interfere with and may prolong successful weaning.[1,4,10,29]

ASSESSMENT

The initial physiological assessment of patients with ISSV or DVWR is the same. Assessment of pulmonary, cardiac, musculoskeletal, and neurological systems is essential for diagnosing patients with ISSV during the preweaning phase of mechanical ventilation and patients with DVWR during the weaning and extubation phases.

Because the patient with ISSV is usually unable to provide historical data, it is important for the nurse to obtain information from the patient's family, other members of the health care team who know the patient, and medical records, The nurse also conducts a thorough baseline physical assessment to identify organs at risk due to increased intrathoracic pressure from mechanical ventilation and/or pulmonary insufficiency. For example, assess measures of oxygen-carrying capacity, including arterial blood gases: pH 7.35–7.45, PaO_2 greater than 50 mm Hg, PcO_2 less than 60 mm Hg, or variation less than 33% from baseline; hemoglobin: 12–15 gm/100 ml; cardiac status: heart rate, arrhythmias, blood pressure, SaO_2, CVP, pulmonary artery pressures, SvO_2 when available. Assess renal function; for example, electrolytes: potassium, 3.5–3.9 mEq/L, magnesium, 1.8–3 mg/dl, phosphates, 2.4–4.8 mg/dl, pH, 7.35–7.45; hydration: hematocrit, 40–50/100 ml, plasma proteins (normals per institution), urinary output, 30 ml/hour or greater, and bowel function. The presence of diarrhea and constipation can be indicative of ileus. Evaluate for the presence of processes that increase metabolic needs, such as systemic or local infection: elevated white blood cell count and configuration; or malnutrition: decreased visceral proteins and decreased albumin.[1,3,4,18]

Nursing assessment of the patient's pulmonary status includes observation of physical parameters and the patient's response to mechanical ventilation. Physical parameters to evaluate the patient's work of breathing include tachypnea, dyspnea, abdominal paradox or asynchrony, spontaneous tidal volume, skin color and turgor, diaphoresis, chest wall expansion, deviation of trachea, auscultation of adventitious breath sounds, arterial blood gases, appearance of the chest X ray.[2-4,18,29]

Parameters for assessing the patient's response to mechanical ventilation include patient comfort, bilateral breath sounds, tidal volume, minute ventilation, ability to breathe "with" the ventilator, and position of the endotracheal tube.[29,33] A complication of mechanical ventilation is an increase in intrathoracic pressure with subsequent decreased venous return and possible liver congestion. Liver function (e.g., LDH, SGOT, and SGGT) is assessed to identify the presence of this complication. Observe for indicators of airway obstruction that can increase the work of breathing, such as pulmonary secretions.[23,33] Review the patient's pulmonary medical history to identify diseases, such as COPD, reactive airway disease, and atelectasis, that interfere with oxygen intake. The neurological exam and a review of the patient's medication history provide the nurse with data for assessment of ventilatory drive.

Assessment of the severity of DVWR (mild, moderate, or severe) determines the patient's ability to progress to the next step in the plan for weaning. Severe Dysfunctional Ventilatory Weaning Response is indicative of physiological factors that will cause Inability to Sustain Spontaneous Ventilation. Unlike the patient with ISSV, the patient with DVWR is able to interact with the nurse and is expected to be an active participant in the weaning and extubation phases of mechanical ventilation. Additional assessment parameters focus on the patient's ability to interact with the health care team. The nurse must determine the most effective mechanism for communicating with the patient (e.g., writing, sign language, or communication board).[5,7] In some instances, the nurse must collaborate with the multidisciplinary team to assess if a tracheostomy is necessary to facilitate communication.[6,8,14] Assess for negative environmental factors that trigger emotional responses and can cause shortness of breath (e.g., the patient's perception of the absence of health care members from the bedside or excessive distractional noise).[7,19] Evaluate the patient's circadian rhythm and identify factors that contribute to sleep deprivation (e.g., unnecessary monitoring during normal sleep hours).[4,8]

Determine the patient's baseline mental status. Assess the patient's cognitive ability (e.g., attention, concentration, and short-term memory) to understand and to remember information about the weaning process and the plan. It is important to use the same assessment criteria for ongoing monitoring of mental status and reporting of findings. The presence of Altered Thought Processes

(acute confusion), such as fluctuations in attention, concentration, and ability to follow commands, is often indicative of underlying physiological abnormalities that can interfere with the weaning process.[13,25] Assessment of the patient's psychological readiness for weaning includes the patient's goals, concerns, and beliefs about the weaning process; the impact of previous attempts to wean; and the patient's perception of a support system. Evaluate for behaviors that are indicative of psychological dependence on the ventilator, such as anticipatory anxiety, expressions of fear of dying, and "tuning out" or blocking discussion of weaning. Find out the patient's past coping techniques for stress reduction that can be incorporated into the weaning process.[8,19]

Inability to Sustain Spontaneous Ventilation

■ Defining Characteristics

The presence of the following defining characteristics indicates that the patient may be experiencing Inability to Sustain Spontaneous Ventilation[1-3,8,18,26]:

- Dyspnea
- Tachypnea
- Increased restlessness
- Increased use of accessory muscles
- Decreased spontaneous tidal volume
- Increased heart rate
- Cardiac arrhythmias
- Apprehension
- Compromised ability to cooperate
- Decreased SaO_2
- Decreased PO_2
- Increased PCO_2
- Increased metabolic rate

■ Related Factors

The following related factors are associated with Inability to Sustain Spontaneous Ventilation*:

- Anemia
- Infection

---

*References 1, 3, 9, 16, 23, 26.

- Increased metabolic requirements to resist nosocomial infections
- Hyperthermia
- Electrolyte imbalance
- Left ventricular dysfunction
- Increased intrathoracic pressure
- Pulmonary edema
- Atelectasis
- Carbohydrate overfeeding
- Abdominal distension (e.g., bowel or obesity)
- Uncontrolled pain
- Activity greater than available energy
- Respiratory muscle fatigue

Dysfunctional Ventilatory Weaning Response

■ Defining Characteristics

The presence of the following defining characteristics indicates that the patient may be experiencing Dysfunctional Ventilatory Weaning Response[*]:

Mild DVWR

- Restlessness
- Slightly increased respiratory rate from baseline
- Responses to lowered level of mechanical ventilatory support may include conveying increased need for oxygen, experiencing breathing discomfort, complaining of fatigue, feeling warm, questioning about possible machine malfunction, exhibiting undue concentration on breathing

Moderate DVWR

- Responses to lowered level of mechanical ventilatory support may include a slight increase from baseline blood pressure, an increase from baseline heart rate, and a baseline increase in respiratory rate
- Hypervigilance to activities
- Inability to respond to coaching
- Inability to cooperate
- Apprehension
- Diaphoresis
- Eye widening, or the "wide-eyed look"
- Decreased air entry on auscultation

- Color changes (e.g., pale, with slight cyanosis)
- Slight respiratory accessory muscle use

Severe DVWR

- Responses to lowered levels of mechanical ventilatory support include agitation, deterioration in arterial blood gases from current baseline, an increase from baseline blood pressure, an increase from baseline heart rate, and a significant increase in respiratory rate from baseline
- Profuse diaphoresis
- Full respiratory accessory muscle use
- Shallow, gasping breaths
- Paradoxical abdominal breathing
- Discoordinated breathing with the ventilator
- Decreased level of consciousness
- Adventitious breath sounds, audible airway secretion
- Cyanosis

■ Related Factors

The following related factors are associated with Dysfunctional Ventilatory Weaning Response[†]:

- Ineffective airway clearance
- Respiratory muscle fatigue
- Multisystem disease
- Neuromuscular chronic disability
- Cardiac failure
- Acute or chronic lung disease
- Electrolyte disorders (e.g., hypophosphatemia)
- Anemia
- Sleep pattern disturbance
- Malnutrition, less than or more than body requirements
- History of multiple unsuccessful weaning attempts
- Inability to communicate effectively
- Adverse environment (e.g., noisy or overly active)
- Negative events in patient's room
- Moderate to severe anxiety
- State anxiety
- Low nurse-patient ratio
- Extended absence of nurse from bedside
- Pharmacological therapy

[*]References 1, 3–8, 10, 11, 15, 18, 21.

[†]References 1, 8, 10, 14, 18, 22–26, 28.

- Obesity
- Infection
- Uncontrolled pain or discomfort
- Uncontrolled episodic energy demands or problems
- Inappropriate pacing of diminished ventilatory support
- History of ventilatory dependence greater than 1 week
- Unfamiliar nursing staff
- Lack of trust in nurse
- Decreased motivation
- Terminal illness
- Inadequate information about role in weaning process
- Perception of futility regarding own ability to be weaned
- Fear
- Clinical depression or prolonged depressed state
- Hopelessness
- Powerlessness
- Decreased self-esteem

DIAGNOSIS

■ Differential Nursing Diagnosis

Nursing diagnoses related to Inability to Sustain Spontaneous Ventilation include but are not limited to Impaired Gas Exchange, Ineffective Airway Clearance, and Ineffective Breathing Pattern.[26] The patient can meet the criteria for all or some of these diagnoses, although when mechanical assistance is required, the appropriate nursing diagnosis is ISSV. For example, if a patient has Impaired Gas Exchange requiring mechanical assistance, the appropriate nursing diagnosis is ISSV. Specific nursing actions focus on initiating and maintaining ventilation with a plan for the earliest removal of ventilatory assistance.

Nursing diagnoses related to Dysfunctional Ventilatory Weaning Response include but are not limited to Ineffective Airway Clearance, Altered Nutrition: More/Less Than Body Requirement, Anxiety, Pain, and Acute Confusion.[26] The patient can meet criteria for all or some of these diagnoses; however, when weaning from mechanical ventilation becomes prolonged or ineffective, the appro-

priate nursing diagnosis is DVWR. Nursing management begins with an accurate nursing assessment and multidisciplinary collaboration to develop and implement a consistent treatment plan to correct all metabolic, physical, psychological, and social factors that interfere with ventilator weaning.

■ Medical and Psychiatric Diagnoses

The diagnosis ISSV indicates a need for mechanical assistance to support breathing. All medical conditions that require assisted ventilation as a therapeutic intervention are related to the nursing diagnosis ISSV. Cardiopulmonary disease or arrest, exacerbated COPD, and trauma are examples of medical diagnoses that usually require the use of mechanical assistance for breathing. ISSV is not typically associated with psychiatric disorders.

The patient with DVWR often has complex medical and psychiatric conditions. Psychiatric diagnoses, such as Anxiety Disorder, Sleep Disorder, and Delirium, can coexist with a general medical condition that requires mechanical assistance for breathing. Multisystem organ failure is an example of a medical diagnosis that coexists with DVWR.

OUTCOME IDENTIFICATION, PLANNING, AND IMPLEMENTATION

Inability to Sustain Spontaneous Ventilation

The desired outcome for patients with ISSV is for them to have the necessary metabolic energy requirements to sustain spontaneous ventilation. The primary nurse or registered nurse case manager plays a pivotal role in the timely assessment of the need for mechanical ventilation, the coordination of a multidisciplinary plan of care, and evaluation of outcomes that are indicative of the patient's ability to sustain spontaneous ventilation.[28,32] Nursing interventions focus on correcting physiological conditions that deplete energy reserves, preventing ventilator-induced complications, and regulating the work of breathing.[1,8,29] Observation for the presence of diaphragm or res-

IV

piratory muscle fatigue is an essential intervention for patients with ISSV because diaphragmatic rest in the presence of diaphragm or respiratory muscle fatigue requires 12 to 24 hours for recovery.[3] Many bedside measures have been described in the literature, but none have been reliable predictors to monitor the presence of diaphragm or respiratory muscle fatigue.[3,4,9] Observation of patient respiratory trends and "knowing" the patient facilitates early recognition of diaphragm or respiratory muscle fatigue.[3,9,28] Despite the fact that patients with ISSV are usually too sick to engage in lengthy interactions with the nurse and other members of the health care team, it is important for caregivers to introduce themselves, explain their role in the patient's care, and to provide the patient with brief ongoing explanations about treatment and procedures.[7] Collaboration with the dietitian and the physician to ensure prompt and adequate nutrition after intubation through gastric or IV supplementation supplies the necessary resources to meet the patient's energy needs during this physically and psychologically stressful time.[7,27,30,31] A supplement that derives its calories from fat and protein is recommended because carbohydrate overfeeding causes excess CO_2 production.[27,30] Gastric feeding is safe and can reduce the potential for infection associated with IV supplementation and decreased intestinal motility.[31]

◢ NURSING CARE GUIDELINES
Nursing Diagnosis: Inability to Sustain Spontaneous Ventilation*

Expected Outcome: The patient will have adequate ventilation as evidenced by oxygenation of tissues and synchronous use of respiratory muscles within 1 hour.

▲ Monitor for complications related to mechanical ventilation such as increased cardiothoracic pressure, decreased venous return, and pulmonary infection *to initiate early intervention regarding complications.*

▲ Observe for presence of diaphragm or respiratory muscle fatigue, increased respiratory rate, minute ventilation, and hypercarbia with respiratory acidosis *to prevent tissue or organ hypoxia.*

▲ Check for correct initial placement of endotracheal tube, and monitor placement according to unit protocols *to ensure optimum oxygen delivery.*

▲ Determine ventilation parameters (e.g., Fio_2, mode of ventilatory assistance, and tidal volume frequency) *to ensure optimum oxygenation.*

▲ Develop a suction protocol that incorporates parameters for hyperoxygenation, hyperinflation, and length of stabilization period between suction catheter passes *to prevent oxygen desaturation.*

■ Observe for trends in the patient's cardiac, renal, and neurological status *to prevent complications related to mechanical ventilation.*

■ Initiate passive or active exercises (e.g., turning, postural drainage, range-of-motion exercises, induced coughing, and deep breathing) *to prevent complications from immobility.*

■ Use sterile technique when removing secretions *to minimize potential for infection.*

■ Position patient comfortably in a manner that allows for full lung expansion *to optimize pulmonary ventilation.*

▲ Use negative inspiratory pressure, positive expiratory pressure, and tidal volume as parameters to regulate activity *to prevent fatigue.*

▲ Establish a schedule for muscle reconditioning, such as mechanically assisted muscle training or graded manual diaphragmatic muscle exercises *to optimize pulmonary ventilation.*

Expected Outcome: The patient will meet metabolic energy requirements as evidenced by maintaining nutritional intake equal to calculated requirements for nutrition within 24 to 48 hours.

▲ Maintain adequate nutrition (e.g., 25–35 kcal/kg with appropriate carbohydrate, fat, and protein) *to ensure sufficient energy supply for tissue oxygenation.*

■ = nursing intervention; ▲ = collaborative intervention.
*References 1–3, 7, 8–10, 16, 22–25, 30, 33.

- Monitor daily weight, intake, and output *to assess fluid and nutrition status*.
- Monitor bowel function (e.g., constipation and diarrhea) *to assess gastrointestinal continuity*.
- ▲ Monitor levels of serum phosphate, potassium, calcium, and magnesium, and collaborate with the physician, the dietitian, or the pharmacist to provide replacement therapy as necessary *to assess optimum nutrients*.
- Regulate environmental activity *to conserve energy and to relieve stress*.
- ▲ Establish a regular schedule for muscle reconditioning that incorporates adequate rest periods *to optimize muscle strength*.
- Schedule rest periods that are congruent with patient's circadian rhythm *to optimize available energy for healing*.
- Revise activity schedule on a daily basis, according to patient's tolerance, *to optimize muscle strength*.

Dysfunctional Ventilatory Weaning Response

Desired outcomes for the patient with DVWR are for the patient to tolerate lower levels of mechanical ventilation, to convey a comfortable and relaxed appearance, and to adhere to the weaning plan. Nursing interventions that optimize the likelihood of the patient's ability to tolerate lower levels of mechanical ventilation include preparing the patient physically and psychologically. The designation of a primary nurse or a registered nurse case manager to collaborate on a consistent basis with the patient, the family and the multidisciplinary team is important.[6,11,20,32] The nurse acts as a communication link between the patient, the family, and the multidisciplinary team in establishing consistent messages to the patient and the family about the plan of care.[4,17] An additional component of the nurse's role in the weaning process is "knowing" the patient's response patterns to lowered levels of mechanical ventilation.[22,28] Because of the enormous communication constraints and social isolation associated with ventilator dependence, it is necessary to establish an effective communication system with the patient.[5,7,12] It is also important for all members of the treatment team to recognize behaviors indicative of Acute Confusion (delirium), which may be manifested by abrupt changes in mental status, such as fluctuations in concentration, attention, and orientation and the inability to follow commands. Assessment for Acute Confusion can be incorporated into routine interactions with the patient as well as at specific, designated times.[13,25] Additional nursing interventions include creating a therapeutic environment, using friends and family as supportive resources, and clarifying family misconceptions about weaning. The development and implementation of a weaning contract (critical pathway) can be an effective intervention in meeting the identified outcomes for the patient with DVWR. The plan should incorporate culturally appropriate positive reinforcers, verbal encouragement, visual progress reports, and therapeutic touch. Consistency among health providers when communicating about the weaning plan is an essential component of the patient's successful weaning.[4-7,13,22,25,32]

◢ **NURSING CARE GUIDELINES**
Nursing Diagnosis: Dysfunctional Ventilatory Weaning Response*

Expected Outcome: The patient will tolerate lowered levels of mechanical ventilation as evidenced by maintaining baseline clinical status at the earliest time.
- Provide the patient with a primary nurse or registered nurse case manager *to facilitate consistent communication and integration of treatment.*
- ▲ Ensure that all caregivers provide consistent explanations about weaning *to promote patient trust in the health care team.*
- Establish an effective means of communicating with the patient *to reduce patient frustration and minimize the negative aspects of mechanical ventilation and maximize the patient's sense of control.*
- Monitor for presence of Acute Confusion (e.g., fluctuations in concentration, attention, or orientation) before initiating the weaning process and throughout the weaning process and collaborate with patient's medical team to search for and treat the underlying cause (e.g., fever, infection, drug therapy, or fluid overload).
- Repeat information until patient conveys an understanding of explanations *to prevent miscommunication.*
- Allow patient sufficient time to respond to information and explanations *to prevent miscommunication and to reduce anxiety.*
- ▲ Reduce ventilatory support in small increments, using one parameter *to maximize weaning success and to minimize the likelihood of weaning failure.*
- Use coaching during weaning process, based on prior agreement with patient (e.g., reminding patient about correct breathing during episodes of shortness of breath) *to support patient's efforts.*
- Collaborate with resource such as psychiatric consultation or liaison clinical nurse specialist for individualized stress management techniques (e.g., relaxation, imagery, and music) during weaning *to ensure optimum weaning plan.*

Expected Outcome: The patient will convey a comfortable and relaxed appearance as evidenced by absence of irritability, restlessness, agitation, or fatigue during the weaning process.
- ▲ Control and minimize noise and activity level in a patient's bedside area; provide privacy; and allow for scheduled rest times *to optimize comfort.*
- Use family or friends as a supportive resource for patient *to reduce anxiety.*
- Prepare family for a supportive role in weaning process by:
  - Providing information about the unit environment (e.g., alarms, monitoring equipment, and nurse call system)
  - Providing information about the weaning plan
  - Introducing all caregivers and explaining their roles in the weaning process
  - Inviting the family to share issues of concern
  - Offering suggestions for appropriate conversation
  - Negotiating visiting times
  - Clarifying the family's role as a supportive resource
- Observe frequently for signs of respiratory muscle fatigue (e.g., increased respiratory rate and minute ventilation, hypercarbia, altered breathing pattern, and increased discomfort) *to ensure optimum oxygenation.*

Expected Outcome: The patient will adhere to the weaning plan as evidenced by participation with primary nurse or registered nurse case manager in implementation of weaning plan and ongoing regimen at all times.
- ▲ Based on individual assessment and collaboration with the patient and the multidisciplinary team, consider use of a formal written weaning contract, mapping, or critical pathway, including the following:
  - Identification of specific goals

■ = nursing intervention; ▲ = collaborative intervention.
*References 1–5, 7, 8, 10, 12–16, 21, 22, 29, 30.

- Timing of weaning interventions
- Expectations regarding adherence to activity and/or exercise protocols
- Patient's participation in self-care activities
- Role of patient and individual team members in achieving weaning goals
- Schedule for reevaluating, renegotiating, and revising the weaning plan *to promote earliest weaning*
- Provide patient and caregivers with a copy of formal written plan and include the copy in patient's chart. Use clear and direct communication (e.g., short, simple sentences) to convey plans for the weaning process *to optimize communication and weaning success.*
- Negotiate the weaning process with patient. Develop a plan for positive reinforcement, such as placing gold stars on a calendar and planning activities outside of the unit, based on individual assessment *to convey visual recognition of the patient's progress.*
- Encourage patient to express thoughts and feelings about perceptions of the weaning process *to reduce anxiety.*
- Encourage patient to convey perceptions of physiological changes (e.g., breathing patterns and recognition of breathing difficulties and presence of secretions) *to reduce complications and increase patient's control over and satisfaction with the weaning process.*
- Use touch, such as a pat on the shoulder, *to offer encouragement and promote trust.*

IV

EVALUATION

Extubation occurs when the patient who has experienced Inability to Sustain Spontaneous Ventilation is able to breathe spontaneously, and parameters that measure oxygenation of tissues are within normal limits or within normal limits for the individual, as determined in collaboration with the multidisciplinary planning team. The synchronous use of respiratory muscles is indicative of normal work of breathing. The patient has normal electrolytes, Pco_2, and visceral proteins. The patient is awake and alert enough to breathe without stimulation or assistance. The patient has no weight gain from water retention or weight loss from muscle or tissue wasting. Continued dependency on mechanical ventilation is indicative of unresolved problems with oxygenation, respiratory muscle fatigue, neurological deficit, drugs, or malnutrition.

The ability of the patient who has experienced Dysfunctional Ventilatory Weaning Response to maintain physiological parameters consistent with his or her baseline clinical status is evidenced by physiological and psychological tolerance to lowered levels of mechanical ventilation. The patient's ability to adhere to the weaning plan is strengthened by early recognition of untoward physiological or psychological events and prompt interventions to resolve these events. Patients who are able to wean from the ventilator convey a comfortable and relaxed appearance and no longer experience irritability, restlessness, agitation, or fatigue. Patients who are unable to tolerate lowered levels of mechanical ventilation should be evaluated for physiological and psychological factors that impede the weaning process. Some patients may never be able to breathe without mechanical assistance. Alternative interventions that address this major lifestyle change are implemented for these individuals.

IV

◤ CASE STUDY WITH PLAN OF CARE

Mr. Joe T., a 64-year-old widower who maintains close contact with his son and daughter who live nearby, was admitted to the surgical intensive care unit on a ventilator following a left upper lobectomy for a large-cell cancerous lesion. His nursing diagnosis was ISSV, and a plan of care directed toward the outcome of meeting Mr. T.'s metabolic needs without the assistance of mechanical ventilation was initiated. His preoperative medical history includes the following data: height, 6′ 1″, weight 154 lb, after a 15-lb weight loss over 4 months; shortness of breath walking from street level to his first- floor apartment; a two-pack-a-day smoking history until the day before surgery; 6 to 7 cups of coffee per day; 8 to 10 beers per week. His employment history indicates that he has been a free-lance writer for the past 20 years for national popular magazines, and he enjoys the traveling associated with his work. Mr. T. experienced three unsuccessful weaning attempts over an 8-day period. These weaning failures were characterized by cardiac arrhythmias (artrial fibrillation, PVCs, and a four-beat run of V-Tach), shortness of breath, asynchronous breathing with the ventilator, abdominal paradox, diaphoresis, and pallor. Mr. T. is frustrated with attempts to communicate with his family and caregivers and has written that he wants to get off the ventilator or die!

◤ PLAN OF CARE FOR MR. JOE T.

Nursing Diagnosis: Dysfunctional Ventilatory Weaning Response Related to Inability to Wean Successfully from the Ventilator after Three Attempts

Expected Outcome: Mr. Joe T. will tolerate levels of mechanical ventilation as evidenced by absence of cardiac arrhythmias; shortness of breath; abdominal paradox; diaphoresis; "fighting the ventilator" during the weaning process.

- Monitor for the presence of diaphragm or respiratory muscle fatigue (atrial and ventricular arrhythmias, shortness of breath, asynchronous breathing with the ventilator, abdominal paradox, and change in concentration).
- ▲ Collaborate with multidisciplinary team to accomplish the following tasks:
  - Determine the best method of weaning for Mr. T.
  - Minimize activities and procedures during weaning trials
  - Remove unnecessary lines (e.g., IVs, central lines, PA catheter)
  - Determine the best method for feeding Mr. T.
  - Ensure that Mr. T. does not receive unnecessary medication that interferes with his ventilatory drive
  - Determine whether methylxanthines are appropriate
  - Determine parameters for discontinuation or continuation of Mr. T.'s weaning plan
- Adopt a low threshold for discontinuation of activities (e.g., bathing or getting out of bed) that increase shortness of breath or reduce SaO_2 less than 90%.
- Establish a daily routine with Mr. T. that allows for his circadian rhythm.
- Coach Mr. T. during the weaning process, using a calm, low voice, to remind him about correct breathing when he experiences shortness of breath.

Expected Outcome: Mr. Joe T. will adhere to the multidisciplinary plan for weaning as evidenced by participating in activities of daily living and cooperating with therapeutic regimens while intubated.

- Collaborate with the psychiatric consultation or liaison clinical nurse specialist in the development of a weaning contract for Mr. T.
- Negotiate weaning plan with Mr. T.
- Arrange with Mr. T.'s son to bring in Mr. T.'s lap-top computer and printer.

■ = nursing intervention; ▲ = collaborative intervention.

- Encourage Mr. T. to keep a daily log.
- Create a personal environment by encouraging Mr. T. to wear his own pajamas and robe during daytime activities, keeping his room door closed with curtain partially open for monitoring, and to decorate the room with his own pictures or posters of other countries.
- Provide a poster board to hang on the wall in Mr. T.'s room and encourage him to have staff and visitors write or draw pictures on it.
- Provide ongoing opportunities for Mr. T. to communicate his thoughts and feelings about his physical and emotional well-being.

■ CRITICAL THINKING EXERCISES

1. How does overfeeding with carbohydrates affect pulmonary ventilation?
2. What were important factors in the nurse's decision to change Mr. Joe T.'s nursing diagnosis from ISSV to DVWR?
3. Why is it important for Mr. Joe T. to have a computer in his room?
4. If activity was minimalized and weaning trials discontinued for 24 hours, why would this be important? Is it important to change activity for 24 hours?
5. Mr. Joe T.'s routine was to stay up late until 2 A.M. and get up late, about 10 A.M. When would be a good time to start weaning trials?

REFERENCES

1. Ahrens TS: Mechanical support of ventilation. In Kinny MR, Packa DR, and Dunbar SB, editors: *AACN's reference for critical care nursing*, ed 3, St. Louis, 1993, Mosby–Year Book.
2. Ahrens TS and Nelsen G: Pulmonary anatomy and physiology. In Kinny MR, Packa DR, and Dunbar SB, editors: *AACN's reference for critical care nursing*, ed 3, St. Louis, 1993, Mosby–Year Book.
3. Burns SM: Preventing diaphragm fatigue in the ventilated patient, *Dimen Crit Care Nurs* 10(1):13–20, 1991.
4. Burns SM and others: Weaning from long-term mechanical ventilation, *Am J Crit Care* 4(1):4–22, 1995.
5. Connolly MA and Shekleton ME: Communicating with ventilator dependent patients, *Dimen Crit Care Nurs* 10(2):115–122, 1991.
6. Gracey DR and others: Outcomes of patients admitted to a chronic ventilator-dependent unit in an acute care hospital, *Mayo Clin Proc* 67:131–136, 1992.
7. Gries ML and Fernsler J: Patient perceptions of the mechanical ventilation experience, *Focus Crit Care* 15(2):52–59, 1988.
8. Grossbach-Landis I: Successful weaning of ventilator-dependent patients, *Top Clin Nurs* 2(3):45–65, 1980.
9. Hanneman SKG and others: Weaning from short-term mechanical ventilation: a review, *Am J Crit Care* 3(6):421–441, 1994.
10. Henneman EA: The art and science of weaning from mechanical ventilation, *Foc Crit Care* 18(6):490–501, 1991.
11. Henneman EA, Lee JL, and Cohen JI: Collaboration: a concept analysis, *J Adv Nurs* 21:103–109, 1995.
12. Holliday JE and Hyers TM: The reduction of weaning time from mechanical ventilation using tidal volume and relaxation biofeedback, *Am Rev Respir Dis* 141:1214–1220, 1990.
13. Inaba-Roland KE and Maricle RA: Assessing delirium in the acute care setting, *Heart Lung* 21(1):48–55, 1992.
14. Jackson NC: Pulmonary rehabilitation for mechanically ventilated patients, *Crit Care Nurs Clin North Am* 3(4):591–600, 1991.
15. Jenny J and Logan J: Analyzing expert nursing practice to develop a new nursing diagnosis, Dysfunctional Ventilatory Weaning Response. In Carroll-Johnson RM, editor: *Classification of nursing diagnoses, proceedings of the Ninth Conference*, Philadelphia, 1990, JB Lippincott Co.
16. Kigin CM: Breathing exercises for the medical patient: the art and the science, *Phys Ther* 70(11):700–706, 1990.
17. Knebel A, Strider VC, and Wood C: The art and science of caring for ventilator-assisted patients, *Crit Care Nurs Clin North Am* 6(4):819–829, 1994.
18. Knebel AR: Weaning from mechanical ventilation: current controversies, *Heart Lung* 20(4):321–331, 1991.
19. Knebel AR: When weaning from mechanical ventilation fails, *Am J Crit Care* 1(3):19–29, 1992.
20. Knebel AR and others: Weaning from mechanical ventilation: concept development, *Am J Crit Care* 3(6):416–420, 1994.
21. Logan J and Jenny J: Deriving a new nursing diagnosis through qualitative research: dysfunctional ventilatory weaning response, *Nurs Diagnosis* 1(1):37–43, 1990.
22. Logan J and Jenny J: Interventions for the nursing diagnosis Dysfunctional Ventilatory Weaning Response: a qualitative study. In Carroll-Johnson RM, editor: *Classification of nursing diagnoses, proceedings of the Ninth Conference*, Philadelphia, 1990, JB Lippincott Co.

IV

23. Lookinland S and Appel PL: Hemodynamic and oxygen transport changes following endotracheal suctioning in trauma patients, *Nurs Res* 40(3):133–138, 1991.

24. McCloskey JC and Bulechek GM: *Nursing interventions classification (NIC)*, ed 2, St. Louis, 1996, Mosby–Year Book.

25. McFarland GK, Wasli EL, and Gerety EK: *Nursing diagnoses and process in psychiatric mental health nursing*, ed 2, Philadelphia, 1992, JB Lippincott Co.

26. North American Nursing Diagnosis Association: *NANDA nursing diagnoses: definitions and classification, 1995–1996*, Philadelphia, 1994, The Association.

27. Perry L: Gut feelings about gut feeding: enteral feeding for ventilated patients in a district general hospital, *Intensive Crit Care Nurs* 9:171–176, 1993.

28. Radwin LE: Conceptualizations of decision making in nursing: analytic models and "knowing the patient," *Nurs Diagnosis* 6(1):16–22, 1995.

29. Shapiro BA and Peruzzi WT: Changing practices in ventilator management: a review of the literature and suggested clinical correlations, *Surgery* 117(2):121–133, 1995.

30. Spector N: Nutritional support of the ventilator-dependent patient, *Nurs Clin North Am* 24(2):407–414, 1989.

31. Sulzbach-Hoke LM and Gift AG: Use of quality management to provide nutrition to intubated patients, *Clin Nurse Specialist* 9(5):248–251, 1995.

32. Thompson KS and others: Building a critical path for ventilator dependency, *Am J Nurs* 91(7):28–31, 1991.

33. Tobin MJ: What should the clinician do when a patient fights the ventilator? *Respiratory Care* 36(5):395–406, 1991.

IV

Sleep Pattern Disturbance

▶ ──────────────────────────────

V

Sleep Pattern Disturbance *is the state in which disruption of sleep time causes discomfort or interferes with an individual's desired lifestyle.*[11]

OVERVIEW

O sleep, O gentle sleep,
Nature's soft nurse! how have I frightened thee,
That thou no more wilt weigh my eyelids down
And steep my senses in forgetfulness?
William Shakespeare
King Henry IV, Part II,
Act 3, scene 1

The comforting, restorative, and healing nature of sleep is referred to often in the literature. Shakespeare describes sleep in *King Henry IV* as "nature's soft nurse" with a quality of gentleness that can be driven away; he then goes on to portray the feeling of frustration experienced when sleep is elusive. It is when sleep is needed the most that we focus on its character, its complexity, and its elusive nature. Henderson[6] has described the inability to rest and sleep as "one of the causes, as well as one of the accompaniments, of disease." The importance of sleep to the well-being of a person is reinforced when sleep is recognized as a basic human need[8] and a survival need.[16]

The North American Nursing Diagnosis Association (NANDA) accepted the diagnostic label Sleep Pattern Disturbance and its definition, defining characteristics, and related factors in 1980.[11] The label is general, encompassing many recognized sleep disorders that must be distinguished from one another to plan an individual-

ized plan of care.[4] An understanding of sleep physiology and sleep architecture, specific sleep disorders, and the cyclical relationship between health problems is critical to making the diagnosis Sleep Pattern Disturbance.

Sleep Physiology and Architecture

Two physiologically and neurologically distinct control mechanisms maintain the sleep-wake cycle: the homeostatic mechanism and the circadian oscillator.[12] The homeostatic mechanism establishes a balance between time spent awake and time spent asleep over a 1- to 2-day period. The balance is set, requiring about 7 to 9 hours of sleep every 24 hours (i.e., 30% to 40% of each day). The circadian oscillator establishes a sleep-tendency variation over the 24-hour day and modulates core body temperature and the levels of many neurological hormones, such as serotonin and cortisol. This mechanism has a 25-hour cycle, requiring time cues (e.g., light sources and television) to be reset daily by 1 hour.

Sleep architecture is the term used to describe the multiple components of sleep. Sleep occurs in two distinct stages: non-rapid-eye-movement (non-REM) sleep and rapid-eye-movement (REM) sleep, as determined by electroencephalography (EEG), electromyography (EMG), and electrooculography (EOG).[2,12] Non-REM sleep is further divided into four distinct stages. The stages of sleep are characterized by physiological, biochemical, and behavioral changes.

A period of sleep begins with non-REM sleep, which progresses from lighter to deeper sleep through the four stages. Stage 1 is a transitional stage between wakefulness and sleep; it may be referred to as *deep drowsiness*. Between 2% and 5% of a young adult's sleep is spent in this stage. During stage 2, the period of *light sleep,* the individual becomes progressively more relaxed. From this stage, the sleeper may revert to stage 1 or may pass into stage 3. A young adult typically spends 45% to 55% of total sleep time in non-REM stage 2 sleep.

Non-REM stages 3 and 4 are characterized by slow-frequency delta waves on the EEG and are differentiated by the relative percentage of these waves; these stages are prominent during the first third of the sleep period. Stage 3, the *deep sleep* stage, constitutes 3% to 8% of a young adult's sleep time. Very deep sleep occurs during stage 4, which occupies 10% to 15% of a young adult's sleep time. These are the restorative stages of sleep, during which much protein synthesis and energy conservation occur.

During REM sleep, or paradoxic sleep, bursts of eye movements can be seen on the EOG. The large muscles of the body become functionally paralyzed. EEG activity increases and resembles the waking state. REM sleep constitutes 20% to 25% of the total sleep time and is the stage during which the individual is most difficult to awaken.

Sleep is cyclical. At its onset the individual normally progresses through repetitive cycles, beginning with non-REM stages 1 through 4 and then returning to stage 2. From non-REM stage 2 the sleeper enters REM sleep, then goes back to stage 2, and the cycle is repeated. These cycles occur at approximately 90-minute intervals, so that four or five cycles are normally completed during the sleep period.

Health problems can decrease the quantity, quality, and consistency of sleep. During illness, sleep is often interrupted or fragmented, altering the normal stages and cycles and producing dysfunctional sleep. With frequent interruptions the patient spends more time in the transitional stages (non-REM stages 1 and 2) and less time in the deeper stages of sleep (non-REM stages 3 and 4 and REM). Thus total sleep time may decrease,

and selective deprivation of the deeper stages of sleep can occur.

Sleep Disorders

The International Classification of Sleep Disorders (ICSD) classifies 88 sleep disorders into four major categories: dyssomnia, parasomnia, medical and psychiatric disorders, and proposed sleep disorders.[1,2] *Dyssomnias* (i.e., disorders resulting in insomnia or excessive sleepiness) are subdivided into three groups: (1) *Intrinsic Sleep Disorders* include those conditions related to excessive sleep or sleepiness (e.g., narcolepsy, idiopathic or recurrent hypersomnia, restless leg syndrome, and sleep-related breathing disorders such as obstructive or central sleep apnea); (2) *Extrinsic Sleep Disorders* refer to disorders caused by exogenous factors (e.g., alcohol-dependent sleep disorder, food allergy insomnia, inadequate sleep hygiene, and environmental sleep disorder); and (3) *Circadian rhythm sleep disorders* refer to disorders resulting from the misalignment of a person's actual sleep time and his or her normal time for sleep (e.g., an irregular sleep-wake pattern, shift work sleep disorder, and time zone change [jet lag] disorder).

The second major classification of sleep disorders, *parasomnia,* includes those disorders related to the occurrence of undesirable phenomena during sleep. Disorders classified as parasomnias include *arousal disorders* (e.g., sleep walking or sleep terrors), *sleep-wake transition disorders* (e.g., rhythmic moving disorder or nocturnal leg cramps), *parasomnias usually associated with REM sleep* (e.g., nightmares or impaired sleep-related penile erections), and *other parasomnias* (e.g., sleep bruxism, sleep enuresis, or primary snoring). Parasomnia disorder can be an indicator that a more serious problem exists (e.g., snoring that results from obstructive sleep apnea).

Sleep disorders associated with medical and psychiatric disorders comprise the third major category. This category includes (1) disorders associated with mental disorders (e.g., mood disorders, anxiety disorders, and alcoholism); (2) disorders associated with neurological disorders (e.g., dementia, Parkinsonism, sleep-related epilepsy, and sleep-related headaches); and (3) disorders associated with medical disorders (e.g., nocturnal cardiac ischemia, chronic obstructive pulmonary disease, sleep-related gastroesophageal reflux, and sleeping sickness).

The last category, *proposed sleep disorders,* includes those conditions or disorders that need to be more clearly defined and described before being classified as a sleep disorder per se. Examples of disorders currently placed in this category include short sleeper, sleep hyperhidrosis, menstruation-associated sleep disorder, and sleep choking syndrome.

It is important to note that some specific sleep disorders might be placed in more than one of the major categories. For example, the sleep disorder experienced by a patient with Parkinsonism would be classified as a sleep disorder associated with a medical/psychiatric disorder as well as a dyssomnia (because the patient experiences insomnia). By focusing on the patient's description of the sleep problem, assessment data can be collected that will support an accurate diagnosis and a realistic plan of care.

ASSESSMENT

The health assessment of every patient should include a sleep assessment. The nurse begins the sleep assessment by gathering information about the patient's most recent sleep experience and then compares that to the patient's previous sleep patterns. If a patient is suspected of experiencing a sleep disorder, an evaluation of the patient's sleep pattern and a comprehensive assessment to identify the defining characteristics and related factors associated with Sleep Pattern Disturbance are warranted.

Patients experiencing Sleep Pattern Disturbance often describe their sleep experience in terms of (1) problems with the quantity or quality of sleep (insomnia), (2) problems in staying awake (hypersomnia), and (3) the presence of abnormal behavior during sleep, as reported by the patient or the patient's sleep partner (parasomnia).[7] Insomnia, hypersomnia, and parasomnia may be symptomatic of a well-defined sleep disorder and therefore must be explored. Regardless of the presenting complaint, the patient's health status, sleep-wake cycle, and factors interfering with the sleep experience should be assessed. Sleep histories, sleep questionnaires, and sleep diaries provide valuable data in determining whether or not the patient is experiencing Sleep Pattern Disturbance.[2,3,12,14]

The patient is considered the authority on evaluating the quantity and quality of the sleep experience. A sleep history can provide valuable information about the usual sleep-wake cycle. The patient should be asked questions that provide information about past and present sleep habits, attitudes toward sleep, effect of the sleep experience on daily functioning, drug and alcohol use or abuse, and emotional and physical illnesses and problems and their treatment.

To estimate the current quantity and quality of sleep, the nurse should ask the patient questions to elicit information. The following questions relate to the quantity of sleep: What time do you go to bed? How long does it take you to fall asleep? What time do you awaken? If you wake during the night, how long does it take to fall asleep? Questions about the quality of sleep include the following: Do you feel rested when you awaken? Do you wake up (without aids, such as an alarm clock) before you feel you are ready? Do you feel sleepy during the day? Do you fall asleep at undesired times? What factors interfere with your getting a "good night's sleep"? The patient's sleep partner should be asked whether the patient snores, seems to stop breathing at times, or kicks or jerks his or her legs during sleep.

Information related to substance use or abuse, medications, diet, sleep hygiene measures, and sleep environment is evaluated to determine whether factors are present that contribute to the presence of a sleep disorder. Alcohol, although it has an acute sedating effect that may help a patient fall asleep, often causes sleep to be fragmented and unsatisfying. This is related to catecholamine release during alcohol withdrawal. The nicotine in tobacco products acts as a stimulant and therefore can interfere with sleep. Cocaine is known to inhibit or fragment sleep, and morphine and heroin can have arousing effects that cause sleep disturbances. Nonsteroidal antiinflammatory drugs, antiarrhythmics, anticonvulsants, corticosteroids, and bronchodilators are just a few of the drugs that can cause insomnia. Many popular over-the-counter remedies, such as diet and cold products, contain stimulating compounds.

Information related to diet is important for the purpose of evaluating whether or not the composition of the diet or the timing of meals contributes to sleep problems. Too much caffeine in the diet —whether in coffee, tea, cola beverages, or products containing chocolate—acts as a stimulant and can delay or interrupt sleep. Ingestion of gas-producing or spicy foods may cause gastrointestinal discomfort that interferes with sleep quantity or quality. The timing of meals before bedtime should also be considered. Ingesting too large a meal close to bedtime can result in discomfort and interfere with sleep onset and maintenance. Ingesting too little food (to the point of going to bed hungry) can also disturb sleep.

Sleep hygiene refers to personal and environmental activities that can affect sleep. The patient should be questioned about daytime sleep periods, activity and exercise routines, and sleep or bedtime rituals and aids. Those activities that interfere with sleep quantity and quality and those activities supportive of sleep are identified. Regularly scheduled naps, although improving sleep latency for patients with narcolepsy (characterized by excessive daytime sleepiness),[13] may create problems for the patient suffering from insomnia. Patients whose daily routines are void of activity and exercise can experience sleep disturbances. Interruption of helpful sleep routines also can alter the patient's sleep pattern.

The first priority in assessing the patient's sleep environment is to determine whether the sleep disturbance occurred as a consequence of a change in the sleep environment. Hospitalization in acute or long-term facilities has been identified as a factor contributing to sleep disorders.[3,5,10,15] A change from the usual home sleep environment to a hotel or someone else's home can also cause a disruption in the sleep pattern and routine. Environmental factors implicated in sleep pattern disruption or disturbances include variables such as noise, light, temperature, and air circulation.[2,12]

When assessing the personal and environmental factors, maturational and cultural factors must be considered. Required sleep time is greatest in infancy, decreases in childhood, stabilizes in adulthood, and then begins to decline in the older adult. Waking during the night is expected during infancy and childhood and tends to occur in the later adult years as well. "Older adults constitute the age group most severely affected by disorders of initiating and maintaining sleep."[10] This age group is also more dependent on the maintenance of a stable sleep environment and the use of sleep aids and rituals.

Cultural factors, in terms of ethnic, racial, and spiritual influences, are also taken into consideration. The sleep environment, sleep rituals, and sleep aids are strongly influenced by culture. The influences may be reflected in an action as subtle as reducing the room temperature or as obvious as chanting prayers while kneeling and bowed in prayer.

When obtaining the sleep history and interviewing the patient to gather information related to personal and environmental factors affecting the sleep experience, the nurse should observe the patient's appearance and behavior. Physical signs, such as dozing during the day, an expressionless face, ptosis of the eyelids, hand tremors, drooping shoulders, and mispronunciation or incorrect use of words, indicate that the patient may have a Sleep Pattern Disturbance. Behavioral signs can include restlessness, lethargy, irritability, agitation, disorientation, and listlessness.

In summary, assessment requires examination of physiological, psychological, and environmental factors, as well as the patient's personal characteristics and lifestyle, to make a diagnosis of Sleep Pattern Disturbance. The nurse must identify the specific factors contributing to the sleep problem and determine whether consultation with other health care providers is needed.

■ Defining Characteristics

The presence of the following defining characteristics indicates that the patient may be experiencing Sleep Pattern Disturbance:

- Verbal complaints of difficulty sleeping
- Verbal complaints of not feeling well rested
- Physical signs (e.g., mild, fleeting nystagmus; slight hand tremor; ptosis of eyelids; expressionless face; thick speech with mispronunciation or incorrect use of words; frequent yawning; changes of posture, namely, sagging or drooping head)
- Fragmented sleep
- Difficulty awakening
- Daytime sleepiness
- Fatigue
- Activity intolerance
- Changes in behavior and performance (e.g., increasing irritability, restlessness, agitation, decreased attention span, disorientation, lethargy, listlessness, and decreased arousal threshold)

■ Related Factors

The following related factors are associated with Sleep Pattern Disturbance:

- Pain
- Impaired oxygen transport (e.g., cardiopulmonary disease and peripheral arteriosclerosis)
- Impaired bowel or bladder elimination
- Impaired metabolism (e.g., hyperthyroidism and hepatic disorders)
- Sleep apnea
- Immobility (e.g., traction, casts, and restraints)
- Inadequate physical exercise
- Change in activity pattern
- Effects of medications or drugs (e.g., tranquilizers, barbiturates, monamine oxidase inhibitors, amphetamines, hypnotics, antidepressants, antihypertensives, sedatives, anesthetics, steroids, decongestants, caffeine, and alcohol)
- Alcoholism

- Stress
- Fear
- Anxiety disorders
- Panic disorder
- Depression
- Change in sleep-wake pattern (e.g., change in work shift, rapid change of time zone, or decrease in sleep time)
- Change in sleep routine
- Unfamiliar or uncomfortable sleep environment
- Hospitalization
- Increased sensory stimulation (e.g., noise or bright lights)

DIAGNOSIS

■ Differential Nursing Diagnosis

Patients diagnosed with Pain (acute or chronic), Impaired Physical Mobility, Activity Intolerance, Urinary or Bowel Incontinence, Anxiety, or Fear could be considered to be at risk for the development of Sleep Pattern Disturbance. Each of the former diagnoses is an etiology or related factor that must be considered when assessing the patient suspected of having an altered sleep pattern. In discriminating the diagnoses Sleep Pattern Disturbance and Fatigue, Fatigue can be a defining character of Sleep Pattern Disturbance, and Sleep Pattern Disturbance is a factor directly related to Fatigue. The patient diagnosed with Fatigue often describes disruptions of the usual sleep pattern over a period of time.

■ Medical and Psychiatric Diagnoses

Any medical diagnosis causing the patient pain or requiring surgical intervention or other invasive treatments puts the patient at risk for experiencing Sleep Pattern Disturbance. Neurological disorders, such as Parkinsonism and dementia, and mental disorders, such as mood disorders and psychoses, are associated with sleep disorders.[1] Narcolepsy and sleep apnea are characterized by disturbances in the patient's sleep pattern. Collaboration between the physician and the nurse is important to assure an ongoing evaluation of the effectiveness of collaborative interventions.

OUTCOME IDENTIFICATION, PLANNING, AND IMPLEMENTATION

The goal in planning care for patients with Sleep Pattern Disturbance is to eliminate or control the alteration in sleep that they are experiencing. Patient outcomes that will help patients achieve this goal are identified. Ultimately the patient is expected to verbalize an increased satisfaction with his or her sleep pattern.

Most essential to eliminating or controlling the sleep alteration is the patient's knowledge of factors that contribute to Sleep Pattern Disturbance as well as those that can contribute to correcting an altered sleep pattern. The patient, if able, should actively participate in (1) identifying problem areas, (2) setting mutually acceptable goals, and (3) implementing measures that will enhance the sleep experience.

Patient education should focus on teaching the patient about the normal sleep-wake cycle and the factors that may delay or interrupt the sleep-wake cycle. These factors include the following: (1) physiological factors such as pain, impaired bladder function, and a recent surgical procedure; (2) psychological factors such as stress, anxiety, and depression; (3) lifestyle factors such as changes in Activity-Exercise Pattern, diet, and changes in usual sleep routines or rituals; and (4) environmental factors such as a noisy or extremely warm sleep environment. Knowledge of the effects these factors can have on the sleep experience will assist the patient in controlling the factors that contribute to the sleep problem.

To assist the patient in identifying and adopting measures that will support an adequate sleep pattern, the nurse should provide the patient with information about specific sleep-promoting techniques (e.g., relaxation exercises or massage[9]) and recommend potential changes in lifestyle that will promote an optimal balance of rest and activity. If the patient's sleep-wake schedule is disrupted, activities should be planned during the day to stimulate wakefulness and comfort measures should be employed at night to promote sleep.

The hospital and home routines and environments should be adapted to support the patient's most effective sleep pattern. Every effort should be made to accommodate the patient's usual sleep time. The patient should be awakened only for essential care or treatment tasks; awakenings should allow for sleep cycles of at least 90 minutes for adequate non-REM and REM sleep time. The environment, especially noise, lighting, and sensory stimulation, should be controlled to support the patient's comfort and to promote sleep. The nurse should use a flashlight rather than the overhead light for patient checks at night whenever possible.

The medications that the patient receives should be evaluated for their effects on sleep. Many sedative and hypnotic medications decrease REM sleep. Drugs that minimally disrupt sleep should be used to complement comfort measures and techniques that promote sleep, and, when possible, drug dosages should be reduced as the medication becomes less necessary. Diuretics may interrupt sleep by increasing the number of awakenings; therefore they should not be scheduled late in the day.

Fluid intake at bedtime may also cause the patient to awaken during the night. The patient can be instructed to take fluids during the day and to restrict intake 2 to 4 hours before retiring. Frequent awakenings during the night to urinate are a problem encountered by many elderly persons. Therefore attention should be directed to this area during the assessment.

Sleep hygiene refers to those personal and environmental activities that affect sleep.[2,12] The following patient guidelines support the maintenance of good sleep hygiene and should be shared with the patient:

1. Maintain a regular sleep-wake schedule; a regular wake-up time leads to a regular time for sleep onset.
2. Avoid afternoon or evening napping if it seems to cause difficulty falling sleep at bedtime.
3. Avoid caffeine, tobacco products, and alcohol in the evening.

4. Avoid stressful activities in the evening, and spend some idle time before going to bed.
5. Do not eat a large meal before going to bed; eat a light snack only if hungry.
6. Eliminate or reduce annoying noise and light.
7. Engage in regular daytime exercise.
8. Don't allow yourself to become frustrated because you cannot fall asleep; rather, get up and do something else, preferably in another room.
9. Discuss sleep medications with your health care provider (some medications, although they increase sleep quantity, can interfere with sleep quality; chronic use of medications to aid sleep may lead to dependence).

◢ NURSING CARE GUIDELINES
Nursing Diagnosis: Sleep Pattern Disturbance

Expected Outcome: The patient will describe (1) factors that contribute to Sleep Pattern Disturbance and (2) factors that promote an optimal sleep pattern.
- Teach the patient and significant other(s) about sleep and rest needs and about factors that contribute to Sleep Pattern Disturbance.
- ▲ Explore with the patient and significant other(s) those physical, emotional, personal, and environmental factors that may be contributing to the patient's sleep problems.
- ▲ Review with the patient any prescription and over-the-counter medications the patient may be taking; discuss the effects the medications may have on the patient's sleep pattern.
- Review with the patient and significant other(s) the sleep hygiene guidelines, discussing how the patient can follow the recommendations included in the guidelines.
- Discuss with the patient and significant other(s) those comfort measures, sleep-promoting techniques (e.g., relaxation training, stimulus control, massage, and positioning), and lifestyle changes that can contribute to optimizing the patient's sleep experience.
  Educating the patient and significant other(s) provides them with the necessary information to become actively involved in implementing recommended interventions and evaluating the effectiveness of those interventions.
- ▲ Evaluate sleep-promoting measures frequently *to determine those that are most helpful to the patient. Ongoing evaluation provides opportunities to refine and to revise interventions so they will be more effective in treating the patient's sleep problem.*

Expected Outcome: The patient will demonstrate an optimal balance between sleep and sleep activity.
- ▲ Assess the patient's past and present sleep and activity pattern. *If the current sleep problem is of long duration it is important to determine how the patient has been coping with the problem and, if of short duration, to identify any recent changes the patient may have experienced.*
- Plan for activities during the daytime *to stimulate wakefulness,* and suggest sleep-promoting measures at night *to enhance the sleep opportunity.*
- ▲ Assist the patient in identifying sleep-enhancing measures (e.g., decreasing lighting and noise and controlling sensory stimulation before and during the sleep time) *to promote maintenance of normal day-night cycles.*
- Assess the value of introducing a nap time into the patient's daytime schedule. If appropriate, schedule nap time for at least 90 minutes *to assist in providing a normal sleep cycle that includes REM sleep and to meet sleep requirements.*

Expected Outcome: The patient will verbalize increased satisfaction with his or her sleep pattern.
- ▲ Encourage the patient to follow the *Sleep Hygiene Guidelines to support sleep onset and maintenance and to enhance the patient's sleep pattern.*

■ = nursing intervention; ▲ = collaborative intervention.   *Continued*

◢ **NURSING CARE GUIDELINES — CONT'D**

- Discuss with the patient those comfort measures that the patient feels important in promoting an optimal sleep pattern (e.g., adjusting the environment, massage, positioning, and relaxation therapy); implement measures if feasible and appropriate. *The patient's perception of the sleep experience and factors that interfere with or promote sleep provide valuable information in identifying measures that will be most supportive in optimizing the patient sleep pattern.*
- ▲ Consult with the physician regarding the need for sleep medications that do not suppress REM sleep *to assure that medication will not alter the quality of the sleep cycle*; explore the patient's feelings about using medications *to involve the patient in making the decision.*
- ▲ Frequently assess the effects of medications on the patient's sleep pattern *to determine if the medication is supportive of maintaining an adequate sleep pattern.*
- With the patient, identify and implement activities that promote comfort, relaxation, and a sense of well-being *to reduce stress that may be interfering with sleep onset and maintenance.*
- ▲ If the patient has to be awakened for medications or treatments (whether in the hospital or at home), work with the patient and significant other(s) to schedule activities to minimize awakenings *to allow for sleep cycles of at least 90 minutes.*
- ▲ Encourage the patient to carry out usual bedtime rituals and routines that help *support sleep onset and maintenance.*

EVALUATION

The nurse should evaluate the care plan and its implementation on an ongoing basis. The patient's perception of the adequacy and effectiveness of the sleep experience should be assessed daily, when possible, to determine the appropriateness of the interventions and changes that should be made. Because the adequacy of sleep is very difficult to evaluate clinically, nurses should use research findings to guide their practice. Cox's extensive study of sleep in hospitalized patients is an example of a study that provides information supportive of developing and evaluating the plan of care for the hospitalized patient who is experiencing Sleep Pattern Disturbance.[3]

The patient's perception of the duration and quality of sleep as well as his or her perception of the assistance provided by the comfort measures,

sleep-promoting techniques, and lifestyle changes are critical to evaluating care. The patient's willingness to control factors that disrupt sleep and to implement measures that enhance sleep should be determined. The patient's ability and desire to participate in his or her own care through mutual goal setting are essential to maintain an adequate and effective sleep pattern on a long-term basis.

If the patient has a sleep disorder that is not responding to medical and nursing interventions, the health care providers should consider referral to a sleep disorders center. To identify centers that are accessible to the patient, contact

The American Sleep Disorders Association
1610 14th Street, N.W.
Suite 300
Rochester, MN 55901-2200
Telephone: (507) 287-6008

■ CASE STUDY WITH PLAN OF CARE

Mrs. Wilma E., a 59-year-old widow, was admitted to the medical unit for treatment of cellulitis of the right arm. On Mrs. E.'s third day in the hospital, the nurse noted that Mrs. E. appeared lethargic and listless. Mrs. E. yawned frequently during the interaction with the nurse and had difficulty concentrating. Mrs. E. was responding to the intravenous antibiotics she had been receiving: over the past 3 days, her temperature went from 102.6°F to 99.6°F, and her respirations, pulse, and blood pressure were within normal limits. The nurse commented to Mrs. E. that she looked tired and asked whether Mrs. E. was having difficulty sleeping. Mrs. E. stated that she hadn't really slept well since she entered the hospital. The assessment revealed that at home Mrs. E. slept 7 to 8 hours each night and maintained an active schedule during the day. She usually drank a cup of hot chocolate and read before she went to sleep, and she stated that she rarely had difficulty falling asleep or staying asleep. In the hospital, Mrs. E. was in a semiprivate room. She stated that she didn't read at night because she feared that the light would keep her roommate awake. She also stated that when awakened at night to have her vital signs taken, she had difficulty falling back to sleep. She said that during the day she tried to take "cat naps" to catch up on her sleep; she had little else to do. She stated, "I'm concerned that my sleeping difficulties will continue when I return home."

■ PLAN OF CARE FOR MRS. WILMA E.

Nursing Diagnosis: Sleep Pattern Disturbance Related to Hospital Environment and Change in Bedtime Routine

Expected Outcome: Mrs. E. will describe factors that contribute to her Sleep Pattern Disturbance and measures that will enhance her sleep pattern while in the hospital and when she returns home.
- Explore with Mrs. E. those factors interfering with her sleep.
- Suggest that Mrs. E. have one of her family members bring a small reading lamp or a book light so that she can feel comfortable reading at night.
- ▲ Encourage Mrs. E. to ask the evening staff to prepare a cup of hot chocolate, if she feels it will help her fall asleep.
- ▲ Evaluate the need to monitor Mrs. E.'s vital signs during the night.
- ▲ Discuss with the evening staff and other care providers Mrs. E.'s sleep problem; review scheduling of intravenous administration, and change it if necessary and feasible; encourage staff to use minimal lighting when monitoring and caring for Mrs. E. during the night.
- Explore with Mrs. E. her concern about not being able to resume her normal sleep pattern when she returns home; review the *Sleep Hygiene Guidelines* with Mrs. E. and discuss how she can introduce sleep-promoting behaviors into her sleep-wake routine when she is at home.

Expected Outcome: Mrs. E. will demonstrate an optimal balance between her activity and her Sleep-Rest Pattern.
- Encourage Mrs. E. to take walks in the hospital corridors during the day.
- Explore with Mrs. E. diversional activities that may interest her and occupy her time.
- Provide Mrs. E. with reading material she might enjoy.
- Assist Mrs. E. in planning a specific nap time (early in the afternoon and at least 90 minutes in duration) to assist in modulating her normal sleep and activity patterns; introduce environmental measures (dimmed light and noise reduction) in and around Mrs. E.'s room during nap time.

Expected Outcome: Mrs. E. will express increased satisfaction with her Sleep-Rest Pattern.
- Evaluate the effectiveness of Mrs. E.'s attempts to implement her usual sleep routine.

■ = nursing intervention; ▲ = collaborative intervention.

Continued

▶ **PLAN OF CARE FOR MRS. WILMA E. — CONT'D**

- ▲ Discuss with Mrs. E. and the evening and night staff the effectiveness of the measures taken to reduce stimuli during nighttime nursing tasks.
- ■ Evaluate with Mrs. E. whether daytime activities have contributed to achieving an adequate and effective sleep experience.
- ■ Discuss with Mrs. E. any changes in the plan of care that would contribute to outcome achievement; if feasible and appropriate, implement changes.

▪▪ CRITICAL THINKING EXERCISES

1. Prepare a patient education booklet that would have been helpful to Mrs. E. Highlight information on sleep hygiene, behavioral management, and pharmacological interventions.
2. If medications were a routine sleep aid for Mrs. E., what implications would that information have on data you should collect during the assessment phase of the nursing process?
3. As you are preparing Mrs. E. for discharge, she states, "If I continue to have problems sleeping when I get home, maybe I should take some medicine to help me sleep." What information should you provide for Mrs. E.?
4. Design a one-page guide that would be helpful to Mrs. E. in understanding the role of pharmacological interventions in treating sleep disorders.

REFERENCES

1. American Sleep Disorders Association: *International classification of sleep disorders: diagnostic and coding manual*, Rochester, Minnesota, 1990, The Association.
2. Bootzin RR, Lahmeyer H, and Lilie JK: *Integrated approach to sleep management: the healthcare practitioner's guide to the diagnosis and treatment of sleep disorders*, Belle Mead, New Jersey, 1994, Cahners Healthcare Communications.
3. Cox K: *Quality of sleep in hospital settings*, Maastricht, 1992, Universitaire Pers Maastricht.
4. Gordon M: *Nursing diagnosis: process and application*, ed 3, St. Louis, 1994, Mosby–Year Book.
5. Gordon M: Report of an RNF study to determine which nursing diagnoses have high frequency and high treatment priority in rehabilitation nursing, part II, *Rehab Nurs Res* 4(2):38–46, 1995.
6. Henderson V: *Basic principles of nursing care*, New York, 1969, Macmillan Publishing.
7. Lacks P and Morin CM: Recent advances in the assessment and treatment of insomnia, *J Consult Clin Psychol* 60: 586–594, 1992.
8. Maslow A: *Motivation and personality*, New York, 1970, Harper & Row.
9. McCloskey JC and Bulechek GM: *Nursing interventions classification (NIC)*, ed 2, St. Louis, 1992, Mosby–Year Book.
10. National Institute of Nursing Research: *Long-term care for older adults: a report of the NINR priority expert panel on long-term care*, NIH Pub No 94-2418, Bethseda, Maryland, 1994, U.S. Dept. of Health and Human Services.
11. North American Nursing Diagnosis Association: *NANDA nursing diagnoses: definitions and classification, 1995–1996*, Philadelphia, 1994, The Association.
12. Neubauer DN, Smith PL, and Early CJ: Sleep disorders. In Barker LR, Burton JR, and Zieve PD, editors: *Principles of ambulatory medicine*, ed 4, Baltimore, 1994, Williams & Wilkins.
13. Rogers AE and Aldrich MS: The effect of regularly scheduled naps on sleep attacks and excessive daytime sleepiness associated with narcolepsy, *Nurs Res* 42(2):111–117, 1993.
14. Rogers AE, Caruso CC, and Aldrich MS: Reliability of sleep diaries for assessment of sleep/wake patterns, *Nurs Res* 42(6):368–372, 1993.
15. Spenceley SM: Sleep inquiry: a look with fresh eyes, *Image* 25(3):249–256, 1993.
16. Yura H and Walsh MB: *The nursing process: assessing, planning, implementing, evaluating*, Norwalk, Connecticut, 1988, Appleton & Lange.

Decreased Adaptive Capacity: Intracranial

▶

Decreased Adaptive Capacity: Intracranial *is a clinical state in which intracranial fluid dynamic mechanisms that normally compensate for increases in intracranial volumes are compromised, resulting in repeated disproportionate increases in intracranial pressure (ICP) in response to a variety of noxious and nonnoxious stimuli.*[6]

OVERVIEW

Increased ICP is one of the most common life-threatening complications affecting patients with intracranial injury. There is considerable risk of secondary brain injury, with long-term disability and even death. By understanding the pathophysiological processes involved in ICP and the defining characteristics of increased ICP, the nurse can be a key player in preventing secondary brain injury.

The seventeenth-century Monro-Kellie hypothesis is helpful in understanding increased ICP. The hypothesis states that the cranium forms a rigid compartment holding three major components: the brain (80%), cerebral spinal fluid, or CSF (10%), and blood (10%).[2] ICP is the pressure that these three components exert inside the rigid cranium. The volume of these three components remains nearly constant in a state of dynamic equilibrium. If the volume of any one component increases, another component must decrease for the overall volume and dynamic equilibrium to remain constant. Otherwise, increased ICP will result. The mechanism by which this reduction in volume occurs is called *compensation*.

Compensation can occur in one of two ways: decreasing CSF volume or decreasing cerebral blood volume. As ICP rises, CSF is channeled from the cranium to the spinal cord. In addition, CSF production can decrease and CSF absorption can increase. Cerebral blood can be reabsorbed into the vascular system outside of the cranium.[1,10] These compensatory mechanisms are limited. When the demands of increased ICP exceed the limits of the compensatory mechanisms (decreasing CSF and blood volume), the third component (the brain) must shift. Thus brain herniation and death may result.

A compensatory mechanism that protects the brain in the early stages of increased ICP is termed *autoregulation*. This adaptive mechanism allows cerebral blood vessels to maintain cerebral blood flow in response to wide fluctuations in systolic arterial blood pressure.[4] In order for autoregulation to function properly, normal carbon dioxide levels and specific pressure ranges of ICP, systolic arterial blood pressure, and cerebral perfusion pressure are needed.[2]

Adaptive compensatory mechanisms fail when a small increase in volume produces a disproportionately large increase in pressure. High elastance (or relative stiffness of the intracranial components) and low compliance (or slackness in response of intracranial components to increased volume) cause compensatory mechanisms to fail.[1,8,9] In terms of autoregulation, if carbon dioxide levels are high, if ICP levels are very high, and if systolic arterial blood pressure and cerebral perfusion pressure are not within a certain range, autoregulation will fail.

Healthy individuals may cough or sneeze, resulting in an increase in ICP. What is the difference between this increase and that of a patient with an intracranial injury? The ICP level should return to normal baseline relatively quickly in healthy individuals. Age also makes a difference. The cranium is not a rigid container in infants and small children because fusion of the sutures has not yet occurred. The intracranial space can thus expand in response to increased volume. In the elderly, some cerebral atrophy occurs, thus creating more space in the cranium for intracranial expansion.

To prevent secondary brain injury from increased ICP, the nurse must understand the underlying pathophysiological process of Decreased Adaptive Capacity: Intracranial and its defining characteristics. Only then will the nurse be able to institute the appropriate interventions to assist the patient's ICP to return to normal.

ASSESSMENT

Assessment includes looking for related factors and defining characteristics of increased ICP. Related factors that may cause increased ICP can be determined through the patient's health history and objective data. The patient may have a brain tumor or have sustained head trauma from a motor vehicle collision. Once this information is known, the defining characteristics can be assessed.

The most important objective data is obtained through the neurological nursing assessment. Assessment of the patient's neurological status can help detect early signs and symptoms of increased ICP. This assessment includes level of consciousness, pupillary response, motor function, sensory function, and cranial nerves. A change in level of consciousness (i.e., irritability, restlessness, or confusion) is the most important sign of increased ICP and needs to be monitored closely and reported immediately. Increased ICP is not constant; thus transient pressure signs may be present, requiring frequent neurological assessments.

Vital signs also need frequent assessment. The nurse must be knowledgeable about Cushing's response, which is a compensatory response designed to provide adequate cerebral perfusion pressure in the presence of rising ICP. Signs and symptoms include a rising systolic blood pressure, a widening pulse pressure, and bradycardia.[2] These signs and symptoms are not common in children.

When the nurse assesses an infant, different signs and symptoms may be present. They include tense or bulging fontanels, a high-pitched cry, an increase in occipital-to-frontal circumference, a change in feeding pattern, and crying while being held. When the nurse assesses an elderly patient, it is important to remember that cerebral atrophy may obscure the signs and symptoms of increased ICP and make detection more difficult. Thus signs and symptoms may differ, depending on the patient's age and the area of insult in the cranium.

An intracranial pressure monitor is an objective way to measure ICP. Moreover, cerebral perfusion pressure can be calculated from knowing the ICP and the mean arterial blood pressure. The nurse must remember that critical values for ICP, mean arterial blood pressure, and cerebral perfusion pressure are lower the younger the child and the older the adult (age over 70).[7]

ICP monitoring involves placing a sensor in the cranium to measure pressure. The transducer converts the raw data into information about the waveform and the pressure value that the monitor can receive and display. There are three types of ICP monitors: intraventricular catheters, subarachnoid bolts or screws, and epidural sensors.[5] In the last few years, fiber-optic catheters have provided direct measurement of brain parenchymal pressures. This type of catheter can be placed into intraventricular, subarachnoid, or intraparenchymal sites.[3]

Waveform patterns noted on the ICP monitor give the nurse additional information for assessing ICP. As noted previously, healthy individuals have transient increases in ICP. When assessing waveform patterns, the nurse looks for trends over time. Normal waveforms have three peaks, declining in a stepdown fashion (noted at P_1, P_2, P_3). As pressure rises, the amplitude of P_2 can exceed P_1, indicating that the patient may be suffering from a loss of compliance and compensation.[10] A variation of the normal waveform, known as a wide-amplitude ICP waveform, or plateau wave, reflects a sharp rise in ICP that plateaus. This type of waveform is indicative of compromised cerebral perfusion pressure, which may result in severe cerebral hypoxia and herniation.[2]

Assessment is critical in preventing secondary brain injury. Health history, physical assessment, and ICP monitoring provide direction for treatment in the patient who is experiencing Decreased Adaptive Capacity: Intracranial. The nurse must know the defining characteristics and related factors to contribute to the interdisciplinary approach of patient care.

■ Defining Characteristics

The presence of the following characteristics[3,6,8,10] indicates that the patient may be experiencing Decreased Adaptive Capacity: Intracranial:

- Repeated increases in ICP greater than 15 mm Hg for more than 5 minutes following any of a variety of external stimuli
- Disproportionate increase in ICP following single environmental or nursing maneuver stimulus
- Elevated P_2 ICP waveform
- Baseline ICP exceeds 15 mm Hg
- Wide-amplitude ICP waveform (plateau wave)
- Early signs and symptoms:
  - Level of consciousness: restlessness, irritability, mild confusion, personality changes, and agitation
  - Pupils: ovoid pupil, slowed reaction, unilateral change in pupil size
  - Vision: blurred, diplopia, visual field deficit, decreased visual acuity, conjugate deviation of eyes
  - Motor function: paresis, paralysis
  - Sensory function: decreased response to light touch and pin prick
  - Headache: occurs in early morning, with nausea and vomiting
  - Speech: slow or slurred
  - Memory: mild memory deficit
  - Vital signs: NO CHANGE
  - Cranial nerves: may show deficits
  - Seizures: may occur

- Late signs and symptoms:
  - Level of consciousness: difficult to arouse, decreased responsiveness, or coma
  - Pupils: unilateral pupil enlarging to fixed and dialted, bilateral fixed and dilated (later), and papilledema
  - Motor function: flexor-extensor posturing
  - Sensory function: may only posture to painful stimuli
  - Headache: increases with severity, accompanied by projectile vomiting
  - Speech: patient may only groan when given to painful stimuli
  - Respiratory: irregular respiration, Cheyne-Stokes respiration, and respiratory arrest
  - Vital signs: Cushing's response, wide fluctuations in temperature
  - Cranial nerves: loss of brain stem reflexes (e.g., cough, gag)
  - Reflexes: decreased or absent (e.g., Babinski's reflex or deep tendon reflex)

■ Related Factors

The following related factors[3,6,8,10] are associated with Decreased Adaptive Capacity: Intracranial

- Sustained increase in ICP greater than 15 mm Hg
- Decreased cerebral perfusion pressure less than or equal to 50–60 mm Hg
- Increased brain volume:
  - Space-occupying masses (e.g., hematomas, abscesses, tumors, aneurysms, emboli, arteriovenous malformations, and parasites)
  - Cerebral edemas (e.g., head trauma or Reye's syndrome)
- Increased CSF volume:
  - Increased production of CSF (e.g., tumor of the choroid plexus)
  - Decreased absorption of CSF (e.g., communicating hydrocephalus and subarachnoid hemorrhage)
  - Obstruction to flow of CSF (e.g., communicating hydrocephalus, subarachnoid hemorrhage, and tumor)
- Increased blood volume:

VI

- Obstruction of venous outflow (e.g., positioning that increases intrathoracic and intraabdominal pressure)
- Hyperemia
- Hypercapnia or hypoxia
- Seizures
- Hyperthermia

DIAGNOSIS

■ Differential Nursing Diagnosis

There are two nursing diagnoses that are closely related to Decreased Adaptive Capacity: Intracranial: Fluid Volume Excess and Altered Tissue Perfusion: Cerebral. Fluid Volume Excess is a state in which an individual experiences an increase of fluid retention and edema. This diagnosis is different from Decreased Adaptive Capacity: Intracranial in that the former tends to refer to Fluid Volume Excess outside of the cranium. Autoregulation keeps cerebral perfusion relatively constant, and the blood-brain barrier is selective in allowing substances to cross into the brain. Thus Fluid Volume Excess does not generally refer to the inside of the cranium.

The second closely related nursing diagnosis is Altered Tissue Perfusion: Cerebral. Cerebral blood flow is just one of three fluctuating volumes that may result in ICP elevations. Moreover, Altered Tissue Perfusion does not necessarily reflect problems primarily managed by independent nursing therapies. Nurses can independently design interventions that decrease the adaptive demands or increase the adaptive capacity in the intracranial system.[8]

■ Medical and Psychiatric Diagnoses

There are many medical diagnoses commonly related to Decreased Adaptive Capacity: Intracranial. Medical diagnoses can be grouped into conditions that increase brain volume, CSF volume, and blood volume. The related factors for this nursing diagnosis include medical conditions related to specific medical diagnoses that could result in Decreased Adaptive Capacity: Intracranial.

OUTCOME IDENTIFICATION, PLANNING, AND IMPLEMENTATION

The specific nursing interventions for patients with Decreased Adaptive Capacity: Intracranial depend on the degree of neurological impairment, but the desired patient outcomes are the same. There are three general outcomes: (1) There will be normal intracranial fluid dynamic mechanisms; (2) factors known to increase ICP will be avoided; and (3) the patient or significant other will state symptoms of increased ICP and employ preventive measures.

Intracranial fluid dynamics can be assessed through an ICP monitor, and interventions can be planned accordingly. Remember that pediatric and elderly populations have lower ICP values. If the patient does not have an ICP monitor, the nurse needs to rely on neurological assessment skills to detect an increase in ICP. The nurse should collaborate with the physician regarding interventions, such as medication administration, to assist the patient in increasing adaptive capacity.

The second outcome focuses on avoiding factors known to increase ICP. If the patient is not attached to an ICP monitor, the nurse needs to assist the patient in avoiding any factors known to increase ICP. The ICP monitor provides the luxury of alerting the nurse as to which noxious and non-noxious stimuli increase ICP in each individual patient. Measures should be employed to maintain oxygenation, maintain proper positioning, prevent Valsalva's maneuver and isometric exercises, limit noxious stimuli, provide frequent rest periods, and prevent hyperthermia and seizures.

The third patient outcome focuses on patient teaching, which begins upon admission. The patient should be taught signs and symptoms of increased ICP as well as measures to prevent ICP. The patient can be observed for compliance in using preventive measures. If the patient cannot comprehend the teaching instructions because of age or decreased neurological status, a significant other can attain this expected outcome.

■ **NURSING CARE GUIDELINES**

Nursing Diagnosis: Decreased Adaptive Capacity: Intracranial

Expected Outcome: The patient will have normal intracranial fluid dynamic mechanisms as evidenced by an intact neurological system, an ICP of 0 to 15 mm Hg, a cerebral perfusion pressure of 60 to 90 mm Hg, normal ICP waveforms, and a CO_2 level less than 45 mm Hg by the time of discharge.

- Monitor neurological status. *Change in level of consciousness is usually the first sign of increased ICP. Changes in vision, motor, and sensory responses, speech, and memory are early signs and symptoms of increased ICP.*
- Measure blood pressure and ICP. *The cerebral perfusion pressure can be calculated by using these measurements. Without normal ranges of blood pressure, ICP, and cerebral perfusion pressure, autoregulation will fail, resulting in increased ICP.*
- Monitor ICP waveforms for elevated P_2 and plateau values. *P_2 elevation is indicative of loss of compliance and compensation. Plateau waves are indicative of compromised cerebral perfusion pressure, which may result in severe cerebral hypoxia and herniation.*
- Monitor CO_2 levels. *Hypercapnia causes vasodilation of cerebral vessels, increasing cerebral blood volume, and thus ICP.*
- Assess for complaints of increased headache, especially in the morning, and nausea and vomiting. *REM sleep, which most often occurs in the morning, increases metabolism, which, in turn, increases cerebral blood flow and ICP. Headache, nausea, and vomiting may be early signs of increased ICP.*
- ▲ Notify the physician regarding any changes in neurological status, abnormal ICP waveforms, and abnormal ICP, cerebral perfusion pressure, and CO_2 values. *Early intervention can prevent secondary brain injury and improve prognosis.*
- ▲ Administer osmotic diuretics, steroids, anticonvulsants, stool softeners, and antipyretics as ordered or needed. *These medications help control increased ICP.*

Expected Outcome: The patient will be assisted in avoiding factors known to increase ICP as evidenced by an ICP greater than 15 mm Hg for less than 5 minutes following exposure to noxious and nonnoxious stimuli until discharge.

- Maintain oxygenation: Maintain a patent airway, assess respiratory depth and pattern, monitor arterial blood gases, limit suction time to 10 to 15 seconds, and hyperoxygenate before and after suctioning. *Hypoxia may further contribute to cerebral ischemia. Hypercapnia leads to increased cerebral blood volume, resulting in increased ICP.*
- Maintain proper positioning: Maintain the patient's head and neck in a neutral position, elevate head of bed to a minimum of 30°, avoid extreme hip flexion, prone position, and Trendelenburg position. *Proper positioning assists in maintaining venous outflow from the cranium.*
- Prevent Vasalva's maneuver and isometric exercises: Prevent initiation of Vasalva's maneuver, cough, gag, vomiting, and sneezing; monitor bowel movements to avoid constipation or impaction; minimize activities that stimulate posturing activities; instruct patient to exhale when turning or moving in bed; and "logroll" the patient. *These activities may increase intrathoracic or intraabdominal pressure, which can obstruct cerebral venous outflow, increasing cerebral blood volume and ICP.*
- ▲ Limit noxious stimuli: Monitor ICP for elevations following nursing care activities and medical therapies, and adjust care as needed. *Unpleasant or painful stimuli increase ICP by activating the sympathetic nervous system, which increases cerebral blood flow and ICP.*
- Provide frequent rest periods: Allow at least 10 minutes' rest between activities. *Spacing activities close together can have a cumulative effect on ICP.*

■ = nursing intervention; ▲ = collaborative intervention.

Continued

VI

◢ **Nursing Care Guidelines — cont'd**

▲ Prevent hyperthermia: Adjust room temperature and patient covering as needed; monitor temperature, and administer antipyretics and cooling blanket as ordered. *Hyperthermia increases ICP by elevating the brain's metabolic rate, which increases cerebral blood volume and ICP.*

▲ Prevent seizures. *Seizures increase cerebral metabolism and may raise intrathoracic pressure, each of which increases cerebral blood volume and ICP.*

Expected Outcome: The patient or significant other will state five signs and symptoms that may be experienced with increased ICP, state three measures to prevent increased ICP, and demonstrate understanding by compliance by the time of discharge.

■ Assess the patient's or significant other's level of knowledge regarding the patient's condition. *Teaching strategies can be determined based on level of understanding.*

■ Discuss with the patient or significant other signs and symptoms that may be experienced with increased ICP (e.g., increased irritability, blurred vision, and weakness). *Signs and symptoms must be identified so that the health care team can be notified and provide early intervention.*

■ Discuss with the patient or significant other measures to prevent increased ICP (e.g., proper positioning, isotonic exercises, and normothermia). (See the interventions listed in the previous expected outcome.) *Measures to prevent increased ICP need to be instituted at home as well as the hospital setting.*

■ Encourage the patient or significant other to demonstrate measures to prevent increased ICP. *By observing the patient demonstrate measures, the nurse can verify that learning has occurred.*

▲ Encourage the patient or significant other to notify the health care team if signs and symptoms indicative of increased ICP are noted. *Early intervention can prevent secondary brain injury and improve prognosis.*

EVALUATION

The first indicator of the effectiveness of nursing interventions, and therefore the attainment of expected patient outcomes, is normal intracranial fluid dynamic mechanisms. This can be determined by an intact neurological system; normal ICP, cerebral perfusion pressure, and CO_2 values; and normal ICP waveforms. However, an intact neurological system as a patient outcome may not be realistic if there is secondary brain injury. The outcome would be changed to reflect the highest level of neurological functioning possible. This outcome should be achieved by the time of discharge.

A second important indicator of the effectiveness of nursing interventions is that factors known to increase ICP need to be avoided. If the increase in ICP is less than 5 minutes in duration, following noxious and nonnoxious stimuli, the patient has achieved intracranial adaptive capacity. Ideally, the achievement of this expected outcome will be continuous during the time nursing care is being provided and after the patient is discharged. If this outcome is not achieved, the nurse needs to reassess implementation of nursing care activities and the patient's or significant other's level of understanding of preventive measures.

A third indicator that patients have achieved expected outcomes is that they can state the signs, symptoms, and measures to prevent increased ICP. The patient or significant other should be observed for demonstrating measures to prevent increased ICP before patient discharge. If this outcome is not achieved, the nurse needs to evaluate teaching methods and the patient's or significant other's level of understanding.

▶ CASE STUDY WITH PLAN OF CARE

Mr. John K., age 68 years, is a white, retired accountant. He has been married for 45 years and has five adult children who live nearby. Mr. K. spends most of his free time golfing. Approximately 6 months ago he had a generalized tonic-clonic seizure on the fifth fairway. MRI revealed a glioblastoma of the right temporal-parietal area. After surgical resection and several chemotherapy and radiation treatments, a subsequent MRI showed no tumor regrowth.

While computing his children's taxes, he noticed a decrease in ability to concentrate. He did not mention this to his wife for fear of upsetting her. Approximately 1 week ago, he had a follow-up MRI, which revealed tumor regrowth. He was then admitted to the hospital for surgical resection of his tumor. Upon admission, the only significant findings on his neurological assessment were his decreased ability to concentrate and his history of one seizure, which has been controlled with Tegretol monotherapy.

The nursing assessment of Mr. K. on his third day after surgery reveals drowsiness, mild weakness of the left arm and leg, pupils unequal in size, with the left = 5 mm and the right = 7 mm, right pupillary reaction sluggish to light stimulus, and complaints of headache.

▶ PLAN OF CARE FOR MR. JOHN K.

Nursing Diagnosis: Decreased Adaptive Capacity: Intracranial Related to Abnormal Intracranial Fluid Dynamic Mechanisms

VI

Expected Outcome: Mr. K. will have normal intracranial fluid dynamic mechanisms as evidenced by an intact neurological system by the time of discharge.
- ▲ Notify the physician immediately regarding any change in neurological status.
- ▪ Monitor neurological status every 2 hours until it returns to baseline level.
- ▪ Assess for complaints of increased headache every 2 hours.
- ▲ Notify the physician if neurological status worsens.
- ▲ Administer osmotic diuretics, steroids, Tegretol, stool softeners, and antipyretics as ordered or needed.

Expected Outcome: Mr. K. will be assisted in avoiding factors known to increase ICP until he is discharged.
- ▪ Assess respiratory depth and pattern every 4 hours.
- ▪ Maintain Mr. K.'s head and neck in a neutral position; elevate head of bed to a minimum of 30°; avoid extreme hip flexion, the prone position, and the Trendelenburg position.
- ▪ Prevent initiation of Vasalva's maneuver.
- ▪ Monitor bowel movements every day for frequency and consistency.
- ▪ Instruct Mr. K. to exhale when turning over or moving in bed.
- ▪ Limit visiting hours of Mr. K.'s wife and five children to 30 minutes at a time.
- ▪ Plan activities of daily living spaced by regular intervals.
- ▲ Observe for seizure activity and administer Tegretol as ordered.

Expected Outcome: Mr. K. and his wife will state five signs and symptoms that may be experienced with increased ICP, will describe three measures to prevent increased ICP, and will demonstrate their understanding of these measures by putting them to use by the time of Mr. K.'s discharge.
- ▪ Assess Mr. K. and his wife's level of knowledge regarding the potential for increased ICP because of his brain tumor.
- ▪ Discuss with Mr. K. and his wife signs and symptoms that may be experienced with increased ICP.
- ▪ Provide Mr. K. and his wife with a written list of signs and symptoms of increased ICP.
- ▪ Discuss with Mr. K. and his wife measures to prevent increased ICP.

▪ = nursing intervention; ▲ = collaborative intervention.

Continued

PLAN OF CARE FOR MR. JOHN K. — CONT'D

- Provide Mr. K. and his wife a written list of measures to prevent increased ICP.
- Observe Mr. K. and his wife for compliance with preventative measures while in the hospital.
- ▲ Reinforce the importance of notifying the health care team if signs and symptoms indicative of increased ICP are noted.

CRITICAL THINKING EXERCISES

1. Is Mr. K.'s expected outcome—having an intact neurological system by the time of discharge—realistic?
2. Mr. K.'s condition worsens and he is transferred to the neurological ICU for ICP monitoring. Would your assessment, outcomes, planning, and interventions be different if you were the ICU nurse taking care of Mr. K.?
3. What would you do differently if Mr. K.'s wife was deceased, if he had no children, and if he could not comprehend the patient teaching by the time of his discharge?

VI

REFERENCES

1. Andrus C: Intracranial pressure: dynamics and nursing management, *J Neurosci Nurs* 23(2):85–92, 1991.
2. Barker E: Avoiding increased intracranial pressure, *Nursing* 20(5):64Q–64RR, 1990.
3. Doyle D and Mark P: Analysis of intracranial pressure, *J Clin Monitoring* 8(1):81–90, 1992.
4. Drummond B: Preventing increased intracranial pressure: nursing care can make the difference, *Focus Crit Care* 17(2):116–122, 1990.
5. Luchka S: Working with ICP monitors, *RN* 54(4):34–37, 1991.
6. North American Nursing Diagnosis Association: *NANDA nursing diagnoses: definitions and classification, 1995–1996,* Philadelphia, 1994, The Association.
7. Pickard J and Czosnyka M: Management of raised intracranial pressure, *J Neurolog Neurosurg Psychiatry* 56(8):845–858, 1993.
8. Rauch M, Mitchell P, and Tyler M: Validation of risk factors for the nursing diagnosis decreased intracranial adaptive capacity, *J Neurosci Nurs* 22(3):173–178, 1990.
9. Treloar D and others: The effect of familiar and unfamiliar voice treatments on intracranial pressure in head-injured patients, *J Neurosci Nurs* 23(5):295–299, 1991.
10. Vos H: Making headway with intracranial hypertension, *Am J Nurs* 93(2):28–39, 1993.

Acute Confusion

▶

Acute Confusion *is the abrupt onset of a cluster of global, transient changes and disturbances in attention, cognition, psychomotor activity, level of consciousness, or sleep-wake cycle.*[20]

OVERVIEW

The nursing diagnosis Acute Confusion refers to an acute, abrupt condition commonly associated with the mental disorder delirium. *Delirium* is described as "a transient, usually reversible dysfunction in cerebral metabolism that has an acute or subacute onset and is manifest clinically by a wide array of neuropsychiatric abnormalities"[28] (p. 312). Identification of the nursing diagnosis Acute Confusion does not depend on confirmation of the diagnosis of delirium. In fact, the nursing diagnosis Acute Confusion may contribute to the recognition of the presence of delirium.

The term *confusion* has often been used inconsistently and ambiguously in nursing and medicine to describe and discuss behaviors that are of an acute and chronic nature.[7,14,18] *Confusion* has been used interchangeably to describe acute behavioral changes characteristic of delirium and behavioral features associated with dementia, another mental disorder.[14,22] The term *Acute Confusion* is used by nurse and physician authors to denote the syndrome of delirium.[2,4,14,19] Acute Confusion is frequently discussed within the context of the elderly population, who often experience undetected brief episodes of delirium.[2] Many authors recognize the frequency of Acute Confusion in the critical care setting, especially in patients who have had cardiovascular surgery.[2,14,19,25,28] Acute Confusion (delirium) is one of the most frequently occurring postoperative complications that occur in the elderly population.[4]

The nursing diagnosis Acute Confusion refers to an acute, abrupt process that is very different from the chronic onset of confusion, which is more characteristically associated with dementia. However, a demented patient with the nursing diagnosis of Chronic Confusion can also become delirious and have the additional diagnosis of Acute Confusion.

The onset of Acute Confusion is indicative of an underlying and potentially catastrophic medical illness that can become life threatening if it is unrecognized and inappropriately treated.[5,14] Abrupt changes in attention, concentration, and orientation signal the onset of Acute Confusion. Literature that addresses Acute Confusion and delirium has focused primarily on the geriatric population.[*] There is a high prevalence of Acute Confusion in the elderly with little factual information about the prevalence of Acute Confusion in children.[14,23,28] Children with a febrile illness or an anticholinergic toxicity can experience Acute Confusion.[1,12] The onset of Acute Confusion in an elderly patient may be the first indication of a previously undetected urinary tract infection or an undiagnosed pneumonia or sepsis.[14,18]

Fluctuations in attention, concentration, levels of alertness, and levels of consciousness are common manifestations of Acute Confusion in patients who have had open-heart surgery.[17] The term *ICU psychosis* is sometimes used to explain acute mental status changes in a critical care setting. The term is inaccurate and misleading, how-

---

[*]References 4, 5, 8, 9, 14, 18, 23.

ever, because it oversimplifies the potential seriousness of the patient's condition by implying that the precipitant is the environment. This limited perspective (ICU psychosis) often results in the lack of searching for the underlying cause(s) of the Acute Confusion and can lead to unnecessary and inappropriate pharmacological management.[19,28] For example, a patient with Acute Confusion who is misdiagnosed with depression may have an antidepressant medication prescribed without an ongoing search for the actual underlying cause of the changes in mental status (e.g., an undetected infection or drug toxicity). The patient with Acute Confusion whose symptoms include anxiety and agitation may be prescribed a long-acting benzodiazepine, such as diazepam (Valium), without further searching for the underlying cause(s). Inappropriate administration of antidepressant and antianxiety drugs (e.g., benzodiazepines) can worsen the underlying confusion and lead to further delay in detecting the actual causes of the confusion, which are usually multifactorial.[5,14,18]

ASSESSMENT

Assessment of the patient's mental status at the time of admission should include a baseline cognitive assessment. Collateral data from family and all care providers can provide additional data regarding the patient's usual cognitive functioning.[8,13] The identification of existing cognitive deficits at the time of admission provides a baseline for comparison if the patient appears to become increasingly confused at a later time.[4,19,25] A cognitive assessment of the elderly patient at the time of admission can also facilitate the early detection of Acute Confusion. Tools such as the Mini-Mental State Examination[6] or the Short Portable Mental Status Questionnaire[21] can be used for formal assessment of cognitive functioning.

Any medical condition that affects brain function (e.g., infection), metabolic encephalopathies (hypoglycemia, dehydration, or vitamin deficiency), myocardial infarction, and substance intoxication

or withdrawal can result in Acute Confusion.[18,25] Recognize that abrupt mental status changes from the patient's usual patterns are indicative of Acute Confusion. Rapid development and fluctuations of symptoms are common. The patient with Acute Confusion may be awake and conversant one moment and then abruptly become unable to complete a sentence in an ongoing conversation. Documentation of changes is important so that health care providers can have an accurate description of the variable and intermittent changes that occur within minutes to hours of each other.[18,23]

Review laboratory data to assess for early signs of organ failure, urinary tract infection, fluid and electrolyte disturbances, decreased oxygen saturation, and toxicity from alcohol, street drugs, or prescribed medications.

Drug toxicity from over-the-counter and prescribed drugs is a common precipitating factor for Acute Confusion, especially in the elderly. It is important to inquire about the patient's use of over-the-counter medications and to review the patient's pharmacy profile, checking to see if a new medication has been prescribed. Assess the patient's response to prescribed medications, and assess for early signs of drug toxicity, especially if psychotropic medications, digoxin, phenytoin, and opioid analgesics are being prescribed. Age-related changes leave the elderly at greater risk for drug toxicity from commonly prescribed drugs.[13,14,27,28] Monitor therapeutic drug levels to determine if they are within acceptable therapeutic limits.

Recognize the probability of Acute Confusion occurring in a patient whose behavior changes from alert, awake, and able to meet self-care needs to hypoactive, less motivated, or somnolent.[14,25] Conduct an informal or formal cognitive assessment that includes the patient's orientation to time, place, and person; ability to attend and concentrate; and accuracy when learning new information (repeating three unrelated words and asking the patient to repeat these words again in 3 to 5 minutes) to help to confirm the presence of Acute Confusion.[13] Consistency of testing—all staff using the same or similar questions—helps to establish ongoing baseline data for comparison of findings to verify accuracy of assessment and for monitoring improvement of confusion.

Observe for the presence of disorganized thinking and patterns of rambling and irrelevant conversation, with abrupt shifting from one topic to another. Is the patient easily distracted? Does the patient have difficulty focusing on conversation or the task at hand?[16,18]

Observe for the postoperative patient's ability to participate in activities such as using the incentive spirometer or initiating coughing and deep breathing after being taught and encouraged to do so.

Assess sleep-wake cycle patterns, recognizing that daytime sleeping and nighttime wakefulness are features of Acute Confusion.[14]

Because the elderly have less functional reserve for tolerating physiological insults, decreased resistance to infection, and increased likelihood to have chronic medical conditions, they are at increased risk for Acute Confusion. Assess for localized infection, elevated body temperature, untreated pain (especially in the demented elderly), injury from undetected falls, urinary retention, or bowel impaction.

Is the patient dehydrated? Is inadequate oxygenation a problem? Are there indications of increased intracranial pressure? Assess for increased autonomic hyperactivity associated with alcohol or drug withdrawal reactions.[3,13,14]

Assess for environmental stressors (e.g., excessive noise from TV, equipment, or staff interactions) that can intensify existing Acute Confusion.

■ Defining Characteristics

The presence of the following defining characteristics° indicates that the patient may be experiencing Acute Confusion:

- Abrupt onset of disturbance and fluctuations in level of consciousness
- Fluctuations in cognition
  - Orientation (time, place, person, and date)

°References 1, 7, 8, 14, 16, 18, 20, 23, 28.

- Attention (hypoalert or hyperalert)
- Concentration (ability to shift, focus, and maintain attention)
- Memory (primarily recent memory)
- Language disturbance, such as *dysnomia* (impaired ability to name objects) or *dysgraphia* (impaired ability to write)
- Fluctuations in sleep-wake cycle (daytime drowsiness and napping and/or insomnia at night)
- Fluctuations in psychomotor activity (hypoactivity or hyperactivity)
- Increased agitation or restlessness
- Fluctuations in emotional responses, such as anxiety, fear, anger, and apathy
- Misperceptions, usually visual, with illusions occurring more often than hallucinations
- Lack of motivation to initiate or follow through with goal-directed or purposeful behavior
- Inability to follow directions
- Exacerbation of cognitive deficits at night

■ Related Factors

The following related factors are associated with Acute Confusion:

Precipitating factors[8,14,18,23,28]

- All infections: systemic (e.g., pneumonia, subacute bacterial endocarditis, and septicemia); intracranial (e.g., bacterial meningitis and viral encephalitis)
- Intoxication from medically prescribed drugs (e.g., anticholinergics, cardiac drugs, antihypertensives, antidepressants, antiparkinsonian agents, benzodiazepines, opioids); specific additional drugs include lithium and disulfiram
- Intoxication from illicit drugs (e.g., cocaine, amphetamines), alcohol, or addictive inhalants
- Intoxication from industrial, animal, or plant poisons
- Drug withdrawal (e.g., from alcohol, sedatives, or hypnotics)
- Metabolic abnormalities (e.g., electrolyte and fluid imbalances, hyperglycemia or hypoglycemia, renal insufficiency, severe vitamin deficiency, or malnutrition)

VI

- Cardiopulmonary conditions (e.g., myocardial infarction, congestive heart failure, pulmonary embolus, and hypoxia from any cardiopulmonary condition, including chronic obstructive pulmonary disease [COPD])
- Cerebral vascular disorders (e.g., transient ischemic attacks or subarachnoid hemorrhage)
- Other medical conditions (e.g., extracranial or intracranial neoplasms, severe anemia, or head trauma)

Facilitating factors[14]

- Bereavement
- Rapid, unplanned relocation to an unfamiliar environment
- Sensory deprivation
- Sensory overload
- Immobilization
- Sleep loss and deprivation

Predisposing factors[14,23,28]

- Age over 60
- Dementia
- HIV or AIDS
- History of brain damage
- Hepatic or renal dysfunction
- Recent surgical procedure, such as postcardiotomy
- Trauma from burns or hip fracture
- Substance abuse or dependence

DIAGNOSIS

▪ Differential Nursing Diagnosis

Nursing diagnoses such as Anxiety, Sensory Perceptual Alterations, Sleep Pattern Disturbance, Ineffective Individual Coping, Noncompliance, and Risk for Injury are inadequate identifications of the phenomenon that the patient is experiencing. These nursing diagnoses do not take into consideration the comprehensive aspects of the patient's response to the underlying medical condition that results in Acute Confusion. Symptoms of Acute Confusion often include anxiety and visual illusions or hallucinations. Daytime somnolence and nighttime wakefulness are indicative of Acute Confusion. Global cerebral dysfunction in the delirious patient can compromise the patient's ability to process and retain information necessary for meeting self-care and learning needs. The lack of participation in goal-directed activities is not volitional. Ineffective Individual Coping and Noncompliance are inappropriate and inaccurate diagnoses at any time for the patient who is delirious. Patients in critical care units who express the wish to die, who pull out IV tubes, and who strike out at staff should be assessed for the diagnosis Acute Confusion.

▪ Medical and Psychiatric Diagnoses

The nursing diagnosis Acute Confusion falls within the diagnostic category of delirium in the American Psychiatric Association's *Diagnostical and Statistical Manual.*[1] Specific subcategories of delirium include delirium due to a general medical condition, substance-induced delirium (intoxication or withdrawal), delirium due to multiple etiologies, and delirium not otherwise specified.[1] Delirium sometimes "mimics" other mental disorders, such as mood disorders (major depressive disorder and bipolar I).[13,14,25] Although the DSM IV diagnostic category of dementia is a risk factor for delirium under certain conditions (e.g., infection or medication toxicity), it is not at all synonymous with delirium. Although a patient who is delirious may have the coexisting diagnosis of dementia, it is critical to recognize that delirium and dementia are two *very* distinct phenomena in terms of their onset, course, and ultimate outcome.[18,25]

OUTCOME IDENTIFICATION, PLANNING, AND IMPLEMENTATION

Nursing interventions for patients with Acute Confusion focus on early and ongoing assessment for contributing risk factors and underlying disease and on early referrals to the medical team for prompt treatment of undiagnosed disorders or iatrogenic conditions.[13,18,25] Early detection of Acute Confusion facilitates prompt and appropriate medical treatment, decreases potential for irreversible brain damage, decreases comorbidities from falls or other self-injury, minimizes the need for restraints, reduces the acuity of nursing care, and is associated with a shorter length of hospital stay, with lower costs.[13] Because Acute Confusion is a fluctuating condition, documentation, feedback, and collaboration from all members of the health care team provide invaluable data about a patient's mental status and usual level of functioning in the community setting as well as in the hospital. Maintaining patient comfort during the time of Acute Confusion may require the use of opioid analgesia, which can worsen the existing confusion. Determining the appropriate dosage can be difficult.[23] Nursing management includes collaboration with the patient's physician and other health care personnel in assessing and managing pain. Patient and family education about what is happening during the time of Acute Confusion and what to expect as the patient recovers from Acute Confusion helps to decrease patient and family anxiety. Patient and family education to enable them to recognize the risk factors and behaviors indicative of the onset of Acute Confusion is a proactive approach that can sometimes prevent the occurrence of Acute Confusion or reduce its severity through early detection. The extent of information provided to the patient and family is based on individual patient and family assessment.[11,16,27]

◢ NURSING CARE GUIDELINES
Nursing Diagnosis: Acute Confusion°

Expected Outcome: The patient will experience no injury to self or others in the environment.
- Observe the patient closely *to reduce risk of injury from falls, extubation, and removal of intravenous lines.*
- Provide adequate staff to be with patient (one-to-one if necessary); place patient close to the nurses' station whenever possible *to ensure close monitoring and to facilitate close observation.*
- Have family member remain with patient (as appropriate) *to increase patient's perception of trust and safety in current environment and to reduce need for restraints. Use of restraints in the patient with Acute Confusion can increase agitation and fear and increase the possibility of deep vein thrombosis and pulmonary embolism.*
- Conceal hospital equipment from patient's direct view *to decrease the likelihood of patient's pulling out lines and disconnecting equipment and to minimize the need for restraints.*
- ▲ Collaborate with the patient's physician to determine need for pharmacological intervention *for ongoing agitation, such as the patient attempting to leave the treatment setting or making verbal threats or threatening overtures to other patients.*

Expected Outcome: The patient will experience increased ability to concentrate and attend to environmental stimuli.
- Assess cognitive functioning at scheduled and unscheduled intervals (checking orientation, attention, and concentration, memory, and thought processes), using informal questions while providing routine care or using standardized mental status assessment tools, such as the Short Portable Mental Status Questionnaire or the Mini-Mental State Examination *to monitor fluctuations in mental status.*
- Reorient patient frequently to date, time of day, surroundings, circumstances for being hospitalized, and names of care providers *because of fluctuations in orientation and short-term memory. Repeating information will assist reality testing.*
- Use large signs on the wall and calendars to inform the patient of location, date, and day of week. Use simple written cues whenever appropriate (e.g., "Use call light to reach nurse; do not get out of bed alone"). *Simple visual cues are necessary because of impaired short-term memory and disorientation.*

■ = nursing intervention; ▲ = collaborative intervention.
°References 2, 8, 10, 11, 13, 18, 20, 21, 23–27.

Continued

◢ **NURSING CARE GUIDELINES — CONT'D**

- Modify environment *to reduce stressors that may increase incidence of misperceptions (e.g., unnecessary equipment or furniture that creates shadows on the wall).*
- Make patient's sensory aides (e.g., glasses or hearing aids) readily available *to reduce misperceptions, visual distortions, and anxiety.*

Expected Outcome: The patient will experience a return of normal sleep-wake patterns.
- Monitor patient for sleep cycle disturbance that includes sleep deprivation *to assess need for environmental interventions.*
- ▲ Collaborate with treatment team in implementation of specific environmental interventions, such as mimicking natural light-dark cycles by having blinds open during the day and closed at night, *to promote normal sleep-wake cycle.*
- Establish a daily schedule for the patient with adequate rest periods *to decrease overstimulation and fatigue and to promote regularity in sleep-wake patterns;* discourage daytime naps.
- ▲ Collaborate with patient and family about usual rituals or activities that patient uses for satisfactory sleep (e.g., soft music and routine hygiene activities) *to minimize need for pharmacological intervention for sleep promotion.*

Expected Outcome: The patient will meet self-care needs to the full extent possible.
- Use simple, short, concrete communication with the patient, including one-step commands, *because patient's ability to concentrate, think abstractly, and recall recent events is impaired.*
- Have patient do as much as possible for self, beginning with hygiene, grooming, and bathing; assist patient as necessary for completion of these activities. Avoid attempting to rush or hurry patient to complete activities. *The patient's compromised medical condition and compromised mental status can affect the ability to participate in or to complete self-care activities.*
- ▲ Collaborate with treatment team to postpone specific patient teaching until any mental status changes have cleared *because the patient's ability to concentrate and attend to new information is limited.*

Expected Outcome: The patient and family will experience decreased anxiety and distress from patient's mental status changes.
- Encourage the family to acknowledge their fears and concerns about patient's condition *to determine appropriate interventions to decrease their anxiety.*
- Teach the family and patient about the transitory nature of the patient's condition *to reduce their initial anxiety;* explain that total clearing of the Acute Confusion may take several days to several weeks *to reduce their uncertainty about its outcome.*
- Encourage the family to maintain ongoing and regular contact with the patient *to help reorient patient, to provide supportive reassurance, and to decrease patient's fears.*
- Determine the need for patient and family debriefing after Acute Confusion has cleared *to reduce possible unnecessary fears and anxiety they may harbor about what happened and to clarify possible distortions that the patient may have of events that occurred during the period of Acute Confusion.*
- Develop a discharge plan that informs other health care providers, the patient, and the family about the patient's recent episode of Acute Confusion *to promote early identification of recurrence of Acute Confusion and to alert them to possible residual effects the patient may still be experiencing.*

EVALUATION

In Acute Confusion, resumption of normal mental status and baseline cognitive functioning should return within hours to weeks after underlying medical conditions are identified and treated. Supportive nursing care includes environmental monitoring for risk factors and assessing mental status every shift to facilitate early detection and prompt treatment of medical problems. A reduction in the severity and duration of symptoms can reduce the potential for physical injury.

Evaluate the patient's ability to remember information and to respond appropriately to his or her environment. Is the patient continuing to experience sensory misinterpretations that leave the patient frightened and mistrustful? Is the patient able to readily orient him- or herself?

Achievement of a satisfactory sleep pattern is an indicator that the episode of Acute Confusion is resolving. Is the patient experiencing normal sleep-wake patterns?

Has the patient returned to a baseline ability to meet self-care needs? If not, continue to evaluate the influence of the patient's medical condition as well as mental status changes on limitations in self-care. Do not assume that lack of satisfactory participation and follow-through is volitional.

Are the patient and family continuing to experience significant anxiety and distress because of the patient's Acute Confusion? If so, continue to encourage them to talk about their fears and concerns, and provide them with appropriate information and explanations about the patient's current status and progress.

Despite attempts to conduct a thorough and comprehensive workup to determine the cause(s) of Acute Confusion, there are times when the underlying causes for the mental status changes are not found. The patient may continue to have a prolonged period of Acute Confusion. Supportive nursing interventions and supportive medical management are important to avoid further potentiation of the existing confusion.

▶ CASE STUDY WITH PLAN OF CARE

Mr. Joe T. is a 61-year-old single patient who sustained a right femur fracture and mild, closed head injury from a motorcycle accident. His blood alcohol level at the time of admission was .225. He has been hospitalized on a trauma/orthopedic floor for 2 days following repair of the right femur fracture. Mr. T. complains of inability to sleep as well as discomfort from leg traction and immobilization. PRN opioid analgesics have been ineffective. Nursing assessment findings indicate that Mr. T. is disoriented, anxious, restless, and mildly tremulous; yells inappropriately; is exposing himself and masturbating; and is attempting to remove one of his intravenous lines.

▶ PLAN OF CARE FOR MR. JOE T.
Nursing Diagnosis: Acute Confusion Related to Closed Head Injury, Alcohol Withdrawal, Surgical Pain, and Immobilization

---

Expected Outcome: Mr. T. will experience no injury to self.
- Maintain a safe environment by ensuring that bed rails are up; use soft waist restraint as circumstances require (prn).
- Conceal IV lines.
- Use soft hand and/or soft waist-restraint prn if patient persists in attempting to remove IV lines.
- Monitor patient for signs of alcohol withdrawal.
▲ Notify physician if findings are indicative of need for alcohol withdrawal protocol.

■ = nursing intervention; ▲ = collaborative intervention.

Continued

▶ **PLAN OF CARE FOR MR. JOE T. — CONT'D**

Expected Outcome: Mr. T. will show decreased restlessness and agitation.
- Monitor for signs of increased intracranial pressure.
- ▲ Based on findings, collaborate with the physician to determine need for head computerized tomography (CT) to rule out intracranial bleeding.
- Provide a low-stimulation environment that includes frequent rest periods.
- Assess patient's response to pain medication, recognizing that the patient may be unable to request medication reliably when experiencing pain.
- Offer prn analgesic at regular, scheduled intervals.
- ▲ Collaborate with physician to determine when timing is appropriate to change from opioid to nonopioid analgesic.

Expected Outcome: Mr. T. will experience improved orientation and reality testing.
- Provide ongoing reorientation that includes reminder of patient's location and circumstances for hospitalization.
- ▲ Have staff introduce themselves by name during each contact with patient.
- Use visible cues for orientation (e.g., clocks, signs, and calendars).
- Remove unnecessary equipment and furniture that could create "frightening" shadows on the wall.

Expected Outcome: Mr. T. will show improved sleep-awake patterns.
- ▲ Collaborate with health care team to schedule times for uninterrupted rest periods.
- Maintain light-dark cycles by opening curtains in the day and keeping lights on and by darkening the room at night.
- Control noise level and flow of staff and visitors interacting with the patient.

■ **CRITICAL THINKING EXERCISES**

1. List common precipitating factors for Acute Confusion in a hospitalized elderly patient.
2. Give examples of questions to ask Joe T. when evaluating his cognitive function.
3. Mr. Joe T. will be discharged to a skilled care facility for rehabilitation. Discuss discharge planning and teaching for Mr. T. and his future caregivers.

REFERENCES

1. American Psychiatric Association: *Diagnostical and statistical manual of mental disorders: DSM-IV*, ed 4, Washington, D.C., 1994, The Association.
2. Blazer D: Geriatric psychiatry. In Hales RE and Yudofsky SC, editors: *The American Psychiatric Press textbook of psychiatry*, ed 2, Washington, D.C., 1994, American Psychiatric Press.
3. Clark S: Psychiatric and mental health concerns in the patient with sepsis, *Crit Care Nurs Clin North Am* 6(2):389–403, 1994.
4. Evans CA, Kenney PJ, and Rizzuto C: Caring for the confused geriatric surgical patient, *Geriatr Nurs* 14(5):237–241, 1993.
5. Farrell KR and Ganzini L: Misdiagnosing delirium as depression in medically ill elderly patients, *Arch Int Med* 155:2459–2464, 1995.
6. Folstein MF and others: Mini-mental state: a practical guide for grading the cognitive state of patients for clinicians, *J Psychiatr Res* 12:189–198, 1975.
7. Foreman MD: Acute confusional states in hospitalized elderly: a research dilemma, *Nurs Res* 35(1):34–38, 1986.
8. Foreman MD: Confusion in the hospitalized elderly: incidence, onset, and associated factors, *Res Nurs Health* 12:21–29, 1989.
9. Foreman MD and Grabowski R: Diagnostic dilemma: cognitive impairment in the elderly, *J Geront Nurs* 18(9):5–12, 1992.
10. Geary SM: Intensive care unit psychosis revisited: understanding and managing delirium in the critical care setting, *Crit Care Nurs Q* 17(1):51–63, 1994.
11. Gerety EK: Acute confusion. In Kim MJ, McFarland GK, and McLane AL: *Pocket guide to nursing diagnoses*, ed 6, St. Louis, 1995, Mosby–Year Book.
12. Hamdan-Allen G and Nixon M: Anticholinergic psychosis in children: a case report, *Hosp Comm Psychiatry* 42(2):191–193, 1991.

13. Inaba-Roland KE and Maricle RA: Assessing delirium in the acute care setting, *Heart Lung* 21(1):48–55, 1992.

14. Lipowski ZJ: *Delirium: acute confusional states,* New York, 1990, Oxford University Press.

15. Matthiesen V and others: Acute confusion: nursing intervention in older patients, *Orthop Nurs* 13(2):21–29, 1994.

16. McFarland GK, Wasli EL, and Gerety EK: *Nursing diagnosis and process in psychiatric mental health nursing,* ed 2, Philadelphia, 1992, JB Lippincott Co.

17. Minarik PA: Cognitive assessment of the cardiovascular patient in the acute care setting, *J Cardiovasc Nurs* 9(4): 36–52, 1995.

18. Morency CR: Mental status change in the elderly: recognizing and treating delirium, *J Prof Nurs* 6(6):356–365, 1990.

19. Neelon VJ: Postoperative confusion, *Crit Care Nurs Clin North Am* 2(4):579, 1990.

20. North American Nursing Diagnosis Association: *NANDA nursing diagnoses: definitions and classification, 1995–1996,* Philadelphia, 1994, The Association.

21. Pfeiffer E: A short portable mental status questionnaire for the assessment of organic brain deficit in elderly patients, *J Am Geriatr Soc* 23:433–441, 1975.

22. Rasin JH: Confusion, *Nurs Clin North Am* 23(4):909–918, 1990.

23. Rummans TA and others: Delirium in elderly patients: evaluation and management, *Mayo Clin Proc* 70:989–998, 1995.

24. Stanley M: Ensuring a safe ICU stay for your confused elderly patient, *Dimen Crit Care Nurs* 10(2):62, 1991.

25. St. Pierre J: Delirium in hospitalized elderly patients: off track, *Crit Care Nurs Clin North Am* 8(1):53, 1996.

26. Sullivan-Marx EM: Delirium and physical restraint in the hospitalized elderly, *Image* 26(4):295, 1994.

27. Tune L and Ross C: Delirium. In Coffey CE and others, editors: *The American Psychiatric Press textbook of geriatric neuropsychiatry,* Washington, D.C., 1994, American Psychiatric Press.

28. Wise MG and Gray KF: Delirium, dementia, and amnestic disorders. In Hales RE, Yudofsky SC, and Talbott JA, editors: *The American Psychiatric Press textbook of psychiatry,* ed 2, Washington, D.C., 1994, American Psychiatric Press.

VI

Chronic Confusion

▶

Chronic Confusion *is an irreversible, long-standing, or progressive deterioration of intellect and personality characterized by decreased ability to interpret environmental stimuli and decreased capacity for intellectual thought processes, manifested by disturbances of memory, orientation, and behavior.*

OVERVIEW

States of chronic confusion, also referred to as dementia, are irreversible if they result from a degenerative type of cerebral pathology.[2,14,19] Elderly individuals experiencing such disease processes generally demonstrate a long and steady deterioration in functional and intellectual abilities as well as a kaleidoscope of behavioral changes. Dementia (Chronic Confusion) affects approximately 10% to 45% of the U.S. population over age 65; those who are 85 and older have a greater incidence of this diagnosis.[20] The cost of health care for individuals with dementia, associated with an extended length of hospital stay, is greater than normal and requires more resources to provide for the special care needs of this population.[17] Approaching care planning often requires the participation of a multidisciplinary team, with the nurse coordinating care to meet patient needs in a consistent and efficient manner.[7]

The individual labeled as confused often displays a behavioral inconsistency with the environment. The ability to respond to environmental stimuli, solve problems, and follow complex instructions is compromised. A confused patient often spends his or her time in a solitary activity, does nothing, or exhibits disruptive behavior that may include wandering, resisting care, and agitation. Many patients are unable to communicate their needs. The dementia patient requires increased time and supervision to provide for personal safety and well-being. Managing and providing care for these individuals can present an overwhelming challenge.[3,6,17,22]

ASSESSMENT

The initial assessment of each patient diagnosed with Chronic Confusion requires a comprehensive evaluation, which includes many factors, such as cognitive status, functional ability, and behavioral history. It is critical that the assessment be multifaceted, taking into account the individual's past and present functional abilities. Nursing interventions are selected by focusing on the individual patient's retained functional, cognitive, and emotional abilities. The process of gathering information about the patient with Chronic Confusion is often time-consuming and difficult. Observation and interaction with the patient will provide clues to the level of cognitive impairment. Ideally the patient would provide information for the interview. However, interaction with a person who has limited communication skills, memory, and insight may be difficult. A caregiver, if available, can provide information about the patient's ability and behavior. Additional information may be obtained from the medical record, other providers, family, and friends.

The assessment beings with observation of the patient. Elements of cognition can be determined by observing the patient's awareness and attention to the person and the environment, ability to follow commands, and ability to communicate. A more formal evaluation of cognitive status can be obtained by administering the Folstein Mini-Mental State Evaluation (MMSE). The instrument is useful for establishing a baseline and provides objective data to indicate acute or progressive change in cognitive status. It must be noted that the MMSE is educationally biased and may not be valid for patients with a limited education. It is also important to determine the patient's reading ability because the provision of simple written instructions or reminders may be a useful cuing technique in the intervention process.[11]

An evaluation of functional status will alert the clinician to issues of mobility and activities of daily living (ADL). Observation of the patient's gait, ambulation, and transfer skill during the initial interview will provide useful information. If there is a tendency for the patient to exhibit wandering behavior, an assessment of speed and endurance is essential. If the patient uses an assistive device, assessment of the device's safety and its use is necessary. Observation of personal hygiene may not reflect the patient's ability to complete self-care activities if there is a caregiver. Collaboration with rehabilitation therapists may be required to complete a comprehensive functional assessment.

Evaluating the historic behavior of the patient is critical to the comprehensive assessment. This information is usually obtained from a caregiver, family member, or friend. Establishing a cooperative relationship with the caregiver is essential to the care of the chronically confused individual. If there is no caregiver in place, an attempt should be made to access the patient's support network.[21] The assessment should include the patient's usual daily routine, sleep-wake pattern, activity preferences, response to overstimulation, and current living situation. Behavior problems often arise when the demented patient is placed in a situation in which the amount, complexity, or intensity of stimuli exceeds the individual's capacity to interpret.[18] The caregiver has usually developed an awareness of the subtle cues and situation that are precursors to aberrant behavior.[16] It is essential to note any change in social skills or personality.

Assessment of the patient's likes and dislikes, personal preferences, comfort items, and pleasurable activities gives a basis for the plan of care.

■ Defining Characteristics

The presence of the following characteristics indicates that the patient may be experiencing Chronic Confusion:

- Clinical evidence of organic impairment
- Progressive or long-standing cognitive impairment
- Altered interpretation of stimuli
- Altered response to stimuli
- No change in consciousness[4]
- Impaired memory (short-term or long-term)
- Impaired orientation to person, time, or place
- Impaired ability for abstraction and conceptualization
- Altered personality
- Impaired socialization
- Depression

■ Related Factors

The following related factors are associated with Chronic Confusion:

- Alzheimer's disease
- Dementia of the Alzheimer's type
- AIDS-related dementia
- Multi-infarct dementia
- Cerebral vascular accident
- Korsakoff's psychosis
- Head injury

DIAGNOSIS

■ Differential Nursing Diagnosis

The nursing diagnosis Chronic Confusion is used for individuals who experience a cognitive impairment lasting longer than 6 months. There are three nursing diagnoses similar to Chronic Confusion. Alteration in Thought Process may be more appropriate for patients with a psychiatric diagnosis. Impaired Memory may be used for patients exhibiting acute or chronic disruptions of memory. Impaired Environmental Interpretation Syndrome

VI

has many of the same elements and interventions as Chronic Confusion. Selection of an appropriate nursing diagnosis may be difficult and is ultimately left to nurse's interpretation. By contrast, Acute Confusion is appropriate for an individual exhibiting signs and symptoms of patient delirium.

■ **Medical and Psychiatric Diagnoses**

Dementia of the Alzheimer's type (DAT) is the psychiatric diagnosis most often associated with the nursing diagnosis Chronic Confusion. Other associated medical diagnoses are Alzheimer's disease, cerebral vascular accident, and head injury. The provision of care for patients with these diagnoses is often complex and requires additional collaboration among disciplines and agencies. Case management is one effective method used to coordinate care delivery to this population.

OUTCOME IDENTIFICATION, PLANNING, AND IMPLEMENTATION

The patient will be able to function in a structured environment is an expected patient outcome. The cognitively impaired patient is able to experience optimum function in a supportive, structured environment. The physical setting and the staff contribute to the milieu that makes up the patient's environment. The staff must interact with the patient using a positive approach and communication skills that demonstrate a high regard for the individual. Controlling the bombardment of external stimuli. (i.e., noise level, traffic activity, and disturbing visual images) that affects the milieu is critical. Activities must be selected on the basis of the unique needs and interests of the patient. The provision of items familiar to the individual (i.e., photographs, furniture, and special possessions) will support a sense of belonging and comfort. Consistency in daily routine and caregivers (staff) play an important part in successful care delivery for this population. It is difficult to complete an evaluation and establish an effective intervention in a 2-week time frame. The focus of treatment is to provide an environment that remains consistent and promotes an opportunity for normalcy.

The patient will demonstrate no increase in episodes of behavioral disturbance is another expected patient outcome. It is important to establish a behavior baseline by interviewing the family or the caregiver. Environmental change may precipitate problematical behavior for patients with cognitive impairment. It may be necessary to initiate a monitor that utilizes systematic observation of episodes of behavioral disturbance over a 24-hour period. Staff must be alert to subtle changes that may affect patient response and record incidents accurately. The family may benefit from reviewing the results of the behavior monitor and validating their own experiences. This discussion may provide opportunities for family or caregiver education.

◢ **NURSING CARE GUIDELINES**
Nursing Diagnosis: Chronic Confusion

Expected Outcome: The patient will be able to function in a structured environment within 2 weeks.

▲ Establish a consistent daily routine. *Patients compensate for inability to plan activities by developing a daily routine that becomes automatic.*[11]

■ Post written daily routine for patient to follow. *Written directions or schedules provide additional cues to the chronically confused individual who retains the ability to read.*[2,18]

■ Provide a consistent caregiver(s). *Patients will experienced increased security when cared for by people they recognize.*[5,16]

■ = nursing intervention; ▲ = collaborative intervention.

- Provide opportunity for 1:1 conversation with caregiver(s). *Providing sufficient time for interacting with the patient reinforces socialization skill and a sense of self-worth.*[10]
- Maintain eye contact, smile, and present a pleasant demeanor when interacting with the patient. *Verbal and nonverbal communication are important in establishing a relationship with a cognitively impaired person.*[18]
- ▲ Place meaningful possessions in the patient's environment (i.e., photographs, mementos, or favorite furniture). *Familiar belongings promote a sense of security.*[16]
- Avoid change in room environment (i.e., reassignment of patient's room, rearrangement of furniture or items, or holiday decorations). *Frequent environment changes may produce conflicting cues.*[5]
- ▲ Provide a daily time for small-group activity that is valued by patient (i.e., music, art, reminiscence group, selected television program, or bible therapy). *Planned activities are beneficial if they are pleasurable and incorporate the patient's culture, habits, values, manners, preferences, and occupation.*[9,11,13]
- Encourage continued interaction with a pet (i.e., allow pet to remain with the patient, allow pet to visit patient if an inpatient, or provide access to animal-assisted therapy). *Pets provide links to the past, encourage conversation, and provide a pleasurable activity option.*[16]
- ▲ Ensure optimal sensory input (i.e., eyeglasses are clean, hearing aid is functional, absence of cerumen impaction). *The cognitively impaired patient is at risk for misinterpretation of the environment when sensory input is not accurate.*[2,5,22]
- Provide adequate nonglare lighting. *Visual perceptions may be altered by glare or shadows.*[5,22]
- Eliminate unnecessary environmental stimuli (i.e., excessive noise level, multiple conversations or activities, and violent or aggressive movies or television programs). *Disturbing visual images or loud noise can precipitate a catastrophic reaction.*[14]
- ▲ Provide instruction as simple one-step commands. *Complex, sequenced instructions are overwhelming to the cognitively impaired individual.*[15,18]
- ▲ Allow sufficient time to complete task. *Completion of an activity promotes self-esteem and satisfaction.*
- ▲ Communicate new or relevant patient information to other staff who see the patient. *Communication among staff is vital to the provision of continuity of care to the cognitively impaired patient.*[18]

Expected Outcome: The patient will demonstrate no increase in episodes of behavioral disturbance within 2 weeks.

- Identify situation or circumstances that may precipitate behavioral disturbance. *There are usually antecedents to behavioral disturbance.*°
- Educate caregiver(s) to possible "triggers" and the appropriate response (e.g., time out, rest, or distraction) to behavioral disturbance. *Early intervention may prevent or modify a behavioral disturbance.*[12]

°References 1, 5, 8, 14, 15, 18.

EVALUATION

The degree of cognitive impairment and the unique qualities of each patient will affect the success of this outcome. Sometimes it is difficult to achieve within a 2-week time frame and may require an extended period of time, ongoing assessment, and tailored interventions. Adaptation to the environment will depend on the amount of time spent in the structured environment (i.e., 1 to 3 days per week in a day care program or a long-term care placement). The patient will have achieved the desired result when he or she is able to participate in activities with the expected amount of cuing. If the patient is not able to function in the environment as expected, collaboration with the multidisciplinary team is indicated. There are a few individuals whose cognitive impairment has progressed to the point that they are unable to maintain any normalcy in their routine.

Collaboration with the family, caregiver, or the patient's support network will yield information about past behavior and circumstances that lead to incidents of behavioral disturbance. The outcome of no increase in episodes of behavioral distur-bance must be measured from the patient's estab-lished baseline. If the patient is at or below the baseline, he or she has met the outcome. If episodes of behavioral disturbance increase, col-laboration with the multidisciplinary team and the formation of a new plan may be necessary.

► CASE STUDY WITH PLAN OF CARE

Bill W. is an 82-year-old white male with a diagnosis of dementia of the Alzheimer's type. Other chronic con-ditions include coronary artery disease, mild hyperten-sion, and posttraumatic stress syndrome. He lives at home with his wife. Bill uses a cane for ambulation. The cane is often hanging from his shirt pocket rather than held in his hand when he walks. His wife reports that he likes to go for walks and that "the neighbors call me if they see him somewhere when they are out driving around." At the Adult Day Health Care he has attended for 3 years, Bill requires assistance to locate the bath-room. Bill was very active in the community as a volun-teer; he frequently asks, "What can I do to help?" His wife reports that he is a religious man and receives com-fort from reading the Bible.

► PLAN OF CARE FOR MR. BILL W.
Nursing Diagnosis: Chronic Confusion Related to Dementia

Expected Outcome: Bill W. will maintain the ability to function in a structured adult day care program environment as evidenced by participating in individual and group activities.
- ▲ Evaluate patient's baseline health and functional and psychosocial status.
- ■ Determine previous activities and interests.
- ■ Ensure that Bill has optimal sensory input (i.e., eyeglasses are clean, hearing aid functions, and there is no cerumen impaction).
- ■ Evaluate Bill's stimulation threshold.
- ▲ Select activities that Bill can complete successfully.
- ▲ Select activities that will have meaning to Bill.
- ▲ Engage in highly structured, repetitive group activities.
- ■ Provide the opportunity for meaningful individual activities (i.e., folding towels, watering plants, and recycling paper).
- ■ Incorporate rest time between activities.
- ■ Use simple, one-step commands when providing verbal cues or instructions.
- ■ Allow time to respond to a command before providing additional information.
- ■ Monitor for changes in behavior or functional status.

Expected Outcome: Mr. W. will not injure himself by wandering from the program.
- ▲ Consult with physical therapy to evaluate Mr. W.'s gait and need for assistive devices.
- ■ Evaluate his potential to wander from program.
- ■ Evaluate for speed and endurance (range) if he exits program area.
- ■ Wear ID bracelet at all times.
- ■ Maintain full-body photograph with information about his height, weight, and distinguishing character-istics in program file.
- ■ Provide an opportunity to sit in a quiet area and read the Bible when Bill begins to seem agitated.

■ = nursing intervention; ▲ = collaborative intervention.

■■ CRITICAL THINKING EXERCISES

1. What information can be obtained from a home visit that would assist the nurse to identify the nurse to identify Mr. W.'s education needs?

2. What communication techniques are important to consider when asking the patient to participate in an activity?

3. How would you evaluate progression of the disease or change in mental status for Mr. W.?

REFERENCES

1. Abraham IL and Reel SJ: Cognitive nursing interventions with long-term care residents: effects on neurocognitive dimensions, *Arch Psych Nurs* 6(6):356–365, 1992.
2. Abraham IL and others: Multidisciplinary assessment of patients with Alzheimer's disease, *Nurs Clin North Am* 29(1):113–128, 1994.
3. Armstrong-Esther CA, Browne KD, and McAfee JG: Elderly patients: still clean and sitting quietly, *J Adv Nurs* 19:264–271, 1994.
4. Barry PP: Medical evaluation of the demented patient, *Med Clin North Am* 78(4):779–793, 1994.
5. Beck CK and Shue VM: Interventions for treating disruptive behavior in demented elderly people, *Nurs Clin North Am* 29(1):143–155, 1994.
6. Bowie P and Mountain G: Using direct observation to record the behavior of long-stay patients with dementia, *Int J Geriatr Psychiatry* 8:857–864, 1993.
7. Daly JM, Maas M, and Buckwalter K: Use of standardized nursing diagnosis and interventions in long-term care, *J Geront Nurs* 21(8):29–36, 1995.
8. Fisher JE, Fink CM, and Loomis CC: Frequency and management difficulty of behavioral problems among dementia patients in long-term care facilities, *Clin Gerontologist* 13(1):3–12, 1993.
9. Forbes EJ: Spirituality, aging and the community-dwelling caregiver and care recipient, *Geriatr Nurs* 15(6):296–301, 1994.
10. Goldsmith SM, Hoeffer B, and Rader J: Problematic wandering behavior in the cognitively impaired elderly, *J Psychosoc Nurs* 33(2):6–12, 1995.
11. Hall GR: Caring for people with Alzheimer's disease using the conceptual model of progressively lowered stress threshold in the clinical setting, *Nurs Clin North Am* 29(1):129–141, 1994.
12. Harvath TA and others: Dementia-related behaviors in Alzheimer's disease and AIDS, *J Psychosoc Nurs* 33(1):35–39, 1995.
13. Khozvam HR: Bible study: a treatment in elderly patients with Alzheimer's disease, *Clin Gerontol* 15(2):71–74, 1994.
14. Nelson J: The influence of environmental factors in incidents of disruptive behavior, *J Geront Nurs* 21(5):19–24, 1995.
15. Rader J, Doan J, and Schwab M: How to decrease wandering, a form of agenda behavior, *Geriatr Nurs* 6(4):196–199, 1985.
16. Rantz MJ and McShane RE: Nursing interventions for chronically confused nursing home residents, *Geriatr Nurs* 16(1):22–27, 1995.
17. Shedd PP, Kobokovich LJ, and Slattery MJ: Confused patients in the acute care setting: prevalence, interventions, and outcomes, *J Geront Nurs* 21(4):5–12, 1995.
18. Stolley JM and others: Managing the care of patients with irreversible dementia during hospitalization for comorbidities, *Nurs Clin North Am* 28(4):767–782, 1993.
19. Ugarriza DN and Gray T: Alzheimer's disease: nursing interventions for clients and caretakers, *J Psychosoc Nurs* 31(10):7–10, 1993.
20. U.S. Bureau of the Census: *Projection estimated from March 1987 Current Population Survey*, Washington D.C., 1987, U.S. Government Printing Office.
21. Webber PA, Fox P, and Burnette D: Living alone with Alzheimer's disease: effects on health and social service utilization patterns, *Gerontologist* 34(1):8–14, 1994.
22. Wolanin M and Phillips L: *Confusion: prevention and care*, St. Louis, 1981, The CV Mosby Co.

VI

Decisional Conflict (Specify)

▶

Decisional Conflict (Specify) *is the uncertainty about which course of action to take when choice among competing actions involves risk, loss, regret, or challenge to personal life values (specify the focus of conflict, such as personal health, family relationships, career, finances, or other life events).*

OVERVIEW

Every day in many clinical settings patients are faced with making choices about alternative actions. Should I have the surgery or not? Should I use condoms or birth control pills? Does my child really need to take medication for hyperactivity? Should I go to the emergency room to have this pain checked out? Should I breastfeed or bottle feed my baby? Is now the time to quit smoking (lose weight, start exercising, do something about my stressful job) or not? Should I move in with my children or go to a nursing home? Decision making is the process of choosing between alternative courses of action (including inaction). Orem[19] describes the process of decision making as the first phase of deliberative self-care. Effective producers of self-care understand the courses of action open to them and the effectiveness and desirability of these courses of action before making a decision about the actions they will take and those they will avoid.

Several models with which to judge the effectiveness and desirability of alternative courses of

The authors are grateful for the advice of the following researchers whose work focuses on decision making: Andrea Baumann, RN, PhD; Lesley Degner, RN, PhD; Hilary Llewellyn-Thomas, RN, PhD; and Marilyn L. Rothert, RN, PhD.

action have emerged in the fields of economics and psychology.[9] Although many theorists disagree about how individuals make or ought to make judgments and decisions, most agree that expectations and values are essential factors in the process.[21] These two elements correspond to Orem's concepts[19] of effectiveness and desirability. *Expectations* are subjective judgments about the probability or likelihood that specific outcomes or consequences will result from a course of action. *Values,* or *utilities,* are the individual's preferences for or the relative desirability of these outcomes. Generally, individuals select alternatives that are likely to produce desirable outcomes and unlikely to produce undesirable outcomes. Conversely, they avoid alternatives likely to produce undesirable outcomes or unlikely to produce desirable outcomes.

Unfortunately, many important decisions have alternatives that are likely to produce desirable and undesirable outcomes. Furthermore, the desired outcomes may partially involve one alternative and partially another. Thus no alternative will satisfy all of a person's personal objectives, and no alternative is without the risk of undesirable outcomes. This situation is known as a *choice dilemma* or a *conflicted decision.*[26] It is characterized by difficulty or uncertainty in identifying the best alternative because of the risk or uncertainty of outcomes, the high stakes in terms of potential gains and losses, the need to make value trade-offs in selecting a course of action,[14] and anticipated regret over the positive aspects of rejected options.[26] Janis and Mann[11] describe Decisional Conflict as the "simultaneous opposing tendencies within the individual to accept and reject a given course of action" (p. 46).

Responses to the Decisional Conflict depend on the degree of conflict inherent in the decision. Sjoberg[26] maintains that a low degree of conflict may be attractive and stimulating, a moderate degree may produce defensiveness, and a high degree may bring about hypervigilance and panic. The intensity of stress symptoms depends in part on the anticipated magnitude of losses resulting from whatever choice is made and the magnitude of the anticipated regret over the positive aspects of rejected options.

Little research has been conducted in clinical practice to examine the prevalence of Decisional Conflict experienced by patients and the variation in responses described by Janis and Mann.[11] Hiltunen's phenomenological study[10] with five clients in a home health setting supported the etiology of loss and the symptoms of uncertainty about the courses of action to take. Degner and Beaton's participant observation study[4] of life-death decisions demonstrated the complexity of Decisional Conflict when decisions are made jointly by clinicians, patients, and families. Disagreement in expectations, values, and decisions occurred within and between groups. These data are supported by Rostain's observations.[22] Continued research in patient decision making in clinical settings is essential because judgment and decision processes vary with the type of decision.[21] Furthermore, concurrent medical problems, emotional distress, and the social influence of health professionals may make the difficulties that patients experience with decision making unique.

ASSESSMENT

The main characteristic manifested by persons having to make a difficult decision is verbalized concern or distress because they are uncertain about which alternative to select. While they are deliberating, they may talk about the undesirable consequences of the choice facing them and question their personal values. Individuals involved in a choice dilemma may demonstrate hesitation, vacillation, and delayed decision making. Self-focusing behaviors and physiological signs of stress (restlessness, increased heart rate, and muscle tension) may be manifested. During some decision-making processes, autonomic indicators of stress increase as individuals move toward a decision and gradually return to the level of the resting state after the decision is made.[11]

Responses to a difficult decision vary according to each individual's perception of the level of risk and the magnitude of loss and regret. For example, people recommended for major surgery find decision making more difficult than those recommended for minor surgery.[16] Other personal and environmental factors will also influence Decisional Conflict. In a Swedish study, women and immigrants found decisions more difficult to make than men and Swedish citizens did; patients with cancer also reported more difficulty in making decisions. Hesitancy about whether or not to have surgery was also associated with uncertainty about the nature, extent, and consequences of the operation and anesthesia.[16] Inexperience, past experience, poor information,[17] and emotional distress may contribute to unclear or unrealistic perceptions about courses of action and their consequences, thereby magnifying the conflict. Hesitation in making a decision may also be influenced by a person's lack of knowledge or skill in implementing the decision once it is made. Social factors can also exacerbate the conflict. Patients may lack the social support from others to assist them in making and implementing a decision. They may also receive unwanted interference from their support network or health professionals.[11,17]

Often a medical diagnosis can lead to Decisional Conflict. With new information about their health, patients must usually consider how they are going to respond to the practitioner's advice regarding their diagnosis, treatment, and lifestyle. Medical problems can also interfere with a person's ability to make decisions by reducing cognitive capacity (as sometimes results from impaired perfusion or trauma to the brain) or by producing emotional distress, which at high levels diminishes a person's ability to think clearly.[7,25] In either case, even simple decisions may generate uncertainty about which course of action to take.

VI

Several assessment guides have been developed to identify a person's perception of a problem and the nature of the conflict, including Janis and Mann's decisional balance sheet[11] and Pender's values clarification exercise.[20] These tools assess the qualitative nature of the conflict. (See O'Connor[17] for a quantitative measure of Decisional Conflict.) Important components to consider are the individual's goals, perceived alternatives and consequences, expectations, and values. From these data the nurse can judge the source of the conflict; the clarity, comprehensiveness, and viability of alternatives; the clarity, accuracy, and realism of the expectations; and the clarity and priority of values. Other contextual data may need to be collected, depending on the situation. The depth and comprehensiveness of data collection will depend on the clinical context and time constraints. Some of the important areas for assessment are outlined below:

1. *Appearance.* Briefly note the patient's sex, race, apparent age, deportment, overt signs of distress, and composure.
2. *Patient's perception of problem.* Ask the patient to explain in his or her own words what seems to be the problem. Validate impressions.
3. *Factors contributing to difficult decision making.* Ask the patient to explain in his or her own words what factors are making the decision difficult. As appropriate to the context, ask questions about personal and environmental factors (e.g., knowledge, experience, support system, other social influences, and personal resources) that are helping or hindering the decision making.
4. *Personal goals and perceived alternatives.* What goals does the patient wish to achieve? In the patient's view, what are the available alternatives?
5. *Expectations.* From the patient's perspective, what outcomes are possible with each alternative? How likely are these outcomes?
6. *Values and utilities.* How desirable or undesirable are these outcomes? Ask the patient to rank their order of desirability.
7. *Resources to implement decisions.* Does the patient perceive difficulty in implementing the

alternatives? Does the patient have the knowledge, motivation, and resources to implement the alternatives?

Quantitative approaches to eliciting the patient's expectations and values have also been developed,[6,15] and some have been tested for reliability, validity, and suitability for clinical practice.[8,10] The need for quantitative assessment will depend on the need for refined judgments of the patient's expectations and values and the acceptability of the assessment to the nurse and the patient. Many studies have illustrated the difficulties encountered in eliciting patient expectations and values. Tversky and Kahneman[31] have found that individuals' expectations or judgments about the likelihood of events do not always correspond to reality. People are influenced by *representativeness*; that is, they have the tendency to ignore what is known about the likelihood of the event and to base expectations of an outcome on how similar it is to the major characteristics of the population or process from which it is generated. For example, patients may judge themselves to be less susceptible to contracting a sexually transmitted disease than the rates reported in the literature if they do not believe that they represent the type of patient who would normally contract the disease. People also tend to judge the likelihood of an outcome by the *availability* (the ease with which instances or occurrences can be brought to mind). Outcomes are often judged more likely than they really are if instances of these outcomes are frequent, recent, vivid, and easily imagined. Conversely, they are judged less likely than they really are if they are rare, remote, bland, and difficult to imagine. Depending on the initial starting point one uses in eliciting information, anchoring or adjusting biases can occur (e.g., "Do you think your chances are greater or less than 50%?" or "Do you think your chances are greater or less than 75%?").

Methodological problems also exist when assessing the patient's values. Preference reversals have occurred, depending on whether outcomes are framed positively or negatively, whether risks involve gains or losses, how much regret was expected, and the reference point from which the person was stating a preference.[12,31] These problems make it difficult to get consistent answers about preferences. Furthermore, Fischhoff, Slovic, and Lichtenstein[6] have found that people have difficulty knowing what they want in making a decision when the outcomes are unfamiliar. Values are clearer for outcomes that are familiar, simple, and directly experienced. Slovic, Fischhoff, and Lichtenstein[28] have stated that in value assessment "there may be no substitute for an interactive elicitation procedure, one that employs multiple methods and acknowledge the elicitor's role in helping the respondent to create and enunciate values." Several of these methods are reviewed by Froberg and Kane.[8]

■ Defining Characteristics

The presence of the following defining characteristics indicates that the patient may be experiencing Decisional Conflict:

- Verbalization of uncertainty about choices
- Verbalization of undesired consequences of alternative actions
- Vacillation between alternative choices
- Delayed decision making
- Verbalization of distress while attempting to make decisions
- Physical signs of distress or tensions (e.g., increased muscle tension, restlessness, and increased heart rate)
- Questioning personal values and beliefs while attempting to make a decision

■ Related Factors

The following related factors are associated with Decisional Conflict:

- Lack of information about alternatives and consequences
- Conflicting or unclear personal values
- Lack of knowledge or skills to implement decisions made
- Interference from others with decision making
- Lack of experience with decision making

- Lack of an adequate support system
- Unrealistic alternatives or expectations
- Threat to values

DIAGNOSIS

■ Differential Nursing Diagnosis

Decisional Conflict may be difficult to distinguish from other diagnoses that exacerbate it (Anxiety, Ineffective Coping, or Knowledge Deficit), or diagnoses that are consequences of Decisional Conflict (Ineffective Management of Therapeutic Regimen or Noncompliance). The major distinguishing characteristic of Decisional Conflict is that the person needs to make a choice and verbalizes uncertainty about what to do. The immediate goal for the person is to make an effective decision. The role of the nurse as a practitioner is to facilitate that choice. With other diagnoses, these problems and goals are not the most salient. For example, (1) if a patient's difficulty managing a therapeutic regimen is due to problems making the changes necessary to do so rather than problems deliberating on the best choice, this is probably Ineffective Management of Therapeutic Regimen; (2) if a new mother has numerous questions about her infant's care and does not focus on a specific decision, this is probably a Knowledge Deficit; (3) if a person states that his anxiety is interfering with his ability to function and relate to others, including making everyday decisions, the predominant problem may be Anxiety; (4) if parents have problems coping with the diagnosis of their son's chronic illness, including dealing with their feelings and solving problems in everyday situations (including decision making), this may be Ineffective Coping; and (5) if a person has made an informed choice to delay recommended surgery for 2 years, this is probably Noncompliance.

■ Medical and Psychiatric Diagnoses

Decisional Conflict may arise in any medical context where therapeutic choices involve making trade-offs between benefits and risks. Decisional Conflict can also be manifested in psychiatric illness such as Antisocial Personality Disorder DSM-

IV 301.7 or Depressive Disorder, major, single, episode DSM-IV 296.20.

OUTCOME IDENTIFICATION, PLANNING, AND IMPLEMENTATION

The expected outcome of Decision Conflict is that the patient will make an effective decision. The difficulty in judging effectiveness is that there is no criterion for judging the correctness of a decision because the decision is based in part on the individual's personal opinions and preferences.[21] Some theorists impose criteria of mathematical or logical consistency on the decision. Prescriptions for consistent behavior have been derived from expected utility theory and Bayesian decision theory, which is based on a combination of probability theory and expected utility theory.[21] These models have been applied to financial decisions[5] and more recently to social and health decisions.[34] They provide a set of rules for combining the patient's expectations and values to determine the alternative with the highest expected value.

Research has demonstrated that human preferences do not correlate well with prescriptive preferences.[24] Proponents of prescriptive models argue that the processing of complex information is beyond human capacity, and they subsequently encourage the use of prescriptive models because they believe that the logic of these models provides the best guide for reaching defensible decisions.[5] On the other hand, opponents of prescriptive theory maintain that a poor descriptive theory should not be used prescriptively.[24]

In spite of the difficulty in establishing criteria for effective decision making, some outcomes need to be specified to guide action, and they are based on the following assumptions: (1) People who have a clear understanding of the nature of the conflict make better decisions; (2) Informed decisions are better than uninformed decisions; (3) Decisions that are consistent with personal values are better than those that are inconsistent; and (4) Decisions that are congruent with subsequent behavior are better than those that are not congruent.

Therefore effective decisions will be defined as those that are informed, consistent with values, and congruent with behavior. An informed decision is one in which patients (1) are aware of relevant alternatives and their outcomes, (2) have clarified expectations of outcomes that are reasonably aligned with reality, and (3) are aware of the nature of the conflict in the decision. A decision that is consistent with personal values is one in which patients (1) are aware of the value trade-offs they need to make, (2) select the alternative consistent with their trade-off preference, and (3) express satisfaction with the decision they have made. Decisions are congruent with behavior when patients implement the action associated with the decision. The decision may change in time, but they have at least attempted to implement the operational phase of the decision.

Assisting individuals to understand and resolve a difficult decision has been compared with psychotherapy[21] and is referred to here as *decision support therapy*. Approaches may range from unstructured counseling to the use of structured decision aids that are based on different theoretical perspectives on how decisions are or ought to be made.[*] Most aids provide an organized approach to examining a decision problem, and some provide methods of combining input (expectations and values) to arrive at an optimal decision. Although the latter function has been debated because of the poor correspondence to actual decision making,[23] the former function is useful in clarifying the individual's perception of the decision and the elements that make the decision difficult.

The effectiveness of decision support therapy and decision aids is just beginning to be explored.[13,18] Pitz and Sach's review[21] identified positive benefits such as clarifying the problem, generating more alternatives through goal-oriented approaches, and recognizing the best action through the use of decision trees. Clancy, Cebul, and Williams[2] found that offering physicians a decision aid to guide their decision about whether to receive the hepati-

---

[*]References 1, 9, 13, 15, 21, 29, 35.

tis B vaccine increased the number of physicians who were immunized. Slimmer and Brown[27] discovered that decision support therapy was no more effective than a conference control therapy in reducing parents' ambivalence about medication for their hyperactive children. However, it was effective in making parents more aware about the importance of deliberating about their decision.

In the first step of decision support therapy,[14] the problem is structured through the specification of the patient's objectives and corresponding attributes and the subsequent generation of proposed alternatives. Next, the possible effect of alternatives is assessed through the determination of the magnitude and likelihood of the outcomes resulting from proposed alternatives (expectations). The third step involves identifying the preferences of decision makers using value- or utility-assessment techniques. Then the alternatives are compared and evaluated to determine the best choice. Finally, plans for implementing the decision are made and carried out.

This process bears a strong similarity to the assessment process, and indeed the data obtained from the assessment are used as a first approximation of the decision problem. It is subsequently revised through a two-way interaction wherein the nurse and the patient fill gaps, clarify, and share expertise. Rothert and Talarczyk[23] have outlined the roles and expertise of the nurse and the patient when making decisions about following treatment regimens. For example, nurses can provide information about the options available, the risk and probability of outcomes, and the health care resources required and available. Patients' expertise includes their preferences or values and personal, social, and economic resources available.

Control over who guides and who is involved in the deliberation process should depend on the patient's preference. For example, patients can be classified into one of three profiles of preference for control: those who want to keep, share, or give away control for decisionmaking.[3] If the patient is a "keeper," he or she may guide the deliberation while allowing nurse input on the scientific facts. "Sharers" may prefer that the nurse begin the guidance, with input and final decision made by the patient, and "givers away" may favor the nurse's adopting an advisory role, with informed consent given by the patient.

When the patient chooses to share the decision-making process with another person, the process is facilitated by (1) the mutual review and clarification of options, consequences, expectations, values, and actions; (2) the revision of elements in which patients lack information by implementing teaching strategies; and (3) the realignment of elements that are unrealistic so that they maintain consistency with current knowledge. The specific interventions depend on the data that the patient provides in the first approximation of the decision problem and the judgments that the nurse and the patient make about how complete, salient, accurate, and parsimonious the first approximation is.

Goals and Alternatives

When options are unclear or patients are uninformed, nurses and patients must explore the alternatives available to meet patients' goals. When options are clear but too numerous, they need to be reduced to a few viable alternatives. When patients' range of options appears too narrow or constraining, it must be expanded to accommodate others that have the potential to meet personal objectives.

A similar process is used for identifying outcomes or consequences of the viable options. There is no need to explore exhaustively all possible consequences of a decision. Rather, the salient outcomes that the patient considers important should be identified. Then expectations of consequences can be clarified and compared with known probabilities. Unrealistic expectations need to be realigned, particularly when patients have exaggerated the chances of negative outcomes. However, the nurse must be more cautious when expectations of positive outcomes (e.g., survival or remission from disease) are exaggerated. Expectations bear a conceptual resemblance to hope.[30] Most nurses would be loath to reduce patients' expectations of survival unless patients requested that they know what their chances are.

VI

Values Clarification

Values clarification can be enhanced through qualitative[11,20] and quantitative[17] exercises. Patients are asked to rank outcomes according to relative desirability; they must also recognize the implicit trade-offs they make when selecting one alternative over the other.

In a study conducted by Ward, Heidrich, and Wolberg,[33] two competing values in the decision about modified radical mastectomy and lumpectomy were the fear of radiation therapy (required after lumpectomy) and the fear of losing a breast.

Decision Selection and Implementation

Once patients are aware of viable alternatives, realistic expectations, and implicit value trade-offs, they are in a better position to make an informed decision consistent with value trade-offs. After selection, they need to act on the decision. Orem[19] refers to the operational phase of the decision as the second phase of self-care. Patients may have briefly considered resources needed before making a decision, but rarely have they worked out all of the operational details. For this part of the therapy, personal and environmental resources to aid in the implementation of the decision are evaluated. If deficits exist, the patient must acquire the self-help skills necessary for implementation and rely on external resources if necessary.

EVALUATION

Expected outcomes are achieved when the patient (1) identifies viable alternatives, (2) expresses realistic expectations of the consequences of alternatives, (3) indicates the relative importance of each consequence, (4) selects a course of action consistent with expectations and values, (5) acquires and uses knowledge and skills to implement the course of action, and (6) expresses satisfaction at having made the best decision under the circumstances. If outcomes are not achieved, reassess the sources of Decisional Conflict and intervene accordingly.

◢ NURSING CARE GUIDELINES
Nursing Diagnosis: Decisional Conflict (Specify)

Expected Outcome: The patient will engage in effective decision making.
- Initiate decision support therapy.

Expected Outcome: The patient will become informed and base his or her decision on this information.
- Aid the patient in clarifying goals, alternatives, and potential consequences. *Lack of information or clarity of these items contributes to Decisional Conflict.*
- Help the patient to clarify the likelihood of potential consequences. Realign unrealistic expectations. *Distortion in expectations often increases conflict (e.g., anticipating a negative consequence when the likelihood is extremely low) or regret (anticipating a positive consequence when the likelihood is extremely low).*

Expected Outcome: The patient will select a course of action that is consistent with his or her values.
- With the patient, clarify desirability of possible consequences of alternatives and their priority. *Unclear values contribute to Decisional Conflict.*
- Identify value trade-offs implicit in making each choice. *Having to make trade-offs contributes to Decisional Conflict. Knowing what makes the decision difficult helps in its resolution.*
- Facilitate alternative selection consistent with personal values. *This increases satisfaction with the decision and the likelihood that the patient will follow through on the choice.*

Expected Outcome: The patient will implement the decision.
- Teach and reinforce self-help skills required for behaviorial implementation of decision. *Individuals have difficulty translating preferences into permanent behavior change without the resources necessary to do so.*

■ = nursing intervention; ▲ = collaborative intervention.

☛ CASE STUDY WITH PLAN OF CARE

Mrs. Nellie G., a 60-year-old postmenopausal patient diagnosed with breast cancer, has recently undergone a modified radical mastectomy. There was no evidence of metastasis, and the results of lymph node biopsy were negative for cancer. The hormone receptor status of the tumor was positive. The medical oncologist informed her that she would need to have adjuvant chemotherapy to reduce her chances of tumor recurrence. She was told that the usual chemotherapy was tamoxifen, an antihormone oral medication that is usually tolerated well with few side effects (e.g., hot flashes and mild nausea that is usually relieved if taken with milk). However, there was a clinical trial in progress to establish the improvement in disease-free survival if a 6-month course of intravenous cylcophosphamide, methotrexate, and 5-fluorouracil (CMF) was given in addition to tamoxifen. The side effects of CMF include nausea, vomiting, fatigue, mouth sores, bladder irritation, and hair loss. Also, the white blood cell count might be depressed, thereby increasing the risk of infection, and occasionally the platelets might decrease, increasing the chances of bleeding. Therefore Mrs. G. would be monitored very closely, and treatment would be delayed or modified if platelets or white blood cell counts dropped too low. Mrs. G. was asked whether she would consider participating in the trial. If she agreed, she would have an equal chance of receiving the tamoxifen alone or the tamoxifen plus intravenous CMF. Mrs. G. was upset that she required treatment in addition to the surgery. She became extremely agitated when intravenous chemotherapy was mentioned. She burst into tears and stated that she was unable to make any decisions at this time. The oncologist gave her the consent form and asked her to talk it over with her family and let him know at the next visit. If she agreed, Mrs. G. would have to receive treatment at that time for her to be eligible in the trial. At the next visit, Mrs. G. still appeared quite distressed. She stated that she had decided to participate in the trial because her family thought she would get more attention from the medical staff, and besides, she had a 50% chance of receiving the oral medication treatment alone. After Mrs. G. signed the consent form, the clinical trial's head office used random procedures to assign her to a treatment plan, and she was allocated to receive tamoxifen plus intravenous CMF. When she learned she would be getting CMF, she started to cry, stating that she did not know whether she could go through with the treatment. The chemotherapy nurse was asked to come and see her.

INTERACTIVE ASSESSMENT

Appearance

A 60-year-old, well-dressed, and well-groomed white woman in emotional state. Swollen red eyes, shaky hand movements, avoiding direct eye contact.

Patient's Perception of Problem

PATIENT: I know I promised I would be in the study, and my family thinks I will get more attention, but I can't bear the thought of taking that chemotherapy. I've seen what it does to people. My mother had it, and it made her sick and miserable—and she died anyway . . . [Stops and cries for a while.] I used to take her to the clinic sometimes, and I saw what it did to some of the other people too. It didn't seem to do much good. I wouldn't have minded if I had been given only the pills, but the chemo . . . I don't know what to do. I've signed the form. The doctor says I have to have the treatment today to be eligible. I know how important it is to study these treatments, and he thinks it could prevent the tumor from coming back. But those side effects. I've been so upset about everything lately . . . I can't think straight.

NURSE: [Validates.] You don't know whether you should take the chemotherapy or not; you're finding it hard to decide.

PATIENT: Yes, that's right.

Factors Contributing to Difficult Decision Making

NURSE: It is a hard decision to make. If you would like, we can discuss the things that make it hard for you to decide. Do you think that would be okay?

PATIENT: Yes. [Pause.] I'm upset, and it's hard to think straight. I wish my husband were here. He's at a meeting, so my neighbor came with me. I don't feel that I can discuss these things with her, and I need to decide now.

Goals and Perceived Alternatives

Patient indicated previously that decision is to take intravenous chemotherapy along with tamoxifen, or to take tamoxifen and refuse intravenous chemotherapy; goals appear to be survival, quality of life, and social approval and will be validated during decision therapy.

Expectations

NURSE: Let's begin by talking about what you think the advantages and disadvantages of taking and not taking

Continued

■ **CASE STUDY WITH PLAN OF CARE — CONT'D**

chemo are. If you took the intravenous chemotherapy, what would be the pluses and minuses of that choice?
PATIENT: Well . . . I know that I would be sick . . . nausea and vomiting and everything. My hair would fall out, and I'd get those mouth sores my mother got . . . awful . . . I would probably get more attention because they will be following me more closely. The drug may stop the tumor from coming back, but then it may not. That's why the need for the study, I suppose. It certainly didn't work for my mother.
NURSE: So from your point of view, taking the chemotherapy may get you more attention but will probably make you sick with nausea, vomiting, hair loss, and mouth sores. It may prevent the tumor from coming back, but it may not.
PATIENT: Yes, that's right.
NURSE: Have I left anything out?
PATIENT: No. I think that pretty well covers it.
NURSE: If you didn't take the intravenous chemotherapy, what would be the pluses and minuses of that choice?
PATIENT: I wouldn't have the side effects from taking just the pills. But my family will be disappointed that I didn't go through with it, and the doctor may get upset. I already signed the form, and I like to keep my word. I wouldn't get the attention, but I suppose I wouldn't need it if I didn't take those strong drugs.
NURSE: So from your point of view, not undergoing chemotherapy will have fewer side effects, but your doctor or your family may disapprove and you may feel bad because you didn't keep your word. You'd get less attention, but maybe that isn't important.
PATIENT: Yes.
NURSE: Any other points about not undergoing chemotherapy?
PATIENT: No.

Values and Utilities
NURSE: So it would appear that, for you, taking intravenous chemotherapy means having unpleasant side effects, but not undergoing chemotherapy means having your family and doctor disapprove of your decision, and you would feel bad for not keeping your word. Do you know which of these consequences would be worse for you: family and doctor disapproval, feeling bad for not keeping your word, or having side effects?
PATIENT: That's hard to say. I don't want the side effects, but I don't want my family or doctor to think badly of me. [The decision appears to involve making trade-offs between toxicity and social approval. Eliciting priorities or trade-offs is deferred until expectations are realigned with reality.]
NURSE: I've listed all the pluses and minuses of the decision you have to make. Maybe we can look these over together. I can let you know from my experience what you can realistically expect from selecting each alternative, and you can let me know how important each of these advantages and disadvantages is to you. Then maybe the best decision for you may be clearer to you.

■ **PLAN OF CARE FOR MRS. NELLIE G.**
Nursing Diagnosis: Decisional Conflict Related to Interference in Decision Making from Anxiety, Time Pressure, Unrealistic Expectations, and Unclear Values About the Relative Importance of the Consequences of Choice

Expected Outcome: Mrs. G. will engage in effective decision making over the next 24 hours.
- Provide Mrs. G. with decision support therapy.

Expected Outcome: Mrs. G.'s expectations of side effects and social disapproval will be realigned as evidenced by her expression of the realistic likelihood of each consequence.
- Reaffirm valid beliefs about alternatives and benefits of treatment.
- Help Mrs. G. realign expectations of side effects (not everyone experiences difficulty, and responses vary by type of treatment; her mother may have had different treatment).
- Remind Mrs. G. that she is free to withdraw from the clinical trial at any time without influencing her care and that her family is unaware of treatment assignment and may have different advice now.

■ = nursing intervention; ▲ = collaborative intervention.

Expected Outcome: Mrs. G. will select a course of action that is consistent with her values as evidenced by her satisfaction in being able to make a difficult decision.
- Help Mrs. G. clarify the priority of the consequences of alternatives (e.g., toxicity, social disapproval, and keeping her word).
- Facilitate alternative selection in light of new information and value clarification.

Expected Outcome: Mrs. G. will implement her decision.
- Review problems implementing decision; support decision implementation (e.g., offer to be there when she informs her family and physician of decision).

▪▪ CRITICAL THINKING EXERCISES

1. Several factors contributed to Mrs. G.'s Decisional Conflict. Classify them as affective (emotional), cognitive (relating to structuring information for problem solving), or social (relating to interpersonal relationships). Rank them according to your estimate of their influence in creating decision difficulty for Mrs. G. Which ones should be tackled first and why?

2. Practitioners need to be aware of their own values when facilitating the decision making of others. What would you do in Mrs. G.'s situation, and on what values would you base your decision? What would you do if your values did not correspond to those of Mrs. G.'s?

3. Patients often ask the nurse's advice when faced with a difficult decision. It is important to identify the reasons behind your opinions, particularly when they may conflict with those of your patient. One strategy is to classify differences in opinions based on (1) different expectations or perceptions of the likelihood of the consequences of the choice and (2) different values or the personal importance placed on consequences. When would it be easier to reach a consensus with your patient: when there are differences in expectations or differences in values?

4. When patients ask for your advice, they are acknowledging your expertise in certain areas. It is important to identify what type of advice your patient is seeking. When do you think patients are more likely to acknowledge your expertise: on the likelihood of consequences or on the values associated with those consequences? How should this affect the way you provide advice to your patients; for example, in Mrs. G.'s case?

REFERENCES

1. Beach LR and Wise JA: Decision emergence: a Lewinian perspective, *Acta Psychol* 45:343–356, 1980.
2. Clancy D, Cebul R, and Williams S: Guiding individual decisions: a randomized, controlled trial of decision analysis, *Am J Med* 84:283–288, 1988.
3. Degner LF and Aquino Russell C: Preferences for treatment control among adults with cancer, *Res Nurs Health* 11:367–374, 1988.
4. Degner LF and Beaton J: *Life-death decisions in health care*, Washington, D.C., 1987, Hemisphere Publishing.
5. Fischer G: Utility models for multiple objective decisions: do they accurately represent human preferences?, *Decision Sci* 10:451–479, 1979.
6. Fischhoff B, Slovic P, and Lichtenstein S: Knowing what you want: measuring labile values. In Wallsten TS, editor: *Cognitive processes in choice and decision behavior*, Hillsdale, New Jersey, 1980, Lawrence Erlbaum Associates.
7. Fitten LJ and Waite MS: Impact of medical hospitalization on treatment decision-making capacity in the elderly, *Arch Int Med* 150:1717–1721, 1990.
8. Froberg DG and Kane RL: Methodology for measuring health-state preferences II: scaling methods, *J Clin Epidem* 42:459–471, 1989.
9. Hammond KR, McClelland GH, and Mumpower J: *Human judgment and decision making*, New York, 1980, Praeger Publishers.
10. Hiltunen E: Decisional conflict: a phenomenological description from the points of view of the nurse and client. In McLane A, editor: *Classification of nursing diagnoses: proceedings of the Seventh Conference*, St. Louis, 1987, The CV Mosby Co.
11. Janis IL and Mann L: *Decision making*, New York, 1977, The Free Press.
12. Kahneman D and Tversky A: The psychology of preferences, *Science* 246:160–171, 1982.

VI

13. Kasper JF, Mulley AG, and Wennberg JE: Developing shared decision-making programs to improve the quality of health care, *Quality Rev Bulletin* June 1992:183–190.

14. Keeney RL: Decision analysis: an overview, *Operations Res* 30:803–838, 1982.

15. Keeney RL and Raiffa H: *Decisions with multiple objectives: preferences and value tradeoffs,* New York, 1976, John Wiley & Sons.

16. Larsson US and others: Patient involvement in decision making in surgical and orthopaedic practice: the project perioperative risk, *Soc Sci Med* 28:829–835, 1989.

17. O'Conner A: Validation of a decisional conflict scale, *Med Decis Making* 15:25–30, 1995.

18. O'Conner A, Llewellyn-Thomas HA, and Drake ER: *Annotated bibliography on shared decision making,* Toronto, 1995, National Cancer Institute of Canada.

19. Orem DE: *Nursing: concepts of practice,* ed 5, St. Louis, 1995, Mosby–Year Book.

20. Pender NJ and Pender AR: *Health promotion in nursing practice,* ed 2, Norwalk, Connecticut, 1987, Appleton & Lange.

21. Pitz GF and Sachs NJ: Judgment and decision: theory and application, *Ann Rev Psychol* 35:139–163, 1984.

22. Rostain A: Deciding to forego life-sustaining treatment in the intensive care nursery: a sociological account, *Perspect Biol Med* 30:117–134, 1986.

23. Rothert ML and Talarczyk GJ: Patient compliance and the decision making process of clinicians and patients, *J Compliance Health Care* 2:55–71, 1987.

24. Schoemaker PJH: The expected utility model: its variants, purposes, evidence, and limitations. In Paelinck JHP and Vossen PH, editors: *The quest for optimality,* New York, 1984, Gower Medical Publishing.

25. Scott D: Anxiety, critical thinking and information processing during and after breast biopsy, *Nurs Res* 32:24–28, 1983.

26. Sjoberg L: To smoke or not to smoke: conflict or lack of differentiation? In Humphreys P, Svenson O, and Vari A, editors: *Analyzing and aiding decision processes,* Amsterdam, 1983, North-Holland.

27. Slimmer LW and Brown RT: Parent's decision making process in medication administration for control of hyperactivity, *J Sch Health* 55:221–225, 1985.

28. Slovic P, Fischhoff B, and Lichtenstein S: Response mode, framing, and information-processing effects in risk assessment. In Hogarth R, editor: *New directions for methodology of social and behaviorial science: question framing and response consistency,* San Francisco, 1982, Jossey-Bass Publishing.

29. Sox HC and others: *Medical decision making,* Boston, 1988, Butterworths Publishers.

30. Stotland E: *The psychology of hope,* San Francisco, 1969, Jossey-Bass Publishers.

31. Tversky A and Kahneman D: The framing of decisions and the psychology of choice, *Science* 211:453–458, 1981.

32. Tversky A and Kahneman D: Judgment under uncertainty: heuristics and bias. In Kahneman D, Slovic P, and Tversky A, editors: *Judgment under uncertainty: heuristics and biases,* Cambridge, 1982, Cambridge University Press.

33. Ward S, Heidrich S, and Wolberg W: Factors women take into account when deciding upon type of surgery for breast cancer, *Cancer Nurs* 12:344–351, 1989.

34. Weinstein MC and Fineberg HV: *Clinical decision analysis,* Philadelphia, 1980, WB Saunders Co.

35. Wilson CZ and Alexis M: Basic frameworks for decisions. In Koontz H and O'Donnell C, editors: *Management: a book of readings,* ed 3, New York, 1982, McGraw-Hill.

VI

Impaired Environmental Interpretation Syndrome

▶
___

Impaired Environmental Interpretation Syndrome *is a consistent lack of orientation to person, time, or circumstances over more than 3 to 6 months, necessitating a protective environment.*

OVERVIEW

Impaired Environmental Interpretation Syndrome is a nursing diagnosis that focuses on patients exhibiting cognitive impairment (i.e., dementia, neurological disease, or substance abuse). The degree of cognitive impairment is moderate to severe and usually necessitates admission or placement in an alternative living situation. Individuals are not able to live alone, The cost of health care for these patients is significant. Continuity of care issues are usually ongoing and require a number of resources to provide for the special needs of this population.[11]

The confused patient displays a behavioral inconsistency with the immediate environment. The patient's response to environmental stimuli, problem-solving ability, and capacity to follow complex instruction are compromised. A confused person often spends his or her time in a solitary activity, does nothing, or engages in behavior such as pacing or wandering. Cognitively impaired patients may not be aware of the change in their behavior or may not recognize a lapse of participation in their usual activities. This population requires increased time and supervision to provide for their safety and well-being. Management and care of these patients can present an overwhelming challenge.[2,4,11]

ASSESSMENT

The initial assessment of the individual for whom the nursing diagnosis Impaired Environmental Interpretation Syndrome is selected requires a detailed review. The areas of focus include cognitive status, living arrangements, support network, and usual daily activity schedule. Family members or friends may provide additional facts that the individual may not recall about his or her life events. Other data sources include community agencies, medical records, and other health providers. A review of medical records may provide information about baseline health, cognition, and functional ability. Comparison of past behavior and routines to present activity is important.

The individual's ability to concentrate, participate in conversation, and respond to commands can be assessed during the initial interview. These skills will reflect the person's ability to interact appropriately with the environment. There are a number of available tools to assist the practitioner in assessing cognition (e.g., the Folstein Mini-Mental State Examination [MMSE]). Referrals to appropriate disciplines (e.g., physical therapy, occupational therapy, audiology, optometry, and psychology) may be necessary to complete the evaluation of the patient's ability to complete activities of daily living (ADL) and instrumental activities of daily living (IADL).[1] Sensory impairment, if not corrected, may cause the individual to misinterpret environmental stimuli. The caregiver, family, or friends must report missing or broken glasses, hearing aids, or dentures, and an attempt

VI

must be made to repair or replace these items. A change or interruption of the sleep-wake pattern or the environment may result in overstimulation and problematic behaviors. Environmental changes include relocation, rearrangement of furniture, different pictures or accessories, daylight-savings time, holiday activities, change in caregiver, or an altered daily schedule. Assessment of the individual's likes and dislikes, personal preferences, comfort items, and pleasurable activities will provide a basis for care.

■ Defining Characteristics

The presence of the following defining characteristics indicates that the patient may be experiencing Impaired Environmental Interpretation Syndrome:

- Consistent disorientation in known and unknown environments
- Chronic confusional states
- Loss of occupation or social functioning from memory decline
- Inability to follow simple directions or instructions
- Inability to reason
- Inability to concentrate
- Slowness in responding to questions

■ Related Factors

The following related factors are associated with Impaired Environmental Interpretation Syndrome:

- Dementia (Alzheimer's disease, multiinfarct dementia, Pick's disease, or AIDS dementia)
- Parkinson's disease
- Huntington's disease
- Depression
- Alcoholism

DIAGNOSIS

■ Differential Nursing Diagnosis

The nursing diagnosis Impaired Environmental Interpretation Syndrome is used for individuals who experience a cognitive impairment lasting longer than 3 to 6 months. There are three nursing diagnoses similar to Impaired Environmental Interpretation Syndrome. The first, Alteration in Thought Process, may be more appropriate for clients with a psychiatric diagnosis. Impaired Memory may be used for patients exhibiting acute or chronic disruptions of memory. Chronic Confusion has many of the same elements and interventions as Impaired Environmental Interpretation Syndrome. Selection of an appropriate nursing diagnosis may be difficult and is ultimately left to the nurse's interpretation. In contrast, Acute Confusion is clearly appropriate for an individual exhibiting signs and symptoms of delirium.

■ Medical and Psychiatric Diagnoses

Dementia of the Alzheimer's type (DAT) is a psychiatric diagnosis often associated with the nursing diagnosis Impaired Environmental Interpretation Syndrome. Other associated medical diagnoses are Alzheimer's disease, cerebral vascular accident, and head injury. The provision of care for patients with these diagnoses is often complex and requires collaboration among disciplines and agencies. Case management is one effective method used to coordinate care delivery to this population.

OUTCOME IDENTIFICATION, PLANNING, AND IMPLEMENTATION

The patient will function in a structured environment is an expected patient outcome. The cognitively impaired patient is able to experience optimum function in a supportive, structured environment. The physical setting and staff contribute to the milieu that makes up the patient's environment. The staff must interact with the patient using a positive approach and communication skills that demonstrate a high regard for the individual. Controlling the external stimuli (e.g., noise level, traffic activity, or disturbing visual images) that affect the milieu is essential. Activities must be meaningful and should be selected according to the unique needs and interests of the patient. The

◢ **NURSING CARE GUIDELINES**

Nursing Diagnosis: Impaired Environmental Interpretation Syndrome

Expected Outcome: The patient will be able to function in a structured environment within 2 weeks.

▲ Establish a consistent daily routine. *Patients compensate for inability to plan activities by developing a daily routine that becomes automatic.*[7]

■ Provide consistent caregiver(s). *Patients will experience increased security when cared for by people they recognize.*[10]

■ Approach and communicate with the patient in a positive manner. *Verbal and nonverbal communication are important in establishing a relationship with a person who is cognitively impaired.*[12]

■ Provide opportunity for 1:1 conversation with caregiver(s). *Providing sufficient time for interacting with patient reinforces socialization skill and a sense of self-worth.*[6]

▲ Place meaningful possessions in the patient's environment (e.g., photographs, furniture, or special possessions). *Familiar belongings promote a sense of security.*[10]

■ Avoid change in room environment (e.g., reassignment of patient's room, rearrangement of furniture or belongings, or holiday decorations). *Frequent environment change may produce conflicting cues.*[3]

▲ Provide a daily time for small group activity that is valued by patient (e.g., music, art, reminiscence group, selected television program, or Bible therapy). *Planned activities are beneficial if they are pleasurable and incorporate the patient's culture, habits, values, manners, preference, and occupation.*[5,7,8]

▲ Ensure optimal sensory input (i.e., eyeglasses are clean, hearing aid is functional, absence of cerumen impaction). *The cognitive impaired patient is at risk for misinterpretation of the environment when sensory input is not accurate.*[1,3]

■ Provide adequate nonglare lighting. *Visual perceptions may be altered by glare or shadows.*[3]

■ Eliminate unnecessary environmental stimuli (e.g., excessive noise level, multiple conversations or activities, and violent, aggressive movies or television programs). *Disturbing visual images or loud noises can precipitate a catastrophic reaction.*[9]

■ = nursing intervention; ▲ = collaborative intervention.

provision of items familiar to the patient (e.g., photographs, furniture, or special possessions) will support a sense of belonging and comfort. Having a consistent daily routine and treatment by caregivers (staff) they recognize plays an important part in successful care delivery for this patient population. It is difficult to complete an evaluation and establish effective intervention in a 2-week time frame. The focus of treatment is to provide an environment that remains consistent.

EVALUATION

The degree of cognitive impairment will affect the success of this outcome. Variation in the milieu or the individual's health status may interfere with the achievement of this outcome. Adaptation to new or unfamiliar surroundings may exceed the 2-week time frame allocated in the care plan. The individual will have achieved the desired result when he or she is able to function within the environment. If the individual is not able to function in the environment as expected, additional collaboration with the multidisciplinary team is indicated. There are a few individuals whose cognitive impairment has progressed to the point that they are unable to maintain a degree of normalcy in their routine.

VI

◤ CASE STUDY WITH PLAN OF CARE

Milton R. is an 80-year-old gentleman who has lived alone since his wife died 6 years ago. The family has been concerned about Mr. R. over the last 6 months. They report that he has had increasing difficulty in remembering if he has eaten, when to put the garbage out, and if he has paid the utility bill. A few weeks ago he phoned the police to report his car had been stolen while he was in the grocery store. The car was found on the opposite side of the parking lot. While on his daily walk in the neighborhood park, he fell and fractured his hip when he tried to avoid a group of skateboarders. He spent a week in the hospital following hip surgery. During this time, the hospital staff reported that he has experienced episodes of confusion. He is being discharged to the rehabilitation unit for mobility training and evaluation. Mr. R. insists that he is going to return to his own home.

◤ PLAN OF CARE FOR MR. MILTON R.

Nursing Diagnosis: Impaired Environmental Interpretation Syndrome Related to Dementia

Expected Outcome: Mr. R. will function in a consistent structured environment.

- ▲ Establish a consistent daily care and therapy schedule.
- ■ Assign primary nurse/therapist(s) to provide care.
- ■ Select room assignment in an area of low environment stimulation.
- ▲ Involve the family in care planning (i.e., preference and past activity patterns).
- ■ Ensure optimal sensory input (i.e., clean eyeglasses, hearing aid, absence of cerumen impaction).
- ■ Adjust lighting to Mr. R.'s preference.
- ■ Eliminated unnecessary environmental stimuli (e.g., excessive noise level or multiple conversations).
- ▲ Communicate new or relevant patient information to other staff and therapists.

■ = nursing intervention; ▲ = collaborative intervention.

▦ CRITICAL THINKING EXERCISES

1. What factors would you consider in assisting the family to participate in the discharge planning process?

2. How would you approach Mr. R. if an alternative living situation is included in the discharge plan?

3. A new nurse floats to your rehabilitation unit. What information would you consider important to communicate to her or him about delivery of care to Mr. R.?

REFERENCES

1. Abraham IL and others: Multidisciplinary assessment of patients with Alzheimer's disease, *Nurs Clin North Am* 29(1):113–128, 1994.

2. Armstrong-Esther CA, Browne KD, and McAfee JG: Elderly patients: still clean and sitting quietly, *J Adv Nurs* 19:264–271, 1994.

3. Beck CK and Shue VM: Interventions for treating disruptive behavior in demented elderly people, *Nurs Clin North Am* 29(1):143–155, 1994.

4. Bowie P and Mountain G: Using direct observation to record the behavior of long-stay patients with dementia, *Int J Geriatr Psychiatry* 8:857–864, 1993.

5. Forbes EJ: Spirituality, aging and the community-dwelling caregiver and care recipient, *Geriatr Nurs* 15(6):296–301, 1994.

6. Goldsmith SM, Hoeffer B, and Rader J: Problematic wandering behavior in the cognitively impaired elderly, *J Psychosoc Nurs* 33(2):6–12, 1995.

7. Hall GR: Caring for people with Alzheimer's disease using the conceptual model of progressively lowered stress threshold in the clinical setting, *Nurs Clin North Am* 29(1):129–141, 1994.

8. Khovsam HR: Bible study: a treatment in elderly patients with Alzheimer's disease, *Clin Gerontol* 15(2):71–74, 1994.

VI

9. Nelson J: The influence of environmental factors in incidents of disruptive behavior, *J Geront Nurs* 21(5):19–24, 1995.

10. Rants MJ and McShane RE: Nursing interventions for chronically confused nursing home residents, *Geriatr Nurs* 16(1):22–27, 1995.

11. Shedd PP, Kobokovich LJ, and Slattery MJ: Confused patients in the acute care setting: prevalence, interventions, and outcomes, *J Geront Nurs* 21(4):5–12, 1995.

12. Stolley JM and others: Managing the care of patients with irreversible dementia during hospitalization for comorbidities, *Nurs Clin North Am* 28(4):767–782, 1993.

VI

Knowledge Deficit (Specify)

▶

Knowledge Deficit (Specify) *is an absence or deficiency of cognitive information*[15] *or the inability to state or explain information or demonstrate a required skill. It is also the inability to explain or use self-care practices recommended to restore health or maintain wellness.*[8] *It may present as a cognitive or psychomotor deficit*[3] *or as a combination of the two.*

OVERVIEW

The nursing diagnosis Knowledge Deficit is the nurse's judgment that the patient lacks the information needed to be an active, informed participant in his or her health care.[16] A deficit in knowledge is commonly experienced by individuals coping with new medical diagnoses, varied pharmacological and treatment regimens, and unfamiliar and often complex procedures and by individuals entering developmental stages or role relationships that demand new patterns of response. Several epidemiological studies have identified Knowledge Deficit as a high-frequency diagnosis among varied patient populations and clinical settings.*

To understand the theory of Knowledge Deficit, one must understand the hierarchy of learning.[12] Knowledge attainment is the most basic type of cognitive learning. It entails receiving and retaining a factual statement long enough to recall it later. Attitudinal learning requires an emotional response rather than a factual one. It involves acquiring information and then personally responding to it.

Psychomotor learning is the behavioral response to internalized information through neuromuscular pathways. It represents the level of learning at which behavior change becomes possible.

The diagnosis Knowledge Deficit is broad and can be applied to deficits in all three learning realms. It may be appropriately applied in circumstances where a person needs increased factual information and in situations where the patient can correctly state the relevant facts but cannot incorporate them into appropriate behavior.

It should be noted that there is a difference between the patient who is unable to translate information into behavior change and the patient who elects not to do so. In the latter case the appropriate diagnosis is not Knowledge Deficit, and assessment must distinguish between the two cases. Differential diagnoses for such patients include Altered Health Maintenance, Noncompliance, Decisional Conflict, and Defensive Coping.

Taxonomy II defines *knowing* as "To recognize or acknowledge . . . to be familiar with . . . to be cognizant of something . . . to understand."[7] Several authors have discussed the broad scope and imprecision of the label and have proposed that it be revised[7] or deleted.[5,7,10,11] Jenny[10] argued that Knowledge Deficit is not a health state or dysfunctional pattern of behavior. She suggested that Knowledge Deficit is more often a risk factor or defining characteristic of another diagnosis. Dennison and Keeling[5] found that its use fostered stereotypical interventions and failed to enhance creative nursing strategies designed to increase information and change behavior. Rakel and Bulechek[17] argued that Knowledge Deficit is valid but too broad in scope and is applied to situations

---

*References 1, 2, 4, 6, 9, 13.

where the problem is alteration in learning, rather than alteration in knowledge. They proposed that two additional diagnoses be included in the Cognitive-Perceptual Pattern, to describe situational learning disabilities.

Because Knowledge Deficit may be a symptom of another problem, the nurse must determine the appropriate clinical weight of the acquired assessment data when he or she formulates the differential diagnosis of every case. The diagnostician must base assessment and diagnosis on an understanding of all types of learning and must recognize that rarely is a simple increase in factual knowledge the optimal outcome of nursing care. Both diagnoses and interventions must focus on facilitating and enhancing health-promoting integration of factual knowledge. Knowledge Deficit will undoubtedly continue to be further refined and specified.

ASSESSMENT

The ability of the nurse to identify and treat a Knowledge Deficit is heavily influenced by his or her understanding of teaching and learning theories and by the scope of assessment in areas that might seem unrelated to knowledge. The impact of such variables as chronological and developmental age, psychological condition, presence of anxiety, socioeconomic status, level of formal education, cultural and language barriers, and interest in learning must be weighed at each phase of the nursing process. Each of these affects the way that the patient's Knowledge Deficit presents and the likelihood that it will be ameliorated.

Validation studies of the defining characteristics of Knowledge Deficit are limited.[5,16] Two studies found the label applied in the apparent absence of any of the published defining characteristics. This may indicate an automatic, rote application of the diagnosis to justify task-oriented patient teaching,[16] or it may reflect the use of defining characteristics as part of the art of providing skilled nursing care, yet to be adequately articulated.

No critical defining characteristics for the diagnosis Knowledge Deficit have been suggested or validated through research.[16] The patient's statements of inadequate recall or understanding of information and of inadequate knowledge are the defining characteristics best supported by the literature.[16] The defining characteristics primarily affect the acquisition of knowledge. Defining characteristics that are behavioral include inaccurately following instructions and inadequately performing a skill or taking a test. Testing, though often used in didactic situations and research, remain an uncommon clinical assessment tool in acute care and community care settings. When applied, often in ambulatory settings, it can provide a useful measurement of knowledge, attitude, and behavioral change.

Assessment must include the broad range of relevant data. These may be cultural factors, socioeconomic factors, developmental stage, intellectual capacity, psychological response to existing illness or wellness, current knowledge, extent to which knowledge is incorporated into behavior, and motivation and readiness to learn. Sensory, neuromuscular, cardiopulmonary, and nutritive integrity must be considered as well.

Both Gordon[8] and the North American Nursing Diagnosis Association (NANDA)[15] list inappropriate or exaggerated behaviors, such as hysteria, apathy, agitation, and hostility, among the defining characteristics of Knowledge Deficit. No other nursing literature supports this, so these behaviors have been omitted from the following list, pending some support for their relevancy.

■ Defining Characteristics

The presence of the following defining characteristics indicates that the patient may be experiencing Knowledge Deficit:

- Verbalization of inadequate information or of inadequate recall of information
- Verbalization of misunderstanding or misconception
- Requesting information
- Instructions inaccurately followed
- Inadequate performance on a test
- Inadequate demonstration of a skill

■ **Related Factors**

The following related factors are associated with Knowledge Deficit:

- Pathophysiological states
- Sensory deficits
- Memory loss
- Intellectual limitations
- Interfering coping strategies (e.g., denial or anxiety)
- Lack of exposure to accurate information
- Lack of motivation to learn
- Lack of readiness to learn
- Inattention
- Cultural or language barriers

DIAGNOSIS

■ **Differential Nursing Diagnosis**

Anxiety, Ineffective Individual Coping, Noncompliance, and Impaired Social Interaction often occur simultaneously with Knowledge Deficit and share defining characteristics or related factors with that diagnosis. A thorough patient assessment should help determine which is the primary problem by considering behavior or verbal statements in light of all the data collected. Often the patient can validate that he or she is anxious because of a lack of critical information versus an inability to recall and use the information he or she has received because of feeling anxious. In some cases it is vital to identify the primary diagnosis because the desired outcome can only be achieved if the primary problem is addressed. In other circumstances the desired outcome can be achieved by treating either diagnosis. Knowledge Deficit may be identified with many other nursing diagnoses.

■ **Medical and Psychiatric Diagnoses**

Many medical diagnoses simultaneously occur with Knowledge Deficit. Among them are hypertension, diabetes mellitus, asthma, and coronary artery disease. Patients with medical and psychiatric diagnoses requiring knowledge for self-care could be considered at risk for Knowledge Deficit. Any illness, developmental stage, or role transition is potentially associated with Knowledge Deficit.

OUTCOME IDENTIFICATION, PLANNING, AND IMPLEMENTATION

Outcome criteria for the patient being treated for Knowledge Deficit can refer to any of the three types of learning: knowledge attainment, attitudinal change, and behavior change. The predominant intervention to treat Knowledge Deficit is patient education. There is a substantial body of literature supporting the contention that varied teaching strategies increase factual knowledge, affect attitudinal changes, and result in behavioral changes.

The outcome criteria and interventions in the standardized care plan represent a continuum. The full spectrum is not necessarily appropriate in all situations. At times the patient's simple demonstration of increased knowledge may be a valid end point for nursing interventions. Because the success of each outcome in the hierarchy depends on the achievement of the lower ones, the interventions identified for the lower outcomes mentioned first in the care plan also apply to the ones mentioned later, but these interventions are not repeated.

Although the categories for outcomes described in the Nursing Care Guidelines can be broadly generalized, the interventions may be quite specific to the particular type of Knowledge Deficit under consideration. These are intended to provide but a few examples of outcomes and rationales.

Simple knowledge attainment or knowledge increase is a first-stage outcome. Patient teaching or patient education is often directed at that goal. A variety of possible techniques have been used to assist the patient to increase knowledge. It is critical that the nurse weigh such variables as culture, developmental stage, acuity or chronicity of the learning need, and the patient's ability and motivation to learn when selecting a particular teaching approach.

Attitudinal change is a second-stage outcome. The patient must evaluate factual knowledge, determine its relevance to his or her own perceived circumstance, and reevaluate personal behaviors in that context. The interventions in this

VI

◢ **NURSING CARE GUIDELINES**
Nursing Diagnosis: Knowledge Deficit

Expected Outcome: The patient will accurately state two facts related to his or her illness within 24 hours.
- Provide accurate and culturally relevant information related to the specific topic, using a teaching technique congruent with the patient's learning need. *The patient must receive accurate information.*
- Involve the patient's family or significant others in the learning process. *The family is able to reinforce and clarify new learning.*

Expected Outcome: The patient will verbally express his or her understanding of information and its usefulness to him or her within 1 to 2 days.
- Discuss and review factual content with patient and family *to assess recall and understanding.*
- Explore the patient's interpretation of the information and its meaning to him or her *to assist the patient to evaluate facts in the context of his or her own life.*

Expected Outcome: The patient will modify his or her behavior based on the acquisition of new knowledge. (The time frame will vary greatly depending on the specific Knowledge Deficit.)
- Identify strategies and resources and behavior change.
- Support and encourage initial and ongoing attempts at change.
- Support the patient through episodes of failure.
- Assist the patient to identify and implement alternative strategies for attaining goals if initial choices are not successful. *The nurse is able to reinforce health-enhancing behaviors positively.*

■ = nursing intervention; ▲ = collaborative intervention.

VI

cluster are designed to assist the patient to evaluate facts in the context of his or her own life.

Behavioral change is a third-stage outcome. Facts and attitudes have been internalized, and the patient is able to demonstrate the value he or she has attached to them by amending a less healthy behavior to one that is more health-enhancing. The rationale for the interventions to promote behavior modification is to reinforce health-enhancing behaviors positively.

EVALUATION

The measures to evaluate success will vary depending on the outcome criteria selected. The patient's acquisition of factual knowledge can be readily measured by written or verbal questioning. This can be done informally as the teaching progresses or formally at the conclusion of a teaching session or series of sessions. Behavioral change is best evaluated by requiring a demonstration of skill or attainment of a specific predetermined goal (e.g., no smoking for 2 days). Attitudinal change is per-

haps the most nebulous and difficult to evaluate. Verbal or written statements indicating an openness to another's viewpoint and an interest in exploring the value of behavioral change (if relevant) indicate that the outcome criteria have been met.

Because of the diversity of clinical situations in which the diagnosis Knowledge Deficit is made, time frames for outcome attainment are difficult to specify. The acuity of the patient's medical condition, his or her learning style and capacity, the amount and nature of the knowledge to be gained, and the setting in which the learning is to occur will all affect the time frame.

Failure to attain the expected outcomes should prompt the nurse to reassess the accuracy of the diagnosis. If it is still felt to be an accurate diagnosis, alternative interventions should be applied. Developmental, cultural, socioeconomic, and interpersonal variables may need reexamination in selecting new techniques. At times a failure to correct Knowledge Deficit occurs because another more fundamental problem must be resolved before the patient is ready or able to learn effectively.

VI

■ CASE STUDY WITH PLAN OF CARE

Mr. Benjamin F., a 22-year-old man, comes to the anonymous test site at the community health center for a human immunodeficiency virus (HIV) antibody test. He is worried that his work situation puts him at risk for exposure to the virus and wants to know his antibody status. He has generally good health and maintains appropriate weight. Mr. F. does not use drugs now, but he did use intravenous heroin for a 6-month period 3 years ago. He has been "clean" since then. He drinks two or three beers on weekends. His Nutritional-Metabolic Pattern, Elimination Pattern, and Sleep-Rest Pattern are all normal and unremarkable. For exercise he uses a stationary bicycle three times a week. He is completely independent in all activities of daily living, and he experiences occasional fatigue that he attributes to working too much overtime. Mr. F.'s vision, hearing, and memory are all excellent. After attending college for 2 years, he now works as a draftsman in an architectural firm. He describes himself as a quick learner, but he responds correctly to only three of the ten questions on the quiz to measure baseline knowledge about HIV infection. Mr. F. says he learns readily from written material and televised programs. Mr. F. is comfortable with his body image and present life, and he hopes to complete college eventually. He lives alone in a one-bedroom apartment, and his family lives in another state. His income is adequate for his needs. He has several close friends nearby. He dates two women regularly and is considering a more serious relationship with the one with whom he is sexually active twice a week. She uses oral contraceptives. Mr. F. is becoming increasingly worried about contracting the HIV infection at work. A co-worker tested HIV positive 6 months ago. Mr. F. and this person use the same telephone, drafting implements, and bathroom facilities. Mr. F. hopes to marry within the next year and believes that it his duty to be sure he does not "bring AIDS home from the office."

■ PLAN OF CARE FOR MR. BENJAMIN F.
Nursing Diagnosis: Knowledge Deficit Related to Lack of Exposure to Correct Information

Expected Outcome: Mr. F. will correctly state three transmission pathways for HIV infections within 1 day.
- Provide accurate information about HIV transmission, using verbal instruction and an AIDS education video.
- Give Mr. F. pamphlets containing the same information to read at home.
- Repeat and reinforce the information at least twice.

Expected Outcome: Mr. F. will correctly state the past behavior (IV drug use) and the present behavior (unprotected sex) that put him at risk for HIV infection within 1 hour.
- Assist him to relate information about risks to his health caused by his own behavior.
- Provide Mr. F. with information to refute misconceptions.
- Support Mr. F. in expressing feelings of anger or guilt, if appropriate.

Expected Outcome: Mr. F. will correctly state the result of his antibody test and its meaning within 1 week.
- ▲ Draw blood specimen and submit to laboratory.
- Inform Mr. F. of the result of the test.
- Explain the significance of the result.
- Ask Mr. F. to repeat the result and its meaning to you.

Expected Outcome: Mr. F. will adopt sexual practices that will reduce his risk of acquiring HIV infection sexually.
- Discuss abstinence as a sexual choice.
- Discuss safer sex practices.
- Demonstrate the proper technique for condom application and allow a return demonstration.
- Maintain an open and nonjudgmental attitude.

■ = nursing intervention; ▲ = collaborative intervention.

■ CRITICAL THINKING EXERCISES

1. What is the differential diagnosis for Mr. F.?
2. Is Knowledge Deficit the primary problem or a defining characteristic of another diagnosis?
3. Is there evidence of other nursing diagnoses that should be addressed?
4. What additional interventions might be used?
5. What alternative strategies might be used if the outcomes are not attained?

REFERENCES

1. Aukamp V: A field study to identify nursing diagnoses for childbearing families. In McLane A, editor: *Classification of nursing diagnoses: proceedings of the Seventh Conference,* St. Louis, 1987, The CV Mosby Co.
2. Burns CE: Field testing of a comprehensive taxonomy of diagnoses for pediatric nurse practitioners. In Carroll-Johnson RM, editor: *Classification of nursing diagnoses: proceedings of the Ninth Conference,* Philadelphia, 1991, JB Lippincott Co.
3. Carpenito LJ: *Nursing diagnosis: application to clinical practice,* ed 5, Philadelphia, 1993, JB Lippincott Co.
4. Collard AF and others: The occurrence of nursing diagnoses in ambulatory care. In McLane A, editor: *Classification of nursing diagnoses: proceedings of the Seventh Conference,* St. Louis, 1987, The CV Mosby Co.
5. Dennison PD and Keeling AW: Clinical support for eliminating the nursing diagnosis of knowledge deficit, *Image J Nurs Sch* 21:142–144, 1989.
6. Fitzmaurice JB, Thatcher J, and Schappler N: High-volume, high-risk nursing diagnoses as a basis for priority setting in a tertiary hospital. In Carroll-Johnson RM, editor: *Classification of nursing diagnoses: proceedings of the Ninth Conference,* Philadelphia, 1991, JB Lippincott Co.
7. Fitzpatrick JJ: Taxonomy II: definitions and development. In Carroll-Johnson RM, editor: *Classification of nursing diagnoses: proceedings of the Ninth Conference,* Philadelphia, 1991, JB Lippincott Co.
8. Gordon M: *Manual of nursing diagnosis, 1993–1994,* New York, 1993, McGraw-Hill.
9. Greenlee KK: The effects of implementation of an operational definition and guidelines for the formulation of nursing diagnoses in a critical care setting. In Carroll-Johnson RM, editor: *Classification of nursing diagnoses: proceedings of the Ninth Conference,* Philadelphia, 1991, JB Lippincott Co.
10. Jenny J: Knowledge deficit: not a nursing diagnosis, *Image J Nurs Sch* 19:184–185, 1987.
11. Kuhn RC: American Association of Critical Care Nurses. In Carroll-Johnson RM, editor: *Classification of nursing diagnoses: proceedings of the Ninth Conference,* Philadelphia, 1991, JB Lippincott Co.
12. Lester PA: Teaching strategies. In Johnson SE, editor: *Nursing assessment and strategies for the family at risk: high-risk parenting,* ed 2, Philadelphia, 1986, JB Lippincott Co.
13. Martin PA and York KA: Incidence of nursing diagnoses. In Kim MJ, McFarland GK, and McLane AM, editors: *Classification of nursing diagnoses: proceedings of the Fifth Conference,* St. Louis, 1984, The CV Mosby Co.
14. Nicoletti A: Nurse's Association of the American College of Obstetrics and Gynecology. In Carroll-Johnson RM, editor: *Classification of nursing diagnoses: proceedings of the Ninth Conference,* Philadelphia, 1991, JB Lippincott Co.
15. North American Nursing Diagnosis Association: *NANDA nursing diagnoses: definitions and classification, 1995–1996,* Philadelphia, 1994, The Association.
16. Pokorny BE: Validating a diagnostic label: knowledge deficit, *Nurs Clin North Am* 20(4):641–655, 1985.
17. Rakel BA and Bulechek GM: Development of alterations in learning: situational learning disabilities, *Nurs Diagnosis* 1:134–146, 1990.

VI

Impaired Memory

▶

Impaired Memory *is the state in which an individual is unable to remember bits of information or behavioral skills. Impaired memory may be attributed to pathophysiological or situational causes that are temporary or permanent.*

OVERVIEW

Memory is the physiological basis of learning and consists of the declarative and procedural systems. The declarative memory system is divided into short-term, recent, and long-term memory. Short-term memory is consciously activated by the individual and requires the ability to focus. Recent memory is not affected by distraction; the individual can attend to other things and not lose recent memory. The recent memory system is important for transferring short-term memory to long-term memory. Storage of information (memories) from days to years is called long-term memory. The procedural memory system includes memory of responses or "how" to do something. Skills and habits are established only by actually performing or engaging in the task. The procedural memory system can be used to compensate for losses in the declarative memory system. Thus learning can be facilitated by conditioning responses or developing patterns to form habits that do not rely on memory.

Loss of memory without apparent physical change or deterioration is often devastating to the individual and difficult for caregivers and family members to comprehend.[6] The inability to perform or neglecting to complete a familiar task, such as grooming, is often the first indication of memory impairment. The onset of memory im-

pairment may be sudden, as in a delirium resulting from an adverse medication reaction, or it may happen more slowly, as in a progression of inability to remember. The deficit may be temporary or permanent.

ASSESSMENT

The initial assessment of the patient with the nursing diagnosis Impaired Memory requires a comprehensive approach. The areas of focus include cognitive status, etiology of memory impairment, coping methods, and usual lifestyle. Family members or friends may provide additional facts that the individual may not recall about his or her life events. A review of medical records may provide information about baseline health, additional diagnoses, cognition, and functional ability. Comparison of past behavior and routines to present activity is important. The patient's ability to participate in conversation, to focus, and to respond to instruction can be assessed during the initial interview. These skills will reflect the patient's ability to interact appropriately. There are a number of tools available to assist the practitioner in assessing memory function and cognition (e.g., the Folstein Mini-Mental State Examination [MMSE]). Referrals to appropriate disciplines (e.g., occupational therapy, speech pathology, and psychology) may be necessary to complete the evaluation.

■ Defining Characteristics

The presence of the following defining characteristics indicates that the patient may be experiencing Impaired Memory:

- Observed or reported experiences of forgetting
- Inability to determine whether a behavior was performed
- Inability to learn or retain new skills or information
- Inability to perform a previously learned skill
- Inability to recall factual information
- Inability to recall recent or past events
- Forgets to perform a behavior at a scheduled time

■ Related Factors

The following related factors are associated with Impaired Memory:

- Acute or chronic output
- Anemia
- Decreased cardiac output
- Fluid and electrolyte imbalance
- Neurological disturbances
- Excessive environmental disturbances

DIAGNOSIS

■ Differential Nursing Diagnosis

The nursing diagnosis Impaired Memory may be appropriate for individuals who are unable to recall information or who are temporarily or permanently unable to complete usual behavioral skills. Alteration in Thought Process is similar and may be more familiar to the practitioner. The nursing diagnosis Chronic Confusion encompasses the elements of the human response to impaired cognition. Impaired Environmental Interpretation Syndrome has many of the same elements and interventions as Chronic Confusion. Acute Confusion is clearly appropriate for the individual exhibiting signs and symptoms of delirium. Selection of an appropriate nursing diagnosis may be difficult and is ultimately left to the nurse's interpretation.

■ Medical and Psychiatric Diagnoses

Acute or chronic hypoxia, anemia, decreased cardiac output, fluid and electrolyte imbalance, and neurological disturbances are medical conditions most often associated with the nursing diagnosis Impaired Memory. Mood disorders may also be associated with this nursing diagnosis. The provision of care for individuals with these conditions and an associated memory loss are often complicated and require extensive evaluation to determine the specific etiology and impairment. Care planning requires collaboration among members of a multidisciplinary team.

OUTCOME IDENTIFICATION, PLANNING, AND IMPLEMENTATION

It is important to establish a rapport with the patient and family. Provide an uninterrupted time and place to allow the individual and family members to discuss treatment goals and concerns. Awareness of the existing impairment is critical to the therapeutic process. The family may benefit from reviewing results of diagnostic testing and validating their observations. This discussion may provide opportunities for family or caregiver education.

The cognitively impaired patient is able to experience optimum function in a supportive, structured environment. The physical setting and the staff contribute to the milieu and provide structure for the rehabilitation process. The staff must interact with the patient using a consistent approach. Activities must be meaningful and should be selected according to the unique preferences of the patient. The provision of items familiar to the individual (e.g., photographs or special possessions) will facilitate memory training. A consistent presentation of information within multiple contexts will promote retention of a new material.[10]

VI

■■ **NURSING CARE GUIDELINES**
Nursing Diagnosis: Impaired Memory

Expected Outcome: The patient will verbalize awareness of memory deficit.

- ■ Provide opportunities for the patient to discuss concerns about Impaired Memory. *Individuals do not necessarily define themselves or their health concerns in terms of disability.*[8] *There is a positive relationship between awareness and treatment outcome.*[10]
- ■ Assure patient that memory impairment is not unusual. *Cognitive difficulty is ranked number one in residual symptoms following brain injury.*[3,7]
- ▲ Collaborate with other disciplines to determine extent of memory impairment. *Comprehensive treatment by multidisciplinary team members is required from a few weeks to 2 years following brain injury.*[5,7]
- ■ Include family members in process of evaluation and rehabilitation. *Individuals with disabilities can set health goals and achieve them; family members are often actively engaged in assisting with therapy and rehabilitation.*[5,9]

Expected Outcome: The patient will participate in the memory rehabilitation process.

- ▲ Assist patient in use of memory book. *Interventions that focus on purposeful activity often improve cognitive function.*[1]
- ■ Cue patient to pair new learning with old (e.g., rather than focus on the task of combing hair, refer to the patient's favorite comb or brush). *It is important to integrate past experiences and individual preferences when designing activities.*[6]
- ■ Frequent cueing and practice of new skills is important. *There is an increased feeling of success when a person can practice and master a task.*[2]
- ■ Present material in different ways (i.e., written, verbally in language(s) understood by patient, pictures, and by demonstration) to determine the individual's preference for learning. *Presentation of educational material should incorporate culture, habits, values, and preferences that have developed over the life span.*[4]
- ■ Be consistent in using memory-training techniques. *Consistent technique applied to multiple contexts facilitates transfer of information.*[10]
- ■ Proceed from simple to complex instruction. *There is risk that a patient will become overwhelmed and withdraw when the amount of information exceeds the capacity to incorporate it.*[10]

■ = nursing intervention; ▲ = collaborative intervention.

EVALUATION

The degree of cognitive impairment and the unique qualities of each individual will affect the success of this outcome. The patient will have achieved the desired result when he or she is able to participate in activities with the expected amount of cueing. If the patient is not able to function as expected, additional collaboration with the multidisciplinary team is indicated. There are a few individuals whose cognitive impairment is severe, and progress will be subtle. These individuals often are unaware of any impairment. Collaboration with the family will yield information about how the patient participates in the home environment in contrast to the therapeutic setting. Involvement of family members in the therapeutic plan plays an important part in the successful accomplishment of goals. Success must be measured against the individual's baseline and expected prognosis. It is difficult to implement all interventions in a 2-week time frame. If the expected outcomes are not met, collaboration with the multidisciplinary team may be indicated.

■ CASE STUDY WITH PLAN OF CARE

Miss D. is a 60-year-old librarian who is working full-time and is active in civic groups. Her health is good except for some arthritic changes. Last month she received a head injury while on the job. The physician at the emergency room advised her to make a follow-up appointment with her physician to make sure everything was okay. Since the injury, she has noticed that there are changes in her ability to recall information and that she sometimes forgets what she is doing if interrupted. Her friends confirm that she sometimes forgets that she called them and repeats the same information to them. Her physician has referred her to a memory-training program.

■ PLAN OF CARE FOR MISS D.
Nursing Diagnosis: Impaired Memory Related to Head Trauma

Expected Outcome: Miss D. will verbalize awareness of memory deficit.
- Provide an opportunity for Miss D. to discuss concerns about Impaired Memory in a supportive environment.
- Assure Miss D. that memory impairment is not unusual after a head injury.

Expected Outcome: Miss D. will demonstrate the ability to use an effective recording system (memory book).
▲ Collaborate with family and significant others to identify previous organizational methods and styles.
▲ Collaborate with other disciplines to determine appropriate therapeutic techniques and approaches.
- Assist Miss D. in selecting a recording system that is meaningful to her, such as a daily calendar, note cards, or a memory book.
- Demonstrate method of recording meaningful information in memory book.
- Assist Miss D. to record data in memory book.
▲ Reinforce use of memory book for reference to attend therapy sessions.
▲ Monitor attendance at therapy sessions.
▲ Provide feedback when therapy sessions are not attended.
▲ Provide feedback and validation as Miss D. gains independence in use of recorded information.

■ = nursing intervention; ▲ = collaborative intervention.

■■ CRITICAL THINKING EXERCISES

1. What questions would you ask Miss D.'s friends that would help you plan appropriate interventions?
2. How would you know Miss D. has incorporated the use of the memory book into her daily routine?
3. What referrals to and interactions with other disciplines would you consider when in care planning?

REFERENCES

1. Abraham IL and Reel SJ: Cognitive nursing interventions with long-term care residents: effects on neurocognitive dimensions, *Arch Psychiatr Nurs* 6(6):356–365, 1992.
2. Becker H and others: Self-rated abilities for health practices: a health self-efficacy measure, *Health Values* 17(5):42–50, 1993.
3. Hall GR: Caring for people with Alzheimer's disease using the conceptual model of progressively lowered stress threshold in the clinical setting, *Nurs Clin North Am* 29(1):129–141, 1994.
4. Harrington DE and others: Current perceptions of rehabili-

tation professionals towards mild traumatic brain injury, *Arch Phys Med Rehabil* 74(6):579–586, 1993.

5. McDowell I and others: Late rehabilitation for closed head injury: clinical psychologists' interventions, *Clin Rehabil* 9: 150–156, 1995.

6. Paulanks BJ and Griffin LS: Behavioral responses of memory-impaired clients to selected nursing interventions, *Phys Occup Ther Geriatr* 12(1):65–78, 1993.

7. Rosenthal M: Mild traumatic brain injury, *Annals Emergency Med* 22(6):1048–1051, 1993.

8. Stuifbergen AK and others: Perceptions of health among adults with disabilities, *Health Values* 14(2):18–26, 1990.

9. Stuifbergen AK and Becker HA: Predictors of health-promoting lifestyles in persons with disabilities, *Res Nurs Health* 17:3–13, 1994.

10. Toglia JP: Generalization of treatment: a multicontext approach to cognitive perceptual impairment in adults with brain injury, *Am J Occup Ther* 45(6):505–516, 1991.

VI

Pain

▶
_____

Chronic Pain

▶
_____

Pain *is an unpleasant sensory and emotional experience associated with actual or potential tissue damage or described in terms of such damage.*[2]

Chronic Pain *is pain that persists a month beyond the usual course of an acute disease or reasonable time for an injury to heal, or pain that reoccurs at intervals for months or years.*[7]

OVERVIEW

The North American Nursing Diagnosis Association (NANDA) includes the diagnoses Pain and Chronic Pain on its official list of approved diagnoses.[25] Inclusion on the list indicates that a diagnosis shows readiness for use and continuing development. The taxonomy or classification system for nursing diagnoses classifies Pain and Chronic Pain under the category of altered comfort, which is included in the human response pattern of feeling, one of the nine organizing patterns of the taxonomy.[25] Pain as a nursing diagnosis is classified on a higher level than Chronic Pain, indicating that Pain is a phenomenon more general than Chronic Pain; thus it lacks the clinical specificity inherent in the diagnosis Chronic Pain.

Acute Pain, although not yet accepted as a nursing diagnosis by NANDA, is considered by pain experts to be distinct from Chronic Pain in terms of definition, signs and symptoms, and management.[2,6,22] For the purpose of this chapter, the phenomenon of Pain is described in general terms, and the phenomenon is operationalized via the nursing process in terms of acute and Chronic Pain.

The Phenomenon of Pain

Pain is a complex phenomenon. Although it is a very real experience to the person who experiences it, its varying characteristics and nebulous quality often makes it difficult for others to comprehend. It can dominate and seem to have an unending nature.[16] "Pain is a subjective experience that can be perceived directly only by the sufferer. It is a multidimensional phenomenon that can be described by pain location, intensity, temporal aspects, quality, impact, and meaning. Pain does not occur in isolation but in a specific human being in psychosocial, economic, and cultural contexts that influence the meaning, experience, and verbal and nonverbal expression of pain."[22]

McCaffery and Beebe offer an operational definition of Pain that is useful in the clinical setting: "Pain is whatever the experiencing person says it is, existing whenever he says it does."[17] This definition implies the personal, subjective nature of Pain and the responsibility of others to infer the presence of Pain based on the patient's communication of the experience. The patient's verbal and nonverbal behaviors—that is, what the patient says and does—become critical in determining whether the patient is experiencing pain. The patient's communications can be used to define and describe further the specific pain experience as it relates to the patient's perception.

To increase understanding of the phenomenon of pain and the pain experience, various theories have been proposed. Three theories are frequently addressed in the literature on Pain: specificity theory, pattern theory, and gate control theory.[8,24,27] Each of these theories addresses pain transmission and therefore could have implications for pain control. The gate control theory, which was proposed in 1965, gained wide acceptance and stimulated significant clinical research related to pain response and control. The theory suggests that the transmission of painful stimuli can be modulated through a gating mechanism located in the substantia gelatinosa in the dorsal horn of the spinal cord. It is thought that activity in the peripheral and central nervous systems could affect the opening and closing of the gate. Studies related to specific pain modulatory systems have supplemented the theory's description of pain transmission and enhanced understanding of the neural mechanisms underlying the variability of the pain experience.[11]

In addressing the variability of the experience, the patient's perception of and reaction to Pain must also be considered. Loeser[15] considers transmission, perception, and reaction in his description of the phenomenon of pain in terms of four components: nociception, pain, suffering, and pain behavior. Nociception involves the brain's detection of tissue damage and physiological transmission of Pain. The second component, pain, is described as the patient's perception of a nociceptive stimulus; this occurs in the brain stem. Suffering refers to the patient's affective response to pain; this involves the higher levels of the brain. Pain behavior includes "anything a person says or does or does not do that would lead one to infer that a noxious stimulus has occurred."[15] Pain behavior is influenced by environmental factors.

Classification of Pain

Because of the multidimensional nature of Pain, clinicians find it useful to classify Pain into two major types: acute and chronic. Such a classification assists the clinician in determining an appropriate plan for pain management. Acute and Chronic Pain typically are differentiated from one another according to the onset, duration, and cause of the pain.

Acute Pain. Bonica[8] defines acute pain as "a constellation of unpleasant sensory, perceptual, and emotional experiences, and certain associated autonomic, psychologic, emotional, and behavioral responses." Acute Pain is an event of recent onset, is usually sudden, and is limited in duration. It is associated with an acute illness or disease, operative or treatment procedures, or trauma. The pain subsides as healing takes place.[2] Other characteristics that distinguish acute pain from Chronic Pain include (1) the pain area is usually identifiable, (2) suffering decreases over time, (3) defining characteristics are more obvious, and (4) there is a likelihood of eventual, complete relief.

Chronic Pain. Chronic Pain is a situation or state of existence. It is characterized by the pain experience continuing a month after the time an acute disease or injury should have healed or recurring at intervals for months or years.[7] Although some clinicians[25] use 6 months as the time frame during which Pain continues before being classified as Chronic Pain, Bonica[7] and others[17,27] consider 6 months to be an arbitrary figure—one that can delay instituting effective therapy and that may result in irreversible processes.

"Chronic pain is an ongoing experience of embodied discomfort that fails either to heal naturally or to respond to normal forms of medical intervention."[14] Arthritis, low back injury,[1] migraine headache, neuralgia, and diabetic neuropathy are examples of conditions that can result in Chronic Pain. Characteristics distinguishing Chronic Pain from acute Pain include (1) the pain area is less easily differentiated, (2) the pain intensity becomes more difficult to evaluate, (3) suffering usually increases over time, (4) defining characteristics are less obvious, and (5) there is little likelihood of complete relief. With Chronic Pain "pain itself becomes the patient's pathology and is considered a syndrome, the primary diagnosis and not just a syndrome."[20]

Chronic Pain is frequently subdivided into two categories: chronic malignant pain and chronic nonmalignant pain.[22] Chronic malignant pain is described as Pain associated with cancer or other progressive disorders. Chronic nonmalignant pain refers to Pain in persons whose tissue injury is non-progressive or healed. This type of Pain is sometimes referred to as *chronic benign pain, resistant pain,* or *persistent pain.* The terms *intractable pain, limited pain,* and *chronic cancer pain* are often used to refer to chronic malignant pain.

The ability to distinguish between acute and Chronic Pain will assist the clinician in making a differential diagnosis that is necessary to identify realistic patient outcomes and appropriate nursing interventions.

ASSESSMENT

A thorough assessment of a patient's pain experience requires the nurse to gather subjective data that present the patient's perspective. The patient should be queried about the location, characteristics (shooting, radiating, deep, superficial), onset and duration, frequency (constant or intermittent), quality (what the pain feels like), and intensity or severity of the pain. It is also important to determine if the patient can identify factors that precipitate or aggravate the pain. Information about the type and effectiveness of pain control measures that have been employed in the past should also be noted. This information will assist the nurse in determining whether the pain is acute or chronic in nature.

In addition to the patient's description of the pain experience, the nurse collects psychological and sociocultural data that will assist in understanding the patient's interpretation of and reaction to the pain experience. Psychological determinants of pain expression can be assessed in terms of (1) affective factors (emotions such as fear, anxiety, and anger); (2) cognitive and behavioral factors (beliefs and behaviors related to the meaning attributed to the pain, learned responses to Pain and injury, and situational factors influencing the patient's overt expression of Pain); and (3) constitutional factors (related to the personality or physiological makeup of the patient and representing tendencies to respond to Pain in normal, exaggerated, or understated ways).[10]

The patient's age, sex, religion, cultural and social background, available family and support systems, and employment responsibilities are influencing factors that can affect the patient's response to Pain.[20,24,27] Culture is of special interest in assessing the individual patient's interpretation of the pain experience and its concomitant emotional arousal. "Because the meaning of any given pain experience is defined by the culture in which it occurs, the total experience differs across cultures."[10]

Data specific to a patient's "pain history" provides valuable information that will contribute to a valid pain assessment and to effective Pain management. The Agency for Health Care Policy and Research[2] identified seven areas that should be explored through the "pain history":

1. Significant previous or ongoing instances of pain and its effect on the patient
2. Previously used methods for pain control that the patient found helpful or unhelpful
3. The patient's attitude toward and use of opioid, anxiolytic, or other medications, including history of substance abuse
4. The patient's typical coping response to stress or pain—the presence or absence of psychiatric disorders such as depression, anxiety, or psychosis are noted under this area
5. Family expectations and beliefs concerning pain, stress, and the postoperative course (or the disease process or healing of trauma)
6. Ways the patient describes or shows pain
7. The patient's knowledge of, expectations about, and preferences for pain management methods and for receiving information about pain management

Assessing Pain in children requires tailoring the assessment strategies to the child's developmental level and personality style and to the particular situation.[3,13] The pain history may be obtained from the child or parents. Information such as the words the child uses to express pain, previous pain experiences, the child's usual verbal and nonverbal reactions to pain, and what works best to decrease or take away the child's pain will be valuable to the ongoing pain assessment as well as determining the most effective interventions.

The subjective data should be complemented by objective data gained through the nurse's careful observations of the patient's behavioral response. These data are especially crucial in assessing for the presence of Pain in infants, small children, and noncommunicative adults. Physiological signs and observed patient behaviors can indicate that a patient is experiencing Pain. These signs and behaviors may differ depending on whether the patient is experiencing acute or Chronic Pain, and they are therefore presented with the discussion of assessment as it relates to each of these types of pain.

A variety of measures that can assist in assessing a patient's pain experience have been developed. Verbal self-reporting instruments range from a listing of questions that require the patient to make a simple "yes" or "no" response to a list of questions that elicit descriptive responses. Pain flowcharts can be used to maintain an ongoing record of the patient's evaluation of the pain's characteristics, intensity, and frequency and the nurse's observation of the patient's physiological and behavioral responses. Visual analog scales provide a relatively simple means to measure the various dimensions of Pain. For example, to measure the intensity of the pain experience, the patient could be asked to mark a point on a horizontal line that represents a continuum of pain intensity that ranges from no pain to unbearable pain, with points in between representing various grades of intensity.

One of the better known pain assessment tools is the McGill-Melzack Pain Questionnaire. The questionnaire, a four-page tool recommended for use during the initial assessment, measures sensory, affective, and evaluative dimensions of Pain. Types of pain experiences, methods of pain relief, and pain patterns can be differentiated through use of the questionnaire.[21,27] One longer version and three shorter versions of the questionnaire are available and are used in clinical practice.[29]

McCaffery and Beebe[17] offer an initial pain assessment tool and a pain flow sheet that are "practical in any clinical situation and easily adapted to an individual patient's needs." The initial assessment tool addresses 10 areas: location;

intensity; quality; onset, duration, variations, and rhythms; manner of expressing pain; what relieves the pain; what causes or increases the pain; effects of pain; other comments; and the plan. The flow sheet provides a means to track the frequency and intensity of pain, the analgesic(s) used to treat pain, changes in the patient's vital signs, the patient's level of arousal, other observations, and the plan.

The choice of a measuring tool to assess the pain experience will depend on the patient's physical response and pain behavior. For example, a patient experiencing intense pain may be restless and irritable and may withdraw from social contact. In such a case, attempts should be made to elicit from the patient only the simplest descriptions of the pain experience. Questions requiring a "yes" or "no" answer would be more appropriate than those requiring complex answers.

Acute Pain

The patient experiencing acute Pain will describe pain that is intense and of short duration. The nurse may observe that the patient is protective of and guards the areas of the body where the pain is focused. The patient's attention may be introverted, and a withdrawal from social contact may occur; thought processes may appear to be impaired, giving the impression that the patient is confused or disoriented. Distraction behaviors such as moaning, whimpering, crying, rubbing, and pacing are often observed; and irritability, restlessness, and agitation may be noted. The patient may assume an unusual posture (e.g., knees drawn to the abdomen).

The face of the patient experiencing acute Pain usually mirrors the pain experience.[27] The "facial mask of pain" reflects a beaten look; facial features may appear pinched, jaw muscles tight, and teeth clenched; eyes may lack luster and be widely open or tightly shut; and eyebrows may be knotted. The portrait of the patient experiencing acute Pain may be vivid, with well-defined characteristics, or blurred, with few defining characteristics.

Physiological signs that indicate the patient may be experiencing acute Pain include changes in blood pressure and pulse rate, increased or decreased respiratory rate, dilated pupils, diaphoresis, and increased muscle tension. The patient may complain of nausea.

Knowledge and understanding of the factor(s) contributing to the acute Pain experience will guide the nurse and the patient in identifying realistic outcomes for the patient and the nursing interventions that will support the patient in the achievement of the outcomes. The related factors for acute Pain are classified into physiological factors and psychological factors. The physiological factors include trauma to tissue as a result of injury, disease, or surgery; invasive diagnostic tests, such as venipuncture and cystoscopic examination; allergic responses that invoke painful sensations, such as "burning" skin; and untoward effects of a therapeutic treatment, such as a tight cast or a dressing exerting pressure that interrupts circulation. Psychological factors include a lack of knowledge of techniques that could suppress pain and control anxiety. Whereas anxious behavior could be considered a defining characteristic, its role in triggering and influencing the intensity of the acute Pain episode indicates inclusion as a related factor.

■ Defining Characteristics

The presence of the following defining characteristics indicates that the patient may be experiencing acute Pain:

- Verbal report of intense, limited pain experience
- Facial mask of pain (e.g., "beaten look," pinched features, tightened jaw muscles, clenched teeth, lackluster eyes, widely open or tightly shut eyes, knotted brows)
- Blood pressure and pulse rate change
- Increased or decreased respiratory rate
- Dilated pupils
- Diaphoresis
- Increased muscle tension
- Unusual posture
- Protective, guarding behavior
- Self-focusing
- Narrowed focus
- Altered time perception
- Impaired thought process

- Distraction behaviors (e.g., moaning, whimpering, crying, rubbing, pacing)
- Irritability
- Restlessness
- Agitation
- Withdrawal from social contact

■ Related Factors

The following related factors are associated with acute Pain:

- Tissue trauma (e.g., injury, disease, or surgery)
- Invasive diagnostic tests (e.g., venipuncture and bone marrow aspiration)
- Allergic responses
- Therapeutic treatment effects (e.g., a cast causing extreme pressure or rabies vaccine)
- Lack of knowledge of pain control techniques
- Anxiety

Chronic Pain

The patient experiencing Chronic Pain is not as likely to report the pain experience as the patient with acute Pain. Chronic Pain has an enduring quality and becomes a stable element in the patient's daily life.[9]

Often a patient haunted by Chronic Pain learns to accept the Pain as a condition of life. The nurse must be alert to the presence of defining characteristics that indicate the patient may be experiencing Chronic Pain. Some of the characteristics of Chronic Pain are the same as characteristics of acute Pain; the difference rests in the more subtle and persistent nature of those characteristics as they relate to Chronic Pain.

Protective, guarding behavior of the area where the pain is concentrated often becomes incorporated into the patient's manner of body positioning and movement. Chronic Pain can consume the patient's energy, and the patient may be overwhelmed by the search for pain relief or the efforts required to cope with the pain sensation. Irritability, restlessness, and depression may be noted more frequently.

The patient may experience an altered ability to maintain involvement in usual activities. As a result, family and social relationships that have

VI

offered the patient support in the past may be disrupted. Weight changes related to anorexia and changes in the patient's sleep pattern often occur. The "facial mask of Chronic Pain" may reveal a "beaten," drawn look, the eyes may lack luster, and the eyebrows may appear knotted.

The factors contributing to Chronic Pain include conditions in which tissue injury is nonprogressive or healed (e.g., low back pain resulting from arthritis or an injury incurred in the past). A chronic physical disability can also contribute to Chronic Pain (e.g., a patient who has an extreme limp as a result of a serious injury to the left leg). The patient may experience Chronic Pain in the right leg related to attempts to compensate for the limp. A deficit in knowledge of the measures that may be used to control Chronic Pain can also contribute to the Chronic Pain experience.

It is important to note that in the discussion of Chronic Pain, the term is used in the context of chronic nonmalignant, nonprogressive pain. Pain associated with cancer or other progressive disorders (chronic malignant pain) requires the nurse to assess for the characteristics of acute and Chronic Pain.[4] The patient with this type of Pain often experiences the intensity of the acute Pain experience and the duration of the Chronic Pain experience. Assessment of psychological function is especially important because the patient must cope with the diagnosis of a progressive disease and the prospect of progressive intensity of Pain.

■ Defining Characteristics

The presence of the following defining characteristics indicates that the patient may be experiencing Chronic Pain:

- Verbal report of pain experience lasting for more than 1 month beyond usual course of acute disease or healing of an injury
- Facial mask of pain (e.g., "beaten look," lackluster eyes, and knotted brows)
- Changes in sleep pattern
- Weight changes
- Protective, guarding behavior
- Self-focusing

- Irritability
- Restlessness
- Depression
- Altered ability to continue previous activities
- Disruption of family and social relationships

■ Related Factors

The following related factors are associated with Chronic Pain:

- Chronic condition or disease
- Chronic physical disability
- Deficit in knowledge of measures used to control Chronic Pain

DIAGNOSIS

■ Differential Nursing Diagnosis

The nursing diagnoses Pain and Chronic Pain are associated with physiological alterations (e.g., tissue damage, trauma or injury, and disease) and should be distinguished from experiences of emotional or psychological pain. Emotional pain is a consideration in other nursing diagnoses (e.g., Ineffective Individual Coping, Self-Esteem Disturbance, Hopelessness, Powerlessness, and Dysfunctional Grieving). The patient diagnosed with Pain or Chronic Pain may also experience emotional pain; if so, a diagnosis reflecting the emotional pain should be made.

■ Medical and Psychiatric Diagnoses

The medical diagnoses associated with acute and Chronic Pain are numerous. In the case of a disease process, the pain experienced may be more directly related to the treatment of the disease (e.g., surgical intervention or invasive treatments). Pain may be the most prominent presenting symptom when a patient seeks medical assistance (e.g., myocardial infarction, cholecystitis, otitis media, pulmonary emboli, renal calculi, and appendicitis). Disease processes or illnesses that are chronic or progressive in nature can cause the patient to experience Chronic Pain. Examples of these include peripheral vascular disease, rheumatoid arthritis, connective tissue diseases, chronic pancreatitis, and cancer.

OUTCOME IDENTIFICATION, PLANNING, AND IMPLEMENTATION

The goal of nursing care for the patient experiencing Pain is to assist the patient in achieving optimal control of the Pain. Regardless of the type of pain experience, the nurse must direct attention toward working with the patient in the exploration and implementation of the Pain control techniques that will be most effective. The extent to which the nurse can support and guide the patient in the quest to control Pain depends on the depth and breadth of understanding of the patient's pain experience.[24] This understanding evolves from the initial and ongoing assessments of the patient's pain experience.

The nurse must know of the current pharmacological and nonpharmacological approaches to pain management. When assisting the patient in choosing pain control measures, the nurse must address the patient's lifestyle support systems, daily routine, and preferences. The patient's willingness to alter his or her lifestyle or daily routine to incorporate pain control measures is critical to the success of a pain management program.

Acute Pain

An important consideration in planning care for the patient who experiences acute Pain is to incorporate nursing interventions that address the pharmacological management of the Pain. The nurse is responsible for administering and monitoring the effects of all medications prescribed for the patient. Often the patient in acute Pain will receive narcotic analgesics. Determining when the patient will receive these medications may depend on the nurse's assessment of the patient's pain experience and the effects that a previous dosage had. It is not uncommon to hear patients state that they continue to have moderate to severe Pain after receiving pain medication. This may be related to the fact that doses of narcotic analgesics are often too low or too widely spread. Inadequate dosing frequently is related to incorrect assessment, insufficient knowledge of the action and effects of the

prescribed drug, and the personal attitudes of caregivers and patients about the drug.[2,19,22]

The route of drug administration should also be considered. Recent developments have added novel routes of drug administration (e.g., transdermal and transmucosal) to the more traditional routes (e.g., oral, intramuscular, and intravenous).[5] As the novel approaches to drug administration are further developed and refined, choices of the most effective and most desirable routes from the patient's perspective will expand. An obvious advantage of the transdermal and transmucosal routes of administration is that patients who fear "needles" and who cannot take medication orally do not have to have injections.

The use of nonpharmacological measures to control Pain must also be considered for the patient experiencing acute Pain.[12,26,30] Often interventions that help the patient relax are most effective before the intensity of pain increases. The nurse may guide the patient in taking slow, deep breaths or in reciting a word or phrase slowly and repetitively. Imagery may be another effective technique. The patient is guided in imagining a relaxing scene, such as a quiet beach or a forest after a rain. The scene can become the patient's "haven" when Pain becomes severe. For children experiencing acute Pain, the use of a distraction has been found to reduce their behavioral distress.[28]

The nurse should assume the responsibility to explore with the patient all possible pain control measures that may provide relief. The nurse should use all members of the health care team as resources in such an exploration.

Chronic Pain

The pain experience of the patient who suffers from Chronic Pain touches the patient's family, significant others, and even social and employment contacts. Thus the nurse must consider the patient's lifestyle, family and employment responsibilities, and daily routines when planning care.

Pharmacological agents may or may not be used in the treatment of patients with Chronic Pain. Because of the long-term nature of this type of Pain, the nurse must exert care to avoid "overtreat-

VI

ment" of these patients. In an effort to control Pain that "just won't go away," the patient may take prescribed drugs or over-the-counter analgesics too often or in excessive doses. The nurse should teach the patient the expected and untoward effects of the drugs being taken, as well as the appropriate amount and frequency of dosing. If the patient has the option to vary the dose and frequency, the information the nurse provides may be critical to the patient's well-being.

Nonpharmacological pain control measures are especially helpful to the patient in Chronic Pain. Such measures can range from activities that require the patient's participation to requirements that the patient avoid certain activities that intensify the pain experience.[18,23] When recommending a specific pain control approach, the nurse must assess its potential effectiveness and the patient's ability and desire to use it. The effectiveness of nonpharmacological measures should be monitored as rigorously as pharmacological approaches are monitored.

The Nursing Care Guidelines list patient outcomes and nursing interventions that can be considered for any patient experiencing Pain, whether acute or Chronic. The guidelines should be tailored to the individual patient and his or her pain experience.

VI

◢ **NURSING CARE GUIDELINES**
Nursing Diagnosis: Pain

Expected Outcome: The patient will describe pain control measures that reduce or eliminate Pain.
- ▲ Using the assessment guidelines, assess the patient's Pain and the characteristics of his or her pain experience. *Ongoing assessment is necessary to detect discrete changes in the intensity, duration, and quality of the patient's Pain; this provides data upon which refinements and revisions in the plan of care are based.*
- ▲ Evaluate with the patient and the health care team the effectiveness of past and present pain control measures (pharmacological and nonpharmacological) that have been employed. *Review of the effectiveness of interventions currently used and used in the past can help identify the most effective approach to managing the patient's Pain.*
- ▲ Review with the patient and family nonpharmacological interventions that may assist in controlling Pain.
    1. Describe the interventions to the patient (e.g., biofeedback, transcutaneous electrical nerve stimulation (TENS), hypnosis, massage or exercise therapy, and behavioral therapy, such as relaxation therapy, guided imagery, music therapy, and desensitization).
    2. Assess the patient's desire and willingness to use a particular intervention.
    3. Support the patient in making a decision regarding pain control measures that can be tried.
    Nonpharmacological interventions can offer patients some control in treating their Pain; such interventions may be used alone or to augment pharmacological interventions.

Expected Outcome: The patient will implement pain control measures to reduce or eliminate Pain.
- ▪ Support and guide the patient in making a decision to choose a particular pain control measure.
- ▪ Discuss with the patient and family lifestyle modifications that may be necessary to implement the pain control measure effectively.
- ▲ Assist the patient and family in determining how lifestyle modifications can be made.
- ▲ Describe the health care system and the community-based resources that are available to guide the patient in using a particular pain control measure (such as physical therapy) or in modifying the lifestyle (such as introduction of diversional activities into the daily routine).
- ▪ With the patient and family, evaluate the effectiveness of the pain control measure after it has been implemented.
    By providing the patient and family adequate information about particular pain control measures and by supporting and guiding the patient in implementing the chosen measures, it is more likely that the patient will be successful in reducing or eliminating Pain.

▪ = nursing intervention; ▲ = collaborative intervention.

Expected Outcome: The patient will reduce or eliminate factors that precipitate or intensify the pain experience.

- Work with the patient and family to identify factors (personal, disease-related, treatment-related, or environmental) that precipitate or intensify the patient's pain experience. *The patient and family's perceptions provide valuable data when attempting to determine factors directly related to the experience of Pain.*
- Encourage the patient to keep a pain diary that will assist in identifying actual and potential precipitating factors. *Use of a pain diary provides the patient with a tool to assist him or her in accurately reporting and evaluating precipitating factors.*
- Describe to the patient and family measures that may be used to control the precipitating factors and discuss them. *Knowledge and understanding of the measures will make the patient and family more comfortable in using such measures.*
- Evaluate the effectiveness of the measures used through ongoing assessment of the pain experience *so that necessary changes in the plan of care can be made in a timely manner.*
- ▲ Introduce the patient to self-help and support groups for persons experiencing Pain; *such groups may provide guidance related to coping with Pain, techniques that can be used to control precipitating factors, and pain control measures.*

EVALUATION

Evaluation of the effectiveness of interventions employed to help the patient reduce or eliminate the pain experience requires the nurse to do an ongoing assessment throughout the implementation phase of the nursing process. Measures that are used to control Pain may or may not be effective for a particular patient. If they are ineffective, the nurse and the patient should continue to seek alternative measures that help the patient achieve the ultimate goal of controlling Pain.

Thus the effectiveness of the nursing interventions must be measured over time. The patient must be patient and wait to feel relief, and the nurse must be patient to observe patient behaviors indicating that the pain is being controlled. The family or significant others can also contribute to the evaluation of the effectiveness of the plan of care. They can provide data related to changes in (1) the patient's pain behavior, (2) the patient's ability to resume activities and social contacts, and (3) the patient's confidence as it relates to the control the patient has over the pain experience.

VI

▶ CASE STUDY WITH PLAN OF CARE

Mr. Bill T., a 55-year-old, independent, dry wall contractor, sustained an injury to the lumbar spine 1 year before this visit. He had attempted to lift and hold a sheet of dry wall. He has come to the outpatient clinic to find out if anything can be done about the "nagging pain" he has been experiencing since the injury. Mr. T. lives with his wife; he has three children and five grandchildren. He states that he is concerned about picking up the grandchildren when they come to visit.

The physical examination and review of Mr. T.'s health history indicate that he is in good general health except for the lower back pain he experiences. The radiographs of the lumbar spine show no abnormalities. An assessment of Mr. T.'s pain experience reveals that the pain is "like a strong, dull ache across the lower back." He states that "the pain is worse when I'm on my feet all day," and he finds himself feeling irritable at work and at home. He states that he was "afraid of being hooked on medicine" but that he takes aspirin "now and then" when the pain intensifies. He says, "The aspirin seems to help a little, but not much." The nurse diagnosed Mr. T. as having Chronic Pain (low back) related to back injury sustained 1 year ago.

■ PLAN OF CARE FOR MR. BILL T.
Nursing Diagnosis: Chronic Pain (Low Back) Related to Back Injury Sustained 1 Year Ago

Expected Outcome: Mr. T. will describe measures that will control his low back Pain.
▲ Include Mr. T. and members of the health team in determining the most appropriate measures for pain control.
▲ Describe to Mr. T. nonpharmacological pain control measures that can reduce or eliminate his Pain and the rationale for using them.[1]
  1. Engaging in a prescribed exercise routine strengthens the abdominal and the back muscles; strong abdominal muscles assist in maintaining correct posture and reduce the stress placed on the back muscles.
  2. Use of TENS can trigger therapeutic endorphin levels (usually recommended in 1-hour cycles several times a day).
  3. Use of relaxation therapy when Mr. T. is irritable or tense; tense muscles increase the pain sensation, and relaxed muscles can decrease the pain sensation.
■ Consult with the physician, and if appropriate, suggest that Mr. T. consider taking acetaminophen or nonsteroidal antiinflammatory drugs.[1] Both medications are available over the counter.

Expected Outcome: Mr. T. will control the factors that intensify his low back Pain.
■ Work with Mr. T. to identify how he can decrease the amount of time he stands each day.
■ Describe and demonstrate appropriate standing, walking, sitting, sleeping, and lifting postures that Mr. T. should use; have Mr. T. return the demonstration.
■ Encourage Mr. T. to explore using posture aids; for example, sacroiliac support (a support cushion that enhances spinal alignment when sitting or driving) and a firm mattress or bed board.

Expected Outcome: Mr. T. will implement pain control measures to reduce or eliminate Pain.
■ Arrange a meeting with Mr. and Mrs. T. to review the pain control strategies Mr. T. can consider.
■ Discuss with Mr. and Mrs. T. the importance of familial support in promoting adherence to the proposed treatment plan.
■ Work with Mr. T. in incorporating the prescribed exercise plan into his daily routine.
■ Evaluate Mr. T.'s initial efforts in using nonpharmacological pain control measures.
■ If Mr. T. is taking medication(s) to help control the pain, provide information about the medication(s) he is taking; offer guidance on appropriate dosing and scheduling of any over-the-counter medications.
■ Provide for regular assessment of the pain experience and the effectiveness of the treatment plan.

■ = nursing intervention; ▲ = collaborative intervention.

■■ CRITICAL THINKING EXERCISES

1. Develop a patient education booklet that would have been helpful to Mr. T. in learning about the nonpharmacological pain control measures. Use drawings, diagrams, and pictures to support the narrative sections of the booklet.
2. Identify the major pharmacological agents used to treat Pain. Compare and contrast their actions and side effects. What information would you provide Mr. T. regarding the pharmacological agents most commonly used to treat back pain?
3. Prepare a list of support or self-help groups located in your city that are available to patients experiencing Chronic Pain and secure information from them. What is the role of these groups in assisting patients experiencing Pain?

REFERENCES

1. Agency for Health Care Policy and Research: *Acute low back problems in adults: assessment and treatment* (AHCR Pub No 95-0643), Rockville, Maryland, 1994, U.S. Department of Health and Human Services.
2. Agency for Health Care Policy and Research: *Acute pain management: operative or medical procedures and trauma* (AHCR Pub No 92-0032), Rockville, Maryland, 1992, U.S. Department of Health and Human Services.
3. Agency for Health Care Policy and Research: *Acute pain management in infants, children, and adolescents: operative and medical procedures* (AHCR Pub No 92-0020), Rockville, Maryland, 1992, U.S. Department of Health and Human Services.
4. Agency for Health Care Policy and Research: *Management of cancer pain: adults* (AHCR Pub No 94-0593), Rockville, Maryland, 1994, U.S. Department of Health and Human Services.
5. Biddle C and Gilliland C: Transdermal and transmucosal administration of pain-relieving and anxiolytic drugs: a primer for the critical care practitioner, *Heart Lung* 21: 115–124, 1992.
6. Bonica JJ: Definition and taxonomy of pain. In Bonica JJ, editor: *The management of pain,* vol 1, ed 2, Philadelphia, 1990, Lea & Febiger.
7. Bonica JJ: General considerations of chronic pain. In Bonica JJ, editor: *The management of pain,* vol 1, ed 2, Philadelphia, 1990, Lea & Febiger.
8. Bonica JJ: History of pain concepts and therapies. In Bonica JJ, editor: *The management of pain,* vol 1, ed 2, Philadelphia, 1990, Lea & Febiger.
9. Chapman CR and Syrjala KL: Measurement of pain. In Bonica JJ, editor: *The management of pain,* vol 1, ed 2, Philadelphia, 1990, Lea & Febiger.
10. Chapman CR and Turner JA: Psychologic and psychosocial aspects of acute pain. In Bonica JJ, editor: *The management of pain,* vol 1, ed 2, Philadelphia, 1990, Lea & Febiger.
11. Fields HL: Sources of variability in the sensation of pain, *Pain* 33:195–200, 1988.
12. Good M: A comparison of the effects of jaw relaxation and music on postoperative pain, *Nurs Res* 44(1):52–57, 1995.
13. Hester NO: Pain in children. In Fitzpatrick JJ and Stevenson JS, editors: *Annual review of nursing research,* vol 2, New York, 1993, Springer.
14. Kotarba JA: *Chronic pain,* Beverly Hills, California, 1983, Sage Publications.
15. Loeser JD: *Pain and its management: an overview,* program and abstracts, NIH Consensus Development Conference on the Integrated Approach to the Management of Pain, Bethesda, Maryland, May 19–21, 1986.
16. Mahon SM: Concept analysis of pain: implications related to nursing diagnoses, *Nurs Diagnosis* 5(1):14–25, 1994.
17. McCaffery M and Beebe A: *Pain: clinical manual for nursing practice,* St. Louis, 1989, The CV Mosby Co.
18. McCloskey JC and Bulechek GM: *Nursing interventions classification (NIC),* ed 2, St. Louis, 1996, Mosby–Year Book.
19. Meehan DA and others: Analgesic administration, pain intensity, and patient satisfaction in cardiac surgical patients, *Crit Care* 4(6):435–442, 1995.
20. Meinhart NT and McCaffery M: *Pain: a nursing approach to assessment and analysis,* Norwalk, Connecticut, 1983, Appleton-Century-Crofts.
21. Melzack R: The McGill Pain Questionnaire: major properties and scoring methods, *Pain* 1:277–299, 1975.
22. National Institutes of Health: *The integrated approach to the management of pain,* National Institutes of Health Consensus Development Conference Statement, vol 6, no 3, Betheseda, Maryland, 1986, The Institutes.
23. National Institutes of Health: *Pain research,* News Features from NIH 86(3), Bethesda, Maryland, 1987, The Institutes.
24. National Institute of Nursing Research: *Symptom management: acute pain—a report of the NINR priority expert panel on symptom management: acute pain* (NIH Pub No 94-2421), Betheseda, Maryland, 1994, U.S. Department of Health and Human Services.
25. North American Nursing Diagnosis Association: *NANDA nursing diagnoses: definitions and classification, 1995–1996,* Philadelphia, 1994, The Association.
26. Tiernan PJ: Independent nursing interventions: relaxation and guided imagery in critical care, *Crit Care Nurse,* October:47–51, 1994.
27. Turk DC and Melzack R: *Handbook of pain assessment,* New York, 1992, The Guilford Press.
28. Vessey JA, Carlson KL, and McGill J: Use of distraction with children during an acute pain experience, *Nurs Res* 43(6):369–372, 1994.
29. Wilkie DJ and others: Use of the McGill Pain Questionnaire to measure pain: a meta-analysis, *Nurs Res* 39:36–41, 1990.
30. Zahourek RP and Larkin D: Hypnosis and therapeutic suggestions for managing pain and stress, *Alt Health Pract* 1(1):43–53, 1995.

VI

Sensory/Perceptual Alterations (Specify): Visual, Auditory, Kinesthetic, Gustatory, Tactile, Olfactory

Sensory/Perceptual Alterations (Specify): Visual, Auditory, Kinesthetic, Gustatory, Tactile, Olfactory is a state in which an individual experiences a change in the amount or patterning of incoming stimuli, accompanied by a diminished, exaggerated, distorted, or impaired response to such stimuli.[13]

OVERVIEW

The sensory/perceptual process is the ability to receive and interpret information from the external and internal environments. It is vital for survival and essential for reflex activity, decision making, knowledge development, and behavioral change. It is necessary for cognition, that is, the process of obtaining and using knowledge about one's world.[7] Mental status or cognitive function can affect sensory/perceptual function. Conversely, a disruption or alteration in the sensory/perceptual process affects behavior and cognitive processes.

The sensory/perceptual process has physiological and psychological components. The physiological or sensory component encompasses the detection of visual, auditory, kinesthetic, gustatory, tactile,[14] and olfactory stimuli by sensory receptors and transmission of these sensations to the brain. The psychological component, perception, is a mental process of selection, integration, and interpretation of sensory data. Because perception is an internal mental process, its presence and development are inferred from behavior. Whereas hearing seems to occur in our ears and seeing in our eyes,

in actuality the impulses coming from the stimulated receptors housed in these organs are interpreted by the cortical areas of the brain. The sensory/perceptual process depends on the function of the peripheral and central nervous systems as well as the neuroendocrine system.

It has been hypothesized that there is a basic need or drive for sensory stimulation and that in a waking state an individual strives to maintain an optimum level and variety of sensory stimulation to the cortex. This need or drive has been labeled *sensoristasis*. The level of required stimulation is thought to vary among individuals and to be influenced by such variables as age, culture, and environment. Individuals seek additional or alternative stimuli if sensory stimulation falls below optimum levels. Inadequate or excessive stimulation for extended periods of time results in disorganization of behavior. Thus the concept of sensoristasis explains the disorganization of behavior that occurs in situations of sensory deprivation or sensory overload.

The concept of sensoristasis helps us to understand a portion of the sensory/perceptual process, but it is not sufficient to explain the entire process. Information-processing theories and transactional, person-centered theories provide further explanations of the process of sensory perception.

Information-processing theories view adaptation to the environment as a basic need.[1] Knowledge of the environment is essential to meeting that need. Knowledge is obtained from information derived from the assortment of sensory stimuli that surrounds the individual, and thinking and

VI

524

learning are used to obtain that information. This process is called *perception*. As learning and thinking modify the individual, the individual modifies perceptions of incoming stimuli. Thus the process of perception is continuously affected by experience with the environment.[2,8]

Transactional theories view perception as a uniquely individual process that is influenced by an individual's needs, goals, cognitive processes, and experiences. Individuals transact with their unique environments to develop sets of ideas or precepts about the sensory stimuli they receive. From these precepts assumptions about reality are formed. Assumptions in turn influence perception so that perception becomes a learned behavior of constructing reality to fit a set of assumptions about it. Brunner and Postman demonstrated this in a classic experiment using playing cards.[3] Experimental subjects were asked to identify a series of playing cards. Most of the cards were normal, but some were altered: a red six of spades and a black four of hearts. Without any apparent awareness of something being different, subjects almost always identified altered cards as if they were normal. It was proposed that the subjects expected the color and shape of the cards to be as they had previously experienced them to be: black clubs or spades and red hearts or diamonds. They distorted either the color or the shape of the altered cards to support the set of assumptions that they had previously formed regarding playing cards. It might be said that our generalizations and expectations filter out and distort most of our sensory experiences to make them consistent with our expectations. Each of us creates a representation of the world around us, and that representation in turn greatly determines our perception of the world.[1,2,4]

The preceding theoretical considerations indicate that perception is universal and individual. The same basic anatomical structure and physiological mechanisms necessary to carry out sensory perception are possessed by all persons. However, individual physiological, psychological, and sociocultural factors affect each individual's perceptual process and interpretation of reality.[1,2,8,11] Drugs, physical fatigue, fever, pain, chemical imbalances,

and biological variance (constitutional makeup, age, and range of sensory modalities) are major physiological factors. Psychological factors include past experiences, maturation level, motivation, beliefs, values, attitudes, and emotional stress. Social class, education, customs, and ethnicity have been identified as sociocultural factors. Although none of us have exactly the same perceptual experiences, we are able to agree on certain perceptions and broad categories of sensory perception.

Perception is also affected by the variety and type of stimuli competing for our attention at any particular time. The intensity, size, repetition, and novelty of stimuli have been identified as characteristics that determine selection and attention during the perceptual process.[16] The sensory/perceptual process is a complex function that can be altered by any number of conditions that interfere with the reception, transmission, or interpretation of stimuli.

ASSESSMENT

Sensory/Perceptual Alterations affect the way reality or the world about us is viewed. Alterations may be mild or severe and acute or chronic. Acute alterations tend to occur abruptly and manifest themselves with more severe defining characteristics, such as confusion, disorientation, or bizarre mood swings. Sudden sensory loss, drug intoxication, and sudden trauma are often related factors for an acute sensory/perceptual alteration. Chronic alterations usually develop gradually and tend to have related factors that are more often long-term or permanent in nature. The defining characteristics initially may be rather subtle but often become more pronounced with time. Chronic alterations are often related to such factors as socially restricted environments, progressive neurological disorders, and decline in sensory function related to aging. Important defining characteristics for this nursing diagnosis are evidence of reality distortion. This evidence is subjective and objective in nature. The nurse obtains evidence regarding reality distortion through interviews, observation, and examination of the patient; through consulta-

VI

tion with other health care providers and family members; and from records and reports. The sensory status of the patient and environmental factors need to be examined. The patient's level of consciousness is obviously a major determinant of the method used to obtain the needed assessment data.

While interviewing or interacting with the conscious patient, the nurse should observe and note any emotional manifestations of apathy, depression, anxiety, apprehension, listlessness, restlessness, rapid mood changes, or hostility. Perceptual distortions such as paranoid statements, illusions, and visual or auditory hallucinations are important findings. Impaired or disorganized thought processes may also manifest themselves. Any difficulty in thinking, concentrating, reasoning, problem solving, or following the therapeutic regimen should be identified. Inappropriate or slow responses to the examiner's questions should also be noted.

The patient's current medical diagnosis and health history will give the nurse information about previous and current injuries or illnesses that may affect perceptual status. The review of the systems portion of the health history provides data about several of the sensory modalities and about sensory/perceptual function. It is important to note whether the patient has or has had visual or hearing problems, and if adaptive devices are used. Problems with vertigo, paresthesia, and hyperesthesia are also noted in this section of the health history. Information about the patient's personal and social history helps the nurse develop an understanding of the patient as an individual and as a member of a family and community. The personal and social history may be obtained from the patient, but in many instances it will be available in existing records. The history should provide information about the patient's occupation and education; leisure activities; habits, including use of drugs, over-the-counter medications, and alcohol; usual sleep patterns; and cultural background. The nurse may need to supplement recorded information with information from the patient or family members.

Objective data assessment includes a neurological and mental status examination. For a detailed presentation of the neurological examination, the reader should refer to a basic book on physical examination. Only a brief overview of the sensory portion of the neurological and mental status examination is presented here.

In addition to the basic visual, auditory, olfactory, and taste tests, the sensory system portion of the neurological examination should include tests for tactile sensation, superficial pain, vibration, and proprioception (kinesthetic sense). For these latter tests, the patient should be told what to expect and should be reassured that the examiner will not inflict pain. Each of these procedures is carried out with the patient's eyes closed. The examination should always start by examining opposite corresponding parts of the body and having the patient compare the sensations on one side with those on the other. Slight differences are not ordinarily significant. If definite differences are noted, the abnormal area should be clearly defined by further testing.

Tactile sensation is examined by lightly touching the body with a wisp of cotton. An organized but unpatterned testing of both arms, the trunk, and both legs is used. The patient is asked to indicate when and where touch is felt. The sensations on opposite sides of the body as well as those on distal and proximal parts of the body are compared.

Pain and temperature sensations are carried out in the same major pathways so that in most circumstances it is not necessary to test for temperature sensation if the pain sensation is intact. Superficial pain is tested by determining sensitivity to a pin prick. The sharp and dull ends of a safety pin are applied with the same intensity to symmetrical areas of the body. The patient is asked to differentiate between sharp and dull sensations. To test temperature sensation two tubes are filled with water: one with hot water and one with cold. The same pattern is followed as in testing for pain, but the patient is instructed to identify the sensation as hot or cold.

Vibration is evaluated by placing the handle of a vibrating low-frequency (128 cycles/sec) tuning fork against a bony prominence. The patient is instructed to tell the examiner when a buzz is felt and to signal when the buzz stops. If the patient does not perceive the vibrations at distal points, the examination progresses proximally until the vibrations are felt. Older patients will usually have decreased vibratory sense in the lower extremities.

Position sense is tested by holding the lateral surfaces of the distal phalanx of the patient's thumb, index finger, or great toe and moving it up or down. The nurse then asks the patient to indicate in which direction it has been moved, and makes side-to-side comparisons. Position sense can also be tested by the Romberg test (the difference in balance when tested with the eyes open and with the eyes closed) or by asking the patient to touch the tip of his or her nose with the eyes closed.

After peripheral sensation has been examined, integration of sensation in the brain is tested. This may be done by two-point discrimination. The patient is touched with two sharp objects simultaneously on opposite sides of the body; he or she should recognize that two points have been touched. If only one point is recognized, the side where the touch is not felt is said to demonstrate extinction. This ability varies over different parts of the body. At the tips of the fingers patients should be able to recognize two points as close as 2 to 3 cm apart, whereas over the back the distance between points will need to be considerably wider.

Additionally, higher cortical integration can be tested through the sensory abilities of stereognosis and graphagnosia. *Stereognosis* is the ability to identify familiar objects (e.g., keys, coins, or paper clips) placed in one's hand. *Graphagnosia* is the ability to recognize numbers or letters drawn by the examiner on the palm of the hand. Again, both tests are carried out with the patient's eyes closed.

Assessment of the patient's mental status is critical to any evaluation of the sensory/perceptual process. Careful observation of the patient during history taking, during physical examination, and while providing care should give the nurse a sound basis for evaluating the patient's mental status. A separate examination is not always indicated. For instance, memory and affect can be assessed when asking patients details about their illnesses and past events. Components of mental status assessment include general appearance and behavior,

sensorium, mood and affect, thought content, and intellectual capacity. In some settings, standardized mental status tests are routinely used. These tests can provide a fairly simple and reliable method of obtaining mental status data and can be repeated at intervals to detect in a consistent manner changes in mental status. Health assessment texts usually provide detailed examples of such tests. However, inherent cultural biases, relevance in long-term care settings, and lack of performance norms for the elderly limit the appropriate use of these tests. Current literature that provides a comparison of the parametric properties and other characteristics of such tests should be reviewed before selecting and using one on a routine basis.

Along with the subjective and objective patient data, environmental data are essential to assessment. Compared with the patient's usual environment, it should be determined if there is sufficient stimulation in the present environment, if the patient is receiving enough social stimulation to maintain an adequate level of meaningful stimuli, and if noise and activity in the environment are creating too many stimuli. Boredom, inactivity, daydreaming, increased sleeping, lack of sleep, disorganization of thoughts, anxiety, or panic may be indicative of too few or too many stimuli in the environment.[6,9,12]

The assessment data not only provide evidence of the defining characteristics for the diagnosis but identify probable related factors. Numerous factors have been identified as being related to the development of Sensory/Perceptual Alterations: Visual, Auditory, Kinesthetic, Gustatory, Tactile, and Olfactory. Factors may be grouped into four categories: altered environment; altered sensory reception, transmission, and/or integration; chemical alterations; and psychological stress.[13] These related factors identify those at risk for Sensory/Perceptual Alterations and determine the nature, extent, and severity of the alteration when it does exist.

Altered environments results in excessive or insufficient stimuli. The use of isolation, special care units, incubators, traction, body casts, bed rest, and physical confinement results in thera-

VI

peutically restricted environments. The quantity, quality, and types of stimuli available to patients in such environments are severely limited. Contact with family and friends is restricted, and familiar sights, sounds, and smells are replaced by meaningless unpatterned or monotonous sensory stimuli.[6,12] Some therapeutic environments, such as intensive care units, are so overloaded with sensory stimuli that are meaningless to the patient that they too affect perception. Persons confined to such environments are apt to exhibit sensory distortions, disorientation, or hallucinations.

Other environments that are not therapeutically restricted may be socially restricted because of living circumstances. Persons of any age who are confined or limited in meaningful social contact (e.g., institutionalized, homebound, aged, chronically ill, or terminally ill patients) or those stigmatized because of mental illness, retardation, or physical handicaps are apt to experience socially restricted environments. An infant or child whose home environment does not provide adequate levels of stimulation also experiences this type of restriction. Impaired emotional, intellectual, and social functioning have been attributed to such socially restricted environments.

The second major category of factors related to Sensory/Perceptual Alterations includes those that result in altered sensory reception, transmission, or integration. They may be pathophysiological, situational, or maturational. Neurological disease, trauma, or deficits, alterations in sensory organs, sleep deprivation, pain, and the inability to communicate, understand, speak, or respond are classified in this category of factors. Stroke, head injury, and spinal cord injuries are some of the medical diagnoses most often associated with neurological disease, trauma, and deficits.[16] Sensory organ alterations may be congenital and may result in malfunctioning or dysfunctional sensory organs, as occurs in congenital deafness and blindness. Alterations may also be acquired as the result of injury, surgery, or other treatment. Burns that alter tactile receptors, radiation therapy that affects olfactory and taste receptors, and cataract surgery that alters the eye are examples of this. Sleep

deprivation often occurs when activities involved in the care and monitoring of patients disrupt sleep patterns and deprive patients of their usual amounts of sleep.[6,9,12] This is a particular problem in intensive care units. Other sensory deficits are attributable to general neurophysiological changes that occur with aging, such as decreases in vision, hearing, and gustatory and olfactory discrimination. Patients may be unable to communicate because of a pathological condition, because of a medical intervention such as intubation or tracheostomy, or because their culture and language are different from those around them.[11]

The third category of factors related to Sensory/Perceptual Alterations is made up of endogenous and exogenous chemical alterations. Hypoxia, electrolyte imbalances, vitamin B deficiencies, and elevated blood urea nitrogen are examples of endogenous factors. Mind-altering drugs and central nervous system stimulants and depressants are classified as exogenous factors. Both endogenous and exogenous chemical alterations affect the peripheral and central nervous systems. The visual and auditory hallucinations seen in alcohol withdrawal and color vision deficiencies with digoxin toxicity are examples of this.

Psychological stress has been identified as a fourth category of factors related to Sensory/Perceptual Alterations. Such things as extreme anxiety, panic, and bereavement narrow our perceptual fields and interfere with attention to and interpretation of stimuli.

■ Defining Characteristics

The presence of the following defining characteristics indicates that the patient may be experiencing Sensory/Perceptual Alterations[13,15]:

- Reported or measured changes in sensory acuity
  - Diminished or distorted visual, auditory, tactile, gustatory, olfactory, and kinesthetic capabilities
  - Motor incoordination
  - Alteration in posture
  - Change in muscular tension
  - Vertigo

- Changes in thought processes
  - Disorientation in time, in place, or with persons
  - Altered abstraction or conceptualization
  - Change in problem-solving abilities
  - Body image alteration
  - Hallucinations
  - Inappropriate responses
- Changes in usual behavior patterns
  - Change in usual response to stimuli
  - Altered communication patterns
  - Complaints of fatigue
  - Altered sleep patterns
- Change in emotional lability
  - Restlessness
  - Irritability
  - Anger
  - Apathy
  - Rapid mood swings

■ Related Factors

The following related factors are associated with Sensory/Perceptual Alterations[13]:

- Altered environmental stimuli (excessive or insufficient)
- Altered sensory reception, transmission, or integration
  - Neurological disease, trauma, or deficits
  - Inability to communicate, understand, or respond
  - Sleep deprivation
  - Pain
- Chemical alterations
  - Endogenous (e.g., electrolytes imbalance)
  - Exogenous (e.g., drugs)
- Psychological stress
  - Anxiety
  - Fear
  - Bereavement

DIAGNOSIS

■ Differential Nursing Diagnosis

The major defining characteristic for the diagnosis of Sensory/Perceptual Alterations is diminished or distorted visual, auditory, tactile, olfactory, or kinesthetic capability. It is not unusual for more than one sensory modality to be affected because the medical and psychiatric problems that result in alteration of the reception, transmission, integration, or interpretation of sensory stimulation often affect more than one sensory modality. For example, a neurological disease simultaneously could affect hearing, vision, and kinesthetic function. Identification of the specific sense modality or modalities affected determines the specificity of the diagnosis. Furthermore, altered sensory/perceptual function may be a related factor for other nursing diagnoses (e.g., Personal Identity Disturbance, Fear, or Anxiety). In these instances, the sensory alteration may be an antecedent or contributing factor to the diagnosis. At times, the altered sensory perception may be a manifestation or defining characteristic of the diagnosis itself. In these instances it is usually one of several defining characteristics and is not critical to the diagnosis. For example, the diagnosis Altered Thought Process might include alterations in sensory/perceptual function as one defining characteristic,[10] but impaired judgment, problem solving, and disturbances of thought flow would be more critical to the diagnosis.

Perhaps the most closely related nursing diagnosis is Unilateral Neglect. In Unilateral Neglect, however, perceptual alterations are limited to one side of the body and sensory alterations may or may not be present. In many instances, where Sensory/Perceptual Alterations have been identified, it might be better to give priority to diagnoses that address the patient's responses to Sensory/Perceptual Alterations. Risk for Injury, Impaired Verbal Communication, and Social Isolation are diagnoses that could provide more direction for independent nursing actions when Sensory/Perceptual Alterations are present.

A major difficulty in using this diagnosis is the lack of research to validate the diagnosis and its defining characteristics.[10]

■ Medical and Psychiatric Diagnoses

Cerebrovascular accidents, spinal cord compression, and head injury are medical diagnoses most often associated with neurological disease,

VI

trauma, and sensory/perceptual deficits. Narrowed perceptual fields and attention to and interpretation of stimuli with subsequent Sensory/Perceptual Alterations are seen in generalized anxiety disorder, depressive state, and psychoactive substance use disorders such as cocaine abuse and intoxication. These are just a few among many psychiatric and medical disorders that alter sensory reception, transmission, integration, or interpretation.

OUTCOME IDENTIFICATION, PLANNING, AND IMPLEMENTATION

Outcomes of nursing interventions for patients with Sensory/Perceptual Alterations will depend on individual patient characteristics, identified related factors, and presenting defining characteristics for a given patient. Nursing interventions are directed toward preventing injury and providing mechanisms to help the patient with the Sensory/Perceptual Alterations. The overall goal is to promote, maintain, and restore optimal sensory/perceptual function as evidenced by elimination of defining characteristics.

Priority should be given to keeping the patient continuously free of unintentional injuries. Nursing interventions should ensure that the patient and/or family understand the safety hazards posed by the specific sensory/perceptual deficit. In addition, safety precautions are instituted to eliminate environmental hazards and to provide the patient with supervision and assistance to protect the patient from hazards posed by the specific alteration.

Second, cognitively intact patients should communicate a sense of familiarity and security with their environment within 24 hours. To accomplish this the nurse should institute measures that orient the patient to the environment, give meaning to sensory stimuli, assist the patient in compensating for Sensory/Perceptual Alterations, and promote the use of intact senses. The success of these interventions is evidenced by a decrease in defining characteristics (e.g., anxiety and disorientation).

Because inadequate sleep or rest can be a major factor in causing or exacerbating Sensory/Perceptual Alterations,[9,12] the third outcome is that the patient should sleep at least two 3- to 4-hour periods every 24 hours. Nursing interventions focus on modifications in the scheduling of treatment and activities and on the control or elimination of extraneous stimuli such as noise and lighting.

The fourth outcome relates to the patient's consistent use of assistive devices and compensatory aids correctly. Assistive devices and aids vary according to the specific Sensory/Perceptual Alteration and the nature of the related factor(s). Nursing interventions focus on assessing the knowledge of the patient and family regarding such devices and their use. Interventions might also require teaching the patient and family about their proper use or obtaining the services of other professionals (e.g., a hearing or vision specialist or a physical therapist). The nurse will also collaborate with other health professionals to ensure appropriate referrals for evaluation and prescription of such devices. In some instances, specific rehabilitation programs are available for patients with auditory, visual, or kinesthetic problems. If sensory/perceptual function is to be maximized, the nurse, in collaboration with the physician and other professionals, must ensure that the patient and family have knowledge about and access to such assistive and compensatory devices and services.

◢ **NURSING CARE GUIDELINES**

Nursing Diagnosis: Sensory/Perceptual Alterations (Specify): Visual, Auditory, Kinesthetic, Gustatory, Tactile, Olfactory

Expected Outcome: The patient will continuously remain free of unintentional injuries (e.g., burns, pressure injuries, and falls).
▲ Instruct patient and/or family about the nature and safety implications of identified alterations.
■ Institute appropriate safety precautions, providing assistance and supervision and eliminating or reducing environmental hazards:
  ■ Remove clutter and unnecessary equipment.
  ■ Place furniture and personal articles consistently in one place.
  ■ Keep assistive devices such as walkers, canes, glasses, and call bell within easy reach of the patient.
  ■ Keep bed in lowest position when patient is unattended.
  ■ Use night-lights.
  ■ Be sure overbed tables and beds have wheel locks engaged.
  ■ Have patient use nonskid slippers or sturdy shoes when ambulating.
  ■ Modify the environment and daily routines to allow for slower response and adaptation.
  ▲ Provide for position change at least every 2 hours and active or passive exercise at least once a day.
Safety precautions and changes in position reduce the risk of unintentional injury and iatrogenic complications.

Expected Outcome: The cognitively intact patient will demonstrate a sense of comfort and security as evidenced by accurate identification of objects, events, and sounds within the environment, a decrease in emotional lability, an increased attention span, and/or maintenance or improvement of orientation to time, person, and place within 24 hours.
■ Use orienting cues:
  ■ Address the patient by the name he or she prefers each time the patient is approached or spoken to.
  ■ Introduce yourself and wear a name tag.
  ■ Using the patient's intact senses, provide orienting information about the routines, objects, events, sounds, and smells in the environment.
  ■ Make frequent references to time and place.
  ■ Place clocks and calendars where the patient can see them; use large size if vision is impaired.
  ■ Put familiar objects in reach of patient.
  ■ Have patient use personal toilet articles and clothing whenever possible.
Orienting cues help maintain and increase orientation to reality, as well as give meaning and pattern to stimuli.
■ Encourage active participation in activities of daily living and treatments. *Active participation provides the patient with a sense of control and adds meaning to stimuli.*
■ Provide the patient with a clear, concise explanation of what will be seen, heard, smelled, or tasted during treatments and routines. *Providing sensory information avoids novelty and surprise and gives meaning to stimuli.*
■ Encourage participation in familiar activities, such as reading, hobbies, conversation, visiting with family and friends, and selective use of radio, television, or other audiovisual devices. *Familiar activities give meaning and variety to stimuli and provide the patient with a sense of control.*
▲ Compensate for deficits with assistive devices and stimulation of alternative senses:

Visual
  ▲ Use visual aids (magnifiers, glasses, low-vision devices, and focused lighting).
  ■ Control glare.
  ■ Use verbal description and touch to provide sensory information.

■ = nursing intervention; ▲ = collaborative intervention.   *Continued*

VI

■ NURSING CARE GUIDELINES — CONT'D

Auditory

- Speak slowly, and articulate clearly without exaggerated mouth movements or shouting.
- Direct sound to patient's better ear.
- Face the patient when speaking, and allow light to illuminate your face.
- Minimize background or competing noise when addressing patient.
- Supplement speech with hand gestures and written information.
- Check that hearing aids are in place and working properly.
- ▲ Check ears for impacted cerumen and arrange for removal if present.

Tactile and kinesthetic

- ▲ Use assistive devices or provide support during ambulation and transfers.
- Use distraction, such as conversation, music, and cool compresses, to alleviate intensity of disturbing sensations.

Olfactory and gustatory

- Control obnoxious or objectionable odors in the environment.
- ▲ Serve foods visually appealing in color,[5] arrangement, and texture.
- ▲ Serve hot foods hot (when they're more odoriferous).
- ▲ Provide variety of condiments.
- Have patient rinse mouth with normal saline several times a day, and use gravies and sauces to moisten food. *A dry mouth reduces gustatory sensitivity.*
- Avoid smoking, alcoholic beverages, and mouthwashes containing alcohol, lemon juice, or peroxide. *These agents dry mucous membranes.*

Assistive devices enhance or compensate for diminished sensory/perceptual abilities. Alternative sensory stimulation compensates for diminished or absent sensory/perceptual abilities.

Expected Outcome: The patient will sleep at least two 3- to 4-hour periods every 24 hours.
- ▲ Provide adequate pain relief if needed.
- Dim lights at night and at specified periods.
- Reduce unnecessary noise, traffic, and personnel.
- ▲ Arrange and space treatments and activities to ensure uninterrupted periods of rest and sleep. *Control of extraneous stimuli promotes adequate sleep and rest.*

Expected Outcome: The patient will consistently use assistive devices and compensatory aids correctly.
- Assess patient and family knowledge related to assistive devices and aids for the specified Sensory/Perceptual Alteration.
- ▲ Provide information and instruction to patient and family related to the alteration and compensatory techniques and devices.
- Check assistive devices for proper functioning.
- ▲ Obtain referrals for further evaluation and sensory rehabilitation, especially of visual, auditory, and kinesthetic alterations.
- ▲ Provide patient and family with information on community services and financial resources that are available to assist in procurement and use of assistive devices and compensatory aids. *The correct use of aids and assistive devices assists the patient to compensate for altered sensory/perceptual function. Many patients do not use such aids, devices, or services because they do not know about them or how to obtain them or because they are financially constrained.*

EVALUATION

The effectiveness of the nursing interventions is determined from objective data that indicate that the goals of preventing injury and promoting, maintaining, and restoring optimum contact with reality have been achieved. The absence of injury and a decrease in or elimination of defining characteristics, such as anxiety and disorientation, should be expected. No specific time frame is designated for the outcome related to freedom from injury in that this outcome must be continuously evaluated while the patient receives nursing care. Achievement of the outcome related to the patient's comfort and security with the environment is evidenced by the patent's orientation to time, person, and place; ability to recall past and recent events; appropriate responses to the environment; and stabilization of emotions. A 24-hour time frame is designated because nursing interventions to achieve this outcome must be instituted as soon as the patient is admitted. Although no research has been found that indicates how long it takes such interventions to take effect, research on the provision of sensory information to patients indicates that cognitively intact patients show some immediate response to these interventions.

The 24-hour time frame is selected for the outcome related to sleep because studies done in the 1960s and early 1970s indicate that sleep deprivation for as little as 24 hours results in Sensory/Perceptual Alterations. No recent studies that indicate otherwise have been located. On the other hand, the outcome related to proper use of assistive devices and compensatory aids is short-term and long-term in nature. If the patient has or is given an assistive device, proper use must begin immediately. When the patient requires referral, the outcome may only be measurable after a longer period of time (weeks or months).

The same methods and techniques used to make the initial diagnosis will provide the needed data for evaluation. If the expected outcomes are not met or are only partially met, reassessment of the patient and environment and modification of nursing interventions may be necessary. The time frame for meeting the outcome criterion may not have been adequate, or the initial diagnosis may not have been correct.

VI

▶ CASE STUDY WITH PLAN OF CARE

Mrs. Clara W. is a 69-year-old, married patient in an orthopedic unit of a general hospital. Mrs. W. had a total left hip replacement for osteoarthritis 3 days ago. From the time of her admission, she has been alert, oriented, and cooperative, but the night nurses report that Mrs. W. was confused and agitated during the night. She insisted that her daughter was calling for help. Her health history indicates no previous hospitalizations except for childbirth. Mrs. W. has osteoarthritis and a visual acuity of 20/70 (uncorrected) bilaterally. However, with the use of bifocals she has corrected vision of 20/30 bilaterally. Her last eye examination was 6 months ago. The patient is a retired secretary and business school graduate.

Mrs. W. has been married for 45 years to a 70-year-old, retired insurance agent. Mrs. W. lives with her husband in a two-bedroom apartment in a retirement community. She has one married daughter and two teenage grandchildren who live nearby and visit frequently. She has a married son and three grandchildren in California. Mrs. W. drives a car and does her own shopping, cleaning, and cooking despite her arthritic hips and knees. She enjoys knitting and television game shows, and she does volunteer work with the American Red Cross and is active in a national secretaries' sorority, Polish-American Club, and church. Mrs. W. is a nonsmoker and an occasional social drinker; she does not use recreational drugs. Before hospitalization, she was taking calcium supplements and Naprosyn, 400 mg three times a day, as prescribed by a physician. Mrs. W. sleeps with her husband, is usually in bed by 10:30 P.M., and sleeps 8 to 9 hours a night.

Her vital signs, hematology, and electrolyte reports are within normal limits. She is conscious and responsive but has poor recent memory and recall, although her past memory is intact. Results of neurological and sensory examinations are within normal limits, except

Continued

■ CASE STUDY WITH PLAN OF CARE — CONT'D

for a slight decrease in light touch and vibratory sensation in the left leg. Mrs. W.'s bed is near the door in a two-bed room, which is across from the nurses' station. Records indicate that she has slept little the past few nights because of pain and noise from the nurses' station. Bed rest was prescribed until yesterday, when she was up in a chair twice, for an hour each time. She had been receiving meperidine hydrochloride (Demerol), 50 mg intramuscularly every 4 hours, for relief of pain until yesterday morning, when she started on Emperin with codeine for relief of pain. Her husband and daughter have not been able to visit because of a snowstorm.

■ PLAN OF CARE FOR MRS. CLARA W.

Nursing Diagnosis: Sensory/Perceptual Alterations: Auditory and Kinesthetic Related to Therapeutically and Socially Restricted Environment, Noise, Pain, Sleep Deprivation, and Recent Hip Surgery

Expected Outcome: Mrs. W. will continuously remain free of falls, wounds, pressure sores, or other unintentional injuries.
- Instruct Mrs. W. and her family about the nature and safety implications of kinesthetic alteration in left leg.
- Institute appropriate safety precautions, providing assistance and supervision during toileting and bed-to-chair transfer and eliminating or reducing environmental hazards:
  - Patient should use nonskid slippers when transferring.
  - Remove clutter and unnecessary equipment.
  - Place furniture and Mrs. W.'s personal articles consistently in one place.
  - Keep Mrs. W.'s assistive devices (walker, glasses, and call bell) within easy reach.
  - Keep bed in lowest position when patient is unattended.
  - Use night-lights.
  - Be sure table over bed and beds have wheel locks engaged.
  - Have Mrs. W.'s husband bring low-heeled, sturdy shoes for use when Mrs. W. ambulates.
  - Provide extra time for toileting and transferring.
  - ▲ Assist Mrs. W. with position change at least every 2 hours (except for specified sleep periods) and active or passive exercise at least once a day.

Expected Outcome: Mrs. W. will demonstrate a sense of comfort and security within the environment as evidenced by accurate identification of objects, events, and sounds; a decrease in emotional lability; an increased attention span; and maintenance of orientation to time, person, and place within 24 hours.
- Use orienting cues:
  - Address Mrs. W. by the name she prefers (i.e., Clara).
  - Introduce yourself and wear name tag.
  - Provide orienting information about the routines, objects, events, sounds, and smells in the environment, especially noises from the nurses' station.
  - Make frequent references to time and place.
  - Place clocks and calendars with large-size print where Mrs. W. can see them.
  - Put familiar objects within Mrs. W.'s reach; have Mr. W. bring small family pictures as soon as he is able to visit.
  - Have Mrs. W. use personal toilet articles and her own robe and slippers.
  - Encourage Mrs. W. to bathe herself, comb her hair, and apply her usual makeup. Have her fill out her own menu.
  - Put up cards from family and friends so Mrs. W. can view them.
- Provide Mrs. W. with a clear, concise explanation of what will be seen, heard, and felt during dressing changes and transfers to and from bed.

■ = nursing intervention; ▲ = collaborative intervention.

- Assign the same nurse to Mrs. W. for the next 3 days.
- Encourage Mrs. W. to work on her knitting while sitting in the chair.
- Put the television on Mrs. W.'s favorite shows (9 A.M. game show and 3 P.M. soap opera).
- Have Mrs. W. speak with her husband and daughter by phone daily until they can visit.

Expected Outcome: Mrs. W. will sleep at least two 3- to 4-hour periods every 24 hours.
- ▲ Check for adequate analgesic control every 3 to 4 hours, but especially at 10 or 11 P.M. and at the time of scheduled transfers from or to bed. If inadequate, seek alternate analgesia.
- Dim lights at night.
- Close Mrs. W.'s door at night to reduce noise from the nurses' station.
- Schedule out-of-bed periods at 11:30 A.M. and 4:30 P.M. If asleep, do not awaken patient between 11:00 P.M. and 3:00 A.M. and between 3:30 and 7:00 A.M.

Expected Outcome: Mrs. W. will consistently use assistive devices and compensatory aids correctly.
- Assess Mrs. W.'s knowledge about use of walker.
- ▲ Provide information and instruction to Mrs. W. and her family related to use of walker.
- Check walker for proper height.
- ▲ Obtain referral for physical therapy.
- ▲ Provide Mrs. W. and family with information about the Arthritis Foundation and Medicare coverage of durable medical equipment.

VI

■ CRITICAL THINKING EXERCISES

1. What is the significance of noting the type and dosage of analgesia Mrs. W. is receiving?
2. How would abnormal hematological or electrolyte reports change the nursing diagnosis or interventions for Mrs. W.?
3. Given Mrs. W.'s recent agitation, confusion, disorientation, and poor recent memory, why or why not consider psychiatric evaluation?
4. What other nursing diagnoses might be formulated from the data on Mrs. W.?
5. What other nursing interventions can you describe that might promote adequate sleep and rest for Mrs. W.?

REFERENCES

1. Bastick T: *Intuition: how we think and act,* Chichester, Great Britain, 1982, John Wiley & Sons.
2. Bray SA: Alterations in special senses. In Mitchel PH and others, editors: *AANN's neuroscience nursing,* Norwalk, Connecticut, 1988, Appleton & Lange.
3. Brunner J and Postman L: On the perception of incongruity: a paradigm, *J Pers* 18:206, 1948.
4. Bunting S: The concept of perception in selected nursing theories, *Nurs Sci Q* 1:168, 1988.
5. Clydesdale FM: Changes in color and flavor and their effect on sensory perception in the elderly, *Nutri Rev* 52: S19, 1994.
6. Easton C and MacKenzie F: Sensory-perceptual alterations: delirium in the intensive care unit, *Heart Lung* 17:229, 1988.
7. Gardephe CD: The 5 senses, *Am Baby* (55)5:A2–A6, 1993.
8. Gibson E: *Principles of perceptual learning and development,* New York, 1969, Appleton-Century-Crofts.
9. Gottlieb GL: Sleep disorders and their management, *Am J Med* 88(Suppl 3A):29S, 1990.
10. Janken JK and Cullinan CL: Auditory/sensory perceptual alteration: suggested revision of defining characteristics, *Nurs Diagnosis* 1:147, 1990.
11. Kloosterman N: Cultural care: the missing link in severe sensory alteration, *Nurs Sci Q* 4:119, 1991.
12. McGonigal KS: The importance of sleep and the sensory environment to critically ill patients, *Intens Care Nurs* 2:73, 1986.
13. North American Nursing Diagnosis Association: *NANDA nursing diagnoses: definitions and classification, 1995–1996,* Philadelphia, 1994, The Association.
14. Stanley C: The healing touch, *Nurs Times* (91)29:36–37, 1995.
15. Valdez M: Evaluation and management of the dizzy patient: an otolaryngology perspective, *ADVANCE for Nurs Practitioners* (3)9:27, 1995.
16. Wyness MA: Perceptual dysfunction: nursing assessment and management, *J Neurosurg Nurs* 17:105, 1985.

Altered Thought Processes

Altered Thought Processes *is a state in which an individual experiences a disruption in cognitive operations and activities.*[8]

OVERVIEW

Altered Thought Processes is a nursing diagnosis that can be assigned to individuals across the life span in a variety of health care settings. Individuals with medical, surgical, or psychiatric conditions can experience a disruption in cognitive operations and activities. Defining characteristics reflect a diagnosis based on thought and cognition.[7]

Cognitive operations and activities are the abilities to imagine, create new ideas, think, learn, retain in memory, know, preserve, and communicate knowledge.[5] Thinking involves the ability to construct ideas in a normal sequential fashion, reason logically, have insight into situations, calculate, make appropriate judgments, demonstrate realistic thinking, make decisions, think in abstract terms, and solve problems.[3] A person with altered thoughts may have impairment in one or more cognitive or thinking abilities.

Through the highly valued abilities of thinking and cognition, people can organize and assign meaning to their experiences in life and master and adapt to their perceived environment. Cognitive processes, particularly thinking and problem solving, are acquired. Their acquisition is most influenced by a person's heredity. Physical maturation and biological functioning, interactions with the environment, social interaction, and internal self-regulation, including emotions, also influence cognitive operations and problem-solving ability.[9]

Glick[6] identified five categories of normal thought processes: (1) attention, (2) memory, (3) language, (4) spatial perception, and (5) higher mental function. *Attention* is the ability to eliminate distractions while focusing on specific types of sensory information. It is important to determine if attention deficit is a related factor in Altered Thought Processes. *Memory,* the retention and storage of sensory information, influences problem solving, new learning, and independence in living. *Language* plays a role in thinking, conceptualization, and problem solving. *Spatial perception* may reveal objective evidence of early brain dysfunction. Deficits in spatial perception lead to difficulty performing self-care activities or an inability to distinguish spatial concepts. *Higher mental functions* includes calculation, categorizing, logical thinking, abstract reasoning, and exercising values and judgment in decision making and problem solving. Attention, memory, language, and spatial perception must be intact to use higher mental functions.[11]

ASSESSMENT

Determining the level of consciousness is a first step in assessing a patient's mental status. Consciousness determines a patient's ability to relate to self and to the environment. A continuum of responsiveness includes five levels: alertness, lethargy or somnolence, obtundation, stupor or semicoma, and coma.

The nurse assesses the patient's cognitive processes by gathering subjective data about the patient, observing the patient, interviewing significant others and caregivers, and using assessment tools to gather information. It is important to assess the cognitive functioning of all patients, regardless of the patient's age, medical or psychiatric diagnosis, or the health care setting. The nurse utilizes observational and communication skills in this assessment process.

To establish Altered Thought Processes as the nursing diagnosis for a particular patient, the nurse must establish rapport with the patient and show empathy, respect, and acceptance. Several meetings between the nurse and the patient might be necessary to gather assessment data and establish the nursing diagnosis accurately.

There are a number of screening tests nurses can use to identify cognitive impairment.[2,13] Examining a patient's mental status is one way a nurse can assess a patient's cognitive processes and thinking to obtain an overview of a patient's here-and-now functioning.[3,12,13,14] To formulate an accurate nursing diagnosis, factors that influence cognition, such as behavior and feelings, are also assessed.

Observe the patient's physical appearance: sex, stated age and apparent age, nutritional status, hygiene, manner of dress, general state of health, and eye contact. Assess the patient's speech for rate, volume, amount, and characteristics. Speech disturbance is seen in patients with medical conditions and psychiatric disturbance. Note the level and type of motor activity. Is there evidence of tension, restlessness, or psychomotor retardation? Are there any abnormal movement patterns? Describe the patient's relationship to you during your assessment. Is the patient cooperative, guarded, withholding, pleasant, hostile, or irritable?

People's feelings influence their moods. *Mood* is defined as a patient's self-report of his or her general mental state and feelings. Patients can be asked to rate their mood on a scale of 1 to 10. By asking direct questions, the nurse can assess the patient for the presence of thoughts about self-harm or harming others. *Affect* is a momentary manifestation of a person's emotional response to internal and external events. Affect is expressed in posture, facial and body movements, tone of voice, vocalizations, and word selection.

Include an assessment of the patient's perception, or the processing of information about one's internal and external environments.[13] Misinterpretations of reality may take the form of hallucinations or illusions. Patients with hallucinations have auditory, olfactory, tactile, gustatory, or visual sensory experiences in the absence of verifiable stimulation. Identify the possible presence of command hallucinations and the risk for danger the patient poses to him- or herself or to others. An *illusion* is a false perception or false response to an existing sensory experience.

Assess the components of thought content and thought process. Thought content refers to the meaning that a person is communicating. Delusions, phobias, and obsessions are examples of alterations of thought content. Thought process refers to how well connected a person's thoughts are. Examples of alteration in thought process include loose associations, flight of ideas, circumstantial and tangential thinking, and thought blocking.

The patient's attention, vigilance, and orientation also must be assessed. *Attention* is the patient's ability to focus on a specific stimulus without distraction by extraneous environmental stimuli. Attention is necessary to the performance of more complex functions such as memory, language, and abstract thinking.[6] *Vigilance* refers to the ability to sustain attention over an extended period of time —the capacity to concentrate. The nurse should observe if a patient is paying attention to what the nurse says or if the patient's attention appears to wander. Slowed or delayed responses, rambling speech, distractibility, and hyperactivity with poor concentration are indications of inattention. *Orientation* is the patient's ability to show awareness of self as a person by stating his or her name correctly, by stating the date, season, and time of day, and by correctly identifying the place.

The process of memory is assessed in terms of whether the patient has immediate recall, recent memory, and remote memory.[6,13] Immediate recall occurs within a range of a few seconds to a few minutes before data is selectively transferred to short-term memory. *Recent memory* is short-term

VI

memory. It functions to hold information for immediate use, rehearsal, or memorization. Failure to retain information in short-term memory can result from anxiety or from pathophysiological conditions. *Remote memory* is long-term memory. A person can use information acquired and stored over a period of weeks, months, or years.

■ Defining Characteristics

The presence of the following defining characteristics indicates that the patient may be experiencing Altered Thought Processes:

- Inaccurate interpretation of environment
- Hypervigilance or hypovigilance
- Altered states of consciousness
- Disorientation as to person, time, or place
- Impaired recent memory and remote memory
- Altered sleep patterns
- Suicidal or homocidal ideation
- Attention deficit
- Distractibility
- Hyperactivity
- Wandering
- Alteration in perception (e.g., hallucinations or illusion)
- Delusions
- Egocentricity
- Inappropriate, non-reality-based thinking
- Disturbed thought flow (e.g., circumstantial thoughts, tangential thoughts, neologisms, flights of ideas, loose associations, word salads, thought blocking, or perseveration)
- Disturbed thought content (e.g., delusions, obsessions, preoccupations, and phobias)
- Inappropriate or labile affect
- Impaired judgment
- Impaired problem solving
- Cognitive dissonance
- Confabulation

■ Related Factors

The following related factors are associated with Altered Thought Processes:

- Anemia

- Hypoxia
- Dehydration
- Hypothyroidism and hyperthyroidism
- Hypoglycemia and hyperglycemia
- Hepatic failure
- Acid-base disturbances
- Azotemia
- Hyponatremia
- Cushing's syndrome
- Hypopituitarism
- Acute myocardial infarction
- Congestive heart failure
- Vascular occlusion
- Pulmonary embolism
- Chronic liver disease
- Head trauma
- Brain tumors
- Infections, viral or bacterial
- Chemical toxicity (e.g., lead, radiation, or medications)
- Hormonal changes
- Chronic renal disease
- Post-heart-lung machine
- AIDS
- Arteriosclerosis
- Chronic hypertension or hypotension
- Chronic obstructive pulmonary disease
- Hereditary degenerative brain disease
- Anxiety
- Alzheimer's disease
- Substance abuse, acute or chronic
- Schizophrenia
- Mood disorders
- Sensory overload or deprivation
- Physical, sexual, or emotional abuse
- Traumatic situational stress (e.g., rape, natural disaster, or combat experience)
- Imprisonment
- Culture shock

DIAGNOSIS

■ Differential Nursing Diagnosis

The nursing diagnosis Altered Thought Processes applies to patients experiencing problems with cognition. The patient must show evidence of inaccurate interpretation of the environment.[2,11] A change in problem-solving ability is also an important defining characteristic. If a patient is experiencing perceptual problems, a diagnosis of Sensory/Perceptual Alterations is more applicable. The nurse must also consider the applicability of other nursing diagnoses, particularly Chronic Confusion, Acute Confusion, Ineffective Individual Coping, and Impaired Environmental Interpretation Syndrome.

■ Medical and Psychiatric Diagnoses

Medical and psychiatric diagnoses related to Altered Thought Processes are psychiatric diagnoses with organic etiologies within the medical class delirium, dementia, amnestic and other cognitive disorders.[1] Amnestic disorders are characterized by memory disturbance and impairment in the ability to learn new information or recall previously learned information. Symptoms can be transient or chronic and may be substance induced. Delirium is a disturbance of consciousness that develops over a short period of time—hours to days—and fluctuates during the course of the day. Symptoms can be induced by medical conditions or substance intoxication or withdrawal. Dementia involves multiple cognitive deficits: memory impairment, loss of intellectual abilities, language disturbance, personality changes, and changes in abstraction, judgment, and other higher cortical functions.

Medical conditions that directly affect cognition, such as those listed as related factors, can result in Altered Thought Processes.

OUTCOME IDENTIFICATION, PLANNING, AND IMPLEMENTATION

In planning nursing care for the patient with Altered Thought Processes, it is important to focus on data collected during the assessment of the patient. It is essential to establish priorities to assist the patient in achieving an optimal level of physiological, psychological, and social functioning. The nurse must consider the patient's perception of his or her experience in the here-and-now as well as information provided by caregivers and significant others. Outcomes are designed with consideration of patient characteristics, related factors, related medical and psychiatric diagnoses, and collaborative interventions and are based on mutual goal setting with the patient. Time frames recommended for achievement of outcomes are estimates based on the general priority of human needs.

The success of interventions will in part be determined by the etiology of the cognitive changes. Nursing interventions are based on providing for patient safety, eliminating or mediating the effect of the etiology, facilitating communication in interpersonal relationships, and establishing structure and routines to protect the patient's sense of self as a person.

◢ NURSING CARE GUIDELINES
Nursing Diagnosis: Altered Thought Processes*

Expected Outcome: The patient will engage in activities that promote basic physical requirements within 2 days.
- ■ Monitor vital signs, neurological status, intake and output, and nutritional status *to promote patient's survival.*
- ▲ Assist with mobility and ambulation *to improve the functional abilities of the patient.*
- ▲ Assist with hygiene and activities of daily living. *Patients with Altered Thought Processes often lose the ability to engage in self-care activities independently.*

■ = nursing intervention; ▲ = collaborative intervention.
*References 4, 10, 11, 12.

Continued

◢ **NURSING CARE GUIDELINES — CONT'D**

- Monitor environmental stimulation *to control external stimuli that could overwhelm patient and to prevent sensory deprivation.*

Expected Outcome: The patient will maintain own safety and will refrain from harming others within 3 days.

- Assess for presence of suicidal thoughts. *Patients with impaired ability to cope are at risk for harm to self.*
- Assess patient for signs of agitation and the potential for aggression. *With impaired thinking, patients cannot effectively solve problems or judge the consequences of their actions.*
- ▲ Provide a calm, safe, familiar, nonthreatening environment in the least restrictive manner possible. Close observation, one-to-one, is a minimally restrictive measure to ensure safety of patient and others. Physical restraints are used only if less restrictive measures are ineffective. *This helps the patient differentiate between internal and external stimuli.*
- Encourage patient to validate thoughts. *This intervention focuses on feelings and thoughts underlying patient distortions, and it identifies needs underlying patient thoughts.*

Expected Outcome: The patient will experience a sense of self-value within 1 week.

- ▲ Identify and focus on patient strengths *to promote patient involvement in care and patient's sense of accomplishment.*
- Orient the patient to reality *to enhance feelings of self-worth and personal dignity.*
- Validate patient's feelings *to gain an understanding of patient's experience and to acknowledge the patient as a person.*
- Provide opportunities for patient to focus on concrete, easy-to-accomplish tasks *to promote a sense of achievement and self-worth.*
- ▲ Approach in a caring, supportive way. *Caring in a relationship promotes self-esteem.*

Expected Outcome: The patient will communicate in a manner that is understandable and responsive to others within 5 days.

- ▲ Control excess environmental stimulation *to allow the patient to process information.*
- Focus on here-and-now *to direct patient's focus to reality-centered situations.*
- Ask patient the meaning of what is said. *Focusing on content gives patients positive support in their efforts to communicate.*
- Validate with the patient your understanding of the meaning of patient's communication. *Rephrasing helps patient identify specific thoughts and feelings and supports patient's efforts to communicate.*
- Tell the patient when you have difficulty understanding what was said. *Asking patient to clarify helps keep communication clear.*
- ▲ Involve significant others in communicating with the patient, *reducing caregiver burden and aiding the caregiver to cope with stress.*

■ = nursing intervention; ▲ = collaborative intervention.

EVALUATION

Evaluation is the process of determining achievement of expected patient outcomes, if actual patient status corresponds to expected outcomes, and the effectiveness of the overall plan of care and specific interventions for the patient.

Evaluation can take place at any point in the nursing process. The desired outcome for Altered Thought Processes is for the patient to achieve the highest level of cognitive functioning that is realistic for the patient.

■ CASE STUDY WITH PLAN OF CARE

Mrs. Sadie P., 81 years old, is a widow currently living alone in a "seniors" apartment building. Her grown daughter, her primary caregiver, lives in her own home close to Mrs. P. The patient's husband died 15 years ago. A geriatrician follows her case, and on her last visit she scored 17/30 on the Mini-Mental Status Examination. Mrs. P. showed non-reality-based thinking, impairment of recent memory, confabulation, distractibility, impaired ability to solve problems, reason, and calculate, and deterioration in her ability to engage in self-care activities. Her medical diagnoses include hypertension, arthritis, and primary degenerative dementia, Alzheimer's type. She was referred for home care psychiatric nursing to assess her safety in the home and to monitor her mental status.

Initial assessment revealed a pleasant, cooperative heavyset female, who appeared younger than her stated age. She was alert and oriented to place and person but not to time (disoriented to month, year, and season). She could not remember three objects after 2 minutes, but she knew her place of birth. She correctly verbalized a direction to breathe through her mouth but could not follow the direction. Alteration in thought flow was evidenced by loose associations and tangential thinking. Mrs. P. was convinced a neighbor was entering her apartment and stealing her belongings. She stated her husband lived with her but was out working on the day of the visit. During the assessment, Mrs. P. was distracted, getting up several times, looking in the refrigerator, and washing dishes in the kitchen. On a subsequent visit the nurse telephoned her to gain entry to the apartment building, and Mrs. P. answered the telephone. When directed by the nurse to use a telephone code to allow the nurse entry, she told the nurse she did not have a telephone.

One week after beginning a new day program, Mrs. P. started wearing soiled clothing and on a second occasion was dressed to leave her apartment wearing three slips, a blouse, and shoes and stockings but had forgotten a skirt. Although she knows her name and has written it correctly, she could not write it accurately. She verbalized frustration with her awareness of this incongruence. She has been putting refrigerated foods in the cupboards, in the freezer, and in the trash and frequently misplaces her apartment keys. Recently she refused to attend the day program. During an outing with her daughter, she walked into the street and oncoming traffic. Her daughter describes feeling exhausted by the burden of care and concern for her mother's safety. She has started the process of locating an assisted living program for Mrs. P.

■ PLAN OF CARE FOR MRS. SADIE P.
Nursing Diagnosis: Altered Thought Processes Related to Alzheimer's Disease

Expected Outcome: Mrs. P.'s environment will support her safety by the end of her first home visit.
- Assess Mrs. P.'s potential for harm to herself and others.
- Protect Mrs. P. from injury within her apartment (by removing environmental hazards) and in the community (by avoiding environmental hazards). Review with Mrs. P. and her daughter potential safety hazards, and identify the means to remove and avoid them.
- Encourage Mrs. P.'s daughter to continue to try to locate living arrangements that will offer Mrs. P. adequate assistance.

Expected Outcome: Mrs. P. will maintain her current level of self-care activities.
- Assess Mrs. P.'s current self-care status.
- Assist Mrs. P. in establishing a predictable daily routine that provides adequate time for and supports completion of self-care activities; provide clear, simple directions.
- Compliment Mrs. P. on her accomplishments in hygiene, grooming, and housekeeping.

■ = nursing intervention; ▲ = collaborative intervention. *Continued*

Expected Outcome: Mrs. P. will engage in activities that promote physiological functioning by the second home visit.

- Monitor physiological stability, medications, food and fluid intake, and activity tolerance; discuss routines with Mrs. P. and her daughter that will optimize Mrs. P.'s physiological well-being; suggest visual stimuli that will assist Mrs. P. in knowing when to take medications.
- ▲ Assess the environmental stimuli at the day program to determine if it creates sensory overload for Mrs. P.; if necessary, recommend alternative programs that are more suitable for Mrs. P.
- Encourage Mrs. P. and her daughter to take daily walks at a regularly scheduled time, following the same route each day.
- ▲ Refer Mrs. P.'s daughter to community social services that can assist in identifying appropriate living arrangements for Mrs. P.

Expected Outcome: Mrs. P. will engage in reality-based communications by the third home visit.

- Orient Mrs. P. to time with visual displays such as a clock and a calendar.
- Redirect Mrs. P. to reality-based interaction as necessary.
- Seek the meaning of what Mrs. P. is trying to communicate.
- Recommend to Mrs. P. and her daughter ways to arrange contact with Mrs. P.'s peers.

Expected Outcome: Mrs. P. will experience a sense of self-esteem and pride by the third home visit.

- Involve Mrs. P. in establishing a daily routine and structure.
- Support Mrs. P.'s personal strengths by complimenting her.
- Validate Mrs. P.'s feelings.
- Provide opportunities for Mrs. P. to experience a sense of accomplishment.

VI

■■ CRITICAL THINKING EXERCISES

1. How do you feel about interacting with a person who is experiencing non-reality-based thinking?
2. What factors would you consider to promote environmental safety for Mrs. P.?
3. What types of community-based support would you recommend for Mrs. P.'s family?
4. Compare and contrast reality orientation and validation of feelings for patients such as Mrs. P., who are disoriented.

REFERENCES

1. American Psychiatric Association: *Diagnostic and statistical manual of mental disorders,* ed 4, Washington, D.C., 1994, The Association.
2. Baker FM: Screening tests for cognitive impairment, *Hosp Comm Psychiatry* 40:339–340, 1989.
3. Deptula D, Singh R, and Pomara N: Aging, emotional states, and memory, *Am J Psychiatry* 150:429–434, 1993.
4. Dixson B: Intervening when the patient is delusional, *J Psychiatr Nurs Mental Health Serv* 7:25–34, 1969.
5. Folstein M, Folstein S, and McHugh P: Mini-Mental State: a practical method for grading cognitive state of patients for the clinician, *J Psychiatr Res* 12:189–198, 1975.
6. Glick O: Normal thought processes, *Nurs Clin North Am* 28:715–727, 1993.
7. Hancock CK and others: Altered thought processes and sensory/perceptual alterations: a critique, *Nurs Diagnosis* 5: 26–30, 1994.
8. North American Nursing Diagnosis Association: *NANDA nursing diagnoses: definitions and classification, 1995–1996,* Philadelphia, 1994, The Association.
9. Piaget J: *The origins of intelligence in children,* New York, 1952, International Universities Press.
10. Schroeder P: Nursing intervention with patients with thought disorders, *Perspect Psychiatr Care* 17:32–39, 1979.
11. Sideleau B: Irrational beliefs and intervention, *J Psychosoc Nurs* 25(3):18–24, 1987.
12. Snyder M: *A guide to neurological and neurosurgical nursing,* ed 2, Albany, New York, 1991, Delmar.
13. Strub R and Black F: *The mental status examination in neurology,* ed 2, Philadelphia, 1985, FA Davis.
14. Trzepacz P and Bahe R: *The psychiatric mental status examination,* New York, 1993, Oxford University Press.

Unilateral Neglect

Unilateral Neglect *is the state in which an individual is perceptually unaware of and inattentive to one side of the body.*[9]

OVERVIEW

Unilateral Neglect is one of a number of perceptual deficits that can be seen after injury to the nondominant hemisphere of the brain.[1] Such an injury can be caused by a cerebrovascular accident (CVA), or stroke, a cerebral aneurysm, a tumor, or, in rare cases, trauma. The effect is inattention to the affected side of the body or to the environment around the affected side.

Perception is the ability to integrate and interpret sensory data. Several cerebral regions provide an integrated network for the mediation of directed attention: the posterior parietal lobe, the frontal eye fields, and the cingulate gyrus.[4] If any of these areas of the brain become damaged, interpretation of data is altered, and perception and attention are impaired. The parietal lobes are supplied by the anterior cerebral, middle cerebral, and posterior cerebral arteries. Because there is great variability in the responses of the human brain, injury or blockage of any of these arteries can cause damage to the parietal lobe.

Perceptual deficits such as neglect may be associated with physical defects such as hemiplegia, sensory deficits, or hemianopsia. These do not have to be present for neglect to occur and can be present without neglect.[3] The nondominant hemisphere is generally on the right side of the brain. Injury to the dominant parietal lobe usually correlates with problems in communication.[12]

Unilateral Neglect may appear with other perceptual deficits in combinations that are not very predictable or related to the magnitude of the injury. The nurse must therefore look for a variety of perceptual deficits when assessing the patient with a lesion of the nondominant hemisphere, even when there are no physical sequelae.

Unilateral Neglect is inattention to the affected side of the body (hemiinattention) or to the environment from the midline toward the affected side (hemispatial neglect). These two types of neglect can be categorized as disorders related to perception of self and disorders related to perception of space.[10] Some studies suggest that Unilateral Neglect is a deficit of attention and exploration that makes it difficult not only to pay attention to the affected side but to disengage attention from the unaffected side.[6] Disorders in perception of self also include anosognosia. Agnosia and apraxia are categorized separately but are related disorders of perception. Unilateral Neglect rarely occurs in isolation and usually is associated with one or more other perceptual deficits.[1] Unilateral Neglect occurring in combination with other related perceptual deficits is known as *neglect syndrome*.

Anosognosia is a denial phenomenon where the patient lacks insight into the presence of deficits or the significance of the deficits.[5] Anosognosia is most prominent in the acute phase after injury. *Agnosia* is the inability to recognize and identify familiar objects through an otherwise intact sense. Agnosia can be visual (not recognizing an object), tactile (not recognizing a familiar object held in the hand when the eyes are closed), or auditory (not recognizing familiar sounds).[10] *Apraxia* is the inability to do a skilled motor function despite adequate muscle power, sensation, and coordination. The patient will not be able to get dressed if handed clothes or to brush his or her teeth if handed a toothbrush. This is due to an inability to conceptualize and plan the task.[10] Different aspects of the neglect syndrome have been related to different regions of the brain.[4] The parietal region is linked with sensory/perceptual aspects (neglect of self and agnosia), the frontal region with exploratory/motor aspects (neglect of space and apraxias), and the cingulate gyrus with the motivational/emotional aspects (anosognosia).

ASSESSMENT

It is during the acute phase after a stroke or other brain injury to the right or nondominant hemisphere that Unilateral Neglect and other components of the neglect syndrome are most severe. Any form of neglect of self or space can severely affect the patient's safety and performance of activities of daily living (ADLs).[6] If neglect is not recognized for what it is, the patient may be thought to be confused, uncooperative, flighty, stubborn, or otherwise cognitively impaired.[11]

Anosognosia is most prevalent in the early phase after the stroke. The patient may completely deny the stroke deficits or the significance of any effects. The patient may state the ability to walk or may confabulate reasons why walking is not possible ("I can't walk because I don't have my shoes on"). The patient may deny ownership of the affected limbs, asking the nurse to "Get this dead body out of my bed" or saying that the limbs belong to someone else.

To assess for anosognosia, ask the patient to state what is wrong or why the patient came to the hospital. Often the patient will state something like "I fell, but now I am fine." If the patient initially denies any deficits, ask about the strength of the affected limbs or the patient's ability to use them. If the patient actively denies a deficit, ask specific questions or give simple commands regarding the affected limbs. This is when the patient may start to confabulate.

The unconcern, unawareness, or denial associated with anosognosia sometimes are related to a general clouding of the sensorium immediately after the injury.[10] As the sensorium clears, the anosognosia usually lessens to the point that the patient can admit to deficits but will still neglect the affected side in some fashion.

Unilateral Neglect of self or space is usually obvious. The patient experiencing neglect of self may roll over or sit on an affected arm, for example. The patient may not groom the affected side, leaving that side unshaved, unwashed, or undressed. The patient may also neglect to hook eyeglasses over the affected ear, leaving them "hanging,"[8] or may sit with the head turned toward the unaffected side.

The person experiencing neglect of space will not respond to stimuli such as people, noises, or light coming from the environment on the affected side. The patient will not be able to find objects placed on a table or nightstand on the neglected side and may not eat food on that side of the plate. When the patient with neglect of space starts to ambulate or move around the unit, he or she may bump into doorjambs or walls because of neglect of that portion of the environment.

To assess more specifically for neglect of space, have the patient draw a stick figure or the face of a clock. The figure will only be one-sided, and the numbers will be drawn on only one side of the clock rather than distributed evenly around it. If the patient is able to read, only words on the side of the page corresponding to the unaffected side will be read, sometimes to the point that the patient only reads half a word. This might be noticed when a patient is asked to fill out a form, such as a daily menu, and only one side of the form is filled out.

Unilateral Neglect is the portion of the neglect syndrome most often associated with homonymous hemianopsia (visual field cut). The patient may need to be assessed by an ophthalmologist or neurologist for the presence or absence of this visual defect. If the patient has hemianopsia and not cortically mediated neglect, the patient can be taught to overcome the visual defects by scanning the affected side. Patients with neglect will have more difficulty learning to scan the affected side.

Agnosia, the failure to recognize and identify objects through an otherwise intact sense, can affect any of the senses. If hearing or language is suspected to be involved, the patient should also be assessed by a speech-language pathologist.

The patient with apraxia will have the muscular and cognitive ability to carry out a task but will be unable to do so when asked. At other times, the patient may do the activity unconsciously. The deficit may become obvious as the patient starts to become more involved in performing ADLs. The patient may be unable to brush his or her teeth or to shave when handed the appropriate utensil. The patient may not eat a meal correctly, as evidenced by pouring coffee in the cereal or using a fork to spread the butter. The occupational therapist can assist the nurse in assessing the exact type of apraxia. Dressing apraxia is different from the dressing problems seen in neglect of self. In neglect of self, the unaffected side is dressed correctly, but the unaffected side is not dressed at all or is dressed incompletely. In dressing apraxia, the patient is unable to figure out which types of clothes go where and may try to put a leg into the sleeve of a shirt or put a shirt on first, then a bra.

Members of the physical medicine and rehabilitation team (physiatry, occupational therapy, and physical therapy) will be involved with the patient from the early days after the injury and will be helpful in assessing the exact constellation of deficits and determining the treatment plan. The nurse must act in collaboration with these other professionals through all phases of the nursing process.[2]

■ Defining Characteristics

The defining characteristics for the nursing diagnosis Unilateral Neglect are outlined, along with those of other aspects of neglect syndrome that a patient may be experiencing. The related factors apply to the entire neglect syndrome.

The presence of the following defining characteristics indicates that the patient may be experiencing Unilateral Neglect:

Unilateral Neglect

- Consistent inattention to stimuli on the affected side

- Patient ignores position of affected side (e.g., sits on hand)
- Does not eat food on one side of plate
- Does not groom, dress, or bathe the affected side
- Ignores stimuli (noises, people, lights) in the environment of the affected side
- Bumps into doorway or walls on affected side while ambulating or self-propelling in a wheelchair

Anosognosia

- Denies deficits
- States physical abilities that no longer exist (e.g., walking)
- Demonstrates poor safety awareness

Agnosia

- Does not recognize familiar objects by sight
- Does not recognize familiar sounds
- Does not recognize familiar objects by feel

Apraxia

- Unable to do previously learned motor tasks in proper sequence

■ Related Factors

The following related factors are associated with Unilateral Neglect[9]:

- Effects of disturbed perceptual abilities (e.g., hemianopsia)
- Neurological illness or trauma

DIAGNOSIS

■ Differential Nursing Diagnosis

Unilateral Neglect is a specific cognitive/perceptual deficit that must be suspected after injury, especially stroke, to the nondominant hemisphere. If there is a possibility that the patient may be experiencing any aspect of the neglect syndrome, the nurse should assess the patient carefully to avoid confusing neglect with other nursing diagnoses such as Altered Thought Processes, Acute Confusion, Impaired Memory, Ineffective Denial, or Sensory/Perceptual Alterations. In the early stages after a stroke, the patient's sensorium may be clouded, leading to these other diagnoses, especially Altered Thought Processes and Acute Con-

VI

fusion, in addition to the diagnosis Unilateral Neglect. The differential diagnosis between Ineffective Denial and anosognosia may be difficult, but anosognosia is most likely if there other components of the neglect syndrome present. A person who is neglecting one side of the body may seem to have Impaired Memory but should be observed carefully for the defining characteristics of Unilateral Neglect. Unilateral Neglect will be one of many Sensory/Perceptual Alterations seen after a stroke.

■ Medical and Psychiatric Diagnoses

The most common medical diagnoses related to the nursing diagnosis Unilateral Neglect are cerebrovascular accident (CVA), cerebral aneurysm, cerebral neoplasia, and traumatic brain injury. Although neglect is often seen after CVA and cerebral aneurysm in the right temporoparietal lobe, it is not seen as commonly after the other diagnoses. If the nurse suspects that a form of neglect is present after neurological trauma or illness, collaboration should occur with the members of the treating team to finalize the diagnosis.

OUTCOME IDENTIFICATION, PLANNING, AND IMPLEMENTATION

Unilateral Neglect and other aspects of the neglect syndrome are seen immediately after the injury and may remain present in some form throughout the acute hospital and rehabilitation stays and even upon discharge to home. *It is key that all members of the health care team collaborate to create a consistent treatment approach,* with similar expected outcomes, to optimize the patient's recovery. The nurse should ensure compliance with interventions that take place on the nursing unit and monitor those outcomes.

Initially, safety and injury prevention are of primary concern. If the patient is displaying signs of anosognosia, he or she will try to do things that he or she cannot, such as ambulate to the bathroom. The patient may also confabulate well, making it easy for the health care team members to overestimate ability. The environment should stay simple and oriented to the patient's unaffected side, so that the patient will not try to search for needed items that are in the neglected space.

As the anosognosia subsides, efforts must be made to direct the patient's attention to the affected side. Not only must attention be drawn to the affected side but the activity must be compelling enough to help the patient disengage from the unaffected side. Interventions should include cueing, immediate feedback, and positive reinforcement.[6]

Throughout the patient's stay, the family or significant others must be included in the plan of care. They must be taught about the aspects of the neglect syndrome that are relevant to the patient. It is not uncommon for the family to think that the patient is being stubborn or forgetful when in fact the patient is displaying the symptoms of neglect. Once the family understands the patient's deficits, they should be included in the patient's care, helping direct the patient to attend to the neglected side.

As the patient's awareness of the neglected side improves, he or she should be able to increase participation in ADLs. If the neglect is very severe, the patient may never fully regain the ability to attend to the affected side and thus may always need assistance. The treatment team, in collaboration with the family, must decide at what point the patient has reached maximum recovery.

The family or significant others must also be included in this portion of the treatment plan because they will need training to assist the patient with ADLs and mobility and because they are crucial members of the discharge planning team.

Once the patient is able to understand the deficits that have resulted from the injury, the nurse will need to assist the patient and family to utilize effective coping strategies. Often these patients were fully independent before the injury and will need much positive reinforcement to regain or maintain their self-esteem. The family will be coping with the changes in their loved ones and their family structure, and they will need the assistance of the team to identify and utilize effective methods of coping.

◣ NURSING CARE GUIDELINES
Nursing Diagnosis: Unilateral Neglect

Expected Outcome: The patient will display safety awareness and prevent injury. Safety awareness should improve once the anosognosia subsides, usually within the first week after the event.
- ▲ Keep all four side rails up while patient is in bed because *the patient may not remember the extent of the deficits.*
- ▲ Approach the patient from the unaffected side and keep call light and personal items on unaffected side so that the patient *is not trying to find things that are in the neglected space.*
- ▪ Keep the environment simple and well lit *to avoid confusion.*
- ▲ Do not rely on the patient's statement of abilities and therefore perhaps overestimate the patient's ability to perform a task or activity. *The patient may still be denying the deficits (anosognosia) and may be confabulating about current abilities.*
- ▲ Reorient the patient as needed; *the patient's sensorium may remain clouded for days to weeks after the injury.*

Expected Outcome: The patient will display increased awareness of affected side. This should start to occur within 1 to 3 weeks of the event.
- ▲ Include activities that attend to both sides of the body *so that the patient may pay attention to the neglected side and disengage from the unaffected side.*
- ▲ Remind the patient to use the affected extremities if motor function remains or to position the extremities properly after turning, sitting, and so on. *These interventions will help direct attention to the neglected side.*
- ▲ As the patient progresses, encourage interaction of staff and visitors with the neglected side because *this will assist patient to disengage from the unaffected side.*
- ▲ Teach the patient to scan the affected side on a regular basis, especially during activities that involve that side *as a method of learning to compensate for the neglect.*

Expected Outcome: The patient will perform ADLs at expected optimal level (based on amount of other physical and cognitive deficits present). This should be evaluated at the end of the acute hospital stay (usually 1 to 2 weeks after the stroke) and again at weekly intervals during rehabilitation. The patient should be making significant gains toward independence by the end of the fourth week after the injury.
- ▲ Place food on the side of the tray that the patient is not neglecting *so the patient will eat all the meal.*
- ▲ While the patient is still completely neglecting one side, assist patient with dressing and grooming while verbally going through the steps of the activity; *this is especially important for patients with apraxia because they will need to relearn tasks.*
- ▲ When the neglect starts to subside, have the patient start to perform own ADLs, with verbal cueing as needed *as part of the relearning process.*
- ▲ Continue to teach the patient to scan the affected side during ADLs. *Teaching the patient to scan is the most important way to help the patient compensate for the neglect.* One way to do this is to center the meal on the tray and have the patient scan the meal periodically to ensure completion.

Expected Outcome: The patient will use effective coping mechanisms to maintain positive self-esteem once the patient is able to recognize the deficits. This should be maximized before discharge to home so that the patient will remain engaged in all aspect of his or her life.
- ▲ Have the patient identify and use positive coping strategies that have been successful in the past *because strategies that have worked before will be the most likely to succeed during the current crisis.*
- ▲ Assist the patient in identifying new coping strategies as needed *because new situations may require different coping styles.*

▪ = nursing intervention; ▲ = collaborative intervention.   *Continued*

■ **NURSING CARE GUIDELINES — CONT'D**

▲ Use positive reinforcement of progress made and, when appropriate, include the patient in goal setting to bolster self-esteem *because patients with new disabilities often can see only what they can't do rather than what they can.*

Expected Outcome: The family or significant others will verbalize understanding of the patient's deficits and demonstrate this understanding by following the treatment plan as set by the health care team. This should start right away, and the family should be fully involved by the end of the first week if there are no other medical complications that would preclude their involvement.

▲ Give the family a realistic assessment of the patient's injury and deficits, demonstrating as appropriate. *The sooner the family understands the deficits, the sooner they will be able to participate in the patient's care and the discharge planning.*

▲ Teach the family the appropriate interventions for each stage of the patient's progress *because the patient's abilities will change as the treatment progresses.*

Expected Outcome: The family or significant others will demonstrate effective coping mechanisms to provide appropriate support for the patient and each other. This assessment needs to occur by the end of the acute hospital stay because it is a key part of discharge planning and because it may be a condition of the patient's entry into rehabilitation.

▲ Use interventions to promote family coping that are similar to those used for the patient; *an injury to a member of the family affects the whole family.*

▲ Encourage the family to eat well and to rest *so they will have the energy to assist the patient and to make decisions as needed.*

▲ Be an empathetic listener *so that the team is aware of all the family's concerns.*

EVALUATION

Just as it is relatively clear when a patient is experiencing Unilateral Neglect, it usually becomes apparent when the neglect starts to subside. However, the nurse must be aware of the extent of the injury and other factors in the patient's history (e.g., previous strokes and age) so that the outcomes and the evaluation of these outcomes do not set the patient or family up to fail. Unilateral Neglect and the other components of the neglect syndrome are usually only a part of the roster of deficits seen after a stroke or brain injury. The evaluation of the patient's abilities in ADL and mobility skills must take into account any other physical and cognitive disabilities that are present. Usually the neglect will substantially improve within the first few weeks after the injury. However, some patients never recover from or fully learn to compensate for their neglect and, as a result, remain severely disabled. Persistence of the neglect, along with physical disabilities, will preclude independent living. It is key that the nurse, along with the rest of the team, monitor the patient carefully for improvement of the neglect so that appropriate discharge planning can start as early as possible.

◤ CASE STUDY WITH PLAN OF CARE

Mrs. Faye B., a 52-year-old, right-handed woman, had an uncomplicated CVA to the right side of her brain 1 week ago. She is in a wheelchair, slumped to the left, with her hand hanging down off the armrest. She does not notice when her husband, who is sitting on her left side, calls her name. She is dressed correctly, except that her left hand is not in her sweater sleeve. Her report notes that she has a dense left hemiplegia with no known visual deficit. Her eating habits are reported as "poor" (she only eats "half" her meal), and she occasionally calls items by the wrong name. Before her CVA she was fully independent. Her medical history includes only hypertension for which she was taking medication regularly. Her treatment team includes her primary care physician, physical therapy, occupational therapy, speech therapy, and the social worker. Mrs. B. has a husband and two grown children, but they live a 2-hour drive from the hospital. She has a large support network of friends and fellow church members. Her insurance plan allows for a total of 30 days of rehabilitation, durable medical equipment, and 25 outpatient visits. The family has few other financial resources.

◤ PLAN OF CARE FOR MRS. B.
Nursing Diagnosis: Unilateral Neglect of Self and Space Related to Right Parietal Stroke as Evidenced by Inattention to Left Side of Body and Environment

Expected Outcome: Mrs. B. will demonstrate awareness of her left side as evidenced by her correctly positioning the left side of her body after movement and her use of items in the left hemispace.
- ▲ Have Mrs. B. position her left arm and leg after every change in body position.
- ▲ Teach Mrs. B. to scan her left side while eating and during other activities.
- ■ Put personal items on Mrs. B.'s left side, and remind her to look to her left when trying to locate these items. (Always keep the call bell on the right side for safety.)
- ▲ Approach Mrs. B. from the left.

Expected Outcome: Mrs. B. will not injure her neglected extremities.
- ■ Have Mrs. B. use a sling on her left arm until she is more aware of its position after activity.
- ▲ Ensure that Mrs. B. and all other team members working with her check the position of her affected extremities on a regular basis.

Expected Outcome: Mrs. B. will perform ADLs at expected optimal levels (Mrs. B.'s ability to perform ADLs will be affected by her hemiplegia as well as her neglect).
- ■ Teach Mrs. B. to scan when eating to ensure that all food is eaten.
- ▲ Assist Mrs. B. with dressing at first, going through step-by-step instructions as to how to doff and don clothing.
- ▲ Have Mrs. B. recite steps for all ADLs and try to follow the steps as they are recited.
- ▲ Teach Mrs. B. to scan to the left when grooming and bathing to ensure that the left side receives the same attention as the right.

Expected Outcome: Mrs. B. will name all objects correctly.
- ▲ Work with the speech therapist to assess and treat any agnosia that is present.
- ▲ Use cueing as needed to assist Mrs. B. in correctly naming objects or people.

Expected Outcome: Mrs. B. will verbalize and use her usual effective coping mechanisms.
- ▲ Assess Mrs. B.'s coping mechanisms and assist her to use them.

Expected Outcome: Mrs. B.'s family will verbalize understanding of Mrs. B.'s deficits and demonstrate this understanding by appropriately assisting Mrs. B. with ADLs and mobility.
- ▲ Arrange family meeting with all members of the team to outline the deficits and plan of care.

■ = nursing intervention; ▲ = collaborative intervention.

Continued

◤ PLAN OF CARE FOR MRS. B. — CONT'D

- Involve the family in the nursing care of Mrs. B. as fits their comfort level; involve the family in all aspects of her care as their comfort level increases.
- ▲ As Mrs. B.'s final needs for assistance in ADLs and mobility become clear, ensure that the family is taught how to care for her and is able to demonstrate these skills.

Expected Outcome: Mrs. B.'s family will demonstrate effective coping mechanisms as evidenced by their ability to provide appropriate physical and emotional support for Mrs. B.
- ▲ Assess family's usual coping strategies; assess premorbid role of each family member.
- ▲ Assess the effect that the long drive to the hospital is having on the family's ability to organize themselves, their ability to deal with daily life issues that cannot be ignored, and their eating and sleeping patterns.
- ▲ Identify community resources that will be available after discharge.

▦ CRITICAL THINKING EXERCISES

1. During your first assessment of Mrs. B., she is confused as to time and states that there is nothing wrong with her. Her husband says that she has never been good at facing difficult issues and just prefers to ignore them. What assessments might you make to differentiate between anosognosia and the nursing diagnosis Ineffective Denial?

2. Three weeks after her stroke, Mrs. B. is still not scanning her neglected side on a regular basis. Her husband, who up until now needed to continue to work, has taken a 1-week vacation. What interventions would you teach Mr. B. to assist in your treatment plan?

3. Mrs. B. now has only 5 days left on her insurance plan, and she is still not fully compensating for her neglect. Her husband has had to return to work. Both her children live near her. What are some community supports that you will want to ensure are in place before Mrs. B. is discharged?

REFERENCES

1. Boothe K: The neglect syndrome, *J Neurosci Nurs* 14:38, 1982.
2. Bronstein KS and others, editors: *Promoting stroke recovery: a research-based approach for nurses,* St. Louis, 1991, Mosby–Year Book.
3. Burt MM: Perceptual deficits in hemiplegia, *AJN* 70:1026, 1970.
4. Daffner KR and others: Dissociated neglect behavior following sequential strokes in the right hemisphere, *Ann Neurol* 28(1):97–101, 1990.
5. Hickey JV: *The clinical practice of neurologic and neurosurgical nursing,* ed 3, Philadelphia, 1992, JB Lippincott Co.
6. Kalbach LR: Unilateral neglect: mechanisms and nursing care, *J Neurosci Nurs* 23:125–129, 1991.
7. McCourt AE and others, editors: *The specialty practice of rehabilitation nursing: a core curriculum,* ed 3, Skokie, Illinois, 1993, Rehabilitation Nursing Foundation.
8. Nicklason F and Finucane P: "Hanging spectacles" sign in stroke, *Lancet* 336(8727):1380, 1990 (letter).
9. North American Nursing Diagnosis Association: *NANDA nursing diagnoses: definitions and classification, 1995–1996,* Philadelphia, 1994, The Association.
10. O'Brien MT and Pallett PJ: *Total care of the stroke patient,* Boston, 1978, Little, Brown & Co.
11. Stone S and Greenwood R: Assessing neglect in stroke patients, *Lancet* 337(8733):114, 1991 (letter).
12. Wyness MA: Perceptual dysfunction: nursing assessment and management, *J Neurosci Nurs* 17:105, 1985.

Anxiety

▶ ──────────────────────────────

Anxiety *is a subjective feeling of apprehension and tension manifested by physiological arousal and varying patterns of behavior. The source of anxiety is nonspecific or unknown to the individual.*

OVERVIEW

Anxiety is a common problem in patients across the life span and has diverse manifestations. Anxiety can impair a patient's coping and learning.[16,18,21,28,38] It can also influence quality of life,[34] immunity to disease,[39] and response to medical treatment,[3,15,27,36] and increase pain.[2,20] Anxiety has been described as a vague, uneasy sense of worry, nervousness, or anguish, often without an awareness of underlying feelings. Stressors are nonspecific or unknown to the individual.[22]

Peplau,[26] in a classic nursing work, characterized Anxiety as an energy that must be defined operationally by behaviors associated with the subjective experience. She described four levels of Anxiety (mild, moderate, severe, and panic), which have effects on physiological functioning, observation, awareness, learning and adaptation, and patterns of behavior.

Several conceptual models have sought to explain the phenomenon of Anxiety. The psychoanalytic model, based on Freud's theories, attributed Anxiety to birth trauma and separation, with subsequent Anxiety resulting from traumatic events in the life cycle. Freud distinguished realistic Anxiety from neurotic Anxiety, which he described as a disproportionate response that required defense mechanisms for management.[19]

Neo-Freudians such as Fromm,[10] Horney,[13] and Sullivan[33] defined Anxiety as an interpersonal phenomenon. Fromm[10] interpreted Anxiety as a culturally based response to freedom and isolation. Horney[13] theorized that instinctual drives were a product of Anxiety and a defense against a hostile world. Sullivan[33] described Anxiety as tension resulting from perceived or anticipated appraisal by others and need for social approval.

Spielberger[32] described two types of Anxiety states: (1) a transitory condition varying in intensity and fluctuating over time (state Anxiety); and (2) a stable personality characteristic that influences a person's perception of the environment (trait Anxiety). Behaviorists and learning theorists explained Anxiety as a conditioned or learned response. May[19] concluded that neurotic symptoms were reinforced because they reduced anxiety.

Using a biological model, researchers have studied Anxiety in terms of genetics and brain neurochemical responses. One explanation for Anxiety centers around the GABA A benzodiazepine receptor complex and abnormal receptor function, leading to decreased inhibitory activity.[9] Benzodiazepine receptors and diazepine binding inhibitors (DBI) are thought to play a major role in steroid production and activation of the hypothalamic-pituitary-adrenal axis in the stress response.[8] Anxiety disorders, such as panic disorder and obsessive compulsive disorder, are now being associated with neurotransmitter and receptor abnormalities with genetic linkage.[5,25] Posttraumatic stress disorder has also recently been associated with noradrenergic dysregulation.[31]

Stress and coping theorists have described Anxiety as one of many stress emotions.[17] Cognitive psychologists theorize that emotional responses are determined by the individual's cognitive appraisal of threats and coping options.[17] Robinson[29] states that Anxiety represents the initial psychophysiological signal of the stress response in a person.

ASSESSMENT

Anxiety is adaptive when arousal is appropriate to the situation and the individual is able to perform activities of daily living (ADLs) and cope with problems. Maladaptive Anxiety occurs when an exaggerated response results in decreased levels of performance and inappropriate behavioral patterns. It may be difficult to identify when defense mechanisms function to protect the individual from the pain of Anxiety in its pure state. Anger, denial, somatic complaints, and withdrawal are some of the behavioral responses used to reduce Anxiety or avoid awareness of it. In all instances the nurse's presence and empathy are important. Empathic understanding, the ability to go beyond the self and experience the other, allows an intuitive knowledge of the patient's experience and may communicate a feeling of connection and caring needed for the patient to disclose his or her thoughts and feelings. However, Anxiety may be transmitted interpersonally, and the nurse must maintain a calm presence while communicating support and concern.

Three separate, interacting response channels for emotional expression are recognized: motor or behavioral, self-report, and physiological arousal. Responses in all channels may not be consistent; that is, behavior may indicate Anxiety, but the emotion may be denied by the patient, and signs of physiological arousal may or may not be present. Individual responses in the expression of Anxiety through these channels vary.

Escape from or avoidance of certain stimuli are behaviors indicating Anxiety. Self-report, measuring the degree of Anxiety usually felt (trait Anxiety), or the response to current specific situations (state Anxiety), may be elicited by questions about current and past concerns, thoughts, and feelings. Physiological arousal may be observed in muscle tension, aimless movements, tremors, or clumsiness and may be measured by indices of auto-

nomic nervous system activation, such as increased heart rate, blood pressure, and respiration and changes in appetite and sleeping patterns.

Using a systematic approach, first identify and describe salient patient behaviors that indicate Anxiety (e.g., "You're shaking"), then ask the patient to describe related thoughts ("Are you worried about something?") and concurrent emotions ("How do you feel about that?"). The patient's ability to recall past events, analyze feelings, and project into the future will not be effective when the individual is highly anxious. The immediate distress of Anxiety must be relieved before the patient can explore the sources and dimensions of Anxiety and identify coping skills and resources.

Behavioral observations are useful in differentiating levels of Anxiety in individual patients as they affect the ability to observe, focus attention, learn, and adapt. Mild Anxiety is described as an alert aware state in which learning may readily occur. Moderate Anxiety is characterized by heightened alertness and selective attention to relevant stimuli that may be directed to focus on specific details when needed. Perceptions are greatly reduced, and behavior such as an exaggerated startle response to environmental stimuli or inattentiveness and staring (into space) without seeing, reflecting dissociative thought processes, may be seen with severe Anxiety. Panic is marked by extreme arousal and may result in fight-or-flight behaviors such as that of a child who screams and cries while clinging to the parent before separation for a surgical procedure.

Patient interactions with family, friends, and health care providers and environmental stimuli may provide data about factors related to Anxiety. The experience and awareness of Anxiety may shift, depending on the social context. Observe whether the patient's affect changes in the presence of family or other significant members of their social network. Environmental variations may affect the degree of Anxiety. Physical features of the environment, such as noise, space, lighting, and temperature, influence Anxiety responses.[24] Determine whether other factors are present that affect autonomic responses and may contribute to or potentiate Anxiety, such as medications,[35] drug withdrawal, delirium, or acute confusional states due to electrolyte imbalance or hypoxia.[4,14]

■ Defining Characteristics

The presence of the following defining characteristics indicates that the patient may be experiencing Anxiety:

- Self-report of apprehension, worry, and nervousness
- Increased heart rate, blood pressure, and respiratory rate
- Palmar sweating
- Increased muscle tension
- Hand tremors
- Repetitive, purposeless movements
- Speech pitch, rate, and volume increased
- Vocal quivering
- Changes in appetite
- Urinary frequency and urgency
- Escape/avoidance behavior
- Narrowed perceptual field: self-focused and inattentive
- Inappropriate behaviors: anger, fear, guilt, and regression
- Hypervigilance
- Denial
- Withdrawal

■ Related Factors

The following related factors are associated with Anxiety:

- Threats to bodily health
- Threats to self-concept
- Threatened social losses: significant others, status, and significant roles
- Unmet needs: security, dependency, and power
- Conditioning
- Uncertainty
- Situational or maturational crisis
- Interpersonal transmission (spread of Anxiety from one person to another)
- Social irresponsibility, guilt, or immaturity
- Lack of control over events

DIAGNOSIS

■ Differential Nursing Diagnosis

Fear and Ineffective Denial may be confused with Anxiety and are closely related phenomena.[22] These diagnoses have in common a response to perceived threats. Fear is distinguished from Anxiety by the patient's awareness and identification of the threatening object and resolution of fearful behaviors when identified threats are removed or resolved. Threats evoking Fear result in an immediate and consistent response marked by physiological arousal with activation of the sympathetic nervous system. The patient's attention and behaviors will be directed toward avoiding, escaping, or removing threatening stimuli and will persist until threats are resolved. Ineffective Denial as a nursing diagnosis is more difficult to discriminate from denial as a symptom of Anxiety. Denial may reduce the level of Anxiety and thus protect the patient for a period of time and allow reappraisal of threats and the search for effective coping options. However, when denial includes behaviors that are detrimental to one's health (e.g., not seeking or following health care advice when needed), the diagnosis Ineffective Denial should be applied.

■ Medical and Psychiatric Diagnoses

Medical diagnoses where Anxiety is a prominent feature include chronic, debilitating conditions, terminal illness, trauma, substance-related disorders, and psychiatric disorders. For example, Anxiety is often seen in patients (or their families) with acute myocardial infarction, cardiac disease, and chronic obstructive pulmonary disease (COPD) because of the life-threatening nature of the illness; recurrent dyspnea; problems with hypoxia; and side effects of medications.[12,23,37] Patients with cancer and AIDS may develop Anxiety, depending on the stage and the prognosis of the illness and the degree of catastrophic stressors.[6,11] Patients with traumatic brain injury or other brain lesions may appear anxious and restless, with increased intracranial pressure, delirium, or emotional lability mimicking Anxiety.[30] Patients with substance intoxication (substance-induced delirium) and

VII

substance withdrawal may develop Anxiety because of the autonomic irritability and effects of the substance on the central nervous system.[1] Patients with Anxiety frequently have psychiatric diagnoses such as posttraumatic stress disorder, panic disorder, phobias, obsessive compulsive disorder, generalized anxiety disorder, or acute stress disorder.[1]

OUTCOME IDENTIFICATION, PLANNING, AND IMPLEMENTATION

Initial interventions should focus on reducing incapacitating Anxiety states and preventing escalation of Anxiety levels. Outcomes include a patient report of reduced Anxiety and overt signs of relaxation, such as reduced physiological arousal indicated by heart rate, blood pressure, respirations, muscular tension, ability to attend to and process new information, and appropriate reaction to stimuli. Anxiety may be relieved or attenuated through strategies that are distracting or relaxing or that change how the patient thinks about threats. These treatments have a common base in their effects on central nervous system control of emotion and behavior. Distraction focuses attention on nonthreatening stimuli that compete with those that elicit Anxiety. This is useful for short-term interventions, such as those used during an invasive procedure. Use of music, touch, or relaxation training elicits the relaxation response. These methods can be especially useful as long-term therapy and can be self-administered or provided by family or friends as well as the nurse. The risks involved are usually minimal to most individuals. However, with relaxation training deterioration in the physical or mental state is possible in patients with a history of cardiac arrythmias, severe depression, or psychosis. Imagery may be used as an adjunctive therapy or by itself, particularly for patients experiencing fatigue or complications in multiple body systems that preclude the use of muscle relaxation techniques.

Anticipating and preventing severe Anxiety through patient education has proven effective.[7] Information should be provided before the patient encounters stressful situations, such as painful or threatening procedures. The timing, type, and amount of information given to patients should vary depending on their expressed needs and preferences. Including effective coping options is important when providing information about future events. In this way patients know what to expect and how to minimize potentially distressful responses. Other specific strategies may be planned to meet basic needs related to security, dependence, and power. Security interventions provide structure and consistency, minimize stress, and build trust. Anticipating needs, nurturing coping behaviors, and increasing attention to the patient will meet dependency needs. Power needs can be addressed by offering patients choices, avoiding needless conflicts, and allowing and accepting honest emotional expressions. Acknowledging these as basic needs in all patients as a guide to care may prevent regressive behavior, which indicates elevated Anxiety states.

The next stage of intervention attempts to assist the patient in meeting emotional self-care needs and coping more effectively with Anxiety. Cognitive strategies include guided problem solving to work through stressful periods; learning to identify sources of Anxiety and underlying feelings; cognitive reappraisal of potential threats and coping options; calming self-talk; and the use of relaxation techniques as part of a daily routine of emotional calibration or when needed. The immediate distress of Anxiety must be relieved before the patient will be able to explore the sources and dimensions of Anxiety and identify coping skills and resources.

■ NURSING CARE GUIDELINES
Nursing Diagnosis: Anxiety

Expected Outcome: The patient will report reduced feelings of Anxiety and will display overt signs of relaxation, indicated by reduced physiological arousal, the ability to attend to and process new information, and appropriate reactions to stimuli immediately following interventions.

- Use distraction (e.g., music), touch (e.g., slow-stroke massage and therapeutic touch), rhythmic breathing (or rebreathing techniques for hyperventilation responses), and imagery *to elicit the relaxation response*.
- Provide instructions and guided practice on muscular relaxation techniques *to reduce tension in striated muscles (musculoskeletal system) and thus smooth muscles (cardiovascular and gastrointestinal systems)*.

Expected Outcome: The patient will not experience severe Anxiety states or panic before, during, or after stressful medical procedures.

- ▲ Collaborate with physician and other care providers before stressful events to provide accurate information (including the sequence of events and the sensations that most patients experience) to the detail preferred by the patient *to reduce uncertainty*.
- Teach coping strategies appropriate for the procedure or anticipated stressful event *to provide patients with a sense of control and ways to minimize stressful responses*.

Expected Outcome: The patient will be able to participate comfortably in care, to report a sense of well-being and satisfaction with care during and following the health-care-giving episode, and to seek health care when appropriate.

- Structure environment as needed by assigning consistent caregivers, modulating stimulation (increasing or decreasing it as appropriate), and attending to safety precautions; be calm and reliable *to provide patient a sense of security*.
- Gain insight into the patient's perspective empathically; anticipate needs; acknowledge feelings as normal; increase attention to patient as needed; provide positive feedback for accomplishments; and foster visitation and patients' interactions with their social support network (family, friends, spiritual advisors, etc.) *to meet patient needs for dependency and belonging*.
- ▲ Develop trust and rapport by being nonjudgmental and authentic in response to patient behaviors; determine priorities based on patients' values; help patient avoid conflicts, especially over trivial matters; offer choices and advocate as needed with other caregivers when deciding or negotiating treatment decisions *to meet patient needs for power and self-control*.

■ = nursing intervention; ▲ = collaborative intervention.

VII

EVALUATION

Ongoing evaluation of patients' responses should be compared to baseline measures immediately following short-term interventions, such as massage or guided imagery. Validate the relaxation response by asking the patient how well the treatment helped him or her to relax. Physiological arousal (heart rate, blood pressure, respirations, and muscular tension) should be monitored before, during, and after stressful procedures. The patient should be able to attend to instructions and cooperate with treatment or diagnostic procedures without evidence of extreme arousal or reports of discomforts. Evaluate patients' feeling states before disengagement (e.g., when transferring to another level of care or at discharge from the hospital). Collaborate with the physician to determine whether there is a need for referral to mental health specialists, psychologists, or psychiatrists for more in-depth assessment and therapy.

◼ CASE STUDY WITH PLAN OF CARE

Mr. Roger K. is a 59-year-old man with chronic obstructive pulmonary disease and hypertension controlled by medication. He has a 3-month history of hoarseness and recent difficulty in swallowing. The patient is diagnosed as having squamous cell carcinoma of the right true vocal cord with subglottic extension. Surgical excision with partial laryngectomy is planned. Physical examination discloses that Mr. K. weighs 204 pounds and is 5′8″ tall. His heart rate is 86 beats/min and blood pressure 160/98. Respiratory rate is 22/min, with soft rhonchi in lung bases. The patient is somewhat barrel-chested. He has a history of smoking two to three packs of cigarettes per day and drinking eight to ten drinks of whiskey per day. Mr. K. lives with his wife in their own home; his son and family live in the same town. Now that he is retired he does not see old friends from work much because of the hypertension. He has a pension and medical insurance. He reports that he is a Methodist but has not been active in church. His father, who is dead, and brother had prostate cancer. Mr. K. reports eating, but without pleasurable taste, and moderate difficulty in falling asleep, with easy wakening. He reports great concern about the proposed surgical intervention, although he is unable to identify anything specific. He repeatedly asks about the possibility that he will not be able to talk after surgery. Mr. K. reports one episode of hallucinations during withdrawal from alcohol during a prior surgery. Mr. K. appears distressed. His apprehension is characterized by generalized muscular tension; alternately clenched and tremulous jaws; hands tightened into fists with jerky, restless movements; and a strained, tense facial expression. His voice pitch is elevated at times. His speech is compatible with a conversational level, but the volume and rate is somewhat increased. He is slightly verbose, giving lengthy answers to questions. He makes frequent eye contact with his wife during the interview.

VII

◼ PLAN OF CARE FOR MR. ROGER K.
Nursing Diagnosis: Severe Anxiety Related to Threats to Biological Integrity and Self-Concept and Uncertainty

Expected Outcome: Mr. K. will exhibit a reduction in the level of Anxiety following interventions.
- Acknowledge concerns and give reassurance of close surveillance by nursing staff.
- Offer relaxation training options before the operation, and begin instruction as soon as possible.
- Encourage wife's presence and support.
- Monitor Anxiety level.

Expected Outcome: Mr. K. will participate in preoperative and postoperative care (especially pulmonary); will ask appropriate questions or report satisfaction with information provided; and will begin guided self-care by fourth day after the operation.
- ▲ Facilitate communications with physician, and validate understanding.
- ▲ Explain preoperative and postoperative procedures. Include expected sensations, and the timing and sequence of events after Anxiety level is reduced.
- ▲ Give information on short-term and long-term alternatives for communication in the postoperative period; consult with physician regarding referral to speech therapist if needed.
- ▲ Anticipate stressful events and plan coping strategies with patient and physician (i.e., recognize and anticipate alcohol and smoking withdrawal after surgery).

Expected Outcome: Mr. K. will be able to identify Anxiety and ways of coping that work.
- Assist Mr. K. to clarify the meaning of stimuli as needed.
- Assist Mr. K. to identify his Anxiety response, related factors, and successful past coping actions; and encourage coping actions that Mr. K. can initiate by himself or that may be supported or initiated by his wife.
- Guide problem solving or reappraisals of problems as needed.

◼ = nursing intervention; ▲ = collaborative intervention.

■ CRITICAL THINKING EXERCISES

1. What physiological manifestations of Anxiety are present in the case of Mr. K., and what related factors may influence them?

2. How might the priority of interventions for Mr. K.'s Anxiety change throughout his hospital stay?

3. How would the nurse monitor Mr. K.'s level of Anxiety following surgery, taking into account his level of consciousness and medications that may affect his state?

REFERENCES

1. American Psychiatric Association: *Diagnostic and statistical manual of mental disorders,* ed 4, Washington D.C., 1994, The Association.

2. Biederman JJ and Schefft BK: Behavioral, physiological, and self-evaluative effects of anxiety in the self-control of pain, *Behav Modification* 18(1):89–105, 1994.

3. Boakes RA and others: Prevalence of anticipatory nausea and other side-effects in cancer patients receiving chemotherapy, *European J Cancer* 29A(6):866–870, 1993.

4. Bowman AM: Relationship of anxiety to development of postoperative delirium, *J Geront Nurs* 18(1):25–30, 1992.

5. Breier A: Panic disorder: clinical features, neurobiology, and pharmacotherapy, *NY State J Med* 91(suppl 11): 435–475, 1991.

6. Breitbart W: Psycho-oncology: depression, anxiety, delirium, *Semin Onc* 21(6):754–769, 1994.

7. Davis TMA and others: Preparing adult patients for cardiac catheterization: information treatment and coping style interactions, *Heart Lung* 23(2):130–139, 1994.

8. Ferrarese C and others: Diazepine binding inhibitor (DBI) increases after acute stress in rat, *Neuropharm* 30(12B): 1445–1452, 1991.

9. Ferrarese C and others: Benzodiazepine receptors and diazepam binding inhibitor: a possible link between stress, anxiety, and the immune system, *Psychoneuroimmun* 18(1):3–22, 1993.

10. Fromm E: *Escape from freedom,* New York, 1941, Rinehart.

11. Gaskins S and Brown K: Psychosocial responses among individuals with human immunodeficiency viral infection, *Appl Nurs Res* 5(3):111–121, 1992.

12. Gift AG and Cahill CA: Psychophysiologic aspects of dyspnea in chronic obstructive pulmonary disease: a pilot study, *Heart Lung* 19(3):252–257, 1990.

13. Horney K: *The neurotic personality of our time,* New York, 1937, WW Norton.

14. Inaba-Roland KE and Maricle RA: Assessing delirium in the acute care setting, *Heart Lung* 21(1):48–55, 1992.

15. Katz RC, Wilson L, and Frazer N: Anxiety and its determinants in patients undergoing magnetic resonance imaging, *J Behav Ther Exp Psychiatr* 25(2):131–134, 1994.

16. Koopman C and others: When disaster strikes, acute stress disorder may follow, *J Traum Stress* 8(1):61–74, 1995.

17. Lazarus RS and Folkman S: *Stress, appraisal, and coping,* New York, 1984, Springer Publishing.

18. Lazarus RS: Coping theory and research: past, present, and future, *Psychosom Med* 55:234–247, 1993.

19. May R: *The meaning of anxiety,* New York, 1977, Pocket Books.

20. McCracken LM and Gross RT: Does anxiety affect coping with chronic pain? *Clin J Pain* 9(4):253–259, 1993.

21. Moore SM: Development of discharge information for recovery after coronary artery bypass surgery, *Appl Nurs Res* 7(4):170–177, 1994.

22. North American Nursing Diagnosis Association: *NANDA nursing diagnoses: definitions and classification, 1995–1996,* Philadelphia, 1994, The Association.

23. Nymathi A and others: Coping and adjustment of spouses of critically ill patients with cardiac disease, *Heart Lung* 21(2):160–166, 1992.

24. Oberle K and others: Environment, anxiety, and postoperative pain, *Western J Nurs Res* 12(6):745–757, 1990.

25. Pauls DL and others: A family study of obsessive-compulsive disorder, *Am J Psychiatr* 152(1):76–84, 1995.

26. Peplau HE: A working definition of anxiety. In Burd SF and Marshall MA: *Some clinical approaches to psychiatric nursing,* New York, 1963, Macmillan Co.

27. Redd WH: Behavioral intervention for cancer side effects, *Acta Oncologica* 33(2):113–117, 1994.

28. Reider JA: Anxiety during critical illness of a family member, *Dimen Crit Care Nurs* 13(5):272–279, 1994.

29. Robinson L: Stress and anxiety, *Nurs Clin North Am* 25(4): 935–943, 1990.

30. Rosenthal M: Mild traumatic brain injury syndrome, *Ann Emerg Med* 22(6):1048–1051, 1993.

31. Southwick SM and others: Psychobiologic research in posttraumatic stress disorder, *Psychiatr Clin N Amer* 17(2): 251–264, 1994.

32. Spielberger CD: Theory and research on anxiety. In Spielberger CD, editor: *Anxiety and behavior,* New York, 1966, Academic Press.

33. Sullivan HS: *The interpersonal theory of psychiatry,* New York, 1953, WW Norton.

34. Trzcieniecka-Green A and Steptoe A: Stress management in cardiac patients: a preliminary study of the predictors of improvement in quality of life, *J Psychosom Res* 38(4): 267–280, 1994.

35. Tune L and others: Association of anticholinergic activity of presented medication with postoperative delirium, *J Neuropsychiatr Clin Neurosci* 5:208–210, 1993.

36. Vasterling J and others: Cognitive distraction and relaxation training for control of side effects due to cancer chemotherapy, *J Behav Med* 16(1):65–80, 1993.

VII

37. Webb MS and Riggins OZ: A comparison of anxiety levels of female and male patients with myocardial infarction, *Crit Care Nurs* 14(1):118–224, 1994.

38. Well ME and others: Reducing anxiety in newly diagnosed cancer patients: a pilot program, *Cancer Prac* 3(2):100–104, 1995.

39. Zorrilla EP, Redei E, and DeRubeis RJ: Reduced cytokine levels and T-cell function in healthy males: relation to individual differences in subclinical anxiety, *Brain, Behav, and Immun* 8(4):293–312, 1994.

VII

Body Image Disturbance

Body Image Disturbance *is a disruption in the perceptions, beliefs, and knowledge possessed about one's own body structure, function, appearance, and limits.*[4,5]

OVERVIEW

Body image can be seen as a distinct aspect of the self-concept. It is generally known as that part of the perceived self that constitutes a personal picture or image of the appearance of the body and its functions.[10] As such, it is contained within the person and subjected to ongoing changes based on life experiences, such as physical illnesses, accidents, and associated social and cultural values.

"A healthy body awareness would be based on self-observation and appropriate concern for one's physical well-being"[15] (p. 379). "Numerous research studies have documented the close positive relationship between self-concept and body image. This association appears to exist both within American society and across other cultures"[15] (p. 374).

Body image may overlap with other aspects of the self-concept, such as personal identity, role performance, and self-esteem, and is an integrated aspect of the global self-concept.[5,11] Life experiences that result in changes in body image can affect values and beliefs inherent in the self-concept and thus influence responses, performance, and thought processes. For example, a change in body structure, such as the loss of a limb, implies a change in body image because appearance and functional capacity are affected. The same change also implies other possible alterations in self-concept because beliefs and values influence self-

worth and may reduce self-esteem, making the adjustment process more complex and difficult.[10,15] The loss of former integration and function may lead to the need to mourn for the change or loss.[13]

The significance attributed to body image, the way a person sees the body and its functions, will vary according to the nature and intensity of values and related emotions invested in that image.[12] In North American society appearance, including dress and makeup, is a highly valued norm. Plastic surgery is not uncommon to alter a nose considered too large or too small or to have one's face "lifted" to eliminate the wrinkles of aging. The magnitude of the cosmetic industry and the "youth cult" seen in the advertising business are further indicators of societal values that determine what is considered desirable or undesirable in appearances. Young people in particular tend to be preoccupied with the ideal of thinness in appearance, which leads to fads in nutritional habits that have possible health risks.[6] The desire to be fashionable in dress and hairstyle exerts subtle pressures for changes in appearance and reflects adjustments to changing norms. Within the context of these influences body image is dynamic and never static. Yet there is an internal consistency shaped by the developmental process and life experiences associated with emotions and social and cultural rewards that gives meaning and value to one's body image. The qualitative aspects of body image, attitudes, and feelings, whether positive or negative, tend to resist change and can lead to a discrepancy in the reality of body image as seen by self and others. The "ideal" image or the "undesirable" image can persist as a mental concept. This persistence can be seen when one dresses in oversized

VII

or undersized clothing based on a mental image of self and in disregard for actual changes in body size. To change one's concept of body image takes time. Furthermore, much of "the editing of the experiences that go into making and modifying the body image is not conscious," and people have difficulty fully describing their body image.[12]

An understanding of body image and its significance in society and therefore in health care must incorporate the developmental process of the early years. Psychosocial and intellectual attributes evolve over time and shape body image in the socialization process, with ongoing associations and assimilated perceptions within the cognitive domain. The maturation process, including the integration of neuromuscular functions, allows for an increasing capacity for activities that lead to the experience of mastery and social rewards associated with body image. The ongoing changes in body size and function are valued or devalued in the social context of peers and family. Therefore early life experiences can have lasting effects on the mental perception of body image. For example, if the family shows a positive attitude to a child with a handicap, the child will gain confidence and maintain a positive body image. On the other hand, exposure to ridicule or social isolation by his or her peers or family will confirm a negative appearance and cause the child to form an undesirable mental image that can persist even after corrective surgery has been done.

Marked changes in body structure and function take place during adolescence. Existing social and cultural norms for appearance are challenged, and peer responses develop standards for conformity in dress and behavior. Growth rates and pubertal maturation can vary considerably at a given age. Being different or smaller or taller than the average height of the peer group can cause ridicule or social isolation, with possible disturbances in body image.

In certain areas of nursing practice attention to possible Body Image Disturbance can be significant in relation to health goals. Generally, patient responses to illness and life events are in part based on the perceived threat to body image and the values and beliefs attached to it. Any surgical intervention and many medical treatments or diagnostic procedures involve temporary or permanent changes in appearance and functional capacity.

In certain age ranges marked in appearance and function occur, and adaptation to and acceptance of these changes can be difficult and may require professional guidance and assistance. Children at the toddler and preschool stages of development exert their energies toward autonomy and initiative in mastering locomotion and self-care tasks. Parental responses that offer positive experiences related to these developmental tasks need to be encouraged. Adolescents experience rapid growth and changes associated with puberty; they can find it difficult to cope with the imbalance and conflicts in self-perception and the need for peer approval. Anxieties and fears related to changes in body image need to be considered when working with adolescents. Similarly, patients in their senior years may require assistance in making necessary adjustments to changes in body image.[7,9]

Certain life events or illnesses may cause drastic or abrupt changes in body image. Examples are accidents with severe trauma, loss of limbs, loss of hair, mutilation or physical abuse, and skin diseases. In these situations an acute disturbance in body image can be assumed, and planned nursing interventions will complement the medical/surgical treatment and assist the patient in making necessary adjustments that promote an experience of self-worth and self-acceptance.[12]

Mental illness can influence the perception of one's body image and the care given in presenting an acceptable appearance to others. For example, in bipolar disorders grooming can be exaggerated. In the extreme situation, the patient may make little effort to present an acceptable appearance, as often is seen in depressed mental states. In such situations behaviors related to body image can guide treatment approaches and result in desired changes.

Patients may come from a cultural background in which norms for body appearance or behaviors differ markedly from those generally held in the

North American culture. For example, in Nigeria women strive to be obese because a corpulent appearance is valued and brings social rewards; whereas in North America obesity, especially in women, can have a negative social value.

Handicaps that affect appearance and make a person different from the acceptable norm of wholeness and perfection can place considerable stress on self-perception and on the formation of a realistic body image. For example, the person with cerebral palsy lacks motor coordination. The person's grimaces and "odd" posture, gait, and speech often cause negative social responses, such as ridicule and stigmatization. The person can form a negative body image that can become the root for other problems, such as social isolation, depression, or violence.

ASSESSMENT

Assessment of physical appearance and body image should be a component of any biopsychological assessment of the patient. The assessment can provide information about the congruence between the patient's mental image and reality.

Any patient who has experienced an illness (e.g., weight loss, edema, or skin rashes) or is experiencing functional losses (e.g., immobility or limitations in self-care) will need to adjust to these alterations.[11] Assessment needs to focus on the patient's abilities or difficulties in making a positive adjustment. Is the patient aware of the change? Does the patient express preoccupation or distress? Does the person have the necessary knowledge to understand the change? Has the patient encountered similar changes before this experience, and how did the patient cope with these? Does the change in appearance or function have special meaning to this person?

In severe trauma, disfigurement or loss of a body part through surgical amputation, as may occur in a burn accident or in the treatment of cancer, changes are often abrupt, with long-term implications for alteration in appearance and function.[11] Adjustments in body image must take place, and ongoing assessment is necessary to determine progress or disturbances in perceptions of what is altered and the meaning of the alteration. Observations and associated exploration of feelings and perceptions are assessment strategies. For example: "Mr. T., I noticed you keep your eyes shut when I do the dressing. Is it that you find it difficult to look at your stump?"

Disturbances in body image may occur during the various phases of growth and development. Transitional phases in which changes in body structure and function take place may present adjustment challenges or difficulties. In early childhood, parenting influences on the development of body image need ongoing assessment. How parents respond to the child's exertion of autonomy or initiative, how they accept or reject the child's appearance and respect the child's capacity to function, or how they praise or scold behavior may indicate positive or negative factors affecting how the child learns to see him- or herself.

The nurse may observe parental responses and interactions with the child during visits to clinics, during hospitalizations, or during health counseling sessions. Observations of the child may show timidity or lack of initiative in social situations. Such behaviors can reflect insecurities related to fears of rejection. Problems adjusting to school as reported by parents or teachers may also indicate experiences of ridicule or rejection by peers, making the child feel unliked and not acceptable to others, thus contributing to a negative self-perception. Questioning the child in the following simple way will aid assessment: "How do you like school? How do you like the other boys and girls? Do you think they like you? Is there something special about you they like? Dislike? Tell me about it—what happened?"

Adolescence requires special attention in assessment of possible difficulties in adjusting to the rapid growth changes, to the appearance of secondary sex characteristics, and to the expectations of peers and adults. Observations should focus on how individuals fit general expectations or norms for height, weight, or features of masculinity or femininity. The young boy or girl who differs widely from expected norms for the age

VII

group may avoid social contacts and peer-related activities such as games and sports. The nurse must determine whether such avoidance is based on the perceived difference in body size and associated social value.

Nutritional assessment can reveal fads related to idealized thinness or overeating resulting in obesity. The nurse can explore eating habits, the frequency and nutritional value of meals, and associated attitudes, especially as these relate to actual or desired changes in body image during adolescence. School health-counseling sessions or visits to clinics provide opportunities for assessment.

During the adult years, pregnancy may cause some women to experience difficulties accepting the changes in body size.[9] Although the changes are temporary, they are unavoidable. They may cause distress about the lost ideal thinness or create a sense of being less attractive to others. Expressions of dislike regarding weight gain and abdominal expansion, repeated concerns about looks, and the wish to avoid others may indicate a preoccupation with body image. Negative statements about these changes during prenatal visits can offer an opportunity to explore perceptions and their associated meanings for the pregnant woman.

As the senior years bring about changes in posture, function, and general appearance, adjustment to these changes need ongoing assessment. With advancing years, contacts with health services are more frequent and offer opportunities to explore whether the person is accepting and adjusting to changes in body image. Dress and makeup may show preoccupation with a youthful appearance. Seeking remedies for normal skin changes, such as wrinkles and discolorations, may indicate a lack of knowledge about normal changes or the inability to make a positive adjustment.

Congenital deformities, such as a clubfoot, cleft lip, or birth injuries resulting in cerebral palsy, present a special challenge for the development of body image. How significant others, especially the parents, respond to and learn to accept the "different" appearance or the "deficit" in function requires ongoing assessment. Can they touch the deformed body part? Are they hiding the child

from social exposure? Do they seek appropriate health counseling for their child? Do they experience prejudices about the deformity? As the child grows, does he or she show awareness of the difference, express dislike, or seek to avoid peer contact? Avoidance of the deformity may indicate difficulties in coping with self-perceptions. The use of figure drawings can aid assessment of body image and show avoidance, lack of inclusion, or oversized or undersized body parts.[17]

Mental illness can be based on distortions or fixations regarding perceptions of body image. Unrealistic perceptions of body size or appearance, expressed in feelings of being too tiny, too fat, or ugly, may indicate negative attitudes toward self. Lack of proper grooming, refusal to engage in self-care, sadness in facial expression, avoidance of social contacts, or open, repeated, negative complaints about body parts, functions, and appearance suggest a possible disturbance in body image affecting mental health. It is important to note that a disturbance in body image can result from a person's perceptions related to an actual change in body part or function or to a perceived change in image although no actual change in body function or part has occurred.

Patients who come from different parts of the world may dress or behave in ways that can cause public ridicule, name calling, or stigmatizing. Wearing head covers, such as a turban, having the face veiled, or wearing a nose ring may be seen as unusual, odd, or inappropriate. Is the patient aware of how others perceive him or her? Does the staring or name calling cause distress or avoidance of public places? Does the patient know how to help others understand his or her personal background or values to gain acceptance? Can he or she make some changes to accommodate social expectations? Assessment in this situation is directed toward finding out if the patient is experiencing difficulties being in a different cultural environment or if the patient has the necessary knowledge and coping skills to adjust and maintain positive self-perceptions.[11]

Assessment of characteristics of Body Image Disturbance is ongoing and part of every encounter with patients of all ages and in any setting in which nurses offer professional services. The nurse can use some instruments, such as "draw a person" and the "Disfigurement/Dysfunction Scale" to obtain measurements of body perceptions.[1] In most instances, however, nurses collect data as they observe and interact with their patients.

Defining Characteristics

The presence of the following defining characteristics[5,8] indicates that the patient may be experiencing Body Image Disturbance:

- Actual loss of body part or change in function
- Verbal or nonverbal indications of distress about changes in body structure or function
- Lack of acceptance of missing body part or change in function
- Failure to look at or touch body part
- Preoccupation with body change or loss
- Failure to adjust to developmental changes
- Lack of self-care
- Improper grooming
- Nutritional fads
- Grieving response
- Distorted perceptions
- Inability to look at altered body site
- Hiding or overexposing body part
- Depersonalization of altered body part
- Increased focus on past strengths, function, or appearance
- Extension of body part to include environmental objects
- Avoidance or refusal of social contact
- Perceptions of being different and unacceptable by peers
- Lack of knowledge or conflict regarding cultural or social norms
- Difficulties adjusting to cultural environment
- Changed lifestyle

Related Factors

The following related factors are associated with Body Image Disturbance:

- Obvious body changes as a result of illness, surgery, accident, or treatment
- Functional loss (especially when loss has high personal and/or social value)

- Deviations from norms of appearance
- Inability to adjust to or integrate body changes or losses
- Mental illness
- Eating disorders (e.g., bulimia nervosa)
- Body dysmorphic disorder
- Transitional life stages, developmental crises
- Age-related changes
- Changes in social values and role expectations
- Rigid ideas about appearance
- Negative perception of self
- Inadequate knowledge
- Social prejudices regarding handicapping conditions
- Negative parenting behaviors
- Lack of problem-solving skills in acculturation
- Cultural factors
- Spiritual factors

DIAGNOSIS

Differential Nursing Diagnosis

Presenting defining characteristics such as hiding an altered body part, lack of acceptance of a missing body part or a change in function, and inability to look at an altered body site need to be carefully evaluated within the context of other presenting characteristics to differentiate between the nursing diagnoses Ineffective Denial and Body Image Disturbance. Likewise, presenting characteristics such as a grieving response need to be further evaluated to distinguish between Anticipatory Grieving, Dysfunctional Grieving, or Body Image Disturbance. Other determinations that need to be made, for example, include whether to identify Self-Care Deficit as a nursing diagnosis separate from Body Image Disturbance.

Medical and Psychiatric Diagnoses

Body Image Disturbance is related to a number of medical diagnoses and conditions (e.g., alopecia, burns—especially second and third degree, cancer —especially of the head and neck, breast cancer, gastrointestinal cancer leading to colostomy, cerebral palsy, dermatitis—especially eczema, elephantiasis, multiple sclerosis, obesity, and conditions leading to paralysis, such as a stroke. Likewise,

VII

Body Image Disturbance is frequently experienced by patients with such mental illnesses as anorexia nervosa, bulimia nervosa, conduct disorder, somatoform disorders, or Tourette's disorder.

OUTCOME IDENTIFICATION, PLANNING, AND IMPLEMENTATION

The onset of Body Image Disturbance can be sudden, with drastic changes induced by losses in body structure or function, such as result from accidental amputation or trauma, or it can be more insidious, occurring over a period of time, as happens with developmental changes, altered perceptions in mental illness, or the deformities of arthritis. Overall goals will focus on alleviating or modifying the Body Image Disturbance, with an emphasis on the patient making a favorable adaptation and showing a return to or development of an integrated, realistic perception of body image. Expectations for patient outcomes are guided by a time frame that indicates a logical progression in the adaptation process.

Four successive yet interrelated phases describe the adaptation process. These are impact, retreat, acknowledgment, and reconstruction.[12] The nurse can develop patient outcomes and related nursing interventions with reference to these phases as the patient experiences them.

Development of awareness of what is altered or perceived as altered is the initial goal. With a sudden change or loss the impact can be experienced as shock, disbelief, denial, and sadness. In cases of significant losses, goals for expression of grief should precede expectations for acceptance and the learning of replacement skills.[12]

Interventions focus on assisting the patient to express perceptions and feelings. Providing privacy for the expression of sadness (having a "cry") or allowing the patient to be alone for a while will facilitate awareness and will offer the patient a sense of care and respect.

With awareness comes realization of what the change of body image implies; that is, how it might threaten social roles, job functions, future goals, or one's values and beliefs. These realizations characterize the retreat phase as the patient tries to sort through the inner turmoil of fears and anxieties. The goal is to support the patient and to help resolve fears and anxieties. Interventions will address showing acceptance of needs such as hiding, avoiding exposure or social contacts, self-care, and wishing to talk—or not talk—about experienced changes. Yet need also exists for gentle persuasion to explore the altered body site. The nurse can first give a description of what he or she sees and then set goals with the patient for when the body part will be viewed or touched.

Significant others can play a role in supporting and assisting the patient; however, they need information on what to expect and how to be helpful. They too need support and assistance to express their own thoughts and feelings.

As the patient gains an understanding, he or she begins to acknowledge changes experienced in body appearance and function. The nurse can facilitate the process of acknowledgment by reinforcing efforts the patient makes in recognizing the realities of the change, such as naming the changed aspect with use of personal pronouns (my stump, my colostomy, my paralyzed side); offering opportunities for social contacts and encouraging the patient to talk with others about the changed appearance or function; introducing information regarding available technical aids for functional losses (such as crutches, makeup, or prostheses); introducing services that can assist in gaining new skills (such as physiotherapy for crutch walking, occupational therapy for managing self-care, or enterostomal therapy in case of a colostomy). With readiness to learn, the reconstruction phase of adjustment can take place. Nursing interventions will then focus on providing information and guidance on possible resources; facilitating relearning such as self-care; learning of new skills in the use of appliances and technical aids or how to dress attractively; encouraging and supporting realistic goals for progress; offering praise and acknowledgment for accomplishments, even for small steps of progress; identifying available support groups and supporting the initiation of contacts; and involving significant others in giving support and encouragement and fostering independence.

◢ NURSING CARE GUIDELINES
Nursing Diagnosis: Body Image Disturbance

Expected Outcome: The patient will show awareness of loss or change and express grief.
- Assess perception patient has of body image.
- Assist the patient to express feelings. *If the nurse shows acceptance and encourages expression of feelings, the patient can learn to accept his or her own responses and gain support in expressing thoughts and feelings.*
- Assist patient through normal grieving.
- Communicate acceptance of expressed feeling.
- Provide privacy for expression of feelings.
- Spend time with patient to show social acceptance. *Spending time with the patient and referring to the altered body aspect by naming it (e.g., your stump, colostomy, rash, or paralyzed arm) will convey social acceptance and provide a reality focus for gradual awareness of the altered body part.*
- Refer to altered body part with proper name.

Expected Outcome: The patient will resolve fears and anxiety.
- Assist the patient to express anger, frustration, and disappointment.
- Facilitate exploration of anxiety and fears.
  Assisting the patient to express and explore feelings of anger, disappointment, and frustration will help identify underlying anxieties or misconceptions.
- Accept initial need for concealment of change.
- Provide gentle persuasion to explore altered body part; for example, encourage talking about it and viewing it.
- As necessary, assist patient to identify distortion of own body image, which is necessary before patient can accept reality and begin to cope with deficit.
- Use cognitive techniques to help change distorted body image.[2]
- Set mutual goals for progressive self-care.
- Assist patient to recognize own strengths and assets in appearance and functions. *Helping the patient to realize strengths, positive efforts, or assets in appearance and function will facilitate holistic perceptions and counterbalance fears and anxieties associated with the change in body image.*
- Help significant others to support and assist the patient.
- Provide information to significant others.

Expected Outcome: The patient will acknowledge changes.
- Facilitate and reinforce efforts the patient makes in recognizing realities. *When the patient is assisted to focus on the realities of the situation and gains a future orientation, he or she can develop readiness to invest energies and efforts toward constructive adjustments.*
- Offer opportunities for social contacts with persons who had similar experiences. *A show of acceptance by significant others can be a trustworthy social reflection on the patient's altered body image from which a positive adjustment can develop.*
- Introduce information about technical aids or replacements.
- Introduce rehabilitative services that can assist the patient; for instance, physiotherapy and enterostomal therapy.
- Teach significant others required care skills.
- Offer praise and encouragement.

Expected Outcome: The patient will express constructive integration of body image.
- Provide information and guidance on how to access and use available services.
- Facilitate learning of new skills.
- Engage in activities that augment a positive self-concept not linked to body image and appearance.[16]

■ = nursing intervention; ▲ = collaborative intervention.

Continued

VII

◢ NURSING CARE GUIDELINES — CONT'D

- Introduce the patient to support groups and facilitate initial contacts.
- Praise and acknowledge appearance and accomplishments for even small steps of progress. *Praise, support, guidance, and encouragement facilitate learning and aid acceptance and integration of changes in appearance and function into a positive perception of one's body image.*
- Encourage the patient to engage in normal social activities.
- Discuss with the patient body image perception.
- Praise constructive problem solving to enhance appearance.
- Encourage significant others in giving support and fostering independence.

EVALUATION

As the patient manifests progressive adaptation to the experienced loss or change in body function or altered appearance, he or she expresses emotions of sadness and anger and names and talks about the change in function or undesired appearance. The patient is able to express feelings of frustration and disappointment (e.g., "This looks awful. How will I ever manage my job? My wife or husband can never love me like this"). In the nurse-patient relationship the patient expresses fears and anxieties. Similarly, significant others show acceptance of fears and encourage the patient to express these. The patient sets goals for self-care and manages to look at or touch the changed body part, uses proper naming, and explores functional abilities.

The patient gradually tolerates social exposure and seeks to resume normal social activities. The patient acknowledges the help of others and can focus on assets in appearance and abilities. He or she learns and manages new skills. Significant others are supportive and refrain from overprotection or unnecessary assistance. The patient shows pride in his or her own efforts to manage new skills and in an attractive appearance. The patient can reflect on the total experience: the initial distress, fears, and anxieties about the altered body image, steps taken to adjust, and the positive and negative aspects of seeing the body in a holistic, acceptable way. Problem-solving skills are evident in knowing how to find needed resources and how to access available health services or support groups to promote and maintain a positive body image.

▶ CASE STUDY WITH PLAN OF CARE

Mrs. Susan L. is a 52-year-old widow who underwent a colon resection for a benign tumor 5 days ago, resulting in a permanent colostomy of the descending colon. Surgery and postoperative recovery were uncomplicated. Mrs. L. is now on a semiliquid diet and requires only occasional relief of pain. She has been fitted with a colostomy pouch that the nurse drains and cleans as needed at regular intervals during the day. Drainage has been moderate and of semiliquid consistency. The release of flatus has been necessary several times during the past day. Mrs. L. shows distress about the colostomy care, stating, "I wish you would go away with that tray. I never want to see you again." During appliance changes she was tearful, turning her face away and pinching her nose to avoid smelling the odor. She refused visitors, permitting only her two daughters to see her. She asked the nurse to deodorize the room before their visits. She feels discouraged and has said, "How can I live with this thing?" She led an active life before surgery, is financially independent, has her own apartment, and has lived alone since her husband's death 3 years ago. She belongs to several social clubs and has many friends. Her two daughters are married and live nearby. Before her marriage she was a fashion model and has always liked to design and sew her own clothes. She has taken great pride in her youthful appearance and in being neat and attractively dressed. She used to keep fit by watching her diet and swimming several times a week.

- ### PLAN OF CARE FOR MRS. SUSAN L.

Nursing Diagnosis: Body Image Disturbance Related to Structural and Functional Changes in Elimination Resulting from Colostomy[1-17]

Expected Outcome: Mrs. L. will show awareness of loss as evidenced by tolerating colostomy care and beginning to inspect the stoma site and appliance over the next 2 days.
- Prepare Mrs. L. for each pouch emptying and stoma care by planning mutually suitable times.
- Use proper name, "stoma care," and describe what is seen and done.
- Acknowledge the need to look away and that it takes time to gather courage to look.
- Show acceptance for the expression of grief and the need for denial.
- Plan with Mrs. L. for a time to inspect the stoma, depending on Mrs. L.'s level of awareness and readiness.
- Show Mrs. L. the equipment that is used without expecting participation.
- Show personal acceptance through attentive care and brief visits not associated with stoma care.

Expected Outcome: Mrs. L. will resolve emotions as evidenced by expression of frustration, anxieties, and fears.
- Encourage expression of feelings about the change in appearance and elimination.
- Assist by mentioning possible threats to Mrs. L.'s social life and her desire to be attractive so these can be explored.
- Offer some initial information on successful management of elimination and available appliances.
- Assist the daughters in their understanding of Mrs. L.'s initial response, stoma care, and management of elimination; stress the importance of their visiting, acceptance, and support.

Expected Outcome: Mrs. L. will acknowledge changes as evidenced by participation in stoma care before discharge from the hospital and by using proper terminology.
- Encourage proper use of terminology; for instance, *colostomy* and *stoma*.
- Encourage gradual participation in stoma care; plan with Mrs. L. daily inspection of stoma, with verbal description of what she sees.
- Offer praise for accomplishments.
- Discuss possible social contacts; encourage plans for visitors.

Expected Outcome: Mrs. L. will manifest constructive integration of body image as manifested by discussing appearance of open stoma as part of self; beginning to manage altered elimination; resuming contacts with friends during visiting hours; planning how to adjust clothing for neat appearance; demonstrating understanding of elimination, ostomy care, and odor control: accepting daughters' involvement in ostomy care; and talking positively about adjustments in lifestyle after discharge.
- Encourage verbalization of stoma appearance.
- Teach ostomy care, management of elimination, and odor control.
- Praise accomplishments.
- Facilitate and assist in discharge planning for attractive clothing and social activities.
- Introduce enterostomal therapist as available resource and support.
- Involve daughters in colostomy care if Mrs. L. agrees.
- Reinforce positive statements about body appearance and management of elimination.
- Discuss participation in recreational and exercise regimen.

■ = nursing intervention; ▲ = collaborative intervention.

VII

■ CRITICAL THINKING EXERCISES

1. What are the defining characteristics that lead to the nursing diagnosis Body Image Disturbance for Mrs. L.?

2. What information could be helpful to Mrs. L.'s daughters in terms of understanding Mrs. L.'s initial response and subsequent stoma care?

3. Identify Mrs. L.'s strengths and resources. How can these be useful to Mrs. L.?

REFERENCES

1. Dropkin MJ: Coping with disfigurement and dysfunction after head and neck cancer surgery: a conceptual framework, *Semin Oncol Nurs* 5(3):213–219, 1989.

2. Dunner DL: *Current psychiatric therapy*, Philadelphia, 1993, WB Saunders Co.

3. Foster RLR, Hunsberger MM, and Tackett-Anderson JJT: *Family-centered nursing care of children*, Philadelphia, 1989, WB Saunders Co.

4. Jourard SM: *Personal adjustment: an approach through the study of healthy personality*, ed 2, New York, 1966, Macmillan Publishing.

5. Kim MJ, McFarland GK, and McLane AM: *Pocket guide to nursing diagnoses*, ed 6, St. Louis, 1995, Mosby–Year Book.

6. Koff E and Rierdan J: Perceptions of weight and attitudes toward eating in early adolescent girls, *J Adolesc Health* 12:307–313, 1991.

7. Mason KJ: Congenital orthopedic anomalies and their impact on the family, *Nurs Clin North Am* 26(1):1–16, 1991.

8. North American Nursing Diagnosis Association: *NANDA nursing diagnoses: definitions and classification, 1995–1996*, Philadelphia, 1994, The Association.

9. Olds SB, London ML, and Warner PA: *Maternal newborn nursing: a family-centered approach*, ed 5, Menlo Park, California, 1996, Addison-Wesley.

10. Olson B, Ustanko L, and Warner S: The patient in a halo brace: striving for normalcy in body image and self-concept, *Orthop Nurs* 10(1):44–50, 1991.

11. Price B: *Body image nursing concepts and care*, New York, 1990, Prentice Hall.

12. Roberts SL: *Behavioral concepts and the critically ill patient*, ed 2, Norwalk, Connecticut, 1986, Appleton-Century-Crofts.

13. Robertson SM: Self-concept disturbance. In McFarland GK and Thomas MD: *Psychiatric mental health nursing: application of the nursing process*, Philadelphia, 1991, JB Lippincott Co.

14. Santopinto MDA: The relentless drive to be ever thinner: study using the phenomenological method, *Nurs Sci Quart* 2(1):L29–L36, 1989.

15. Stuart GW and Sundeen SJ: *Principles and practice of psychiatric nursing*, ed 4, St. Louis, 1991, Mosby–Year Book.

16. Townsend MC: *Psychiatric/mental health nursing: concepts of care*, Philadelphia, 1993, FA Davis.

17. Wong DL, Wilson D, and Whaley LF: *Whaley & Wong's nursing care of infants and children*, ed 5, St. Louis, 1995, Mosby–Year Book.

VII

Fear

Fear *is the feeling of dread related to an identifiable source that the person validates.*[6]

OVERVIEW

Fear is an uncomfortable, ominous feeling caused by conscious recognition of a source of danger. A survival mechanism, Fear is a protective emotion that mobilizes the individual for "fight or flight" to cope with a potential or actual threat.

As a normal, adaptive response to danger, Fear follows a specific sequence in human development.[10] The newborn infant is frightened by loud noises or by a sudden loss of support. The toddler at the age of 2 to 5 years—a particularly fearful period in human development—may fear ghosts, animals, the dark, or separation from significant others. These Fears are replaced in the school-age child by more realistic fears, such as Fear of bodily injury, war, and death. The adolescent is more often frightened of failure in school, rejection by peers, pain, and disease. Generally, developmental Fears are diminished by maturation and by simple measures that reassure the child, such as a night light for Fear of darkness. Elderly clients often express fears of sensory impairment, loneliness, or poverty.

ASSESSMENT

A nursing diagnosis of Fear results from subjective and objective data obtained from three areas of observation: physiological responses, behavioral manifestations, and the subjective experiences of the patient. Neuroendocrine-stress-response acti-

vation signifies the physiological signs and symptoms of Fear. The resulting "fight or flight" response is initiated when a threat is perceived in the cortex of the brain. A signal via the sympathetic branch of the autonomic nervous system stimulates the adrenal glands to release epinephrine and norepinephrine. The resulting cardiovascular excitation is characterized by increased heart rate, increased blood pressure, and the shunting of blood from the skin and gastrointestinal tract to the heart, central nervous system, and skeletal muscles. The nurse may observe pupil dilation, pallor, increased or irregular respiratory rate, and palmar sweating in the frightened patient. The patient may report insomnia, anorexia, and urinary frequency.

Behaviorally the fearful individual may "flee" by withdrawing from social interaction or "fight" with aggressive or hostile actions. The patient may direct anger toward the nurse or significant other as a convenient or safe alternative to confronting the real source of Fear. The patient may exhibit increased alertness to "it, out there," as an additional behavioral manifestation. Intellectual functioning may also be affected, resulting in impaired attention, decreased learning ability, and frightening visual images.

Subjective data include reports from the fearful individual of tension, apprehension, uncertainty of self, fear, terror, panic, or jitteriness. The patient may express a desire to "run away from it all" or "pulverize" the source of the threat.

Few valid, reliable, and useful instruments are available to measure patients' Fear in clinical settings. The Fear Survey Schedule,[3,7] which is reliable and valid, measures Fear of animals, illness, death, and interpersonal events. The Fear Thermometer[10] works by having patients indicate their level of Fear by placing a mark on a scale 1 to 10. Because this instrument is simple and efficient, it can be adapted to many clinical situations for comparison measurements over time. Most often, however, a nursing diagnosis of Fear results from the nurse's observing the defining characteristics while providing care for the patient.

A variety of related factors increase the chances for a nursing diagnosis of Fear. Natural (developmental) or innate fears occur during specific developmental stages. In addition, individuals (particularly children) may learn to fear specific stimuli when they observe this response in role models or significant others. When a mother reacts in terror to spiders, her young children will likely adopt a similar response. Hospitalized patients, who are separated from their support systems in a potentially threatening situation, develop a risk for Fear. Unfamiliarity with the hospital environment or a language barrier may compound the threat experienced by the patient. Sensory impairments, such as blindness or diminished hearing, also increase the likelihood that individuals will develop Fear, especially during hospitalization, when they must depend on unfamiliar hospital personnel for assistance in meeting basic safety needs. Although environmental stimuli may provoke a Fear response in many settings, this reaction is more likely to require nursing intervention in critical care units, where sensory overload is common, familiar support systems are present infrequently, and the threat to survival is frighteningly real. Furthermore, the neuroendocrine physiological response to Fear in patients with compromised adaptive abilities can lead to cardiac dysrhythmias, fluid and electrolyte imbalances, seizures, and other serious complications.

The nursing diagnosis Fear occurs more commonly with life-threatening illnesses; conditions requiring mechanical ventilation or other life support; situations where the patient's ability to communicate is disrupted (as with a tracheostomy or facial trauma); and in patients with sensory losses (e.g., blindness or deafness).

▪ Defining Characteristics

The presence of the following defining characteristics indicates that the patient may be experiencing Fear[9,12]:

- Sympathetic stimulation—cardiovascular excitation, superficial vasoconstriction, and pupil dilation
- Sleep disturbance
- Irritability
- Facial tension
- Terrified appearance
- Jitteriness
- Apprehension
- Increased tension
- Impulsiveness
- Increased alertness
- Wide-eyed expression
- Episodes of crying
- Focus on "it, out there"
- Fight behavior—aggression
- Flight behavior—withdrawal
- Persistent questioning
- Reassurance-seeking behaviors
- Decreased self-assurance
- Concentration on source

▪ Related Factors

The following related factors are associated with Fear[6]:

- Natural or innate origins (e.g., sudden noise, loss of physical support, heights, pain)
- Sensory impairment
- Threatening environmental stimuli
- Phobia (e.g., social phobia)
- Learned response (e.g., conditioning and modeling from or identification with others)
- Knowledge deficit or unfamiliarity
- Separation from support system in a potentially threatening situation (e.g., hospitalization, treatments)
- Language barrier

DIAGNOSIS

■ Differential Nursing Diagnosis

Several authors have addressed the need to differentiate between the nursing diagnoses Fear and Anxiety.[9,11-13] Although similar to Anxiety, Fear occurs in response to an identifiable danger or threat.[11,13] Anxiety on the other hand is a vague, diffuse uneasiness occurring in response to unidentifiable threats to the individual's essential values. They are closely related, however, because underlying every Fear is the anxiety of being unable to preserve one's own being. The presence of a Fear-Anxiety Syndrome has been suggested to reflect the interactive nature of the two diagnoses.[9,12]

■ Medical and Psychiatric Diagnoses

The psychiatric diagnosis specific phobia[1] should be differentiated from the common Fear response experienced by everyone. A phobia is a specific type of Fear that is exaggerated and often disabling.[1] It is characterized by an intense desire to avoid the feared object or situation—a situation that objectively poses little or no threat of danger. Acrophobia, or Fear of heights, is a common phobia.

OUTCOME IDENTIFICATION, PLANNING, AND IMPLEMENTATION

Expected outcomes for the diagnosis Fear include patient recognition of this response, verbalization of fearful feelings, and the development of effective coping mechanisms. The ultimate goal is resolution of the problem with decreased signs and symptoms of Fear. Once the nurse identifies a nursing diagnosis of Fear, the nurse should validate this assessment with the patient. The patient must learn to recognize and acknowledge the signs and symptoms of Fear as the "fight or flight" response to danger. At this stage, verbalization of feelings may help the patient lessen the intensity and duration of the powerful emotions accompanying Fear. The nurse should listen actively while encouraging the patient to discuss a fearful event or situation to assess the patient's ability to cope with Fear. Together with the patient, the nurse should explore the source of the Fear and evaluate the extent to which the patient's Fear is valid.

When the source of the Fear has been clearly identified, the nurse may assist the patient in avoiding the danger, decreasing the danger, or ameliorating the Fear response.[4,8] Discussing advantages and disadvantages of alternative approaches with the patient may enhance this process. Although it is often impossible to eliminate the danger, such as an uncomfortable treatment or life-threatening surgery, providing the patient with information about what to expect (particularly on a sensory level) decreases the threat.[5] Whenever possible, allowing the patient to have some form of control over the situation also helps diminish the degree of Fear.

The nurse provides emotional support for the fearful patient by remaining with him or her, explaining the situation as indicated, by touching and comforting, and by assuring the patient that Fear is a normal human response to danger. Instructing patients on health care or referring them to other health professionals or social service agencies may be indicated. The nurse should discuss with parents the appropriate age-related fears in children.[2]

In addition to adjusting the threatening situation to cope with Fear, patients can learn to manage the emotional distress that accompanies Fear. Progressive muscle relaxation exercises, visual imagery, halting the fearful thoughts, and progressive desensitization to feared objects and situations all work by ameliorating the patient's fearful response.[2] Physical exercise can serve as a healthful outlet to dissipate the tension accompanying Fear. Distress may also be alleviated by the presence of significant others and by music, religious objects, security blankets, or other sources of comfort.[8]

VII

◢ **NURSING CARE GUIDELINES**
Nursing Diagnosis: Fear

Expected Outcome: The patient will recognize and express feelings of Fear.
- Assist patient in recognizing signs and symptoms of Fear and acknowledging them as a response to a threat. *Acknowledging a problem is basic to resolving it.*

Expected Outcome: The patient will verbalize the source of the Fear, will express a realistic perception of danger and will evaluate his or her coping ability and need for assistance.
- Using therapeutic communication, encourage patient to verbalize subjective feelings, personal perception of danger, perception of own coping skills and limitations, and the need for assistance from the nursing staff. *Verbalizing feelings can lessen the intensity and duration of Fear.*
- Reduce distorted perceptions by educating patient and encouraging specifics rather than generalizations. *A realistic appraisal promotes effective problem solving to decrease danger.*
- Initiate teaching the patient as needed to decrease lack of knowledge and unfamiliarity. *Knowledge of what to expect, particularly on a sensory level, decreases Fear of the unknown.*

Expected Outcome: The patient will use coping mechanisms effectively to decrease Fear.
- Help patient identify resources and develop skills to cope with Fear, such as systematic desensitization or strategies to avoid or overcome danger. *Progressive desensitization and avoidance of fearful situations can prevent or ameliorate fearful responses.*
- Use patient's support system to increase comfort and relaxation. *Familiar sources of comfort and support can alleviate the distress that accompanies Fear.*
- ▲ Teach additional coping techniques as needed, such as progressive muscle relaxation, visual imagery, and physical exercise. *Progressive muscle relaxation and visual imagery can modify the response to Fear. Exercise can dissipate effects of "fight or flight" hormones.*

Expected Outcome: The patient will verbalize a decrease in feelings associated with Fear and display a decrease in behavioral manifestations and physiological signs of Fear.
- Continually monitor level of Fear and degree of coping *to assess the need for changes in the plan of care.*

■ = nursing intervention; ▲ = collaborative intervention.

EVALUATION

Evaluation involves measuring the progress toward the expected outcomes and the reduction in the defining characteristics of Fear. Does the patient verbalize a decrease in the physical symptoms of Fear? Display a decrease in the behavioral manifestations of Fear? Verbalize recognition of the Fear response in self? Describe the source of the threat? Does the patient effectively deal with Fear and relieve the distressing effects of Fear? Are the observable defining characteristics of Fear reduced or absent? The nurse should continue to monitor the patient's level of Fear and degree of coping by assessing the patient for changes in the subjective and objective defining characteristics of Fear. If the expected outcomes are not achieved in a reasonable period of time, the nurse should consider referring the patient for more intensive, specialized treatment of the Fear response.

■ CASE STUDY WITH PLAN OF CARE

Mr. Jerry S. is a 60-year-old bank manager with extensive coronary artery atherosclerosis. He is admitted to the coronary care unit for a cardiac catheterization and evaluation after repeated bouts of angina. Mr. S. has been generally healthy throughout his life, and his only previous hospitalization was for an appendectomy as a child. He remembers it as frightening. His knowledge of coronary artery disease is somewhat limited. Although he attempts to follow a low-fat, low-cholesterol diet, he admits he has difficulty adhering to the diet. Expressing Fear of the anticipated cardiac catheterization procedure, he describes an acquaintance whose "heart stopped and had to be restarted" during a cardiac catheterization. Mr. S. has had some difficulty sleeping since being hospitalized and often awakes in the early morning thinking about the cardiac catheterization. Mr. S. experiences chest pain almost daily, resulting from stressful situations and physical activity. He reports that his job is often stressful, and parenting is occasionally stressful. Mr. S. deals with stress by talking with his wife about his concerns or listening to classical music.

■ PLAN OF CARE FOR MR. JERRY S.

Nursing Diagnosis: Fear Related to the Separation from Support System in a Potentially Threatening Situation

Expected Outcome: Mr. S. will identify and discuss specific fears about cardiac catheterization.
- Encourage expression of feelings about cardiac catheterization.
- Explore aspects of the procedure that threaten Mr. S.
- ▲ Explain the catheterization procedure and what Mr. S. can expect—include sensory information.
- ▲ Take Mr. S. to catheterization lab the day before surgery to meet the staff and ask them questions.

Expected Outcome: Mr. S. will verbalize feelings about separation from support systems.
- Encourage expression of feelings by using active listening.
- Allow and encourage wife and family to visit whenever possible.

Expected Outcome: Mr. S. will use situational support to reduce Fear and increase comfort.
- ▲ Suggest visit by personal priest or hospital chaplain.
- Remain with Mr. S. during catheterization procedure.
- Suggest music as a diversion during hospital stay.
- Teach Mr. S. other coping techniques (e.g., muscle relaxation and visual imagery) to use during catheterization procedure and whenever necessary.

Expected Outcome: Mr. S. will verbalize and demonstrate decreased signs and symptoms of Fear.
- Monitor Fear levels and vital signs, especially cardiac rate and rhythm and chest pain, providing relief from pain if it occurs. Report and document.

■ = nursing intervention; ▲ = collaborative intervention.

■ CRITICAL THINKING EXERCISES

1. What is the difference between Anxiety and Fear?
2. What nursing intervention can reduce signs and symptoms of Fear in a fearful patient?
3. How can the nurse evaluate the effectiveness of interventions to reduce Fear?
4. How might Fear be considered beneficial?

VII

REFERENCES

1. American Psychiatric Association: *Diagnostic and statistical manual of mental disorders,* DSM-IV, ed 4, Washington, D.C., 1994, The Association.
2. Carpenito LJ: *Nursing diagnosis: application to clinical practice,* ed 6, Philadelphia, 1995, JB Lippincott Co.
3. Geer JH: The development of a scale to measure fear, *Behav Res Ther* 3:45, 1965.
4. Grainger RD: Conquering fears and phobias, *Am J Nurs* 91(5):15, 1991.
5. Hartfield MT, Cason CL, and Cason GJ: Effects of information about a threatening procedure on patient's expectations and emotional distress, *Nurs Res* 31(4):202, 1982.
6. Kim MJ, McFarland GK, and McLane AM: *Pocket guide to nursing diagnoses,* ed 6, St. Louis, 1995, Mosby–Year Book.
7. Klieger DM: The non-standardization of the Fear Survey Schedule, *J Behav Ther Exp Psychiatr* 23(2):81, 1992.
8. McFarland GK and Mock VL: Fear. In Kim MJ, McFarland GK, and McLane AM: *Pocket guide to nursing diagnoses,* ed 6, St. Louis, 1995, Mosby–Year Book.
9. Taylor-Loughran AE and others: Defining characteristics of the nursing diagnoses *fear* and *anxiety*: a validation study, *Appl Nurs Res* 2(4):178, 1989.
10. Whaley LF and Wong DL: *Nursing care of infants and children,* ed 5, St. Louis, 1995, Mosby–Year Book.
11. Whitley GG: Concept analysis of fear, *Nurs Diag* 3(4):155, 1992.
12. Whitley GG: Expert validation and differentiation of the nursing diagnoses, *fear* and *anxiety, Nurs Diagnosis* 5(4):143, 1994.
13. Yocum, CJ: The differentiation of fear and anxiety. In Kim MJ, McFarland GK, and McLane AM, editors: *Classification of nursing diagnoses: proceedings of the Fifth National Conference,* St. Louis, 1984, The CV Mosby Co.

VII

Hopelessness

▶

Hopelessness *is a subjective state in which a patient sees limited or no alternatives or personal choices available and is unable to mobilize energy on his or her own behalf.*[34]

OVERVIEW

Hopelessness, defined as a profound sense of the impossible, has been identified as a cardinal symptom of depression and a precursor to suicide.[13] Researchers have noted associations between Hopelessness and unresolved losses, feelings of helplessness, physical frailty, and an increased incidence of physical illness, particularly cancer.[11,18] Recent studies suggest that hope and Hopelessness may affect immune system function[49]; high levels of hope may promote wound healing.[31] Although Hopelessness and depression are positively correlated, Hopelessness more strongly predicts suicidal intent and eventual suicide.[4,15,22,46] Research supports that counteracting Hopelessness is critical in alleviating painful despair, mobilizing psychic energy needed for healing, creating an expectation for enjoying a positive future, and preventing self-invitation to physical decline and death.[51] The presence of Hopelessness on a long-term basis threatens a patient's physical, psychological, and spiritual health and quality of life.[13] Nurses, in their strategic positions, are charged with fostering or nurturing the development or preservation of hope.[13]

Nurse researchers have completed a number of studies of hope and Hopelessness involving children and adolescents,[30,48] older adults,[16,27,38] critically ill adults,[35,39] chronically ill adults,[45] mentally ill older adults,[36] terminally ill adults,[23,24] and family caregivers of the terminally and critically ill.[26,40] Findings suggest that Hopelessness is a feeling of despair and discouragement (the affective component), a thought process that expects nothing from self or others (the cognitive component), and a way of acting in which the patient attempts little or takes inappropriate action (the behavioral component).[13] Hopelessness signals that one's needs or goals have not been met or that life or one's situation has become difficult or unbearable.[13]

Hopelessness may operate as a disposition (an ingrained individual trait) or state (a temporary condition).[48] Dispositional Hopelessness remains consistent and less malleable in response to changes over time and life events. Contrary to this dispositional perspective, state Hopelessness refers to the thoughts that the patient experiences at a particular time and in a given situation; moreover, such a state may change over time or life events.[48] Hopes can be fluid, transient, or intermittent. Serious illness or loss or multiplicity of losses can severely test hope and may lead to Hopelessness. Hope and Hopelessness are not mutually exclusive; hope is not the complete absence of Hopelessness.[35] Recent work by Ersek[12] exploring the process of maintaining hope in adults undergoing bone marrow transplantation for leukemia supports that a delicate interplay exists between dealing with the potential for Hopelessness and keeping hope in place and that this interplay enables the patient to maintain hope while still acknowledging the potential for Hopelessness.[12]

Theoretically hope and Hopelessness share four central attributes—experiential, spiritual/transcendent, rational, and relational processes.[14] The experiential process addresses how one accepts "trial, captivity, and suffering" as integral parts of self. Experts notes that it is not so much the experience itself that determines whether patients become hopeful or hopeless but the number of difficult life events, the ability to interpret and process these difficult life experiences, personal values, and internal and external resources.[13] It is the multiple intrapersonal, interpersonal, and environmental/sociological experiences and current situational determinants that lead one to hope or Hopelessness. Situational determinants of hope and Hopelessness, particularly in health care settings, are further determined by the patient's life stage; the symptoms, stage, and duration of illness; and the particular treatment setting.[27] Patients who are hopeless cannot imagine the possibility of help outside themselves, whether afforded through some form of deity, inner transcendence, or relationships with others (transcendent process). Patients experiencing Hopelessness have an inability to trust others or difficulty imagining that others can provide any gratification or support, or they experience the absence of others who can love and support them (relational process). It is in the rational thinking process, however, that Hopelessness is most distinguishable from hope. Patients experiencing Hopelessness generally have difficulty in one of three areas: (1) articulating their desires and thinking about goals for themselves or their future; (2) setting goals that aren't rigid, inflexible, unattainable, or unrealistic; or (3) possessing available internal or external resources to meet their realistic goals.[13]

In Hopelessness the continuity between one's past, present, and future is generally disrupted.[13] Hopelessness may occur when patients do not have the cognitive, affective, and behavioral internal resources or strengths necessary to hope. In Hopelessness the individual's motivational system is generally inhibited in some way. Rotter's[47] work on internal and external locus of control provides a framework for further examining the role of control as it relates to Hopelessness. Internal control suggests that patients perceive events as contin-

gent on their own behavior. A high or low sense of internal control can be a component of Hopelessness. Often patients who feel hopelessness have a low sense of personal control. In other situations, however, patients have a high but unrealistic sense of personal control.[47] External control suggests that patients perceive events as contingent on factors outside of themselves. A patient with high external control may unrealistically anticipate that help from others or the external environment will resolve the dilemma, thus assuming little, if any, personal control. On the other hand, patients who are hopeless may have a low sense of external control because others have so frequently failed or frustrated them.[47]

Patients with serious chronic illnesses frequently experience Hopelessness. It is estimated that 70% of suicide victims suffer from one or more active, mostly chronic, illnesses at the time of death.[32] The vulnerability to Hopelessness in individuals with chronic illness can be directly proportionate to the severity of their losses. Losing health status, control of bodily functions or body parts, self-esteem, attractiveness, social relationships, independence, finances, and significant roles in the family and the work setting can all cause grief in the chronically ill patient that, if not resolved, can lead to Hopelessness.[41]

The elderly may be predisposed or even developmentally vulnerable to Hopelessness.[5,16,38] Aging is generally accompanied by psychosocial and physiological changes, and frequently those changes involve losses. Physiological losses include diminished visual acuity, impaired hearing, a marked decrease in the sense of taste, loss or graying of hair, reduction in muscle mass, and significant skeletal changes. Energy generally diminishes, and efficiency and speed of task completion may be compromised.[5] Social roles may be dramatically revised as former caretakers become cared for by their children, as financial resources shrink, and as peers die. These losses and changes may result in feelings of powerlessness that, if not contained, may become a self-destructive cycle leading to depression and Hopelessness that could hasten death.[38,41] The nurse should be aware of the population at risk for the development of Hopelessness, as well as the nature of their feeling state and etiological factors.

Hope is essential for families of critically and terminally ill patients to facilitate coping and adjustment. Recent findings support the importance of hope in family caregivers and suggest that hope within others, particularly close family members, may have a reciprocal (interdependent) role in maintaining the ill family member's hope.[26,39,40] Conversely, Hopelessness of the patient or the family affects the other in the relationship.

Children and adolescents are particularly vulnerable to Hopelessness. Early childhood experiences influence a person's ability to hope.[48] Hopeful thinking is typically established by toddlerhood and reinforced throughout the subsequent years of childhood. A person learns to hope if a trusting environment is promoted. Hopes in children are often unrealistic and fragile but become more realistic as the child matures. The loss of trust in significant others, abandonment by caregivers, loss of bodily functions, or inability to achieve developmental tasks may make the child or adolescent more prone to Hopelessness. To achieve adulthood, an adolescent must first achieve hopefulness. Hinds and Martin[30] identified that adolescent hopefulness differs from adult hopefulness in that adolescents experience a wider range or greater intensity of hopefulness. Adolescents believe in the value of forced effort; that is, identifying an area of hope and fostering it. Forming an attachment, providing consistent boundaries, and modeling are common processes that adult caregivers need to provide to children and adolescents to bolster hopeful thinking.

There has been little research focused on understanding hope from the viewpoint of people from other cultures, people living in extreme poverty, or people who are homeless. The minimal data set that is available suggests that hope is influenced by its cultural interpretation.[13] For those cultures that are not future oriented, Hopelessness may not be relevant. Hopelessness focuses on an inability to achieve goals, which is future oriented. Averill[2] found that Koreans conceived of hope as controllable, voluntary, intellectual, and a permanent part of one's personality. In contrast, Americans linked hope to faith, a reliance on God's will and individual effort, with hope being more of a transitory emotional state influenced by the situation. In the American Indian culture the reaction to stressful conditions involves merely waiting out the circumstances; importance is placed on "living with the environment," with a natural expectation that the environment will eventually offer a solution.[43] In this situation, the passivity is not Hopelessness but hopefulness. Similarly, Asians have a fatalistic belief system, which leads them to accept events as predetermined.[43] These individuals believe they have little control over their lives and accept what is given to them in life. Nurses must be aware of and sensitive to the various cultural orientations to hope, and then plan appropriately.

Hope involves a delicate balance of experiencing the pain of difficult life experiences, sensing an interconnectedness with others, drawing upon one's spiritual or transcendent nature, and maintaining a rational or mindful approach for responding to these life events.[13] Many health care professionals believe that hope is capable of influencing physical, psychological, and spiritual health, and the patient's ability to hope facilitate healing. Hope-inspiring strategies and threats to hope have been identified in critically ill,[35,39] chronically ill,[45] and terminally ill[23,24] persons. Hope emerges from many different sources, including a patient's faith, relationships with others, feeling of being needed, and sense that he or she has a task to accomplish.[41,43,50,51] Threats to hope include overwhelming fatigue, isolation, concurrent losses, and poorly controlled symptom management. The nurse must assess each patient's hope sources and actual or potential threats so that hope-inspiring strategies can be planned.

Dufault and Martocchio[9] describe hope as a multidimensional, dynamic force of life characterized by a confident yet uncertain expectation of achieving a future good that, to the hoping person, is realistically possible and personally significant. Hope is conceptualized as consisting of two spheres with six dimensions. The first sphere—generalized

VII

hope—has a broad scope and includes a sense of a future beneficial (but presently indeterminate) development and is characterized by the belief that things will somehow work out. Generalized hope provides a person deprived of a second sphere (particularized hope) with protection against despair and the ability to continue with life's demands. Particularized hope is the expectation that the present can be improved, what is missing can be attained, desired circumstances will occur, and unfavorable outcomes will not happen. This sphere of hope provides incentive for coping with life's obstacles.[9]

ASSESSMENT

Assessment of hope and Hopelessness in the clinical population is extremely complex and needs to take place within a guiding framework. Two frameworks that are particularly useful are those of Dufault and Martocchio's[9] six dimensions of hope (affective, cognitive, behavioral, affiliative, temporal, and contextual) and Farran, Wilken, and Popovich's[14] four central attributes of hope and Hopelessness (experiential, relational, spiritual/transcendent, and rational thought processes). Hopelessness is a subjective emotional state that must be validated by the nurse with the individual. It is essential that the clinician determine the patient's general level of hope or Hopelessness and whether the patient's present health is challenging his or her hope structures (experiential process).[13] Emotional and cognitive areas must be assessed carefully by the nurse to make the inference that the patient is experiencing Hopelessness. The nurse should gather data about the patient's knowledge of his or her medical condition and prognosis; the effect of the disorder on self-care capacity; mental status, particularly mood and cognitive ability; availability of support systems; past experience with illness; frequently employed coping mechanisms; and any history of psychiatric illness.[10,44,51] Health care professionals may have difficulty acknowledging that suicidal intent is present. The nurse must be aware of his or her own feelings about suicide to develop an effective

helping relationship and plan nursing interventions. Gathering of subjective data includes assessing for defining characteristics (activities of daily living, energy and motivation, meaning and purpose in life, choice or control in situations, and future options) and for related factors, including presence of illness or treatment (chronic, prolonged, deteriorating, or exhausting) and significant relationships.[6] It is important to determine the patient's connectedness with other persons, a spiritual being, nature, pets, and the inner self (relational process).[13] Assessment must be made of the patient's sources of hope, availability of a support system, and perceived meaning and purpose in life (spiritual/transcendent process).[13] Assessment of goals needs to include an identification of the patient's goals, if present, their specificity, the probability of their attainment, their flexibility, and whether they are reality based, as well as the availability and adequacy of internal and external resources (rational thought process).[13] Objective data include assessing for defining characteristics of general appearance (grooming, posture, and eye contact) and level of activity.[6]

Another source of data includes observation of the patient's behavior and thematic analysis of his or her comments and described indicators of hopelessness: (1) hypoactivation—the patient reports feelings of emptiness or has difficulty identifying feelings; (2) general psychological discomfort—a sense of loss, deprivation, tension, irritability, and feeling of constriction in the throat; (3) social withdrawal—emotional distance; (4) a sense of incompetence—expressions of vulnerability, helplessness, or inability to accomplish anything or feeling overwhelmed by life.[41] To analyze conversations with the patient, screen for words and themes that indicate despair. Gottschalk[20] developed a system for content analysis in which the following themes represent Hopelessness: (1) not receiving good fortune, luck, or God's favor, (2) not receiving help, sustenance, or esteem from others or self, (3) pessimism, (4) discouragement from self and others, and (5) lack of ambition or interest. Other indicators include (1) feeling at the end of one's rope or at an impasse; (2) losing gratification from roles and relationships; (3) sensing disrupted continuity between the past, the present, and the future; and (4) recalling former incidents of helplessness.[7,8]

Survey instruments designed specifically to measure hope or Hopelessness offer potentially more precise measurements of hope and Hopelessness. There are currently eleven survey instruments with which to measure hope; three have been translated collectively into four languages (Spanish, Thai, Swedish, and Chinese).[13] Only the Herth Hope Index has been specifically designed for use by clinicians in the clinical setting.[25] This abbreviated scale (12 items) is designed specifically to address the factors of fatigue and decreased attention span that are frequently present in ill individuals. Miller[39,40] suggests using a one-item rating scale to screen quickly an individual's feelings of hopefulness. Several other hope and Hopelessness scales have been found reliable and valid in the measurement of hope with specific populations, but their length may inhibit their usefulness in measuring hope and Hopelessness in the clinical populations. Ten of the eleven survey instruments are designed to measure hope in the adult population. The only instrument designed specifically to measure hope in the adolescent is the Hopefulness Scale for Adolescents—a 24-item visual analogue scale designed to measure the degree of positive future orientation an adolescent feels at the time of measurement.[29]

There are currently three tools designed specifically to measure Hopelessness: the Beck Hopelessness Scale,[3] the Hopelessness Scale for Children,[33] and the Geriatric Hopelessness Scale.[17] The Beck Hopelessness Scale[3] is a brief (20-item) self-report index of the negative expectations that adults hold toward the present or the future. The Hopelessness Scale for Children,[33] patterned after the Beck Hopelessness Scale, is a 17-item self-report scale, for use with children 7 years of age or older. The Geriatric Hopelessness Scale is a 30-item self-report scale that is based on the premise that elderly patients often perceive some pessimism and futility in projecting themselves into the future.[17]

It is important to remember that hope and Hopelessness are complex and multidimensional, so that exploration should not stop with one observation, one survey, or one interview, especially if the data are unclear or conflicting or if life events are changing. A combination of methods is the most effective strategy to measure hope or Hopelessness for many patients. Observation must always be an ongoing process. The clinician may need to reevaluate the reliability and validity of the methods chosen in relationship to the patient's age, mental abilities, attention span, and cultural beliefs and values.[13] Measurement over time is necessary, particularly for the adolescent, whose hopes are in a constant state of change. Clinical assessment of hope and potential Hopelessness should be done upon initial contact with each patient and family, with ongoing assessments at periodic intervals. The timing of the reassessment may be fixed (i.e., weekly or monthly) or flexible, based on observed changes in the patient's physical, emotional, or spiritual state or in relation to change in experiences or life events. Further collaboration with the family or significant others may be particularly important to gain a greater understanding of the patient's hope(s).

■ Defining Characteristics

The presence of the following defining characteristics indicates that the patient may be experiencing Hopelessness[34]:

Major (must be present)
- Slowed response to stimuli
- Passivity
- Decreased affect
- Decreased vocalization
- Verbal cues (indicating despondency, "I can't," or sighing)

Minor (may be present)
- Decreased appetite
- Increased or decreased sleep
- Weight loss
- Lack of initiative
- Lack of involvement in care
- Closing eyes

VII

- Decreased problem-solving and decision-making capabilities
- Turning away from speaker
- Shrugging in response to speaker
- Conveying negative or slowed thought processes
- Decreased ability to recall events from the past
- Suicidal thoughts

■ Related Factors

The following related factors are associated with Hopelessness[34]:

- Failing or deteriorating physiological condition
- Prolonged treatment that causes discomfort, disfiguration, or has no positive results
- Prolonged activity restriction, creating isolation
- Long-term physiological or psychological stress
- Abandonment of or separation from significant others, or isolation
- Loss of belief in transcendent values or God

DIAGNOSIS

■ Differential Nursing Diagnosis

Major competing diagnoses include Powerlessness, Ineffective Coping, and Reactive Situational Depression. Carpenito[6] differentiates Hopelessness from Powerlessness in that a hopeless person sees no solution to the problem or way to achieve what is desired, even if he or she has control of his or her life. A powerless person may see an alternative or answer to the problem yet be unable to do anything about it because of perceived lack of control and resources. Ineffective coping is the state in which an individual experiences or is at risk of experiencing an inability to manage an internal or external stressor effectively because of inadequate resources.[34] A hopeless person can see no solution or even act when the resources are adequate.[13] Gordon[19] differentiates Reactive Situational Depression from Hopelessness. Reactive Situational Depression involves "feelings of sadness, despair, or dejection regarding a particular situation. . . ." The condition is usually transitory and responds to nursing interventions. Hopelessness, in contrast, involves "an all-pervading sense of no hope, choices, or alternatives."[13]

■ Medical and Psychiatric Diagnoses

Hopelessness has been associated with suicidal behaviors in depression, bipolar disorder, alcoholism, schizophrenia, and panic disorder[1,6,7] and also with many different medical diagnoses, including AIDS, Alzheimer's disease, burns, carcinomas, end-stage renal disease, stroke, and spinal cord injuries with paralysis.[6] It is imperative that the nurse carefully assess each patient for behaviors reflecting defining characteristics and related factors of the nursing diagnosis in these specific medical or psychiatric disorders and in other health conditions.

OUTCOME IDENTIFICATION, PLANNING, AND IMPLEMENTATION

The role of nurses in engendering hope in their patients is well documented in the literature.[13,18,21,42] The Iowa Nursing Classification System Project was the first attempt to classify potential nursing interventions designed to promote instillation of hope; use and perceived effectiveness of the activities have yet to be validated.[37] A recent study evaluated the use and effectiveness of hope interventions in the home care setting from the perspective of the nurse.[28] The top five interventions identified by the home health care nurse and the hospice nurse were reflective of the four attributes of hope and were consistent with hope-enhancing strategies identified in qualitative studies with critically ill, chronically ill, and terminally ill elderly individuals.

The six dimensions of hope described by Dufault and Martocchio[9] provide a framework for planning nursing strategies. Interventions in the affective dimension include encouraging patients to express feelings and concerns about their health and the future and conveying empathy when the patient expresses fears, doubts, and worries. In the cognitive dimension, interventions can be used to assist the patient in clarifying or modifying reality perceptions. In the behavioral dimension, the nursing interventions focus on enabling the patient to take action, to recognize and use resources, and to accept support when necessary.

The affiliative dimension allows the nurse to plan strategies regarding the patient's sense and manner of relatedness to others. The nurse can help the patient explore ways of maintaining or strengthening relationships with others. In the temporal dimension, the patient and the nurse can review past achievements and develop correlations between past, present, and future goals. In the final dimension of hope, the contextual dimension, nursing interventions can focus on creating an environment that will provide opportunities for exploration and communication of desired goals, readjustment of plans, and reflection on the meaning of life and death.[9]

A variety of nursing interventions and strategies can be implemented by the nurse to achieve the expected outcome of decreased Hopelessness and increased hopefulness.[13] The success of the nursing intervention strategies can be measured by the patient's ability to make decisions, to participate actively in his or her own care, and to express an expectation of enjoying a positive tomorrow.

Providing self-care assistance when indicated, encouraging the patient's curiosity and interest in self-care, teaching to increase knowledge and competence, and creating or modifying the environment to facilitate active patient participation support attainment of the expected outcome of self-care maintenance. The nurse who provides empathic listening, conveys an understanding of the patient's affect, explores reality perceptions, assists the patient to capitalize on achievements, and helps the patient to develop and modify as needed short- and long-term goals facilitates reaching the expected outcome of identification

and expression of feelings, concerns, and goals for him- or herself and enhances the potential for overcoming despair.

Providing physical and emotional comfort and supporting internal resources (courage, endurance, and patience), combined with asking about and observing for intent to commit suicide are essential to achieving the expected outcome of eliminating suicidal intent. Hackett and Stern[22] indicate that asking about suicidal thoughts, ideas, wishes, motives, intent, and plans will not plant the intent; in fact, most patients are grateful to discuss the issue. Collaborating with mental health experts is essential in working with the suicidal patient.

Hope is interdependent; therefore strategies that involve the family and the patient will lead toward the expected outcome of maintaining a positive relationship with significant others. Colt[7] stresses that significant others can provide a source of physical and emotional assistance to the patient engaged in overcoming feelings of Hopelessness and should not be afraid to show the patient that they care. The nurse can teach the family their role in sustaining hope and provide needed supportive counseling for family members. The patient may need to be taught by the nurse ways to foster, maintain, and strengthen relationships with others.

The nurse's continuing support of the patient's use of effective coping mechanisms, facilitating opportunities for reminiscing and renewing values, and teaching the patient life awareness activities, mental imaging, and cognitive reframing techniques facilitate the patient's attainment of the expected outcome of integrating the therapeutic regimen into his or her lifestyle.

VII

◢ **NURSING CARE GUIDELINES**
Nursing Diagnosis: Hopelessness

Expected Outcome: The patient will maintain adequate self-care within 1 week.
▲ Create or modify the environment to facilitate the patient's active participation in self-care.
■ Give positive feedback for successful attempt at self-care.
■ Encourage the patient's curiosity and interest in the different aspects of care.
▲ Provide teaching and support when indicated.
▲ Schedule and plan with the patient to increase his or her involvement in decision making, and allow for adequate rest.
■ Demonstrate confidence and technical competence in equipment usage.
Mastery over self-care needs inspires confidence in one's personal capacity for coping.

Expected Outcome: The patient will identify and express feelings, concerns, and goals for self within 1 week.
▲ Identify reasons for living.[44]
▲ Provide opportunities for the patient to express feelings about self and illness.
■ Facilitate expression of feelings by using active listening, asking open-ended questions, and reflecting on the patient's answers.
■ Provide opportunities for patient to express positive emotions (e.g., hope, faith, the will to live, and a sense of purpose).
■ Assist the patient to understand that he or she can deal with the hopeless aspects of life by separating the hopeless aspects from the hopeful aspects.
■ Acknowledge and accept the patient's angry feelings as a manifestation of distress.
■ Explore reality perceptions with patient and clarify or modify them if necessary by providing information and correcting misinformation.
■ Convey an empathic understanding of the patient's fears, worries, and family concerns.
■ Assist patient to recognize and capitalize on achievements and derive meaning from past success and failures.
■ Assist patient to recognize that Hopelessness is a part of everyone's life and demands recognition. It can be used as a source of energy, imagination, and freedom, which encourages a patient to consider alternative choices.[6]
■ Clarify the patient's values to determine what is important.[44]
▲ Give the patient permission to return to former healthy sources of comfort (e.g., gardening or music).
■ Assist patient to develop realistic short-term and long-term goals, progressing from simple to more complex ones; maybe use "bench markers" to indicate time frame for achieving small steps toward reaching the goals.
■ Guide and support the patient to reset, modify, redefine, or refocus goals when appropriate.
Verbalization of feelings, concerns, and goals allows for validation and catharsis, promotes the establishment of trusting relationships with caregivers, and provides an opportunity to enhance self-worth.

Expected Outcome: The patient will demonstrate absence of suicidal intent within 1 week.
▲ Provide physical and emotional comfort.
▲ Observe for signs of suicidal intent (e.g., sudden change in mood behavior, conversation about death, or expressing the futility of life).
■ Assist the patient and family in valuing strengths such as courage, endurance, and patience.
Observation for and assessment of self-harm potential are legitimate nursing roles in providing protection for patients and relief from distress.

■ = nursing intervention; ▲ = collaborative intervention.

VII

Expected Outcome: The patient will maintain positive relationships with significant others within 3 weeks.
- Promote attachment ideation by active discussion of significant relationships.
- ▲ Encourage having someone or something to care about (e.g., pets, family members, or hobbies).
- ▲ Explore with patient ways to foster, maintain, and strengthen relationships with others.
- Encourage closeness and reaching out to others for support.
- Provide privacy for family visits so that intimacy needs can be met.
- Teach the family their role in sustaining hope through a supportive, positive relationship.[27,44]
- ▲ Provide supportive counseling for family members if indicated so that they in turn convey support to the patient.
- Help patient to accept assistance from others, if needed.
The promotion of a psychosocial support system is a valid role for the nurse in enhancing the patient's coping capabilities.

Expected Outcome: The patient will integrate the therapeutic regimen into his or her lifestyle within 3 weeks.
- Review with the patient that he or she is loved, cared for, and important to others.
- Support the patient's use of effective coping mechanisms.
- Maximize esthetic experiences.
- Teach the patient to anticipate experiences he or she can delight in each day (e.g., reading a favorite book, writing letters, or taking a walk).
- Implement life awareness activities to help patient find own meanings in the situation.
- Teach, encourage, and support use of cognitive reframing: posting positive notes, positive self-talks, envisioning hopeful images.
- Encourage mental imaging to promote positive thought processes.
- ▲ Provide opportunities for reminiscing, renewing values, and reflecting on the meaning of life and death.
- ▲ Encourage creative expression of hope through taking or sharing photographs or pictures of hope.
- ▲ Assist patient in renewing his or her spiritual self and belief in transcendent values.
- Create an environment in which patient feels free to express spiritual beliefs.
- Foster lightheartedness and the sharing of uplifting memories.[24]
- ▲ Encourage energizing strategies (e.g., listening to music or reliving favorite activities).[27]
- ▲ Assist the patient and family to identify, assess, select, mobilize, and access external resources within the community, both human (i.e., social support network and support groups) and material (i.e., inspirational books, images, and sounds of hope).
Ultimately the goals of nursing care are to enable the patient to adapt and adjust to lifestyle changes, if necessitated by the presence of illness.

VII

EVALUATION

The success of nursing interventions to inspire hope and alleviate despondency may be apparent or subtle. Patient compliance with the therapeutic regimen and mastery of self-care demands can be readily observed by the nurse or obtained by interviewing significant others. Interviewing the patient will elicit his or her experience of the illness and capacity to employ coping mechanisms. The patient's expression of hope for the future, acceptance of the health situation, and capacity to put the situation into perspective will also validate the nursing interventions. If a successful outcome is not achieved, the nurse should consider making a referral for mental health–counseling services.

▶ CASE STUDY WITH PLAN OF CARE

Mr. Dodd A. is a 74-year-old recently diagnosed with early cancer of the prostate. Mr. A.'s wife died approximately 1 year ago, and he lives alone, although his daughters live near him and visit regularly. Before the death of his wife, Mr. A. had been active in several community organizations but jokes that he "goes to more funerals than meetings" these days. He has lost interest in his favorite activities, reading and completing cross-word puzzles, and has difficulty sleeping at night. He is receiving outpatient radiation therapy and complains of extreme fatigue and loss of appetite. He has missed several morning radiation therapy appointments and relates this to his lack of energy and having to drive 25 miles. He states that he does not believe treatment will help and that soon he will join his wife.

▶ PLAN OF CARE FOR MR. DODD A.

Nursing Diagnosis: Hopelessness Related to Prostate Cancer and the Demands of the Therapeutic Regimen

---

Expected Outcome: Mr. A. will verbalize feelings about the cancer diagnosis and its effect on his life.
- ▲ Encourage expression of feelings about the diagnosis and its effect on Mr. A.'s lifestyle.
- ▪ Explore fears related to mortality.
- ▲ Provide information on treatment outcomes, emphasizing success rate in early stage of cancer.

Expected Outcome: Mr. A. will reestablish an effective sleep-rest pattern and eating pattern.
- ▪ Suggest morning and afternoon nap times to promote adequate rest.
- ▪ Encourage frequent small meals.
- ▲ Suggest daughters bring him food that he particularly enjoys.

Expected Outcome: Mr. A. will comply with therapeutic regimen by receiving radiation therapy as scheduled.
- ▲ Plan an afternoon schedule for radiation therapy appointments.
- ▲ Encourage Mr. A. to contact his children or friends for assistance with transportation.

Expected Outcome: Mr. A. will identify reasons for living and express positive emotions.
- ▲ Implement life awareness activities to help Mr. A. find his own meaning in the situation.
- ▪ Assist Mr. A. to anticipate experiences he can delight in each day (e.g., reading favorite book and working crossword puzzles).
- ▪ Explore with Mr. A. what hope means to him and what strategies he has used in the past to maintain his hopes.
- ▲ Teach and support Mr. A. in the use of envisioning hopeful images.
- ▲ Encourage sharing of uplifting moments with his daughters.
- ▪ Provide opportunities for reflecting on the meaning of life and death.
- ▪ Help Mr. A. identify the significant role he continues to play in his daughters' lives.

Expected Outcome: Mr. A. will maintain positive relationships with his daughters and significant others.
- ▪ Explore with Mr. A. ways he can demonstrate his support and love for his daughters.
- ▪ Teach Mr. A.'s daughters about the important role they play in assisting Mr. A. to maintain hope.
- ▪ Provide opportunities to reminisce and share pictures from the past.

Expected Outcome: Mr. A. will maintain active participation in his community organizations.
- ▲ Promote continued involvement with community organizations by expressing an interest and by encouraging attendance in meetings.
- ▪ Encourage Mr. A. to call close community organization members for an update on community activities and a ride to meetings.

▪ = nursing intervention; ▲ = collaborative intervention.

■ CRITICAL THINKING EXERCISES

1. What factors or events predispose Mr. A. to experiencing Hopelessness?
2. What additional information would be needed about Mr. A. to determine if he is experiencing dispositional or state Hopelessness?
3. What assessment data should the nurse gather to determine suicidal intent in Mr. A.?
4. What internal or external resources may be helpful to Mr. A. in assisting him to move from Hopelessness to hopefulness?

REFERENCES

1. American Psychiatric Association: *Diagnostic and statistical manual of mental disorders,* ed 4, Washington, D.C., 1994, The Association.
2. Averill J, Catlin G, and Chon K: *Rules of hope,* New York, 1990, Springer-Verlag.
3. Beck A and others: The measurements of pessimism: the hopelessness scale, *J Consult Clin Psychol* 42:861–865, 1974.
4. Beck A and others: Hopelessness and eventual suicide: a 10-year prospective study of patients hospitalized with suicidal ideation, *Am J Psychiatry* 142:559–563, 1985.
5. Busse E and Pfeiffer E: *Behavior and adaption in late life,* Boston, 1969, Little, Brown & Co.
6. Carpenito L: *Nursing diagnosis,* ed 6, Philadelphia, 1995, JB Lippincott Co.
7. Colt G: *The enigma of suicide,* New York, 1991, Simon and Schuster.
8. Daly B: Futility, *AACN Clin Issues Crit Care Nurs* 5(1):77–85, 1994.
9. Dufault K and Martocchio B: Hope: its spheres and dimensions, *Nurs Clin North Am* 20(2):379, 1985.
10. El-Gamel V: The usefulness of hope for a nursing assessment on the oncology unit, *J Cancer Care* 2:22–30, 1993.
11. Elliot R and others: Negotiating reality after physical loss: hope, depression, and disability, *J Personality Soc Psychol* 61(4):608–613, 1991.
12. Ersek M: The process of maintaining hope in adults undergoing bone marrow transplantation, *Oncol Nurs Forum* 19(6):883–889, 1992.
13. Farran C, Herth K, and Popovich J: *Hope and hopelessness: critical clinical constructs,* Thousand Oaks, California, 1995, Sage Publications.
14. Farran C, Wilken C, and Popovich J: Clinical assessment of hope, *Iss Ment Health Nurs* 13:129–138, 1992.
15. Flanders S: *Suicide,* New York, 1991, Oxford University Press.
16. Forbes S: Hope: an essential human need in the elderly, *J Geront Nurs* 20(6):5–10, 1994.
17. Fry P: Development of a geriatric scale of hopelessness, *J Counseling Psychol* 31(3):322–331, 1984.
18. Gaskins S: The meaning of hope: implications for nursing practice and research, *J Geront Nurs* 21(3):17–24, 1995.
19. Gordon J: *Nursing diagnosis: process and application,* ed 3, St. Louis, 1994, Mosby–Year Book.
20. Gottschalk L: A hope scale applicable to verbal samples, *Arch Gen Psychiatry* 30:779–785, 1974.
21. Haase J and others: Simultaneous concept analysis of spiritual perspective, hope, acceptance, and self-transcendence, *Image* 24(2):141–147, 1992.
22. Hackett T and Stern T: Suicide and other disruptive states. In Cassem N, editor: *Handbook of general hospital psychiatry,* St. Louis, 1991, Mosby–Year Book.
23. Hall B: Ways of maintaining hope in HIV disease, *Res Nurs Health* 17(4):283–293, 1994.
24. Herth K: Fostering hope in terminally ill people, *J Adv Nurs* 15:1250–1259, 1990.
25. Herth K: An abbreviated instrument to measure hope: development and psychometric evaluation, *J Adv Nurs* 17:1251–1259, 1992.
26. Herth K: Hope in the family caregiver of terminally ill people, *J Adv Nurs* 18:538–548, 1993.
27. Herth K: Hope in older adults in community and institutional settings, *Iss Ment Health Nurs* 14(2):139–156, 1993.
28. Herth K: Engendering hope in the chronically and terminally ill: nursing interventions, *Am J Hospice Palliative Care* Sept/Oct:31–39, 1995.
29. Hinds P and Gattuso J: Measuring hopefulness in adolescents, *J Pediatr Oncol Nurs* 8(2):92–94, 1991.
30. Hinds P and Martin J: Hopefulness and the self-sustaining process in adolescents with cancer, *Nurs Res* 37:336–340, 1988.
31. Jackson B: Hope and wound healing, *J Enterostom Ther Nurs* 21(2):73–79, 1993.
32. Kaplan H and Sadock B: *Study guide and self-examination review for synopsis of psychiatry,* ed 3, Baltimore, 1989, Williams & Wilkins.
33. Kazdin A and others: Hopelessness, depression, and suicide intent among psychiatrically disturbed inpatient children, *J Consult Clin Psychol* 51(7):504–510, 1983.
34. Kim M, McFarland GK, and McLane A: *Pocket guide to nursing diagnoses,* ed 5, St. Louis, 1995, Mosby–Year Book.
35. Le Gresley A: Validation of hopelessness: perceptions of the critically ill. In Carroll-Johnson R, editor: *Classification of nursing diagnoses: proceedings of the Ninth Conference,* Philadelphia, 1991, JB Lippincott Co.
36. Mayers K and Gardner J: Hope in a geriatric psychiatric state hospital population, *J Alzheimer's Care Related Disorders Res* Nov/Dec:308, 1992.
37. McClosky V and Bulechek G: *Nursing interventions classification,* ed 2, St. Louis, 1996, Mosby–Year Book.
38. McGill J and Paul P: Functional status and hope in elderly people with and without cancer, *Oncol Nurs Forum* 20(8):1207–1213, 1993.

VII

39. Miller J: Hope-inspiring strategies of the critically ill, *App Nurs Res* 2(1):23–29, 1989.

40. Miller J: Developing and maintaining hope in families of the critically ill, *AACN Clin Iss* 2(2):307–315, 1991.

41. Miller J: *Coping with chronic illness: overcoming powerlessness,* ed 2, Philadelphia, 1992, FA Davis.

42. Notwotny M: Every tomorrow a vision of hope, *J Psychosoc Oncol* 9(3):117–126, 1991.

43. Pederson P and others, editors: *Counseling across cultures,* ed 4, Thousand Oaks, California, 1996, Sage Publications.

44. Poncar P: Inspiring hope in the oncology patient, *J Psychosoc Nurs* 32(1):33–38, 1994.

45. Raleigh E: Sources of hope in chronic illness, *Oncol Nurs Forum* 19(3):443–448, 1992.

46. Rich C and others: Suicide, stressors and the life cycle, *Am J Psychiatry* 148(4):524–527, 1991.

47. Rotter J: Generalized expectations for internal versus external control of reinforcement, *Psychol Monographs: Gen Applied* 80(1) Whole No 609:1–18, 1966.

48. Synder C and others: The will and ways: development and validation of an individual-differences measure of hope, *J Personality Soc Psychol* 60(4):570–585, 1991.

49. Udelman D and Udelman M: Affects, neurotransmitters, and immunocompetence, *Stress Med* 7:159–167, 1991.

50. Yates P: Towards a reconceptualization of hope for patients with a diagnosis of cancer, *J Adv Nurs* 18(5):701–706, 1993.

51. Wake M and Miller J: Treating hopelessness: nursing strategies from six countries, *Clin Nurs Res* 1(4):347–365, 1992.

VII

Risk for Loneliness

▶ ————————————————————————————————————

Risk for Loneliness *is a subjective state in which an individual is at risk of experiencing vague dysphoria.*

OVERVIEW

Loneliness is part of the human experience. It is intimately connected with the way in which human beings interact and care for one another. Recognized as a universal phenomenon, it has been studied by scientists from various disciplines and written about by poets and novelists. When present, loneliness can have a profound impact on an individual's health and well-being.

Human beings can be described as social animals.[4] They are born into a group, the family, and live within a network of social relationships. As they grow to adulthood, human beings learn, develop, and find meaning and self-worth through these social relationships and group memberships. Through social interaction and the sense of belonging or connectedness to others, individuals fulfill their different needs, which is the basis for well-being.[18] Without the avenues for assistance provided by social relationships, individuals may be unable to fulfill their needs.

However, human beings do not live within groups constantly. For various reasons individuals may find themselves outside group life or unable to contact (connect with) important others. Some individuals may withdraw for reasons of their own, whereas others may be forced through life events into different circumstances. Life events, such as death, divorce, rejection, or separation, can influence one's social interactions, rendering significant

relationships no longer available. For the individual living outside the group life or disconnected from significant others the social network resources may be lacking or deficient.

Loneliness may result when real or perceived deficiencies exist in social network resources. For some, the deficiency may be a temporary situation, eliciting a temporary response of loneliness. For others, the deficiency may be ongoing or permanent, leading to the development of a chronic or permanent sense of loneliness. The state of loneliness is unpleasant and, in turn, may motivate the individual to action. The action, however, may take various routes, from trying to change the situation to trying to escape or defend against the emotional feelings.[4] Changing the situation might include finding new relationships, whereas escaping or defending might lead to alcoholism, mental illness, and suicide.

Conceptualizing Loneliness

Several theoretical approaches have been used to conceptualize loneliness. These approaches include psychodynamic, phenomenological, existential-humanistic, sociological, interactionalist, cognitive, privacy, and systems theory.[34] Much of the theoretical description regarding loneliness has emerged from clinical work. All theories see loneliness as an unpleasant, aversive experience, but only a few see it as a pathological response. Most see the phenomenon as normal and experienced by a cross section of people with current life factors playing a large role in its development. Only the psychodynamic tradition exclusively stresses childhood factors as having a role in the development of loneliness. For the purposes of this chapter, several theoretical approaches will be highlighted.

Within the psychodynamic tradition, the origins of loneliness are traced to childhood experiences[16,45,50] and reflect the basic traits of narcissism, megalomania, and hostility. The driving need for human intimacy, if thwarted during the early childhood years, can lead to harmful consequences later in life. For example, an adolescent who does not develop social skills through early interaction with parents may experience difficulties forming strong attachments or friendship ties. Sullivan argues that loneliness is an integral component of all psychopathology and that the struggle to find relief from loneliness is a central motivating factor in much of human behavior. The psychodynamic theorists base their ideas on their clinical work and are prone to see loneliness as pathological.

In contrast, Rogers[38] attributed loneliness to current forces rather than childhood experiences. He assumes that society pressures an individual to act in certain restricted, socially approved ways. These pressures could lead an individual to feel a discrepancy between the true inner self and the self shown to others. Merely performing society's roles, no matter how well, leads to an empty existence. If an individual fears rejection by others for his or her real self, that person may continue to project a self to others that is not the true self. The person maintains a social facade and continues to feel empty and unfulfilled. Such discrepancies between the actual and idealized self can result in loneliness.[30]

From a sociological perspective, Bowman[3] hypothesizes that three social factors lead to increased loneliness in contemporary society. These factors include (1) a decline in primary group relations, (2) an increase in family mobility, and (3) an increase in social mobility. Particularly in North American society, the stances of individualism, independence, and competition serve to erect barriers to community, engagement, and dependence on one another. The increased use of technology contributes to decreased human interaction, relations, and dependence on one another. Thus current social values and forces can influence feelings of connectedness, boredom, and loneliness.

Weiss,[46] one of the most prominent theorists regarding loneliness, states that "loneliness appears always to be a response to the . . . absence of some particular relational provision" (p. 17). In this interactionist approach, loneliness is the product of the combined (interactive) effect of personality factors and situational factors. Loneliness results when one's social interactions are deficient in supplying crucial social requirements. Weiss described two types of loneliness: emotional and social. Emotional loneliness is seen as resulting from the absence of a close, intimate attachment and resembles the separation anxiety of a child followed by anxiety, restlessness, and emptiness. Loneliness has been linked to personality variables such as low self-esteem[17]; being less extroverted[43]; being more depressed, anxious, and neurotic[20] and perceiving situations and interactions more negatively.[23] Social loneliness is seen in response to deficits in the environment and the response to the absence of meaningful friendships or a sense of community. It is experienced as boredom and feelings of being socially marginal. Certain situations (i.e., divorce, death, and living in a new city) are particularly conducive to social loneliness and can be considered a normal reaction for any individual in that situation.

Weiss argues that multiple relationships are needed to meet the many social needs an individual possesses. Confidants are required to satisfy needs for intimacy and emotional security. Needs for sociability and identity are best met by a group of friends or peers. Within Weiss's view, well-being depends equally on having a confidant and a social group of peers. This notion has been supported by the recent work of Gupta and Korte.[18]

The leading advocates for a cognitive approach to understanding loneliness have been Peplau and Perlman.[34] These authors emphasize cognition as a mediating factor between deficits in sociability and the experience of loneliness. Cognitive approaches suggest that loneliness occurs when the individual perceives a discrepancy between the desired level of social contact and the achieved level of social contact. It occurs when there is a mismatch between the individual's actual social relationships and needs for social contact. It is a subjective experience not synonymous with objective social isolation. A person may feel lonely when no one else is present, when a particular person is absent, when interactional partners treat him or her differently than desired, or when aspects of the situation make the person feel alienated from those with whom he or she could develop a satisfying relationship. Loneliness in this model could be attributed to personality, situational, historical, and current influences.

Moustakes[31] defines two types of loneliness. First, there is the loneliness of self-alienation, which is experienced as a vague and disturbing sense of anxiety. This is called *loneliness anxiety*. Francis refers to this type as *secondary loneliness,* a phenomenon experienced as a result of separation from persons or objects that the individual has invested with meaning or energy.[14] The act of attaching significance to important persons or objects is called *cathectic investment*. The second type of loneliness is called *existential, cosmic,* or *primary loneliness*. It is an intrinsic and organic part of human life and involves the pain and joy of emergence from a long period of desolation. Existential humans are fully aware of themselves as isolated and solitary individuals, whereas persons suffering loneliness anxiety are separated from their feeling and knowing selves.

Existential loneliness is the real experience of the individual. The individual has a conscious awareness of being singular. There is no one else exactly like that person, with his or her thoughts and experiences. Loneliness anxiety is more diffuse and may be experienced after a crisis event. There is a difference in the intensity of these two experiences. Existential loneliness is the real experience of the here and now, perhaps best expressed in the question, "Will I live or die?" Loneliness anxiety involves more focus on fear of aloneness and fear of future implications. Existential loneliness may lead to new insight, creativity, and moti-

vation, whereas loneliness anxiety may isolate and separate the individual from his or her experience. In the words of Moustakes, "Fear, evasion, denial and the accompanying attempts to escape the experience of being lonely will forever isolate the person from his own resources so that there is no development, no creative emergence, no growth or awareness, perceptiveness or sensitivity."[31]

Differentiating Among Concepts

Although related, the concepts of lonesomeness, aloneness, and loneliness are different. The feeling of lonesomeness is not an unusual experience for most individuals. It implies being without the company of others but recognizing a wish to be with others.[34] The individual acknowledges the need to feel close to other people, can express this feeling, and frequently takes steps to reverse the feeling. Aloneness or solitude implies being without the company of others, but it also signifies a singular position, such as being alone to make certain decisions with regard to living. Individuals will choose to be alone to work or to think. They may consciously withdraw to accomplish a goal. In these situations, individuals can be alone but not experience lonesomeness or loneliness.

In contrast, loneliness "is the conscious experience of separation from something or someone desired, required, or needed. It is not solitariness, for there the separation is not felt; nor is it the lack of physical or social contact, for the presence of people will not assuage it. So there must be experienced a need, a desire for contact, and an inability to make it."[22] Rook[40] describes loneliness as "an enduring condition of emotional distress that arises when a person feels estranged from, misunderstood, or rejected by others, and/or lacks the appropriate social partners for desired activities, particularly activities that provide a sense of social integration and opportunities for emotional intimacy" (p. 1391).

Loneliness may be categorized as transient, situational, or chronic. Loneliness may be the product of situational change (e.g., divorce or loss of a spouse) or transitional change (e.g., adolescence) and may be experienced as transitory mood

VII

swings.[49] It may also become chronic as a result of long-term behavioral and affective disorders and last 2 or more years. Whereas transient and situational loneliness are generally the result of environmental events, chronic loneliness is thought to be related to internal factors, such as dysfunctional cognition and affective states that interact with the environment or personality characteristics (e.g., shyness). For example, individuals who are not adequately able to reflect on and learn from their social interactions may experience chronic loneliness.[6]

Experiencing Loneliness

The potential for loneliness, then, exists within any situation in which an individual experiences separation from others because of physical space, ideology, or life events. The situation could mean a change in the person's actual social relations or changes in the person's social needs or desires. Experiencing hospitalization, institutionalization, a move to a new location, death, conversion to new religious beliefs, physical or mental illness, a role change, communication barriers, and sensory isolation could place an individual at Risk for Loneliness. Researchers have reported loneliness in various populations, including those who are widowed,[35] never married,[9] deaf,[4] visually impaired,[13] chronically ill,[24] hospitalized elderly,[37] HIV-positive,[26] psychiatrically ill,[27] spousal caregivers,[2] and in long-term rehabilitation.[2] In particular, the elderly[10] and adolescent[28] populations have been the focus of much of the work regarding loneliness.

The potential for loneliness also exists in any situation where factors are present that predispose individuals to becoming lonely, to persist in remaining lonely over time, or to experience difficulties reestablishing social relations. Lonely people may be shy, introverted, or less willing to take social risks. Inadequate social skills may make it difficult to establish or maintain satisfactory relationships. A predisposition for self-disclosure and privacy requirements for intimacy may also influence the establishment of relationships.[34] Cultural factors may also be important. For example, private schools or corporations may emphasize rugged individualism and success through competition, which might foster loneliness, or the unrealistic expectations for relationships created through the popular media may contribute to feelings of loneliness. Even the physical setting in which an individual lives or works could contribute to feelings of isolation and loneliness. Generally, loneliness is affected by the mismatch between an individual's needs, desires, and skills and the reality of his or her social environment.

Loneliness is quite prevalent in today's society, affecting 25% to 50% of the population.[44] West, Kellner, and Moore-West[47] in their review of the literature report that loneliness occurs throughout the life span. It is most frequent during adolescent and young adult years and least frequent among respondents 65 years of age and older. In general, loneliness increases with age as the number of social contacts decreases. However, recent evidence supports the view that older adults may proactively manage their social relationships to enhance emotional ties and to offset loneliness as their social networks decrease in size.[25] In general, females report a greater degree of loneliness than males, a function perhaps of the way in which women utilize social relationships.[2] Odell[32] found 55% of the 51 hospitalized adults studied to be lonely, whereas Foxall and Ekberg[12] reported only 31% of chronically ill individuals who remained at home to be lonely. Patients who are able to be at home may have different opportunities to maintain relationships and social roles than individuals who are in institutional settings.

A number of variables have been linked with loneliness, including depression, suicide, suicide ideation, hostility, passiveness, inadequate social skills, alcoholism, poor self-concept, and psychosomatic illness.[29] In adolescents, loneliness is negatively associated with self-esteem and has been linked to drug abuse, alcoholism, and delinquency.[5] Lonely people frequently feel worthless, incompetent, and unlovable. In a study of 379 elderly people living at home significant relationships were found between the size of the older adult's social network, health status, and perceived loneliness.[8] Perceived loneliness was the strongest predictor of health status when all the social variables were considered. If the loneliness remains unresolved, the individual may experience social isolation, a decreased ability to function, and ultimately a diminished sense of self-esteem. The experience of loneliness may easily intensify as the individual is separated from the person or things to which he or she had attached meaning or significance.[36]

Overall there is agreement that loneliness is a variable phenomenon that can be potentially devastating. If left unchecked, it can have a significant impact on individuals,[14] undermining self-esteem and the sense of well-being. Research is still required to understand fully the incidence and prevalence of loneliness in various populations and to differentiate loneliness clearly from other phenomenon such as grief.[36,37] Clearly, however, loneliness can occur when a person's needs for intimacy are not met and when the relationships for which a person is striving are lacking.

ASSESSMENT

The observations previously outlined have contributed to the development of the nursing diagnosis Risk for Loneliness. Loneliness is a subjective state described as "a vague, dysphoric, reactive response to the more or less temporary separation from persons and things one has endowed with meaning, import and energy; that is, cathectic investment."[14]

The experience of loneliness may result in a range of mental and emotional responses that on the whole are not pleasant and can be distressful. Based on empirical evidence, loneliness is a vague feeling of psychic discomfort and uneasiness, extremely difficult to describe and undesirable.[14] It is a "depressing" feeling that leads to introspection and worry about those persons or things from whom one is separated. Lonely people are often not aware of the reasons they do what they do when they experience loneliness. There is often an unnoticed inability to do anything while alone. What is felt is not labeled loneliness but a feeling of unexplained dread, of desperation, and of extreme restlessness.[34] It is a subjective feeling of being apart from others.

The meaning of loneliness varies from person to person. To say "I feel lonely" may imply an experience of awkwardness in initiating social contacts, deep feelings of inferiority and inadequacy or an experience of existential separatedness and alienation. Horowitz, French, and Anderson[21] investigated the features all lonely individuals might experience as a way of understanding the common meaning of loneliness. The subjects in this research strongly agreed (.71 to .90) that the lonely person would feel isolated, excluded from activities, not part of a group, inferior, worthless, inadequate, depressed, sad, and unhappy and would think "Something is wrong with me" and "I am inferior." They also agreed, though not as strongly (.57 to .70), that the features of the lonely person would include feeling separated and different from others and thinking "I am different from everybody else" and "I don't fit in." Finally, features of feeling unloved and not cared for; thinking "Others don't like me," "I want a friend," and "I don't know how to make friends"; avoiding social contacts; and isolating oneself from others and working or studying hard for long hours were also seen as part of the prototype of a lonely person.

Following a national newspaper survey, Rubenstein and Shaver[41] were able to describe the feelings associated with loneliness in the general population. When people labeled themselves as lonely, the feelings they mentioned having most often included sadness (66%), depression (60%), boredom (55%), self-pity (50%), and longing to be with one special person (56%). A factor analysis of the feeling data revealed four reliable factors. Desperation was characterized by feeling desperate, panicked, helpless, afraid, without hope, abandoned, and vulnerable. Depression was characterized by feelings of being sad, depressed, empty, isolated, sorry for oneself, melancholy, alienated, and longing to be with one special person. Impatient boredom was characterized by feeling impatient, bored, a desire to be elsewhere, uneasy, angry, and unable to concentrate. Self-deprecation was characterized by feeling unattractive, down on oneself, stupid, ashamed, and insecure. The first factor, desperation, accounts for the largest variation (76.5%) in loneliness.

The reasons individuals identified the feelings associated with loneliness were also studied as part of Rubenstein and Shaver's work. A factor analysis of these reasons revealed five factors. "Being unattached" consisted of items such as having no spouse, having no sexual partner, and breaking up with one's spouse or partner. "Alienation" consisted of feeling different, being misunderstood, not being needed, and having no close friends. "Being alone" consisted of coming home to an empty house and being alone. "Forced isolation" consisted of being housebound, being hospitalized, and having no transportation. "Dislocation" consisted of being far from home, in a new job or school, moving too often, and traveling often.

Assessing Loneliness

Based on the notion that loneliness emerges in response to a perceived discrepancy between a desired level of contact and the actual level of contact with a significant person or object, the assessment process must consider several domains. Very broadly these domains may be grouped as antecedents to the situation, critical attributes of the situation, and consequences of the loneliness response.

The antecedents to the situation encompass what has occurred in the past. The individual brings to the situation a set of human needs, personality characteristics, past experiences, knowledge, skills, and coping predisposition. In particular, each individual brings an innate desire for interpersonal intimacy. This desire varies from person to person but stays with an individual throughout his or her lifetime. As an individual grows and develops the person constantly strives to meet this need by connecting with others. Each person builds a network of social relationships that help that individual feel loved, cared for, and part of a system of mutual obligation. Living within this network of social interactions allows an individual to learn ways of interacting with others and to bolster self-esteem. Emotional support, comfort, and tangible assis-

tance emerge through the social network ties. Individuals create connections to seek relief from adverse experiences and to meet the desire for interpersonal intimacy. As an individual confronts each of life's situations, the person brings with him or her the learning and expectations developed throughout a lifetime concerning social interactions and how to use those relationships. The individual also bring his or her past experiences regarding the loss of relationships and the feelings surrounding those losses.

The critical attributes of the situation encompass the experiential aspects of that situation for the individual concerned. The individual must experience feelings of separation from another, a response to a perceived or real disruption of social relationships, and a discrepancy between the actual relationship with another and the desired relationship.[7] Situations in which an individual feels shame, grief, alienation, or lack of trust may create tension in relationships and promote feelings of separatedness. Similarly, social obstacles (e.g., poverty, family dysfunction, or friendship changes), cultural roles and values, and pain or suffering may also create feelings of tension in relationships. The risk for loneliness increases when individuals are not able to use their resources and opportunities to overcome these various tensions. Sadness, resignation, despair, emptiness, and meaninglessness can result from the occurrence of loneliness.[34]

The clinical observations that reflect the consequences of loneliness include lack of or problems with social relationships, self-labeling, time- or space-oriented problems or complaints, inability to make decisions, and a focus on weakness in oneself or others.[7] Problems with social relationships may be identified through comments about lack of human companionship, the absence of or separation from loved ones, and lack of or perceived lack of human support. Self-labeling refers to negative self-talk, which reflects decreased feelings of self-worth and self-esteem and helplessness. Time- or space-oriented complaints are based on feelings of being confined, deserted, or alone when a person verbalizes the desire for companionship. The inability to make decisions is seen when a person vacillates, hesitates, or is indecisive in dealing with events. Peplau and Perlman[34] described this behavior as planlessness, or living life without a plan. The focus on weaknesses in oneself or others implies that the individual sees the world as mistrusting, sad, powerless, or lacking meaning.

Measuring Loneliness

Standardized instruments have been developed to measure loneliness as a unidimensional concept and as a multidimensional concept. A unidimensional measure assumes all loneliness is the same and any variation is only in intensity. A multidimensional measure assumes there are various types of loneliness across different groups (i.e., children, adolescents, adults, and elders) caused by different factors.

The most widely used loneliness scale is the revised UCLA Loneliness Scale. The original UCLA Loneliness Scale was based on a conceptualization of loneliness as the felt lack of meaningful personal relationships.[42] Continued refinement of the instrument resulted in a 20-item scale that purports to provide a global measure of the subjective experience of loneliness.[43] Extensive reliability and validity testing of the instrument has been completely successfully in student populations.

The other well-known instrument to measure loneliness is the Schedules for the Measurement of Loneliness and Cathectic Investment.[14] It is a 25-item, focused interview with a reported test-retest reliability of 0.98 ($p < 0.001$). Validity was reasonable using responders' self-determined placement on a lonely/not-too-lonely visual analog. Psychometric properties were established in populations of persons separated from their homes and loved ones (i.e., hospitalized medical patients, jail inmates, residents in homes for the aged, or patients in nursing homes).

Assessment Data

The actual data gathered for clinical assessment will depend in large measure on the context of the situation and the time constraints. Ultimately the goal of the assessment is to understand the individual's perception of the situation in which he or she is living. The Risk of Loneliness exists in relation to the tensions one is feeling with regard to social relationships.

It is important to remember that loneliness is an intensely personal, subjective experience. There are no foolproof, objective signs of loneliness. One must depend on patients' statements about their internal experiences or infer loneliness from a cluster of observations. The task may be further complicated because individuals may be unwilling to acknowledge their loneliness to themselves or to others or because they may find it an embarrassment and try to hide their inner pain. However, loneliness stems in some measure from a mismatch between a person and a situation.

Important areas for data collection include the following:

1. The nature of recent life of situational changes. Determine if recent life events or situational changes have created or the potential for change in the patient's social interactions or connectedness with significant persons or things.
2. The patient's perception of the change(s). Explore the patient's perception of the change(s) in terms of (1) feelings of being separated because of the change, (2) experiencing disruption in social relationships, and (3) desiring the relationships to be different than they presently are.
3. The patient's behavior and deportment. Note the patient's age, gender, ease of deportment, overt signs of distress or composure, activity level, rest and sleep patterns, and eating patterns. Explore the patient's feelings of loneliness and when they are intense and when they are lessened.
4. The patient's sense of self. Ask the patient to describe his or her sense of self, including self-worth, personal competence, and aspirations.
5. The context of the situation. Determine the patient's past experience with similar situations. Identify available social relationships (tangible and supportive) and the quality of support. Identify any barriers to accessing social support.

VII

6. The patient's repertoire of skills. Determine the patient's communication skills and interaction patterns with others. Determine the patient's skills in problem solving. Determine the patient's pattern in controlling emotions, and deal with uncertainty or tension.

A key aspect of this assessment is understanding the patient's cognitive appraisal or perception of the situation. The interview environment must be supportive and nonjudgmental for the individual for the patient to reveal the information.

■ Risk Factors

The presence of the following behaviors, condition, or circumstances renders the patient more vulnerable to Risk for Loneliness:

- Changes in relationships through loss, distance, or circumstances (e.g., death, divorce, relocation, retirement, role changes, or hospitalization)
- Changes in relationships because of physical or emotional illness (e.g., Alzheimer's, schizophrenia, HIV positive, disability, or odor)
- Changes in financial status limiting previous activity and movement
- Change in beliefs, values, traditions, or cultural practices (e.g., no longer interacting with referent group)
- Changes in personal control, independence, and independent activity
- Changes in self-esteem, body image, feelings of inadequacy and insecurity

NURSING DIAGNOSIS

■ Differential Nursing Diagnosis

Several nursing diagnoses are closely related to Risk for Loneliness. There could be difficulty discriminating one from another. These diagnoses include Social Isolation, Impaired Social Interaction, Self-Esteem Disturbance (especially chronic low self-esteem), and Relocation Stress Syndrome. In the event these diagnoses are made, Risk for Loneliness should also be considered. These situations place a patient at Risk for Loneliness, and some of the clinical observations of loneliness overlap with the clinical observations for these diagnoses.

■ Medical and Psychiatric Diagnoses

Risk for Loneliness can be observed in a wide range of medical diagnoses. Acute and chronic illnesses may separate a patient from significant others or objects. Hospitalization, changes in lifestyle due to illness, disability, or changes in self-image can place a patient at Risk for Loneliness.

Loneliness is associated with or a component of many psychiatric illnesses. Patients with mental illnesses may experience loneliness resulting from as well as contributing to compromised functional abilities and social problems. Depression and loneliness are frequently interrelated.

OUTCOME IDENTIFICATION, PLANNING, AND IMPLEMENTATION

Ideally the identification of patients at Risk for Loneliness would lead to the implementation of strategies to prevent loneliness. Research is still needed in many instances to identify the specific interventions that are effective with different populations to prevent loneliness.[36] The recommended interventions have been developed in working with patients who experienced loneliness. When loneliness symptoms are present, interventions may be offered to alleviate feelings of isolation. However, if factors are present that make a patient vulnerable to the development of loneliness, interventions could be implemented with a view to its prevention.

Nursing interventions regarding loneliness are based on assisting the patient to identify and deal with the specific situational conditions contributing to loneliness. The assessment process can be used to focus the patient on the context of the situation, the tensions he or she may be feeling, and the outcomes the patient wishes to achieve. After the desired outcomes or goals have been identified, the dialogue needs to focus on the options or approaches that can be used to achieve the outcomes. Assisting the patient to solve problems, determine goals, make decisions, and become familiar with how human interactions work is critical in working with those who are at risk for or experiencing loneliness.[7] Given the nature of loneliness, assessment and intervention may need to be repeated when the patient faces new or additional situations.

The specific nature of the intervention needs to be based on the assessment of the patient's specific situation. Given that loneliness is a subjective state, interventions that may be effective for one patient may not be helpful to another. For example, the specific interventions for lonely hospitalized patients will be different than the intervention for lonely widows living at home. The interventions for the hospitalized patient may need to focus on creating a familiar environment and encouraging the presence of cathectic objects, such as pictures or personal items.[37] Or hospital visitation policies may need to be altered to allow for frequent and meaningful contact with significant others and diminish the effect of separation. The interventions for widows may focus on initiating strategies to increase their comfort with being alone and redesign their notions of companionship.[35]

Determining whether one is intervening in a situation of chronic, situational, or transitional loneliness is important. Chronic loneliness results from long-term deficits in a patient's ability to relate to others and may benefit most from desensitization of social anxiety or social skills training. Situation loneliness occurs from a major disruption of the individual's pattern of social relationships. These individuals may benefit most from reassurance and assistance in identifying social situations in which new relationships can be explored. Transitional loneliness refers to occasional feelings of loneliness most people experience from time to time. Transitional loneliness is most frequently handled by the person rather than requiring intervention from a health care professional.

Identifying the specific nature of a social contact deficit is also critical to selecting the appropriate intervention. Not all social deficits may relate to loneliness.[39] Weiss[46] specified social deficits related to loneliness as being emotional and social.

Interventions aimed toward emotional loneliness must focus on attachment figures, confidants, and intimate partners. Interventions aimed toward social loneliness must focus on ties within a community. Additionally, determining short-term and long-term interventions may be useful. Reading a book or watching television may be useful to offset loneliness in the short term, but if the real issue is a deficit in social network ties, a different approach is required for long-term gains.

In the research by Rubenstein and Shaver,[41] subjects reported what they did when they felt lonely. The most common answers included reading (50%), listening to music (57%), and calling a friend (55%). A factor analysis of this data revealed four factors concerning responses to loneliness. "Sad passivity" contained the items cry, sleep, sit and think, do nothing, overeat, take tranquilizers, watch television, drink, or get "stoned." "Active solitude" included the items study or work, write, listen to music, exercise, walk, work on a hobby, go to a movie, read, or play music. "Spending money" included the items spend money and go shopping. "Social contact" included the items call a friend and visit someone. Of the four response factors, sad passivity was correlated most strongly with loneliness ($r = 0.42$, $p = 0.001$). It is a state of lethargic self-pity that may contribute to a vicious cycle of low self-esteem and social isolation. It is negatively correlated with age ($r = -.23, p < 0.001$), suggesting that this response is characteristic of the young. In some regards, its interpretation could mean, "I am helpless and dejected; love me and take care of me."

In work by Peplau and Perlman,[34] three general ways that patients cope with loneliness were identified: (1) changing the patient's actual social relations, (2) changing the patient's social needs or desires, or (3) reducing the perceived importance of the social deficiency. The first approach is the most direct and can be accomplished by the formation of new relationships, using one's existing network more fully or creating "surrogate" relationships (e.g., pets, television personalities, or talk show hosts). Reducing one's desires for social contact may be accomplished by selecting tasks

VII

and activities one can enjoy alone rather than activities one only enjoys with others. Reexamining one's standards or expectations regarding social relations may also be beneficial. Finally, reducing the importance of a social deficit may occur through denial or devaluation of the relationship. People also try to distract themselves by working longer hours, by using alcohol, or through other such activities. Intervention with patients who are using denial or distraction strategies, which have long-term consequences, must be approached carefully. Creating further insult to self-esteem or leaving a patient without defenses against emotional pain is not helpful.

Russell, Peplau, and Cutrona[43] report behavioral and cognitive strategies that college students found helpful in dealing with loneliness. Commonly students tried behaviors to improve their social life such as being friendlier to others, helping someone else, or improving their physical appearance. They also engaged in nonsocial activities in which they were skilled, perhaps to counteract the potentially negative impact of loneliness on self-esteem. Many reported that they worked hard to succeed at something in which they were good when they felt lonely or that they distracted themselves by mental and physical activity. Cognitive strategies they used included problem solving (thinking about the causes of their feelings and what could be done to overcome them) and distraction (purposely thinking about other things).

Intervention Guidelines

Despite the caution regarding the need to focus interventions specifically, several general guidelines have merit across populations and could be incorporated in nursing practice.[44] Each will be described briefly.

1. Offer support by active listening. Active listening involves trying to understand the issues a patient is describing as well as the person's feelings about the issues. The intervention serves to communicate caring and concern, thus directly addressing the need for meaningful interpersonal interaction. Additionally, as the patient talks about problems there may be a lessening of the preoccupation with the problem, a release of energy for considering solutions, and an enhanced ability to solve problems.

2. Promote development of positive relationships. Involvement in groups has been identified as an effective method for treating loneliness.[1] Groups may be designed as therapeutic groups or self-help groups.[19] Group membership offers avenues for enhanced learning or problem solving and increased social contacts.[48] Establishing ties to a meaningful group can enhance personal feelings of relatedness. New relationships may also emerge from visitor programs or "buddy" programs. Additionally, forming relationships with pets[15] and finding avenues for creativity[33] have been useful in forming new attachments.

3. Facilitate maintaining relationships with others. When an individual's usual methods for interaction are not available, he or she may need assistance to identify different approaches. For example, the patient in isolation may need to be encouraged to talk on the telephone or to write letters. Some lonely patients may need to be encouraged to tell family and friends they would like company or contact. The nursing intervention may need to be directed toward acknowledging the value of social contacts, normalizing the desire for social interaction, and helping the patient discover ways of requesting the contact from those he or she considers significant. Additionally, there may be value in direct conversation with family and friends about the types of actions they might perform that would help meet the needs of a lonely patient. Family members and friends could be encouraged to visit, write, or telephone.

4. Encourage positive reminiscing and cognitions. Reflecting on past events can help a patient recapture previous feelings of strength and self-worth. Reminiscing is a specific approach used to promote ego integrity and hope in elders.[11] Personal items, pictures, art, and music can be used effectively as stimulus to reminiscing. Additionally, helping patients identify negative

patterns of thinking ("I'll never be able to do that") and explore their validity can be useful.

5. Promote effective problem solving and coping with change. As life events unfold and circumstances alter social interactions, patients may require assistance in understanding the nature of the events and their responses. They may also require assistance in identifying how to meet the specific demands of the situation and achieve the outcomes they desire. Access to information and services may need to be facilitated or coordinated by the nurse. Additionally, the patient may require help in setting realistic goals and making concrete plans to accomplish the goals.

6. Promote involvement in activities. Involvement in activities serves a number of purposes. It keeps patients busy and active, increases their contact with others, and can contribute to feelings of self-worth. Activities may also serve to direct attention toward the outside world rather than toward oneself. Specific suggestions may need to be made to a patient regarding types of activities as well as plans organized to make participation possible.

◢ **NURSING CARE GUIDELINES**
Nursing Diagnosis: Risk for Loneliness

VII

Expected Outcome: The patient will understand the factors influencing feelings of loneliness.
▪ Support the patient's humanness, uniqueness, and right to be involved in decision making.
▪ Seek to understand the patient's perspective on the present situation.
▪ Explore the patient's perspective regarding alterations in social relationships, feelings about the alterations, and desire for a different relationship.
▪ Discuss the risk factors for loneliness, and explore their application to the current situation with the patient.

Expected Outcome: The patient will verbalize a sense of personal integrity and movement toward desired goals.
▪ Establish realistic and concrete goals with the patient.
▪ Identify specific strategies for achieving the selected goals.
▪ Review capabilities for achieving the goals.
▪ Identify if additional resources are required to achieve the goals.
▪ Establish realistic time frames for reaching the goals.

Expected Outcome: The patient will engage in activities to decrease the barriers to social interaction and to promote social contact.
▪ Assist the patient to identify barriers to desired social interaction.
▪ Assist the patient to explore options for achieving desired social contacts (reducing the barriers and taking action).
▪ Teach patient necessary knowledge or skills.
▪ Encourage the patient to express his or her desire for social contact and to maintain his or her existing social network.
▪ Acknowledge progress toward desired goal(s).

Expected Outcome: The patient will experience a decrease in feelings of loneliness.
▪ Encourage the expression of worries and concerns.
▪ Explore patterns of thinking (especially self-defeating thoughts).

▪ = nursing intervention; ▲ = collaborative intervention.

EVALUATION

The nurse uses observation of and interaction with the patient to evaluate the effectiveness of the nursing interventions. The desired effect must be defined in the context of the particular situation and the desired outcome identified by the individual patient.

In general it is anticipated that the patient would gain an understanding of the factors contributing to the feelings of loneliness. He or she would discuss and engage in activities to decrease barriers to social contact and to promote social contacts. Eventually the individual would feel a lifting or resolution of the discomfort and unease associated with loneliness. The individual would be able to overcome or cope with the tensions in the situation that exacerbate the loneliness, to make decisions, to establish goals, and to achieve the desired outcomes. Ultimately the individual would experience a personal connectedness with a significant other.

◢ CASE STUDY WITH PLAN OF CARE

Ms. Sally M. is a 35-year-old mother of two. Her daughter is $3\frac{1}{2}$ years old and her son is $1\frac{1}{2}$ years old. Ms. M. has recently separated from her husband and moved to a new city to start a new job. She left behind her immediate family relatives, with whom she was very close and spent a lot of time. However, she felt she had to make the move for the employment and "to get a new start." Her former husband also moved to the other side of the country for work reasons and does not plan on seeing the children for some time. He is committed to providing some financial support for their care.

Ms. M. has been in her new environment for a month and is due to start work in 2 weeks. She finds she can't settle down to do anything around her house, although there is a great deal to do. She is restless and sad and keeps thinking about how things used to be. When asked how she is feeling, she finds it hard to describe exactly how she is feeling, other than she does not like it. She does acknowledge that she feels "all by her self" and "not really connected to anything." "Drifting" is another word she uses to describe her activity at home. She states, "I do not want to go on like this."

◢ PLAN OF CARE FOR MS. SALLY M.
Nursing Diagnosis: Risk of Loneliness Related to Separation from Husband and Relocation to a New City

Expected Outcome: Ms. Sally M. will understand the factors that place her at Risk for Loneliness.
- Encourage Ms. M. to talk about the changes in her situation.
- Encourage Ms. M. to discuss her perception of the changes.
- Share information about the factors that place an individual at Risk for Loneliness, and help Ms. Sally M. apply them to her situation.

Expected Outcome: Ms. M. will identify goals for herself regarding social contacts and will engage in appropriate activity to accomplish those goals.
- Explore with Ms. M. what she would like to be different regarding her social interaction.
- Explore ways her goals could be achieved on a short-term and a long-term basis.
- Identify with Ms. M. if resources are required for her to begin to meet her goals (i.e., child care).
- Explore the type of information Ms. M. needs to acquire about the community and its resources, especially activities where mothers and young children gather.

Expected Outcome: Ms. Sally M. will experience a growing sense of connectedness within her new situation and a decrease in the unpleasant feelings of restlessness, drifting, and sadness.
- Set specific timelines to meet, and monitor how Ms. M. is managing.
- Encourage Ms. M. to continue to share her feelings, concerns, and worries.

■ = nursing intervention; ▲ = collaborative intervention.

■ CRITICAL THINKING EXERCISES

1. What types of situations could place an individual at Risk for Loneliness?
2. What clinical observations are indicative of loneliness?
3. What factors should be taken into account in deciding what interventions to select when an individual is at Risk for Loneliness?

REFERENCES

1. Acorn S and Bampton E: Patients' loneliness: a challenge for rehabilitation nurses, *Rehab Nurs* 17(1):22–25, 1992.
2. Bergman-Evans BF: Alzheimer's and related disorders: loneliness, depression, and social support of spousal caregivers, *J Geront Nurs* 20(3):6–16, 1994.
3. Bowman CC: Loneliness and social change, *Am J Psychiatry* 112:194–198, 1955.
4. Brackenroth GAM: Loneliness in the deaf community: a personal or an enforced choice?, *Int J Rehab Res* 16:331–336, 1993.
5. Brage D, Meredith W, and Woodward J: Correlates of loneliness among midwestern adolescents, *Adolescence* 28(111):685–693, 1993.
6. Carr M and Schellenbach C: Reflective monitoring in lonely adolescents, *Adolescence* 28(111):737–747, 1993.
7. Copel LC: Loneliness, *J Psychiatr Nurs* 26(1):14–19, 1988.
8. Cox CL, Spiro M, and Sullivan JA: Social risk factors: impact on elders' perceived health status, *J Comm Health Nurs* 5(1):59–73, 1988.
9. Dalton ST: Lived experience of never-married women, *Iss Ment Health Nurs* 13:69–80, 1992.
10. Dugan E and Kivett VR: The importance of emotional and social isolation to loneliness among very old rural adults, *Gerontologist* 34(3):340–346, 1994.
11. Farran C and Popovich J: Hope: a relevant concept of geriatric psychiatry, *Arch Psychiatr Nurs* IV(2):124–130, 1990.
12. Foxall MJ and Ekberg JY: Loneliness of chronically ill adults and their spouses, *Iss Ment Health Nurs* 10:149–167, 1989.
13. Foxall MJ and others: Predictors of loneliness in low vision adults, *Western J Nurs Research* 14(1):86–99, 1992.
14. Francis GM: Loneliness: the syndrome, *Iss Ment Health Nurs* 3:1–5, 1981.
15. Fraser C: Pets meet the needs of the lonely elderly, *Nurs RSA Verpleging* 7(6):17–18, 40, 1992.
16. Fromm-Reichmann F: Loneliness, *Psychiatry* 22:1–15, 1959.
17. Goswick RA and Jones WH: Loneliness, self-concept and adjustment, *J Psychology* 107:237–240, 1981.
18. Gupta V and Korte C: The effects of a confidant and a peer group on the well-being of single elders, *Int J Aging Human Develop* 39(4):293–302, 1994.
19. Hochberger JM and Fisher-James L: Discharge group for chronically mentally ill, *J Psychosoc Nurs* 30(4):25–27, 1992.
20. Hojat M: Loneliness as a function of selected personality variables, *J Clin Psychol* 38:137–141, 1982.
21. Horowitz LM, French R, and Anderson CA: The prototype of a lonely person. In Peplau LA and Perlman D, editors: *Loneliness: a sourcebook of current theory, research and therapy,* New York, 1982, John Wiley & Sons.
22. Hoskisson JB: *Loneliness,* New York. 1965. Citadel
23. Jones WH, Freeman JE, and Goswick RA: The persistence of loneliness: self and other determinants, *J Personality* 49:27–48, 1981.
24. Keele-Card G, Foxhall MJ, and Barron CR: Loneliness, depression and social support of patients with COPD and their spouses, *Pub Health Nurs* 10(4):245–251, 1993.
25. Lang FR and Carstensen LL: Close emotional and relationships in late life: further support for proactive aging in the social domain, *Psychology Aging* 9(2):315–324, 1994.
26. Laryea M and Gien L: The impact of HIV-positive diagnosis on the individual, part I, *Clin Nurs Res* 2(3):245–266, 1993.
27. Lee H, Coenen A, and Helm K: Island living: the experience of loneliness in a psychiatric hospital, *Applied Nurs Res* 7(1):7–13, 1994.
28. Mahon NE, Yarcheski A, and Yarcheski TJ: Differences in social support and loneliness in adolescents according to developmental stage and gender, *Pub Health Nurs* 11(5):361–368, 1994.
29. McWhirter BT: Loneliness: a review of current literature with implications for counseling and research, *J Counsel Develop* 68:417–422, 1990.
30. Moore JA: Loneliness: self-discrepancy and sociological variables, *Canad Counsellor* 10:133–135, 1976.
31. Moustakes C: *Loneliness,* Englewood Heights, New Jersey, 1961, Prentice-Hall.
32. Odell SH: Someone is lonely, *Iss Ment Health Nurs* 3(2):7–12, 1981.
33. Peden AR: Music making: the connection with persons who are homeless, *J Psychosoc Nurs* 31(7):17–20, 1993.
34. Peplau LA and Perlman D, editors: *Loneliness: a sourcebook of current theory, research and therapy,* New York, 1982, John Wiley & Sons.
35. Porter EJ: Older widows' experience of living alone at home, *Image* 26(1):19–24, 1994.
36. Profitt C and Byrne M: Predicting loneliness in the hospitalized elderly: what are the risk factors? *Geriatr Nurs* 14(6):311–314, 1993.
37. Rodgers BL: Loneliness: easing the pain of the hospitalized elderly, *J Geront Nurs* 15(8):16–21, 1989.
38. Rogers CS: The loneliness of contemporary man as seen in "the case of Ellen West," *Ann Psychother* 3:22–27, 1961.
39. Rook K: Promoting social bonding: strategies for helping the lonely and socially isolated, *Am Psychologist* 39:1389–1407, 1984.

VII

40. Rook K and Peplau LA: Perspective on helping the lonely. In Peplau LA and Perlman D, editors: *Loneliness: a sourcebook of current theory, research and therapy,* New York, 1982, John Wiley & Sons.

41. Rubenstein C and Shaver P: The experience of loneliness. In Peplau LA and Perlman D, editors: *Loneliness: a sourcebook of current theory, research and therapy,* New York, 1982, John Wiley & Sons.

42. Russell D, Peplau LA, and Ferguson M: Developing a measure of loneliness, *J Personality Assess* 42:290–294, 1978.

43. Russell D, Peplau LA, and Cutrona CE: The revised UCLA loneliness scale: concurrent and discriminant validity evidence, *J Personality Soc Psychol* 39:472–480, 1980.

44. Shearer R and Davidhizar R: Loneliness and the spouse of the geriatric patient, *Geriatr Nurs* 14(6):307–310, 1993.

45. Sullivan HS: *The interpersonal theory of psychiatry,* New York, 1953, WW Norton.

46. Weiss RS: *Loneliness: the experience of emotional and social isolation,* Cambridge, Massachusetts, 1973, Massachusetts Institute of Technology.

47. West DA, Kellner R, and Moore-West M: The effects of loneliness: a review of the literature, *Comprehensive Psychiatry* 27(4):351–363, 1986.

48. Windriver W: Social isolation: unit-based activities for imIpaired elders, *J Geront Nurs* 19(3):15–21, 1993.

49. Young JE: Loneliness, depression and cognitive therapy: theory and applications. In Peplau LA and Perlman D, editors: *Loneliness,* New York, 1982, John Wiley & Sons.

50. Zilboorg G: Loneliness, *Atlantic Monthly,* pp. 45–54, January, 1938.

VII

Personal Identity Disturbance

▶

Personal Identity Disturbance is the inability
to define oneself as a unique human being living in
a social environment, or to recall one's personal
characteristics and life history.

OVERVIEW

A person's identity is more than a name and a
social security number. A person's identity is
equated in the most fundamental sense with existence and *being*. A Personal Identity Disturbance
results from confusion about who one *really* is or
from assuming an identity or personality that
clashes with individual or societal expectations. A
serious threat to the self-concept, the nature of the
Personal Identity Disturbance varies with the
cause of the condition and the surrounding circumstances. The intensity may range from relatively mild to severe—from someone experiencing
a mid-life crisis to someone suffering from a prolonged episode of psychosis or severe cognitive
deficits.

Less extreme but still painful disturbances in
personal identity may occur with maturational and
situational crises. Confusion about "who I really
am" is a normal part of growth as one proceeds
through various developmental stages.[5] However,
in transition between stages, people often experience strong feelings of anxiety, conflict, ambivalence, and frustration related to their fears about
the loss of familiar roles and responsibilities and
the challenges of new ones.[2,4,11] Their sense of
identity is shaken as they respond to their own
expectations and those of others about their evolving selves. They must struggle to reformulate
their identities as they accomplish developmental

and occupational tasks and continue their life's
work.[4,5,11]

Life circumstances also dictate the adjustment
of personal identity. Some examples of events that
affect identity are the death of a spouse, the loss of
a job,[4] status as a minority member of society,[8] immigration or relocation to a different cultural setting, such as a nursing home,[9,12] sexual abuse,[3,13]
and the onset of debilitating illness.[7] Some people
experience little disturbance in personal identity,
and others have great difficulty as they try to cope
with crises and change.

More extreme disturbances in identity are characterized by severe confusion about or even denial
of one's identity.[3,7,10] Mental illnesses such as
dementia, schizophrenia, mania, depression, and
borderline personality and dissociative identity
disorders may result in severe disturbances in
personal identity.[1] In these disorders a combination of physiological, psychological, sociocultural,
and spiritual factors interact to disrupt personal
identity, cognition, affect, and functional behavior.
Affected individuals lose the ability to perceive
themselves and the environment realistically.[14] It
is as if they view the interaction between self and
environment through a distorted lens. This distortion of reality transforms their sense of knowing
who they are into their being strangers to themselves, a condition of being "not me." The strange-
ness becomes reinforced by others who react in a
puzzled, anxious, or rejecting way to the "strange
identity." As the disturbed individuals become
more and more estranged from their original identities, they become highly anxious and confused
about the world. Unable to integrate their behavior with the demands of society, their fragmented,

diffuse sense of self leads to the total disintegration of their personalities.[3,7,10,15]

In addition to interpersonal dynamics, pathophysiology can cause a Personal Identity Disturbance. Any disruption in the brain's normal structure and function may affect the sense of personal identity. Psychoactive drugs such as cocaine, narcotics, hypnotics, hallucinogens, and alcohol, may cause extreme but usually temporary changes in identity.[6] Memory loss, as seen in posttraumatic stress disorder and Alzheimer's disease, has grave and permanent effects on identity.[3,12,13] Traumatic injuries to the brain and cerebrovascular accidents may cause identity disturbances. Virtually any insult to the brain that affects perception, cognition, or motor functioning may ultimately result in a Personal Identity Disturbance.[1]

ASSESSMENT

The nurse begins to assess the patient's sense of personal identity while taking a thorough nursing history and conducting a health assessment. The nurse must obtain information from the patient about Functional Health Patterns, particularly the Cognitive-Perceptual and Self-Perception—Self-Concept Patterns. A comprehensive assessment of the individual, including the physical, psychological, sociocultural, and spiritual dimensions, is necessary because the possible causes of a Personal Identity Disturbance are so varied and because related factors are crucial in determining treatment and outcomes. The nurse uses therapeutic communication techniques to guide the assessment of the patient's sense of personal vulnerability and perceptions of threat from within the self or in the environment. Asking about major stressors and recent traumatic events may help to pinpoint the cause of significant changes in perception and behavior.[14]

Establishing a therapeutic relationship is key to decreasing the patient's anxiety and permitting exploration of sensitive topics. The nurse continues the in-depth assessment by asking open-ended questions, which provide the patient an opportunity to share thoughts and feelings about his or her sense of self and usual coping patterns. As the nurse talks to and observes the patient, the patient will reveal his or her sense of identity or lack of identity through verbal and nonverbal behavior.[14] The nurse then evaluates this information about personal identity in terms of the patient's age, gender and sexual preference, ethnicity, developmental stage, family relations, socioeconomic status, social roles, value system, and community.[7,10,13] The nurse also considers the appropriateness to the time and place of the patient's behavioral responses, the congruence between verbal and nonverbal behavior, and the intensity of accompanying emotions, particularly the level of anxiety. Because a person's identity is so unique and because a disturbance may be manifested in such a variety of ways, there is no *single* question or observation of behavior that will provide sufficient evidence for the nurse to make this diagnosis. Examples of assessment questions are in the box on page 603.

The nurse may need to examine other sources of data that influence or have an impact on the patient's sense or personal identity, such as school performance, work role, social support, environmental stimulation, and community events. The patient's family and friends may provide important information about the patient's recent and past behavior that contribute to and validate the nurse's clinical impressions.

A thorough assessment may not be necessary, however, when the patient exhibits obvious disorientation or confusion or has sustained a head trauma or a period of unconsciousness. Then a screening question such as "What is your name?" may be sufficient to diagnose a Personal Identity Disturbance when the patient's response is compared to known facts or a given history.

■ Defining Characteristics

The presence of the following defining characteristics indicates that the patient may be experiencing Personal Identity Disturbance:

- Ambivalence
- Confusion
- Disorientation
- Memory loss

- Hallucinations
- Sense of "not being myself"
- Depersonalization
- Alienation
- Blurred boundaries
- Narcissism
- Anxiety
- Fear
- ~~Secretiveness~~
- Delusions
- Social withdrawal
- Incongruent verbal and nonverbal behavior
- Inappropriate behavior
- Change in appearance or routine
- Loss of meaning in life

■ Related Factors

The following related factors are associated with Personal Identity Disturbance:

- Biochemical imbalances in the brain
- Structural changes in the brain
- Traumatic injury to the brain
- Impairment of sensory organs
- Use of psychoactive drugs
- Ingestion or inhalation of toxic chemicals
- Bodily injury or illness

- Stages of growth and development
- Role conflict and strain
- Conflict in values and morals
- Situational crises
- Disrupted interpersonal relationships
- Dysfunctional family processes
- Cultural discontinuity
- Discrimination and prejudice
- Deviant lifestyle
- Homelessness
- Cult indoctrination

DIAGNOSIS

■ Differential Nursing Diagnosis

A primary nursing diagnosis of Personal Identity Disturbance is indicated when the patient is unable to comprehend and communicate accurately who he or she *is*. The diagnosis of Personal Identity Disturbance is based on the nurse's assessment of the patient's thoughts, affect, and behavior expressed within the context of interview and examination. With a disturbance in identity, the patient will emphatically communicate some degree of anxiety—from moderate discomfort to overt panic—depending on the cause and extent of disturbance.[3,15] The nurse uses emphatic com-

VII

QUESTIONS TO ASSESS PERSONAL IDENTITY

- How would you describe yourself?
- How would you compare your *real* self to your *ideal* self? (How you really are, compared to who you would like to be.)
- Is the way you see yourself *now* different from the way you saw yourself in the *past*? If so, what are the differences? What caused the changes?
- How do you see yourself changing the future? What would you like to change about yourself?
- Do you feel comfortable with who you are? If not, what makes you feel comfortable about yourself?
- Are the important people in your life comfortable with who you are? If not, what makes them uncomfortable?
- Do you sometimes feel uncertain or confused about who you really are? If so, when do you feel this way? Give me an example.
- Do you ever experience a sense of unreality about who you are or about where you fit in the scheme of things? If so, when do you feel this way? Tell me about this feeling.
- Do you ever have a sense of being "not me"? If so, when do you feel this way? Do others tell you about times when you are acting strange or not at all like yourself? Give me an example.
- Do you ever feel as if you are really some other person or as if you do not really exist? If so, when do you feel this way? Tell me about one time.

munication to distinguish whether Anxiety should be designated as the primary nursing diagnosis or as secondary to Personal Identity Disturbance. (See pages 552 to 553 for assessment of Anxiety.) If, in the nurse's clinical judgment, the disturbance in personal identity is more directly attributable to a psychobiological trauma and somewhat transient, the patient's primary diagnosis may be Anxiety.[3,13] Once the anxiety is managed or worked through, the Personal Identity Disturbance will resolve. However, if the loss of identity is pervasive and prolonged, Anxiety may be secondary to the patient's recognition of a progressive and permanent disability affecting cognition and memory. When the underlying medical condition cannot be reversed, the patient's identity will continue to erode, with an increase in the accompanying anxiety and disorientation.[7,15]

■ Medical and Psychiatric Diagnoses

Personal Identity Disturbance is most commonly associated with: (1) psychiatric disorders that manifest signs and symptoms of severe psychological distress; (2) organic brain disorders that reflect dysfunction in the areas of memory, cognition, and ability for self-care; and (3) medical conditions that interrupt the normal neurophysiology of the brain.[1] Posttraumatic stress disorder, dissociative identity disorder, and brief psychotic disorder are examples of psychiatric diagnoses based on the patient's reactions to stress and trauma. The loss of identity or "creation" of a new identity is a protective mechanism to withstand the overwhelming stress of traumatic situations. Dementia of Alzheimer's type and dementia due to HIV disease are examples of psychiatric diagnoses based on the behavioral changes that accompany the destruction of brain tissue due to infection or unknown etiology. Delirium from alcohol withdrawal, toxic chemical poisoning, and hyperthermia may also produce signs and symptoms of confusion, disorientation, and hallucinations. The changes to the person's identity and personality may be temporary or permanent, gradual and subtle, or sudden and dramatic, depending on the nature of the causative agent or event. Medical diagnosis and treatment decisions will be made with the disorder's characteristic pattern of onset, duration, and trajectory in mind. The nurse participates with the health care team in establishing a differential diagnosis by comprehensively evaluating the patient's pattern of behavioral symptoms and contributing factors.

OUTCOME IDENTIFICATION, PLANNING, AND IMPLEMENTATION

After a diagnosis of Personal Identity Disturbance is made and the related factors are determined, the nurse works with the patient and health care team to determine the expected outcomes of treatment. The patient's level of awareness about the health problem must be determined first. Patients with a disturbed sense of identity will vary in self-awareness, but most are sufficiently uncomfortable that they acknowledge there is a problem and willingly accept some assistance from the nurse. In the absence of severe organic damage, the nurse should consider the patient as an active partner in designing an appropriate plan of care. In cases of dementia, the nurse should strive to engage the patient in the care plan to the full extent of his or her capabilities, taking note of the patient's personal preferences, habits, and patterns of daily living. Through the nurse-patient relationship, the nurse may preserve and strengthen the patient's sense of self while working with the health care team to address the physical and physiological symptoms of the underlying disease process or psychiatric disorder.

The overall outcome for a person with a Personal Identity Disturbance is to restore and maintain a coherent sense of identity. To reach the primary outcome, the nurse and the patient must focus on several intermediate outcomes. The first outcome is that the patient will relate feelings of distress or anxiety to a sense of "not being myself" or a loss of identity. Having a sense of depersonalization or self-alienation engenders a high level of anxiety. Therefore reducing the anxiety that accompanies a disturbed sense of identity takes priority. Interventions to decrease anxiety are based on the understanding that when the patient's needs are not met and his or her usual ways of coping do not work, the patient may resort to less functional behavior to obtain relief or may dissociate the self from painful feelings or the stressful environment. The patient may manifest anxiety in many different behaviors, such as passivity and withdrawal, extreme nervousness, hallucinations and delusions, bizarre behavior, or incoherent thoughts. The nurse will work to develop a trusting relationship and decrease anxiety by conveying acceptance and respect, listening for clues about the relation between the patient's distress and ways of coping, using every opportunity to confirm the patient's identity, and meeting the patient's needs as much as possible. The nurse must help the patient to identify unmet needs and to examine the relationships among unmet needs, ineffective coping, and the resulting uncomfortable feelings. Throughout the process of decreasing the patient's anxiety, the nurse uses his or her own healthy sense of self to convey acceptance, empathy, and respect for the patient's unique way of "being in the world."

Next, the predominant factors—developmental, psychosocial, and physical—related to the Personal Identity Disturbance must be considered. An outcome that addresses developmental issues is that the patient will understand the evolution of self in terms of developmental stages, past ways of coping, stressors in the current situation, and personal life goals. The nurse uses a crisis intervention approach within a limited time frame to focus on the present situation and surrounding circumstances. The nurse explores the patient's perception of self, evaluates the effectiveness of the patient's coping behaviors, and determines the availability of social supports. Drawing on knowledge of growth, development, and normative process (such as the grief process), the nurse educates the patient about the thoughts and feelings others commonly experience during similar maturational and situational crises.

When psychosocial factors are most prominent, the nurse's best approach is an ongoing, one-to-one therapeutic interaction. The outcome is that the patient will identify competencies and resources to strengthen his or her personal identity. This is accomplished through exploration of the patient's major roles, relationships, significant life events, and valuable past experiences. The patient's problem with identity may be long-standing, with negative feelings about the self and maladaptive social interactions entrenched in his or her own psyche. However, with the nurse's help the patient can explore thoughts, feelings, and events related to self and formative relationships. As family dynamics and significant childhood experiences are discussed, the nurse may help the patient to work through the associated pain and trauma. Creating a supportive environment, the nurse encourages the patient to explore different facets of the self, inner conflicts, boundaries between the self and the environment, and the meaning of personal existence. Over time the patient comes to a new understanding of his or her part in family dramas and the social community and begins to appreciate the corresponding parts and responsibilities of significant others. The patient is encouraged to test perceptions of reality and to learn new coping behaviors. Specifically, the nurse uses therapeutic communication techniques, such as active listening, clarifying unclear meanings, validating perceptions, modeling self-disclosure, and expressing genuine interest. These interventions facilitate the patient's use of interpersonal competencies, ways of coping, and social resources to build a healthy identity.

To achieve the primary outcome, a restored coherent personal identity, the patient will articulate a clear sense of self. With the nurse's help the client learns to verbalize thoughts, wishes, and feelings using "I" statements to convey a sense of differentiation between self and nonself and the presence of intact ego boundaries. The nurse designs interventions to clarify the patient's self-conception, including the difference between the real self and the ideal self. The nurse engages the patient in role play, role modeling, and role rehearsal. The patient learns to match verbal with nonverbal behavior, to practice presentation of self in simulated social situations, and to elicit social support from others. As the patient exhibits a coherent personal identity, the nurse reinforces new learned behavior and encourages the patient to seek validation from others in the environment for the healthy self and to mobilize social support.

When disturbances in personal identity are caused by physical factors, the disturbance tends to be progressive and permanent or chronic in nature. A successful outcome for the patient with Alzheimer's disease or HIV-related dementia is that the patient will live in a respectful, caring, protective environment and ultimately have a peaceful death. The nurse's interventions must focus on respecting the patient as a unique human being, orienting the patient to the environment, providing appropriate stimuli and activities for the patient, managing the patient's difficult behaviors, and maintaining the patient's personal safety and the safety of others on the unit. The use of memory devices, orienting materials, sensory stimuli, structured activities, exercise, and environmental barriers may be helpful when the brain is severely damaged or cognitive functioning is impaired. In some situations the use of behavioral techniques, such as modeling of targeted behaviors and positive reinforcement, may support the less severely affected patient's sense of self. However, there are often no interventions that will enable the impaired person to regain a true sense of identity. This may be devastating when the individual's self-awareness is still somewhat intact. In this instance, the nurse must be sensitive to the patient's pervasive sense of confusion. Interventions include anticipating the patient's needs, repeating concrete information and specific directions as necessary, providing environmental stimulation, using distraction to avoid conflicts, eliminating environmental hazards, protecting the patient's dignity in social situations, and respecting the patient at all times. In addition, the nurse may need to assess and plan for the needs of the patient's caregivers to prevent their becoming overwhelmed with the tremendous burden of the patient's need for full-time care.

◀ NURSING CARE GUIDELINES

Nursing Diagnosis: Personal Identity Disturbance

Expected Outcome: The patient will relate feelings of distress or anxiety to a sense of "not being myself" or a loss of identity within 24 hours.

- Use therapeutic communication techniques *to establish a trusting relationship that conveys acceptance and caring and facilitates exploration of the patient's identity, needs, and problems.*
- Use crisis intervention techniques *to determine whether the patient presents a risk to self or others because of anxiety, disorientation, confusion, or other symptoms of Personal Identity Disturbance.*
- Elicit the patient's perceptions of identity and reality, ways of coping, and available support systems *to establish a baseline and plan for future interventions.*
- ▲ Meet the patient's needs as much as possible to decrease anxiety *because a highly anxious patient is acutely uncomfortable and unable to engage in problem solving and other therapeutic tasks.*

Expected Outcome: The patient will begin to understand the evolution of self and identity in terms of developmental stages, life experiences, and personal goals before discharge from the unit or the midpoint in outpatient treatment.

- Encourage the patient to verbalize distress or anxious feelings *to gain an understanding of the relationships among his or her own perspective of identity, needs, current symptoms, and stressful situations.*
- Clarify the patient's expectations about self and others, ways of coping, and unmet needs *to comprehend the dynamics of the patient's identity disturbance and to identify alternative ways* to address the patient's needs and restore a coherent identity.

■ = nursing intervention; ▲ = collaborative intervention.

- Do a genogram with the patient *to explore family dynamics and discover patterns of interaction and historical events that influence identity development.*
- ▲ Discuss perceived stressors and the dynamics of a stressful situation with the team and the patient *to help the patient make corrections among situations, events, interactions with family and other people, and the patient's evolving perceptions of identity and sense of self.*

Expected Outcome: The patient will identify competencies and resources to strengthen his or her personal identity before the end of treatment.
- Explore positive attributes, negative self-conceptions, ego strengths and weakness, and major roles and achievements with the patient *to determine the areas of competence and confidence on which to build a coherent identity.*
- Assist the patient to identify life priorities, important values, and sources of motivation *to give directions to identity-enhancing activities and future plans.*
- Assist the patient in exploring personal goals, competencies, and life expectancies *to determine whether they are realistic and appropriate, given the patient's age, gender, sexual orientation, developmental stage, ethnicity, and socioeconomic circumstances.*
- Teach the patient about developmental stages, tasks, and other normative life processes *to provide a context for the patient to understand and cope with his or her own struggles and crises as part of the human condition.*
- ▲ Work with the health care team to provide reinforcement and consistent feedback to the patient *to support realistic expressions of personal identity and to strengthen new adaptive behaviors.*

Expected Outcome: The patient will demonstrate a restored sense of personal identity 1 year after completion of treatment.
- Use self-efficacy and communication techniques such as role play, role modeling, and role rehearsal with the patient *to develop the interpersonal skills and social behaviors that are the basis of a strong sense of personal identity and competency.*
- Assist the patient in testing alternative identities and in practicing new behaviors in a safe, accepting, interpersonal environment *to form realistic expectations for personal competence and to prepare the patient for the reactions of others in the "real world."*
- Give positive affirmations of the patient's identity and competent behaviors *to increase insight, expand self-awareness, build ego strength, and reinforce adaptive coping.*
- ▲ Prepare the patient for the termination of treatment with the team *so that the patient has the tools to continue to practice and strengthen new interpersonal skills that reflect a coherent sense of identity.*

Expected Outcome: The patient with dementia will live in a respectful, caring, and protective environment that meets his or her need for a dependent lifestyle.
- Assess the patient's cognitive, affective, and behavioral competencies *to make plans for and determine appropriate expectations of the patient's reality orientation, functional behavior, emotional status, social interaction, and self-care activities.*
- Provide a consistent, safe environment and routine of daily activities that take into consideration the patient's preferences, habits, and present capabilities *to minimize the patient's need to make decisions or deal with changes that may be upsetting, decrease the feelings of isolation and unreality, support his or her sense of identity and normalization, and prevent accidents or self-harm.*
- Use reminiscence therapy *to preserve long-term memory function as long as possible and to provide a pleasant means of social exchange between the patient and others.*
- ▲ Work with the team to communicate a compassionate and caring attitude *to reassure the patient and family that, despite the patient's loss of personal identity, the team will continue to provide care that affirms the patient's sense of worth and dignity.*

VII

VII

EVALUATION

The hallmarks of a healthy identity are the person's affirmed self-differentiation, coherent presentation of self, appropriate role behavior, and well-articulated value system. When the nurse's interventions are successful, the patient exhibits a clear sense of identity, a reduction in anxiety and other distressful feelings, consistency in presentation of self, patterns of behavior that are appropriate to the sociocultural situation, and the ability to relate to others in a way that can be validated consensually.

When the person has a Personal Identity Disturbance, it takes time to integrate fully a coherent sense of self and act accordingly. Crisis interventions are designed to help the patient recognize personal distress, assess the stressful situation, and mobilize support within a short period of time. If the patient is unable to respond to the nurse's use of crisis intervention, further attention must be paid to decreasing the patient's anxiety. In addition to providing a reassuring presence, the nurse may use measures such as reducing the demands for information and decision making, identifying the safety needs of the patient to protect against self-harm or harm to others, and assessing complicating factors or underlying pathology to make the patient more comfortable.

The patient shows an understanding of the evolutionary process of personal identity when he or she can review family history, childhood development, and life experiences with the nurse and begins to connect the pieces and extract meaning about his or her sense of self and way of being. Patients who lack insight, have impaired memory function, or are too threatened by the memories of past traumas may not be able to engage in this type of life review. The nurse should take a cue from the patient and respond to the feeling tone of the patient's discourse, affirming the patient's identity and conveying positive regard. A longer time frame may be necessary to allow the patient to develop enough trust in the nurse-patient relationship to confront painful past events.

Patients who make positive statements about themselves do not view themselves as victims, confront feelings of guilt, anger, and depression, reexamine negative self-conceptions, set priorities, and manage anxiety in a constructive way have the tools to access inner resources and interpersonal skills. Gradually patients develop more self-awareness of these personal competencies, which provide internal self-consistency, foster goal attainment, and allow meaningful interaction with others. Patients who do not make progress may need more time and more opportunities to explore personal issues and to practice interpersonal skills in a nonthreatening environment.

In addition to working with the patient, the nurse must interact with the family and others in the community. Building a strong identity involves group and family participation as the patient reestablishes boundaries, redefines roles, resolves interpersonal conflicts, and reenters the community in a meaningful way. Through interactions with the patient and family, the nurse may detect behavioral signs that reflect gains or losses in the patient's personal identity and movement toward health or illness.

The patient with dementia who has a dependent lifestyle because of cognitive impairments will gradually lose his or her sense of identity. The nurse must revise the plan of care in light of the patient's remaining capabilities and progressive disability. Providing comfort, a safe environment, and recognition of the patient's unique identity throughout the rest of the patient's life are appropriate goals.

◼ CASE STUDY WITH PLAN OF CARE

Tanya B., an African-American 16-year-old girl, was walking home from school with her friend Tina. As they passed the playground, shots rang out from a "drive-by" shooting. Tanya turned to find Tina slumped unconscious on the ground, with blood seeping from a wound in her head. When the police and the ambulance came, the EMS team pushed Tanya aside, and they administered emergency care before rushing Tina to the hospital.

The next day, the nurse noticed Tanya sitting quietly in a corner in the ER waiting room. Tanya was whispering to herself and shaking her head. She was clutching a large plastic bag stuffed with clothes. When the nurse asked Tanya her name, she would not or could not volunteer it. She said, "I've come to take Tina home. Tina is my true self and we can never be separated. Give Tina her clothes, and tell her we got to go home right now! I've waited long enough." The nurse remembered that a young girl had died in the ER the day before of a massive brain injury from a bullet wound. As compassion-

ately as she could, she told Tanya about her friend's death. Tanya just stared at the nurse for several minutes; then she became incoherent and disorganized. She jumped up and began to pace about the room, mumbling under her breath. Suddenly she lunged at the nurse, screaming, "You're a liar! Did you kill her? I AM Tina . . . How could I be dead? I hate you. Tanya's going to kill you! Tina, help me!" The nurse called for assistance as she stayed in the room with Tanya.

▛ PLAN OF CARE FOR TANYA B.
Nursing Diagnosis: Personal Identity Disturbance Related to a Traumatic Event

---

Expected Outcome: Tanya will express her feelings of anxiety and grief related to the trauma of witnessing her friend's violent death.
- Use a calm, reassuring approach toward Tanya and remain in the room with her.
- Assess Tanya's level of anxiety and meet her needs for safety and comfort.
- Orient Tanya to her surroundings and the present context of her situation.
- Obtain identifying information and confirm Tanya's identity by addressing her by name.
- Ask open-ended questions to help Tanya describe the traumatic event.
- Help Tanya to acknowledge and describe her feelings of distress, fear, and guilt.
- ▲ Notify Tanya's family and request that they come to the ER to meet with the team.

Expected Outcome: Tanya will examine her sense of self and perception of reality.
- Create a supportive atmosphere to facilitate trust.
- Encourage Tanya to talk about her relationship with Tina.
- Support Tanya's use of appropriate defense mechanisms.
- Use assessment questions and therapeutic communication to help Tanya focus on her sense of self and the reality of her friend's traumatic death.
- Explore Tanya's feelings of alienation, unreality, and confusion about her boundaries.
- ▲ Enlist support for Tanya from family, peers, and her community, church, and school.

Expected Outcome: Tanya will identify personal resources and areas of competence to sustain her while she works through her grief reaction.
- Assist Tanya to identify personal strengths and abilities that can help her resolve her feelings related to the traumatic event.
- Teach Tanya how to enhance her self-awareness of inner strengths, positive attributes, and usual adaptive responses to difficult situations.
- Discuss Tanya's previous ways of coping and their effectiveness.
- Identify other losses Tanya has suffered and how she responded to them.
- Assist Tanya to discuss other situations that make her feel anxious, guilty, or depressed.
- ▲ Introduce Tanya to a support group of adolescents with a similar cultural background who have experienced traumatic events.

Expected Outcome: Tanya will regain her personal identity and an accurate perception of reality.
- Instill hope for Tanya to develop a positive outlook toward her future.
- Help Tanya expand her spiritual sense of self and practice her religion, as appropriate.
- Explore ways to help Tanya incorporate the meaning of her friend's into her life experience.
- ▲ Teach Tanya how to seek support from family, friends, and the community.

■ = nursing intervention; ▲ = collaborative intervention.   *Continued*

▪ PLAN OF CARE FOR TANYA B. — CONT'D

▲ Provide reality checks on Tanya's perceptions of events, her interactions with others, and their responses to her.

▲ Check "homework" assignments (e.g., writing in her diary, telling her mother about her achievements in school, and inviting a friend to go the movies) to evaluate Tanya's progress toward recovery and integration of her personal identity.

▪ CRITICAL THINKING EXERCISES

1. Tanya is in the ER waiting room with the nurse. Which of Tanya's verbal and nonverbal behaviors indicate that she has a Personal Identity Disturbance? On the basis of what you observe, could you differentiate whether these behaviors were caused by a psychological or physiological condition? Would that differentiation affect the way you interacted with Tanya at that moment? Why or why not?

2. How should the nurse respond to Tanya's threatening behavior? If you were the nurse, what would you do first, and why? What would you say to Tanya? Why do you think Tanya is being so aggressive? How does her behavior relate to the traumatic event?

3. Tanya's favorite teacher has asked you to design an intervention to deal with violence among adolescents in the school. What would be the main goal of your intervention? How would you get Tanya and her classmates to participate in the activities you planned? What would you need to know to make the intervention culturally sensitive? When would be the best time to do the intervention? How would you measure the desired outcome? Who would pay for your time and materials?

REFERENCES

1. American Psychiatric Association: *Diagnostic and statistical manual of mental disorders,* ed 4, Washington, D.C., 1994, The Association.

2. Bradby M: Status passage into nursing: another view of the process of socialization into nursing, *J Adv Nurs* 15(10): 1220–1225, 1990.

3. Burgess AW, Hartman CR, and Clemens Jr PT: Biology of memory and trauma, *J Psychosoc Nurs* 33(3):16–26, 1995.

4. Dorn FJ: Occupational wellness: the integration of career identity and personal identity, *J Counsel Dev* 71(2):176–178, 1992.

5. Erikson EH: *Identity: youth and crisis,* New York, 1968, WW Norton.

6. Glod CA: Major uses of psychopharmacology in the emergency department, *J Emerg Nurs* 20:33–37, 1994.

7. Harvath TA and others: Dementia-related behavior in Alzheimer's disease and AIDS, *J Psychosoc Nurs* 33(1): 35–39, 1995.

8. Johnson D: Stress, depression, substance abuse and racism, *Amer Indian Alaska Native Mental Health Res* 6(1): 29–33, 1994.

9. Kovatch CR: Evolving images of human dignity, *J Geront Nurs* 21(7):5–6, 1995.

10. Littrell KH and Freeman LY: Maximizing psychosocial interventions, *J Amer Psychiatr Nurs Assn* 1(6):214–218, 1995.

11. Nicholls JG, McKenzie M, and Shufro J: Schoolwork, homework, life's work: the experience of students with and without learning disabilities, *J Learning Disabilities* 27(9): 562–569, 1994.

12. Rentz CA: Reminiscence: a supportive intervention for the person with Alzheimer's disease, *J Psychosoc Nurs* 33(11): 15–20, 1995.

13. Shea CA: Management of violence in society. In Haber JA and others, editors: *Comprehensive psychiatric nursing,* ed 5, St. Louis, in press, Mosby–Year Book.

14. Stein KF: Affect instability in adults with borderline personality disorder, *Arch Psychiatr Nurs* X(1):32–40, 1996.

15. Volicer L, Hurley AC, and Mahoney E: Management of behavioral symptoms of dementia, *Nurs Home Med* 3(12): 300–306, 1995.

VII

Powerlessness

▶ _____

Powerlessness *is the perception that one's own action will not significantly affect an outcome or that one lacks control over a current situation or immediate happening.*[9]

OVERVIEW

Every individual, whether well or ill, has a desire for control.[4,22] Averill[2] discusses three types of personal control: behavioral, cognitive, and decisional. These types of control are reflected in a recent definition of *Powerlessness* as a state in which an individual perceives a lack of personal control over certain events or situations, which impacts the individual's outlook, goals, and lifestyle.[4] Nurses frequently encounter individuals within their practice who are experiencing control issues that adversely affect their health.

Most individuals are subject to feelings of Powerlessness in varying degrees in various situations. An individual's response to loss of control depends on the meaning of loss, on individual patterns of coping, on personal characteristics (psychological, sociological, cultural, and spiritual), and on the response of others.[4,16] The diagnostic category of Powerlessness can be used to describe individuals who respond to loss of control with apathy, anger, or depression.[4] Feelings of Powerlessness may be obvious or subtle, conscious or unconscious, related to long-standing personality traits, or influenced by the immediate situation. Miller[10] has identified seven personal power resources—physical strength and reserve, psychological stamina and support network, positive self-concept, energy, knowledge, motivation, and belief system (hope)—and suggests that compromise of one

or more of these resources may result in Powerlessness.

Powerlessness can have deleterious effects on an individual's physical and emotional states. According to an extensive body of research reviewed by Miller,[11] Powerlessness adversely affects acquisition and retention of material, results in reduced tolerance for aversive stimuli, impairs task performance under adverse environmental conditions, alters mood with manifestations of depressive symptoms, increases stress levels, and may lead to maladaptive coping responses and even death.

Powerlessness is thought to exist on a helplessness and hopelessness continuum.[11] Helplessness is a response learned from repeated exposure to events that one cannot control.[19] This response can apply generally across various situations and can be unlearned. For some persons repeated, unremitting hardships can cause helplessness, but for others seemingly minor mishaps may evoke the feeling. With the continued perception that outcomes are independent of responses, the individual fails to initiate effective interventions and a feeling of Powerlessness ensues. Miller[11] postulates that if Powerlessness is not contained, a cycle of lowered self-esteem and depression occurs, followed by hopelessness.

The behavioral significance of Powerlessness has been established primarily with respect to social learning. Rotter's[17] Social Learning Theory has contributed to the locus of control concept through the proposition that, with time, relatively stable personality characteristics develop and influence the individual's perception of a given situation. Internal and external loci of control can be differentiated. A person high in internal locus of control perceives that events are contingent on the individual's own behavior, actions, and characteristics. One who believes that fate, chance, luck, powerful people, and unpredictable, complex forces dictate life events is generally high in external locus of control. Confronted with illness, a person with a high internal locus of control might educate him- or herself to regain the sense of control, whereas a person high in external locus of control might be unable to perceive his or her actions as affecting the outcome. A person with an external locus of control seems to be more prone to developing Powerlessness.[4] An individual's general expectancy for controlling an outcome governs his or her attention to and acquisition of available information.[19] Powerlessness leads to poor learning of information that would increase the individual's control. Powerlessness is viewed as a form of alienation, as are meaninglessness, normlessness, and estrangement from culture and self.

Johnson[8] introduced the concept of Powerlessness to nursing, noting that the concept may assist in the understanding of patient behavior. Johnson used Seeman's[18] definition of Powerlessness—the expectancy or probability held by the individual that his or her own behavior cannot determine the outcomes or reinforcements he or she seeks—and identified an association between Powerlessness and Rotter's[17] Social Learning Theory.

Two types of Powerlessness have been described: trait and situational.[21] Trait Powerlessness is all-encompassing, including the general affect, lifestyle, and attitude of the individual. Situational Powerlessness may occur in any individual who lacks control in a specific event or circumstance and is probably short lived. Carpenito[4] suggests that the nursing diagnosis Powerlessness may be more clinically useful when used to describe a person experiencing trait Powerlessness rather than situational Powerlessness.

A sense of power and control is normally gained gradually through developmental achievements across childhood and adolescence. Young children are usually externally controlled and Powerlessness is expected. As the child matures, an internal sense of control emerges with an increasing sense of power. Adolescence, however, is a very challenging time as the questions of control and power become central issues. Children and adolescents are particularly vulnerable to Powerlessness during times of illness and hospitalization and at such other times when their coping mechanisms are challenged.[11] Children can gain mastery over stressful situations by participating in play activities while ill or hospitalized.

There is considerable research evidence that points to the importance of power or control in the lives of older adults.[11] For the elderly, vulnerability to Powerlessness increases through the often cumulative multiple losses and stresses that the older generation experiences.[12] Many elderly persons have fewer intact resources such as stamina, resiliency, physical strength, support systems, energy, financial resources, and the motivation to improve their health and adhere to treatment regimens. Psychological stressors, such as the death of loved ones, retirement, relocation, and the physiological changes that accompany aging, may heighten the tendency of the aging person to feel powerless. The added stressors of illness and institutionalization only compound feelings of Powerlessness.

The potential for Powerlessness is often present during acute illness, irrespective of age, particularly when the symptoms are intense and unrelenting, when the illness is particularly debilitating, when the individual has not had much experience with illness, or when the evaluation and diagnosis are extended or intrusive. When chronic illness imposes lifelong adaptation along with a fluctuating health state, ongoing deterioration, intrusive diagnostic and treatment measures, and technology that may be unfamiliar and difficult for the patient to understand, the nurse should again be alert to the risk of increased vulnerability and Powerlessness.[11,25] Eighty-five percent of persons 65 years of age and older have at least one chronic illness.[14] Strain[22] lists eight categories of psychological reaction to chronic illness: (1) the perceived threat to self-esteem and body intactness that challenges the belief that the individual controls his or her own body; (2) fear of losing approval or love, which evolves from the patient's fears that illness and dependence on others will lead to withdrawal; (3) fear of losing control of body parts and their functions with resulting loss of independence; (4) anxiety resulting from separation from loved ones and a familiar environment that provided support, gratification, and a sense of intactness; (5) fear of injury to or complete loss of body parts; (6) guilt and fear of retaliation for incurring the health problem or losing control; (7) fear of pain; and (8) fear of strangers providing intimate care. These experiences can potentiate the feeling of Powerlessness in the chronically ill patient.

Feelings of Powerlessness may be experienced not only by the patient but by family members, particularly those members directly involved in caregiving. Davidhizar[5] found that, although most family members struggle to cope and often focus singlemindedly on the needs of the ill member, overwhelming feelings of Powerlessness often result. Davidhizar suggests that Powerlessness exists on a continuum from occasional feelings of Powerlessness to pervasive and overwhelming feelings of Powerlessness. The precise contribution of individual factors to feelings of Powerlessness is seen as unique to each situation. Three factors provide a conceptual framework for understanding feelings of Powerlessness in family members[5]: the person (personal characteristics, coping strategies, knowledge of illness and resources), the environment (socioemotional support and financial and caregiving resources), and the situation (the patient's degree of uncertainty and degree of anticipation, the characteristics of the illness, and exposure to chronic illness).

The diagnosis of Powerlessness can be particularly challenging in planning care for individuals from other cultures. In Latin America and Asia certain behaviors we would define in our culture as Powerlessness would be an accepted response in their culture. For example, the concept of fatalism, that events are predetermined (e.g., what will be, will be) and that individuals are powerless and have little control over their own lives is accepted and not perceived as a problem. This may pose a challenge to a nurse who is trying to initiate a lifestyle change for better health.[15] Accepted practices in

other cultures, such as *enytro* in the Japanese culture and *yin-nor* in the Chinese culture, may also greatly challenge the nurse's efforts to initiate health-promoting activities to address the diagnosis of Powerlessness.[15,24] The Japanese value of *enytro* (self-control) requires in the individual a humbleness in expectations and an unwillingness to intrude on another's time, energy, or resources. The Chinese practice *yin-nor* is showing an uncomplaining attitude in the face of adversity and displaying tolerance under painful conditions. *Enytro* and *yin-nor* are expected and accepted in both cultures and would not be diagnosed as Powerlessness in those cultures. American Indians, particularly the Sioux-speaking people, deal with problems by invoking a form of "cultural time out" (*wacinko*).[15] During *wacinko* the individual withdraws from society and slows down physically and socially. In the Anglo-Saxon culture, *wacinko* would be diagnosed as a reactive depressive illness, when, in fact, *wacinko* is the solution, not the problem, in the American Indian culture. Powerlessness may be a purposeful act by refugees, particularly the Cambodian people, who have experienced or witnessed torture and rape and have remained alive in their country by practicing *Tiing moovng*, "a dummy personality."[15] To survive in their home country, individuals acted as if they were stupid, deaf, and dumb and learned to obey rules without questioning. Now, in a new country they continue to portray *Tiing moovng* because they are afraid to express their feelings. These cultural beliefs and others pose a challenge for the nurse in diagnosing Powerlessness and in developing effective strategies to work with these individuals.

ASSESSMENT

Powerlessness is a subjective state; therefore all inferences made concerning a patient's feelings of Powerlessness must be validated by the nurse through interview and observation of the patient's actual participation in care and through a review of historical and diagnostic data obtained from the medical record. Skill is required in collecting information from nonverbal cues and inferences and in pulling together diverse bits of information.

Discussion with family members and significant others may reveal additional information about the patient's coping style and personality characteristics. Subjective and objective data may be gathered from the patient through the use of closed and open-ended questions and through observation. The nurse needs to assess each individual to determine his or her usual level of control and decision making and the effects that losing elements of control have had on the person.

In addition, the effect of the person's developmental and cultural practices on control issues needs to be assessed. The nurse should carefully assess the patient for the presence of defining characteristics of Powerlessness (e.g., verbal expressions of passivity and having no control).[13] The nurse may hypothesize the degree of Powerlessness that exists by tracking the frequency and persistence of certain behaviors. For example, withdrawal and lack of participation in care can provide clues to underlying and pervasive feelings of Powerlessness. Related factors have been identified that may contribute to the likelihood of a patient's developing Powerlessness (e.g., health care environment, interpersonal interaction, illness-related regimens, and lifestyle of helplessness) and their presence needs to be determined.[7]

In the actual health care environment, technology and language may be unfamiliar to the patient. Staff members may dehumanize the patient by removing personal possessions, ignoring privacy needs, limiting access to authority figures, watching over him or her excessively, and restricting access to needed equipment. The occurrence of such interpersonal interactions must be determined because they may discourage the patient's involvement in self-care, deny the patient's participation in scheduling, reinforce previous interpersonal failures, or diminish the patient's fragile sense of control over his or her health care. Another significant related factor for which the patient must be assessed is the actual illness-related regimen, which may include progressive physical deterioration that threatens physical integrity; alteration in body appearance and/or mental status; changes in sexual, social, and occupational functioning; and constant adaptation to

the demands of the illness. The patient must also be assessed for a history of helplessness, dependence on others, and poor self-esteem. Medical illness and prognosis and the patient's past experiences with illness, level of knowledge, commonly employed coping strategies, and availability of support systems complete the assessment parameters.[23,26,27]

Interviewing by the nurse can include questions such as "How would you describe your ability to control or cure your present health problem (high, moderate, fair, or poor)? To what do you attribute your ability to control (preventive measure, others, no control, or fate or luck)?" Nurses must also examine their own habits of professional practice for evidence of unconscious reinforcement of dependency and for failure to allow sufficient opportunity for patients to participate in decisions about their care. Miller[12] coined the term *nurse-induced dependency* for this specific type of dependency.

There are two tools currently available to guide the nurse in the assessment of potential or actual powerlessness. Carpenito[4] developed a guide for systematically obtaining relevant objective patient data (participation in grooming and hygiene care; information-seeking behaviors; response to limits placed on decision making and self-control behaviors) and subjective patient data (decision-making patterns, role responsibilities, and perception of control). This guide is helpful in determining a patient's level of control and decision making and the subsequent effects on the individual if these are lost or given up. Miller and Oertel[12] developed a behavioral assessment observational guide that helps systematize patient assessment related to the diagnosis of potential or actual Powerlessness. The tool was developed through field work with the elderly, although it is felt to be applicable to adults of all ages. The guide contains four categories of assessment data: verbal response (expressions of lack of control, giving up, or fatalism); emotional response (withdrawal, pessimism, anger, or submissiveness), participation in activities of daily living (nonparticipation or disinterest), and lack of involvement in learning about self-care responsibilities (lack of knowledge, lack of motivation, or lack of questioning).

It is important to note that factors affecting Powerlessness are very complex and vary from patient to patient. What seems like overwhelming stress for one person may appear to precipitate only a mild reaction, what seems like minimal stress for others may cause a pervasive feeling of Powerlessness.[5] Longitudinal assessment is necessary to take into account possible changes in stressors and the patient's responses to these changes and losses.

■ Defining Characteristics

The presence of the following characteristics indicates that the patient may be experiencing Powerlessness[9]:

Severe

- Verbal expressions of having no control or influence over situation or outcomes
- Apathy
- Verbal expressions of having no control over self-care
- Depression over physical deterioration that occurs despite patient compliance with regimens

Moderate

- Nonparticipation in care or decision making when opportunities are provided
- Expressions of dissatisfaction and frustration over inability to perform previous tasks and/or activities
- Absence of monitoring of own progress
- Expression of doubt regarding role performance
- Reluctance to express true feelings, fearing alienation from caregivers
- Inability to seek information regarding care
- Dependence on others, which may result in irritability, resentment, anger, and guilt
- Lack of defense of self-care practices when challenged

Low

- Expressions of uncertainty about fluctuating energy levels
- Passivity

■ Related Factors

The following related factors are associated with Powerlessness[9]:

- Illness-related regimen
- State of development
- Lifestyle of helplessness
- Interpersonal interaction
- Health care environment

DIAGNOSIS

■ Differential Nursing Diagnosis

Major competing diagnoses include Self-Care Deficit, Noncompliance, Helplessness, and Hopelessness. Differentiation must be made by the nurse between diagnoses if appropriate nursing interventions are to be initiated. Self-Care Deficit is the state in which the patient experiences an impaired motor function or cognitive function, causing a decreased ability to perform self-care activities.[3] Noncompliance describes the patient who desires to comply but is prevented from complying by the presence certain factors.[3] Helplessness is experienced when the patient is beset by a situation in which he or she perceives that his or her response will not affect the outcome. The Learned Helplessness Model hypothesizes that, with the continued perception that outcomes are independent of responses, the patient begins to fear taking any action.[6] Powerlessness builds on the concept of Helplessness with the individual responding to loss of control with apathy, anger, or depression. Hopelessness differs from Powerlessness in that a hopeless person sees no solution to his or her problem or no way to achieve what is desired, even if he or she feels in control of this life. A powerless person may see an alternative or answer to the problem yet be unable to do anything about it because of the perception of lack of control and resources. Prolonged Powerlessness may lead to hopelessness.

■ Medical and Psychiatric Diagnoses

Any disease process or mental condition, acute or chronic, can cause or contribute to Powerlessness. Common sources are related to inability to communicate secondary to cerebrovascular accident; inability to perform activities of daily living secondary to myocardial infarction and pain;

inability to perform role responsibilities secondary to arthritis or systemic lupus erythematosus; or related to progressive debilitating disease secondary to multiple sclerosis and cancer. Common mental conditions that may contribute to feelings of Powerlessness include substance abuse, schizophrenia, Alzheimer's disease, and AIDS.[1,4]

OUTCOME IDENTIFICATION, PLANNING, AND IMPLEMENTATION

The nurse in partnership with the patient identifies expected outcomes to be achieved within specified time frames and initiates multidimensional interventions to achieve them. Setting specific time frames for reaching the specified outcomes provides benchmarks for the patient, thus facilitating more control. Because feelings of Powerlessness usually result from various stressors, a variety of treatment approaches should be planned. Successful intervention with a patient who experiences Powerlessness requires a multidisciplinary team effort, including family, significant others, allied health care professionals, physicians, and social service and community agencies.[5]

The nurse employs nursing interventions and strategies to achieve the expected patient outcomes. The long-term expected outcome, of course, is integration of the therapeutic regimen into the individual's everyday life. Nursing strategies for alleviating Powerlessness and enhancing aspects of patient control are basic to nursing practice. They include (1) modifying the environment; (2) assisting the patient in setting realistic goals and expectations; (3) increasing the patient's knowledge; (4) increasing the sensitivity of health care team members and significant others to the patient's imposed Powerlessness; and (5) encouraging verbalization of feelings.[20] Interventions that allow patients to participate in their care enhance their behavioral control. Interventions that provide patients with knowledge, that solicit their input into situations, and that provide feedback increase patients' cognitive control. Interventions that allow the patient to make choices provide decisional control. Zerwekh[28] describes the role of the nurse as that of a partner and catalyst, empowering the "powerless patient" through the application of six strategies: (1) power through attention: the nurse as active listener; (2) power through identity: the nurse fosters insight; (3) power through knowledge: the nurse as teacher; (4) power through active choice: the nurse as advocate; (5) power through sustained network support: the nurse as facilitator; and (6) power through imagination: the nurse as visionary.

The expected outcome of an increased sense of control of one's situation and activities can be achieved using several strategies. Progress toward this outcome should begin to be evident within a short period of time, usually 2 weeks. The nurse can provide opportunities for the patient to express feelings about him- or herself and illness, provide appropriate information, engage the patient in decision making whenever possible, and modify the environment to increase patient involvement in self-care.

The expected outcome of identifying situations in which Powerlessness is felt is extremely important if appropriate strategies are to be initiated. The nurse can encourage a sense of partnership with the health care team, reinforce the patient's right to ask questions, and assist the patient to develop an awareness of events over which he or she has control and to examine situations in which Powerlessness is felt.

The expected outcome of enabling the patient to engage in problem solving behaviors that increase feelings of mastery often takes the longest period of time to accomplish and follows successful attainment of previous outcomes. Nursing interventions may include the alleviation of physical discomfort, teaching self-monitoring, providing relevant learning materials, evoking interest in mastering aspects of care, and providing positive reinforcement for increased patient involvement in self-care. It is imperative that the nurse employ strategies to involve family members and significant others, to utilize available support systems, to provide opportunities for the expression of positive emotions (hope, faith, a sense of purpose, and the will to live), and to support the patient's involvement in self-help groups, when indicated.

◢ NURSING CARE GUIDELINES
Nursing Diagnosis: Powerlessness

Expected Outcome: The patient will verbalize an increased sense of control over situation and activities within 2 weeks.

- ▲ Provide opportunities for the patient to express feelings about self and illness.
- ■ Explore reality perceptions and clarify if necessary by providing information or correcting misinformation.
- ■ Provide information and allow time to prepare for procedures.
- ▲ Provide consistent caregivers.
- ▲ Modify the environment, if necessary, to facilitate the patient's active involvement in self-care.
- ■ Engage the patient in decision making whenever possible (e.g., the selection of roommate or wearing apparel).
- ■ Provide children with opportunities to make decisions (e.g., getting time for bath or holding still for injection) and specific play therapy before and after a traumatic situation.
- ■ Set goals that are short-term, behavioral, practical, and realistic. Provide daily recognition of progress.
- ■ Help patient anticipate realistic sensory experiences that accompany procedures. Provide reality-oriented cognitive images that bolster a sense of control and coping strategies.
- ▲ Provide opportunities for family to express feelings and participate in care.
  These interventions enhance the potential for mastery over self-care and inspiring confidence in patient's personal capacity for coping.

Expected Outcome: The patient will identify situation in which Powerlessness is felt within 1 week.

- ■ Encourage sense of partnership with health care team.
- ▲ Limit incidents that may induce feeling of Powerlessness (e.g., staff use of medical jargon or focusing on unpredictability of procedural outcomes).
- ■ Reinforce the patient's right to ask questions.
- ■ Acknowledge and accept expression of angry feelings as manifestation of the patient's distress.
- ■ Help patient develop awareness of care aspects that are patient-controlled and separate from uncontrollable events.
- ■ Eliminate unpredictability of events by informing patient of scheduled tests and procedures.
- ■ Provide opportunities for privacy.
  These interventions provide opportunities for reinforcing cognitive control and enhancing interpersonal relationships with health care providers.

Expected Outcome: The patient will engage in problem-solving behaviors by the end of 2 weeks.

- ■ Encourage the patient's curiosity and interest in care.
- ■ Provide positive reinforcement for increasing involvement in self-care.
- ■ Teach self-monitoring (e.g., encourage the patient to keep a diary or records).
- ■ If contributing factors are pain and anxiety, provide information on how to use behavioral control techniques (e.g., relaxation, imagery, humor, and deep breathing).
- ■ Help patient communicate effectively with other health team members.
- ■ Provide relevant learning materials,
- ■ Alleviate physical discomfort that diminishes energy reserve.
- ■ Emphasize the positive; shift emphasis from what patient cannot do to what patient can do.
- ■ While being realistic, point out positive changes.
- ▲ Be alert for signs of health care providers making all decisions for patients.
- ▲ Give permission to use other power sources (e.g., prayer, stress reduction techniques, and self-help groups).
  These approaches focus coping capacities on specific care aspects, thus enabling the patient to adapt to lifestyle changes imposed by illness.

VII

■ = nursing intervention; ▲ = collaborative intervention.

EVALUATION

Powerlessness is not a state of being that develops quickly; therefore it is unrealistic to expect that reversing the factors contributing to Powerlessness will be simple. However, focusing on the day-to-day activities of the patient's world and setting day-by-day goals for increasing frequency of choice provide ample opportunity to measure progress toward enhancing the individual's control.

Self-reporting by the patient will provide the nurse with the most definitive evaluation of the success or failure of nursing interventions. The nurse should also be alert to patient behaviors that indicate feelings of gain, mastery of knowledge, increased skill in performing technical tasks, improved capacity and willingness to meet self-care demands, development of positive relationships with health care team members, actual compliance with the treatment regimen, and capacity to state present and future goals for him- or herself. Observation of self-care and reports of coping and adaptation by significant others will enhance the nurse's ability to evaluate the outcome. After the outcome criteria have been accomplished or feelings of Powerlessness are diminishing, the nurse and/or other members of the health care team need to discuss the process used to relieve Powerlessness with the patient, family members, and significant others. It is important to explain how factors contributed to the Powerlessness, to review why certain strategies were effective, and to discuss how the person will manage feelings of Powerlessness in the future. It is essential that the nurse advocate within the system to eliminate policies and routines that contribute to Powerlessness. Failure to achieve the outcome(s) may indicate underlying personality issues that may necessitate a referral for mental health counseling.

VII

◼ CASE STUDY WITH PLAN OF CARE

Mrs. Lucille B. is a 75-year-old ambulatory female experiencing her sixth hospitalization for uncontrolled diabetes and severe congestive heart failure. She is overweight, complains of frequent episodes of dyspnea, and has a restricted social life because of her diet. Her husband reports that she frequently does not take her medication, often eats what she wants, and no longer attends her program for weight control. Mrs. B. states that weight control and keeping away from sweets has been a "losing battle" since her adolescent years, and she denies that she does not take her medication.

◼ PLAN OF CARE FOR MRS. LUCILLE B.
Nursing Diagnosis: Powerlessness Related to Illness-Related Regimen

Expected Outcome: Mrs. B. will identify aspects of her current situation that make her feel powerless.
- ◼ Explore with Mrs. B. her concerns about her diabetes, congestive heart failure, and treatment regimens.
- ▲ Clarify perceptions and provide information as needed.
- ◼ Encourage discussion about body image, diabetic diet maintenance, and weight control.
- ◼ Explore concerns related to effect of illness on Mrs. B.'s social life.
- ▲ Point out positive changes that have occurred and are occurring.
- ◼ Help her to identify things that can be controlled and that are separate from uncontrollable events.

Expected Outcome: Mrs. B. will comply with medication schedules.
- ◼ Encourage self-monitoring and use of a daily dispenser for medications.
- ◼ Explore current daily medication schedule and suggest Mrs. B. coordinate medication with daily schedule.
- ◼ Encourage Mr. B. to provide positive reinforcement.

◼ = nursing intervention; ▲ = collaborative intervention.

Expected Outcome: Mrs. B. will integrate illness into her lifestyle.

- Help Mrs. B. to set short- and long-term goals that are realistic and attainable.
- ▲ Encourage a return to the weight-control group.
- ▲ Refer Mrs. B. to a dietitian for diet planning.
- ▲ Encourage participation in a diabetes support group.
- ▲ Encourage Mr. B. to support any positive gains his wife makes.
- ▲ Teach Mrs. B. the use of imagery and other relaxation techniques.

■ CRITICAL THINKING EXERCISES

1. What factors, conditions, and events have predisposed Mrs. B. to Powerlessness?
2. What personal power resources are compromised in the case of Mrs. B.? What strategies can the nurse use to empower Mrs. B.?
3. What potential role can Mrs. B.'s husband play in addressing Mrs. B.'s feeling of Powerlessness?
4. What referral to other health care providers, in addition to the dietitian, would you discuss with Mrs. B. to help her change her lifestyle and prevent complications?

REFERENCES

1. American Psychiatric Association: *Diagnostic and statistical manual of mental disorders,* ed 4, Washington, D.C., 1994, The Association.
2. Averill J: Personal control over aversive stimuli and its relationship to stress, *Psychol Bull* 80:286, 1973.
3. Carpenito L: *Handbook of nursing diagnosis,* ed 4, Philadelphia, 1991, JB Lippincott Co.
4. Carpenito L: *Nursing diagnosis,* ed 6, Philadelphia, 1995, JB Lippincott Co.
5. Davidhizar R: Understanding powerlessness in family member caregivers of the chronically ill, *Geriatr Nurs* (2): 66–69, 1992.
6. Drew B: Differentiation of hopelessness, helplessness, and powerlessness, using Erik Erikson's "roots of virtue," *Arch Psychiatr Nurs* IV(5):332–337, 1990.
7. Frick-Helms S: You make the diagnosis . . . *Nurs Diagnosis* 4(4):139, 166, 1993.
8. Johnson D: Powerlessness: a significant determinant of patient behavior? *J Nurs Ed* 6(2):39–44, 1967.
9. Kim M, McFarland GK, and McLane A: *Pocket guide to nursing diagnoses,* ed 6, St. Louis, 1995, Mosby–Year Book.
10. Miller J: *Coping with chronic illness: overcoming powerlessness,* Philadelphia, 1983, FA Davis.
11. Miller J: *Coping with chronic illness: overcoming powerlessness,* ed 2, Philadelphia, 1992, FA Davis.
12. Miller J and Oertel C: Powerlessness in the elderly: preventing hopelessness. In Miller J: *Coping with chronic illness: overcoming powerlessness,* Philadelphia, 1983, FA Davis.
13. Mullin D: Powerlessness: concept analysis and validation of the defining characteristics. In *North American Nursing Diagnosis Association,* Philadelphia, 1994, JB Lippincott Co.
14. O'Heath K: Powerlessness. In Mass M, Buckwalter K, and Hardy M, editors: *Nursing diagnoses and interventions for the elderly,* Redwood City, California, 1991, Addison-Wesley.
15. Pederson P and others, editors: *Counseling across cultures,* ed 4, Thousand Oaks, California, 1996, Sage Publications.
16. Rose K: An issue of powerlessness: psychosocial issues affecting breast cancer care, *J Clin Nurs* 3(3):155–158, 1994.
17. Rotter J: *Social learning and clinical psychology,* New York, 1954, Prentice-Hall.
18. Seeman M: The meaning of alienation, *Am Sociolog Revis* 24:783–791, 1967.
19. Seligman H: *Helplessness: on depression, development and death,* San Francisco, 1975, WH Freeman.
20. Stapleton S: Decreasing powerlessness in the chronically ill: a prototype. In Miller J: *Coping with chronic illness: overcoming powerlessness,* Philadelphia, 1983, FA Davis.
21. Stephenson C: Powerlessness and chronic illness: implications for nursing, *Baylor Nurs Educ* 1(1):17, 1970.
22. Strain J: Psychological reactions to chronic illness, *Psychiatr Quart* 51:173, 1979.
23. Walding M: Pain, anxiety, and powerlessness, *J Adv Nurs* 16(4):388-397, 1991.
24. Wallerstein N: Powerlessness, empowerment and health: implications for health promotion programs, *Am J Health Promo* 6(3):197–205, 1992.
25. Weisman A: Coping with illness. In Cassem N, editor: *Handbook of general hospital psychiatry,* St. Louis, 1991, Mosby–Year Book.
26. White B: Powerlessness and the pulmonary alveolar edema patient, *Dimen Crit Care Nurs* 12(3):127–131, 1993.
27. Zauszniewski J: Nursing diagnosis and depressive illness, *Nurs Diagnosis* 5(3):106–114, 1994.
28. Zerwekh J: Empowering the no longer patient, *Washington St J Nurs* 12:12–17, Summer/Autumn 1983.

VII

Self-Esteem Disturbance

▶ ──────────────────────────────────────

Situational Low Self-Esteem

▶ ──────────────────────────────────────

Chronic Low Self-Esteem

▶ ──────────────────────────────────────

Self-Esteem Disturbance *is a disruption in an individual's perceptions—an unrealistic self-evaluation or unrealistic feelings about the self or personal capabilities, which the individual may express directly or indirectly.*[13]

Situational Low Self-Esteem *is a negative self-evaluation or negative feelings about the self that develop in response to a loss or a change in an individual who previously had had a positive self-evaluation.*

Chronic Low Self-Esteem *is a long-standing negative self-evaluation or negative feelings about the self or personal capabilities.*

OVERVIEW

A review of the literature indicates that self-esteem can be viewed from more than one perspective and that it is a very complicated process, for which we are just beginning to identify behavioral consequences. Maslow[13] developed a hierarchy of five needs that an individual strives to meet. Self-esteem he noted as belonging to the fourth level of the hierarchy, esteem needs. He further asserted that everyone in society needed to have a high level of self-esteem that was stable and firmly based. Why does everyone need to feel valuable (to have high self-esteem)? One investigator con-

cluded that high self-esteem protects the individual from anxiety when facing a threat.[7]

However, the variables affecting self-esteem vary according to the individual and the circumstances. For instance, the cultural norm may vary from one country to another and within a given culture. One study of college students from 31 nations found that a greater correlation existed between financial satisfaction and life satisfaction for students from poor countries, whereas those in wealthier nations were influenced less by financial satisfaction. Finances would be considered a security need at the second level of Maslow's hierarchy. From this same study, men and women from the U.S. were above neutral for life satisfaction (83% and 82%, respectively) and self-esteem (82% and 72%, respectively), whereas men and women from Turkey reported low life satisfaction scores (39% and 47%, respectively) and higher self-esteem scores (78% each). Three other countries followed this pattern. Two oriental countries reported lower life satisfaction and self-esteem scores.[5] Although life satisfaction and self-esteem were highly correlated in the U.S., the strength of the relationship varied considerably in some cultures. In another study, which focused on oriental, black, and white women in the U.S., different variables were associated with high self-esteem. The positive variables for oriental women included the number of children, the unconflicted network size, and the number of positive events. For black women, education had a positive effect and a conflicted network size had a negative effect on self-esteem associations. For white women, the positive associations included nontraditional attitudes toward women's roles and higher income, whereas the number of negative life events and conflicted network size had negative effects. This study underscored the importance of the women's social networks for enhancing self-esteem (oriental women) or eroding self-esteem (black and white women).[18] Another study found differences between men and women who were HIV-seropositive. For women, satisfaction with life and a sense of purpose influenced their self-esteem. For men, self-esteem was associated with personal distinguishing achievements.[1] The findings of these studies emphasize that different individuals and cultures utilize different parameters for developing a positive sense of self-esteem. Additional studies are needed to verify and refine the relationship of variables such as these to self-esteem.

What is self-esteem? Rosenberg[15] defined self-esteem as the favorable or unfavorable attitude that an individual develops toward the self. Inherent within this definition are two factors to be considered. First, the individual *learns* to value the self, whether favorably or unfavorably. Basic self-esteem is learned during early life experiences and is relatively unchangeable. However, there is an aspect called *functional self-esteem* that can fluctuate greatly from one point in time to another. This aspect results from ongoing evaluations of the individual's interactions with his or her environment.[4] The second factor consists of the cognitive and attitudinal processes the individual uses in learning to value the self. Because these are interior processes occurring within the individual, the nurse validates with the patient the meaning of a given behavior or attitude. For instance, we usually think of people at risk for suicide as having low self-esteem. Yet a recent study found that frail people over the age of 85 in nursing homes were at greater risk for suicide if they expressed

high self-esteem and had a need to control their lives.[8]

The study cited previously indicated that high self-esteem may not always have positive consequences or be superior to low self-esteem. In some instances, those with very high self-esteem focus all of their energy and effort on enhancing their self-image. In life these people may bite off more than they can chew and thus place themselves at risk for physical and emotional problems.[2] Because of this they may not acknowledge self-defeating behaviors, such as nonacceptance of performance criticism, and they may exhibit poor self-regulation and reality testing. They may also persist in a task after they had succeeded at it or avoid a task after a humiliating failure. So they have difficulty changing maladaptive behavior because they overestimate their capacities and are overconfident.[2,17]

Those with low self-esteem want the same things that those with high self-esteem do: success, someone to love and admire them, fame, wealth, and so on. However, they have fewer resources to accomplish these wants; so they focus on avoiding failure, rejection, humiliation, or other disasters. Whereas individuals with high self-esteem use strategies to enhance credit for potential success, people with low self-esteem may use similar strategies for protection against implications of failure.[2,17] Similar behaviors by those with very high or very low self-esteem may have different reasons for being initiated.

Very high and very low self-esteem depend on distorted perceptions that frequently have been learned from past experiences. Such experiences by themselves do not cause a Self-Esteem Disturbance but do provide the parameters in which the distorted perceptions develop. A patient's past experiences become cues alerting the nurse to explore the individual's perceptions regarding those experiences and their effect on self-esteem. The same type of experience for two individuals may strengthen the self-esteem of one individual and contribute to a Self-Esteem Disturbance in another. The criteria that individuals use to de-

VII

velop their self-esteem are those to which they subscribe based on their cultural or ethnic background, age, sex, and familial and community mores and values.

In many instances, the Self-Esteem Disturbance encountered by nurses pertains to those involving low self-esteem. The expression of a negative self-evaluation or negative feelings may result from a specific situation (Situational Low Self-Esteem), or it may be the result of a long-standing negative self-evaluation (Chronic Low Self-Esteem).

Situational Low Self-Esteem occurs when individuals report the negative self-evaluation or negative feelings as a temporary event.[2] Usually it can be traced to a specific situation and frequently involves a significant loss to the person, such as a loss of an interpersonal relationship, perceived status, or perceived competency; difficulty in meeting expectations, and/or inability to reach a goal. Sometimes a biological or biochemical disturbance can precipitate such feelings until that abnormality is corrected. For example, strokes in certain parts of the brain, drugs that precipitate abnormal thinking or feeling patterns, or biochemical imbalances have been known to initiate Situational Low Self-Esteem.

Chronic Low Self-Esteem occurs when patients are unable to report or describe positive self-evaluations or positive feelings about the self on a long-standing basis.[2,16] The situation develops as the result of negative reinforcers from childhood or from significant losses later in life to which the patient cannot adjust. The extent to which genetics influences this disturbance has not been determined.

Any of life's experiences may adversely affect a patient's self-esteem or a component of it, depending on how a given individual evaluates the meaning personally.[3] Because of the complexity of the human personality, these factors interact with each other in a uniquely human way, so the effect of an event on a patient's self-esteem must be individually verified. Physiological parameters, which can also affect a person's self-esteem, include physical losses, medical illnesses, and some psychiatric illnesses.[6,11] Physical losses include but are not lim-

ited to areas of sexuality and reproduction, physical disfigurement, incapacity, or dismemberment. For example, a man who becomes impotent may think he is no longer a man and feel worthless. Another man, who is a good heavy-equipment operator, and who loses an arm and a leg in an accident, may think he is a failure because he can no longer work in construction. Or a woman may decide that she is no longer worthwhile because she is so crippled with arthritis that she can no longer care for herself. Chronic medical problems that create a permanent change in a patient's lifestyle or ability to function and that are perceived as having a negative consequence for that individual, can also disrupt a patient's self-esteem. Such problems include but are not limited to chronic renal problems, including the need for dialysis; traumatic injury to the spinal cord resulting in paralysis; chronic pulmonary or coronary diseases; any of the degenerative neurological or skeletal diseases; and cancers. Although a patient is at risk for developing Self-Esteem Disturbance as a consequence of a chronic medical problem, it is also possible to develop enhanced self-esteem because of accomplishments in spite of the problem.

Patients with mental disorders frequently exhibit Self-Esteem Disturbance.[6,16] Although many of these are considered to be primarily psychological in nature, several have physiological parameters as well. Examples of this include the dementias or drug and alcohol intoxication. Although dementias have physiological parameters, the problems these individuals experience in communicating their perceptions present the nurse with difficulties in accurately assessing their level of self-esteem. Some substance abusers may have distorted high self-esteem because they are frequently satisfied with themselves and see no need to change their behavior or their thinking.[12] In fact, they may insist that it is the responsibility of others to change. Only when they become dissatisfied with themselves by incorporating self-esteem that accurately reflects reality will they be motivated to change.

Psychologically related factors frequently pertain to disrupted or distorted thinking and feeling. These include but are not limited to expressions negating the self after a failure, a loss of role or lifestyle, or even success. If failure is attributed to the intrinsic worth of the patient, the feeling and attitude this fosters may prevent a patient from trying anything new or at least severely restrict the amount of risk the individual is willing to take.[2,17]

A loss of role or lifestyle could also lead to a low self-esteem disturbance. Examples include the loss of job, illness, changes in the ability to care for the self, and changes within the family.[13] For instance, a patient who is laid off from work and is unable to secure a new position may feel that he or she is no longer a valuable member of the family because of the inability to provide for the family. Or a patient may need to take a position with a lower salary and status, which can decrease that individual's self-esteem. Or a mother may feel that she is no longer providing a useful service when her last child leaves home so that she experiences lowered self-esteem until she has resolved the change in her role. If the individual cannot resolve the situationally lowered self-esteem, it may become chronically low.

One of the more insidious situations is the perception that the patient no longer has any control over a situation; that is, no matter what is done, the situation cannot be changed. This perception in its varying degrees immobilizes the patient and becomes devastating to his or her self-confidence and self-reliance and thus lowers self-esteem. Examples of such situations are those where an individual feels victimized (e.g., rape, abuse, robbery, or a violated confidence). Depending on the circumstances, the individual may generalize the experience(s) to all areas and develop Chronic Low Self-Esteem.

Social parameters can affect one's self-esteem and include all types of interpersonal interactions. Any statement or behavior indicating abnormally high or low self-esteem in relation to interpersonal relationships needs to be explored for Self-Esteem Disturbance. Only a few examples are given here to help identify areas where a patient might develop Self-Esteem Disturbance. Some patients develop low self-esteem, either chronic or situational, because of a lack of approval, respect, or love from others.[2,13,17] That lack, either real or a distorted perception of reality, decreases the individual's ability to function as effectively as he or she could if provided with adequate positive reinforcements. For example, children who do not receive adequate reinforcement for their positive attributes and whose parent(s) repeatedly inform them that they are bad, no good, or unable to do anything right will learn to express negative attitudes and feelings about the self that frequently result in Chronic Low Self-Esteem. Other psychological factors include negative interpretations of life events, such as involvement in environmental disasters, a change in living condition or residence, or assumption of guilt. Another example is the patient who is kept so dependent on another person that he or she does not learn the skills necessary for successful adjustment to life. This individual lacks self-confidence or self-reliance and experiences Chronic Low Self-Esteem as a result.

At some time or another, everyone will interact with someone who exults the self at the expense of others. Such an individual may be experiencing Situational or Chronic Low Self-Esteem. For example, an upper level manager comes into the hospital with an ulcer. During an interview, he says that he has worked his way up through the ranks and has worked hard to get where he is. He considers his former co-workers "bums" for not demonstrating a little initiative in trying to improve themselves. Depending on the length of time this misperception has been held, that individual might be expressing Chronic or Situational Low Self-Esteem.

Situational Low Self-Esteem may develop when an individual perceives that a significant other is emotionally distancing him- or herself. As a result, that individual may feel that he or she is not worthy of being loved and experiences a lowered self-esteem. Other changes in interpersonal relationships, such as the death of a significant other, can bring about the development of Situational Low Self-Esteem. For example, a family may lose a young child to an incurable illness, but the father, mother, or both may believe they failed as parents even when they did all that they could. Death,

VII

divorce, and separation are changes in interpersonal relationships that may be categorized as losses. Although they may start as factors in the development of Situational Low Self-Esteem, they can be influential in the development of Chronic Low Self-Esteem when a patient cannot reconstitute the previous positive self-evaluation by experiencing positive events.

Many of a patient's values and beliefs are developed in response to his or her cultural and spiritual expressions. The degree to which that patient thinks he or she meets the standard for these values and beliefs frequently related to that patient's level of self-esteem. A patient's self-esteem is also influenced by his or her perceptions of worth to the community, which may take into account his or her positive or negative characteristics or belief in the ability to function. For example, a physician and a trash collector may each believe they are valuable members of the community because they both contribute to the maintenance of health within a community. Or the trash collector may believe that he or she is not as valuable as the physician because of a lack of education or a perceived lack of status. The individual who places a lower value on his or her actions, thoughts, and feelings than on those of others, based on cultural and spiritual factors, may experience lowered Self-Esteem Disturbance. In another situation, a patient may think he or she is more important than others. The patient who thinks that an institution cannot survive without his or her support may experience unrealistically high self-esteem.

One factor that is not always assessed pertains to the purpose of an individual's life. The patient who has lost or never developed a purpose in life may believe there is no reason for his or her continued existence and that life no longer has much meaning or value. Without such a purpose, a Self-Esteem Disturbance exists. It may be Situational Low Self-Esteem or Chronic Low Self-Esteem, depending on the length of time the situation has existed.

Discrimination or acculturation pressures also can influence the development of an individual's self-esteem, either positively or negatively. Immigrants who have not been able to acculturate can develop serious physical or psychiatric conditions and may have a decreased life expectancy, particularly if they do not have a culturally significant support group. Within this group, the nurse needs to assess for posttraumatic stress syndrome[16] and the strength of the individual's self-esteem in relation to the culture of origin.

Basically, a Self-Esteem Disturbance could develop when a patient perceives any loss as important, regardless of what that loss was. The severity of the lowered self-esteem will be directly related to the perceived value or its meaning to the patient, whether or not there is a perceived replacement, and the degree to which that patient is willing to let go. Such losses may pertain to the body, to a patient's role or lifestyle, or to changes in interpersonal relationships.[1-3,6,8,14-18]

The complexity of self-esteem presents numerous problems in accurately and specifically assessing the extent and severity of Self-Esteem Disturbance and its role in health. For a tool to be useful to nursing, it needs to provide information and be easy to administer and score. One tool that meets these criteria is Rosenberg's Self-Esteem Scale (RSI).[15] Rosenberg's Self-Esteem Scale consists of 10 items with scores ranging from 0 (high self-esteem) to 6 (low self-esteem). The items address the individual's perceptions of worth, of being not good, of satisfactions with the self, of self-respect, of ability to function as well as others, of pride in something pertaining to the self, of possessing any good qualities, of feeling useful, and of attitude toward the self and whether the individual is a failure.

Two recent nursing studies used the RSI. One study used it to confirm aspects of low self-esteem from self-reports by pregnant substance abusers.[9] The other one used it for identifying differences in HIV-seropositive men and women.[1] So the RSI has a demonstrated relevance to clinical studies with implications for nursing practice.

In summary, an individual's self-esteem protects him or her against anxiety when threatened. It develops as a result of an individual's perceptions regarding life events. Therefore a multiplicity of related factors can contribute to the development of Self-Esteem Disturbance. In Situational Low Self-Esteem the related factors have occurred during the recent past. In Chronic Low Self-Esteem the related factors have occurred over time with little or no improvement. For a diagnosis of Chronic Low Self-Esteem, the defining characteristics indicating lower-than-average self-esteem must be present for an extended time or the important related factors must have occurred in the distant past.

ASSESSMENT

Self-Esteem Disturbance

In general, any verbalizations by the patient that indicate the individual has a negative perception about the self or personal capabilities can be used as evidence to support a diagnosis of Self-Esteem Disturbance.[4,6,8,15-17] The nurse also needs to validate the meaning of any given behavior with that patient because a specific behavior can express different meanings.[2,17]

Self-Esteem Disturbance can be suspected when individuals verbalize feelings of inferiority, such as not being as good as most people, or being worthless, no good, or inadequate. Patients also may make statements indicating that they feel adrift, with no direction to their lives, that nobody appreciates them, or that others treat them as if they are insignificant. Patients may verbalize negative feelings about the self, such as feeling disappointed or dissatisfied with themselves, unlovable, or unhappy. They may specify that they cannot experience pleasure, live up to expectations, feel useful, amount to anything, contribute anything, or think positively about the self. They may indicate one of the following: they have lost control of their lives; they have nothing in which they can take pride; nothing ever goes right for them; they have only contempt for themselves; or they are no good. Other statements that may indicate Self-Esteem Disturbance include expressions of feelings of being violated, such as after a rape, abuse, robbery, or betrayal of confidence. Verbalizations indicative of Self-Esteem Disturbance also include constant rumination about past failures, defeatist thinking, minimization of strengths, and critical or negative statements about the self. All of these verbalizations express negative feelings and attitudes about the self and indicate low self-esteem.[2,6,9,15,16]

The nurse needs to complete a very careful assessment of the patient's overall self-perceptions to discriminate between Situational or Chronic Low Self-Esteem and unrealistically high self-esteem. Statements indicating unrealistically high self-esteem include grandiose statements that elevate the patient above others and statements indicating that the patient can do better than what he or she realistically can be expected to do. A patient who appears to be satisfied with the self and indicates that there is no need to make *any* changes, even though he or she cannot function in the community, may report high self-esteem.[6,12] These could reflect a defense against low self-esteem. However, the clinician needs to start where the patient is, acknowledging the patient's perceptions, and plan interventions to assist the patient to change distorted perceptions in the desired direction.

Several behaviors may be indicative of Self-Esteem Disturbance, particularly if they form a pattern rather than occurring occasionally. Such behaviors include rigid, narrowly focused, or constricted thinking; lack of or refusal to participate in prescribed therapy or therapeutic activities; inability to follow through on treatment or other activities; or setting unrealistic goals that the patient cannot achieve. In addition, the patient may hesitate to offer opinions and viewpoints or to initiate activities. The patient may demonstrate a decrease in interpersonal interactions, for example, with the family or significant others; or even a decrease in involvement in life. A few patients may bully others to feel better about the self.

Patients with Self-Esteem Disturbance may reduce spontaneous behaviors and experience difficulty in defining the self or engaging in independent activity. They may also find it difficult to seek out new situations. Such patients may be underachievers or chronic procrastinators or may take

VII

longer than usual to relax in a situation. Sometimes body language may indicate that a patient is guarded and trying to protect the self; for example, eye contact may be poor, or the shoulders may curl inward, as if to protect the body. A patient's appearance also might indicate Self-Esteem Disturbance. The patient who does not but is able to perform activities of daily living, such as bathing, grooming, feeding, and toileting, may be expressing feelings of unworthiness, a manifestation of Self-Esteem Disturbance. Or perhaps the patient persists in dressing very inappropriately for the activity in which he or she is engaged (e.g., wearing formal attire, jewels, and furs while gardening). Again, behaviors indicative of Self-Esteem Disturbance should be verified by verbal statements that the patient is actually experiencing a disturbance in self-esteem. As noted earlier, any of these behaviors can have more than one meaning. It is only by validating the patient's perception of the behavior that the nurse can make an accurate assessment of Self-Esteem Disturbance.[1-3,6,9,14,16]

In addition to assessing for verbalizations and behaviors indicative of Self-Esteem Disturbance, the nurse needs to assess for the presence of this nursing diagnosis when other disturbances of self-perception or self-concept occur. These include but are not limited to Fear, Anxiety, Hopelessness, Powerlessness, body Image Disturbance, and Personality Disturbance. Some of the same defining characteristics for other nursing diagnoses, such as Hopelessness, also pertain to Disturbed Self-Esteem. Research is beginning to identify the role of self-esteem in other diagnoses.[2,16]

■ Defining Characteristics

The presence of the following defining characteristics indicates that the patient may be experiencing Self-Esteem Disturbance[6,11,14-16]:

- Anorexia or obesity
- Decrease in sexual relationships and drive
- Frequent expression of body aches and pains
- Overconcern with somatic woes
- Inability to assume responsibilities for self-care
- Homicidal or suicidal behaviors

- Timid, seclusive, pessimistic, unassertive, and/or unable to initiate, follow through, or complete a task in a timely fashion
- Despair, guilt, inferiority, inadequacy, failure, defeatism, frustration
- Denial of past or present successes and accomplishments
- Lack of eye contact, energy, attention to appearance, or initiative in problem solving
- Verbalizations of being unworthy of God's love and forgiveness
- Feelings of hopelessness, helplessness, powerlessness, disappointment, worthlessness, isolation, and depression
- Emotional distancing from significant others
- Withdrawal from activities and interpersonal social relationships
- Reluctance to engage in social interactions
- Resentment of others
- Perception of minimum strengths and assets with refusal to accept positive feedback
- Inability to accept criticism or extremely sensitive to it
- Lack of confidence in social situations
- Difficulties in job performance or perfectionism
- Fear of handling change, making decisions, taking risks, expressing anger, and relating to others

■ Related Factors

The following related factors are associated with Self-Esteem Disturbance[2,6,15,16]:

- Physical losses
- Medical illness
- Inability to adjust to alterations in body function
- Psychiatric illness
- Cognitive or perceptual problems
- Traumatic experiences
- Unresolved emotionally traumatic experiences
- Loss of control
- Negative interpretations of experiences
- Unrealistic expectations of self
- Inadequate knowledge or problem-solving skills for coping with life's stresses
- Loss of role or lifestyle
- Early loss of parent or significant other

- Lack of adequate positive feedback
- Repeated negative interpersonal experiences
- Ridiculed by others excessively
- Inadequate social support
- Perceived loss of relationship with God

Situational Low Self-Esteem

Situational Low Self-Esteem includes any of the general characteristics indicative of Self-Esteem Disturbance that are currently present but were not present before a given situation, and it may include expressions of shame and guilt or evaluation of the self as unable to handle situations and events. For example, a mother may state that since her child was seriously injured she has believed she is not an adequate mother. Or there may be a distinct change in behavior resulting from feelings of insufficiency. For example, a young man may have enjoyed flirting and talking with young women. He stopped this behavior when a girl he had asked for a date 2 months ago laughed at him and told him not to be ridiculous.

■ Defining Characteristics

The presence of the following defining characteristics indicates that the patient may be experiencing Situational Low Self-Esteem[2,11,16]:

- Episodic, negative self-appraisal in response to a sudden loss or change
- Negative verbalization about self in response to a sudden loss or change
- Difficulty making decisions caused by a sudden loss or change
- Expressions of shame or guilt and evaluating self as unable to handle situations or events in response to a sudden loss or change
- See also defining characteristics of Self-Esteem Disturbance

■ Related Factors

The following related factors are associated with Situational Low Self-Esteem:

Major loss(es) of

- Body part or functions

- Significant others
- Job, work, or role
- Pet
- Material goods
- Reputation

Major stress or change in life

- Marriage or divorce
- Prison term
- Addition or loss of a family member
- Failure in school, work, or a significant life event
- Financial problems
- Promotion or demotion
- Adolescent adjustment
- Sexual difficulties
- Hospitalization
- Occupational changes or other major moves
- Change in religious affiliation or practice

Environmental factors

- Disasters (natural or manmade)
- Poverty
- Change in residence or living conditions
- Discrimination
- Acculturation

Chronic Low Self-Esteem

Chronic Low Self-Esteem includes any of the previously cited characteristics of Self-Esteem Disturbance that are long-standing or cannot be traced to a specific situation (e.g., a frequent lack of success in life's activities, hesitation in trying new things or situations, alienation from others, and ruminations about past problems).*

■ Defining Characteristics

The presence of the following defining characteristics indicates that the patient may be experiencing Chronic Low Self-Esteem:

- Long-standing, low self-evaluation and feelings about self and abilities
- Frequent lack of success in life events or work

---

*References 2, 3, 6, 11, 14, 16.

- Pattern of hesitating to try new things or situations
- Long-term alienation from network of community resources
- Pattern of passivity and withdrawal from others
- Frequent ruminations about past problems over time
- See also defining characteristics of Self-Esteem Disturbance

■ Related Factors

The following related factors are associated with Chronic Low Self-Esteem:

- Long-standing negativity as a fixated life response
- Maladaptive fixated life response
- Isolated lifestyle pattern
- Long-term adverse childhood experiences

DIAGNOSIS

■ Differential Nursing Diagnosis

Within the cluster of Self-Esteem Disturbance diagnoses, Chronic Low Self-Esteem is used only if the disturbance is of an extended duration, whereas Situational Low Self-Esteem is used only if a specific situation within the recent past can be identified as the trigger for the disturbance. These areas have been highlighted because they have been identified as occurring more often than the others. In all other instances, the generic diagnosis Self-Esteem Disturbance can be applied as Self-Esteem Disturbance: Excessively High or Self-Esteem: Fluctuating/Labile. Several nursing diagnoses may include elements of Self-Esteem Disturbance that may be Chronic or Situational Low Self-Esteem: Dysfunctional Grieving, Hopelessness, Personal Identity Disturbance, Ineffective Individual Coping, Powerlessness, Sexual Dysfunction, and Risk for Violence: Self-Directed or Directed at Others.

■ Medical and Psychiatric Diagnoses

Situational Low Self-Esteem can be assessed with certain medical conditions that affect the self-concept, such as 607.84 male erectile disorder related to a medical problem. Or Chronic Low Self-Esteem may be diagnosed in psychiatric conditions such as 296.3x major depressive disorder recurrent, 300.4x dysthymic disorder, and eating disorders such as 307.1 anorexia nervosa and 307.51 bulimia nervosa. However, 301.6 borderline personality might have a Self-Esteem Disturbance that reflects an excessively high or fluctuating/labile disturbance.

OUTCOME IDENTIFICATION, PLANNING, AND IMPLEMENTATION

Self-esteem is learned as a result of the interaction between an individual's internal processes and the external environment. Patients can confirm or alter an existing perception of the self based on their perceptions of how they interact with the external environment.

Self-Esteem Disturbance

Nurses can use several techniques or approaches to help provide positive patient-nurse interactions from which the patient can learn to perceive the self positively. These include but are not limited to those specified in this chapter.

First, the nurse must use a nonjudgmental and empathic attitude at all times. This means that the nurse accepts the patient's expressed negative feelings about the self without belittling, criticizing, or demeaning the patient for expressing such feelings. Another technique is for the nurse to express unconditional regard for the patient, which communicates that the patient is of value or worthwhile and offers positive reinforcement for actual achievements. This also occurs when the nurse is congruent and genuine and demonstrates real interest, concern, and understanding without offering false praise. Improvement can also occur when the nurse recognizes the patient's experiences and knowledge while discouraging repeated conversations about past problems or failures.[2,11,14] With these approaches, the nurse provides a climate or external environment conducive to perceiving the self positively.

If the patient recognizes that a problem exists with self-esteem, the patient, the nurse, and the treatment team can identify and work through causative factors. The nurse and the team work with the patient to develop realistic goals and plans to change thinking, feeling, and behavior patterns. Changing entrenched habits of thinking, feeling, and behaving can be difficult and fraught with lapses. It is vital to be patient, to persevere, and to continue to reinforce the progress the patient makes.

Nurse-led groups and one-to-one relationships can provide patients with a nonthreatening, supportive environment in which they learn to respect themselves. The act of collaborating with patients to set realistic, mutually agreed upon goals can itself foster realistic, positive self-esteem. Exploring recurring family themes and patterns to correct misconceptions and to allow the development of newer, more positive conceptions also can enhance positive self-esteem. Groups provide a supportive environment to practice new behaviors and positive language patterns, to validate perceptions regarding self, and to identify maladaptive interpersonal interaction patterns.

Topics for the preceding types of interventions may include clarifying values and beliefs within a positive framework, developing assertiveness skills, learning how personal behavior influences the behavior of others, developing congruence between body language and feelings, and learning to accept and use positive criticism for growth and development. Patients also can validate perceptions of the emotions, statements, and behavior of others.

Sometimes it is necessary to intervene with the significant others to teach them appropriate interaction techniques. Significant others are not always aware how negative statements and lack of positive verbal and behavioral reinforcements on their part assisted the patients to develop disturbed self-esteem. If they develop interaction techniques that are positively reinforcing, the patient has a healthier interaction climate for maintaining the gains reached during treatment.

As noted previously, any situation or intervention can maintain and improve or can decrease a patient's self-esteem, depending on that patient's perception of the event. Nurses infer those changes based on the patient's self-reports and their interpretations of the patient's visible emotions and behaviors.

Volunteer and creative activities in which patients participate can also be used to improve distorted perceptions about the self and can reinforce the concept of making positive contributions to others and to the culture or to improve some aspect of themselves, such as physical fitness.

VII

◢ NURSING CARE GUIDELINES
Nursing Diagnosis: Self-Esteem Disturbance

Expected Outcome: The patient will perceive self in a positive light, as evidenced by making positive statements about the self and exhibiting congruent behavior; by identifying positive relationships and making an effort to maintain and improve them; and by setting realistic goals, initiating the required activities, and following through to reach them.
- Keep a nonjudgmental, empathic attitude.
- Express unconditional regard for the patient.
- Listen actively.
- Be congruent and genuine
  These four interventions provide a safe interpersonal environment for the patient.
- Recognize the patient's past experiences and knowledge.
- Discourage repeated conversations about past problems and failures.

■ = nursing intervention; ▲ = collaborative intervention.

◢ NURSING CARE GUIDELINES — CONT'D

- ▲ Facilitate patient involvement in activities such as helping others, contributing to the community, participating in creative arts and physical activities, and attending support or self-help groups. *These activities validate past experiences and provide the patient an opportunity to practice new behaviors.*
- ▲ Collaborate with patient in setting goals.
- ▲ Teach patient to use new language patterns, using positive statements.
- ▲ Facilitate patient education to clarify values and beliefs, to perceive negative influences, to behave assertively, to identify how personal behavior influences others, to develop congruence between feelings and body language, to learn to accept and use positive criticism, to validate perceptions, to improve interpersonal techniques, and to identify situations that damage self-esteem. *These activities or strategies facilitate personal and interpersonal growth and self-esteem.*
- ▪ Explore recurring family themes or patterns to correct faulty perceptions of self.
- ▪ Teach significant others appropriate interaction techniques.
- ▲ Help patient identify and participate in experiences that are satisfying and rewarding.
- ▲ Encourage patient to engage in individual or group psychotherapy.
- ▲ Increase opportunities for social interaction.
- ▲ Help patient accept responsibility for personal opinions and behavior and then evaluate their outcome in relation to options available.
- ▲ For patients with unrealistically high self-esteem, teach them to evaluate their failures and use that evaluation to set realistic goals for activities to correct distorted perceptions and to value the self accurately.

VII

Situational Low Self-Esteem

In those instances where the patient's self-esteem is higher than his or her capacity, teach the patient to learn from failures and to set realistic goals for his or her activities.

Interventions for Situational Low Self-Esteem include any of those used for Self-Esteem Disturbance but with a focus on changing distorted perceptions concerning a specific situation. Such interventions include an analysis of the situation, problem-solving techniques, and values clarification. Reality-based perceptions of a situation provide the mechanism for developing self-esteem that is congruent with a patient's capabilities and values.[2,11,14]

◢ NURSING CARE GUIDELINES
Nursing Diagnosis: Situational Low Self-Esteem

Expected Outcome: The patient will perceive the situation realistically, will acknowledge factors that decreased his or her self-esteem in the past, and will engage in corrective activities to restore or improve self-esteem.
- ▪ Use interventions specified in Self-Esteem Disturbance as appropriate.
- ▪ Assist patient to analyze situational factors to clarify values and correct distorted perceptions.
- ▲ Assist patient to develop strategies to help cope with loss, stress, or environment factors that can cause low self-esteem.
- ▪ Assist patient to engage in problem-solving activities and to identify behaviors that will help restore self-esteem.
  These strategies reduce length of time to return to previous or better self-esteem or to prevent Chronic Low Self-Esteem.

▪ = nursing intervention; ▲ = collaborative intervention.

Chronic Low Self-Esteem

Interventions for Chronic Low Self-Esteem include any of those used for Self-Esteem Disturbance but with a focus on changing deep-seated and long-term distortions about the self.[11,14] This focus assists patients to examine their life patterns over time and to determine the priority of modifying behaviors. Progress for these patients will be in small increments with a probability of relapses, which can engender discouragement. The nurse should continue to reinforce progress and acknowledge setbacks while supporting the concept that the patient can change.

■ **NURSING CARE GUIDELINES**
Nursing Diagnosis: Chronic Low Self-Esteem

Expected Outcome: The patient will increase frequency of positive statements pertaining to the self and will engage in corrective activities to restore/improve self-esteem.
- Use interventions specified in Self-Esteem Disturbance as appropriate.
- Assist patient to analyze situational factors to clarify values and correct distorted perceptions.
- Assist patient to engage in problem-solving activities and to identify behaviors that will help restore self-esteem.
- Plan for change to occur in small increments.
▲ Assist patient to identify family and community resources that will help improve his or her self-esteem.
These interventions support patient in making efforts to change self-concept in small increments.

■ = nursing intervention; ▲ = collaborative intervention.

VII

EVALUATION

To evaluate the effectiveness of the interventions, validate the patient's feelings and thoughts about the self. If these are realistically positive— at least more so than previously—the interventions brought about change in the desired direction. Observations of the patient's interactions with others can provide cues concerning the desired change and can help the nurse identify what to validate with the patient. If a tool was used to assess the patient's initial level of self-esteem, changes in the scores since then can also demonstrate the effectiveness of the interventions. The evaluation process can be a learning experience for the patient by identifying continuing problems and by providing information for the development of realistic goals concerning future activities.

Interventions for Situational Low Self-Esteem can be evaluated like those for Self-Esteem Disturbance are. If the interventions have been effective, the patient's self-esteem will return to the previous level or will improve. If this does not occur within a reasonable time, the diagnosis may need to be reevaluated and changed to Chronic Low Self-Esteem.

Chronic Low Self-Esteem also can be evaluated the way Self-Esteem Disturbance is. However, the changes toward more positive and realistic self-esteem may take place more slowly and to a lesser degree. There also may be lapses in progress when something occurs to trigger the old, low self-esteem thinking, emotional, and behavioral patterns. If this happens, the nurse should evaluate with the patient what occurred and should help identify approaches or activities to ameliorate the effects of the current traumatizing event.

▶ CASE STUDY WITH PLAN OF CARE

Mrs. Maria M. was admitted to the hospital for a cholecystectomy. She married at 17 and is now 21 with three preschool children. She and her family immigrated from Colombia 2 years ago and now live in a small two-bedroom apartment while they try to save money to purchase a house. During the past 3 months, the children have taken turns at being sick and fussy. Their medical expenditures have significantly reduced the family's savings. Mrs. M. is a nonsmoker, abstains from alcohol, and has no known physical problems other than the one for which she was admitted. Her vital signs are: blood pressure, 130/76; temperature, 99°F; pulse, 88 beats/min; respirations, 24/min; height, 5'4"; and weight, 160 lb. Her abdominal muscles are flaccid, with a tense body. She states that she has not regained her figure or lost the additional weight after her last pregnancy. Her activities include managing the family's finances and the house as well as caring for the children. She attends Mass on Sunday, and occasionally the family will go on a special outing. Her husband is too tired to do anything other than work at his job during the week. On weekends he also works at a part-time job to increase their meager income. They do not believe in using babysitters, so they don't go anywhere they can't take the children. Mrs. M. has one fairly close friend within the apartment complex who speaks Spanish and has two preschool children. Although both can speak some English, neither could be considered fluent in the language. She writes to her mother in Colombia and occasionally receives a letter from her. They have no other relatives in the United States.

During the course of several interactions with the nurse, Mrs. M. stated that she was not really worth the attention the nurse was giving her. As the nurse explored this statement, Mrs. M. stated that her husband was working too hard to support them and to help them get ahead and that she was endangering this because she let the children get sick so much, and now she needed surgery. She felt as if she could not do anything right because the children's illnesses and her surgery were using up all of their savings. She felt so tired after her third delivery and just did not have the energy to care for the children as she should have. Then just before she was admitted to the hospital her husband had stumbled on the children's toys when coming in from work. He could have seriously hurt himself, and then where would they be? Her husband was doing his part, but she was endangering their dreams because she could not keep the children and herself healthy. Also she had been unable to monitor the children's activities to ensure that no one would get injured. One of the nursing diagnoses the nurse formulated was Situational Low Self-Esteem related to the children's illnesses and her surgery, depleting the family's savings.

▶ PLAN OF CARE FOR MRS. MARIA M.

Nursing Diagnosis: Situational Low Self-Esteem Related to the Children's Illnesses and Her Surgery, Depleting the Family's Savings

Expected Outcome: Mrs. M. will experience improved self-esteem as evidenced by verbalizing positive statements regarding her ability to care for children and self and regarding her value and worth to her family and husband; by identifying and verbalizing to her husband her need for rest and expressions of appreciation for her contributions; and by involving herself in culturally related support, peer-group activities and other social or religious activities.

- Be nonjudgmental and empathic of Mrs. M.
- Be genuinely interested and concerned about Mrs. M.
- Discourage repetitious talking about inability to function as a wife and mother.
- Explore with and help Mrs. M. identify her strengths.
- Help Mrs. M. analyze her situation and identify actions she can take to improve it, such as talking with her priest to find out if there are church activities she would enjoy.
- Have Mrs. M. realistically evaluate the demands of caring for three preschool children.

■ = nursing intervention; ▲ = collaborative intervention.

- Provide Mrs. M. with an opportunity to learn assertive behavior within her cultural context.
- Explore assumptions behind Mrs. M.'s self-perceptions, and reinterpret them with a positive frame of reference.
- Assist her in exploring appropriate culturally relevant community supports (e.g., peer groups or religious activities).

■ CRITICAL THINKING EXERCISES

1. What factors were used to determine a nursing diagnosis of Situational Low Self-Esteem?
2. What information would be needed to change the diagnosis to Chronic Low Self-Esteem?
3. Which nursing interventions could use the assistance of Mr. M. in helping to modify Mrs. M.'s feelings about herself?
4. How would you evaluate the effectiveness of the nursing interventions pertaining to Mrs. M.?
5. What changes would you make in the nursing plan of care for Mrs. M.?

REFERENCES

1. Anderson SEH: Personality, appraisal, and adaptational outcomes in HIV-seropositive men and women, *Res Nurs Health* 18:303–312, 1995.
2. Baumeister RF, editor: *Self-esteem: the puzzle of low self-regard,* New York, 1993, Plenum Press.
3. Combs AW and Snygg D: *Individual behavior: a perceptual approach to behavior,* rev ed, New York, 1959, Harper & Row Publishers.
4. Crouch MA and Straub V: Enhancement of self-esteem in adults, *Family Community Health* Aug:65–78, 1983.
5. Diener E and Diener M: Cross-cultural correlates of life satisfaction and self-esteem, *J Personality Soc Psychol* 68(4):653–663, 1995.
6. Fitts W: *The self-concept and psychopathology,* Nashville, Tennessee, 1972, Counselor Recordings and Tests.
7. Greenberg J and others: Why do people need self-esteem? converging evidence that self-esteem serves an anxiety-buffering function, *J Personality and Soc Psychol* 63(6):913–922, 1992.
8. Haight BK: Suicide risk in frail elderly people relocated to nursing homes, *Geriatr Nurs* 16:104–107, 1995.
9. Higgins PG, Clough DH, and Wallerstedt C: Self-esteem of pregnant substance abusers, *Maternal-Child Nurs J* 23(3):75–81, 19—.
10. Josephs RA, Markus HR, and Tafarodi RW: Gender and self-esteem, *J Personality Soc Psychol* 63(3):391–402, 1992.
11. Kim MJ, McFarland GK, and McLane AM: *Pocket guide to nursing diagnoses,* ed 6, St. Louis, 1995, Mosby–Year Book.
12. Larson L: *Trust and self-esteem of psychiatric patients as perceived by the patients and psychiatric nurses,* Ann Arbor, Michigan, 1985, University Microfilms International.
13. Maslow AH: *Motivation and personality,* ed 2, New York, 1970, Harper & Row Publishers.
14. McFarland GK, Wasli EL, and Gerety EK: *Nursing diagnoses and process in psychiatric mental health nursing,* ed 2, Philadelphia, 1992, JB Lippincott Co.
15. Rosenberg M: *Society and the adolescent self-image,* Princeton, New Jersey, 1965, Princeton University Press.
16. Segal ZV and Blatt SJ: *The self in emotional distress,* New York, 1993, Guilford Press.
17. Tice DM: Esteem protection or enhancement? Self-handicapping motives and attributions differ by trait self-esteem, *J Personality Soc Psychol* 60(5):711–725, 1991.
18. Woods NF and others: Depressed mood and self-esteem in young Asian, black and white women in America,

VII

Risk for Self-Mutilation

▶

Risk for Self-Mutilation *is a state in which an individual is at risk to perform an act upon him- or herself to injure but not kill, which produces tissue damage and tension relief.*

OVERVIEW

Self-mutilation includes an array of behaviors, the essence of which is deliberate destruction of tissue without conscious suicidal intent. Moderate pathological self-mutilation is manifested as behaviors of self-biting, self-scratching, self-hitting, and hair pulling. Major self-mutilation includes eye enucleation, facial skinning, and amputation of limbs, breasts, or genitals.[3,15] The underlying dynamics and meaning of these behaviors are multiply determined and complex. The most common feelings reported by patients preceding self-mutilation include tension, self-anger, powerlessness, numbness, and overwhelming guilt, loneliness, and boredom.[3]

Self-mutilation has been correlated with childhood experiences of sexual or physical abuse and stormy or violent family interactions.[13,15,16] The loss of a parent from death or divorce and the occurrence of mental illness in family members, especially alcoholism, is also correlated with self-mutilation in adults.[11] In a study of 89 patients referred to an intensive case management program, 29 practiced self-mutilation. Of these patients, 71% reported being the victim of sexual abuse and 79% experienced physical abuse. Seventy-one percent of the self-mutilating patients were adult children of alcoholics.[11]

The reasons most often given by patients for these behaviors are to relieve tension, to vent anger, to relieve alienation, and to regain control over racing thoughts, fluctuating emotions, and unstable environments.[3,12,14] Patients engaging in major self-mutilation often indicate biblical influence, demonic possession, heavenly commands, atonement for sin, and sexual determinants for their behavior.[15]

ASSESSMENT

When assessing Risk for Self-Mutilation, the nurse should analyze the patient data for the presence or absence of early developmental correlates of adult self-mutilation, as well as current behaviors associated with this diagnosis. Sources of data include a nursing history, the nurse's observations of and interaction with the patient, the patient's perceptions of self and interaction with others, and feedback from significant others about the patient. Correlates of and current behaviors associated with self-mutilation must be significant in amount or severity to result in a diagnosis of Risk for Self-Mutilation.

In taking a history, the nurse must gather data regarding the patient's family history of violence, alcoholism, and physical and sexual abuse. The nurse must use effective interviewing and communication skills to elicit sensitively the patient data needed to plan nursing care. Studies have documented diffidence about abuse by the mental health system.[5,15] However, inquiry concerning these events validates the experience of the patient and opens up discussion and expression of feelings.

The nurse must assess the patient's ability to express feelings. Expression of feelings such as anxiety, anger, or depression can reduce the Risk of Self-Mutilation. However, the manner in which feelings are expressed must allow for management or resolution of the feeling.[1,9]

Impulse control is another critical assessment parameter. The patient experiencing stress who is able to utilize problem-solving abilities and evaluate his or her behavior increases personal control over impulsive behavior and reduces the Risk for Self-Mutilation.[1,9]

The patient's success and comfort with interpersonal relationships is another essential assessment parameter. Patients at risk for self-mutilation experience a personal identity disturbance, lack of self-differentiation, and impaired communication. These difficulties can affect interpersonal relationships. The patient at Risk for Self-Mutilation has difficulty acquiring the knowledge, attitudes, and skills for positive interactions with others, including family.

■ Risk Factors

The presence of the following behaviors, conditions, or circumstances in certain risk groups renders the patient more vulnerable to Risk for Self-Mutilation[6]:

Behaviors, conditions, or circumstances
- History of physical, emotional, or sexual abuse
- Inability to cope with increased psychological or physiological tension in a healthy manner
- Feelings of depression, rejection, self-hatred, separation anxiety, guilt, and depersonalization
- Fluctuating emotions
- Command hallucinations
- Need for sensory stimuli
- Parental emotional deprivation
- Dysfunctional family

Groups at risk
- Clients with borderline personality disorder, especially females 16 to 25 years of age
- Clients in psychotic state—frequently males in young adulthood
- Emotionally disturbed or battered children
- Mentally retarded and autistic children
- Clients with a history of self-injury

DIAGNOSIS

■ Differential Nursing Diagnosis

The nursing diagnosis Risk for Injury is differentiated from Risk for Self-Mutilation in that Risk for Injury is present when the patient is at risk as a result of the interaction of environmental conditions with the individual's adaptive and defensive resources. Self-mutilation differs from suicidal behavior with respect to intent and the nature of the injury. With self-mutilation the intent is relief from tension, and the wounds are superficial, numerous, and involve a portion of the body. In suicidal behavior the intent is to kill, and the wound is singular and deep.

The nursing diagnosis Risk for Self-Directed Violence differs from Risk for Self-Mutilation in that many of the identified risk factors for self-directed violence do not apply to individuals who injure themselves.

■ Medical and Psychiatric Diagnoses

Self-mutilating behavior occurs in patients with a variety of diagnoses. Self-mutilation is reported in patients with personality disorders, such as narcissistic and antisocial personality disorder, and is a diagnostic criterion for borderline personality. Self-mutilation may also occur in psychiatric diagnoses of obsessive-compulsive disorder, schizophrenia, and major depression, as well as in mental retardation and organic conditions.[3,9,12]

OUTCOME IDENTIFICATION, PLANNING, AND IMPLEMENTATION

Nursing interventions for patients at Risk for Self-Mutilation focus on the appropriate expression of feelings, control of impulses, and positive interactions with significant others. When selecting nursing interventions, consideration must be given to the specific risk factors, such as the presence of psychotic, character, or organic disorders; violence and sexual or physical abuse in the family; and destructive feelings that are present. Environmental, developmental, and cultural

VII

◢ NURSING CARE GUIDELINES
Nursing Diagnosis: Risk for Self-Mutilation*

Expected Outcome: The patient will express feelings appropriately.
- Develop trust through consistency and reliability. *Trust is essential to establishing an interpersonal relationship conducive to expressing one's feelings.*
- Designate same staff as much as possible to work with patient. *A sense of consistency facilitates expression of feelings.*
- Create a nonthreatening environment. *A sense of being safe in the environment enhances the patient's ability to express feelings.*
- Teach patient to name the feeling state being experienced. *Identification of feeling is the precursor to description of feeling state.*
- Assist patient to identify situations that precipitate feelings. *Teaching the patient to analyze situations for precipitants facilitates his or her ability to express feelings appropriately.*
- Support the use of appropriate defense mechanisms and expression of feelings *to reduce acting-out behaviors.*

Expected Outcome: The patient will experience fewer episodes of impulsive behavior.
- Assist patient to replace faulty interpretations of perceived stressors with reality-based interpretations. *Improving patient's ability to interpret stressors accurately reduces Risk for Self-Mutilation.*
- Explore with patient past successes in reducing stress *to capitalize use of patient's strengths.*
- Develop with patient a plan to reduce stress. *An increase in stressors can precipitate self-mutilation.*
- Instruct patient on stress reduction techniques and assertive skills. *Reducing patient's stress increases his or her control over impulsive behavior.*
- Set limits on inappropriate behavior *to assist patient in differentiating appropriate from inappropriate responses.*
- Demonstrate and teach problem-solving skills. *Increasing patient's ability to solve problems and to think through consequences of actions expands the patient's range of behavioral responses.*
- Assist patient to identify advantages and disadvantages of alternatives for behaviors *to lessen patient's sense of entrapment and to widen his or her perspective on the situation.*
- Teach patient to evaluate personal behavior. *Increasing the patient's ability to solve problems and to think through the consequences of actions expands the patient's range of behavioral responses.*

Expected Outcome: The patient will interact positively with significant others.
- Relay unconditional positive regard for patient *to raise patient's self-esteem.*
- Assist patient in identifying positive attributes of self. *Identification of strengths and repeated positive interactions with others and the environment improve the patient's self-regard.*
- Engage patient in values clarification, self-appraisal, and identification of ideal self *to develop a clearer sense of self-identity.*
- Explore situations in which patient overidentifies with others. *Self-differentiation enhances self-identity.*
- Assess degree to which patient's self-perception is affected by dysfunctional relationships. *Correlation exists between self-mutilation and disrupted or dysfunctional relationships.*
- Demonstrate interpersonal skills through role playing. *Improvement in interpersonal skills contributes to mastery of the environment.*
- Encourage patient to carry out familial roles and responsibilities that reinforce positive feelings and interaction *to decrease stressors or threats to self.*

■ = nursing intervention; ▲ = collaborative intervention.
*References 1, 2, 4, 6–9, 13, 15, 16.

factors may also affect the selection of nursing interventions.

The appropriate expression of feelings reduces the patient's Risk for Self-Mutilation. The feelings preceding self-mutilation most commonly reported by patients include tension, depression, self-anger, powerlessness, depersonalization, numbness, and overwhelming guilt, loneliness, and boredom.[3,9,10] These feelings mount according to the patient's perception of the situation. Often, before the patient is aware of the situation and the related feelings, an emotional outburst occurs.[8]

An essential feature of self-mutilation is lack of impulse control. The patient believes that he or she is trapped in a stressful situation and experiences a narrowed perspective of the situation and the alternatives.[3] The patient experiences an absence of or an inability to use problem-solving skill. Because an increase in stressors may precipitate self-mutilation, improving the patient's ability to interpret and reduce stressors accurately decreases the risk for self-mutilation.

Instability of self-image, identity disturbance, and the resulting dysfunctional relationships are characteristic of the person who self-mutilates. Instability of self-image is often experienced as chronic feelings of boredom or emptiness. Identity disturbance is pervasive and is demonstrated by uncertainty about sexuality, career choice, selection of friends, and values. Interpersonal relationships are intense, unstable, and overidealized or devalued. A focus for nursing interventions is providing the patient the experiences and feedback that foster self-regard.

EVALUATION

Evaluation of the nursing interventions to reduce the Risk for Self-Mutilation is determined by the patient's attainment of the identified expected outcomes. Achievement of the patient outcomes is assessed through the nurse's observation of and interaction with the patient, the patient's evaluation of his or her tendency toward self-mutilation, and feedback from others. If the identified limitations are no longer present and the patient demonstrates the ability to express feelings appropriately, control impulses, and interact positively with others, the expected patient outcomes have been achieved, and the Risk for Self-Mutilation has been reduced. If expected outcomes have not been achieved, the patient is assessed for presence of risk factors. A revised plan for care is developed, implemented, and evaluated.

VII

◼ CASE STUDY WITH PLAN OF CARE

Sandra P. is 20 years old and unemployed and currently lives with her mother. She has been brought to the mental health clinic by her younger sister, who states, "I have had it. If you don't do something, someone is going to be hurt at home." Ms. P. is described by her sister as moody, with frequent outbursts of anger often directed at her parents. Their father recently entered a residential facility for the treatment of chronic alcoholism.

There is a history of violence within the family. Ms. P. was taken several occasions to the emergency room for treatment of injuries inflicted by her father. Ms. P. reports feelings of anxiety, emptiness, and boredom. "I can't seem to hang on to friends or a job. Every time I think I have figured out who I want to be with and what I want to do, something happens, and I lose my friends and my job."

▶ PLAN OF CARE FOR MS. SANDRA P.
Nursing Diagnosis: Risk for Self-Mutilation

Expected Outcome: Ms. P. will express her feelings appropriately as evidenced by managing anxiety, naming feelings, and matching her feeling state to other people and the context.
- Establish a nurse-patient relationship, building trust through consistency and reliability.
- Request that Ms. P. monitor and report on situations that precipitate feelings.
- Analyze situations reported by Ms. P. for identification of precipitants and labeling of feelings.
- Explore with Ms. P. alternative for expressing feelings, utilizing hypothetical situations, or actual situations described by Ms. P.
- Encourage expression and exploration of feelings that Ms. P. experiences during nurse-patient interactions.
- Support Ms. P.'s appropriate use of defense mechanisms.

Expected Outcome: Ms. P. will experience fewer episodes of impulsive behavior as evidenced by her use of stress reduction techniques, identification of consequences of behavior, and use of problem-solving skills.
- Teach stress-reduction techniques (e.g., meditation and progressive neuromuscular relaxation).
- Discuss techniques that Ms. P. found useful in the past to reduce stress, and encourage them.
- Assist Ms. P. to identify alternatives for obtaining and maintaining employment.
- Discuss advantages and disadvantages of each alternative identified for obtaining and maintaining employment.
- Assist Ms. P. to make a plan for obtaining a job.
- Evaluate implementation of plan with Ms. P., identifying consequences of behaviors.

Expected Outcome: Ms. P. will interact positively with others as evidenced by making positive statements about herself, describing a clearer sense of self, and reporting satisfaction from interactions.
- Point out Ms. P.'s strengths.
- Engage Ms. P. in clarification of values, self-appraisal, and identification of ideal self.
- Analyze Ms. P.'s description of troublesome relationships for their impact on Ms. P.'s self-definition.
- With the patient, role-play positive strategies for interaction.
- Provide feedback to Ms. P. regarding positive interaction strategies utilized in nurse-patient relationship.
- ▲ Discuss family or group therapy with Ms. P.

■ = nursing intervention; ▲ = collaborative intervention.

▦ CRITICAL THINKING EXERCISES

1. Patients at Risk for Self-Mutilation may elicit strong feelings from staff. Describe how the nurse may effectively resolve feelings of anxiety, guilt, anger, and inadequacy.
2. The reasons most often given by patients for self-mutilating behaviors are to relieve tension, to vent anger, and to regain control over thoughts, emotions, and unstable environments. Identify alternative behaviors to explore with the self-mutilating patient for relief of tension, expression of feelings, and control of self and the environment.
3. How do environmental, developmental, and cultural factors affect selection of nursing interventions for the patient at Risk for Self-Mutilation?

REFERENCES
1. Anderson M: Clients with altered impulse control. In McFarland G and Thomas M: *Psychiatric mental health nursing practice: application of the nursing process,* Philadelphia, 1991, JB Lippincott Co.
2. Emerson J and Walker E: Self-injurious behavior in people with a mental handicap, *Nurs Times* 86:43–46, 1990.
3. Favazza A: *Bodies under siege: self-mutilation in culture and psychiatry,* Baltimore, 1993, Johns Hopkins Press.

4. Godfrey M: Clients with personality disorders. In McFarland G and Thomas M: *Psychiatric mental health nursing: application of the nursing process,* Philadelphia, 1991, JB Lippincott Co.
5. Jacobson A and Herald C: The relevance of childhood sexual abuse to adult psychiatric in-patient care, *Hosp Comm Psychiatry* 41:154, 1990.
6. Kim M, McFarland G, and McLane A: *A pocket guide to nursing diagnoses,* ed 6, St. Louis, 1995, Mosby–Year Book.
7. McCloskey J and Bulechek G: *Nursing interventions classification,* ed 2, St. Louis, 1996, Mosby–Year Book.
8. McFarland G, Wasli E, and Gerety E: *Nursing diagnosis and process in psychiatric mental health nursing,* ed 2, Philadelphia, 1992, JB Lippincott Co.
9. Naschinski E: High risk for self-mutilation. In Thompson J, McFarland G, Hirsch J, and Tucker S: *Mosby's clinical nursing,* ed 3, St. Louis, 1993, Mosby–Year Book.
10. Oldham J: *Personality disorders: new perspectives on diagnostic validity,* Washington, D.C., 1991, American Psychiatric Press.
11. Rose S, Peabody C, and Stratigeas B: Undetected abuse among intensive case management clients, *Hosp Comm Psychiatry* 42:499, 1991.
12. Russ M and others: Subtypes of self-injurious patients with borderline personality disorder, *Am J Psychiatry* 150: 1869–1871, 1993.
13. Sabo A and others: Changes in self-destructiveness of borderline patients in psychotherapy, *J Nerv Ment Diseases* 183(6):370–375, 1995.
14. Sansone R, Sansone L, and Wiederman M: The prevalence of trauma and its relationship to borderline personality symptoms and self-destructive behaviors in a primary care setting, *Arch Fam Med* 4:439–442, 1995.
15. Sebree R and Popkess-Vawter S: Self-injury concept formation: nursing diagnosis development, *Perspec Psych Care* 27(2):27–35, 1991.
16. Shearer S: Phenomenology of self-injury among inpatient women with borderline personality disorder, *J Nerv Ment Diseases* 182(9):524–526, 1994.

VII

ROLE-RELATIONSHIP PATTERN

Caregiver Role Strain

▶

Risk for Caregiver Role Strain

▶

Caregiver Role Strain *is difficulty experienced by a caregiver in performing the caregiver role.*

Risk for Caregiver Role Strain *is a caregiver's risk for experiencing difficulty in performing the caregiver role.*

OVERVIEW

The provision of health care within the family system is a tradition in this country. The national trend toward increased longevity,[9] increased chronicity of health conditions, containment of spiraling health care costs, and a decrease in the length of hospital stay all place an increased emphasis on the informal caregiving system. *Caregiver burden* and *caregiver stress* are terms that arise frequently in the literature in reference to the physical, psychological, social, and financial concerns associated with the caregiving role. Another term for this is *Caregiver Role Strain*.

Caregiving spans generations, cultures, values, and lifestyles.[11,13,15,18,22] The care recipient may be of any age. Current literature focuses primarily on the elderly. The caregiver is most often female, usually a spouse, daughter, or daughter-in-law. These women frequently experience conflict with other roles, such as wife, mother, employee, or community participant.[3,4] Generally this group of female caregivers is involved with direct in-home care. Spousal caregivers tend to provide a greater total number of hours of care, use fewer formal care resources, have greater restrictions of health and physical stamina, and report increased social isolation.

Other family members, neighbors, friends, or individuals from the community may be involved in the provision of care to the care recipient. This group participates at a level of caregiving that accomplishes goals through contracting for services or by provision of intermittent or supervisory care. The length of time in the caregiver role and the caregiver's attitude toward the role can influence the caregiver's relationship with the care recipient and the quality of care provided.

Entering into the role of caregiver often follows another person's crisis, such as an unexpected surgery, a fall, or a change in health status. It is not a role that people plan to undertake. There is little if any time to prepare for this role. Most individuals have had no previous caregiving experience. The uncertainty and guilt that surround the circumstances of care begin to set the stage for caregiver role strain.[20,23,31]

The response to the caregiver role varies. Tasks may be simple, such as assisting with meals or medications, or they may be more complex, such as using technical equipment or dealing with problematic behaviors. Although the literature reports that the psychological aspects of stress are perhaps more prevalent and amenable to intervention, the caregivers may not always perceive the stress when present. The stress of caregiving is multidimensional and unique to each individual. The caregiver is unique and must be assessed on a continuum over time.

Research to date has examined multiple dimensions of the caregiving response. Studies look at subjective and objective portions of the burden of care. However, many studies focus on a limited period of time. Additional longitudinal research studies are needed. Little is known about the long-range effects that caregiving might have on marriage, career, or family dynamics.[31]

ASSESSMENT

Each caregiving situation has unique qualities.[3] A suggested evaluation of this cluster of nursing diagnoses might include gathering a nursing history of the care recipient, a nursing history of the caregiver, a formal in-home evaluation, available community resources, and other supports. The assessment must focus on the strengths of the caregiver and also examine ever-changing environmental factors, such as circumstances of care and financial demands. By using this approach to assessment, an appropriate match of interventions can be achieved.

The nursing history of the care recipient must be comprehensive. Assessment of activities of daily living, cognitive status, and any behavioral or psychological issues is needed to create a baseline from which to measure change. Determination of the care recipient's prognosis is useful in facilitating the caregiver's planning process. It is useful to ascertain the recipient's perception of illness, relationship with the caregiver and support system, and willingness to accept help. Reassessment at intervals is necessary because changes in care demands, mental status, or behavioral problems influence susceptibility to Caregiver Role Strain.

The health status of the caregiver often serves as a barometer for role strain. A careful history of the caregiver needs to be obtained. Information to gather includes a baseline medical history with particular attention to chronic conditions. It is useful to determine usual health care practices, such as how frequently the caregiver has medical and dental check-ups, which over-the-counter medications are used and for what purpose, and how minor illnesses are handled. A discussion of major illness or disability within the family or support network may provide the nurse with additional insight.

The usual roles in which the caregiver is active need to be identified and prioritized by time and importance. Conflict between competing roles is a frequent occurrence. The quality and history of the relationship between the caregiver and the care recipient requires note. An unsatisfactory or inadequate relationship may be a contributing factor to role strain. The relationship to the community and support systems must be identified. The caregiver's willingness to ask for and accept assistance with care is paramount to the intervention process.

Depression is prevalent in those experiencing role strain. The caregiver may be unable to report a change in mood or activity because his or her sole purpose has become providing care to the care recipient. It is appropriate to administer a depression scale to the caregiver at intervals to assess change over time. The level of stress that the caregiver might experience may also be misperceived.

The nurse must assess other parameters related to the caregiver role. It is important to determine the caregiver's sense of spirituality and use of spiritual resources.[27] Baseline information about current and past socialization patterns is useful when planning interventions.

The home provides an opportunity to view the actual caregiving arena and quite often to see the interactions of the key players. In addition to the usual safety and access concerns, areas to note are the presence of adaptive equipment and whether or not it is being used correctly. A survey of the home will help the health care team to know if there is space for additional assistive equipment. The home visit is also a good time to learn about plans for emergency situations, such as falls, or caregiver absence.

Caregiver Role Strain
■ Defining Characteristics
The presence of the following defining characteristics indicates that the individual may be experiencing Caregiver Role Strain:

- Feeling exhausted
- Inability to complete caregiving tasks
- Declining health status
- Sleep pattern disturbance
- Feeling depressed
- Feeling loss of usual or expected relationship with care receiver
- Grieving
- Increased stress or nervousness
- Increased emotional lability
- Preoccupation with care routine
- Low self-esteem
- Withdrawal from social contacts
- Change in leisure activities
- Family conflict
- Change in expression of spirituality

■ Related Factors

The following related factors are associated with Caregiver Role Strain:

- The severity of care recipient's illness
- Increasing care needs of care receiver
- Caregiver health impairment
- Caregiver not developmentally ready for caregiving role
- Providing direct, long-term in-home care
- Discharge of family member with significant home care needs
- Unpredictable illness course or instability in the care recipient's health
- Substance abuse or codependency of caregiver or care recipient
- Developmental delay or retardation of the care recipient or caregiver
- Marginal family adaptation or dysfunction before caregiving situation
- Marginal coping patterns of caregiver
- Psychological or cognitive problems in the care receiver
- Past history of poor relationship between caregiver and care recipient
- Care recipient exhibits deviant, bizarre behavior
- Conflicting role demands
- No previous experience with caregiver role
- Spiritual belief system

Risk for Caregiver Role Strain
■ Risk Factors

The presence of behaviors, conditions, or circumstances like the related factors for Caregiver Role Strain render the patient more vulnerable to Risk for Caregiver Role Strain.

DIAGNOSIS
■ Differential Nursing Diagnosis

The nursing diagnosis Caregiver Role Strain is the felt difficulty in performing the family caregiver role, and Risk for Caregiver Role Strain is the vulnerability for feeling that difficulty. The focus is on actual caregiving; resources to support the caregiving process; the relationship between the caregiver and the care recipient; and the caregiver and family response to issues of caregiving (i.e., conflict, stress, communication, loss, emotional response). Two similar diagnoses are Parental Role Conflict and Altered Role Performance. Parental Role Conflict is the state in which a parent experiences role confusion and conflict in response to a crisis. This diagnosis focuses on the traditional family unit and a specific relationship between parent and child. Altered Role Performance is disruption in the way one perceives one's role performance. This is being developed but appears to focus entirely on the patient's response to a role. Other nursing diagnoses that could be associated with Caregiver Role Strain include Ineffective Individual Coping, Knowledge Deficit, and Social Isolation.

■ Medical and Psychiatric Diagnoses

Diagnoses that are commonly related to Caregiver Role Strain/Risk for Caregiver Role Strain are dementia of the Alzheimer's type, cerebral vascular accident, neurological conditions (i.e., multiple sclerosis and cerebral palsy), pulmonary disease (i.e., chronic obstructive pulmonary disease), psychiatric conditions (i.e., schizophrenia), and birth defects (i.e., mental retardation, developmental disorders, or spina bifida). These conditions are often irreversible and may require ongoing care lasting months or years. The clinical presentation of these diagnoses extends across physical, cognitive, functional, emotional, and social domains that are often interrelated in a complex pattern of problems or issues. Alzheimer's disease and related dementias usually present as a behavior disorder characterized by impaired memory with related functional problems. Cerebral vascular accidents, although primarily associated with the elderly, are occurring more frequently among young and middle-age adults. The associated clinical presentation is varied and often includes interrelated physical, psychosocial, and functional issues. Neurological and pulmonary conditions occur throughout the life span. The individual's stage of development may be an additional factor to consider in planning care. A child who is mentally or physically challenged may require ongoing in-home services and specialized educational intervention. Congenital deformities, although often corrected with surgery and/or other medical interventions, affect the psychosocial and economic integrity of the family unit, which may require counseling and intervention. A multidisciplinary approach to care planning provides expertise in assessment, intervention, and evaluation of care delivery. With the current health care focus on reducing costs and increasing life expectancy, more people are being cared for in the home environment. A case management model is often utilized to provide continuity of care through collaboration with various disciplines and services for efficient use of resources. The case manager may have credentials in any one of the health disciplines. The initial home visit usually includes a nursing assessment of the caregiver and care recipient health care needs.[4] This is integrated into the comprehensive assessment and treatment planning process by the case manager. Nursing may provide ongoing in-home assessment and evaluation to support treatment interventions and revision of the plan as appropriate. Although frequent in-home contact with the caregiver and care recipient is required initially, after an effective plan has been established the case management model allows the care situation to be monitored by telephone. This provides the supportive link to

health care providers for the caregiver and reduces costs for the health care system.

OUTCOME IDENTIFICATION, PLANNING, AND IMPLEMENTATION

Caregiver Role Strain

One expected outcome is that the caregiver will state appropriate informal or formal resources. Communities have a myriad of resources to offer the caregiver, but the task of learning where they are, how to access them, and which are appropriate for an individual situation is overwhelming. Caregivers come to the role with little or no previous experience, and they frequently express uncertainty about their performance and care expectations. There are a number of distinctions between out-of-home services and in-home services. To use out-of-home services the patient will require transportation to the location where they are provided. Patients must have some degree of mobility, be able to complete personal care activities independently or with assistance, and behave appropriately in group interactions. In-home services are designed primarily to assist with personal care dependencies and those with mobility limitations. Patients who exhibit mental impairment or behavior disruptions or who have difficulty accepting assistance from a person other than the primary caregiver would benefit from in-home services. The caregiver and the care recipient can benefit from referral to appropriate services. Evaluation of cultural beliefs will influence the selection of appropriate services. Those who do not choose to access formal services may prefer family support or their own network of social support from neighbors and friends.

Another expected outcome is that the caregiver will verbalize and participate in stress-reduction strategies. There is a tendency among caregivers to neglect self-care activities and to experience an increased level of psychological stress. This inattention to their own health status can translate into aggravated health problems, increased somatic complaints, and depression. Each caregiving experience is unique in terms of the emotional response and life transitions experienced by the caregiver. Therefore stress-reduction methods and strategies for coping with the demands of caregiving must include an array of choices. Although caregivers tend to identify the physician as their information resource, nursing provides the initial and ongoing contact with the health care system. The nurse is instrumental in monitoring the caregiver for changes in health status, validating emotional expressions, and providing education and referrals for strategies to reduce stress related to the caregiving role.

Another expected outcome is that the caregiver will identify changes in his or her role expectations. The many roles and competing demands for the caregiver's time, resources, and energy may result in increased stress within the family unit. There is a tendency for caregivers to attempt to be all things to all people as they try to maintain all of their usual roles in addition to their new caregiving role. Assistance and reassurance in prioritizing roles and establishing realistic time management strategies is critical to alleviating some of the perceived strain. Once the tasks of caregiving are identified they can be negotiated with other family members or the support network or met by incorporating other resources into the plan of care.

Risk for Caregiver Role Strain

An expected outcome is that the caregiver is able to state appropriate community resources and how to access them. When a new caregiving situation arises or when a stable one changes, there is a need to reexamine available resources within the immediate support system and within the community. The caregiver may initially need assistance determining how to meet the needs of the care recipient, how to access community resources, and how to select appropriate services. Often the family dynamics and history designate the primary caregiver, usually a spouse or female family member. If no close family unit exists, friends or a significant other may assume the task of caregiving. If the designated caregiver is unable to acknowledge the need for formal or informal support with the caregiving role or is unwilling to accept help, it is difficult to enlist additional resources.

A second expected outcome is that the caregiver is able to identify existing strengths and weaknesses in family dynamics. The nurse will assist the caregiver to identify the existing strengths and weaknesses of the family unit. The relationship between family members, particularly the primary caregiver and the care recipient, affects the care situation. The "family" may consist of a spouse, significant other, traditional family members, friends, or neighbors, who make up the care recipient's support network. Families, the primary caregiver, and the care recipient may find that psychotherapy is helpful to work through unresolved issues or to learn more effective communication techniques.

■ **NURSING CARE GUIDELINES**
Nursing Diagnosis: Caregiver Role Strain

Expected Outcome: The caregiver will state appropriate informal/formal resources within a time frame of 2 weeks.
- Assess caregiver and family experience or strengths in caregiving. *Increasing preparedness and competence of care participants for caregiving activities may yield a decreased sense of burden.*[4]
- Establish a therapeutic relationship with the caregiver. *Interventions are more likely to succeed when a therapeutic relationship exists between the nurse and the caregiver.*[4]
- Identify issues of caregiving from a family perspective. *Families have specialized insight about the care recipient and the caregiving situation.*[19]

■ = nursing intervention; ▲ = collaborative intervention.

- Assess caregiver's knowledge of availability of resources. *Families need an introduction to and information about how to use public or private service programs.*[6]
- Determine caregiver and care recipient willingness to accept resource support. *Many families do not use in-home or out-of-home services because of perceived barriers.*[5]
- ▲ Collaborate with the family to resolve identified caregiving issues. *Interventions require the cooperative efforts of family members.*[4]
- Select and offer referrals (i.e., in-home services, respite care, support group, or psycho education group) according to the unique caregiving situation. *The competency level of the caregiver can be enhanced by increasing his or her pool of resources as well as skill level.*[16,28]
- Provide education about care recipient's disease and care needs; support family's development of caregiving skills as appropriate. *Educating the family and helping them learn caregiving skills is an important strategy.*[10,17]
- ▲ Establish access to advice or an information resource that will be available on a continuing basis following discharge. *Increased predictability and control reassures the family about their ability to manage their caregiving situation (i.e., transition from hospital to home).*[4]

Expected Outcome: The caregiver will verbalize and participate in stress-reduction strategies within a time frame of 4 weeks.

- Discuss caregiver concerns that may affect his or her perception of the burden of caregiving. *Availability of informal or formal support services (i.e., assistance with medications, bathing, relief caregiver, or hours of informal support) may affect the ability of the caregiver to continue in that role.*[7]
- Explore stress-reduction methods appropriate to the caregiver (e.g., participation in pleasurable activities, massage, relaxation tapes, guided imagery, exercises, meditation, or biofeedback techniques). *Interventions should be individualized to account for the uniqueness of each caregiving situation and the stage in the caregiving process.*[4,21,29]
- Explore renewed or continued involvement in church and social activities. *Social and spiritual support has been found to play a significant role in stress reduction among caregivers.*[27]
- Provide information about community support groups. *Education and support groups can provide information about the disease process, provision of care, and mutual support and can address caregiver isolation.*[6,12]
- Review the importance of monitoring the health status of the caregiver. *Caregiving is a stressful activity that may affect the caregiver's health.*[26]
- Explore and validate emotional expressions related to burden of care with caregiver. *The period of transition through the caregiving experience includes loss, rediscovery of a sense of self, and feelings of satisfaction or frustration.*[4,22,31]

Expected Outcome: The caregiver will identify changes in his or her role expectations within a time frame of 8 weeks.

- ▲ Examine the caregiver's usual role and priorities within the family system; compare past and present relationships within the family unit. *Dynamics associated with increased role strain include relationships within the family system, living arrangements, and the quality of interpersonal relationships with the care recipient.*[2]
- ▲ Educate the family about the process of caregiving. *Focused educational sessions can be efficient and a relatively inexpensive method of treatment that can be offered by a variety of health care professional.*[16]
- Assist caregiver to anticipate the need to reprioritize or renegotiate within family and support network as caregiving demands change. *Education and counseling with families and caregivers should be ongoing throughout the caregiving experience.*[25]

VIII

◢ **NURSING CARE GUIDELINES**
Nursing Diagnosis: Risk for Caregiver Role Strain

Expected Outcome: The caregiver is able to state appropriate community resources and how to access them within 1 week.

■ Evaluate family and social networks and spiritual beliefs. *Families have specialized insight about care recipient and caregiving situations.*[19,14]

▲ Discuss financial eligibility requirements for resources. *Amount of available finances or insurance influences decisions about discharge dispositions.*[7]

■ Discuss the range or availability of community resources appropriate for present and future needs. *Families need an introduction to and information about how to use public or private service programs.*[6]

■ Evaluate willingness of caregiver to access resources. *Many families do not use in-home or out-of-home services because of perceived barriers.*[5]

■ Discuss and evaluate circumstances in which resources might be incorporated in the care regimen. *Education and support can provide information about the disease process, provision of care, and mutual support and can address caregiver isolation.*[6,12]

▲ Establish access to advice or information resource that will be available on continuing basis following discharge. *Increased predictability and control measures the family of their ability to manage their caregiving situation (i.e., transition from hospital to home).*[4]

Expected Outcome: The caregiver is able to identify existing strengths and weaknesses in family dynamics within 1 week.

■ Identify the dynamics between caregiver and care recipient. *The quality of the former relationship is likely to influence the caregiving situation.*[8]

■ Identify past patterns of dealing with caregiving and illness. *Caregiving reflects an individual's life history (i.e., their experience in caregiving situations, personal disposition, and commitment to the care recipient).*[24]

■ Offer family or individual therapy for resolution of conflict or unresolved issues. *Focused educational sessions can be an efficient and a relatively inexpensive method of treatment that can be offered by a variety of health care professional.*[16]

■ = nursing intervention; ▲ = collaborative intervention.

EVALUATION

The progress of a patient with this nursing diagnosis is measured by the caregiver selecting appropriate resources for care, after evaluation and discussion with the nurse. Note that the time line for this will be dictated by the average length of stay in the program; the degree to which outcomes are achieved will be influenced accordingly. The success of this plan depends on the nurse's collaboration with other health care professionals and a trusting relationship between the caregiver and nurse. The achievement of the expected outcomes depends on holistic assessment of the dynamics of the caregiving situation.

Caregiver Role Strain

Generally the caregiver will be able to state appropriate informal and formal resources he or she has selected within a 2-week time frame. Each care situation has unique aspects, and selection of appropriate resources will vary. Success is evident when the caregiver outlines an initial plan that supports the caregiving role. When the caregiver is unable to identify appropriate resources, additional assessment focused on the willingness or ability to assume the caregiver role and utilize resources must be initiated. It may be necessary to seek an alternative plan to meet the care recipient's needs.

VIII

Within 4 weeks the caregiver should be able to verbalize and demonstrate participation in stress-reduction activities. Each caregiver has unique preferences that will influence the selection of an appropriate stress-reduction strategy. Collaboration with other disciplines may offer the greatest variety of stress-reduction strategies. The caregiver will benefit from discussion of techniques for setting priorities and for time management that allow pursuit of pleasurable and self-care activities. Attainment of the expected outcome is evident when the caregiver states that he or she has participated in a pleasurable activity and expresses satisfaction with the choice of strategy. When the caregiver is unable to participate in stress-reduction activities, he or she may be overwhelmed by the caregiving role. Further assessment may be necessary to determine unresolved issues; referral to counseling may be indicated.

The caregiver should be able to identify changes in role expectations within an 8-week time frame. This will be evidenced by the caregiver's ability to prioritize activities and the demands of various life roles. The caregiver may verbalize perceived value and satisfaction from the caregiving experience. The caregiving role is often long-term; reassessment of competing roles may be indicated in anticipation of the changing needs in the care situation. When the expected outcome has not been achieved, additional assessment is indicated. Collaboration with the multidisciplinary team may be necessary to determine appropriate interventions.

Risk for Caregiver Role Strain

The caregiver will be able to state appropriate community resources and how to access them within the first week. The resources selected should be appropriate to the finances and needs of the caregiving situation. Education should address access to available resources along the continuum of caregiving. When the caregiver is unable to identify appropriate resources, additional assessment focused on the willingness or ability of the caregiver to assume the caregiver role and to utilize resources must be initiated. Within the first week, the caregiver should focus on identifying existing strengths and weaknesses in family dynamics. The "family" may consist of a spouse, significant other, traditional family members, friends, or neighbors who make up the care recipient's support network. Selection of appropriate resources depends on knowledge of family dynamics. When there is limited awareness of existing strengths and weaknesses, there is a possibility that the primary caregiver will be unable to succeed in the caregiving role or will experience stress. Additional family or individual therapy may be required to resolve conflict and to identify strengths within the family unit.

VIII

▶ **Case Study with Plan of Care**

Mr. Lennie P. is a 45-year-old African-American male. The admitting diagnoses are adjustment disorder, spinal cord injury, and decubitus ulcer. Mr. P. has experienced many problems in his previous living situation. He is paraplegic and dependent on caregivers for assistance with lower body dressing, transfers, bathing, elimination, and health status monitoring. He has demonstrated impaired ability to solve problems, poor judgment, and difficulty in social interactions. He is alienated from his family. Mr. P. sold his hospital bed when he was admitted to the hospital so his family "wouldn't have the chance to sell it and get the money." Currently he has two close friends who have been designated as conservators for his health care and financial management. Mr. P. has assured his friends that he will be discharged to his home and that he can be cared for there with "some-body to come in to help." Both conservators are employed full time and live some distance from Mr. P.'s home. They are supportive of his desire to live at home but are uncertain how they could avoid the "hassle we heard about when he manipulated the people taking care of him last time. . . . Things got out of hand because the caregivers could not be there all the time." The conservators have no experience in direct care, dressing changes, elimination management, or transfer techniques. They agreed to be conservators because of a long-standing though distant friendship. They are overwhelmed with the unassembled hoyer lift that Mr. P. had delivered to his home while he was in the hospital. The conservators have met with the social worker but have additional questions and concerns related to actual care needs.

▪ **PLAN OF CARE FOR CAREGIVERS OF MR. LENNIE P.**
Nursing Diagnosis: Risk for Caregiver Role Strain Related to Inexperience with Caregiving and Complexity of Caregiving Tasks

---

Expected Outcome: The conservators will develop an appropriate plan for continuity of care following discharge.

▲ Determine financial eligibility for in-home services.

▪ Complete arrangements for home evaluation by therapist(s) and conservators before discharge to evaluate equipment needs, safety issues, and availability of space for in-home caregiver.

▲ Assist the conservators to select a live-in caregiver (i.e., review applicant references, assist with interview questions, advise them to complete a background check of selected applicant before hiring).

▪ Discuss alternate plan for interrupted caregiving (i.e., illness, vacation, resignation of caregiver).

▪ Establish access to advice and information that will be available to them on a continuing basis following Mr. P.'s discharge.

▪ = nursing intervention; ▲ = collaborative intervention.

▦ CRITICAL THINKING EXERCISES

1. How would the nurse help the conservators expand opportunities for Mr. P.'s social interaction in the community?

2. What consideration are important in developing an alternate plan for care delivery should the live-in caregiver be unavailable?

3. What are the appropriate disciplines to include in the discharge planning process?

4. What stress-reduction strategies would you recommend for the conservators who are in a coordinating role rather than direct-care delivery activities?

5. What information can be obtained from the home visit that will help the conservators participate in the discharge planning process?

REFERENCES

1. Abraham IL and others: Multidisciplinary assessment of patients with Alzheimer's disease, *Nurs Clin North Am* 18:3–16, 1995.

2. Anderson CS, Linto J, and Stewart-Wynne EG: A population-based assessment of the impact and burden of caregiving for long-term stroke servivors, *Stroke* 26(5):843–849, 1995.

3. Archbold PG and others: Mutuality and preparedness as predictors of caregiver role strain, *Res Nurs Health* 13:375–384, 1990.

4. Archbold PG and others: The PREP system of nursing interventions: a pilot test with families caring for older members, *Res Nurs Health* 18:1–16, 1995.

5. Biegel DE and others: Predictors of in-home and out-of-home service use by family caregivers of Alzheimer's disease patients, *J Aging Health* 5(4):419–438, 1993.

6. Christenson D and Moore I: Intensive case management in Alzheimer's disease home care: an interim report on the Cincinnati (Ohio) Medicare Alzheimer's project, *J Long-Term Home Health Care* 13(4):43–52, 1994.

7. Cox C and Verdiec MJ: Factors affecting the outcomes of hospitalized dementia patients: from home to hospital discharge, *Gerontologist* 34(4):497–504, 1994.

8. Davidhizar R: Understanding powerlessness in family member caregivers of the chronically ill, *Geriatr Nurs* 13(2):66–69, 1992.

9. Decker SE and Young E: Self-perceived needs of primary caregivers of home-hospice clients, *J Comm Health Nurs* 8(3):147–154, 1991.

10. Deutsch LH and Rovner BW: Agitation and other noncognitive abnormalities in Alzheimer's disease, *Psychiatr Clin North Am* 14(2):341–351, 1991.

11. Dyson LL: Families of young children with handicaps: parental stress and family functioning, *Am J Ment Retard* 95 (6):623–629, 1991.

12. Farran CJ and Keane-Hagerty E: Interventions for caregivers of persons with dementia: educational support groups and Alzheimer's association support groups, *Appl Nurs Res* 7(3):112–117, 1994.

13. Folkman S and others: Caregiver burden in HIV-positive and HIV-negative partners of men with AIDS, *J Clin Consult Psychol* 62(4):746–756, 1994.

14. Forbes EJ: Spirituality, aging, and the community-dwelling caregiver and care recipient, *Geriatr Nurs* 15(6):297–302, 1994.

15. Fredman L, Daly MP, and Lazur AM: Burden among white and black caregivers to elderly adults, *J Gerontol* 50B(2): S110–S118, 1995.

16. Gallagher-Thompson D and DeVries HM: Coping with frustration classes: development and preliminary outcomes with women who care for relatives with dementia, *Gerontologist* 34(4):548–552, 1994.

17. Hall GR and others: Managing Alzheimer's patients at home, *J Gerontol Nurs* 21(1):37–47, 1995.

18. Hardy VL and Riffle KL: Support for caregivers of dependent elderly, *Geriatr Nurs* 14(3):161–164, 1993.

19. Harvath TA and others: Establishing partnerships with family caregivers: local and cosmopolitan knowledge, *J Gerontol Nurs* 20(2):29–35, 1994.

20. Karmilovich SE: Burden and stress associated with spousal caregiving for individuals with heart failure, *Prog Cardiovasc Nurs* 9(1):33–38, 1994.

21. Keady J and Nolan M: A stitch in time. Facilitating proactive interventions with dementia caregivers: the role of community practitioners, *J Psychiatr Ment Health Nurs* 2:33–40, 1995.

22. Langner SR: Finding meaning in caring for elderly relatives: loss and personal growth, *Holist Nurs Pract* 9(3):75–84, 1995.

23. Loukissa DA: Family burden in chronic mental illness: a review of research studies, *J Adv Nurs* 21:248–255, 1995.

24. Opie A: The instability of the caring body: gender and caregivers of confused older people, *Qual Health Res* 4(1):31–50, 1994.

25. Raia PA: Helping patients and families to take control, *Psychiatr Ann* 24(4):192–196, 1994.

26. Reese DR and others: Caregivers of Alzheimer's disease and stroke patients: immunological and psychological considerations, *Gerontologist* 34(4):534–540, 1994.

27. Robinson KM and Kaye J: The relationship between spiritual perspective, social support, and depression in caregiving and noncaregiving wives, *Schol Inq Nurs Pract* 8(4):375–396, 1994.

28. Robinson KM and Yates K: Effects of two caregiver-training programs on burden and attitude toward help, *Arch Psychiatr Nurs* 7(5):312–319, 1994.

29. Suwa-Kobayashi S, Yuasa M, and Noguchi M: Nursing in Japan: caregivers of elderly family members with dementia, *J Gerontol Nurs* 21(2):23–30, 1995.

30. Thompson EH and others: Social support and caregiving burden in family caregivers of frail elders, *J Gerontol* 48(5):S245–S254, 1993.

31. Wuest J, Ericson PK, and Noerager-Stern P: Becoming strangers: the changing family caregiving relationship in Alzheimer's disease, *J Adv Nurs* 20:437–443, 1994.

VIII

Impaired Verbal Communication

▶

Impaired Verbal Communication *is the state in which an individual experiences a decreased or absent ability to use or understand language in human interaction. Difficulties experienced in verbal communication must occur over time and be evidenced by observable signs or reported symptoms for a nursing diagnosis of Impaired Verbal Communication to be valid.*

OVERVIEW

Communication is a dynamic, complex, continuous series of reciprocal events through which messages are exchanged, primarily to produce a response from a person or a group. It includes all conscious and unconscious behavior that affects another person. Therefore communication is essential in interpersonal relationships. The communication process is continuous; that is, it has no beginning or end.

The four major component of the communication process are sender, message, receiver, and feedback.

The sender generates and transmits a message. A message is triggered by internal or external stimuli, such as ideas, events, or situations, that are mediated by the senses. The sender can focus consciously on only a few of the many stimuli available at any one point in time. The selected stimuli are analyzed and evaluated before a message is developed. This process involves the sender's review of his or her self-perception and perceptions of others and the rehearsal of possible actions and expected reactions. It is mediated by such psychosocial factors as self-concept, values, mood, and culture and by the parts of the central nervous system that connect input with output (e.g., sensory end organs, nerve fibers, and the cerebral cortex). After internally rehearsing alternative messages, the sender transmits the one evaluated as potentially the most successful.

The message is derived through the translation of ideas, purpose, and intention and is formulated into a code that is carried to the receiver through a channel.

The two basic systems of codification of a message are the *analog* and the *digital systems*. The analog system is nonverbal and is based on similarities in form, color, or proportion between the actual communication and the event represented.[10] Nonverbal communication is as effective and significant as verbal communication and, in some circumstances, even overrides the verbal message. Nonverbal communication fulfills a variety of purposes, such as augmenting or replacing verbal communication, displaying feelings, regulating the speed of verbal messages, and reflecting the relationship between the sender and the receiver.

Nonverbal communication encompasses[11] *kinesics* (the study of body movement, especially such nonverbal behaviors as facial expression, eye contact, and gestures); *paralanguage,* including such vocal phenomena as pitch and range of voice, vocal differentiators (e.g., crying and laughing), vocal identifiers (e.g., "ah" and "uh-hum"), and the conveyance of emotions through the voice quality; *proxemics,* which includes the study of the relationship of space and social interaction (e.g., four main distances are intimate, personal, social, and public, each indicating the distance, relationship, appropriate messages, and activities between sender and receiver); *touch* (i.e., the physical contact between sender and receiver, which is a significant form of nonverbal communication); and *cultural artifacts,* such as items or substances that reflect a given culture or subculture (e.g., the use of cosmetics, jewelry, and clothing).

Cultural considerations are very important in the analog system of codifying a message. For example, culture influences the interpretation of eye contact. Eye contact often reflects a willingness to interact. However, extended eye contact can indicate aggression and the deliberate intent to induce anxiety. An absence of eye contact can communicate disinterest, lack of self-esteem, competitiveness, embarrassment, or hurt. Gestures express or emphasize the communicated ideas. How a person feels about another can be indicated through gestures, including body position and the placement and movements of eyes, hands, and feet. Because gestures are learned through imitation, culture determines the meaning of the gesture. The personal zone ranges from 12 inches to 36 inches. Confidential or personal information is communicated in this zone. Americans use this zone at parties and in close friendships. The effectiveness of touch is influenced by the meaning of touch to a given person within a given culture. The mores of a culture must also be considered when interpreting cultural artifacts. For example, the use of perfume may be interpreted in one culture as an invitation for interaction. However, in another culture that values the body's natural odors, perfume would be considered offensive.

In the digital system of message codification, signs and symbols represent concepts and objects. Language is created through manipulation of these signs and symbols. Verbal communication depends on a digital system. To communicate, persons must have the same meanings for words. This involves more than a common language because each word has both a *denotation* and a *connotation*. A denotative meaning is the one that is most generally used and the connotative meaning is an additional meaning specific to a person. The connotative meaning includes associations, referents, and emotions derived from personal experience

that add to the denotative meaning. Because effective communication depends on similar meanings, the selected words must convey the intended meaning and be understood by the other person.

The receiver perceives and interprets the message based on stimuli in his or her perceptual field. These stimuli include those in the sender's verbal and nonverbal communication and the immediate environment (context). As with the sender, the receiver's stimuli are selectively received, reviewed, and interpreted. The receiver's perception is affected by such psychological factors as concept of self and others, feelings, and social and cultural factors.

To organize the complex and dynamic series of events into a communication sequence for interpretation and response, the receiver "punctuates" the interactional sequence by organizing it into a beginning and an end.[5] Disagreement between the sender and the receiver about the punctuation of a communication sequence often results in conflict and impaired communication. For example, a student claims that he cheated on an examination because he believes the teacher does not trust him. "I may as well do what I'm accused of," the student states. The teacher views the situation differently. She is distrustful and suspicious in response to the student's behavior.

The receiver responds according to his or her perceptions and interpretations, thereby providing feedback and becoming a sender. *Feedback* is the receiver's communicated reaction to the sender's message. Feedback regulates the communication process by stimulating modification or correction. Feedback should be clearly and tactfully stated, relevant to the person, culture, and context, and be appropriately timed to facilitate understanding and agreement between communicators. In providing feedback, the original receiver becomes a sender, thereby perpetuating the communication process.

The characteristic of successful communication include the following[8,11,12]:

1. The sender and the receiver are physically able to receive, analyze, and send messages.

2. Appropriate input is selectively analyzed.
3. Consistent verbal and nonverbal communication are used.
4. The sender and the receiver have similar meanings for words.
5. The message is appropriate to the context and complete (not overloaded or insufficient in information).
6. The timing of the message coincides with its meaning and the context.
7. The sender and the receiver agree on the punctuation of a communication sequence.
8. If indicated, the feedback is clearly stated, relevant to the person, context, and culture, and appropriately timed.
9. The sender can correct the information or the message.
10. Concordant information is established between the sender and the receiver, both of whom attain confirmation and gratification.

Many variables can positively or negatively affect the communication process. When these variables consistently exert a negative influence on a person's communication, a pattern of impaired communication results.

ASSESSMENT

When assessing the patient's communication pattern, the nurse should analyze the patient data for the presence or absence of characteristics of successful communication. Sources of data include the nurse's observation of and interaction with the patient, the patient's perceptions of his or her communications with others, and feedback from significant others about the patient's communication ability.[8] Limitations in verbal communication must be significant in amount and frequency to result in a diagnosis of Impaired Verbal Communication.

Several factors affect the communication process and are related to Impaired Verbal Communication. These include *growth and development, physical condition, stress, emotional state, perception, culture,* and *communication skills*.

Communication is a major human function, mastery of which involves learning a series of pro-

gressive tasks over time. Each stage of human *growth and development* includes physical, social, psychological, and cultural events that can enhance or interfere with the development of effective communication. Some examples are the rapid physical and cognitive development of a child, the growing independence of the adolescent, the complexity of an adult's roles, and the effects of the aging process.

Physical conditions or medical treatments may affect a person's ability to communicate. Those directly affecting communication include conditions and treatments that interfere with the physical ability to receive and process sensory input or generate output, such as blindness, cerebrovascular accident, cleft palate, endotracheal intubation, laryngectomy, and wired jaws. Communication may be indirectly influenced by physical conditions, such as social withdrawal resulting from embarrassment about physical symptoms.

Stress also affects communication. Stress, a complex phenomenon, is precipitated by internal or external demands that result in neurocognitive, affective, physiological, and behavioral responses.[12] A moderate level of stress enhances learning and increases motivation and productivity. However, excessive stress can cause mental, social, or physical dysfunction, including impaired communication.

Feelings or *emotional states* are states of mind or being that can enhance or impede communication. The expression of feelings, such as anxiety, anger, or depression, can facilitate communication and interpersonal relationships by allowing others to know us and our feelings. However, the expression of feelings can also impair communication, most often through the manner used to express the feeling. For example, a staff nurse may be angry that her supervisor frequently reminds her about her tasks. If she expresses her anger by throwing the temperature chart on the desk and storming out of the nurses' station when the supervisor reminds her to take temperatures, communication has ceased because of her emotional outburst. If she instead responds by saying, "I appreciate and share your concern about getting the work done, but I feel angry when you continually remind me to do my work. I would prefer to be informed of my assignments only once. I will ask for assistance when I need it." The supervisor in this example has more information on which to base her supervision of this staff nurse, and the channels of communication remain open.

A person's behavior depends on his or her perceptual field at the moment. *Perception* is a process that includes reception, selection, organization, and interpretation of sensory data. Each component of the communication process is affected by perception. The receiver will only perceive input considered relevant and will then only respond to *some* of the perceived input. The resulting messages sent and received are mediated by perception of self, the environment, the culture, and the receiver. The nervous system, past experiences, values, needs, and the emotional state of the individual all influence perception. Whenever perception is limited because of distortion, omission, or falsification of sensory input, impaired communication results.[12]

Culture also influences the communication process. The culture of the communicators determines the meanings of verbal and nonverbal communication and governs where, what, how, why, and with whom a person communicates. Impaired communication can result from not understanding or considering cultural influences.

Effective communication also depends on *communication skills*. A variety of effective communication styles and skills have been described in the literature.[9,11,12] Impaired communication may result when the communicator has not learned or fails to use the style and specific skills that enhance the communication process.

■ Defining Characteristics

The presence of the following defining characteristics indicates that the patient may be experiencing Impaired Verbal Communication:

- Inability to speak dominant language
- Refusal or inability to speak
- Stuttering or slurring
- Impaired articulation
- Dyspnea

- Difficulty with phonation
- Inability to speak in sentences
- Disorientation
- Inability to modulate speech
- Inability to find words
- Inability to name words
- Inability to identify objects
- Loose association of ideas
- Flight of ideas
- Incessant verbalization
- Hyper- or hypovigilance
- Distorted perception
- Inappropriate feedback
- Inappropriate expression of feelings
- Disparate verbal and nonverbal messages
- Disagreement in punctuation of communication

■ Related Factors

The following related factors are associated with Impaired Verbal Communication:

- Decrease in circulation to the brain
- Physical barrier (e.g., intubation)
- Psychological barriers or psychosis
- Faulty perception
- Anatomical deficit (e.g., cleft palate)
- Developmental or age-related physical problems
- Sensory organ impairment
- Afferent or efferent nerve impairment
- Cerebral cortex impairment
- Excessive stress
- Emotional state
- Inadequate self-perception
- Poor communication skills
- Social isolation
- Cultural differences

DIAGNOSIS

■ Differential Nursing Diagnosis

The nursing diagnosis Sensory/Perceptual Alteration (verbal) is defined as a change in the amount or the pattern of incoming stimuli, accompanied by diminished, exaggerated, distorted, or impaired responses to such stimuli. Interruption in the process of forming accurate perceptions in turn

VIII

has a direct or indirect effect on subsequent emotions and behavior. Altered communication patterns are one example of such an effect. Anxiety is a vague, uneasy feeling, the source of which is often nonspecific or unknown to an individual. Behavioral manifestations are related to the level of anxiety experienced. Moderate to severe levels of Anxiety affect the communication process. The range of perception is reduced or disrupted, and verbalization may change in amount, difficulty, and appropriateness.

■ Medical and Psychiatric Diagnoses

Medical diagnoses most commonly related to Impaired Verbal Communication are those that reflect dysfunction of language and speech systems. Language involves the comprehension and transmission of ideas and feelings through the use of conventional signs, sounds, and gestures, including the sequential ordering of them according to accepted rules of grammar, whereas speech is the articulatory and mechanistic aspects of verbal expression.[2] Examples of these medical diagnoses are Bell's palsy, cerebrovascular accident, craniocerebral trauma, Parkinson's disease, and tracheotomy. Examples of psychiatric diagnoses that commonly manifest themselves as Impaired Verbal Communication include schizophrenia and the anxiety, bipolar, depressive, and psychoactive-substance-use disorders.

OUTCOME IDENTIFICATION, PLANNING, AND IMPLEMENTATION

Nursing interventions for patients with Impaired Verbal Communication can be organized according to which of the four major components of the communication process they treat: sender, message, receiver, or feedback. When selecting nursing interventions, the nurse must consider related factors, such as physical condition, emotional state, and perceptions, that may negatively influence the communication process.

To generate and transmit a message, the patient (either the sender or receiver) must notice, perceive, and process stimuli. The physical, developmental, and psychosocial conditions of the patient as well as environmental and cultural factors can interfere in this stage of communication, thereby becoming the foci of nursing interventions.

Extremely physically ill patients may be unable to participate in assessment or in trials of a communication system, and their acceptance of communication disabilities may be unstable. The environment can be manipulated by the nurse to reduce or to increase available stimuli, such as providing music or pictures for the patient in an intensive care unit. The patient's ability to identify and to focus on relevant stimuli can be aided directly through the nurse's teaching these skills. Indirect interventions include reducing excessive stress and the emotions affecting identification of and attention to stimuli. The nurse can also intervene to prevent or to correct the patient's distortion, omission, or false perception of stimuli.

Effective communication also depends on the ability to send precise, succinct, and understandable messages. The nurse should refer the patient for assistance in correcting, modifying, or preventing physical conditions that interfere with the transmission of messages. The nurse can assist the patient in this stage of communication through demonstrating, teaching, and supporting the patient's use of effective communication techniques. The nurse must identify the patient's cognitive skills and interpretation of nonverbal communication. The nurse should also assist the patient in mastering any developmental tasks or overcoming cultural differences that interfere with the transmission of clear messages. Attempts at communication (verbal and nonverbal) should be encouraged.

The message component of communication involves the translation of ideas, purpose, and intent into congruent verbal and nonverbal communication. A number of communication aids may be used to assist a patient unable to speak[1,2] (e.g., signing systems, individualized communication charts, electronic aids, and writing or drawing). Any aid used should be introduced early in treatment to avoid the patient's rejection of it as second

◼ **NURSING CARE GUIDELINES**
Nursing Diagnosis: Impaired Verbal Communication*

Expected Outcome: The patient will notice, perceive, and process relevant stimuli.
- ▲ Refer patient for help correcting, modifying, or preventing physical conditions that interfere with communication. *Speech pathologists or others working in conjunction with the nurse are valuable partners who can assist with assessment and intervention strategies.*
- ◼ Manipulate environment to increase or decrease stimuli. *Perception and interpretation of communication is based on stimuli within the perceptual field.*
- ◼ Teach patient to discern and focus on relevant stimuli. *A person can consciously focus on only a few of the many stimuli available.*
- ◼ Assist in correcting faulty perceptions. *The reception and selection of appropriate stimuli depend on an individual's perception.*
- ◼ Teach methods to reduce stress. *Excessive stress can result in inaccurate perception and impaired communication.*

Expected Outcome: The patient will send precise, understandable messages.
- ◼ Assist patient in mastering tasks appropriate for the individual's age or developmental level. *Communication involves learning a series of progressive tasks over time.*
- ◼ Assist patient in increasing or modifying language skills. *Words that describe intended meaning and that the other person understands must be selected.*
- ▲ Include family members in speech therapy program. *Inclusion of family members increases their sense of positive involvement and acceptance of the patient following discharge.*
- ◼ Demonstrate, teach, and support patient's use of effective communication techniques. *Use of effective communication techniques results in transmission of understandable messages. The nurse promotes further communication and serves as a role model through use of these techniques.*
- ◼ Point out discrepancies in the patient's verbal and nonverbal behaviors. *The message component of communication depends on translation of ideas, purpose, and intent into congruent verbal and nonverbal communication.*
- ◼ Point out discrepancies in the message sent and the context within which it is sent. *The connection between message and context is explained, and the patient's perception is corrected.*
- ◼ Demonstrate, teach, and encourage expression of feelings. *Appropriate expression of feelings facilitates communication.*

Expected Outcome: The patient will transmit and receive feedback.
- ◼ Provide opportunity for and encourage interaction with others. *Communication occurs within the context of relationships, which all have variables that affect the process of communication.*
- ◼ Help patient understand the dynamics of relationships. *Evaluating the effects of one's behavior on others and understanding interpersonal relationships are necessary to send and receive feedback.*
- ◼ Describe, demonstrate, and encourage use of active listening skills. *Listening communicates concern, interest, or acceptance.*
- ◼ Support the patient's attempts to provide feedback to and accept feedback from others. *Communication is modified or corrected through the regulatory process of feedback.*

◼ = nursing intervention; ▲ = collaborative intervention.
*References 1–4, 6–9, 11, 12.

VIII

best if speech is not regained. The patient must be taught how to use a communication aid and must be encouraged to do so. An essential starting point is establishing a reliable yes or no response. Any movement that the patient can use consistently may be used. Written instructions posted near the patient's bed are helpful. A patient must be assured that assistance will arrive quickly. Beeper alarms sensitive to minimal pressure may be placed near any body part that the patient can reliably control. The nurse can intervene by indicating to the patient discrepancies in nonverbal and verbal behaviors. The patient's cultural background must be considered when selecting nursing interventions. A cultural assessment may be obtained by interviewing the patient, family members, or significant others. Interactions to reduce stress or to modify the feeling states that interfere with congruent messages should be also used.

Feedback is the regulatory process by which communication is modified or corrected, thereby establishing understanding between communicators. Therefore interventions that enhance the patient's ability to provide clear, relevant, and timely feedback should be used by the nurse. In the context of the nurse-patient relationship, the nurse can assist the patient in evaluating strengths and limitations in communication and in under-

standing the dynamics of relationships. The nurse should demonstrate, teach, and support the use and acceptance of feedback as well as the use of effective communication techniques, including active listening.

EVALUATION

The nursing interventions to alleviate Impaired Verbal Communication are evaluated by determining the patient's ability to identify expected outcomes. Achievement of the expected outcomes is assessed through the nurse's observation of and interaction with the patient, the patient's evaluation of his or her communication with others, and feedback from significant others about the patient's communication ability. If the previously identified limitations are no longer present and if the patient reports satisfaction from communication, the expected patient outcomes have been achieved and the problem of Impaired Verbal Communication has been resolved.

If expected outcomes are not achieved, the patient is assessed for the presence of the defining characteristics of Impaired Verbal Communication. A revised plan of care is developed, implemented, and evaluated.

▶ CASE STUDY WITH PLAN OF CARE

Mrs. Marilyn A. has recently been transferred to a medical unit from intensive care, where she was admitted with the diagnosis cerebrovascular accident (CVA). Her treatment on the medical unit focuses on supportive care and initial rehabilitation, one aspect of which is correction of an alteration in communication resulting from dysarthria. Dysarthria is a condition in which the musculature used in speaking is paralyzed, weak, or uncoordinated after a stroke or other neurological problem.[10] Mrs. A.'s speech is slow and halting and lacks variation in pitch and inflection. She often expresses herself nonverbally through behaviors indicating anger and frustration whenever she attempts to communicate. A

65-year-old, retired elementary school teacher, Marilyn is married and has two daughters and three grandchildren. She has adequate financial resources and an attentive, supportive family. Her medical history includes hypertension, which she has had for 20 years; she smokes one pack of cigarettes per day but has had no previous cardiovascular illness or hospitalizations. Her physical and emotional health before the CVA were good. Mrs. A. stands 5′4″ and weighs 145 pounds. Her diet is balanced but somewhat high in calories and cholesterol. Her activities include maintaining the home, reading avidly, volunteering as a tutor for children with reading difficulties, and traveling with her husband.

■ **PLAN OF CARE FOR MRS. MARILYN A.**
Nursing Diagnosis: Impaired Verbal Communication Related to Dysarthria

Expected Outcome: Mrs. A. will accurately process perceived stimuli as evidenced by verbal and non-verbal responses pertinent to the environment, the self, and other persons.
▲ Refer Mrs. A. to speech pathologist for differential dysarthria diagnosis to confirm unimpaired selection and processing of stimuli.

Expected Outcome: Mrs. A. will communicate her needs and wants clearly as evidenced by congruent verbal and nonverbal communication, speech that varies in pitch and inflection, and lack of anger and frustration when attempting to communicate.
■ Provide adequate time for Mrs. A. to initiate or respond to communication from others.
■ Ask Mrs. A. to overemphasize words she is trying to say.
■ Initially ask questions that Mrs. A. can answer with few words.
■ Provide alternatives for expressing needs and wants, such as paper and a pencil or a communication board that includes pictures Mrs. A. can point to.
▲ Teach Mrs. A.'s husband the alternate communication system and encourage him to use it.
■ Demonstrate and encourage nonverbal behaviors that replace or emphasize verbal expression of needs and wants.
■ Praise patient's use of effective communication techniques.
■ Obtain books on tape from library.
■ Acknowledge and encourage appropriate expression of anger and frustration that Mrs. A. encounters in communication.

Expected Outcome: Mrs. A. will transmit and receive feedback as evidenced by her request for response to communication, acceptance of response, clarification or elaboration of idea, and use of effective communication techniques.
■ Establish a nurse-patient relationship.
▲ Provide opportunity for and encourage interaction with others in the medical unit and with family members.
■ Provide feedback to Mrs. A. concerning her strengths and limitations in communication.
■ Provide opportunities to practice effective communication techniques.
■ Use Mrs. A.'s strengths and offer unconditional positive regard to help her accept positive and negative feedback.
■ Instruct Mrs. A. to request feedback so that she can judge whether she is accurately understood.

■ = nursing intervention; ▲ = collaborative intervention.

VIII

■ CRITICAL THINKING EXERCISES

1. A person cannot not communicate. What does this statement mean? What implications does this have on assessment of the patient's communication pattern?
2. To communicate, the message sent must be the message received. How can the nurse assist the patient in determining that the message sent is the same as the message received?
3. Impaired communication can result from not understanding or considering cultural influences. Describe how culture may influence the four major components of the communication process: sender, message, receiver, and feedback.
4. Because communication occurs within the context of relationships, collaborative care is essential for the patient with Impaired Verbal Communication. Name and describe the role of the key collaborators in the care of such a patient.

REFERENCES

1. Adkins E: Nursing care of clients with impaired communication, *Rehab Nurs* 16:74–77, 1992.
2. Boss B: Managing communication disorder in stroke, *Nurs Clin North Am* 26(4):985–990, 1991.
3. Buckwalter K and others: Family involvement with communication-impaired resident in long-term care settings, *Applied Nurs Res* 4(2):77–83, 1991.
4. Burgess A: *Psychiatric nursing in the hospital and the community*, ed 5, Norwalk, Connecticut, 1990, Appleton & Lange.
5. Crowther D: Metacommunications: a missed opportunity, *J Psychosoc Nurs Ment Health Serv* 29(4):13–16, 1991.
6. Kim M, McFarland G, and McLane A: *Pocket guide to nursing diagnoses*, ed 6, St. Louis, 1995, Mosby–Year Book.
7. McCloskey J and Bulechek G: *Nursing interventions classification (NIC)*, ed 2, St. Louis, 1996, Mosby–Year Book.
8. McFarland G, Wasli E, and Gerety E: *Nursing diagnoses and process in psychiatric mental health nursing*, ed 2, Philadelphia, 1992, JB Lippincott Co.
9. Palmer J and Yantis P: *Survey of communication disorders*, Baltimore, 1990, Williams & Williams.
10. Ruesch J and Bateson G: *Communication: the social matrix of psychiatry*, New York, 1987, WW Norton.
11. Stuart G and Sundeen S: *Pocket guide to psychiatric nursing*, ed 3, St. Louis, 1995, Mosby–Year Book.
12. Thompson JM and others: *Mosby's clinical nursing*, ed 3, St. Louis, 1993, Mosby–Year Book.

VIII

Altered Family Processes: Alcoholism

▶

Altered Family Processes: Alcoholism *is the condition in which psychosocial, spiritual, and physiological functions of the family unit are chronically disorganized, leading to conflict, denial of problems, resistance to change, ineffective problem solving, and a series of self-perpetuating crises.*

OVERVIEW

There is a growing body of nursing literature that supports the idea that the family, rather than the individual, should be a central focus of concern for the nursing discipline.[4,8,9,40,41] Persons who abuse alcohol also affect others in their environment, especially family members. Alcoholism is an illness that alters intimate relationships within the family and impairs functioning of the nonalcoholic as well as the alcoholic members of the family. When one member of a family becomes dependent on alcohol, the family organization must change for the family to survive. For many families, alcoholism is a condition that becomes the central organizing principle around which family life is structured. In this way, alcoholism becomes inseparable and integral to the fabric of family life.[35]

In a Gallup poll in 1987, one in four families reported a problem with alcohol in the home.[31] An estimated 15.4 million Americans exhibit some symptoms of alcoholism or alcohol dependence.[27] It is estimated that alcohol imposes an $85.8 billion burden on the U.S. economy.[27] Drug abuse costs are estimated at $58.3 billion.[26] Alcoholism is such a common problem that it touches the lives of almost everyone. *Alcohol abuse* is defined by DSM-IV as a maladaptive pattern of [alcohol abuse] leading to clinically significant impairment

or distress, as manifested by one or more of the following occurring within a 12-month period:

1. Recurrent [alcohol] abuse resulting in a failure to fulfill major role obligations at work, school, or home (e.g., repeated absences or poor work performance related to substance abuse; suspensions or expulsions from school related to substance abuse; and neglect of children or household)
2. Recurrent [alcohol] abuse in situations in which it is physically hazardous (e.g., driving an automobile or operating a machine when impaired by [alcohol])
3. Recurrent [alcohol-related] legal problems (e.g., arrests for [alcohol]-related disorderly conduct)
4. Continued [alcohol] use despite having persistent or recurrent social or interpersonal problems caused or exacerbated by the effects of [alcohol] (e.g., arguments with spouse about the consequences of intoxication, physical fights)[1]

An important distinction must be made between families with alcoholism and families with an alcoholic member. Families with alcoholism are families in which one or more family members are abusing alcohol and alcoholism has become the central organizing principle. The term *alcoholic system* or *alcoholic family* describes families in which chronic alcoholism is the central organizing feature. In contrast, a family with an alcoholic member still faces the challenges of alcoholism, but the family has not reorganized in substantive ways to accommodate the alcoholic member.[34] From a nursing perspective, the term *families with alcoholism* is preferred. Although the phrase *alco-*

holic family is more common in the research literature, it connotes a disease-based perspective or a medical model of the family rather than the health-and-wellness approach that is more consistent with nursing's philosophical base.

The diagnosis Altered Family Processes: Alcoholism centers around the concept of an alcoholic system. The family systems model provides a framework for understanding patterns of family dysfunction associated with alcoholism.[3,17,20,35] The family system has dysfunctional behaviors and interactions that inhibit differentiation and support continuation of the alcohol abuse. In general, if the member of the family with alcohol abuse is kept within the family constellation, the family must fulfill the roles and responsibilities that were previously done by the member abusing alcohol. Isaacson[17] identified five dysfunctional characteristics of alcoholic families. First, the family resists change, and interactions of its family members support the stability of the dysfunctional system. Second, the individuals in the family behave and interact in ways that maintain a rigid, closed system, limiting interaction with the outside environment. Also, family problems are repeated over generations. In addition, the alcohol use covers up other family problems. Last, Isaacson[17] asserts that the family has rigid interaction patterns that do not change in response to changing circumstances.

As the alcohol abuse progresses, subtle changes in the family system occur while the family adjusts to the insidious progression of the illness. Steinglass[34] describes "regulatory behaviors" that reorganize the family around alcoholism to structure the pattern of everyday life, set family priorities, and ensure stability. Three areas that are restructured around the family's alcoholic member are daily routines, family rituals (e.g., holidays, vacation, and dinnertime), and short-term problem solving. The focus on the family's regulatory behaviors serves as a vehicle for assessment in determining the role that alcoholism has in family life.

According to an extensive study of families with alcoholism, Steinglass and others[35] found that existing daily routines become skewed and adapted to fit more closely with the drinking pattern of the alcoholic member. Daily routines include behaviors related to the home, work, school, and local communities. The behaviors in the home, however, are the most important for the family. In describing the effect of alcoholism on daily routines, Steinglass and others suggest focusing on the rhythmicity, intensity, and variability of the behaviors. The family's use of space and time also reflect the patterning or organization of the home and further describe the subtle qualitative characteristics of the daily routines. Thus such behaviors as food preparation, mealtimes, social activities in the home, and housekeeping are often arranged to minimize the likelihood of interference with the alcoholism or to interfere minimally with the drinking behavior.

Alcoholism easily disrupts the carrying out of family rituals. Holiday times, vacations, rites of passage (e.g., birthdays, weddings, and funerals), and family reunions are often undermined by the intrusion of alcoholic behavior or the need to accommodate an alcoholic member. The family often has to work at preserving its rituals so that they do not become disrupted. Most often, family rituals are altered to ensure that the alcoholic member can remain a full participant in the ritual. For example, the time and site of a Christmas dinner may be changed from a relative's home to the family's home so that the intoxicated alcoholic member can join in for at least part of the activities.

The third category of observable regulatory behavior in families includes patterns of short-term problem solving centered around alcohol-related crises. When a family member is intoxicated, the behavior of the alcoholic member is a threat to the family's stability. A threat to the family's stability is a problem to which the family must respond to solve the problem. The degree of predictability in problem-solving strategies, the degree of affective expressiveness, and the degree of cohesion between family members when engaged in short-term problem solving around the alcoholic member's behavior are three areas to assess for the impact of alcoholism on the family system. Steinglass[34] points out that there are two unique problem-solving aspects in alcoholic families. First is the great sensitivity to destabilization and the vigorous response of the family to any challenge. Thus the alcoholic family often responds disproportionately to the magnitude of the problem at hand. Second, the problem-solving activities are only activated when active drinking occurs. For example, if a family member's heightened expressiveness is important to family problem solving, the heightened expressiveness only will occur when the member is intoxicated.

Coleman[5] describes relationships within alcoholic families. There is a dysfunction with intimacy as members of the family have difficulty developing close relationships with others. Specifically, intimacy dysfunction is related to difficulty with boundaries. Boundaries are defined by rules that delimit appropriate behavior in relation to one another.[37] Healthy boundaries are flexible and open at times but become rigid and closed depending on the circumstances. Coleman[5] describes three characteristics of boundaries in families with alcohol abuse. Family members are too invasive of one another's boundaries. Boundaries may also be distant and rigid, or they are so ambiguous that family members do not know their standing with other family members. Emotional bonds with others outside of the family are often weak because family members are frequently disconnected from the extended family and from the community.

Another characteristic of the family with Altered Family Processes: Alcoholism is the system of denial.[3,5,34,37] Denial and family secrets permeate the family. The denial system distorts reality to avoid dealing with the problems in the family associated with the alcoholic behavior. Denial permits the addicted person to continue using alcohol by negating the adverse effects of the alcoholism from their awareness. Children often become partners in the family denial as a means of keeping the secret within the family. Family members act as if everything is normal.

Dysfunctional family patterns also include changes in role functions. Role changes serve to disguise the illness and to distract family members from the real problems and from their feelings. Because family members repress, suppress, or deny feelings, emotional growth for family members is thwarted. Most role behaviors revolve around the substance abuser. Spouses and children feel emotionally abandoned as the alcohol becomes the primary relationship for the addicted family member. The addicted person's behavior is unfamiliar, unacceptable, and unpredictable and includes angry outbursts, rages, and selfish, demanding behaviors.[37] The family atmosphere is tense and fearful. Parenting becomes inconsistent or even nonexistent. Parenting roles become reversed because children may need to take on the role of parent to care for one another or even to care for their parents because attention is absent.

Wegscheider[39] identifies five common role patterns in families with alcoholism. The "chief enabler" is usually a spouse or parent. The chief enabler protects the abuser and compensates for the loss of control. The protection and compensation enables the illness to continue within the family. The enabler has been more recently described as the "codependent." The codependent is a person who allows another's behavior to affect him or her while being obsessed with controlling the other person's behavior. The codependent develops an unhealthy pattern of relating to others, low self-esteem, a need to be needed, a strong urge to change others, and a willingness to suffer as a result of being closely involved with someone who has a drug or alcohol problem.[43]

The "family hero" is usually the oldest child, who takes on the role of hero through hard work, achievement, and success in school. The family hero provides self-worth for the family and has an overdeveloped sense of accomplishment, responsibility, and perfectionism. The family "scapegoat" is the third role described by Wegscheider.[39] The scapegoat is the child who acts out or abuses alcohol or drugs, thereby deflecting focus away from the family problems. Underneath the scapegoat's acting-out behavior, he or she feels loneliness, deep hurt, and pain. The "lost child" is often the third or middle child. These children often withdraw and are quiet and independent, avoid confrontation, are lonely, feel inadequate, and have difficulty emotionally connecting to others. The

VIII

last role behavior is the family "mascot." The mascot is often the youngest child, who provides the fun and humor to distract family members from the tension of alcohol abuse. The mascot is often an underachiever, senses the tension, and feels insecure, frightened, and lonely. The roles described by Wegscheider[39] are defensive personalities that represent survival strategies for family members living in what is experienced as a frightening family environment. However, each family is unique, and the complex dynamics of family should not be simplified to fit these categories.

Disruption of the family because of alcoholism is a serious, complex, and pervasive family problem. Characteristics of alcoholic families include concealment of true feelings and needs; deterioration of relationships within and outside of the family; separation and divorce; marital sexual dissatisfaction; role reversal; role ambiguity; family disorganization; family dissatisfaction; and resistance to change.[7,25,28,42]

Lindeman, Hawks, and Bartek[22] have made a major contribution in developing the nursing diagnosis Altered Family Processes: Alcoholism. The staggering figures involved in the financial cost of alcoholism can also be viewed from a family perspective in that they represent the loss of income and jobs. Alcoholism has been linked to family violence, child abuse,[13] incest,[12,33] disrupted family roles and functions, family conflict, impaired family communication, and certain physical and psychological illnesses.[21,23,25,32,36] Nurses are in a prime position to identify family members who are abusing alcohol to help families face and deal with the problem, to decrease enabling behaviors, and to motivate the person to seek treatment.[37]

ASSESSMENT

Diagnostic and treatment considerations for Altered Family Processes: Alcoholism include (1) the level of impairment in the identified patient, (2) the extent that the family is organized around alcohol, and (3) the degree that alcohol has disrupted family growth and development. Mild, moderate, and severe pathology of family processes often parallel the progressive early,

middle, and late stages of alcoholism.[38] A family with early-stage alcoholism will engage in normal problem solving and will attempt to adjust. Signs of an emerging problem (e.g., alcohol-related accidents and increasing use of alcohol to cope with normal stress) may be outside the family's awareness and denied or rationalized. The family with middle-stage alcoholism may develop a pattern of habitual, self-defeating coping responses. Enmeshment with alcoholic behaviors is reflected in repeated and unsuccessful attempt to control the drinker's behavior. The family with late-stage alcoholism may collapse as a result of escalating stress and a breakdown in all spheres of family function.[11] Alternately, families may reach a stable, dysfunctional status that permits the family unit to exist while the alcohol-impaired individual continues to drink him- or herself to death.[35]

The impact of alcohol on the family is determined by assessment of the alcohol-impaired individual and other significant family members (i.e., the marital dyad, the immediate family, and the important extended family). Conjoint interviews are recommended to gain different perspectives of the problem.[34] Separate spousal interviews (or separate parent and child interviews if the drinker is an adolescent or older adult) should be allowed to elicit concerns that either may be reluctant to address in the presence of the other (e.g., violence, sexual abuse, or planned separation).[29]

The nurse may encounter families with direct or indirect presentations of alcohol-related problems.[24] Direct presentations occur when the family requests help for an alcohol-impaired member or when the family becomes involved to support the individual drinker's request for help. Commonly, an alcohol-related crisis (e.g., major financial or legal problems) precipitates the request for assistance and may require immediate attention and referral before assessment can proceed. Indirect presentations of alcohol-related problems occur when assistance is sought for problems ostensibly unrelated to alcohol, such as marital and relationship problems, depression, and behavioral problems with children. These families often require a more gradual approach to alcohol assessment and intervention.

Families affected by alcoholism often experience profound denial, shame, and a sense of failure. Extensive psychological defenses (e.g., repression and denial) may be in place for the purpose of avoiding painful feelings. It is important therefore that the nurse project an open, caring, nonjudgmental attitude and avoid blaming or reinforcing criticism of the drinker or other family members. Sensitivity to cultural factors, such as age, gender, ethnicity, economic status, and religion is also required. For example, women often experience more guilt than men about their drinking and experience lower self-esteem[10]; older adults' ability to ask for and receive help may be hindered by lifelong attitudes and beliefs about alcohol[14]; and children may feel unduly responsible for family problems.

The alcohol-impaired individual is assessed for readiness to change and for drinking history. A number of alcohol screening and assessment tools are available to the nurse to assist with data collection.[2,18] The duration and pattern of patient use can be established by determining the onset of alcohol use, the amount used, and the frequency of use (e.g., daily weekly, monthly, or binge versus maintenance drinking). Alcohol abuse is differentiated from alcohol dependence by the presence of tolerance (more of the substance required to get the same effect) and withdrawal symptoms (e.g., autonomic hyperactivity; insomnia; tactile, auditory, or visual hallucinations; and seizures).[1] The abuse of other substances is common and patients should be questioned about it. Inquiries on the psychological aspects (e.g., thoughts and feelings about their use), the social context (e.g., drinking situations), and the cultural context (e.g., acceptability) of drinking provide clues for specific cognitive, emotional, and behavioral changes necessary to establish sobriety. Questions regarding the patient's view on the relationship of his or her current problems to alcohol use, the patient's drinking goals (abstinence, reduced drinking, or continued drinking), previous attempts to reduce or quit drinking, and experiences with 12-step groups and/or professional treatment help identify motivations for change, insight, and strength as well as potential barriers to treatment.

Family assessment includes identifying data about the family, a family history, and family regulatory behaviors, relationships, role functions, and communications. Family self-assessment instruments, such as the Family Assessment Device, the Family Assessment Measure, the Family Adaptability and Cohesion Evaluation Scales, and the Family Environment Scale, can be utilized adjunctively by the nurse to collect large amounts of family information before or after the initial interview.[30]

Identifying data includes the family's composition, ethnic and cultural background, religious affiliation, employment status, income, and developmental stage. A family history may be gathered utilizing a genogram (a diagram of 3 or 4 generations) to identify family relationships, substance abuse patterns, and intergenerational influences. Concurrent substance abuse in other family members should be determined and, if present, recognized as an obstacle to individual and family recovery. Conversely, recovering members should be identified and praised because they represent potential sources of support for sobriety.

The family's understanding of their current situation should be explored. Questions should elicit their views of the relationship of current and past problems to alcohol abuse, the role of other factors contributing to current problems, and what changes they expect will improve the situation. Current and past coping responses to intoxicated behaviors should be identified. Family members may engage in ultimatums, threats, avoidance, sexual withdrawal, or indulgence, or they may seek help. What strategies in the past resulted in less drinking or more drinking or had no effect? Behaviors that enable drinking or activities that sabotage abstinence should be investigated. For instance, have family members ever encouraged drinking by loaning money to, buying alcohol for, or drinking with the patient? Previous efforts to obtain help should be identified as well as outcomes. What goals do family members identify for themselves and the family as well as the alcohol-impaired person?

The extent to which the family is organized around alcohol is assessed by exploring the role of

VII

alcohol in daily routine and family rituals and traditions. Family members may be asked what adjustments or accommodations are made for the alcohol-impaired individual during the daily routines of food preparation, mealtimes, social activities, home maintenance, and sleep-wake cycles. The effects of alcohol on family rituals and traditions can be discerned by asking about alcohol-related considerations for vacations, birthdays, holidays, and religious celebrations; the presence of alcohol as these events; and the extent to which these activities have been disrupted by alcohol. Families organized around alcohol will describe myriad disruptive effects associated with the alcohol-impaired individual's behavior and/or numerous measures undertaken by the family to ameliorate these effects.

Family roles and relationships are assessed for competence factors such as happiness, optimism, problem-solving abilities, allowance for individuality, acceptance of individuals, and love in the home.[16] Families impaired by alcoholism will often experience low satisfaction, poor self-esteem, crisis-orientation, rigid role expectations, and tension. Flexible family controls may be lacking and may be replaced with rigid, laissez-faire, or chaotic rules and structure. Impaired control may be manifested in emotional, physical, and sexual abuse, and family members should be asked about it directly. Marital conflict is prevalent. Inquiry should be made about past, present, or planned separations. Sexual problems are common and should be reviewed. Spouses and children frequently overfunction to compensate for the underfunctioning, alcohol-impaired individual. Inconsistent parenting may be present, and parental responsibilities, such as child care and home maintenance, may be inappropriately assumed by the children. Emotional neglect of the children may be evidenced in poor parent-child communication and lack of parental affection. Ask the children about school, behavioral, and health problems.

Family communication is assessed for the presence of direct, open discussions and open conflict resolution. Families with alcoholism may exhibit controlling, contradictory, indirect, or closed communication patterns. Triangulation, or the inclu-

sion of a third family member (often a child) to manage dyad conflict (often between parents), is common, as is blaming or scapegoating select members for all of the family problems. Patterns of pursuing and distancing may be apparent.[6] For example, the spouse, attempting to cope with anxiety caused by drinking, relentlessly berates or coaxes the alcoholic to change his or her behavior. This stimulates anxiety in the alcohol-impaired individual, who then distances him- or herself by drinking.

Family affective involvement and expression is assessed for open expressions of warmth, caring, and closeness. Altered family emotional processes may be described as uninvolved, lacking in feeling, narcissistic, or enmeshed.[37] Appropriate range, quality, and quantity of emotional expression may be limited and is reflected in patterns of avoiding, denying, or repressing feelings. The family may demonstrate diminished interest in the activities of individual family members. A marked lack of nurturance and support for one another may be evident, coupled with rigid expectations for each member. Poor parent-child communication and lack of affection may indicate the emotional neglect of children. Emotional bonds with extended family and society are often weak or absent.

■ Defining Characteristics

The presence of the following defining characteristics indicates that the family may be experiencing Altered Family Processes: Alcoholism[22]:

- Loss of drinking control
- Denial of problems
- Alcohol abuse
- Substance abuse other than alcohol
- Impaired communication
- Ineffective problem-solving skills
- Limited understanding of alcoholism
- Enabling behaviors
- Rationalization
- Alcohol-centered family occasions
- Refusal to ask for help
- Escalating conflicts
- Deterioration of family relationships
- Disturbed family dynamics

- Marital problems
- Sexual dysfunction
- Inconsistent parenting
- Family denial
- Closed communications
- Rigid family rules
- Impaired family controls
- Over- or underfunctioning
- Disturbed academic performance in children
- Decreased self-esteem
- Anger
- Depression
- Anxiety
- Guilt
- Shame
- Loneliness
- Insecurity
- Avoiding, repressing, denying emotions
- Responsibility for the alcoholic's behavior
- Resentments

■ Related Factors

The following related factors are associated with Altered Family Processes: Alcoholism:

- Alcohol misuse
- Alcohol abuse
- Alcohol dependence
- A family history of alcoholism
- Lack of problem-solving skills
- Impaired interpersonal skills
- Unresolved developmental stages
- Insufficient instrumental or expressive resources

DIAGNOSIS

■ Differential Nursing Diagnosis

Three NANDA nursing diagnoses need differentiation from Altered Family Processes: Alcoholism: Altered Family Processes; Ineffective Family Coping: Disabled; and Ineffective Family Processes: Compromised. Many of the defining characteristics of Altered Family Processes are applicable to Altered Family Processes: Alcoholism; however, the definition and related factors do not apply. The definition of Ineffective Family Coping: Disabled partially addresses the situation

that may exist in families with alcoholism; however, the related factors of this diagnosis do not adequately describe the etiology of alcoholism in the family as a whole. In addition, the defining characteristics of Ineffective Family Coping: Disabled do not include problems such as the chronicity of the situation and the inability of family members to meet and express emotional needs. Last, Ineffective Family Processes: Compromised is even less appropriate for families with alcoholism because it is most concerned with temporary situations resulting from illness or disability.[22] Most importantly, Altered Family Processes: Alcoholism is distinguished from all other diagnoses by its emphasis on the family as a whole and the presence of alcoholism.

■ Medical and Psychiatric Diagnoses

Related psychiatric diagnosis alcohol dependence and alcohol abuse. Specifiers to each diagnosis include the following: with physiological dependence, without physiological dependence, early or partial remission, sustained partial or full remission, and on agonist therapy. Personality disorders and affective disorders are common.[1] Alcoholism is associated with a wide variety of medical complications, including malnutrition and gastrointestinal, neurological, hematological, coronary, and skeletal muscular disorders. Nicotine addiction is endemic. High rates of alcohol consumption are involved in motor vehicle accidents, general aviation crashes, drownings, suicides, and homicides.[27] Current trends in collaborative care include prevention, screening, brief intervention, comprehensive biopsychosocial assessment, and treatment matching.

OUTCOME IDENTIFICATION, PLANNING, AND IMPLEMENTATION

Outcomes for families experiencing alcoholism include reduced or eliminated drinking, a modified family atmosphere conducive to the alcoholic's efforts to change, and readjustment of family processes toward recovery and wellness. Nursing interventions seek to empower the family with

VIII

information about the effects of alcohol on the individual and family, to assure for safety, to guide the family in establishing an alcohol-free environment, and to support them in accessing family recovery resources.

Assessment findings are reviewed with the family and include confirmation of alcohol abuse or dependence; discussion of denial, enabling, or sabotaging behaviors; destructive use of anger, rationalization, and projection; and maladaptive alcohol-related interaction patterns. The nurse should respond carefully to family concerns and questions, with support for accurate perceptions, clarification of misperceptions, and validation of feelings. Family strengths and resources should be highlighted. For instance, the family may be commended for their efforts in seeking treatment.

Alcohol education is provided to correct knowledge deficits, clarify values, shift attitudes, and prepare the family for change.[29] Factual information on the effects of alcohol should be given and myths about alcohol dispelled (e.g., beer is safer than hard spirits, or alcohol helps with sleep). Values clarification is facilitated by discussing the importance placed on alcohol for socialization, stress management, and problem solving. Attitudes toward alcohol (e.g., alcohol helps coping) may be changed by comparing the relative advantages and disadvantages of drinking. Reframing alcohol abuse as a family problem introduces the need for family members to begin focusing on themselves instead of the alcohol-impaired person. Alternate behaviors to alcohol interactions may be explored. For example, time-outs may be identified as a strategy to interrupt escalating conflicts.

Treatment recommendations usually include individual alcohol treatment of the identified patient and referral of family members to education groups, individual or family counseling or therapy, and/or self-help groups (e.g., Al-Anon). The potential for violence or abuse is a serious matter, and recommendations for the management and cessation of physical, emotional, sexual abuse must be made. An empathetic stance is helpful while assisting the family to establish a plan for safety or when informing them of obligations to report suspected abuse.

The family is assisted in establishing an alcohol-free environment. Necessary anticipatory guidance about the tasks of early recovery is provided. For example, roles can be expected to change and new behaviors required as the family shifts from a drinking-focused organization to a recovery-focused organization. Disappointment that chronic problems and conflicts do not magically disappear once alcohol is removed may be experienced. Resentments can occur as the alcoholic reasserts him- or herself in family functioning. The time required by members to attend treatment and support groups may conflict with individual expectations for time spent together.

A written behavioral contract is a useful technique that specifies the goal of abstinence and the responsibilities of each family member toward attaining the goal.[29] The alcohol-impaired person may be required to attend professional treatment and a specific number of Alcoholics Anonymous (AA) meetings per week and to avoid alcohol-related situations. Family members may be required to eliminate alcohol from the home, to limit criticism of the drinker, and to support attendance at treatment and AA meetings. Drinking lapses are common, and a plan of action should be identified for this possibility. Contracts ideally are realistic, mutually agreed upon, and achieved by active participation of all family members.

If the alcohol-impaired individual is unwilling to stop drinking, the nurse may assist the family to confront the alcoholic further or disengage from the alcoholic. The classic Johnson intervention[19] is a planned confrontation by a specially trained therapist, carried out in a caring manner to confront the alcoholic and to convince him or her to accept treatment. Consequences for failing to accept treatment are spelled out and may include loss of employment or being asked to leave the home.

◢ NURSING CARE GUIDELINES
Nursing Diagnosis: Altered Family Processes: Alcoholism

Expected Outcome: The family will maintain a safe environment.
- Assess for abuse in the family. *Abuse is often common in families with alcoholism.*
- If abuse is present, take steps to assure safety for the client, significant other, or the children. *A family may require outside help to assure the safety of its members.*

Expected Outcome: Family members will identify the presence of alcoholism and its effects on individual and family functioning.
- Assess individual drinking history and family consequences or complications. *Assessment forms the basis for treatment planning and intervention.*
- Use a nonjudgmental, accepting, and empathetic stance to facilitate family members' expression of thoughts and feelings. *Alcohol-impaired families experience painful feelings and stigma.*
- Discuss evidence of denial, sabotaging, or enabling behaviors; use of anger, rationalization, and projection; role impairment; and alcohol-related interaction patterns. *The nurse shares observations to increase family insight and awareness of alcohol-affected family dynamics.*
- Reframe alcohol-related problems as a family issue. *Family members begin self-change and recovery by differentiating their needs from those of the alcohol-impaired individual.*

Expected Outcome: The family will establish an alcohol-free environment to begin recovery and improve treatment engagement.
- Provide alcohol education as needed. *Education is provided to reduce knowledge deficits, change attitudes, and improve coping skills.*
- Teach alternate behaviors to alcohol-interaction patterns (e.g., assertiveness and anger management). *Negative interactions may precipitate further abusive drinking.*
- Identify family strengths and individual recovery responsibilities. *Identification of strengths assists in mobilizing family resources.*
- Provide anticipatory guidance regarding effects of removing alcohol from the family system. *Removal of alcohol from the family system challenges patterned communication and family roles.*
- Develop family contract specifying the goal of alcohol cessation and actions required of the drinker and individual family members. *Alcohol abstinence is improved when goals are clearly stated and actions to support goals are specific.*
- Include specific consequences and a plan of action if drinking resumes. *A plan of action assists family if relapse occurs. Relapse is a common occurrence.*
- Encourage involvement in self-help groups, education groups, and family therapy as appropriate. *Group work and family therapy offer support and guidance during the process of change.*
- Assist the family in increasing positive interchanges, planning for shared recreational and leisure activities, and reestablishment of family core rituals. *Alcohol cessation shifts family homeostasis and requires new relational skills.*

■ = nursing intervention; ▲ = collaborative intervention.

VIII

EVALUATION

Evaluation of nursing interventions related to Altered Family Processes: Alcoholism is determined by (1) the extent the individual and family can establish and maintain sobriety and (2) the adjustment of altered family processes toward a more functional level. Potential outcomes include the following: the drinker and the family both change; the drinker changes but the family does not change; the drinker does not change but the family does; and neither the drinker nor the family changes.[15] The plan of care is modified accordingly for each outcome. When the family and the drinker establish sobriety and embark on mutual change, short-term and intermediate care may focus on relapse prevention, increasing positive interchanges, planning shared recreational and leisure activities, conflict resolution, and problem solving.[29] Long-term care may include counseling and assistance with role adjustment, sex and intimacy, and parent-child relationships.[29]

The individual may accomplish sobriety; however, the family may demonstrate resistance to changing destructive interaction patterns. For example, some family members may continue to keep alcohol in the home or be unable to disengage from running conflicts. Family interventions and goals then require reassessment. The individual may be encouraged to develop sources of sober support outside the family and may be offered skills training to cope with ongoing family dysfunction.

Introduction of sobriety into an alcohol-impaired family system may also precipitate marital breakup in couples who determine they have irreconcilable differences. O'Farrell and Cowles[29] state that the therapist can assist the family to negotiate separation and divorce "without requiring the alcoholic to fail again and be the scapegoat for the breakup."

If the alcohol-impaired person is unable to establish sobriety but family members are willing to engage in efforts toward change, interventions can focus on individual coping abilities, family functioning, and strategies to encourage sobriety and professional treatment.[29] If the family and the alcohol-impaired person are unwilling to attempt change, the goals of continued treatment are discussed and renegotiated. A referral or open offer for future assistance can be made if the family chooses to terminate therapy.

CASE STUDY WITH PLAN OF CARE

Jack C. is meeting with a nurse case manager at an alcohol treatment center to discuss concerns about his wife's drinking. Jack recently received a phone call from the pediatrician's office expressing concern that his wife has smelled of alcohol during a recent visit for their 6-year-old son. Jack reports that his wife had been a social drinker for the entire 8 years of their marriage, with increased use in the past year. She seems more preoccupied with drinking. There has been decreasing contact with each other's families and increased absences from her job, for which Jack has called in. Jack describes the family atmosphere as tense, and his son has seemed more withdrawn. Recently there have been more arguments about money concerns. Lately he has been alarmed that his wife has lost control while disciplining the children. He has tried to control his wife's drinking by getting her to agree to only two drinks after dinner and by removing alcohol from the house. The nurse intake coordinator assesses for and makes the diagnosis Altered Family Processes: Alcoholism and arranges for Mr. C. to bring his wife in for a couple's interview.

PLAN OF CARE FOR THE C. FAMILY
Nursing Diagnosis: Altered Family Processes: Alcoholism Related to Alcohol Abuse

Expected Outcome: The C. family will have a safe environment after the first session.
- Assess for presence of abuse and relationship to intoxication.
- If abuse is found, take steps to ensure safety of children.
- Teach parenting skills if needed.

Expected Outcome: The C. family acknowledge the presence of alcoholism and its effects on family functioning within one to two sessions.
- Assess individual and family functioning.

■ = nursing intervention; ▲ = collaborative intervention.

- Determine the role of alcohol in the family.
- Provide feedback to family regarding evidence of Altered Family Processes: Alcoholism.

Expected Outcome: The C. family will establish an alcohol-free environment within two or three sessions.
- Provide education about the effects of alcohol on individual and family functioning.
- Provide guidance about the effect of removing alcohol from the family.
- Develop contract with Mr. and Mrs. C. specifying goal of alcohol cessation and actions required by each family member (e.g., outpatient treatment 3 days a week for Mrs. C.).
- Identify plan of action if Mrs. C. resumes drinking.
- Encourage involvement in self-help groups, AA, or Al-Anon.

Expected Outcome: Mr. C. will demonstrate understanding of his role in his wife's drinking in four to eight sessions.
- Elicit from Jack ways in which he attempts to control her drinking.
- Assure Jack that he neither causes the drinking nor controls it.
- Help Jack distinguish between destructive aspects of enabling behavior and genuine motivation to help his wife.
- Teach Jack communication and problem-solving skills as appropriate.

■ CRITICAL THINKING EXERCISES

1. How does the enabler's role influence the abuser's use of alcohol?
2. How does the pattern of alcohol use affect the children in the family?
3. What are the effects of alcohol on intimacy in the family?
4. How do the role structures and functions change in the family with alcoholism?
5. How will removing alcohol from the family potentially affect the stabilization of family dynamics?

REFERENCES

1. American Psychiatric Association: *Diagnostic and statistical manual of mental disorders,* ed 4, Washington, D.C., 1994, The Association.
2. Babor TF: Alcohol and drug use history, patterns, and problems. In Rounsaville B, Tims F, Horton F, and Sowder B, editors: *Diagnostic sourcebook on drug abuse research and treatment,* Rockville, Maryland, 1993, U.S. Department of Health and Human Services.
3. Bowen M: Alcoholism as viewed through family systems theory and family psychotherapy, *Ann New York Acad Sci* 233:115–122, 1974.
4. Clements IW and Roberts FB: *Family health: a theoretical approach to nursing care,* New York, 1983, John Wiley & Sons.
5. Coleman E: Marital and relationship problems among chemically dependent and codependent relationships. Special issue: Chemical dependency and intimacy dysfunction, *J Chem Depend Treat* 1(1):39–59, 1987.
6. Eell MAW: Interventions with alcoholics and their families, *Nurs Clin North Am* 21(3):493–504, 1986
7. El-Guebaly H and others: Adult children of problem drinkers in an urban community, *Brit J Psychiatry* 156:349–355, 1990.
8. Friedmann M-L: Closing the gap between grand theory and mental health practice with families, Part 1: the framework of systematic organization for nursing of families and family members, *Arch Psychiatr Nurs* 3:10–19, 1989.
9. Gilliss CL and others: *Toward a science of family nursing,* Menlo Park, California, 1989, Addison-Wesley.
10. Gomberg ES: Women with alcohol problems. In Estes NJ and Heinemann ME, editors: *Alcoholism: development, consequences, and interventions,* St. Louis, 1986, The CV Mosby Co.
11. Gorski T and Miller M: *Staying sober: a guide for relapse prevention,* Independence, Missouri, 1986, Herald House/ Independence Press.
12. Herman JL: *Trauma and recovery,* New York, 1992, Basic Books.
13. Hindman M: Family violence, *Alcohol Health Res World* 1:1–11, 1979.
14. Hoffman A and Heinemann M: Alcohol problems in elderly persons. In Estes NJ and Heinemann ME, editors: *Alcoholism: development, consequences, and interventions,* St. Louis, 1986, The CV Mosby Co.
15. Howe B: *Alcohol education: a handbook for health and welfare professionals,* London, 1989, Tavistock/Routledge.

VII

16. Hulgus YF, Hampson RB, and Beavers WR: *Self-report family inventory,* Dallas, 1985, Southwest Family Institute.

17. Isaacson EB: Chemical addiction: individuals and family systems, *J Chem Depend Treat* 8(1):7–27, 1991.

18. Jacobson GR: A comprehensive approach to pretreatment evaluation: detection, assessment, and diagnosis of alcoholism. In Hester RK and Miller WR, editors: *Handbook of alcoholism treatment approaches: effective alternatives,* New York, 1989, Pergamon Press.

19. Johnson V: *I'll quit tomorrow,* New York, 1980, Harper & Row.

20. Kaufman E: Family systems and family therapy of substance abuse: an overview of two decades of research and clinical experience, *J Studies Alcohol* 42:466–482, 1985.

21. Kua E and Ko S: Family violence and Asian drinkers, *Forens Sci Int* 50:43–46, 1991.

22. Lindeman M, Hawks JH, and Bartek JK: The alcoholic family: a nursing diagnosis validation study, *Nurs Diagnosis* 5(2):65–73, 1994.

23. McGann K: Self-reported illnesses in family members of alcoholics, *Family Med* 22:103–106, 1990.

24. McIntyre J: Family treatment of substance abuse. In Straussner S, editor: *Clinical work with substance-abusing clients,* New York, 1993, Guilford Press.

25. McKay J and others: Family dysfunction and alcohol and drug use in adolescent psychiatric inpatients, *J Am Acad Child Adolesc Psychiatry* 30:967–972, 1991.

26. National Council on Alcohol and Drug Dependence: *The war on drugs: failure and fantasy,* Washington, D.C., 1991, The Council.

27. National Institute on Alcohol Abuse and Alcoholism: *Eighth special report to U.S. Congress: alcohol and health,* DHHS Pub No AMD 281-88-003, Alexandria, Virginia, 1993, Editorial Experts.

28. O'Farrell T, Choquette K, and Birchler G: Sexual satisfaction and dissatisfaction in the marital relationships of male alcoholics seeking marital therapy, *J Studies Alcohol* 52: 441–447, 1991.

29. O'Farrell TJ and Cowles KS: Marital and family therapy. In Hester RK and Miller WR, editors: *Handbook of alcoholism treatment approaches: effective alternatives,* New York, 1989, Pergamon Press.

30. Olson D and Tiesal JW: Assessment of family functioning. In Rounsaville B and others, editors: *Diagnostic sourcebook on drug abuse research and treatment,* Rockville, Maryland, 1993, U.S. Department of Health and Human Services.

31. Raskin MS and Daley DC: Overview of addiction. In Daley DC and Raskin MS, editors: *Treating the chemically dependent and their families,* Newbury Park, California, 1991, Sage Publications.

32. Reich W, Earls F, and Powell: A comparison of the home and social environments of children of alcoholics and non-alcoholic parents, *Brit J Addictions* 83:831–839, 1988.

33. Sheinberg M: Navigating treatment impasses at disclosure of incest: combining ideas from feminism and social construction, *Family Process* 31:201–216, 1992.

34. Steinglass P: Family therapy: alcohol. In Galanter M and Kleber HD, editors: *Textbook of substance abuse treatment,* Washington, D.C., 1994, American Psychiatric Press.

35. Steinglass P and others: *The alcoholic family,* New York, 1987, Basic Books.

36. Stoker A and Swadi H: Perceived family relationships in drug abusing adolescents, *Drug Alcohol Depend* 25:293–297, 1990.

37. Sullivan EJ: *Nursing care of clients with substance abuse,* St. Louis, 1995, Mosby–Year Book.

38. Washousky R, Levy-Stern D, and Muchowski P: The stages of family alcoholism, *EAP Digest* 13(2):38–43, 1993.

39. Wegschieder S: *Another chance: hope and health for alcoholic families,* Palo Alto, California, 1981, Science & Behavior Books.

40. Whall AL: *Family therapy theory for nursing: four approaches,* Norwalk, Connecticut, 1986, Appleton-Century-Crofts.

41. Whall AL and Fawcett J: *Family theory development in nursing: state of the science and art,* Philadelphia, 1991, FA Davis.

42. Wills E: *Perceived health status, perceived stress, and family satisfaction of wives of alcoholics and non-alcoholics.* Unpublished doctoral dissertation, Austin, 1990, University of Texas.

43. Zerwekh J and Michaels B: Co-dependency: assessment and recovery, *Nurs Clin North Am* 24(1):109–120, 1989.

VIII

Altered Family Processes

▶ ────────────────────────────────────

Altered Family Processes *is the state in which a family that normally functions effectively experiences a dysfunction.*[10]

OVERVIEW

In spite of major societal changes in recent years, the family remains the basic unit in American society. Families vary significantly in lifestyles, structure, power relationships, values, social and intellectual competence, and health status. A variety of theoretical perspectives have contributed to a greater understanding of the family as a unit of care in practice and research. These perspectives include family social science theories, nursing theories, and family therapy theories. Commonly used family social science frameworks include developmental, interactionist, and systems theories. *Family* is defined in many different ways, depending on the particular theoretical perspective being used. For this discussion, *family* is defined as "two or more persons who are joined together by bonds of sharing and emotional closeness and who identify themselves as being part of the family."[4] This family systems definition is broad enough to include traditional and nontraditional variant family forms.

Although family forms may vary, families share common characteristics. Families are social systems with cultural attitudes, beliefs, and values. Each family has its own set of rules, structure, communication styles, and basic functions.[8] Families also move through developmental stages during the family life cycle.[3] However, given the changing nature of family forms in today's society, no rigid pattern of family life cycle stages is descriptive of every family. Developmental theory is useful as a component of comprehensive assessment and intervention because it provides a guideline for family growth and health promotion.

Duvall[3] identifies eight stages in the family life cycle: (1) the married couple, (2) the childbearing family, (3) the family with preschoolers, (4) the family with school-age children, (5) the family with teenagers, (6) the launching center family, (7) the middle-age family, and (8) the aging family. During each of these stages, family members accomplish certain stage-critical family developmental tasks. For example, during the eighth stage the parents may need to cope with living alone or adjust to retirement. These adjustments are considered normal or developmental. Family developmental tasks refer to growth responsibilities that families must carry out during each stage to meet biological requirements, cultural imperatives, aspirations, and values.

Families perform certain functions in society, including the provision of affection, security, affiliation, socialization, and control. Friedman[4] identifies the five basic functions of the family as (1) the affective function (maintenance of each member's personality), (2) the socialization and social placement function, (3) the reproductive function, (4) the economic function, and (5) the health care function (provision and allocation of physical necessities and health care). By performing these effectively, the family meets the needs of its members and society.

Healthy, well-functioning families demonstrate certain characteristics or strengths.[11] Identification of family strengths is important to consider when planning nursing interventions with the family. For example, if a family is deeply religious, then using this resource as a source of support should be encouraged. Otto[11] provides a framework for assessing the strengths that indicate a well-functioning family system. The absence of one or more of these characteristics may indicate an Alteration in Family Processes. Otto's 12 family strengths are the following:

1. Fulfillment of the family member's physical, emotional, and spiritual needs
2. Sensitivity to the needs of the family members
3. Effective communication of thoughts and feelings
4. The provision of support, security, and encouragement
5. The initiation and maintenance of growth-producing relationships and experiences within and outside of the family
6. The creation and maintenance of constructive and responsible community relationships
7. Growth with and through children
8. Flexibility in the performance of family roles
9. Helping oneself whenever possible and accepting aid when self-help does not suffice
10. Mutual respect for the individuality of family members
11. Growth-through-crisis experiences
12. Family unity, loyalty, and intrafamily cooperation

Family therapy theories are practice theories that provide a foundation for working with dysfunctional or troubled families.[4] Family therapy theories are generally pathology-oriented in contrast with family social science theories, which are primarily oriented toward normal families. Most family therapy theories have been influenced by systems theory. Specific theoretical approaches to family therapy may focus on family crisis interventions, behavior, psychodynamics, structure, experiences, or communication. In the family systems model, a healthy family is viewed as not only withstanding stress but changing and growing with the experience.[15] A dysfunctional family is unable to meet this challenge. In the structural model, alter-

ations in family processes result when the family structure becomes unbalanced. The communication-strategic model postulates that family dysfunctions occur as a result of inadequate communication and interaction patterns.

In summary, the family remains the basic social unit in society. Although families vary in form, structure, roles, cultural and religious values, coping styles, and communication patterns, commonalities exist. Healthy, well-functioning families demonstrate cohesion, flexibility, stability, role reciprocity, and mutuality. Effective family functioning is influenced by internal and external forces. Through the nursing process, nurses assist families in improving, maintaining, and promoting healthy family processes.

ASSESSMENT

Given the complexity of family phenomena, a combination of several family theories and assessment tools may be indicated as a basis for a comprehensive systematic approach to family assessment. Some of these theories include systems, developmental, structural-functional, and interactional approaches. Sources of family assessment data include objective observations of the home, its internal and external environment, and the interaction of family members; subjective responses of family members; and information from other health care team members.

Several approaches to family assessment are identified in the literature. Analysis of structural characteristics of the family, such as family type, organization, differentiation, boundaries, specialization, and territoriality is one approach. Internal and external processes would be analyzed from an exchange theory perspective. Another approach is the structural-process approach, which focuses on family division of labor and power, communication, boundaries, relationships with others, means of giving and obtaining emotional support, rituals and symbols, and personal roles. The process parameters focus on decision making, performance of family functions, and structural changes within the family system. The family process parameters are the methods families use to meet members' needs and to maintain communication for mutual growth and maturation. The six major categories of assessment described in the Friedman Family Assessment Model include the family's specific identifying data, present and past family developmental stages, environmental data, family structure, family functions, and family coping abilities.[4]

Two useful tools that can facilitate the data collection process are the genogram and the ecomap. The *genogram* is a diagram of the family constellation that shows the intergenerational relationships among family members. Genograms are schematically similar to family trees and provide a means for obtaining information about family relationships, the health status of family members, and family reactions to sociocultural and spiritual variables affecting their lives. The *ecomap* graphically depicts the family's relationships and interactions with the external environment. These tools assist the family in visualizing how internal or external forces may be affecting the family's health and well-being. Additionally, families with long-standing problems with their relationships may be aided by further assessment, using Satir's family life chronology model.[14]

A number of other family assessment tools are available to assist the nurse in data collection. These include the family Apgar,[15] the Family Functioning Index,[13] the Family Environmental Scale,[9] and the Family Dynamics Measure.[7]

Given the pluralistic nature of our society, cultural perspectives on health and illness vary in families. To provide culturally appropriate nursing care, an understanding of factors that affect family behaviors regarding health and illness is warranted. Cultural assessment provides meaning to behaviors that might otherwise be perceived negatively.[8] The family's patterns also influence how it copes with crises. Because the family unit is viewed as a primary source in the development of its members' attitudes, beliefs, values, and patterns of behaviors, conducting a cultural assessment would assist the nurse in planning culture-specific care with the family.[1,5] Cultural assessment is often a component of the comprehensive family assessment instrument.

Many stressors can affect family functioning and family well-being. Some of these stressors originate within the family itself, whereas others develop externally. For some families, certain events may precipitate a crisis. A *crisis* is defined as an upset in a previously steady state. Crises may be maturational or situational.[12] *Maturational* (developmental) *crises* are "normal" crises or transition points during physical, social, psychological, and intellectual growth. Examples of maturational crises are marriage, parenthood, adolescence, middlescence, and retirement.

Situational crises also occur throughout life but do not occur during specific maturational processes and are generally not anticipated. A situational crisis is sudden, external, and unexpected. Therefore the family's risk for developing distress increases because the members are unprepared to deal with changes accompanying situational events. The occurrence of a family crisis is determined by the family's perception of the event, the availability and adequacy of family support, and the family's ability to cope.[2] Situational and developmental crises may occur simultaneously, thereby increasing the chances for stress in the family system even more. Adolescent parenthood is an example of this.

Because one of the primary goals of nursing is the promotion and maintenance of health and the prevention of disease in families, a comprehensive assessment of the family health care function is indicated. Families play a major role in the provision of health care for family members. There is significant variation in families regarding perceptions and knowledge about health and illness, health care practices and beliefs, and lifestyle behaviors. The family's health history, use of health services, and adequacy of health insurance are important factors affecting family health. Environmental hazards, dietary practices, medication usage, and exercise level are additional areas for assessment. Thorough assessment will help identify behaviors that place the family at risk for ill-

VIII

ness, injury, or disease. Intervention strategies, such as health education and counseling, may be indicated to improve the family's level of health.

■ Defining Characteristics

The presence of the following defining characteristics indicates that the patient may be experiencing Altered Family Processes:

- Family unable to meet physical, emotional, spiritual, or security needs of its members
- Family fails to accomplish current or past developmental task
- Inability to express or accept wide range of feelings
- Inability to express or accept feelings of members
- Inability to adapt to change or to deal with traumatic experiences constructively
- Inability to accept or receive help
- Inability of family members to relate to each other for mutual growth and maturation
- Parents do not demonstrate respect for each other's child-rearing practices
- Rigidity in function and roles
- Ineffective family decision-making process
- Family does not demonstrate respect for individuality and autonomy of its members
- Failure to send and receive clear messages
- Inappropriate family boundaries
- Unexamined family myths
- Inappropriate or poorly communicated family rules, rituals, or symbols

■ Related Factors

The following related factors are associated with Altered Family Processes:

Situational transition and/or crises
- Disaster
- Economic crisis
- Change in family roles
- Trauma

Developmental transition and/or crises
- Birth of an infant with a defect
- Loss of a family member

- Addition of a family member
- Retirement

DIAGNOSIS

■ Differential Nursing Diagnosis

Related nursing diagnoses include Ineffective Family Coping: Compromised; Ineffective Family Coping: Disabling; Dysfunctional Grieving; Parental Role Conflict; and Altered Parenting. Generally these related diagnoses are focused on more specific health concerns or alterations within the broader area of family processes. Alteration of Family Processes focuses on the inability of the family to meet needs of members, to carry out family functions, or to maintain communications for mutual growth and maturation. Validating the critical defining characteristics with the family will clarify which diagnosis is most accurate. Often there will be several nursing diagnoses identified. Ongoing family assessment is indicated.

■ Medical and Psychiatric Diagnoses

Medical diagnoses that may be related to Altered Family Processes include any disease or illness that results in long-term disability or incapacitation, such as dementia, AIDS, cancer, traumatic injury, chronic renal failure, and terminal illness. Psychiatric diagnoses that are commonly related to Altered Family Processes include dementia, schizophrenia, and psychoactive substance use disorders. The illness or injury of a family member impacts the larger family system. Frequently, collaborative health care services are indicated to facilitate more effective family health outcomes.

OUTCOME IDENTIFICATION, PLANNING, AND IMPLEMENTATION

Nursing interventions for patients with Altered Family Processes are directed at acknowledgment of and adaptive responses to change in family roles, identification of effective coping patterns, participation in decision-making processes, and identification and utilization of community resources. Nursing interventions focus on the reduction of defining characteristics and the promotion of effective family processes. Time estimates for attainment of anticipated outcomes need to be negotiated with the family.

Initial nursing interventions will assist the family in reducing or resolving the crisis. The use of a systematic assessment tool will provide adequate background information about the family as a unit, the ill family member, and the health care environment. An understanding of family theory and family nursing research is crucial to plan interventions that are conducive for the family. The nurse and the family develop plans and goals together. In general, healthy families demonstrate the traits of good self-esteem; a sense of nurturance, acceptance, encouragement, and support; good communication; commitment to family; spending quality time together; problem-solving skills; and a shared religious orientation.[3] Family strengths should be reinforced and used in times of stress.

Because of the family crisis or situation, the division of labor and role responsibilities may be altered. To promote smooth role transition, nursing interventions may address the competence, knowledge, and skills needed for a particular family role. How the family defines its situation is a major factor in how it responds to crisis or illness.[8] Family assessment data provide cues about previous family coping strategies. Families have their own schedules for coping and for accepting extrafamilial help. Family coping over time is very complex; function or dysfunction is not a simple linear cause-and-effect outcome.[12] Because many factors influence family functioning, rigid intervention regimens based on assumptions of family care may not be effective. Interventions that work with one family may alienate another. Families cope in different ways at different times. Factors that influence family coping include the characteristics of the event, a perceived threat to the family, available resources, and past experiences. It is important to note that the family's perspective on crisis and illness may be very different from the nurses' or the ill family member's perspective. Nursing interventions should focus on the family as the unit of care and address the family's need for information, confidence, hope, and assurance of good care for the ill family member.

Many factors influence family functioning and decision making, including past unresolved issues, repeated hospitalization of an ill family member, and depletion of economic, physical, and emotional resources. The ill family member's need to maintain control may be in opposition to the family's need to care for the ill member. Families need to negotiate role division and to clarify how decisions will be made. Nursing interventions that promote the maintenance of family control and self-esteem, that provide information for informed decision making, and that facilitate open lines of communication may ease the distress and dysfunction in the family unit. Teaching the family practical coping skills, strategies for caring for the ill family member and for themselves, and how to negotiate with the health care delivery system may also be indicated. Family conferences with health care personnel will enhance communication and decision making.

Assessment of the family's support system is essential to mobilize assistance when needed. Some families who have closed rigid boundaries may not know how or may not have the desire to seek extrafamilial support. Other families desire assistance but lack the knowledge and skills needed to obtain support. Nursing interventions can promote utilization of intrafamilial and extrafamilial support through education, referral, and consultation with other health care providers and community agencies. For the family experiencing Altered Family Processes, continuity of care and follow-up are essential nursing activities.

VIII

■⌐ **NURSING CARE GUIDELINES**
Nursing Diagnosis: Altered Family Processes

Expected Outcome: The family will reduce or resolve the crisis or situation within 2 months.
- Assist family in clarifying the impact of the present situation on the family unit and its ability to meet the situational demands effectively.
- Assist the family in prioritizing family health care needs.
- Respect each family member's responses to the situation.
- Assist family to identify family strengths and coping abilities.
- Guide family in developing alternative strategies to reduce the crisis.
- Provide concrete opportunities for members to be actively involved in resolution of the situation.
- Teach family members skills required for care of ill member.
- Promote wellness for all family members through health education and counseling.
- Encourage family to participate in activities that promote feelings of competence and self-esteem.
  Families experiencing a crisis need to preserve and identify the normality of the experience and maintain competency, mastery, and self-esteem.[16]

Expected Outcome: The family will express feelings openly and honestly and will direct energies toward a purpose within 2 months.
- Promote an open, trusting relationship with family.
- Create a supportive therapeutic environment for family, where members feel accepted and affirmed.
- Support use of regularly scheduled family meeting times.
- Support family in goal formulation directed toward resolution of crisis.
- Provide opportunities for family to practice effective communication techniques.
- Encourage members to share feelings and perceptions openly and honestly.
  Expediting communication within the family and promoting mutual goals facilitates meeting reciprocal needs in a family crisis and promotes effective family coping.[6]

Expected Outcome: The family will become involved in problem-solving processes that are directed at resolution of the crisis within 2 months.
- Support family attempts at problem solving.
- Provide opportunities for family to discuss past and present coping strategies that might be used in the current situation.
- Encourage regular family meetings to clarify goals and role expectations of each member.
- Praise family achievement of goals.
- Assist family to identify effective decision-making patterns.
- Encourage time for rest and relaxation for all family members.
  Family-centered nursing care promotes self-care capabilities and decision making about health care matters.[5]

Expected Outcome: The family will experience cohesion and will adapt to change within 2 months.
- Encourage mutual support of family members by identifying family strengths and competence.
- Provide positive reinforcement of effective coping strategies and communication techniques.
- Assist family in setting realistic goals, monitor progress, and provide regular feedback.
- Assist family to identify intrafamilial and extrafamilial support systems.
- Support family members' individual need for privacy.
- ▲ If indicated, initiate and coordinate referrals to social service, financial counselors, support groups, home health care, and other community resource agencies.
  Access to additional coping resources will increase family self-confidence and competence and will decrease isolation and low self-esteem.[12]

■ = nursing intervention; ▲ = collaborative intervention.

VIII

EVALUATION

The evaluation process is ongoing and is shared by the nurse and the family. The family's outcomes must be examined to determine the effectiveness of the interventions. For families with Altered Family Processes resulting from illness of a family member, behaviors indicating that predetermined objectives have been realized include the following:

1. The family expresses feelings freely and appropriately.
2. Family members are involved in problem-solving processes directed at appropriate solutions for the situation or crisis.
3. Energies are being directed toward a purpose.
4. The family expresses an understanding of illness or trauma, treatment regimen, and prognosis.
5. Family members are allowing and encouraging the ill member to handle the situation in his or her own way.
6. Family members acknowledge a change in family roles and assume responsibility for those changes.
7. Family members identify coping patterns.
8. Family members identify and contact available resources as needed.

If family goals are not met within the mutually agreed upon time period, then interventions strategies need to be reevaluated. Were the goals reasonable and attainable for the family? What does the family perceive as obstacles to goal attainment? Alternative interventions should be implemented if defining characteristics of Altered Family Processes continue to be present. Referral to other health care team members may be indicated. Further assessment of the family's ability and readiness to accept assistance is also indicated.

▶ CASE STUDY WITH PLAN OF CARE

Mr. Elmer B., a 78-year-old male, resides with his 76-year-old wife in their own home in the country. Mr. B. recently suffered a cerebrovascular accident, which has left him with partial paralysis of the left side. He needs assistance with activities of daily living and is confined to a wheelchair at this time. Family finances are limited. Mrs. B. is a very proud woman who prefers to manage her husband's care by herself and has refused assistance up to this point. Although Mr. and Mrs. B. were involved in many community organizations and activities before Mr. B.'s illness, Mrs. B. has discontinued all activities and interests outside the home to care for her husband. Although Mr. B.'s health status continues to improve daily, Mrs. B. fears that something may happen if she spends time away from him. Mr. and Mrs. B. have an adult daughter who is married and lives in the same town. She has offered to assist her parents financially and physically. Mrs. B. refuses to discuss these issues with her daughter. Mrs. B. feels that her husband's care is her responsibility and does not want her daughter to take on this "burden." The family physician is concerned about a deterioration in Mrs. B.'s health. Her blood pressure is elevated; she complains of insomnia; and she has recently lost weight. Mrs. B. states that she is exhausted but does not want her husband or daughter to know how she feels. She has always taken care of her husband and does not want to change that now. The family physician refers the B. family to the community health nurse.

▶ PLAN OF CARE FOR THE B. FAMILY
Nursing Diagnosis: Altered Family Processes Related to Illness of a Family Member (Situational Crisis)

Expected Outcome: The B. family will express feelings freely and honestly within 2 months.
- Assess situation or crisis for causative factors.
- Provide a supportive therapeutic environment where members feel accepted and affirmed.

■ = nursing intervention; ▲ = collaborative intervention.　　　　　　　　　　　　　　　*Continued*

VIII

► PLAN OF CARE FOR THE B. FAMILY — CONT'D

- Provide opportunities for family to practice effective communication techniques.
- Encourage family members to express feelings openly.
- Support regular family meetings to clarify goals and role expectations.
- Assist the family to clarify the impact of Mr. B.'s illness on the family unit and members' ability to meet the situational demands.

Expected Outcome: The B. family's energies will be directed toward a purpose within 2 months.
- Assist family to identify problems and work toward goal resolution.
- Support family involvement in care of Mr. B. through health teaching.
- Teach or guide problem-solving methods.
- Provide opportunities for all family members to be involved in resolution or reduction of crisis situation.
- Support family in developing alternative strategies related to division of labor and communication patterns within family unit.
- Provide feedback about family progress and summarize realistic goals for the future.

Expected Outcome: The B. family will express understanding of the illness, treatment regimen, and prognosis within 2 months.
- Provide health education concerning Mr. B.'s health status and progress; clarify any misinformation.
- Provide health education regarding health promotion and maintenance for all family members.

Expected Outcome: The B. family will identify and mobilize their support system within 2 months.
- Assist the family members to identify family strengths and coping abilities.
- Assist the family to identify intrafamilial and extrafamilial support networks.
- Assist the family in setting realistic goals for individual members and for the family as a unit.
- Acknowledge Mrs. B.'s feelings of role strain and encourage problem solving.
- Provide information about community resources and coordinate services if needed.
- ▲ Family members will contact community agencies, friends, support groups as needed.

■ CRITICAL THINKING EXERCISES

1. What are the specific family strengths of the B. family and how might these be used to promote health and well-being?
2. Because the family assessment is an ongoing process, what particular sociocultural aspects of the B. family warrant further investigation?
3. Identify specific health promotion activities that would benefit the B. family.
4. How would a nursing assessment from a family perspective differ from a nursing assessment focused only on Mr. B.?

REFERENCES

1. Anderson JM: Health care across cultures, *Nurs Outlook* 38(3):136–139, 1990.
2. Clemen-Stone S, Eigsti DG, and McGuire SL: *Comprehensive family and community nursing*, ed 4, St. Louis, 1995, Mosby–Year Book.
3. Duvall EM: *Marriage and family development*, ed 5, Philadelphia, 1977, JB Lippincott Co.
4. Friedman MM: *Family nursing: theory and assessment*, ed 3, Norwalk, Connecticut, 1992, Appleton & Lange.
5. Giger JN and Davidhizar RE: *Transcultural nursing: assessment and intervention*, ed 2, St. Louis, 1995, Mosby–Year Book.
6. Hill R and Hansen D: The family in disaster. In Baker G and Chapman D, editors: *Man and society in disaster*, New York, 1962, Basic Books.

VIII

7. Lasky and others: Developing an instrument for the assessment of family dynamics, *Western J Nurs Res* 7:40–57, 1985.

8. Leininger M: *Qualitative research methods in nursing,* Orlando, Florida, 1985, Grune & Stratton.

9. Moos R, Insel P, and Humphrey B: *Preliminary manual for family environmental studies,* Palo Alto, California, 1974, Consulting Psychologists Press.

10. North American Nursing Diagnosis Association: *NANDA nursing diagnoses: definitions and classification, 1995–1996,* Philadelphia, 1994, The Association.

11. Otto HA: Criteria for assessing family strength, *Fam Process* 2(2):329–337, 1963.

12. Parad HJ: *Crisis intervention: selected readings,* New York, 1965, Family Services Association of America.

13. Pless IB and Satterwhite B: A measure of family functioning and its application, *Int J Epidemiol* 1:271–277, 1973.

14. Satir V: *Conjoint family therapy,* Palo Alto, California, 1967, Science & Behavior Books.

15. Smilkstein G: The family Apgar, *J Fam Pract* 6:1231–1239, 1978.

16. Young R: The family-illness intermesh: theoretical aspects and their application, *Soc Sci Med* 17:395–398, 1983.

VIII

Anticipatory Grieving

▶

Dysfunctional Grieving

▶

Anticipatory Grieving *is a multidimensional process that includes intellectual and emotional responses and behaviors an individual experiences before a perceived potential loss, grieving before an actual loss occurs.*[21-23]

Dysfunctional Grieving *is a process that includes maladaptive intellectual and excessive or prolonged emotional responses and behaviors that are intensified to the degree that an individual is unable to progress through the process of normal grieving after experiencing a significant loss.*[16,21]

OVERVIEW

Familiarity and knowledge of responses associated with normal grieving are essential for the recognition and understanding of Anticipatory Grieving and Dysfunctional Grieving. Normal grieving encompasses a range of feelings, moods, and behaviors that follow a significant loss of someone or something that was meaningful to the person (e.g., the death of a significant other, the death of a pet, the loss of a job, or the loss of a home).

Normal grieving is experienced as subjective distress, tension, or mental pain. The span of grief reactions encompasses infancy through old age. Normal grieving is characterized by feelings of sadness, anger, guilt, self-reproach, anxiety, loneliness, fatigue, helplessness, shock, yearning, emancipation, relief, and numbness. Additional features include sensations of somatic distress (e.g., tight-

ness in the throat, shortness of breath, digestive problems, an empty feeling in the stomach, or lack of physical strength.[19,23,24] *Chronic sorrow,* "operationally defined as pervasive sadness and/or other emotions commonly associated with grief that is permanent, periodic, and potentially progressive in nature"[8] (pp. 78 and 79), is recognized as a normal grieving response. Families of the chronically mentally ill and parents of mentally retarded children often experience chronic sorrow. This grief response has also been identified in chronic situations that result in a lifestyle disruption (e.g., people with progressive chronic disease and cancer as well as caregivers for these people).[8,13]

The process of normal grieving begins with shock and disbelief and progresses to developing awareness of the loss, restitution, and eventual resolution of the loss.[9,23] The process of anticipatory grieving, according to Kubler-Ross,[17] includes denial and isolation, anger, bargaining, depression, and acceptance. Kubler-Ross emphasizes that these behaviors do not necessarily occur in sequential order and that successful preparatory grief work does not require the individual's experiencing each of these "stages" or behaviors. Reestablishment of equilibrium and successful completion of mourning after a significant loss depend on the patient's ability to (1) accept the reality of the loss; (2) experience the pain of grief; (3) adjust to an environment without the lost object (e.g., person, prized possession); (4) withdraw emotional energy and reinvest it in another relationship, activity, or possession.[23]

Anticipatory Grieving refers to a grieving process that occurs before the actual loss. This response, viewed by some as preparation for the actual loss, includes grieving for past, present, and anticipated future losses.[10,22]

Any kind of change—physical, psychological, or social—may be perceived as a loss. Potential significant losses include loss of body part(s), function(s), or image or the impending loss of one's own life. Other potential losses include loss of a significant other because of geographical separation, change in marital status, or diagnosis of a terminal illness. Bowlby[4] believes that the loss of a loved one is one of the most painful experiences a human can suffer. The perceived potential loss of a valued possession, employment, status, or social role can result in Anticipatory Grieving.[10,15,20]

Lindemann[19] recognized anticipatory grief as a response to separation when a family member left for military service during World War II. He described this form of grief as a syndrome in which concern for adjustment after the potential death of a loved one is so great that the person experiences the same process of grieving as though an actual death had occurred.

Loss is a subjective experience. The intensity of response to a potential loss is influenced by the meaning of the loss for the individual. The very same loss can be of great significance to one person and of little consequence to another.[10] Previous experiences with loss, cultural and spiritual beliefs, and socioeconomic background influence an individual's responses to an anticipated loss. Emotional, cognitive, behavioral, and somatic patterns of grief and mourning during Anticipatory Grieving are similar to responses that occur with normal grieving.[6,10,22]

Resolution and restitution of the losses associated with Anticipatory Grieving, however, differ from the resolution and restitution that occur with normal grieving. Anticipatory Grieving related to terminal illness has a definitive end point—death, whereas grieving after a loss can be prolonged. During Anticipatory Grieving, there is the hope that action can be taken to prevent the actual loss

from taking place. This is in contrast to the experience of normal grieving in which there is no action that can alter the fact that the loss has occurred. The terminally ill person who experiences Anticipatory Grieving does not reach a period of reestablishment, such as in normal grieving. Resolution occurs with the acceptance and recognition of impending death.[10,17]

Anticipatory Grieving may facilitate adjustment to the actual loss by lessening the intensity of grieving that the person feels after the loss takes place. Anticipatory Grieving related to the impending death of a significant other can allow for preparation to cope with grief and to begin to let go of a relationship. However, it has also been observed that Anticipatory Grieving can intensify attachment behaviors and that the actual death of a significant other is still felt as a shock. The repeated cycle of Anticipatory Grieving, preparing for a potential loss while striving to live in the present, may compromise the survivor's ability to cope effectively with the grieving process.[4,10,22]

Shock and disbelief are characteristic behaviors during the period of recognizing the anticipated loss.[4,9] Denial displayed as initial intellectual acceptance and extremely appropriate behaviors is a common mental mechanism that occurs at this time. Overt attempts to block out factual information related to the loss represent the use of denial as a temporary defense that precedes partial acceptance.[17]

Emotional responses of acute sadness, anxiety, helplessness, and hopelessness are common during the period of developing awareness of the loss.[9] Tearfulness may accompany feelings of anguish and despair. Kubler-Ross[17] identifies anger, bargaining, and depression as additional behavioral manifestations during this time.

Dysfunctional Grieving occurs when an individual fails to accomplish the "tasks of mourning" after experiencing an actual or perceived loss.[23] Avoidance of the intense distress and other emotions associated with the grief experience is a major obstacle to the completion of grief work. Lindemann[19] used the term *morbid grief reactions*

VIII

to denote distortions of normal grief. Personality factors such as difficulty tolerating dependency and needing to be the strong one in the family can prevent a person from experiencing feelings that facilitate adequate resolution of a loss.[23]

The term *pathological grief* has been used to describe grief that has intensified to a degree at which the patient is overwhelmed and resorts to maladaptive behavior. Or the person remains in an interminable state of grieving without further progression of the mourning process toward completion of the tasks of mourning.[15] The inability to accept the fact that a loss has occurred can lead to prolonged, excessive denial as well as prolonged depression.[20]

ASSESSMENT

The perceived potential loss of a significant object that is of value is the central related factor for the response of Anticipatory Grieving. Assessment begins with determining the patient's perception of the anticipated loss of an object, possession, or person that is of value and the significance of this loss for the person.

Assessment of Anticipatory Grieving includes the recognition that medical, surgical, and obstetrical conditions can represent perceived potential losses for the identified patient and the patient's family. Medical conditions such as cancer, end-stage renal disease, myocardial infarction, chronic obstructive pulmonary disease, and diabetes can activate the process of Anticipatory Grieving because of the potential losses that are associated with these conditions. Recognize the threat that surgical interventions pose to the patient (e.g., loss of satisfaction with body image, loss of body functions, and loss of life itself). Assess for prenatal complications and fetal abnormalities that can result in Anticipatory Grieving.

The defining characteristics of Anticipatory Grieving include the expression of distress with the recognition of the potential loss of a significant object. The nurse should assess the patient's perception of his or her strengths or weaknesses for coping with the perceived loss. Recognize that

the responses by the patient and family to the current situation are influenced by past experiences with loss, illness, and death. Past problem-solving abilities, socioeconomic and educational background and cultural and spiritual beliefs also influence the patient's ability to cope with a potential loss.[6,10,22] How much time has elapsed since the individual learned of the potential loss? What are the patient's behavioral patterns since he or she first learned of the loss? What disruptions have the patient and family experienced in their current lifestyle because of the loss? Monitor the impact of the potential or actual loss on patient and family finances, living arrangements, and transportation.

Denial of a potential or actual loss is a defining characteristic that frequently occurs during the period of shock and disbelief. Denial is characterized by behaviors directed toward insulating and protecting the patient from the intensity of feelings that are generated by the potential or actual loss.[9] Denial may also occur during later phases of the Anticipatory Grieving experience. Observe for the influence of denial by health care providers on the patient's use of denial.[19]

Ambivalence is another defining characteristic of Anticipatory Grieving.[10,22] During the early period of Anticipatory Grieving, the element of hope that is held by significant others may be associated with feelings of ambivalence toward the patient. Sleep and appetite disturbances and changes in activity level and communication patterns may occur in the patient and significant others.

The patient and family often differ in their ability to recognize and accept the actual or potential loss, and they often differ in their manner of communicating their grieving. Observe for possible conflicts that may occur among the patient, the family, and the treatment team because of these differences.

Recognize that the process of Anticipatory Grieving includes progression as well as regression as the patient and family attempt to achieve the realization and resolution of the anticipated loss.[22]

The initial assessment for Dysfunctional Grieving begins with assessment of the individual's progression through specific tasks of mourning. To what extent has the patient progressed? Obtain information about the causes and circumstances of the loss. When did the loss occur? What is the patient's perception of the loss? What is the patient's perception of his or her adaptation to the loss? What are the patient's past life experiences and past problem-solving skills?[11,19,21,23]

Look for indications of inhibition, suppression, or absence of emotional reactions to the loss. To what extent has the patient assumed the social role of the strong one in the family? Has the patient been forced to deal with important tasks related to the loss to the extent that his or her own grieving needs have been ignored? The absence of Anticipatory Grieving may be a related factor in the absence of emotional reactions to a loss.[18,21,23]

Bowlby[4] believes that avoidance of conscious grieving in response to the death of a significant other eventually results in some form of depression. Assessment for possible precipitants of this depression includes an anniversary of a death that has not been mourned; another loss, of an apparently minor kind; reaching the same age as the significant other who died; and a loss suffered by a compulsively cared-for person with whose experience the failed mourner may be identifying.

Assess for indicators of prolonged normal grieving (e.g., excessive reliving of past experiences, feeling that the loss occurred "only" yesterday) and general themes of loss. Assess for specific factors that can contribute to Dysfunctional Grieving. For example, social negation of a loss can occur when an individual has an abortion or miscarriage and the experience has not been defined as a loss by members of the person's social network. Look for *socially unspeakable losses* that are mourned by the bereaved but are not seen as socially appropriate to discuss.[2] Examples include suicide, abortion, miscarriage, children lost to adoption, and the death of an illicit lover.

Social isolation can contribute to Dysfunctional Grieving. Precipitants of social isolation are geographical separation from significant others, a breakdown of the extended family, diminished importance of religious institutions, and the loss of an entire support system through death.[12]

The elderly are at risk for complicated grief reactions because of factors that include decreased cognitive capacity and change in familiar routines after loss of spouse.[11] They are also at risk for a diminished social network. Limited financial resources, loss of vision, and decreased mobility can affect their ability to drive. Assessment of cognitive ability and the actual or potential social network and resources is important. Assess for the absence of a social network for the nonelderly as well.

Excessive or distorted emotional reactions are an indication of Dysfunctional Grieving. Assess for extreme anger or hostility or prolonged or excessive denial. Severe hopelessness, excessive guilt, and self-blame may lead to suicidal ideation and intent.

Observe for alterations in eating habits, sleep patterns, activity level, and libido. Increased illness in a previously well person may be indicative of Dysfunctional Grieving. Increased smoking and excessive alcohol consumption may also be indicative of bereavement difficulty.[12] It is important to rule out the presence of an actual medical condition. Although increased somatization is common among some ethnic groups and some symptoms are equated with grief behaviors, persistent somatic complaints may be indicative of an underlying medical condition that requires medical intervention.[12,23]

Parental Dysfunctional Grieving processes and unconscious family maneuvers can contribute to unresolved grief in children (e.g., disrupted communication or the expectation that the surviving child will replace the deceased family member).[3,19] Recognize that children often express their need for help in coping with loss by displaying disruptive, aggressive or hostile behavior, having problems in school performance, or exhibiting regressed behavior, and somatic complaints.[12]

Assessment of Dysfunctional Grieving must include consideration of the effect of the loss on the entire family system. Unresolved grief can be a key factor in family pathology and can contribute to pathological relationships across generations.[23]

VIII

Anticipatory Grieving

■ Defining Characteristics

The presence of the following defining characteristics[17,21-23] indicates that the patient may be experiencing Anticipatory Grieving:

- Appetite disturbance, decrease more common
- Emptiness, hollowness in stomach
- Choking sensation
- Decreased energy, fatigue
- Sleep disturbance
- Altered libido
- Expression of distress at the potential loss
- Denial of potential loss; shock, disbelief, and avoidance of focus on loss
- Increased anxiety
- Anger
- Guilt
- Self-accusation of negligence
- Feelings of loss and loneliness
- Absent-mindedness
- Preoccupation with self
- Sense of unreality
- Ambivalence
- Hope for preventing loss
- Realization or resolution of impending death or loss
- Disinterest in or difficulty carrying out activities of daily living
- Altered communication patterns
- Social withdrawal
- Hostility or irritability toward others
- Increased reliance on spiritual counselor
- Anger toward God
- Disavowal of spiritual beliefs

■ Related Factors

The following related factors[4,12,16,19,22] are associated with Anticipatory Grieving:

- Perceived potential loss of significant object that is of value, as, for example, the following:
  - Physiopsychosocial well-being
  - Body part(s)
  - Body function(s)
  - Impending death of self
  - Significant other
  - Social role

- Personal possessions
- Pet
- Griever's own physical health
- Unique meaning of anticipated loss
- Nature of relationship and roles to be lost
- Degree of unfinished business
- Griever's coping skills
- Griever's ethnic, religious, and cultural background
- Griever's fears about death
- Griever's attitude toward illness
- Griever's knowledge of illness
- Griever's ability to communicate

Dysfunctional Grieving

■ Defining Characteristics

The presence of the following defining characteristics[1,16,19,21,23] indicates that the patient may be experiencing Dysfunctional Grieving:

- Alterations in eating habits, sleep and dream patterns, activity level, or libido
- Somatic expression of fear (e.g., choking sensations, difficulties in breathing)
- Somatic symptoms representing identification with the person who died
- Physical distress under upper half of sternum accompanied by expressions such as "There's something stuck inside"
- Refusal to follow a prescribed treatment regimen
- Inhibition, suppression, or absence of emotional reactions, including difficulty expressing loss and delayed emotional reaction
- Prolongation of normal grieving
  - Excessive reliving of past experience
  - Interference with life functioning
  - Prolonged alterations in concentration and/or pursuit of tasks
  - Feeling that loss occurred only yesterday
  - Unabated search behavior for lost person or object
- Excessive or distorted emotional reactions
  - Extreme anger or hostility
  - Prolonged or excessive denial
  - Developmental regression
  - Extreme feelings of low self-esteem
  - Severe feelings of identity loss

- Excessive idealization of dead person or lost object
- Excessive guilt and self-blame
- Suicidal ideation
- Prolonged depression
- Recurrence of depressive symptoms and searching behavior on specific dates
- Diminished participation in religious and ritual activities

■ Related Factors

The following related factors[1,4,16,18,23] are associated with Dysfunctional Grieving:

- Absence of Anticipatory Grieving
- Stressful and prolonged anticipated loss
- Chronic illness in self or family member
- Multiple losses with unresolved grief
- History of delayed or prolonged grief
- Unexpected or sudden loss of significant person, animal, or prized possession
- Ambivalent relationship with lost object (i.e., a person)
- Secondary gains from grieving
- Inability to attend to grieving because of other tasks
- Socially unspeakable loss(es)
- Negation of the loss by others
- Social isolation
- Loss of or change in significant social role
- Inadequate social support
- Unconscious family maneuvers for coping with loss

DIAGNOSIS

■ Differential Nursing Diagnosis

It is important to recognize the intensity of normal grieving to avoid misdiagnosis of Dysfunctional Grieving, Ineffective Denial, and Ineffective Individual Coping for the patient and family who are experiencing normal grieving or normal Anticipatory Grieving.[8,13,18,21,23] The initial perception of feeling overwhelmed when a person faces a potential loss is common in normal grieving. Observe for behaviors that include compliance with recommended important diagnostic tests and nursing and medical interventions, recognizing that a degree of initial denial serves to protect the grieving person from being overwhelmed from a potential or actual loss. Ineffective Individual Coping refers to an overall impairment of adaptive behaviors and problem-solving abilities. Individuals with chronic sorrow, a manifestation of normal grieving, use constructive coping strategies for dealing with their recurring feelings of sorrow; people with chronic, unresolved grief, Dysfunctional Grieving, have a limited coping repertoire for managing their loss(es). Differentiation between Ineffective Denial and Dysfunctional Grieving may be difficult at times; obtaining a loss history from the patient and family can help clarify diagnostic accuracy. Differentiation between Hopelessness and Dysfunctional Grieving includes assessment of the patient's appraisal of the loss, the duration or extent of emotional responses, and looking for indication of unfinished tasks of grieving to help clarify the accuracy of the diagnosis. Differentiation between Anticipatory Grieving and Powerlessness includes assessment and evaluation of the patient's perception of control. Sometimes it is helpful to discuss the actual diagnoses with the patient and family to ensure accuracy of problem identification, outcomes, and interventions.

■ Medical and Psychiatric Diagnoses[2,5]

Psychiatric disorders commonly related to Anticipatory Grieving fall within the category of adjustment disorders, where an individual experiences a psychosocial stressor or stressors that precipitate the onset of emotional or behavioral symptoms, such as depressed mood, tearfulness, worry, and anxiety. For the most part, these symptoms resolve within 6 months after the stressor or the related consequences have ended.[2] Specific adjustment disorders related to Anticipatory Grieving include adjustment disorder with depressed mood, adjustment disorder with anxiety, and adjustment disorder with mixed anxiety and depressed mood. The diagnostic category bereavement is used when the individual who has experienced the death of a loved one views a depressed mood as "normal." The person experiencing bereavement (normal grieving) may choose to seek professional help for temporary management of sleep and appetite disturbances and may participate in some sort of bereavement counseling. Psychiatric disorders commonly related to Dysfunctional Grieving fall within the category of mood disorders, such as major depressive disorder, where the patient experiences continuation of symptoms of depression for more than 2 months after a significant loss. Specific symptoms include depressed mood or loss of interest or pleasure as well as ongoing guilt about one's role and actions taken in relation to the deceased; recurrent thoughts of death (to be with loved one); marked psychomotor retardation; and significant impairment in role responsibilities and functioning.[2] People who are grieving are at risk for exacerbation of existing medical conditions and for developing new medical conditions.

OUTCOME IDENTIFICATION, PLANNING, AND IMPLEMENTATION

Nursing interventions for patients facing an anticipated loss are directed toward their participating in constructive anticipatory grief work. The overall goal for patients who are experiencing Dysfunctional Grieving is to facilitate the normal grieving process. Nursing interventions should be based on the unique needs of each individual patient.

Anticipatory Grieving

Discussion of thoughts and feelings related to the perceived potential loss is one outcome that indicates that the patient and family are participating in constructive anticipatory grief work. Grieving spouses have emphasized their need to verbalize and ventilate their feelings.[14]

Verbalization of information needs also contributes to constructive anticipatory grief work. Grieving spouses and families of terminally ill patients place a high priority on the need for ongoing information.[14] Nursing interventions that encourage the ongoing identification of information needs and avoid defensive and judgmental responses to criticisms of health care providers facilitate successful resolution of the grieving process.

The ability to make informed decisions is another component of constructive anticipatory grief work. People facing a potential loss are also confronted with decisions related to the loss. Interventions that facilitate exploration and discussion of available options increase the likelihood of the patient's making informed decisions.

Interventions that promote the use of appropriate resources are essential. The crisis nature of an anticipated loss may result in the patient and family overlooking familiar, already existing resources (e.g., other family or clergy). The patient and family may be unaware, however, of the existence of formal and self-help support groups that serve to decrease the initial sense of loneliness and isolation that often accompanies the experience of loss. Access to assistance from legal and financial resources can decrease stress associated with the loss and allow the patient and family to continue to focus on constructive grief work.

■⌐ **NURSING CARE GUIDELINES**
Nursing Diagnosis: Anticipatory Grieving °

Expected Outcome: The patient will discuss thoughts and feelings related to the anticipated loss.
- Encourage the patient to describe perceptions of the potential loss, including fears and concerns *to assist in assessment of the patient's understanding of the reality of the impending loss; also, patients who are able to verbalize their thoughts and feelings about a loss are less likely to experience Dysfunctional Grieving.*
- During the period of shock and disbelief, provide a quiet and private environment *for the expression of emotions.*
- Assure the patient that it is normal to experience intense feelings and reactions *to allay possible fears of losing his or her mind.*

■ = nursing intervention; ▲ = collaborative intervention.
°References 5, 6, 18, 22.

- Avoid defensive and judgmental responses to criticisms directed at health care providers, *recognizing that common responses to perceived loss and feelings of helplessness include the displacement of anger and blame on the health care team.*
- During the stage of developing awareness of the loss, encourage the patient to discuss thoughts and feelings with significant others; *family support can reduce the patient's sense of despair; the ability of the patient and family to talk together increases the likelihood of the patient integrating positive and negative aspects of the perceived loss.*
- Encourage the patient to reminisce and to explore the possible positive and negative aspects of the anticipated loss *to facilitate movement toward eventual restitution and resolution of the loss.*

Expected Outcome: The patient will verbalize information needs on an ongoing basis.

- Encourage the patient to describe his or her understanding of the current health situation *to help identify where he or she might benefit from being provided with additional information and to clarify possible misconceptions patient might have about current situation.*
- Recognize variation in information needs during period of mourning *as patient begins to accept the reality of the impending loss.*

Expected Outcome: The patient will make informed decisions.

- Facilitate patient's exploration and discussion of available options *to minimize patient's feeling forced to make decisions.*
- ▲ Provide opportunity for contact with others who have experienced a similar loss or who are facing a future similar loss. *Sharing mutual concerns in a supportive setting can contribute to the process of making informed decisions.*
- ▲ Promote patient's contact with appropriate members of the health care team *to ensure that patient obtains adequate information for making decisions.*

Expected Outcome: The patient will use appropriate resources.

- ▲ Facilitate exploration of available assistance from family, friends, clergy, and other community resources. *The perception of social support decreases likelihood of Dysfunctional Grieving.*
- ▲ Encourage patient to consider participating in groups with others who have experienced similar losses (e.g., ostomy groups, laryngectomy groups, Reach for Recovery, and I Can Cope). *Participation with others who are anticipating or have experienced a similar loss can decrease feelings of aloneness and isolation.*
- ▲ Inform the patient and significant others of resources for financial assistance or for legal consultation. *The patient and family may be unaware of community resources that can assist with financial or legal problems related to the anticipated loss.*

Expected Outcome: The patient will maintain constructive interpersonal relationships.

- Acknowledge to the patient and significant others that the pattern of their past relationships with each other will be similar to their present relationships with each other as they experience their anticipated loss. *This is to increase their awareness of what to expect from each other.*
- Offer hope for their ability to cope with potential loss *to promote mobilization of coping strengths.*
- Encourage and teach the patient and significant others good health habits (e.g., adequate dietary intake, rest, and activity). *Health practices that promote a sense of well-being have a direct effect on patient's and significant others' ability to maintain constructive interpersonal relationships.*

Dysfunctional Grieving

Although somatic symptoms are a common major presentation in the patient with Dysfunctional Grieving, they can also be indicative of an underlying medical condition that requires a medical evaluation and treatment.[23] Untreated medical conditions interfere with the patient's ability to experience normal grieving. Identification of the unfinished tasks of mourning provides the basis for specific interventions for the patient. Has the patient accepted the reality of the loss?

VII

Has the patient experienced the pain of grief? Has the patient been able to adjust to an environment without the lost object (e.g., a person or prized possession)? Are there indications that the patient has been able to withdraw emotional energy and reinvest it in another relationship, activity, or possession?[23]

The demonstration of nonexcessive and nonprolonged emotional reactions is an expected outcome for the patient experiencing Dysfunctional Grieving. Referral to a mental health provider for further evaluation and treatment may be necessary, especially for patients with suicidal ideation and intent. Interventions that encourage and permit an open expression of feelings without the nurse becoming

defensive facilitate the patient's ability to understand possible reasons for emotional responses.

It is essential that the patient who has experienced Dysfunctional Grieving be able to develop goals that are congruent with the loss. Nursing interventions that encourage description of future expectations and that promote the patient's recognition of past and present coping strengths contribute to the development of congruent goals. Interventions that coordinate referrals and resources to help the patient develop new skills, make readjustments in lifestyle, and make new emotional investments also contribute to the patient's ability to develop goals that are congruent with the loss.

■ **NURSING CARE GUIDELINES**
Nursing Diagnosis: Dysfunctional Grieving°

Expected Outcome: The patient will work through phases of normal grieving.
▲ Assess for themes of physical complaints and symptoms *to determine need for referral for evaluation and treatment of coexisting medical conditions that can interfere with the patient's participation in constructive grief work.*
■ Assess the present stage of grieving, the grief tasks that are not completed, and barriers to the grieving process *to determine appropriate subsequent nursing interventions, recognizing that grieving does not proceed in a linear fashion and that "phrases and tasks" are not necessarily sequential in their occurrence.*
■ Encourage patient to describe current objects of value or facts that are related to the loss *to help the patient begin to experience thoughts and feelings that have been avoided.*
■ Encourage the patient to describe perceptions of current adaptation *to elicit information for assessing the extent to which the patient is able to acknowledge awareness of the loss and to stimulate patient's conscious recognition of the grief process.*
■ Assess for patient's intellectual acceptance of the reality of loss with absence of emotional acceptance *to determine the extent of patient's need to protect him- or herself from the reality of the loss.*
■ Observe for responses from health care providers that could be reinforcing maladaptive denial. *This information is necessary for planning continuing appropriate collaborative interventions.*
■ Point out reality in a nonthreatening manner—without arguing with the patient or significant others—*to help the patient and family begin to recognize that the painful reality of the loss is inescapable.*
■ Present the patient with increasing factual information *to clarify possible differences in perception of what happened and to increase patient's realization of the extent of the loss.*

Expected Outcome: The patient will demonstrate nonexcessive and nonprolonged emotional reactions.
■ Encourage the patient to describe current and anticipated problems related to the loss, including feelings and coping patterns, *to encourage patient's conscious recognition of the grieving process and subsequent feelings to assess for current coping strengths and deficits and to plan appropriate interventions for the patient to engage in constructive grief work.*

■ = nursing intervention; ▲ = collaborative intervention.
°References 1, 5, 7, 9, 20, 23.

- Assess for suicidal thoughts or plans. *It is not uncommon for people experiencing excessive and prolonged emotional reactions to a loss to have suicidal ideation or intent.*
- ▲ Initiate referral (based on individual assessment) for psychiatric mental health evaluation by advanced practice nurse (e.g., clinical nurse specialist, nurse practitioner, or another mental health professional) *to evaluate the need for medication and/or formal grief therapy to assist in the resolution of excessive and prolonged emotional reactions.*
- Support verbalization of ambivalence *to help patient become more aware of angry feelings and to begin to recognize that anger does not negate positive feelings for a lost person or possession.*
- Help the patient begin to test the reality of guilt that is associated with the loss *so that the patient can begin to differentiate between guilt that is part of normal grieving and guilt that is irrational.*
- Prepare the patient for potential sudden onset of intense emotional responses that may be activated by holidays, anniversaries, or other triggering stimuli such as smells or places associated with the lost person or object *to increase patient's awareness and understanding of emotional responses.*

Expected Outcome: The patient will develop goals that are congruent with the loss.
- Have the patient discuss recognition of changes in his or her own life *to increase awareness of adaptations since the loss.*
- Promote patient's recognition of past and present strengths that can be used for coping with the current loss *to increase patient's sense of control over future directions.*
- Assist patient to mobilize his or her support system *to prevent social isolation during the time of change.*
- Encourage the patient to set realistic daily goals *to increase the sense of control of ability to make constructive changes.*
- Consider the use of role playing *to facilitate the patient's awareness of possible alternatives and consequences of decisions.*
- Encourage discussion of plans for transition from a focus on grief-related support to a focus on moving on with life *to decrease reliance on grief support.*
- ▲ Promote the coordination of community resources (e.g., senior centers, widow-to-widow groups, church groups, adult day care programs, and parents without partners) *to help the patient develop new skills, make readjustments in lifestyle, and make new emotional investments.*

VII

EVALUATION

Evaluation of Anticipatory Grieving and Dysfunctional Grieving must take into consideration that grieving does not proceed in a linear fashion and that there are no "set" times for resolving grief. Anticipatory Grieving for the family member of a patient with a slowly progressing fatal illness can extend over a period of years. Two years is not an undue length of time to recover from the death of a loved one. Recognize that normal grieving includes intense responses that are sometimes misinterpreted as abnormal or dysfunctional. Evaluation of Anticipatory Grieving and Dysfunctional Grieving should take into consideration the cultural beliefs and practices that influence the manner in which people grieve.

Anticipatory Grieving

One indicator of the patient's participation in constructive anticipatory grief work is the ability to discuss thoughts and feelings related to the potential loss. The patient and family should also be verbalizing their information needs on an ongoing basis. Are the patient and family making informed decisions in relation to the potential loss? The ability to use appropriate resources and to maintain constructive interpersonal relationships is another indicator of participation in constructive anticipatory grief work.

Dysfunctional Grieving

The patient should be experiencing less or no Dysfunctional Grieving. Is there an absence or reduction of the defining characteristics of Dysfunctional Grieving? Be sure that excessive, prolonged, distorted, or delayed emotional reactions are no longer present. Has the patient been able to establish and begin to work toward achieving realistic goals that are congruent with the loss? Look for indications that the patient is moving toward reinvesting emotional energy in other people or objects and is experiencing gratification in adapting to new activities and roles.

⚑ CASE STUDY WITH PLAN OF CARE

Mr. Max M. is a 51-year-old widowed man. He maintained an extremely stoic demeanor when he was admitted to the head and neck surgical service for a partial pharyngectomy and laryngectomy approximately 2 weeks after a diagnosis of squamous cell cancer was made. His preoperative evaluation included a speech pathology observation that he was an excellent candidate for using an electrolarynx. His postoperative treatment plan included a series of radiation treatments. Approximately 3 weeks before the conclusion of his radiation therapy, he began to avoid using the electrolarynx, stating "Everybody I know who uses one of these makes themselves a complete bore." He resorted to using his note pad to communicate. Nurses observed him to be increasingly impatient with various members of his treatment team. For example, one day he threw his electrolarynx at his speech patholo-gist. He walked slowly with his head held down. There was minimal eye contact, and he appeared to be reluctant to "open up" with staff and other patients. The patient has had non-insulin-dependent diabetic disease for 15 years and a 20-year history of alcohol abuse but has been "dry" for 5 years. He has smoked one pack of cigarettes per day for 30 years. Mr. M. has worked in various aspects of radio broadcasting since the age of 21. Before admission, he was employed by a local station as a newscaster and part-time disc jockey. He has been a widower for 1 year, since his wife died suddenly of a myocardial infarction. His only daughter was killed in a car accident 5 years ago. The patient describes himself as somewhat of a loner since his wife's death. He is an agnostic with a personal philosophy of "enjoy life while you can." He enjoys model plane building, traveling, and playing golf.

⚑ PLAN OF CARE FOR MR. MAX M.

Nursing Diagnosis: Dysfunctional Grieving Related to Absence of Anticipatory Grieving and Actual Loss of Body Part (Larynx), Prized Possession (Voice), and Multiple Previous Losses

Expected Outcome: Mr. M will demonstrate nonexcessive and nonprolonged emotional reactions to recent losses as evidenced by engaging in normal grieving.
- Encourage Mr. M. to describe perceptions of his current postoperative adaptation.
- Encourage description of experiences that preceded the loss of Mr. M.'s voice, including the sudden death of his wife.
- Promote discussion of other factors that Mr. M. perceives to be related to his current loss.
- Assess for possible suicidal ideation or intent.
- Permit open expression of feelings of anger, and assist Mr. M. to begin to try to understand possible reasons for these feelings.
- Point out the need for universal grieving. Evaluate the need for referral for grief therapy to provide further opportunity for Mr. M. to discuss his adaptation to his recent losses.

Expected Outcome: Mr. M will agree to resume use of his electrolarynx.
- Encourage Mr. M. to describe current and anticipated problems related to the loss of his voice.
- Evaluate the influence of denial on Mr. M.'s avoidance of using the electrolarynx.
- Collaborate with the health team to clarify factual information of Mr. M.'s health situation in terms of diagnostic findings and prognosis.

■ = nursing intervention; ▲ = collaborative intervention.

- Convey recognition that Mr. M.'s knowledge of communication skills as a broadcaster (such as enunciation) will assist in his adaptation to the electrolarynx.

Expected Outcome: Mr. M will develop goals that are congruent with his losses.
- Encourage Mr. M. to describe his plans for the future, including employment and social and recreational activities.
- Encourage Mr. M. to contact the radio station to investigate alternative employment possibilities.
- Encourage Mr. M. to explore possibilities for decreasing the social isolation he had experienced before his surgery.

■■ CRITICAL THINKING EXERCISES

1. Give examples of Max M.'s defining characteristics of Dysfunctional Grieving.
2. Give examples of specific behaviors that indicate that Mr. M. is engaged in normal grieving.
3. Why is it important for Mr. M. to work toward decreasing his social isolation?
4. Describe additional nursing interventions and rationales that would be appropriate for Mr. Max M.

REFERENCES

1. Almeida CM: Grief among parents of children with diabetes, *Diabetes Educator* 21(6):530–532, 1995.
2. American Psychiatric Association: *Diagnostical and statistical manual of mental disorders,* ed 4, Washington, D.C., 1994, The Association.
3. Baker JE, Sedney MA, and Gross E: Psychological tasks for bereaved children, *Amer J Orthopsychiatry* 62(1):105–116, 1992.
4. Bowlby J: *Attachment and loss,* vol 3, New York, 1980, Basic Books.
5. Browning MA: Depression, suicide, and bereavement. In Hogstel MO, editor: *Geropsychiatric nursing,* ed 2, St. Louis, 1995, Mosby–Year Book.
6. Carson VB: Losses and endings in the nurse-client relationships. In Arnold E and Boggs KU: *Interpersonal relationships: professional communication skills for nurses,* ed 2, Philadelphia, 1995, WB Saunders Co.
7. Curry LC and Stone JG: Moving on: recovering from the death of a spouse, *Clin Nurs Spec* 6(4):180–190, 1992.
8. Eakes GG: Chronic sorrow: the lived experience of parents of chronically mentally ill individuals, *Arch Psychiatr Nurs* 9(2):77–84, 1995.
9. Engel G: *Psychological development in health and disease,* Philadelphia, 1968, WB Saunders Co.
10. Gerety E: Grieving, anticipatory grieving, dysfunctional grieving. In McFarland GK and Thomas MD: *Psychiatric mental health nursing,* Philadelphia, 1991, JB Lippincott Co.
11. Glass BC: The role of the nurse in advanced practice in bereavement care, *Clin Nurs Spec* 7(2):62–74, 1993.
12. Green M: Roles of health professional and institution. In Osterwies M, Solomon F, and Green M, editors: *Bereavement reactions, consequences, and care,* Washington, D.C., 1984, National Academy Press.
13. Hainsworth MA and others: Chronic sorrow in women with chronically mentally disabled husbands, *J Am Psychiatr Assoc* 1(4):120–124, 1995.
14. Hampe S: Needs of the grieving spouse in a hospital setting, *Nurs Res* 24:113–120, 1975.
15. Horowitz MJ and others: Pathological grief and the activation of latent self-images, *Am J Psychiatry* 137:1157–1162, 1980.
16. Kim MJ, McFarland GK, and McLane AM: *Pocket guide to nursing diagnoses,* ed 6, St. Louis, 1995, Mosby–Year Book.
17. Kubler-Ross E: *On death and dying,* New York, 1969, Macmillan Publishing Co.
18. Lasker JN and Toedter LJ: Acute versus chronic grief: the case of pregnancy loss, *Am J Orthopsychiatry* 61(4):510–524, 1991.
19. Lindemann E: Symptomatology and management of acute grief, *Am J Psychiatry* 101:141–148, 1944.
20. McFarland GK, Wasli EL, and Gerety EK. *Nursing diagnosis and process in psychiatric mental health nursing,* ed 2, Philadelphia, 1992, JB Lippincott Co.
21. North American Nursing Diagnosis Association: *NANDA nursing diagnoses: definitions and classification, 1995–1996,* Philadelphia, 1994, The Association.
22. Rando TA: A comprehensive analysis of anticipatory grief: perspectives, processes, promises, and problems. In Rando TA: *Anticipatory grief,* Lexington, Massachusetts, 1986, Lexington Books.
23. Worden J: *Grief counseling and grief therapy,* ed 2, New York, 1991, Springer Publishing Co.
24. Xiaoqin SL and Lasker JN: Patterns of grief reaction after pregnancy loss, *Am J Orthopsychiatry* 66(2):262–271, 1996.

VIII

Risk for Altered Parent/Infant/Child Attachment

▶

Risk for Altered Parent/Infant/Child Attachment *refers to the disruption of the interactive process between parents or significant others and the infant that fosters the development of a protective and nurturing reciprocal relationship.*[9]

OVERVIEW

The process of parent/child attachment is a critical concept in maternal-child health nursing. *Attachment* can be defined as "the unique relationships between two people that is specific and endures through time."[4] Understanding this concept involves not only how the relationship between a parent and child is established but the factors that influence the development of the relationship.

Klaus and Kennell describe maternal/infant attachment as an interaction of responses between a parent and child that begins in pregnancy, continues through the newborn period, and culminates in a bond between a mother and her infant.[4] However, the process does not end at the time a bond is formed; the reciprocity and interaction continue to nurture and maintain the relationship. Reva Rubin in her seminal work on attachment and maternal role attainment asserts that the process occurs in stages. She also maintains that the process of maternal role attainment occurs concurrently with and is dependant on the process of attachment between a mother and her infant.[10]

Paternal/infant attachment may follow a similar pattern, but there are important differences. Fathers are not socialized into parenthood in the same way mothers are, nor do they experience the physiological changes associated with pregnancy and childbirth. Both of these factors affect attach-ment. In addition, the mother often controls the father's access to the infant; this may affect the spontaneity of the interaction and ultimately the attachment.[2]

There are critical periods in the development of parent/infant/child attachment. The first of these is the period before pregnancy. A woman's previous experiences related to motherhood can be powerful predictors of the quality of the attachment with their own infant.[5] The woman's relationship with her mother, her socialization in caring for infants and children (e.g., babysitting or playing with dolls), and the observation of maternal behaviors in others all serve as model behaviors that a woman can add to her repertoire to use in nurturing her infant and child. If a woman has not had these experiences or if they have been problematic, this may affect her ability to form an attachment with her child. For men, previous relationships with and socialization to infants are early influences on their later attachments. Deficiencies in earlier relationships with infants and children may hamper the attachment to their own infants.

Pregnancy is a more pronounced period in the development of feelings of attachment. It is characterized as a time of great change, physically and psychologically. Once the pregnancy is confirmed, the man and woman begin to think of themselves as parents—taking on the new role of mother and father. When a woman hears the fetus' heartbeat or feels movement, she begins to accept the new role she is taking on, and sees the fetus as a part of her as well as an individual. These milestones strengthen the process of attachment. This is further enhanced by fetal movement, which a woman may internalize and regard as a response to her actions. Prenatal attachment has been linked to maternal attachment after birth and may provide the structure for postpartum attachment.[8] This stage is called *binding in*.[10]

After delivery, reciprocal behaviors stimulate and enhance the attachment between the parents and the infant. Infant behaviors elicit a response in the parents. Likewise, the parents' behavior elicits a response in the infant. Immediately after delivery, when the infant cries and the mother holds and strokes the infant, the infant is soothed and becomes quiet. This reinforces the mother's self-confidence in her maternal abilities. After delivery, the infant is alert and attentive. This encourages the parents to make eye-to-eye contact. Mutual gazing is an important behavior that facilitates attachment. Parents interact with their infant using voices and movement in getting acquainted with their infant, eliciting a response from the infant. This is referred to as *entrainment*. This stage, during the first 2 to 3 days, is called the *taking in* stage.

In the neonatal period, the attachment bonds formed through early parent-infant interactions are strengthened as the relationship develops. The infant should be with parents as much as possible to increase the parents' competence in care-taking skills, to enhance the identification between parents and infant, and to continue the attachment process.

At 4 to 6 weeks parents begin to notice the responsiveness of their infant in terms of visual tracking, smiling, laughing, and visually fixating on people and objects. Parents often will consider their infant's behavior as a response to something the parent has done. The reciprocity seen in the early postpartum period continues throughout the parents' relationship with their infant. This stage is referred to as *taking hold*.

At about 7 to 9 weeks, parents verbalize that their infant recognizes them by visual tracking, ceasing to cry when picked up, and having different reactions to other adults, indicating a preference for the parents. This parental identification is an important facet of the reciprocity of attachment.

By the end of the third month, parents are strongly attached to their infant. This is evident by the infant's consistent parental preference and by parents verbalizing fear or guilt about leaving or losing their infant. The interaction between the parents and their infant gradually has become synchronous and rhythmic, like a well-rehearsed dance.[3]

Transition to the parental role, whether maternal or paternal, is an important component of parent/infant attachment. Achievement of parental role identity is a cognitive, social, and developmental process characterized by a sense of competence and satisfaction with the role and the infant's attachment.[10]

Rubin theorized that maternal identity develops as the pregnant woman accomplishes four tasks: (1) seeking safe passage for herself and her infant during pregnancy and childbirth; (2) securing the acceptance of the infant by significant others; (3) giving of oneself and taking from others for the well-being of the infant; and (4) bonding to the infant by imagining being a mother.[10]

In paternal role attainment, men also have experiences that transform their identities during the partner's pregnancy. It has been suggested that men develop an emotional involvement and attachment to an infant in stages, progressing from a period of noninvolvement and disbelief (early in pregnancy) through the time when the pregnancy is becoming more real (following the second trimester, until delivery) and ending with an acceptance of the role of "father" as the infant begins to grow and interact.[6]

ASSESSMENT

When assessing a family for Risk for Altered Parent/Infant/Child Attachment, the nurse should interview the family members to obtain information about the family's history and to identify the critical events that characterize the attachment process. The answers to the following questions may assist the nurse in determining how the process of parent/infant attachment has been progressing. The mother and father should both be interviewed.

VIII

1. Did the mother and father have any experience with infants before this child?
2. How does the infant's mother describe her relationship with her own mother?
3. How do the mother and father describe the pregnancy?
4. How do the mother and father describe the delivery and birth experience?
5. How do the mother and father describe their infant (e.g., fussy, easy to care for, sleepy)?
6. Has the infant experienced any illnesses, or has the infant's growth and development pattern caused the parents concern?
7. Who does the mother identify as her support person(s)?
8. How do the mother and father feel about their new role as parents?
9. Was the pregnancy and delivery easier or harder than they expected?
10. Is the parental role easier or harder than they expected?

In addition to interviewing the family members, interactions between all members of the family should be observed. The nurse can ask him- or herself the following questions to focus the observations of family interactions: How does the infant act while being held or spoken to? Does the infant stop crying while being held? Do the parents make frequent eye contact with the infant en face (i.e., the position in which the mother, father, and infant are face to face with eye contact)? Do the parents speak to their infant while holding or stroking the infant (entrainment)? Do the parents appear comfortable caring for their infant?

Many factors have been identified that can influence the attachment process positively or negatively. For example, perceived stress or anxiety influences attachment by diverting the parents' attention from the attachment process to resolve the stressful situation. Parental stress or anxiety can be related to the infant's temperament and/or the parent's concept of themselves as parents. If an infant is fussy or sleepy most of the time, meaningful interaction between the infant and parents may be limited. The infant's behavior may result in

the parents thinking that they are doing something wrong or are not being good parents.[1,7]

A positive parental self-concept is critical in fostering parent/infant attachment. If either parent feels unworthy or incapable of interacting with the infant, this will adversely affect the development of the parental role and the attachment process. Similarly, if the parents have unrealistic expectations related to the prenatal, intrapartal, and postpartum periods as well as unrealistic perceptions of what parenthood will be like, they are likely to experience disappointment. This could cause them to be anxious and consequently interfere with their response to the infant.

Social support is crucial in facilitating attachment by buffering the stress the parents may feel when confronted by an unfamiliar or difficult situation. The support network provides physical and emotional resources and is comprised of significant others (i.e., the nuclear and extended family, friends, and health care providers). The absence of social support can affect the attachment process in that the parents' needs may be unfulfilled, causing anxiety and consequently making it difficult for the parents to attend to the needs of their infant.

If a parent is separated from the infant because the parent or the infant is ill or if the parents have little privacy when with the infant, the attachment process can be disrupted. If one parent is unavailable to the infant or is unable to interact with the infant, the parent/infant attachment can become one-sided between the available parent and the infant.

Through the assessment phase of the nursing process, it is important for the nurse to identify healthy parent/infant attachment behaviors and to identify those factors that can interfere with further development of behaviors supportive of parent/infant/child attachment.

■ Risk Factors

The presence of the following behaviors, conditions, or circumstances renders the patient more vulnerable to Risk for Altered Parent/Infant/Child Attachment:

- Premature birth or immature infant
- Illness of infant or child, limiting interaction with parents
- Infant with altered behavioral organization
- Illness of parent, resulting in separation
- Inability of parents to meet the personal needs of the infant
- Lack of confidence in parenting skills
- Ineffective coping skills
- Anxiety related to the parental role
- Separation
- Lack of privacy, limiting quality time between parents and infant or child
- Absent or weak support network

DIAGNOSIS

■ Differential Nursing Diagnosis

The diagnosis Risk for Altered Parent/Infant/Child Attachment is pertinent to families in the childbearing period. It addresses those processes that begin early in the parent-infant relationship and continue as the child matures. Throughout pregnancy and during the neonatal period, the attachment bonds are formed; it is during this period that the diagnosis is most frequently made. This diagnosis is centered on the parents and the infant or child, because attachment is a reciprocal process between and among family members. In contrast, the diagnosis Altered Parenting specifically addresses parental behaviors only. Diagnoses related to Risk for Altered Parent/Infant/Child Attachment are Risk for Disorganized Behavior and Disorganized Behavior. These diagnoses imply that the infant is at risk for or has some limitations in the ability to interact without some consequence to his or her own self-regulation. If one or both parents are diagnosed with Ineffective Coping: Compromised or Ineffective Coping: Disabling, the parent/infant/child attachment process could be at risk of being altered.

■ Related Medical and Psychiatric Diagnoses

Infant prematurity or immaturity and any medical or psychiatric diagnosis that causes the interaction between a parent and the infant or child to be limited are associated with Risk for Altered Parent/Infant/Child Attachment. The infant, child, or parent who has a chronic disease that requires frequent hospitalization or complex treatment could be separated from the family for a long time. A parent diagnosed with a communicable disease may have to keep a distance from the infant or child for a period of time. Psychiatric diagnoses such as bipolar depression and substance abuse can interfere with the quantity and quality of interactions between the parent and the infant or child.

OUTCOME IDENTIFICATION, PLANNING, AND IMPLEMENTATION

The desired outcome for the family diagnosed as being at Risk for Altered Parent/Infant/Child Attachment is that the family (parents/infant/child) will display behaviors that enhance the attachment process. The interventions identified in the plan of care include strategies that minimize the effect that the identified risk factors can have on the family and strategies that enhance the attachment process. Interventions also incorporate, when possible, attachment behaviors that have been or currently are effective for the family.

Before the birth of the infant, anticipatory guidance can be used to instruct the parents explaining (1) what to expect during pregnancy and after the infant's birth; (2) the "normalcy" of their experiences; and (3) what is helpful to have in place before the delivery (e.g., support from family and friends and necessary equipment and clothing for the baby). Specifically, the demands of the parental role, baby care, infant behaviors, and coping strategies to help adjust to the new role should be addressed.

At the delivery, an environment that supports the mother's birth plan and facilitates parent/infant/child attachment should be provided. Interventions should be directed toward dimming lights, controlling extraneous noise, and giving the infant to its mother as soon as possible after birth. The father or other support persons can be involved in comforting the mother and the baby. The

VIII

nurse should demonstrate how to hold the infant, using the en face position and entrainment.

Throughout the newborn period, support and education is offered to the family to increase interactions between the parents and the infant. The mother should be encouraged to get adequate rest and to spend as much time as possible with the infant. Overzealous family members and friends may interfere with the routine the parents are attempting to establish for themselves and their infant by offering an abundance of advice. They may even take over the care of the infant. It is important to discuss with the parents how they will handle these situations to decrease the stress that the situations may cause.

EVALUATION

For the family at Risk for Altered Parent/Infant/Child Attachment, evaluation of the effectiveness of the plan of care must continue until the identified risk factor(s) is eliminated or adequately controlled. The nurse should observe parent and infant behaviors. The effectiveness of the family's coping strategies and support networks in dealing with specific associated risk factors can be evaluated in terms of the family's ability to introduce behaviors that enhance attachment and to avoid behaviors that contribute to delaying or deferring attachment.

◢ NURSING CARE GUIDELINES
Nursing Diagnosis: Risk for Altered Parent/Infant/Child Attachment

Expected Outcome: The family will display behaviors that enhance attachment between the parents and the infant.

Prenatal Period
▲ Provide the expectant parents information about pregnancy, childbirth, infant care, and infant birth behavior *to educate them about the attachment process and to assist them in that process.*

Intrapartal Period
■ Provide an environment conducive to interaction and attachment between the parents and the newborn infant. This includes involving the father or other support persons, ensuring the mother that she will have as much control of the birth as possible, dimming lights to encourage the infant to open its eyes, and allowing the mother to hold and feed the infant as soon and as much as possible. *These activities promote interaction and the development of attachment.*
■ Provide the mother with information about infant behavior *to increase her understanding of the maturing infant and the interactions that can be expected from the infant.*
■ Reinforce positive attachment behaviors by both parents *to encourage them to incorporate such behaviors into their care of the infant.*

Postpartum Period
■ Assess parent-infant interactions during each home visit or during parent-infant office or clinic visits *to determine if attachment behaviors continue to be adequate.*
■ Encourage parents to discuss any concerns they may have related to parent-infant interactions and the quantity and quality of time spent with their infant. *This provides an opportunity to offer strategies for potential problems immediately, rather than waiting until the problem interferes with parent/infant attachment.*
■ If a separation between a parent and the infant is anticipated, discuss ways for the absent parent to remain in contact with the infant (e.g., a tape recording of the parent singing a lullaby or talking softly to be played for the infant or new pictures of the infant to be shared with the absent parent) *to mediate the effects of parent-infant separation as much as possible.*
▲ Discuss with the parents the support networks available to them (e.g., family, friends, and care providers) *to assist them in identifying assistance they may need to control the stressors they may be experiencing.*

■ = nursing intervention; ▲ = collaborative intervention.

▐ CASE STUDY WITH PLAN OF CARE

Mrs. Susan W. is a 32-year-old primigravida at 38 weeks gestation in active labor. She was raised by a single mother and is an only child. This pregnancy was complicated by preterm labor and bleeding at 28 weeks; bed rest and tocolysis have been prescribed until delivery. Her birth plan includes having her husband and mother in attendance, receiving no anesthesia, and de-livering in a birthing room. During labor, the baby's fetal heart tones have been variable, and occasionally they drop below 100 beats/min. She is receiving oxygen by mask and is positioned left-side lying to increase placental perfusion. Mrs. W. states, "My husband and I are so afraid that things will not be as we planned. We're worried for the baby's safety."

▐ PLAN OF CARE FOR MRS. SUSAN W.

Nursing Diagnosis: Risk for Altered Parent/Infant Attachment Related to Anxiety about Labor Complications

Expected Outcome: The family will display behaviors that will enhance the parent/infant attachment process.

- ▲ Discuss with the physician and the patient's family the feasibility of Mr. W. and Mrs. W.'s mother staying in the birthing room, despite complications.
- ▪ Involve Mrs. W.'s husband and mother in the labor coaching
- ▪ Assist Mrs. W. with the oxygen mask and left-sided positioning, explaining why both interventions are being used.
- ▪ Explain to Mrs. W. that after Baby W. is delivered she can take off the oxygen mask and return to lying on her back to see her infant better.
- ▪ Explain to Mr. and Mrs. W. that the pediatrician will examine Baby W. after delivery because of the fetal bradycardia, and Baby W. will be returned to them as soon as possible.
- ▪ After delivery and once Baby W. is stable, place the infant on Mrs. W.'s chest to facilitate eye-to-eye contact and breastfeeding.
- ▪ Demonstrate to Mr. and Mrs. W. how to hold and speak to Baby W. to maintain Baby W.'s alertness.
- ▪ Explain to Mr. and Mrs. W. that after the first 30 to 60 minutes, Baby W. will be sleepy and difficult to arouse. Despite this, Mrs. W. should attempt to breastfeed every 3 hours.
- ▪ Dim the lights after delivery to enhance Baby W.'s alertness and responsiveness.
- ▪ Observe the interaction between Mrs. W., her husband, and her mother to assess the support that is provided for Mrs. W.
- ▪ If feasible, keep Baby W. with Mrs. W. rather than having Baby W. go to the nursery.
- ▪ Document the nursing interventions you provide and the attachment behaviors you observe to assure continuity of care among the care providers.
- ▲ Make a referral to the hospital home care agency to reassess the family's attachment behaviors after discharge.

▪ = nursing intervention; ▲ = collaborative intervention.

▦ CRITICAL THINKING EXERCISES

1. Describe specific parent-infant activities that Mr. and Mrs. W. and Baby W. should engage in at home to stimulate development of parent/infant attachment.

2. Design a family education booklet that provides information that would have been help-ful to Mr. and Mrs. W. before and immediately after delivery and will be useful to them at home.

3. Explore at-home factors that can be supportive and those that can interfere with development of optimal parent/infant attachment. Give recommendations for enhancing supportive factors and eliminating those that interfere.

VIII

REFERENCES

1. Coffman S, Levitt MJ, and Guacci-Franco N: Infant-mother attachment: relationships to maternal responsiveness and infant temperament, *J Pediatr Nurs* 10:9–18, 1995.
2. Ferketich SL and Mercer RT: Paternal-infant attachment of experienced and inexperienced fathers during infancy, *Nurs Res* 44:31–37, 1995.
3. Kang R: Early parent-infant attachment. In *Early parent-infant relationships,* ed 2, 1991, March of Dimes.
4. Klaus MH and Kennell JH: *Maternal-infant bonding,* St. Louis, 1976, The CV Mosby Co.
5. Koniak-Griffin D: Maternal role attainment, *Image* 25(3): 257–262, 1993.
6. May KA: Three phases of father involvement in pregnancy, *Nurs Res* 31:337–342, 1982.
7. Mercer RT: A theoretical framework for studying factors that impact on the maternal role, *Nurs Res* 30(2):73–77, 1981.
8. Muller ME: Prenatal and postnatal attachment: a modest correlation, *JOGNN* 25:163–172, 1996.
9. North American Nursing Diagnosis Association: *NANDA nursing diagnoses: definitions and classification, 1995–1996,* Philadelphia, 1994, The Association.
10. Rubin R: Attainment of the maternal role, *Nurs Res* 16(3):237–245, 1967.

VIII

Parental Role Conflict

▶

Parental Role Conflict *is the state in which a parent experiences role confusion and multiple demands in response to a crisis.*

OVERVIEW

The current approach to caring for a hospitalized child involves acknowledging the stress of the hospitalization on the child and family and the benefits of family-centered care. The concept of family-centered care includes 24-hour parental visiting and increased parental participation in the child's care. Survival of children with complex chronic conditions and shorter hospital stays has increased parental responsibility for caregiving in the home.

Hospitalization of children is a source of considerable stress for the parents. Studies have identified this stress as a crisis for the family, whether the illness is acute, critical, or chronic. Parents' ability to manage a crisis directly affects their child's ability to cope with the illness and hospitalization. Although a crisis may be for a limited time, ongoing mastery of its impact requires adaptation for successful coping to occur.

Initially parents of a hospitalized child may experience shock, followed by denial, anger, and guilt. Adaptation to the crisis event includes developing an understanding of the significance of the crisis, responding to the demands of the crisis, and developing a sense of mastery.[7] This mastery or adaptation is accomplished through a variety of strategies that focus on problem solving or the use of emotion.[6,7]

Sources of parental stress have been explored in the critical care setting.[4,7] Identified stressors include the physical environment, the provision of information, responses of children to the environment and the underlying condition, and uncertainty about the child's condition. In addition, concerns regarding alteration of the parental role have been consistently identified as a significant source of stress.[4,7] Graves and Ware[5] explored perceptions by parents and the hospital staff regarding sources of parental stress during a child's hospitalization. Thirty-six mothers, 14 fathers, 27 nurses, and 23 physicians responded to an inventory that focused on uncertainty, annoyance, child discomfort, negative emotional states, and change. Mothers perceived all of the components of the inventory as more stressful than the health professionals did. Interestingly, fathers identified child discomfort and negative emotional states as less stressful than the health professionals did. In Ogilvie's[10] qualitative study, parents (*n* = 9) identified the child's fear, pain, emotional responses, and behavioral responses to the surgery as stressful. Aspects of the physical environment, the use of technology, certain procedures related to surgery, and postoperative care were identified as well.

Parents of chronically ill children have their own unique struggles to cope with their children's conditions. Initially parents may experience acute grief at the loss of a healthy child. Subsequently many children and their families experience repeated hospitalizations, lengthy hospitalization, or home-based, technology-dependent care. The chronicity of caregiving is a challenge for parents learning to cope with their child's illness experience.[15] Parents of children who require technology-based care in the home have particular stressors, such as loss of privacy, loss of parental control over the child, and lifestyle differences between the professional and the family.[14]

Lazarus and Folkman[8] describe coping as a process of managing the demands produced by the situation that are viewed as stressful and the emotions that these stressors generate. What is seen as stressful can be quite distinctive to each individual or family. This unique view is based on the meaning or significance that the stressor has in terms of its potential threat to one's well-being. Factors from the individual and the environment determine how a stressor is appraised and managed. Personal factors, such as age, gender, ethnicity, anxiety, and locus of control, will determine the balance between resources and demands. Situational factors, such as previous experience with crisis, physical and environmental aspects, and available support are also important.

Parents have been found to use a variety of coping strategies during a child's critical illness and hospitalizations for surgery.[7, 10] Problem-focused methods include information seeking and developing a plan of action. Emotion-focused methods include denial, intellectualization, distancing, or focusing on the positive aspects of the situation.

Palmer describes the parental role as having many facets, such as supporter/comforter, teacher/learner, and provider of direct physical care.[11] Although the parent is generally effective in these roles in usual situations, the tacit rules and needs of the child can change in a significant way during hospitalization and illness. Whereas some parents wish to be involved in caring for their child, nurses may not encourage this because of their differing beliefs and expectations about the parental role.[1, 2] Conversely, some parents may not be comfortable being involved in their child's care to the extent that the child's nurse expects. These issues highlight the need for nurses and parents to negotiate roles they are comfortable with. Brown and Ritchie[1] studied 25 nurses on a pediatric unit. Nurses determined the level of parental involvement and expected parents to attend to the routine physical needs of the child. Several studies have found that nurses themselves could not agree on what was an appropriate level of parental involvement.[1,15]

Callery and Smith suggest that issues of power and control influence the nurses' negotiations with parents.[2] Whereas nurses function in a familiar environment and are cognizant of rules and regulations, parents must function from a base of less power and control. Additionally, parents must deal with stress, anxiety, uncertainty, and possibly decreased confidence in their own parenting abilities. An imbalance of power and control between the parenting and nursing roles may result.[2] The potential outcome is role confusion and conflict because of a lack of information, unclear expectations, or minimal involvement in care decisions. Parent's wishes to be involved in their child's care will vary and need to be clarified. Parents need clear communication about their role in their child's care and the importance of their support.[15]

In home-based care, the issues of parental involvement, power, and control vary significantly from the hospital setting. The health professional is viewed as a guest in the home and can be seen as a source of relief and help or as a strain. The family's knowledge and insight into their child's needs and care must be respected to maintain family boundaries and to promote empowerment.[12]

In summary, studies have shown that serious childhood illnesses and hospitalization create considerable stress for parents. Additionally, technology-dependent, home-based care has its own distinctive set of stressors. Parents can experience confusion and incongruity with the health care team related to their parenting role with a child who is ill. Systematic preparation and support for their new role may help minimize this conflict.

ASSESSMENT

When a child is hospitalized or experiences a critical illness, the entire family is affected. Research indicates that parents experience significant stress and concern during this period. Parents may experience a variety of emotions, ranging from guilt because of a sense of responsibility for the child's illness to fear and uncertainty toward the course of treatment, the outcome of the illness, or hospitalization. In addition to parental fears and concerns regarding the illness are issues related to usual family functioning. These concerns include care of siblings, financial considerations, and employment concerns. Moreover, a child's illness, particularly if it is critical or chronic, can intensify unresolved conflicts in the marital relationship. For single parents, stressors may be magnified because they are the primary persons shouldering the burden of responsibility. All of these factors work singly or together to influence parents' responses to the situation in which they find themselves. Nurses need to consider all of these aspects when contemplating the nursing assessment.

Assessment also needs to address the composition of the family and the roles that family members play within the family unit. It is important to know each individual's responsibility and the impact of the hospitalization on these responsibilities. Family members need to clarify who is willing to participate in caregiving.[16]

The major characteristic of a parent experiencing Parental Role Conflict is the expressed concern or the feeling of inadequacy about providing for the child's emotional or physical needs during hospitalization or in the home setting. Parents describing disruptions in caretaking practices and routines may be identifying concerns about changes in their own role, their family's functioning, their communicating, and in general their family's well-being. Discussion of these concerns will help clarify individual parents' beliefs, values, and cultural expectations regarding their role. Parents experiencing Parental Role Conflict may express a sense of loss in decisions about their child's well-being. Some parents may withdraw from being involved in the routine care of their child even after considerable encouragement and support is given by others. Some parents may express feelings of guilt, anger, fear, anxiety, or frustration about the effects of the child's illness on the whole family. The extent to which these characteristics are evidenced in any parent may well be a function of several related factors and of the effect the illness has on the family as a whole.

The degree of Parental Role Conflict is a function of the interplay of a number of factors. The age and developmental level of the child can influence the parent's response. Situational factors, such as the type of admission, the seriousness of the diagnosis, and the transition from hospital to home can also influence parents' responses. Parental resources can also have a significant impact, such as the nature of the marital relationship, support by other family members, cultural beliefs about health, illness, and parenting, and financial concerns about housing and employment. The context or the physical environment is another layer of interaction. Environmental stressors include intimidation by invasive or restrictive treatment methods (e.g., isolation or intubation) and by the nature of the specialized care centers (e.g., the sights and sounds of equipment and the policies of the institution). In the home these stressors include intimidation by equipment and procedures required to meet particular patient needs (e.g., apnea monitoring or chest physiotherapy). Access to and support from the health care system can influence all levels of interaction. Parental responses can be influenced by the availability and quality of professional support and by the professionals' willingness to allow parental involvement.

The following principles are important to consider when assessing parents' needs:

- Parents will have unique perceptions of the situation
- They will display varying levels of tolerance to the crisis of illness or hospitalization
- Parents will have diminished anxiety when they receive information on a continuous basis about their child's condition and management
- Parents will need time to develop coping strategies[6]

Other principles for the professional to consider include a nonjudgmental approach to the expression of parents' feelings and the need to support parental involvement in their child's care according to the degree of their desire to do so.[6] Stress, coping, and role theory provide a baseline framework to consider Parental Role Conflict.

Subsequent important areas for assessment include the following:

- Appearance. Briefly note the patient's apparent age, sex, race, and deportment and any overt signs of distress or composure.
- Parents' perception of the problem. Ask parents to explain in their own words their perception of the situation as they experience it.
- Factors influencing the situation. Assess parents regarding the nature of the stressors that influence their situation. What are the environmental factors (e.g., the physical environment, the child's condition, and the procedures to be performed)? What are the contextual issues (e.g., the child's level of development, parental understanding of the condition, and the effectiveness of using the health care system)? Also include, if appropriate, individual factors (e.g., family composition, support systems, past methods of coping, and financial resources).

After eliciting the data, ask parents to describe how their "usual" parental role has been compromised by these stressors and to identify their needs and expectations at this time. Provide parents with an environment that allows them to express their fears and concerns openly, with little fear of recrimination.

■ **Defining Characteristics**

The presence of the following defining characteristics indicates that the parent may be experiencing Parental Role Conflict:

- Lack of confidence about physical care
- Decreased involvement in physical care
- Anxiety or uncertainty about diagnosis and prognosis
- Decreased involvement in decision making
- Concerns about cultural practices not considered
- Concurrent stressors concerning multiple role demands
- Concerns about the effect on family dynamics

■ **Related Factors**

The following related factors are associated with Parental Role Conflict:

- Unclear diagnosis
- Inadequate knowledge of procedures
- Ineffective symptom management
- Multiple health care professionals
- Parental health
- Invasive procedures
- Unrealistic staff expectations
- Decreased decision making
- Multiple roles
- Decreased parental role
- Concurrent family stressors
- Cultural practices conflicting with health care system beliefs
- Inadequate social supports
- Disrupted family routines
- Financial concerns
- Marital conflict
- Uncertainty
- Religiosity
- Hope

DIAGNOSIS

■ **Differential Nursing Diagnosis**

Different points of the illness experience–hospitalization continuum can elicit a variety of parental responses to the situations. Often at the time of diagnosis, a parent will experience an acute grief reaction; however, this stage is usually for a limited time, although the limit is difficult to predict. When grief becomes prolonged, with periods of depression, a diagnosis of Dysfunctional Grieving is more appropriate. Characteristic evidence of this diagnosis are significant alterations in concentration of the ability to carry out normal parenting tasks over a period of time and distancing by the parent from routine family functions and from social or religious activities. The diagnosis Anxiety is more frequently used to describe responses to short-term, unplanned hospitalizations or the diagnosis of a critical illness. Anxiety is characterized by denial, withdrawal, apprehension, and reports of worry by the parent. This diagnosis may occur in tandem with or result in Parental Role Conflict.

Chronic conditions, prolonged hospitalizations, or home-based technology-dependent care may result in the diagnoses Altered Family Processes and Caregiver Role Strain. Chronic illness or a congenital defect in a child necessitates changes in family roles and leads to Altered Family Processes. Characteristically, the prolonged burden of caring for a chronically ill child often occurs in the home setting. Parents experience feelings of depression, grief, increased stress, family conflict, and withdrawal from social supports. These diagnoses also can occur in tandem with Parental Role Conflict.

■ Medical and Psychiatric Diagnoses

Depression, schizophrenia, and confusional states can significantly alter the parents' ability to be involved with their child's care or to cope emotionally with the stress of an ill child. Parents themselves may be experiencing an acute or chronic condition, such as AIDS, a seizure disorder, multiple sclerosis, rheumatoid arthritis, cancer, and cardiac or cerebrovascular conditions. The parents' own health status can have a serious impact in the short term on their ability to participate in their child's care. This difficulty is especially true if parents are experiencing an acute exacerbation of their own health problems.

OUTCOME IDENTIFICATION, PLANNING, AND IMPLEMENTATION

The overall outcome anticipated with a diagnosis of Parental Role Conflict is a reduction in factors compromising role functioning and expressed satisfaction with role functioning. The first expected outcome is that the parents verbalize an understanding of their child's condition and treatment plan. The benefits of providing clear, concise, and timely information have been well documented.[7,9,10] Information provided in appropriate terminology for parents on an ongoing basis can assist them to reduce the individual, situational, and contextual stressors. Similarly, in home-based care, the family continues to require ongoing explanations, including resources available to them. During initial periods of crisis, information needs to be repeated because the assimilation of infor-

mation may be difficult in response to the crisis.[6] It may be helpful to encourage parents to write down the questions they wish to ask. Written information can help enhance verbal explanations but should not replace them.

The second expected outcome is the parents' ability to manage effectively the care required by their child's illness. Providing direct care is one way that parents can cope with anxiety and guilt about their child's illness and that they can use to gain a sense of control over the environment. Nurses can coach parents in appropriate activities and can consistently provide information that allows parents to make informed decisions. This helps parents maintain their sense of competence in their parenting abilities. Melnyk[9] gave mothers ($n = 108$) of young children with unplanned hospitalizations information about what behaviors to expect of their children and how to maintain their parental role. This intervention reduced the mothers' anxiety, increased their level of participation, and increased their level of support for their children. Parents of technology-dependent children require continual reassurance about their parenting skills. Parents need to be involved in developing the plan of care; this includes parents of children cared for at home to enhance their role, particularly where children have chronic conditions and require repeated hospitalizations or home-based care.[13,16] Families need to be active participants in multidisciplinary team conferences as well.

Parents will need assistance to help their child understand and cope with the illness and its treatment. Understanding the normal expected behavioral and emotional reactions of children in various age groups to hospitalization is necessary. Parents familiar with the range of emotional and behavioral responses they may encounter will be better able to cope with such behavior if it occurs. Melnyk[9] found that children displayed fewer negative behavioral changes if the mother received teaching about what to expect of her child and on ways to cope with it. Parents can assist the staff in interpreting their child's normal reaction to stressful situations and in using this information to determine how far in advance to prepare the child

VIII

◾ **NURSING CARE GUIDELINES**
Nursing Diagnosis: Parental Role Conflict

Expected Outcome: The parents will demonstrate an understanding of their child's condition and treatment plan by the time of discharge from the hospital and on an ongoing basis as needed.
- ▪ Assess the parents' readiness to learn.
- ▲ Assess the parents' current level of understanding before any teaching or information sharing.
- ▲ Reinforce and clarify any previous explanations regarding the child's condition and treatment plan.
- ▲ Repeat teaching or review as needed.
  Baseline assessment of parent's knowledge base is necessary to teach at an appropriate level. Teaching parents before they are ready will result in poor or no understanding or recall of information provided. Parents experience considerable emotional disorganization during a crisis, and this will hamper efforts to absorb new information. Therefore reinforcement and review are required, as needed.
- ▪ Establish a therapeutic relationship by assuming a nonjudgmental attitude and by communicating concern for the well-being of the parents and the child. *A therapeutic relationship will facilitate the establishment of trust, which will enhance communication between the nurse and the parent.*

Expected Outcome: The parent will demonstrate the ability to manage the child's illness effectively by the time of discharge from the hospital and on an ongoing basis as needed.
- ▪ Negotiate caregiving roles with the parent in a nonjudgmental manner. *Parents may be unsure as to what type of care they can be involved in, or they may desire to be involved in only specific types of care.*
- ▪ Coach and guide the parents in the negotiated care as needed.
- ▲ Explain the normal reactions of children to illness and hospitalization.
- ▪ Enlist the parents' help in explaining the treatment plan and procedures in an age-appropriate approach.
- ▲ Educate the parents in the value of play therapy, and encourage its use. *Research suggests that providing support to maintain the parenting role and providing child behavioral information will help the parent to support their child more effectively during hospitalization and at home after discharge from the hospital.*

Expected Outcome: The parent will demonstrate the ability to meet the needs of all family members and the ill child by the time of discharge and on an ongoing basis as needed.
- ▲ After developing a therapeutic and trusting relationship, provide support and encouragement for the parents to explore stressors that affect them and their needs. *A therapeutic relationship will facilitate the establishment of trust, which will enhance communication between the nurse and the parent.*
- ▲ Identify past successful coping techniques.
- ▲ Identify hospital and community resources as appropriate.
- ▲ Assist the parents to plan and implement strategies to reduce stress and to meet personal needs. *Parents will use coping strategies that are consistent with their values, beliefs, and cultural background. Often in a crisis parents will need support in initiating problem-focused strategies. The use of effective support systems can add an additional layer of support to meet the needs of the whole family. In chronic conditions, the use of support groups can be invaluable in meeting the needs of the family. A long-term illness will create a set of demands on parents different from those of an acute event, and parents must be reminded to pace themselves.*
- ▲ Begin to explore the effect of a critical or chronic illness on the family unit and the future implications of that effect; refer patient for psychotherapeutic counseling as needed. *Long-term changes will often need to be made by the family, and psychotherapeutic counseling can be beneficial in supporting long-term coping strategies.*

▪ = nursing intervention; ▲ = collaborative intervention.

for specific procedures and how much detailed information to give. Parents need to be coached on the value of play in helping the child deal with feelings they cannot put into words.

The third expected outcome is the parents' demonstrated ability to meet the needs of all family members and those of the ill child. The family as a whole must be taken into consideration because the illness of a child affects the entire family. The parental response will be influenced by the specific attributes and stability of the family unit. Short-term illnesses tend to be limited in duration, and the crisis that is generated often is managed effectively by the family with support from nursing. Critical or chronic illnesses demand a more complex and sustained response to a prolonged crisis. Parents need to be made aware of the possible emotional needs of the siblings of the hospitalized child. Siblings may experience a variety of emotional responses, including fear of becoming ill, anger, jealousy, separation effects, and guilt.[16] Strategies for supporting the siblings can include loosening the visiting policies where possible, making psychological preparation programs available for elective procedures, presenting age-appropriate explanations on an ongoing basis, and involving older siblings in the plan of care for the ill child. Other therapeutic strategies such as bibliotherapy and therapeutic play also may be helpful. It is essential to assist parents to find ways of spending "special" time with the siblings.

To assist the parents in identifying the nature and magnitude of their current stressors, the nurse needs to establish an environment of trust by adopting a nonjudgmental approach, by using therapeutic communication skills, and by demonstrating to parents that their concerns are important. Parents can be helped to identify previously successful strategies to manage stress in their current situation. Where the child's care is chronic or critical, parents need to be reminded of their own health needs and helped, if they need it, with balancing their own personal needs and the multiple role demands.

Social support systems are crucial for the family of a chronically or critically ill child for several reasons. Families require ongoing information, advice, clarification of fears and concerns, and understanding from professional help. Social networks can be invaluable at this time because they provide linkages with family, friends, community, and spiritual resources. However, assessment of a parent's readiness for group involvement is important before a referral to a support group.

EVALUATION

The nurse will use observations and interaction with the parents to evaluate the extent to which the nursing interventions have been successful. Reasonable achievement of expected outcomes by the time of discharge includes (1) parents verbalizing a basic understanding of the child's condition, plan of treatment, and care after discharge, including the effective of emotion-focused strategies; (2) parents demonstrating comfort with routine parenting tasks, including management of their child's behavioral responses to hospitalization; and (3) parents verbalizing, communicating, or evaluating problem-focused strategies used to cope with the family members' needs. Referral for appropriate health care follow-up and home health care would need to occur if these outcomes cannot be demonstrated by the time of discharge from the hospital. For chronic conditions, family demands are ongoing and the patient's condition or treatment plans can change. Therefore ongoing reassessment and revision of the plan of care is crucial in long-term, follow-up care.

VIII

▶ CASE STUDY WITH PLAN OF CARE

Mrs. My L. is a 32-year-old mother of three who resides in a small town. She has to drive 2 hours to the nearest large medical center. Her children range in age from 3 to 14 years, and the family has not had any major health problems. Mrs. L. is a full-time homemaker and takes pride in her role. She came from Vietnam 8 years ago and speaks minimal English. Mr. L. is fluent in English and is employed by a firm that requires much business travel during the work week. Mrs. L. has the major responsibilities for the family and the home. Over the past year, Mrs. L. has noted that their youngest child, a daughter (Hong), has appeared pale and lethargic and has been losing weight. She has been seen by the family physician several times in the past year, only to be told that she has a virus that rest will cure. Experiencing frustration, Mrs. L. has demanded a referral to a pediatrician. The pediatrician admitted Hong to the pediatric unit of a teaching medical center in a large city nearby, where she is sharing a room with three other children. After an initial workup, a diagnosis of rheumatic fever with kidney involvement was made, and a course of IV antibiotics was started. Although Mrs. L. is quite pleased that Hong is receiving full medical attention, she does not understand the diagnosis, the test, the proposed length of hospitalization, or the prognosis. She has been finding it very difficult to manage her home and other children and to spend enough time at the hospital. Hong has been crying persistently since admission because of pain, loneliness, and separation from her family. Today Mrs. L. took a 5:00 bus to the city to spend the day with Hong. She found Hong whimpering, withdrawn, and refusing to acknowledge her presence. The nurse approached Mrs. L. and said, "I'm glad you're here. I'm so busy this morning. Can you give Hong her bath?" and left the room. Another nurse found both of them crying. Mrs. L. stated through an interpreter that she is exhausted and doesn't know whether she can carry on. She doesn't know how to help Hong, doesn't understand much of what is happening, and thinks she is not doing a good job of anything.

The assessment yielded the following findings: (1) In appearance the 32-year-old mother of three children looks exhausted and is crying. (2) Mrs. L.'s perception of the problem is that she is frustrated with the previous medical management of Hong's condition, is pleased that Hong is now receiving full medical attention, feels exhausted and unsure if she can carry on, is unsure how to help Hong, and feels she is not doing a good job with anything. (3) The factors influencing the situation are situational or environmental; contextual; and personal. The situational or environmental factors include unplanned admission; hospital at some distance from the home; shared hospital room; intrusive and invasive diagnostic workup and treatment; potentially serious medical diagnosis because of complications; lack of interpreter services, making Hong significantly upset. The contextual factors are that developmentally Hong's thinking is preoperational; she is suffering separation anxiety, experiencing pain, and was not prepared for admission because of its unplanned nature; Mrs. L. lacks understanding of Hong's condition, the treatment plan, and her prognosis and length of stay, and she has no previous experience with hospitalization. The personal factors are that Mrs. L. is the mother of three dependent children, visits alone, takes great pride in her homemaking role, and has limited spousal emotional support because of her husband's business travel. The mother has the sole responsibility for the home and family; experiences guilty feelings because of her inability to visit frequently; feels the stress of the nurses' expectations; suffers feelings of inadequacy; and has a limited understanding of English.

▶ PLAN OF CARE FOR MRS. MY L.
Nursing Diagnosis: Parental Role Conflict Related to Unfamiliarity with Hong's Illness and Frustration in Meeting Needs of Self and Family

---

Expected Outcome: Mrs. L. will demonstrate understanding of Hong's illness and treatment plan.
- Assess Mrs. L.'s readiness to learn and her current understanding of Hong's condition and treatment plan. (An interpreter is needed.)

■ = nursing intervention; ▲ = collaborative intervention.

▲ Provide clear, concise information at timely intervals and ask for feedback regarding Mrs. L.'s understanding. Repeat and clarify explanations as needed.

■ Encourage Mrs. L. to write down her questions and concerns. Provide written information with interpretation or in native language as much as possible.

▲ Reassure Mrs. L. that confusion and the need for ongoing information are a usual part of the stress response.

Expected Outcome: Mrs. L. will demonstrate an appropriate ability to manage Hong's coping with the illness and hospitalization.

■ Assess and respect Mrs. L.'s readiness to be involved in Hong's daily activities. Reassess on an ongoing basis.

▲ Explain how children of Hong's age normally respond to the stress of illness and hospitalization.

■ Coach and assist Mrs. L. in providing comfort through communication and touch.

▲ Role model the use of play as a means of helping Hong cope.

▲ Acknowledge increased parental anxiety during invasive or intrusive procedures.

■ Assess the degree of involvement Mrs. L. wishes to have. Prepare Mrs. L. for what she will see during invasive procedures. Coach Mrs. L. in providing comfort during these procedures (if she desires to do so) and after.

▲ Role model and coach Mrs. L. in age-appropriate preparation of Hong for procedures.

Expected Outcome: Mrs. L. will express satisfaction with her ability to meet her needs and those of her family and Hong.

▲ Establish a therapeutic relationship through use of acknowledgement of parental concerns, active listening, and a nonjudgmental approach.

▲ Recognize Mrs. L.'s past and current stressors and coping skills. Assess her beliefs about illness and her previous coping strategies from a cultural perspective.

▲ Plan with Mrs. L. how she can modify her role expectations to manage her current stresses successfully and to offer resources when necessary.

▲ Discuss with Mrs. L. the siblings' responses to Hong's hospitalization. Explain to her about their possible emotional responses, and provide guidance about possible strategies.

VII

■ CRITICAL THINKING EXERCISES

1. Discuss the strategies you would use if Hong were hospitalized in the pediatric intensive care unit. How would the setting affect Mrs. L.'s ability to meet the expected outcomes in the plan of care?

2. What alteration in the plan of care would need to occur if Hong were an adolescent?

3. Develop an altered plan of care if Mrs. L. were a single parent employed outside the home and unable to visit very frequently.

REFERENCES

1. Brown J and Ritchie JA: Nurses' perceptions of parent and nurse roles in caring for hospitalized children, *Children's Health Care* 19(1):28–36, 1990.

2. Callery P and Smith L: A study of role negotiation between nurses and parents of hospitalized children, *J Adv Nurs* 16:772–781, 1991.

3. Coyne IT: Parental participation in care: a critical review of the literature, *J Adv Nurs* 21:716–722, 1995.

4. Curley MAQ and Wallace J: Effects of the nursing mutual participation model of care on parental stress in the pediatric intensive care unit—a replication, *J Pediatr Nurs* 7(6):377–385, 1992.

5. Graves JK and Ware ME: Parents' and health professionals' perceptions concerning parental stress during a child's hospitalization, *Children's Health Care* 19(1):37–42, 1990.

6. Kruger S: Parents in crisis: helping them cope with a seriously ill child, *J Pediatr Nurs* 7(2):133–140, 1992.

7. LaMontagne LL , Johnson BD, and Hepworth JT: Evolution of parental stress and coping processes: a framework for critical care practice, *J Pediatr Nurs* 10(4):212–218, 1995.

8. Lazarus RS and Folkman S: *Stress, appraisal and coping*, New York, 1984, Springer Publishing.

9. Melnyk BM: Coping with unplanned childhood hospitalization: effects of informational interventions on mothers and children, *Nurs Res* 43(1): 50–55, 1994.

10. Ogilvie L: Hospitalization of children for surgery: the parents' view, *Children's Health Care* 19(1):49–56, 1990.
11. Palmer SJ: Care of sick children by parents: a meaningful role, *J Adv Nurs* 18:185–191, 1993.
12. Patterson JM and others: Caring for medically fragile children at home: the parent-professional relationship, *J Pediatr Nurs* 9(2):98–100, 1994.
13. Perkins MT: Parent-nurse collaboration: using the caregiver identity emergence phases to assist parents of hospitalized children with disabilities, *J Pediatr Nurs* 8(1):2–9, 1993.
14. Scannell S and others: Negotiating nurse-patient authority in pediatric home health care, *J Pediatr Nurs* 8(2):70–78, 1993.
15. Watt-Watson J, Everendon C, and Lawson C: Parents' perceptions of their child's acute pain experience, *J Pediatr Nurs* 5(5):344–349, 1990.
16. Wells PW and others: Growing up in the hospital: part II. Nurturing the philosophy of family-centered care, *J Pediatr Nurs* 9(3):141–149, 1994.

VIII

Altered Parenting

▶

Risk for Altered Parenting

▶

Altered Parenting *occurs when the nurturing figure(s) experiences an inability to create an environment that promotes the optimum growth and development of another human being.*[16]

Risk for Altered Parenting *occurs when the nurturing figure(s) is at risk for experiencing an inability to create an environment that promotes the optimum growth and development of another human being.*[16]

OVERVIEW

Parenting is a learned behavior, primarily based on the observations and perceptions of child rearing in one's own childhood home and those of friends. The mobility of families in today's society has often separated the nuclear family from the resources available in the extended family, which used to provide opportunities to observe and participate in infant and child care. In response to the loss of primary experiences of child rearing in developmental years, many communities have developed support groups to provide knowledge regarding the birth process and parenting skills.[3] In addition, situations related to ineffective individual or family coping may contribute to potential or actual alterations in parenting behaviors.

The characteristics of an adequate family environment include basic support for the physical survival of the child; stimulation of the child's emotional, social, and cognitive achievements; promotion of the psychological development of the child to ensure adequate control over impulses and emotions; reality testing; and moral stability and the ability to disengage from the family constellation as part of a process of life-long individuation.[17] Adequate parenting is the ability to provide such an environment for all the children of the family.

The roles of parent within the structure of the family system are set by the culture surrounding it. The stereotype of the "typical American family," based on an idealized view of the nuclear family, is a development of the mid-twentieth century owing more to the power of American advertising than to reality based on census statistics. The type of family structure where the parents live together with two or three children and carry out the "traditional" roles of father leaving for work daily in a successful career and mother functioning as homemaker and nurturer of the family is increasingly a thing of the past.[6] Although this structure has been offered as the model for viewing the family in sociological and political arenas, the nuclear family may function erratically in the long-term process of child rearing. Several additional family structures, such as blended families, foster families, communal families, and single-parent families, should be considered as alternatives to the nuclear family in today's society. Within any of these types of family structure there may be deviations from the accepted norms of the community. The most common deviations today are school-age parents, in single- or two-parent families, and homosexual parents.

The primary task of parenting is the socialization of the child.[3] This includes providing an environment that offers sufficient food, shelter, and safety for adequate growth as well as stimulating the cognitive and social skills needed for interaction with others. It is the parent's job to reflect reality to the child and teach what is acceptable and unacceptable behavior.[18] The specific needs change as the child matures.[9] Nurturing, as evidence by frequent holding, touching, smiling, and talking, is needed during infancy. Toddlers and preschoolers need firm, consistent (yet flexible) control strategies as well as expanded play activities and a cognitively rich physical and social environment. Children of all ages need a parent who is a mediator of environmental stimulation and responds to their behavior, being available and sensitive to and accepting of their emotions.

Although many people assume that parenthood is a natural phenomenon and that all adults instinctively react to the presence of a child in a nurturing fashion, becoming a parent creates a period of instability in a family system that requires transitional behaviors. The period of transition to parenthood may be divided into four phases: the anticipatory phase, the honeymoon phase, the plateau phase, and the termination phase.[12] The anticipatory phase begins with the commitment to form a stable family unit and ends with the birth of the first child. During the early part of this phase, various activities prepare the adults to assume parenting responsibilities. Among these are the revision of each partner's roles, the redefinition of family rules, the reassignment of tasks necessary to the survival of the family, and the development of behaviors expressing intimacy and individuality.

When pregnancy occurs, the couple begins to demonstrate specific preparations for parenting. An increase in passive and dependent behaviors of one or both parents has been noted in the literature. This has been interpreted as a final testing opportunity to take on a dependent role before becoming the one on whom the infant will depend.[12] If the dependency needs of the potential parent are not accepted and met by significant others, a sense of insecurity or inability to meet the dependency needs of the child may develop.

Another behavior occurring during this time is an increase in fantasies and the recall of unresolved childhood conflicts. These are connected with the task of resolving the separation from one's own parents before becoming a parent. The couple is dealing with the fact that although each is still a son or daughter of his or her respective parents, they are no longer children. At the same time, they are developing a relationship with the unborn infant and beginning to identify parenting behaviors they wish to display.[12] Additional tasks during the late anticipatory phase concern concrete preparation for the care of the child: obtaining clothing and furniture and making decisions about how the child will be fed and which partner will care for the infant during specific periods of the day. Failure to deal with these issues may reflect inability to understand the specific requirements of parenthood in providing for the basic needs of the child.

The honeymoon phase is the period after the birth of the child when the attachment between parent and child is formed through intimacy and prolonged contact.[12] This is a period of intensity, with each parent exploring the relationship with the new individual now present. Ambivalence is a result of the changes in lifestyle created by the helplessness of the infant, the tremendous energy required to meet its needs, the disparity between the "idealized" child and the actual child, and the feelings of helplessness and vulnerability produced by the need to care for the infant's total needs. One study[13] has shown significant differences between expectations and the actual process of parenting during the first 3 weeks after birth.

Balancing the individual ambivalence created during this phase with the other individual needs and those of the relationships between parent and child and between the parent's need as a couple requires direct or indirect support from external sources.[12] Friends, relatives, community or church support groups, and other resources offer validation of the universality of the new parent's perceptions and reactions. They provide occasional release from the responsibilities and intensity of the parent-child relationship; function as emotional sounding boards to help in the acceptance of concerns and self-doubts; give concrete information about child care, care of the self, and resources in the community; and enhance the parents' enjoyment of the child by sharing these experiences. When external support resources are not available to the parents during this honeymoon phase, the likelihood of inability to make a successful transition to parenting increases, and professional interventions may be necessary to promote a family system that can nurture the optimum growth and development of all its members.

The plateau phase may be described as the protracted middle phase of the child's dependency where parental roles are refined and exercised. Although the term *plateau* gives rise to an image of stability, the act of parenting through the various stages of childhood and adolescence is one of constant change. The parents must learn to juggle the ever-changing balance of dependence and independence within the child and maintain the environment to provide for the physical needs of the family. The ambivalence created during the honeymoon phase may remain to some extent throughout the entire parenting experience. Children rarely meet the expectations of their parents, frequently create situations in which the parents feel helpless, and continue to require the expenditure of physical and emotional resources that produce scarcity in other aspects of the family systems. The stresses that develop during the extended period of parenting may increase to the point that survival of the family system or of individuals within the system is threatened.

Two principles of survival are altruism and reciprocity.[5] Altruism is related to the cost-benefit ratio. When benefits are given to another, it involves a cost to the giver. The parent-child relationship is assumed to include giving without considering the cost; thus parenting is perceived to be based on altruism. However, even an altruistic relationship is based on reciprocity. Reciprocity may be of three types: generalized, balanced, or negative.[5] *Generalized reciprocity* is defined as a one-way flow that requires nothing in return to continue and may be viewed as an altruistic expression. This type of reciprocity is expected in parents of infants and young children, who depend on the adults in their environment for survival.

The cost of helping a child grow and develop is sufficiently balanced by the growth and development of the child. *Balanced reciprocity* is a direct and real exchange of resources, and it occurs between the parent and the child as the child becomes older and develops a degree of independence. Balanced reciprocity may be expressed directly in terms of requiring the child to perform certain tasks to receive spending money or indirectly in terms of the child offering statements of appreciation or gifts, which represent an emotional expenditure. *Negative reciprocity* is an attempt to get something for nothing. Persons who perceive themselves never to have experienced sufficient altruistic reciprocity may approach parenthood with the expectation of having this need met by their children. The child's role then becomes that of provider rather than receiver, and a situation of negative reciprocity has been instituted in which parent and child expect needs to be met without having to give in return. During this prolonged phase of parenting it is essential that internal and external sources of support for the family system be available as the potential for developmental and situational crises recurs.

The final phase of parenthood is disengagement, in which parent-child roles are revised.[12] As children assume independent roles in the adult world, parents must reassess the allocations of emotional and physical resources they have made in the past. More resources are now available to be placed in the parental dyad and in meeting individual needs. Removing these resources from the children initiates feelings of loss and may reawaken former ambivalent feelings. The children may be unable to accept the total loss of dependence and may expect to have available the same level of generalized reciprocity that existed in childhood. Negotiating the balance between dependence and independence with adult children becomes as threatening to the survival of the family system as any earlier crisis, and the need for sufficient internal and external supports still exists.

No single style of parenting has been shown to be an "ideal" to be emulated in all situations. Whereas in the past parents tended to rear their children as they had been reared, current societal trends have produced an overwhelming number of books, pamphlets, instructional courses, and self-help groups aimed at providing answers to difficult parent-child interactions. Parenting styles have usually been classified on two continuums: the permissive-restrictive or the democratic-authoritarian.[4,19] An alternative is a multidimensional model that reflects the need to consider the parents' natural behavior as well as the characteristic behavior of the child. Thus permissive parenting behavior may be indicative of an overindulgent or indifferent parent or one who values creativity and responsible freedom. In such a multidimensional model, parenting behaviors that express love may range from permissive to democratic to authoritative and finally to possessive and overprotective. These behaviors are child-centered and accepting in nature. Behaviors that are essentially hostile to the child may range from indifferent and neglectful to demanding and antagonistic to authoritarian and dictatorial. These behaviors are centered on the needs of the parent and reject the child.

Although family systems and specific parenting behaviors may have changed as communities have become more mobile and urban, the basic parenting functions remain. Parents continue to have the responsibility to provide for the physical survival of the child, to protect the child from dangers to his or her safety, to help the child develop a sense of security and self-esteem, and to function as a socializing agent to encourage the child to participate in the community and to seek continuity. Meeting the responsibilities of parenting requires access to physical, social, and emotional resources within the family structure and the community. When the resources or the access to them is limited, the ability to function as a parent is compromised and intervention from health care professionals may be required.

ASSESSMENT

Altered Parenting

Although Altered Parenting may occur in any family structure, some individuals or families are perceived to be at higher risk for developing or experiencing difficulties in parenting. Any situation or condition of the parent or the child that intensifies the stress within the family unit increases the risk for Altered Parenting.

Because parenting behaviors are the result of the interaction of many factors in the history of individual parents, the parents' relationship to each other, and their relationship to their own parents and to their children as well as the multiplicity of factors within the current situation, it is difficult to assess the degree to which parenting is successful. All aspects of the Functional Health Patterns need to be assessed. However, some should focus on the child, whereas others should focus on the parent(s) or on the relationship between the parent(s) and the child. Information about the Nutritional-Metabolic, Elimination, Activity-Exercise, and Sleep-Rest Patterns of the child may be essential in identifying the presence of maltreatment. Assessment of the Health-Perception—Health Management, Cognitive-Perceptual, and Value-Belief Patterns of the parent(s) will provide information relating to etiology and intervention strategies. The nurse should assess the child and the parent(s) in the areas of their Self-Perception—Self-Concept, Role-Relationship, and Coping—Stress-Tolerance Patterns. The nurse should emphasize the assessment of social and economic factors because these have been demonstrated to be significant in contributing to the maltreatment of children.

Assessment of parenting behaviors should include the parent-child relationship and the resources available.[5] The initial element to be assessed within the relationship is the attachment capacity of the parent and the child. Attachment capacity must be present to some extent or this distortion will result in rejection. Assessment of the attachment behaviors is conducted by obtaining historical information and by observing current behaviors related to pregnancy, bonding at birth, and the progressive expansion of reciprocity in the parent-child relationship. The ability and willingness of the parent to consider the child's needs before his or her own is an indication of altruism within the relationship, and the ability to respond appropriately to the child's cues also demonstrates an increasing reciprocity.[8]

Assessment of the resources available to the parent-child relationship is the next step. The presence or absence of resources and their appropriate use can predict the degree to which parenting behaviors may be successful. Resource assessment has three elements: physical resources limitations, social support systems, and the emotional resources of the parent and the child. Physical resources include not only the physical health and capacity of each member of the family but aspects of the physical environment, such as economic resources and their use to provide physical means of survival for the child. Assessment of the social support systems available explores the extended family, neighborhood, and community resources available and used by the family to survive stressors. The third element to be assessed is the emotional resources present in the parent and the child. Emotional resources represent the extent to which a person is able to respond to another in a generalized or a balanced reciprocal relationship. This resource pool may be a result of the parent's childhood, the parent's or child's personality characteristics, or factors present in the current relationship. This element also includes the educational variables of intellectual ability and the fund of parenting alternatives available.

Many assessment tools have become available within the last 10 years. Hansen and MacMillan[10] reviewed a wide selection of these, grouping them into categories corresponding to the specific behaviors known to be associated with maltreatment of children. The categories identified were identification of abuse and neglect; child management; anger and arousal; knowledge and expectations; problem-solving and coping skills; and social support. The use of multiple assessment procedures or information sources is emphasized. For example, the Parenting Risk Scale describes the key dimensions of parenting as emotional availability, control, psychiatric disturbance, knowledge base, and commitment, and it offers a tool based on a systematic semistructured interview designed to clarify relevant information, which is generally accepted as appropriate to discover problems in the care and development of children.[15]

■ **Defining Characteristics**

The presence of the following defining characteristics indicates that Altered Parenting may be occurring:

- Inappropriate caretaking behaviors (e.g., feeding, elimination, rest)
- Physical or psychological abuse
- Inappropriate visual, tactile, or auditory stimulation of the child
- Growth and developmental lag in the child
- Frequent accidents or illnesses of the child
- Lack of parental attachment behaviors
- Inattention to infant or child needs
- Frequent verbalizations of dissatisfaction or disappointment with the child
- Frequent identification of negative characteristics of the child
- Frequent attachment of negative meanings to characteristics or behavior of the child
- Verbalization of resentment toward the child
- Signs of depression, apathy, and disturbed or bizarre behavior in the child
- Rejection of caregiver or overcompliance by the child
- Verbalization of frustration with parenting role or role inadequacy
- Inappropriate or inconsistent discipline
- Abandonment

■ **Related Factors**

The following related factors are associated with Altered Parenting:

- Little or no prenatal care
- Parental absence or inability to function because of illness
- Unwanted child displays undesired characteristics or is physically or emotionally ill
- Inability or unwillingness to assume parenting responsibilities
- Ineffective coping with anger
- History of ineffective or abusive relationships with own parents
- Chaotic or inappropriate role relationships

VIII

- Lack of external resources, such as contact with or support from own parents or others in the extended family, or contact or support from community resources
- Daily stressors secondary to poverty, unemployment, or financial hardship
- Unrealistic expectations of self, spouse, or child
- Lack of knowledge, cognitive functioning, or role identity as a parent
- Lack of available role model
- Situational or developmental crises (e.g., financial or emotional)
- Poor problem-solving skills
- Poor education level (high school or less)
- Verbalizations (e.g., of not being able to control child)
- Noncompliance with health appointment for self or for the child
- Compulsively seeking role approval from others
- Involvement with the police

Risk for Altered Parenting

The following risk factors are associated with Risk for Altered Parenting:

- Unwanted child displays undesired characteristics or is physically or emotionally ill
- Inability or unwillingness to assume parenting responsibilities
- Ineffective coping with anger
- History of ineffective or abusive relationships with own parents
- Chaotic or inappropriate role relationships
- Lack of external resources, such as contact with or support from own parents or others in the extended family, or contact or support from community resources
- Daily stressors secondary to poverty, unemployment, or financial hardship
- Unrealistic expectations of self, spouse, or child
- Lack of knowledge, cognitive functioning, or role identity as a parent
- Lack of available role model
- Situational or developmental crises (e.g., financial or emotional)
- Poor problem-solving skills
- Poor education level (high school or less)

- Verbalizations (e.g., of inability to control child)
- Noncompliance with health appointment for self or for the child
- Compulsively seeking role approval from others
- Involvement with the police

DIAGNOSIS

■ Differential Nursing Diagnosis

Altered Parenting and Risk for Altered Parenting should be differentiated from Altered Family Process, Ineffective Family Coping, and Parental Role Conflict. Altered Family Process would be appropriate if the behaviors indicate an inability to function within the role of a member of the family group, not specifically that of parent, and this diagnosis usually involves a dysfunction of the entire family. Ineffective Family Coping is most often used when key family members are unable to facilitate adaptive behaviors during a crisis. Parental Role Conflict is applicable when previous effective functioning is challenged by external factors, such as illness or divorce, and role confusion may be expected.

■ Medical and Psychiatric Diagnoses

Altered Parenting and High Risk for Altered Parenting may occur when either parent is experiencing an illness episode. Chronic medical or psychiatric illness, such as cancer, tuberculosis, COPD, schizophrenia, bipolar disorders, substance abuse, or personality disorders, often results in the inability of the parent(s) to provide for the basic physical and psychological needs of the child because all energy is directed toward maintaining their own physical experience. Children diagnosed with Attention Deficit Disorder or Conduct Disorders, or children who experience multiple episodes of illness or trauma may be part of a family system where Altered Parenting behaviors exist.

OUTCOME IDENTIFICATION, PLANNING, AND IMPLEMENTATION

Outcomes expected from interventions into Altered Parenting or Risk for Altered Parenting are provision of a safe environment for the child; promotion of parent-child attachment behaviors; provision of an adequate knowledge base for effective parenting; development of realistic expectations for self, spouse, and child within the family system; and development of role identity as a parent. These overall goals are continuous throughout the parenting process. The specific goal will change with the age of the child and whether the setting for nurse-parent interactions is an inpatient setting, an outpatient clinic, or the home environment.

The provision of a physically and psychologically safe environment for the child is the basic function of a parent. Child abuse and neglect are the extreme deviations on a continuum of parenting adequacy. Deficiencies in this area may range from routinely ignoring a child's diet or personal hygiene to running a home with multiple safety hazards to severe physical abuse. Lutzker[14] describes specific interventions designed to focus the parent's awareness of the child's need for personal hygiene, adequate nutrition, and home safety and cleanliness. In situations where the parent(s) cannot provide for the minimum safety and physiological needs of the child, mechanisms designed by the community must be engaged to remove the child to a safer environment.

Bonding and attachment are two concepts that have received much attention in recent years and may be seen as the two most significant parenting abilities.[5] *Bonding* may be defined as a unidirectional process, flowing from parent to child, that begins during pregnancy and peaks during the first few days after birth. The process of bonding begins with planning, confirming, and accepting the pregnancy and progresses through the steps of feeling fetal movement, accepting the fetus as an individual person, giving birth, hearing and seeing the baby, touching and holding the baby, and caring for the baby.

Attachment is a process that develops during the first year of the child's life and depends on a successful bond being in place.[5,7] Attachment activities appear to be based on the need to maximize opportunities for survival, and the process reflects the growing trust and security the child finds in the parents. The attachment relationship is reciprocal, containing elements of generalized and balanced reciprocity. Little consideration is given to the cost of parenting, but small actions undertaken by the child, such as smiling in response to the parent's voice, provide sufficient reward.

The majority of interventions found in the literature focus on some aspect of providing an adequate knowledge base for effective parenting.[1,2,20] Lack of information, lack of role models, lack of external resources, and ineffective coping skills may all be decreased through appropriate patient education methods. It is essential to develop the specific teaching strategy based on the parent's needs, cognitive level, previous information, previous life experiences, and emotional and psychological development. Attempting to teach *techniques* to parents without understanding the underlying dynamics may be ineffective. In many cases, the interactions may not appear genuine, and children are quick to sense this. Dependence on a technique to solve the problem may also lead to further blame of self or the partner if the desired results are not obtained. Hardy and Streett[11] have demonstrated the effectiveness of a well-designed family support and parenting education program.

Many parents have unrealistic expectations for their role and abilities as parents, of their spouse's role and abilities, or the role and abilities of the child in the relationship. This may lead to increased frustration and anxiety as the expected behaviors are not manifested. Since anxiety is frequently transformed into anger, the potential for disruption of the parenting function is great. Helping the parent to identify the source of the anger and to develop more realistic expectations defuses the anxiety and offers an opportunity to develop alternative behaviors.

The role of the parent is one of the most complex in our society. Understanding and accepting the parenting role is not an automatic reaction to becoming a parent. Parenting is a learned behavior. In many communities the opportunity for observing parenting behavior is limited, and persons are forced to rely on their perceptions of how they were parented. Interventions that provide information about alternative parenting behaviors and opportunities to discuss the changes in lifestyle

VIII

required as a parent broaden the perspective of the parent and aid in internalizing the parenting role.

Many of the defining characteristics of Altered Parenting are the result of insufficient emotional, social, or physical support. Parents whose own basic needs for safety, nutrition, or love have not been met will be unable to meet the needs of another. Once specific areas of deficiencies have been identified, the nurse may offer information about services available to provide the support needed.

EVALUATION

Evaluation of the extent to which specific interventions help the parent meet the identified goals must be ongoing. Each interaction between the nurse and the parent contains the opportunity to assess and evaluate the change in attachment behaviors, expectations, and role identity. Descriptions of parent-child interactions, parental reactions to new disciplinary procedures, and parental experiences with community support agencies or groups provide the data from which evaluations can be made. When evaluation shows that one stage of a goal, such as identification of alternative caretaking activities, has been reached, nursing interventions need to be designed to support the next stage, thereby stabilizing and consolidating the behavior. Including the parent in the process also reinforces the positive changes and becomes a valuable part of the treatment interventions.

◢ **NURSING CARE GUIDELINES**
Nursing Diagnosis: Altered Parenting and Risk for Altered Parenting

Expected Outcome: The parent will provide a safe environment for the child as evidenced by the child remaining physically and psychologically safe.
- Monitor degree of risk to child's physical and psychological safety.
- Contact other family members or appropriate authorities if child's safety seems jeopardized.
  The provision of a physically and psychologically safe environment for the child is the basic function of a parent. In situations where the parent(s) cannot provide for the minimum safety and physiological needs of the child, mechanisms designed by the community must be engaged to remove the child to a safer environment.

Expected Outcome: The parent will demonstrate parent-child attachment behaviors.
- Encourage touching behaviors by parents.
- Encourage play activities between parent and child.
- Encourage age-appropriate caretaking activities by parents.
  When a lack of attachment behaviors is observed, helping the parent learn to enjoy play activities and the natural developmental achievements of the child will create the feeling of successful parenting and lead to better bonding.

Expected Outcome: The parent will demonstrate adequate knowledge base for effective parenting behavior by providing for child's physical, psychological, emotional, and social needs.
- Assist parent(s) to identify knowledge deficits related to caring for child.
- Identify learning readiness and learning capability of parent(s).
- Provide information and opportunity for parent(s) to test out new information.
  Lack of information, lack of role models, lack of external resources, and ineffective coping skills may all be decreased through appropriate patient education methods.

■ = nursing intervention; ▲ = collaborative intervention.

VIII

Expected Outcome: The parent will achieve role identity as a parent as evidenced by identifying socially expected parenting behaviors and incorporating the concept of "parent" as an integral part of his or her role identity.

- Assist parent to identify major components and priorities of the role identity (i.e., child of one's parents, spouse, or career identity) and the source of "ideal" parenting behavior.
- Observe parent-child interactions and encourage parent to verbalize incongruence between verbalized "ideal" of parent behavior and actual behavior.
- Provide an opportunity for parent to explore role identity through individual counseling or group interaction.
- Provide an opportunity for parent to observe and experience effective parenting behaviors.
- Provide an opportunity for parent to implement alternative parenting behaviors.
- Give positive reinforcement for additional parenting behavior that will support incorporation of concept of "parent" into role identity.

  Parenting is a learned behavior. In many communities the opportunity for observing parenting behavior is limited, and persons are forced to rely on their perception of how they were parented. Interventions that provide information about alternative parenting behaviors and an opportunity to discuss the changes in lifestyle required as a parent broaden the perspective of the parent and aid in internalizing the parenting role.

Expected Outcome: The parent will develop realistic expectations of self, spouse, and infant or child.

- Assist parent to identify present expectations of self, spouse, and infant or child.
- Assist parent to identify areas of failure to meet expectations of self and others.
- Provide an opportunity for the parent to express feelings about unmet expectations.
- Encourage parent to speculate on reasons for expectations being unmet.
- Encourage parent to acknowledge own responsibility for attempting to meet expectations as well as set realistic limits of self and others.
- Help parent to develop realistic expectations as a result of increased knowledge of normal development and basic needs.
- Help parent to develop strategies that increase the possibility expectations will be met (e.g., discussing expectation with spouse or child or identifying steps that must occur to meet expectations).

  Helping the parent to identify the source of the unrealistic expectations and develop more realistic ones diffuses the anxiety and offers opportunity to develop alternative behaviors.

Expected Outcome: The parent will recognize realistic limitations of self and of support systems and will activate additional support systems as needed.

- Assist parent to identify specific areas of needed emotional, social, or physical support.
- Assist parent(s) to identify specific strengths of self and of support systems.
- Encourage parent to express feelings about areas of need.
- Provide information about available resources.
- Assist parent to select appropriate resources.
- Act as liaison or advocate as needed.

  Many of the defining characteristics of Altered Parenting are the result of insufficient emotional, social, or physical support. Persons whose own basic needs for safety, nutrition, or love have not been met will be unable to meet the needs of another. Once specific areas of deficiencies have been identified, the nurse may offer information about services available to provide the support needed.

VII

VIII

■ Case Study with Plan of Care

During a routine postpartum home visit, the nurse discovered Alan, a 6-week-old infant, crying in a locked bedroom while his mother appeared to be asleep with the TV on in another room. Mrs. Angie A., his mother, explained that she had been unable to quiet him. He had cried all morning, although she had fed him, changed him, and rocked him. He usually enjoyed his bath, and she had thought that might calm him. However, his crying increased until it was intolerable, so she put him in the bedroom and turned on the TV to "drown him out" because she was tired and needed to sleep.

Mrs. A. states that Alan was a wanted child of a planned pregnancy. She and her husband had participated in natural childbirth classes and had decided to use a birthing room because there had been no difficulties with the pregnancy. However, the labor lasted longer than anticipated, and she required medication, which made it safer for the baby to use the delivery room. Mr. A. was present at the delivery, and both parents were able to hold Alan soon after his birth. Mrs. A. reported positive feelings about caring for Alan, although she expressed some nervousness because he seemed so little. She also stated that she had a good relationship with her parents and was particularly close to her father, who was available to help with problems. She was the youngest child and did not remember any experience of taking care of infants.

Mrs. A. stated that she had never had any physical problems and enjoyed participating in active sports, which she had missed during the later stages of her pregnancy, and that she was "always too tired now" to do anything. Alan appeared to be a healthy child, and his weight fell within normal limits.

Both of Mr. and Mrs. A.'s parents were still living, but in distant cities. They had visited for a few days after Alan was born, but they had not been able to stay. They called frequently, and Mrs. A. stated that she believed she could usually call her mother or her mother-in-law if she had any "real" problems. Mr. A. has a good job, with income sufficient to support the family in comfort. However, his job includes extensive travel at times, and he has been away from home for the last 5 days. Mr. and Mrs. A. moved to their present home a few months before Alan was born, and Mrs. A. stated that she didn't know the neighbors very well.

Both parents are college graduates and participated in "expectant parent" classes. Mrs. A. stated that even though she and Mr. A. had never been around small children, they had read child-rearing information and thought that they knew what to expect from children at different ages.

■ Plan of Care for Mrs. Angie A.

Nursing Diagnosis: Altered Parenting Related to Unrealistic Expectations of Self and Child, Lack of Support from Significant Others, and Unmet Social and Emotional Needs

---

Expected Outcome: Mrs. A. will provide a safe environment for Alan as evidenced by consistent, routine observation of him.

- Assist Mrs. A. to describe the need for consistent observation of Alan, especially when awake.
- Discuss additional reasons for Alan to cry and appropriate responses to determine if the baby is ill or hurt.

Expected Outcome: Mrs. A. will verbalize realistic expectations of herself, her spouse, and Alan in relation to expected infant behavior and nurturing responses.

- Assist Mrs. A. to identify present expectations of herself, Mr. A., and Alan, such that she can stop Alan's crying or her husband is available to help her as she believes her father had been.
- Assist Mrs. A. to identify areas of failure to meet expectations of herself and others so that she can understand Alan's need and thus be able to stop his crying.
- Provide the opportunity for Mrs. A. to express her feelings of anxiety and anger when Alan continues to cry.
- Help Mrs. A. develop strategies that increase the possibility that expectations will be met (e.g., discussing her expectations with Mr. A. or identifying steps that must occur for her to meet expectations).

■ = nursing intervention; ▲ = collaborative intervention.

Expected Outcome: Mrs. A. will recognize realistic limitations of herself and of support systems and will activate additional support systems.
- Assist Mrs. A. to identify specific areas of needed emotional, social, or physical support, such as help with child care when Mr. A. is away for several days.
- Provide information about additional resources available to meet her areas of need.
- Assist Mrs. A. to select appropriate resources to supplement her own and those of her support system.
- Act as liaison and advocate as needed in obtaining help from appropriate resources.

■ CRITICAL THINKING EXERCISES

1. For Mrs. A., what are some of the limited resources that contribute to Altered Parenting?
2. What are Mrs. A.'s strengths that nursing care can build on?
3. What teaching plan could be developed for Mrs. A. for her to understand possible physical symptoms that might lead to crying?

REFERENCES

1. Ammerman RT: Etiological models of child maltreatment: a behavioral perspective, *Behav Modif* 14:230–254, 1990.
2. Azar ST and Siegel BK: Behavioral treatment of child abuse: a developmental perspective, *Behav Modif* 14:279–300, 1990.
3. Bigner JJ: *Parent-child relations: an introduction to parenting,* New York, 1989, Macmillan Publishing Co.
4. Black MM and others: Parenting style and developmental status among children with nonorganic failure to thrive, *J Pediatr Psychol* 19:689–707, 1994.
5. Bolton FG: *When bonding fails: clinical assessment of high-risk families,* Beverly Hills, California, 1983, Sage Publications.
6. Campbell JM: Parenting classes: focus on discipline, *J Comm Health Nurs* 9:197–208, 1992.
7. Denehy JA: Interventions related to parent-infant attachment, *Nurs Clin North Am* 27:425–443, 1992.
8. Fleming BA and others: Assessing and promoting positive parenting in adolescent mothers, *Maternal-Child Nurs J* 18:32–37, 1993.
9. Halpern R: Poverty and early childhood parenting: toward a framework for intervention, *Am J Orthopsychiatry* 60:6–17, 1990.
10. Hansen DJ and MacMillan VM: Behavioral assessment of child-abusive and neglectful families: recent developments and current issues, *Behav Modif* 14:255–278, 1990.
11. Hardy JB and Streett R: Family support and parenting education in the home: an effective extension of clinic-based preventive health care services for poor children, *J Pediatr* 115:927–931, 1989.
12. Hrobsky DM: Transition to parenthood: a balancing of needs, *Nurs Clin North Am* 12:457–468, 1977.
13. Klinnert MD and others: Marriages with children at medical risk: the transition to parenthood, *J Am Acad Child Adolesc Psychiatry* 31:334–342, 1992.
14. Lutzker JR: Behavioral treatment of child neglect, *Behav Modif* 14:310–315, 1990.
15. Mrazek DA, Mrazek P, and Klinnert M: Clinical assessment of parenting, *J Am Acad Child Adolesc Psychiatry* 34:272–282, 1995.
16. North American Nursing Diagnosis Association: *NANDA nursing diagnoses: definitions and classification, 1995–1996,* Philadelphia, 1994, The Association.
17. Pfeffer CR: Development issues among children of separation and divorce. In Stuart IR and Abt LE: *Children of separation and divorce: management and treatment,* New York, 1981, Van Nostrand Reinhold.
18. Simon J: The single parent: power and the integrity of parenting, *Am J Psychoanal* 50:187–198, 1990.
19. Steinberg L and others: Impact of parenting on adolescent achievement: authoritative parenting, school involvement, and encouragement to succeed, *Child Devel* 63:1266–1281, 1992.
20. Webster-Stratton C: Enhancing the effectiveness of self-administered videotape parent training for families with conduct-problem children, *J Abnorm Child Psych* 18:479–492, 1990.

VIII

Relocation Stress Syndrome

▶

Relocation Stress Syndrome *is a problem of transition and adaptation to a new physical or cultural environment. It is characterized by physiological and psychosocial disturbances related to changes in physical surroundings and the social environment following transfer from one location to another.*

OVERVIEW

Changes in one's residential environment are common in our highly mobile culture and may occur throughout the life span. These changes are multifaceted in nature and often occur within the context of events such as hospitalization, admission to a nursing home, voluntary or involuntary residential moves, job relocation, geographical moves within national boundaries, cross-cultural migration and resettlement, voluntary or involuntary institutionalization, transfers between facilities, discharge from the hospital to the community, intrahospital transfers of patients between wards, room changes within a ward, out-of-home placement for young children, and changes in foster homes.

Responses during the adjustment period following a move from one environment to another have been referred to in the literature as *culture shock,*[24] *relocation shock,*[28] *acculturation stress,*[15] *migration stress,*[17] *life transition and crisis of transfer response,*[31,36] *separation anxiety,*[42] *separation conflict,*[33] and *transfer anxiety.*[7]

Barnhouse and others have summarized the defining characteristics of Relocation Stress Syndrome.[4] Often this syndrome is characterized by grieving, anxiety, uncertainty, and crisis coping as the individual strives for mastery of a new situation and resolution of multiple losses. The adaptation process is a continuum and includes reactions to the event of relocation and ongoing efforts by the individual to establish new relationships and achieve equilibrium in a new environment. Relocation adjustment is influenced by personality factors, coping style, family developmental levels, cultural norms, social support and resources and the person's perceptions about the changes.

For some individuals, relocation is experienced as a stimulating, morale-boosting, growth-producing, and positive process.[9] For some elderly people, a transfer to a new environment may have minimal impact, with age and the presence of stress-buffering social support affecting health status.[16,27,34] In others, relocation may actually improve their daily functioning level and morale, provided that adequate pretransfer preparation and greater involvement in decision making have occurred.[14,18,19] For other individuals, relocation threatens their self-integrity and triggers anxiety and psychological stress during the process of reorganization.[26] For the elderly patient or the chronically institutionalized individual, transfer to a new environment may result in Acute Confusion and cognitive deterioration[22,23] as well as increased aggression and the reemergence of symptoms.[44,47]

Frequently relocation occurs within the context of other life stressors, such as trauma, chronic illness, hospitalization, financial and social losses, altered role performance, retirement, admission to a nursing home, placement in a foster home, developmental and family crises, job transfers, political upheaval, persecution, war, and transcultural migration.° The cumulative effects of these multiple and often interacting stressors frequently contribute to emotional upheaval and changes in health status, and they may challenge the individual's adaptive capacity.

Coping successfully with relocation stress is influenced by the presence of an adequate social support system for the individual,[34] a history of previous, successful transfers, some degree of perceived personal control over the move (versus a sudden, unanticipated move),[39] the predictability of the stressor, the ability to manipulate some aspect of the environment, and pretransfer preparation for the move by caretakers.[8,14] In one study, quality of the new environment, perceived choice, social support, predictability, and cognitive appraisal of the move as threat of challenge were correlated significantly with adjustment to relocation.[2]

Postrelocation adjustment is often characterized by progression through the grieving process because relocation creates loss, disruption, and change in such things as familiar surroundings, caretakers, the social network, activities of daily living, schedules, living arrangements, roles, status, personal identity, and personal comforts. Psychosocial adaptation may also include establishing new cues for orientation and accommodation to another culture, language, or lifestyle. These dual tasks of grieving and adapting to the multiple demands of an unfamiliar environment constitute the major work of relocation adjustment and mastery.[3]

Symptoms of relocation stress are varied. They have included increased disorientation, anxiety, and behavioral management difficulties in the elderly[23,26]; increased levels of aggression in institutionalized psychiatric patients[21,32,44]; decreased school functioning, withdrawal, disordered attachment, negativity, and anger in young children and adolescents†; exacerbation of other developmental problems[20]; marital stress[46]; and posttraumatic stress disorder in refugees.[41]

Relocation stress alone does not necessarily increase morbidity and mortality in the elderly, but it may interact with other variables to produce changes in health status. The age of the elderly patient may also affect their adjustment to relocation.[27] Some studies have reported actual improvements in cognitive responses or stabilization of mood in the elderly after relocation when residents were prepared for relocation.[18]

Hospitalized patients frequently respond to relocation stress with increased helplessness, powerlessness, and anxiety. For example, a patient transferred out of the intensive care unit to the general nursing floor may experience distress when separated from supportive staff and constant monitoring by life-saving equipment.[40,42,43] In studies of other intrahospital relocations, there were few adverse effects when the hospital stays were brief and there was pretransfer preparation.[11] Other patient outcomes after room transfers within nursing homes have been described by Everard, Rowles, and High, who outlined a decision-making model.[12]

ASSESSMENT

The diagnosis Relocation Stress Syndrome is most closely associated with acute external stressors of changes in the patient's environment and social network. However, the nurse is encouraged to explore multiple precipitating factors and to assess the patient and the family's responses from a systems point of view. Because the patient's responses are mediated by multifactorial influences, consideration must be given to the combined impact of concomitant stressors brought about by the hospitalization experience, changes in health status and roles brought about by illness, alterations in cognitive functioning, and the degree of acculturation mastery for the immigrant patient.

The coping capacity and adaptation needs of patients with this potential diagnosis can be determined by interviewing the patient and family at the time of admission to the hospital or nursing home and from medical record information docu-

°References 1, 5, 6, 13, 17, 25–27, 36, 37, 44, 45.
†References 10, 33, 35, 37, 38, 45.

VII

menting the course of the illness, the patient's emotional responses, and the need for special support (e.g., language translators). Assessing the patient and the family's perceptions about the move and changes in the environment and caretakers is important in determining the degree of disruption and vulnerability.

The nurse should also assess the time frame in which patients undergo relocation. Rapid, unplanned moves, for example, may compromise a patient's adjustment and increase the likelihood of developing Relocation Stress Syndrome if pretransfer preparation is overlooked. In caring for the elderly and for critical care patients being transferred from the intensive care unit to a general nursing floor, the nurse should assess what the patient understands about the changes that will occur in the personnel, acuity level, staffing, equipment, and other aspects of the new environment.

For cognitively impaired patients, the elderly, or chronic psychiatric patients, the nurse should obtain a baseline, pretransfer assessment of mental status and functional status (e.g., the ability to participate in activities of daily living). History provided from family or other caregivers familiar with the patient before the transfer is a valuable source of collateral information useful in evaluating coping skills, activity level, posttransfer cognitive functioning, and overall adaptation to the new environment. This information will be invaluable if the patient is an unreliable historian.

Nursing assessment for the potential diagnosis Relocation Stress Syndrome should also include attention to the patient's grieving and comfort level. Grieving may be delayed when energy is focused on the external, logistical details of reorganization within a new setting. Because relocation involves adjustment to various type of loss (e.g., personal identity loss, social or cultural loss, loss of familiar routines and structure, and loss of cherished belongings and personal space), the nurse should observe the patient for dysfunctional or delayed grieving responses.

For the immigrant patient adjusting to a transcultural move, admission to the hospital may heighten acculturation issues and relocation stress. The nurse should assess the patient's cultural identity, degree of acculturation, and fluency with the English language and should identify the patient's beliefs about health and health practices and ethnic preferences that could promote comfort and personalized, culturally sensitive care.

For children and adolescents affected by major geographical moves with their families, or for those experiencing transfer between foster home placements or out-of-home placements, it is useful for the nurse to assess for a history of recent, multiple moves and to determine the type, frequency, and significance of major attachment losses (e.g., siblings, biological parents, extended family, schoolmates, playmates, neighbors, grandparents, and pets). Assessing parental or caretaker coping with relocation issues may also provide information about other stressors within the home context and the amount of support available to the child or adolescent.

The nurse should also assess the developmental level of the child or adolescent to facilitate better understanding of age-appropriate coping and the emotional expression of relocation stress. A history taken from parents or caretakers, schools, and other health care professionals familiar with the child or adolescent may provide valuable information that can be useful in determining the child or adolescent's support and learning needs.

■ **Defining Characteristics**

The presence of the following defining characteristics indicates that the patient may be experiencing Relocation Stress Syndrome:

- Appetite and weight changes
- Increased confusion (elderly)
- Sleep disturbance
- Anger and increased aggression
- Anxiety
- Dependency
- Feelings of displacement
- Grieving
- Loneliness

- Loss of identity
- Powerlessness
- Uncertainty about the future
- Unfavorable comparison of posttransfer and pretransfer settings and staff
- Verbalization of being upset or concerned about transfer
- Lack of acculturation behaviors (e.g., learning new language or new customs)
- Alienation and detachment
- Reluctance to establish new emotional attachments
- Status ambiguity
- Performance problems in school (child)
- Regressed behavior (child)

■ Related Factors

The following related factors are associated with Relocation Stress Syndrome:

- Intensive care patient being transferred from the intensive care unit to a step-down unit of the general nursing floor
- Hospitalized patients being transferred between wards or rooms within a ward
- Hospital admission of the elderly
- Admission of the elderly to a nursing home
- Chronic psychiatric patient transferred between wards
- Chronic, institutionalized psychiatric patients being discharged to the community
- Repeated moves
- Young children and adolescents making geographic moves with their families
- Young children and adolescents undergoing foster home placement
- Migrant worker status
- Traumatic departures from homeland (political refugees)
- Cross-cultural migration
- Foreign student status
- Advanced age
- Dementia
- Delirium
- Chronic physical or mental illness

- Childhood
- History of repeated moves

DIAGNOSIS

■ Differential Nursing Diagnosis

Relocation Stress Syndrome may be confused with the diagnosis Anxiety, which is a common psychosocial response during changes in social or geographical environments.[29] Anxiety can be distinguished from Relocation Stress Syndrome by the fact that the individual is often unable to identify the specific threat, which may be internal as well as external. Resolution of anxious feelings and behavior occurs when the stressor is removed or the crisis is resolved. In Relocation Stress Syndrome, stressors are primarily external in nature, with culture-bound responses to a changed environment. The nursing diagnosis Ineffective Individual Coping is similar to Relocation Stress Syndrome but is broader in scope and includes more than adaptation to a new physical or cultural environment.[29] In Ineffective Individual Coping, adaptive difficulties impair problem solving and coping with major life changes, physical or mental illness, and role changes, often without major external crises affecting the individual. The perceived ability to cope with these demands is also reduced.

■ Medical and Psychiatric Diagnoses

Medical diagnoses most commonly related to Relocation Stress Syndrome include psychiatric conditions associated with acute, situational crises; cognitive disorders; and physical disabilities that limit adjustment to a changed environment. Patients with Relocation Stress Syndrome may progress in their symptomatology and develop adjustment disorders with mood, conduct, and physical complaints as well as posttraumatic stress disorder. Patients with compromised cognitive functioning, as in AIDS, traumatic brain injury, dementia, delirium, and other cognitive disorders, are more prone to Relocation Stress Syndrome and may adjust poorly to changes in routine,

VII

environment, and caregivers. Patients with sensory-motor deficits (e.g., blindness, deafness, or paralysis) are also at risk for similar responses.

OUTCOME IDENTIFICATION, PLANNING, AND IMPLEMENTATION

Initial nursing interventions for Relocation Stress Syndrome are aimed at reducing anxiety, supporting the patient through grieving, adjusting to the changes, and increasing a sense of control. As adjustment to relocation extends beyond a discrete event, interventions must continue after the patient has been transferred to a new setting, with ongoing assessment of patient responses. In addition, the nurse should assess the impact of other stressors on the patient during this adjustment period.

Reducing anxiety and preventing the escalation of existing distress is a primary intervention for Relocation Stress Syndrome. Outcomes include the patient reporting reduced anxiety; having the ability to focus and assimilate new information; showing the ability to solve problems and learn new skills in the changed environment; and having reduced physiological arousal as evidenced by a decrease in heart rate, respirations, blood pressure, and muscle tension within 1 month following relocation. Interventions include establishing a supportive relationship with the patient; helping the patient identify sources of anxiety and verbalize his or her own perception of stressors; orienting the patient to the new environment; and initiating pretransfer preparation. Avoiding multiple caregivers before and after the transfer and allowing the patient time to establish relationships with staff in the new setting will help reduce anxiety. Pretransfer preparation of the patient and the family, such as orienting them to the new environment, teaching about withdrawal of equipment, and introducing them to new caregivers, whenever possible, are other examples of anxiety-reducing interventions to mitigate the potential negative aspects of relocation.

The nurse should plan and implement strategies to support the patient through the normal grieving process associated with Relocation Stress Syndrome. This process may be anticipatory in nature but may continue after the transfer occurs. Outcomes include patient progression through a normal grieving process, indicated by the patient acknowledging losses associated with relocation, a self-report of decreased emotional distress, reduced preoccupation with losses, and a daily reinvestment of energy into relationships and activities in the new environment. Interventions include strategies to ascertain the patient's perception of losses; encouragement of the expression of emotional distress to a supportive listener; identification and mobilization of support systems in the new environment; identification of coping strengths within him- or herself; and assessment of the patient for dysfunctional grieving responses.

◢ **NURSING CARE GUIDELINES**
Nursing Diagnosis: Relocation Stress Syndrome

Expected Outcome: The patient will report reduced anxiety indicated by the ability to focus and to assimilate new information; by the ability to solve problems and to learn new skills in the changed environment; and by reduced physiological arousal within 6 to 8 weeks following interventions.

- Establish a supportive, nonthreatening relationship with patient *to build trust, a sense of security, and continuity in the new setting.*
- Orient patient to the new environment and new caregivers *to reduce disorientation and to increase a sense of control.*
- Maintain structure in schedule and activities, and arrange for consistent caregivers whenever possible *to foster predictability and familiarity.*

■ = nursing intervention; ▲ = collaborative intervention.

- Assist patient in identifying stressors associated with relocation and in verbalizing concerns about changes *to assess patient's perception of events, coping needs, and degree of cumulative stress.*
- ▲ Collaborate with the patient, family, and health care team members to initiate early pretransfer preparation, such as explaining planned changes, describing the new setting, and introducing the patient to new caregivers *to minimize stressors, to allow for anticipatory grieving, and to increase a sense of control over events.*

Expected Outcome: The patient will progress through normal grieving within 6 to 8 weeks after relocation, as indicated by a self-report of decreased emotional distress, reduced preoccupation with losses, and daily reinvestment of energy into relationships and activities in the new environment following interventions.

- Elicit patient's perceptions of relocation adjustment, including difficult aspects of the move, concerns, dissimilar aspects of the environment, and cumulative stressors *to assess the degree of loss and vulnerability for dysfunctional grieving responses.*
- Assist patient in acknowledging feelings of loss and discomfort associated with relocation and adjustment to a new environment *to decrease anxiety, isolation, and internalization of distress.*
- Determine patient's support systems, and assist him or her in mobilizing resources and identifying resources and strengths within him- or herself *to promote personal coping and problem solving.*
- Assess patient for dysfunctional grieving responses *to determine the need for psychiatric referral and treatment.*
- Assist patient in setting realistic social and personal goals in the new setting *to increase self-esteem and a sense of mastery.*

EVALUATION

Evaluation of interventions for Relocation Stress Syndrome should be validated with the patient and caregivers in the posttransfer environment. Successful strategies will decrease anxiety, promote normal grieving, and reduce the loss of control associated with a changed environment. Resolution of the crisis of relocation could be expected within 6 to 8 weeks following the event. The patient should report reduced anxiety, demonstrate an ability to solve problems, establish new social attachments, and participate in activities in his or her new environment. The patient should also report reduced grieving and preoccupation with losses and increased energy. If the Relocation Stress Syndrome persists, timely referral to a mental health professional is indicated for further evaluation and therapy.

VIII

▶ CASE STUDY WITH PLAN OF CARE

Mrs. Alice R. is an 89-year-old trauma patient who is married and lives with her 90-year-old husband in their own home. While driving, Mrs. R. apparently suffered a syncopal episode, resulting in a single-vehicle accident, during which time she sustained multiple spinal and rib fractures. Mrs. R. and her husband were hospitalized on the same nursing unit but not in the same room. After one uneventful day of hospitalization in the surgical intensive care unit, Mrs. R. was moved to a step-down unit. Her husband remained in critical condition.

Nurses on the step-down unit reported that Mrs. R. seemed anxious, especially because she had to share a nurse with several other patients, and that she seemed panicky whenever the nurse left the room, used the call light excessively, complained constantly of pain, and seemed withdrawn and resistant to activity. In addition, she stated that she preferred the "other unit" and talked about the better care that she received there. Mrs. R. frequently talked about feeling "disconnected from home" mentioning that she and her husband had recently planned to move into a retirement center and had already partially relocated some of their belongings there.

▶ **PLAN OF CARE FOR MRS. ALICE R.**
Nursing Diagnosis: Relocation Stress Syndrome Related to Transfer from the Intensive Care Unit to a Step-Down Unit and Recent Partial Move from Own Home to a Retirement Center

Expected Outcome: Mrs. R. will report a reduced level of anxiety and show increased participation in her own care and ward activities following interventions.
- Support Mrs. R. after the transfer by acknowledging her emotional distress in an unfamiliar setting.
- Allow Mrs. R. to verbalize feelings and concerns associated with the ward transfer and her changed environment.
- Orient Mrs. R. to the new ward, introduce her to new caregivers, and explain changes in equipment and staffing patterns.
- Provide the same caregivers as much as possible.
- Accompany Mrs. R. if she is going off the unit for procedures, and explain any changes planned.
- Maintain a calm environment and promote comfort for Mrs. R.
- ▲ Encourage the family to bring in Mrs. R.'s favorite afghan and bedroom slippers.
- ▲ Confer with Mrs. R. about her preferences and daily routines, and maintain her usual schedule as much as possible.

Expected Outcome: Mrs. R. will show an improved mood and increased coping with anticipated relocation events following discharge from the hospital by participating in decision making about her placement, by verbalizing feelings about temporary placement in an extended care facility, and by describing future plans to move to a retirement center.
- Assess Mrs. R.'s understanding of the need for the placement and of planned multiple moves versus discharge to home directly.
- ▲ Initiate an early discharge planning conference with Mrs. R.'s caregivers before hospital discharge.
- ▲ Teach the family strategies to support Mrs. R. during the relocation process (e.g., bringing favorite familiar belongings from home to personalize the environment).
- Assist Mrs. R. in identifying support systems and planning realistic future goals for herself in the new settings.
- Promote Mrs. R.'s autonomy by allowing her control over some decisions regarding her care, space, and privacy.

■ = nursing intervention; ▲ = collaborative intervention.

▦ CRITICAL THINKING EXERCISES

1. What differences in adjustment might occur between young children and their parents following relocation?
2. List examples of questions appropriate for young children during assessment of Relocation Stress Syndrome.
3. In a cognitively impaired elderly patient, describe how to monitor nonverbal early symptoms of Relocation Stress Syndrome.

REFERENCES

1. Anderson JM and others: On chronic illness: immigrant women in Canada's work force—a feminist perspective, *Can J Nurs Res* 25(2):7–22, 1993.

2. Armer JM: Elderly relocation to a congregate setting: factors influencing adjustment, *Iss Ment Health Nurs* 14:157–172, 1993.
3. Aroian KJ: A model of psychological adaptation to migration and resettlement, *Nurs Res* 39(1):5–10, 1990.
4. Barnhouse AH, Brugler CJ, and Harkulich JT: Relocation stress syndrome, *Nurs Diagnosis* 3(4):166–168, 1992.
5. Bashir MR: Issues of immigration for the health and adjustment of young people, *J Pediatr Child Health* 29(suppl 2): S42–S45, 1993.
6. Beiser M and Edward RG: Mental health of immigrants and refugees, *New Directions Ment Health Serv* 20(61):73–86, 1994.
7. Bokinskie JC: Family conferences: a method to diminish transfer anxiety, *J Neurosci Nurs* 24(3):129–133, 1992.
8. Brugler CJ, Titus M, and Nypaver JM: Relocation stress syndrome: a patient and staff approach, *J Nurs Admin* 23(1): 45–50, 1993.
9. Dimond M, McCance K, and King K: Forced residential

VIII

relocation—its impact on the well-being of older adults, *Western J Nurs Res* 9(4):445–464, 1987.

10. Eagle RS: The separation experience in children in long-term care: theory, research, and implications for practice, *Am J Orthopsychiatry* 64(3):421–434, 1995.

11. Eisen SV and Grob MC: Patient outcomes after transfer within a psychiatric hospital, *Hosp Commun Psychiatry* 43(8):803–806, 1992.

12. Everard K, Rowles GD, and High DM: Nursing home changes: toward a decision-making model, *Gerontol* 34(4): 520–527, 1994.

13. Fein E: Issues in foster family care: where do we stand, *Am J Orthopsychiatry* 61(4):578–583, 1991.

14. Gass KA and others: Relocation appraisal, functional independence, morale, and health of nursing home residents, *Iss Ment Health Nurs* 13:239–243, 1992.

15. Gil AG, Vega WA, and Dimas JM: Acculturative stress and personal adjustment among hispanic adolescent boys, *J Commun Psychol* 22(1):43–54, 1994.

16. Grant PR, Skinkle RR, and Lipps G: The impact of an interinstitutional relocation on nursing home residents requiring a high level of care, *Gerontol Soc Amer* 32(6): 834–842, 1992.

17. Hertz DG: Bio-psycho-social consequences of migration stress: a multidimensional approach, *Isr J Psychiatry Relat Sci* 30(4):204–212, 1993.

18. Hobbs MS: A study of the characteristics and needs of people transferred from acute hospitals to nursing homes, *Med J Australia* 159(6):385–388, 1993.

19. Holzapfel SK and others: Responses of nursing home residents to intrainstitutional relocation, *Geriatr Nurs* 13(4): 192–195, 1992.

20. Horwitz SM, Simms MD, and Farrington R: Impact of developmental problems on young children's exits from foster care, *J Behavior Peds* 15(2):105–110, 1994.

21. Jones EM: Interhospital relocation of long-stay psychiatric patients: a prospective study, *Acta Psychiatr Scand* 83:214–216, 1991.

22. LeFroy RB and others: A study of the characteristics and needs of people transferred from acute hospitals to nursing homes, *Med J Australia* 159(6):385–388, 1993.

23. Lindesay J, Macdonald A, and Stark I: *Delirium in the elderly,* Oxford, England, 1990, Oxford University Press.

24. Lipson JG: The health and adjustment of Iranian immigrants, *Western J Nurs Res* 14(1):10–24, 1992.

25. Magzawa AS: Migration and psychological status in South African black migrant children, *J Genet Psychol* 155(3): 283–288, 1994.

26. Mikhail ML: Psychological responses to relocation to a nursing home, *J Geront Nurs* 18(3):35–39, 1992.

27. Mirotznik J and Lombardi TG: The impact of intrainstitutional relocation on morbidity in an acute care setting, *Gerontol* 35(2):217–224, 1995.

28. Netting FE and Wilson CC: Accommodation and reloca-

tion decision making in continuing care retirement, *Health Soc Work* 16(4):266–273, 1991.

29. North American Nursing Diagnosis Association: *NANDA nursing diagnoses: definitions and classification, 1995–1996,* Philadelphia, 1994, The Association.

30. O'Conner BP and Vallerand RJ: Motivation, self-determination, and person-environment fit as predictors of psychological adjustment among nursing home residents, *Psychol Aging* 9(2):1891–1894, 1994.

31. Oleson M: Application of Moos and Schaefer's (1986) model to nursing care of elderly persons relocating to a nursing home, *J Adv Nurs* 18:479–485, 1993.

32. Osborne OH and others: Forced relocation of hospitalized psychiatric patients, *Arch Psychiatr Nurs* 4(4):221–227, 1990.

33. Palmer SE: Group treatment of foster children to reduce separation conflicts associated with placement breakdown, *Child Welfare* 69(3):227–238, 1990.

34. Patterson BJ: The process of social support: adjusting to life in a nursing home, *J Adv Nurs* 21:682–689, 1995.

35. Penzerro RM and Lein L: Burning their bridges: disordered attachment and foster care discharge, *Child Welfare* 74(2):351–366, 1995.

36. Porter EJ and Clinton JF: Adjusting to the nursing home, *Western J Nurs Res* 14(4):464–481, 1992.

37. Puskar KR and Dvorsak KG: Relocating stress in adolescents: helping teenagers cope with a moving dilemma, *Pediatr Nurs* 17(3):295–298, 1991.

38. Puskar KR and Martsolf DS: Adolescent geographic relocation, *Iss Ment Health Nurs* 15(5):471–481, 1994.

39. Reinardy JR: Decisional control in moving to a nursing home: postadmission adjustment and well-being, *Gerontologist* 32(1):96–103, 1992.

40. Saarman L: Transfer out of critical care: freedom or fear, *Crit Care Nurs Q* 16(1):78–85, 1993.

41. Sack WH, Clark GN, and Seeley J: Post-traumatic stress disorder across two generations of Cambodian refugees, *J Am Acad Child Adolesc Psychiatry* 34(9):1160–1166, 1995.

42. Schactman M: Transfer stress in patients after myocardial infarction, *Focus Crit Care* 14(2):34–37, 1987.

43. Swarczinski C and Graham P: From ICU to rehabilitation: a checklist to ease the transition for the spinal cord injured, *J Neurosci Nurs* 22(2):89–91, 1990.

44. Thomas MD and others: Intrahospital relocation of psychiatric patients and effects on aggression, *Arch Psychiatr Nurs* 4(3):154–160, 1990.

45. Vercruysse NJ and Chandler LA: Coping strategies used by adolescents in dealing with family relocation overseas, *J Adolesc* 15(1):67–82, 1992.

46. Wamboldt FS, Steinglass P, and Kaplan De-Nour A: Coping within couples: adjustment two years after forced geographic relocation, *Fam Process* 30(3):347–361, 1991.

47. Wells DA: Management of early postdischarge adjustment reaction following psychiatric hospitalization, *Hosp Commun Psychiatry* 43(8):803–806, 1992.

VIII

Altered Role Performance

▶

Altered Role performance *is a disruption in role functioning (e.g., inadequate role transition, role distance, role conflict, or role failure) as perceived by self and others.*

OVERVIEW

The social context of life and living requires that each person function in a variety of roles. Each role is characterized by a set of behaviors that guide interactions and transactions involving the self and others. Roles are influenced by social forces, norms, and values that affect conduct in a given situation, society, or culture. A basic principle is that any role held by an individual will have a relationship to roles held by others. Some roles are more clearly defined and enacted in circumscribed, time-limited situations, such as that of a tennis player. Others, such as the role of father, are more diffuse and change with growth and development, family structure, and general shifts in social norms and values.[14]

Roles and role performance are learned and acquired. The functionalists view roles as persisting over time in any given society, with socialization guiding role development with positive and negative reinforcements. On the other hand, the interactionists see society as a framework within which people interact dynamically. Each person is simultaneously involved in interpreting another's behavior and constructing responses based on perceived cues, such as expectations, feelings, and beliefs, transmitted in the interaction.[4] Together these two perspectives explain major forces that contribute to persistent general expectations for role behavior as well as those influences that individualize role performance and give rise to change.

In nursing, it is important to understand how social roles develop and evolve because they influence a sense of well-being in the person and influence life goals and health. Roles give meaning and value to life, and they foster a sense of belonging and contributing to society. Roles are action- and interaction-oriented and can be viewed as motivating forces in stimulating biopsychosocial integrity.

Life experiences, including role expectations, can affect the development of coping skills.[16] Roles are associated with shared beliefs and values and with personal likes or dislikes about social behavior, and they are an integral part of the self-concept.[13] Nurses, in recognizing the significance of role performance and its relevance to health, can promote learning and coping when patients encounter role changes.

The various roles an individual performs can be classified as *primary, secondary,* or *tertiary*.[14] *Primary roles* are based on sex and relate to age and to stages in the developmental process. The individual rarely has a choice in being male or female and is expected to perform according to his or her developmental stage (e.g., being in the social position of a child). Social norms and expectations shape primary roles, and role behavior must meet generally recognized social standards.

Transitional life stages, such as adolescence, are characterized by changes in age-related role behavior that can be stressful and confusing. Children and families may require professional guidance during transitional periods of development.

Secondary roles have an element of choice and tend to be task-oriented to fulfill certain functions associated with life stages (e.g., the role of husband and wife or father and mother). Other secondary roles are based on achieved positions, such as being a teacher. These roles relate to work or occupations that require specified skills and knowledge for role competence, and they are instrumental in providing sustenance for self and others. Roles in general have an affective component in that they meet personal ambitions for success and recognition and give meaning and satisfaction to life and living. Life circumstances may require changes. The experience of role loss or role acquisition can be traumatic, with the grieving process resulting from role loss. Or the person may need to learn new sets of behaviors with associated feelings of uncertainty, anxiety, and insecurity about role expectations. Because secondary roles have an element of choice and usually persist over long periods of time, individuals invest personal energies that are achievement-oriented to yield material rewards and personal growth and satisfaction. When life changes occur, such as promotion, unemployment, marriage, divorce, or illness, the individual must master significant role changes and may require professional services to make a healthy adjustment.

The third category of roles, *tertiary roles,* is more transitory. These tend to be associated with responsibilities or obligations taken on by choice for a limited period of time (e.g., being president of a club). Tertiary roles are often linked to secondary roles. When such a role is changed or lost, considerable stress can occur, affecting other roles and possible leading to negative self-perception.

A number of conditions influence each role as it is learned, acquired, or maintained. Goals designated to meet perceived expectations, to gain social rewards, or to reap other personal gains direct role behavior. Role performance requires a set of circumstances, such as artifacts, tools, or designated space. Furthermore, any role requires the participation of others to complement and facilitate role performance. Added to external cir-

cumstances are feelings of success and accomplishment based on immediate feedback or recognition shown by others. There are also feelings of confidence that certain external circumstances can lead to success and that others are interested and willing to offer support, thus making the performances worthwhile. If circumstances do not facilitate role performance, conflicts, insecurities, and role failure may arise, resulting in a disturbance of role performance. Felt obligations and perceived expectations are powerful forces that constantly shape, guide, and give purpose to role behavior. Thus the circumstances of illness or altered health may create stressful changes in roles and role-determined relationships.

In a multicultural society such as that of North America, cultural attitudes, values, and beliefs may prescribe role behavior that can be quite different for similar social positions.[4] To expect role sharing in cases of illness or disability may not be acceptable or compatible with the existing belief system and ethnic orientation. The secondary role of husband, wife, parent, or child may have cultural sanctions or taboos that regulate behavior during childbirth or when a death has occurred. For example, a Vietnamese family may not be able to provide home care for an aging mother with a terminal cancer because their duty would be to keep doors and windows open at all times regardless of the severe winter coldness. Similarly, a Jewish husband may not be able to coach his wife during labor and delivery because at that time he must attend to certain religious practices associated with birth. Cultural and religious beliefs and practices have a strong influence on role performance and must be recognized when role functions are threatened by illness and when the health care system is organized and dominated by majority rules and standards for role performance.

Altered Role Performance can be described as one of four types, each involving stress: *altered role transition, role distance, role conflict,* and *role failure.*[12]

Role transition occurs in developing new roles or when existing roles change because of altered

VIII

circumstances that affect role behavior. Developmental crises occur when growth and maturation bring about changes in capabilities and expectations for roles and role mastery and the individual is not prepared to cope with or cannot cope with the changes experienced. Developmental periods of role transition usually are anticipated, but the guidance for role mastery may be insufficient or inadequate or expectations may be unrealistic. Altered Role Performance can then occur.

An individual may have adequate role behavior (e.g., mothering an infant), but when this role behavior differs from socially prescribed expectations, this is described as role distance.

One of the more common alterations in role performance arises in role conflict. Conflict can arise when expectations for role performance are incompatible or incongruent within a certain role. This situation would be considered intrarole conflict. Another type of intrarole conflict can arise when role expectations are incongruent with beliefs and values the individual holds. Other sources of role conflict the individual can encounter are incompatibility or incongruity between different roles that a person plays.[4] Such role stress is defined as *interrole conflict*. In these situations the person cannot meet certain role expectations for one role because another role requires behaviors that are incompatible or incongruous with the first role.

In role failure there is evidence of absence or ineffectiveness in performing the functions of a role or in experiencing role satisfaction. Failures in secondary roles are usually more serious because important life goals may be threatened. However, failure in any role may be very stressful to the individual experiencing it. Many reasons may exist for role failure. The person's ability to function in a given role may change when injuries or illness (including mental illness) impose limitations or when age-related factors indicate a lack of maturity in younger years and limitations in senior years. Conditions in the environment may also change, resulting in a lack of resources, support, or even purpose for a given role. Roles may be vaguely defined or ambiguous, leading to uncertainty and confusion about role expectations, which contribute to perceived role failure. Inability to function in a role as a result of illness or disability may require relinquishing a valued role, and role loss may be experienced.

ASSESSMENT

Changes in health status or transitional periods of development are likely to affect role performance. As the ability to perform a given role is altered or if the individual cannot meet expectations for role performance, role stress arises and he or she will experience role strain.[1,4] This strain can further compromise the individual's ability to cope with physical and mental illness or with developmental expectations. Family members often assume the caregiver role, affecting role functions within the family. Caregivers may experience considerable role strain during family illness or when disability occurs in the family.[15] What changes in role functions have occurred, and how are caregivers coping with these? The patient's physical condition, the age of the caregiver, the health of the caregiver, family commitments, and loss of work (income) can be important causes of caregiver stress.[2]

Assessment requires knowledge about the significance of role performance to the self-concept and knowledge about the person's perceived health and well-being. Knowledge is also needed about what to expect in terms of cultural beliefs, social norms, and the individual's life stage, level of development, and actual role performance. In the assessment process, the nurse must consider ethnic and cultural beliefs, values, and norms. These can play a significant part in the perceptions of role ambiguities and associated stresses.[5] For example, an Italian mother insists on feeding her convalescent child pasta, although the child is on a medical regimen at home requiring a modified diet. Assessment must include the mother's knowledge base, her values and beliefs, and her perception of her role as care provider in this new context. The presence of the defining characteristics of inadequate role performance must be determined.

Assessment requires effective interactive skills to elicit the nature of what the patient is experiencing related to personal perceptions of how role performance is affected and what this means for attainment of life goals or personal ambitions. The nurse who offers an opportunity to discuss the patient's primary, secondary, and tertiary roles will convey (1) an interest in role performance, (2) a holistic approach to the patient's life situation, and (3) an understanding of expressed views or concerns. In clarifying role perceptions with the patient, the nurse can determine the hierarchy of importance of secondary and tertiary roles as perceived by the patient. Apart from eliciting information about role perception from the patient, the nurse may also have an opportunity to observe role behavior in certain situations.

The nurse must assess role transition, role distance, role conflict, and role failure. In regard to role transition, for example, during the early teen years a transition from childhood to adolescence is expected. The secondary role of becoming a high school student and making decisions about participation in certain sports, such as playing hockey—a tertiary role—require supportive circumstances from peers and guidance from teachers and parents. Assessment must consider whether the individual has completed previous studies at primary school, indicating readiness to cope with a higher level of education. In case of enrollment in sports, the nurse needs to assess the student's previous experience and his or her physical abilities along with access to sports activities, time schedules, needed equipment, and parental supports. Focusing on how the student perceives encountered role changes is important; for example, "Now that you are in high school, do you see that the way you used to learn is different? In what ways? What makes being in high school so fun? How do you think the others in your class want you to behave? What about the teachers? What do they expect?" Such questions can determine whether the student has a sense of orientation to the changed role and is coping to make needed adjustments. Or the nurse may find that the student has fears and unrealistic perceptions based on a lack of preparation or knowledge.

How a woman perceives and performs her role as a mother caring for an infant may satisfy the infant's and the mother's needs. However, the expectations regarding the mothering of the infant, based on prescribed cultural and social norms, are different. The mother may swaddle her infant, yet the cultural norm prescribes freedom of movement as a developmental prerequisite. Thus the mother will experience role strain when her behavior meets with disapproval and she receives instructions to change her way of caring for the infant. The nurse can assess role distance by observing role functions and by questioning role perceptions. When functions and perceptions both differ from prescribed norms, the nurse can make a diagnosis of Altered Role Performance (role distance).

An example of role conflict is the teacher who is expected to attend regular afternoon meetings of the teachers' association and also supervise students during afternoon sports activities. Conflict will result because these two expectations are incompatible. Assessment must identify the kinds of expectations exerted on role behavior and how and why conflict arises. The individual teacher may experience conflict because he or she is unaware of regulations or policies that could resolve the conflict, or the teacher may lack problem-solving skills that can meet both responsibilities—attending meetings and supervising students. A nurse working in a hospital is expected to care for patients admitted for induced abortions. The nurse knows that such patients require supportive nursing care, yet the nurse might find abortions to be unacceptable on moral grounds. This nurse will experience conflict related to a personal belief that is perceived as incongruent with expected role functions. Assessment will need to focus on identifying the nature of the conflict and on exploring how the person is trying to cope with the experienced role strain. Coping may be inadequate if it is characterized by avoiding expected role functions. The nurse may have somatic complaints, such as headaches, which may be evidence of subconscious

VIII

avoidance that does not deal with the sources of conflict. The nurse may lack problem-solving skills in seeking alternatives for satisfactory role performance. The nurse in the intrarole conflict situation above could seek to work on a unit where he or she will not encounter abortion cases. During acute or chronic illness, the patient role may be in conflict with many other roles the person holds.

Assessment will need to center on eliciting the patient's perceptions of role expectations for secondary and tertiary roles. As different roles are discussed, the nurse needs to listen for evidence of experienced role strain. Expressions such as "I want to be a good mother or father and a good teacher, but it does not seem to work" or "Having to stick to my diabetic diet will never work when I am back in my business" may indicate frustration and possible role conflict. To determine the person's ability to function in a variety of roles, the nurse may need to assess the patient's level of knowledge about available alternatives and problem-solving skills for conflict resolution.

The nurse must assess role failure and its causes. For example, the college student may fail to perform in the student role because of a reading disability, immaturity, lack of support, or lack of a goal for studies.

Characteristic behaviors may be expressed as dissatisfactions with a role (e.g., "I do not like being a mother" or "I do not wish to return to my job as a secretary"). The patient (a mother) may be observed as performing role expectations ineffectively (e.g., feeding or diapering the infant improperly). If she neglects the infant, this may indicate the absence of expected mothering behavior. Patients may express their felt inadequacies by saying "I am no good at this" or "I can never learn to do this right." The patient may express felt confusion and ambiguity about role performance in statements such as "My mother told me to lie down when breastfeeding, and now you tell me to sit up when breastfeeding. How am I supposed to know what is right?" Questioning the patient about role expectations may reveal a lack of knowledge about role functions. Assessment also should focus on needed equipment, social supports, and envi-

ronmental factors that promote comfort when role functions are performed. The mother may fail in breastfeeding if her husband does not approve of this function or if she has no role model for learning. To assess adequacy or inadequacy for a given role, a checklist of role expectations can be developed that can assist the nurse in conducting a comprehensive assessment of role performance.

■ Defining Characteristics

The presence of the following defining characteristics[6,11] indicates that the patient may be experiencing Altered Role Performance:

Role transition

- Feelings of anger or depression
- Change in self-perception of role
- Change in usual pattern of responsibility
- Change in capacity to perform role
- Inability to achieve desired role
- Refusal to participate in role
- Change in others' perception or expectations of role

Role distance

- Uncertainty about role requirement
- Lack of knowledge of role
- Different role perceptions

Role conflict

- Confusion
- Frustration in role (intrarole or interrole conflict)
- Ambivalence about role
- Inadequate problem-solving skills
- Incongruent, incompatible role expectations

Role failure

- Withdrawal
- Loss of role skills
- Inability to achieve desired role
- Refusal to participate in role
- Difficulty in learning new role

■ Related Factors

The following related factors are associated with Altered Role Performance:

- Physical illness (e.g., cancer[8] or stroke[3])

- Decline in physical strength or ability
- Alcohol or drug abuse
- Mental retardation
- Cognitive difficulties
- Low self-concept
- Crisis
- Developmental crisis
- Severe stress during change in occupation
- Inability to deal with changed expectations in new role
- Role incompatibility
- Lack of adequate role model
- Role ambiguity or incongruity
- Inability to learn new role requirements
- Inadequate social support
- Inadequate resources
- Stressors in salient social roles[7]
- Very frustrating social situations
- Cultural transition

DIAGNOSIS

■ Differential Nursing Diagnosis

Several NANDA nursing diagnoses are closely related to Altered Role Performance. Parental Role Conflict, "the state in which a parent experiences role confusion and conflict in response to crisis"[11] (p. 48), is a specific type of Altered Role Performance. It is appropriately used when parents have concerns and feel inadequate in caring for the child's needs, provide evidence of disrupted caretaking behavior, and express concern about family functioning. Likewise, Caregiver Role Strain, "a caregiver's felt difficulty in performing the family caregiver role"[11] (p. 44), could be viewed as a more specific type of Altered Role Performance. Other examples include Altered Parenting.

■ Medical and Psychiatric Diagnoses

Physical illness, especially severe chronic illness, such as AIDS, Alzheimer's disease, multiple sclerosis, or severe osteoporosis, can lead to a disruption in role functions. The same can be said for chronic mental illness, such as major depressive disorder, mental retardation, substance-induced delirium, vascular dementia, and anorexia nervosa.

OUTCOME IDENTIFICATION, PLANNING, AND IMPLEMENTATION

In setting goals for desired role mastery or required role changes, the patient, significant others, and the nurse are mutually involved in the planning process. It is the patient who has to attain perceived satisfaction in role adjustments to meet personal goals, ambitions, or social expectations.

Inadequate Role Transition

The experience of stressful role transition may occur during developmental stages or when life events, such as illness or disability, require role changes. The patient is expected to relinquish previous role behavior and master new role behavior. The nurse can assist the patient in identifying losses of previously held and valued role functions, with a focus on why these are no longer feasible related to altered capabilities or changes in life situations. In determining the type of role that is changed and its importance to the patient, the nurse can anticipate a grieving response. Encouraging the expression of emotions and verbalization of perceived losses will facilitate grieving.[9] The patient may require information about changed capacity as well as the role options available for consideration. For example, a letter carrier with a hip disorder may need to understand how his or her decreased walking capacity affects the current role and may need to know that letter sorting is a possible employment alternative. The nurse can encourage the patient to seek needed information and to explore options.

Anticipating life stages and associated roles, such as becoming a mother or reaching retirement age, will focus nursing interventions on anticipatory guidance and preparatory teaching. Prenatal classes provide a group setting for discussion of expectations regarding infant care and the demands of the mothering role on a woman's time and energy. Nurses as group leaders can facilitate the expression of concerns and can give direction to focus discussion on known expectations, norms, and values related to the role. The community

VIII

nurse may suggest group sessions for older people nearing retirement age or offer counseling regarding assessment of capabilities and interests and encourage development of new and meaningful secondary or tertiary roles. Knowledge and skill enhance confidence in role perception and mastery in role performance.

Because roles are interdependent and complementary, significant others may need assistance to focus on their functions in clarifying role behaviors and expectations when patients experience role transitions. For example, the roles of husband and wife are complementary. With the experience of a myocardial infarction, both roles require adjustments and clarification.[10] The nurse can encourage significant others to communicate recognition of desired role behavior. The nurse can support them in their efforts to discuss anticipated behaviors, sentiments, sensations, and goals involved in the patient's role change and their own complementary functions. Increased role awareness and effective communication will facilitate role transitions.

Role Distance

When Altered Role Performance is recognized as role distance, nursing interventions will be designed to reduce or alleviate role distance. Because cultural beliefs and values can play a significant part in the patient's orientation toward a given role, such as mothering, the nurse must make an effort to understand the patient's value system. To do this, the nurse explores the reasoning and perceptions associated with the observed role function, such as the previously mentioned swaddling of the infant. By showing respect for the practice in its cultural context, the nurse can then guide the patient into discussing and comparing traditions of the past with current methods of infant care and their rationale.

Another example of role distance occurs when the mother of a premature infant treats the infant as—and expects the infant to behave as—a normal full-term infant. The nurse may need to focus first on the mother's wish to perceive her infant as full-term to avoid her felt disappointment. When the nurse shows acceptance of the mother's feelings and encourages the expression of disappointment, the patient will then be ready to focus on the infant's actual needs and the mother's ability to meet them. Strategies for teaching may include role clarification with discussion and presentation of information on role expectations and role modeling with demonstrations of handling the premature infant as well as a referral to reference groups of other parents with premature infants.

Role Conflict

When role conflicts are encountered, resolution of conflict becomes the expected patient outcome for planned nursing interventions. As a first step, conflict situations require a thorough exploration of the type of conflict the patient experienced. As the nurse and the patient together identify conflicting expectations, perceptions can be clarified, rectified, or reinforced. For example, the teacher experiencing intrarole conflict can be advised to plan with colleagues to share the responsibilities of supervising sports activities and attending association meetings.

For interrole conflicts, the nurse can assist the patient in assessing the felt demands on his or her time and efforts in relation to both roles. For example, the mothering role that requires play time with the children may be given a higher priority than the teaching role that requires "extra time" for pupils. Reflective counseling can help the patient accept differences in role perception, thus reducing felt strain about conflicts.

Incompatibilities and incongruities of roles may require joint family or group meetings in which the nurse facilitates the discussion and exploration of conflicts and assists the group in clarifying mutual expectations. Verbalization of felt strain and experienced stress can foster mutual understanding, acceptance, and goal setting for the resolution of experienced conflict.

Role Failure

In role failure, planned interventions will address the lack of knowledge and skills for a given role and assist the patient to achieve satisfactory role competence. Assessing the patient's readiness to learn and setting mutually acceptable goals are prerequisites for all teaching strategies. Role failure implies that the patient has tried to achieve a role and has not succeeded or that the patient's ability or health status has changed, resulting in role failure. The patient is most likely feeling disappointment and distress. Facilitating the expression of these feelings and at the same time recognizing the strengths and abilities that the patient possesses for achieving the desired role can mobilize confidence and energies for the learning task.

A jointly developed list of tasks for expected role performance (e.g., mothering an infant) may provide guidance for focusing on definable tasks and associated knowledge and skills. By discussing each task (e.g., feeding an infant) the nurse can assess and reinforce existing knowledge and provide additional information. The nurse can demonstrate how to hold the infant for spoon-feeding while he or she discusses the position and utensils that facilitate the feeding process. Because many role functions cannot be fully described because they involve social interactions, role modeling becomes an important teaching strategy. Using opportunities to model interaction with the infant may stimulate the mother to interact similarly. Interpreting the infant's behavior may sensitize the mother in recognizing the cues the infant gives for her behavior. The nurse should also seek every opportunity to praise the mother's efforts and effectiveness in appropriate role behavior. Recognition and praise reinforce learning and build confidence and competence in role performance.

When role failure is related to a change in ability to meet expectations, the nurse may assist the patient and others within the role set to examine whether modifications in role performance are feasible and acceptable to all concerned. For example, a teacher with early Alzheimer's disease may be able to perform selected teaching responsibilities with small groups or individual students while avoiding large groups and public speaking responsibilities.

The nurse also can use role rehearsal as a teaching strategy. The nurse can act as the designated role partner to provide the patient with responses and cues for experimental learning. This teaching strategy may be particularly useful in working with teenagers who fail to assume an appropriate student role or with parents who fail to work out their respective roles in raising children. In most cases of role failure the nurse can facilitate learning to overcome inadequacies. The nurse's support and assistance can help the patient gain satisfaction from competent role behavior.

VIII

◢ **NURSING CARE GUIDELINES**
Nursing Diagnosis: Altered Role Performance

Expected Outcome: The patient will experienced less stressful role transition as evidence by verbalizing role loss and expressing satisfaction about functioning in a changed or new role and by demonstrating appropriate knowledge and skill for role mastery.
- Assist the patient in identifying role loss or change.
- Explore with patient what has changed. *So that they can develop realistic goals for adjustment, the nurse and patient need to explore the patient's perceptions of what has changed and how this change is affecting different roles.*
- Facilitate grieving response to experienced role loss. *Grieving requires expression and resolution before the patient can recognize the need for a new role and direct energies toward learning it.*
- Inform the patient about altered functional capacity and how it affects role performance.
- Explore available options for role change or adjustments.
- Offer anticipatory guidance for life-stage role transitions. *Anticipatory guidance and preparatory teaching will facilitate role transition and can prevent stresses when role changes do take place.*

■ = nursing intervention; ▲ = collaborative intervention.

Continued

◢ **NURSING CARE GUIDELINES — CONT'D**

- Offer assistance to patient's significant others when patient is undergoing a role transition. *By assisting expression of altered role perception and possible role strain and by facilitating clarification of expectations for complementary role functions, the nurse can offer guidance and reduce or prevent role insufficiency.*

Expected Outcome: The patient will demonstrate reduced or alleviated role distance as evidenced by the expression of awareness and ability to meet role expectations.

- Explore and clarify perceptions of role performance. *Because the patient may not be aware that role functions differ from expected cultural or social norms, the nurse will need to focus on clarifying perceptions and fostering awareness of prevailing expectations.*
- Show respect for existing belief systems and values that support role expectations. Explore perceptions associated with observed role functions.
- Demonstrate role behaviors that patient needs to learn. *Added knowledge and skill can reduce role distance.*
- Make referral to appropriate reference group.

Expected Outcome: The patient will demonstrate resolution of role conflict as evidenced by reduced stress and frustration and by verbalization of a resolution of role conflicts.

- Assist the patient in exploring encountered role conflict and in identifying sources of stress. *The patient needs to recognize sources of stress to determine incompatibility or incongruities causing conflict.*
- Offer clarification and rectify misunderstandings.
- Assist the patient in reaching a compromise, if necessary. *Mutual efforts and compromise may allow for time to meet role-related activities and thus reduce frustrations arising from a felt conflict.*
- Offer supportive guidance for determining priorities. *Supportive guidance may help the patient recognize priorities in relation to felt ambitions or desired goals for role performance.*
- Suggest family or group meetings to clarify conflicting role expectations.
- Foster effective communication and problem-solving skills. *As the nurse facilitates open communication among all participants in role sets, they learn to solve problems and become prepared to prevent or resolve future role conflicts.*[17]

Expected Outcome: The patient will resolve role failure as evidenced by satisfactory role competence.

- Assess the patient's readiness to learn required role functions.
- Assist in identifying reasons for role failure. *The reasons for the patient's inability to meet role expectations must be explored and mutually acknowledged so that realistic learning goals can be developed.*
- Facilitate expression of disappointment about encountered failure.
- Assist the patient in recognizing strengths and abilities.
- Teach the patient knowledge and skills by using role modeling and role rehearsal. *This approach allows the patient to anticipate role behaviors and sentiments and try out behaviors that can correct previously identified inadequacies in imaginary role play without actual pressures or obligations for role performance.*
- Involve others in clarifying expectations and giving feedback.
- Offer praise for accomplishments.

EVALUATION

Evaluation of the resolution of Altered Role Performance is ongoing and requires participation by the patient and significant others. The nurse and the patient together assess which goals are met and which need modifications. In case of role transition, the patient relinquishes previous role behavior and shows role mastery, with expressed satisfaction in accomplishing role expectations. In case of role distance, the patient expresses awareness of role expectations and shows the ability to assume expected role functions. In case of role conflict, the patient identifies sources of conflict and engages him- or herself and others in problem-solving activities that set realistic priorities or find acceptable compromises for mutually satisfying role expectations. In case of role failure, the patient learns to perform role behaviors competently and expresses confidence and satisfaction about role attainment.

■ CASE STUDY WITH PLAN OF CARE

Mrs. Mary M. was looking forward to the birth of her second child; however, in her thirty-second week of gestation she went into premature labor and gave birth to a son who weighed 1.9 kg. The infant was transferred to the neonatal intensive care unit (NICU). The medical diagnosis was prematurity, with a good prognosis for normal development. Mary made infrequent visits to the NICU. The nurse observed that she did not want to touch the infant. She was tearful during some visits and did not initiate questions about the infant's care. She said, "He looks so tiny. How can I take care of him? He is so different from the way Susie was. I am afraid of him; he seems so fragile. He needs a lot of extra care and all these feedings!" Mary has a supportive husband and a 3-year-old daughter. Both are looking forward to having the baby at home. She considers herself a "good mother" for her daughter but has had no previous experience in caring for a premature infant. She was hoping to remain active in her career as a teacher by doing substitute teaching.

■ PLAN OF CARE FOR MRS. MARY M.

Nursing Diagnosis: Altered Role Performance (Inadequate Role Transition) Related to Stressful and Frustrating Role Changes Encountered in Mothering a Premature Infant

---

Expected Outcome: Mrs. M. will experience a less stressful role transition as evidenced by expressing grief and disappointment about the loss of the expected mothering role.
- Encourage regular visits to the NICU, and plan to stay with Mrs. M. during visits, making her feel welcome.
- Facilitate expression of sadness, and show acceptance of Mrs. M.'s disappointment.
- Assist Mrs. M. in comparing her previous full-term child with the premature infant to identify similarities and differences in role expectations.

Expected Outcome: Mrs. M. will engage in learning to care for her premature infant.
- Introduce Mrs. M. to the equipment surrounding her infant, and explain its function in assisting her infant to grow.
- Allow time to observe and model the caregiving, and simultaneously discuss and interpret the infant's behavioral cues.
- Encourage gradual engagement in care tasks (diapering, feeding, and comforting).
- Explain the special needs of the infant.
- Provide contact with other mothers who care for their infants in the NICU.
- Offer praise for accomplished care, and reflect on the infant's responses that indicate comfort and progressive growth.

Expected Outcome: Mary M. will demonstrate confidence and satisfaction in mastery of her mothering role for the infant before he is discharged.
- Encourage visits by both parents, and facilitate the husband's involvement and positive reinforcement of mothering skills.
- Provide opportunities to discuss concerns, and provide information on the infant's anticipated progress and development.
- Make referral to community nursing service for needed support or counseling after discharge.
- Assist Mrs. M. to verbalize satisfaction and confidence in her mothering role.

■ = nursing intervention; ▲ = collaborative intervention.

VIII

■■ CRITICAL THINKING EXERCISES

1. What is the rationale for working through feelings such as sadness and for exploring Mrs. M.'s perceptions of differences in role expectations in caring for her premature infant?

2. What are the important aspects of a teaching plan for Mrs. M., and why is this so important?

3. What discharge planning and information will need to be shared with the community nursing service to facilitate ongoing services?

REFERENCES

1. Burns C and others: New diagnosis: caregiver role strain, *Nurs Diagnosis* 4(2):70–76, 1993.

2. Caradoc-Davies TH and Dixon GS: Stress in caregivers of elderly patients: the effect of an admission to a rehabilitation unit, *NZ Med J* 104:226–228, 1991.

3. Evans RL and others: Post-stroke family function: an evaluation of the family's role in rehabilitation, *Rehab Nurs* 17(3): 127–132, 1992.

4. Hardy ME and Conway ME: *Role theory: perspectives for health professionals*, ed 2, Norwalk, Connecticut, 1988, Appleton & Lange.

5. Hernandez GG: Not-so-benign neglect: researchers ignore ethnicity in defining family caregiver burden and recommending services, *Gerontologist* 31(2):271–272, 1991 (letters).

6. Kim MJ, McFarland GK, and McLane AM: *Pocket guide to nursing diagnosis*, ed 6, St. Louis, 1995, Mosby–Year Book.

7. Krause N: Stressors in salient social roles and well-being in later life, *J Gerontol* 49(3):1237–1248, 1994.

8. Lancee WJ and others: The impact of pain and impaired role performance on distress in persons with cancer, *Can J Psychiatry* 39(10):617–622, 1994.

9. McFarland GK, Wasli EL, and Gerety EK: *Nursing diagnosis and process in psychiatric mental health nursing*, ed 2, Philadelphia, 1991, JB Lippincott Co.

10. Musolf JM: Easing the impact of the family caregiver's role, *Rehab Nurs* 16(2):82–84, 1991.

11. North American Nursing Diagnosis Association: *NANDA nursing diagnoses: definitions and classification, 1995–1996*, Philadelphia, 1994, The Association.

12. Nuwayhid KA: Role transition, disturbance, and conflict. In Roy SC and Andrews HA: *The Roy adaptation model, the definite statement*, Norwalk, Connecticut, 1991, Appleton & Lange.

13. Robertson SM: Self-concept disturbance. In McFarland GK and Thomas MD: *Psychiatric mental health nursing, application of the nursing process*, Philadelphia, 1991, JB Lippincott Co.

14. Roy SC and Andrews HA: *The Roy adaptation model, the definite statement*, Norwalk, Connecticut, 1991, Appleton & Lange.

15. Titler MG, Cohen MZ, and Craft MJ: Impact of adult care hospitalization: perceptions of patient, spouses, children, and nurses, *Heart Lung* 20(23):174–182, 1991.

16. Warda M: The family and chronic sorrow: role theory approach, *J Pediatr Nurs* 7(3):205–210, 1992.

17. Whitlatch MS, Zarit SH, and Eye A: Efficacy of interventions with caregivers: a reanalysis, *Gerontologist* 32(1):9–14, 1991.

VIII

Impaired Social Interaction

▶

Impaired Social Interaction *is the state in which an individual participates in an insufficient or excessive quantity or ineffective quality of social exchange.*[10]

OVERVIEW

People have an innate need for relationships. From the moment of birth, a person learns to relate with others. The ongoing learning process continues until death. Relating with others requires social skill and social sensitivity. Throughout life, a person learns to handle the needs of dependence and independence by maintaining interpersonal relationships. The ability to relate interdependently with others is one indicator of maturity.

Throughout life, people engage in social interactions, which allow them to know themselves more fully. If a person feels inadequate or unable to handle social interactions, the potential for loneliness, isolation, depression, and withdrawal increases. Nursing focuses on the ability of patients to enter in growth-producing relationships.

Effective social interaction occurs when the involved persons maintain a sense of self during mutual interaction. People related with each other for a variety of purposes. To understand how people maintain social interactions, three main areas must be studied: (1) positive self-concept, (2) accurate perception of reality, and (3) the need for interdependence.

A positive self-concept is essential to maintaining healthy social interactions. A person's self-concept incorporates all the beliefs and convictions that constitute self-knowledge and that influence interpersonal relationships.[11] The self-concept includes (1) self-awareness, (2) the validity of one's self-concept, (3) feelings about oneself, and (4) one's sense of identity.[5] Self-awareness is defined as a person's consciousness of his or her beliefs, ideals, and goals. The validity of one's self-concept is the capacity to see oneself realistically and, to the degree possible, objectively.[5] Feelings about oneself relate to one's self-acceptance, including personal strengths, limitations, and ability to evaluate realistically the potential for personal change and growth. One's sense of identity involves a positive self-regard and the capacity to know oneself and not doubt that inner identity. The self-concept develops from relationships with significant others throughout the life span, and it influences human behavior. One must therefore understand a person's situation through his or her frame of reference.

A person's perception of reality will also affect social interaction. The perception of reality is healthy when it corresponds to reality. This criterion for positive mental health includes (1) freedom from need distortion and (2) social sensitivity.[5] *Freedom from need distortion* is defined as a correct perception of one's reality. It is the ability of the person to assess reality, make assumptions, validate assumptions, and draw conclusions that enable him or her to take appropriate action. *Social sensitivity* means treating the inner life of another person with concern and attention. Social sensitivity implies that conclusions drawn about another person are free from need distortion. A person's ability to perceive is influenced by degrees of anxiety or threat. A perceived threat can heighten anxiety; chronic anxiety can narrow a person's ability to perceive and can heighten need distortion. The person acts to protect him- or herself, which in turn inhibits social interaction.

Social interaction is also influenced by the human need for interdependence in relationships. This is the capacity for people to give and to receive in relationships. Interdependence can be viewed as the point of balance between dependent and independent behavior. Inherent in the concept of independence is the human need for autonomy. Autonomy is the capacity to act for oneself. It is only when a person is clear about his or her own boundaries and separateness from the other that effective interdependent social interaction can occur. As a criterion for positive mental health, autonomy involves regulating behavior from within; that is, making decisions based on one's own internalized standards and values.[5]

In summary, persons with a positive self-concept can perceive reality better, free from need distortion, resulting in an increased ability to explain their world, inquire into the nature of their world, and take risks. Their interdependence with others enables them to learn and to gain satisfaction through their self-competence. Effective social interactions are influenced by a person's interdependence with others. One's self-concept and perception of reality affect social interactions. Through the nursing process, nurses frequently assist patients to correct, maintain, or enhance their social interactions.

ASSESSMENT

The defining characteristics of the nursing diagnosis Impaired Social Interaction include subjective and objective data. Subjective data include the patient's verbalizations of discomfort in social situations or verbalizations of an inability to receive or communicate a satisfying sense of belonging, caring, interest, or shared history.[6] The nurse also assess a patient for Impaired Social Interaction by listening for expressions of anxiety. How does the patient experience anxiety in social interactions?

Under what circumstances does this occur? How does the patient perceive him- or herself when relating with others? The nurse should ask the patient how time is spent each day and assess the patient's quality of relaxation time, close friendships, and his or her degree of comfort in meeting new people. Is the patient threatened by close interactions? What defenses are used? Is it possible that the patient never learned adequate communication and interpersonal skills to feel competent in social interactions? Perceived incompetency can cause patients to feel a threat to the self and heightened anxiety and to experience narrowed perceptions, leading to a preoccupation with self-protection. The nurse should observe whether the patient explores his or her world openly and freely. Anxiety can immobilize a patient's social interaction. A patient's interaction with the nurse reflects how he or she interacts in other social situations. The nurse must assess the nurse-patient interaction to understand the patient's situation more fully.

Subjective data revealing the patient's self-concept, perception of reality, and interdependence are key areas of assessment. To assess the self-concept, the nurse listens for the patient's expressions about him- or herself. What messages are heard? Are these messages ambivalent, negative, or positive? The nurse listens for themes and patterns of response that indicate the patient's self-views. Does the patient verbalize disappointment with him- or herself? Does the patient describe personal strengths and limitations? Patients with the diagnosis Impaired Social Interaction may share an underlying fear of rejection. For a variety of reasons, repeated rejections in social situations can be generalized to all interactions. Therefore the patient struggles with the ability to trust him- or herself and others. What are the patient's beliefs about him- or herself, and how do these influence interactions? Can the patient verbalize his or her beliefs, values, goals, strengths, and limitations? Can the patient begin to view him- or herself more objectively? What is the potential for a positive self-regard?

In assessing the patient's perception of reality, the nurse can consider the following questions: Is the patient's perception of reality accurate? Does the patient see options that are available? Are his or her perceptions free from need distortion? Does the patient use defenses that cause need distortion? When does this happen? Does it occur in interactions with the nurse? Does the patient demonstrate social sensitivity toward others? Are conclusions about others free from need distortion? Does anxiety interfere with the patient's ability to perceive accurately?

The nurse assesses interdependence by observing how a patient assumes responsibility for him- or herself in social interactions. A patient's sense of self may be so anxiety laden that it inhibits awareness of beliefs, values, and standards. When this occurs, social interactions can become impaired. The patient is unable to maintain a clear boundary between the self and the other. This inhibits the patient from viewing the other person as valued and separate and can promote excessive dependence. Because the sense of self is intertwined with anxiety and poor learning experiences, the patient doubts his or her sensitivity to others. The patient may fear self-exposure and avoid relationships. The assessment might include questions such as the following: Is the patient able to take responsibility for him- or herself in social situations? Can he or she make decisions and live by them? Is the patient able to respect his or her own rights and the rights of others? Can the patient give and receive in relationships? Can the patient make decisions according to his or her own internalized standards? What tolerance does the patient demonstrate in handling needs for togetherness and for individuality? Does the patient seem to borrow strength or a sense of self from others?

Assessment of objective data includes observing patient behavior, such as discomfort in social situations or an inability to communicate or use interpersonal skills effectively. Objective data may be obtained from observations of the patient in a clinical setting, reports by significant others, or the patient history. Assessment is important to establish patterns of patient limitations and strengths and to define deficits that inhibit the patient from healthy functioning. Assessment provides a valid basis for the nurse to establish interventions that will enable the patient to attain specific goals. Assessment also provides an opportunity for the nurse to share with the patient the behavior that has been observed so that both can understand the patient's perceived need. Assisting the patient to working with the nurse toward therapeutic goals is in itself a measure to correct Impaired Social Interaction.

Nurses frequently encounter patients in many settings who are struggling with social interactions. For example, a patient with an unexpected illness may have stress that causes him to relate negatively with others. An adolescent in school may face an adjustment problem that disrupts his or her ability to interact effectively. Because nurses function in many settings, they must recognize the potential for Impaired Social Interaction so they can intervene to prevent actual impairment and provide a corrective learning experience to struggling persons. Sensitivity to cultural and family factors is important in nursing assessment because cultural and family practices affect the beliefs, norms, and values the patient embraces.[7]

■ Defining Characteristics

The presence of the following defining characteristics[10] indicates that the patient may be experiencing Impaired Social Interaction:

- Verbalized or observed discomfort in social situations
- Verbalized or observed inability to receive or communicate a satisfying sense of belonging, caring, interest, or shared history
- Observed use of unsuccessful social interaction behavior
- Dysfunctional interaction with peers, family, or others
- Family report of change in style or pattern of interaction

- Presence of a pattern of mild, moderate, or severe anxiety in social interactions
- Presence of a pattern of dependent behavior in social interactions
- Presence of a pattern of superficiality in relationships

■ Related Factors

The following related factors[10] are associated with Impaired Social Interaction:

- Limited physical mobility
- Loss of body function
- Hearing or visual deficits
- Chronic illness
- Terminal illness
- Knowledge deficit about ways to enhance mutuality
- Communication barriers
- Therapeutic isolation
- Environmental barriers
- Self-concept disturbance
- Anxiety
- Altered thought process
- Absence of available significant others or peers
- Sociocultural dissonance
- Language or cultural barriers

DIAGNOSIS

■ Differential Nursing Diagnosis

Two nursing diagnoses closely related to Impaired Social Interaction are Social Isolation and Ineffective Individual Coping. Differential diagnosis among the three can be thought of in terms of the focus of each diagnosis. Social Isolation focuses on the aloneness experienced by a person, along with the perceived meaning of the experience. Impaired Social Interaction, on the other hand, focuses on the quality of social exchange. The person is able to carry on interaction, but in a limited way, or is struggling to enhance the quality of the relationship. A pattern of Impaired Social Interaction can lead to Social Isolation. The goal of nursing intervention is to address the need defined in the diagnosis and to prevent Social Isolation. The second related diagnosis is Ineffective Individual Coping. The focus of this diagnosis is the adaptive behavior demonstrated by an individual in meeting the demands of life. This diagnosis addresses the overall pattern of coping that defines how a person functions over time. Impaired Social Interaction can be a result of or can lead to Ineffective Individual Coping. The focus of Impaired Social Interaction is specific in terms of the quality of the interaction and the relationship. Goals and plans to assist a person to learn about and experience relationships based on trust and mutuality promote growth and a sense of identity. This positive health outcome contributes to individual coping. The distinction among the three diagnoses is important in addressing assessed needs and desired health outcomes.

■ Medical and Psychiatric Diagnoses

Three psychiatric diagnoses commonly related to the diagnosis Impaired Social Interaction are adjustment disorder, mood disorders, and schizophrenia.[1] These diagnoses represent a sampling of disorders among the mental health–mental illness continuum from least to most severe. The interdisciplinary and collaborative approach to the treatment of mental disorders is a model of practice that is time tested and effective in the mental health field. The nursing diagnosis is an important component of an interdisciplinary treatment plan. Adjustment disorder is a short-term, maladaptive reaction to an identifiable stressor. Stressors may come from multiple sources related to situational and developmental crises. The potential for Impaired Social Interaction is possible. Health outcomes related to this nursing diagnosis can occur through therapeutic relationships that support a person's strengths as the patient learns new ways of coping and sustaining relationships.[2]

Mood disorders range along a continuum from mania to depression. These disorders affect social interactions because of the inappropriate judgments made while a person is in a manic state or because of the detrimental effects of a depressed state. Symptoms of major depression include depressed, sad, and hopeless feelings, along with a loss of interest and pleasure in activities and relationships. Negative self-evaluations and feelings of worthlessness can precipitate suicidal attempts. Depression can be treated effectively. It is frequently found in patients who receive health care in primary care settings.[8] Effective screening and early diagnosis facilitate treatment and health outcomes associated with the diagnosis Impaired Social Interaction. Schizophrenia, the most severe of the disorders discussed, involves characteristic psychiatric symptoms, such as delusions, hallucinations, and disturbances of affect, thought, and perception. A person diagnosed with schizophrenia often experiences impaired work and role functioning, including impaired interpersonal functioning. Efforts to reduce the negative symptoms of schizophrenia are often targeted in social skill training programs, which aim to increase social competence and the patient's overall quality of life.[3,9] The nursing diagnosis Impaired Social Interaction is particularly relevant to the diagnosis of schizophrenia.

OUTCOME IDENTIFICATION, PLANNING, AND IMPLEMENTATION

Nursing interventions for patients with Impaired Social Interaction address three key areas: (1) developing a positive self-concept, (2) building social skills, and (3) establishing mutual relationships.

A five-level approach to facilitate growth toward a positive self-concept includes (1) self-awareness, (2) self-exploration, (3) self-evaluation, (4) realistic planning, and (5) a commitment to action.[11] This approach requires time to meet with the patient on a regular basis. This can be accomplished through short-term intervention on an outpatient or home care basis. Assisting a patient to become self-aware and to explore how self-perception influences social interaction can cause anxiety. The nurse must plan interventions that assist the patient to work through feelings and beliefs about him- or herself to develop a positive self-concept. The nursing interventions must also

focus on assisting the patient to determine the significance of experiences, to clarify perceptions of him- or herself and others, and to explore personal strengths and limitations. The nurse must support patient strengths while assisting the patient with behavioral limitations. As the patient becomes increasingly objective in viewing him- or herself, goals, options, and planned change can be explored and used as a basis of action. The nurse supports the patient's decision-making and goal-planning actions toward growth.

Deficits in social skills are revealed as the nurse assesses patient strengths and limitations; the patterns of behavior inhibiting the patient in social situations are established. After these deficits are identified, the nurse can assist the patient in recognizing and dealing with them. It is possible for new social skills to be learned and integrated into patterns of behavior. Realistic goals for the patient guide the nurse's actions. Ideally the patient is involved in the goal-setting process. The nurse and the patient develop a plan in which social skills can be taught. Within the nurse-patient relationship, social skills can be practiced. The nurse observes the patient's use of social skills and assists in considering other approaches to the interaction. Problem situations can also be role-played with the nurse for problem solving, discussion, and practice. It is often beneficial for the nurse and the patient to reverse their roles to help the patient learn new ways of interacting. Supportive feedback and encouragement helps the patient gain confidence and a sense of independence. What the patient learns in role-playing can be applied to other social situations.

Establishing a mutual working relationship with the nurse is one method for the patient to develop and learn how to maintain a new sense of self. The nurse does not assume responsibility for the patient; rather, the patient is viewed as a person of worth capable of self-care and self-direction. The patient is invited and encouraged to enter a mutual relationship with the nurse. The patient is supported to use the strengths that subsequently develop in other relationships. Interventions that promote mutuality in the therapeutic relationship include

VIII

assisting the patient to observe patterns of behavior (dependent, independent, and interdependent) in relationships, to describe and discuss feelings associated with the dynamics of identified behaviors, to choose to alter existing behaviors positively, to make decisions, and to accept responsibility.[4]

Ideally the nurse seeks supervision to assess the nurse's own position in the therapeutic relationship. The nurse's consistent goal is to assist the patient to act for him- or herself while maintaining effective social relationships.

◢ NURSING CARE GUIDELINES
Nursing Diagnosis: Impaired Social Interaction

Expected Outcome: The patient will attend outpatient sessions with the nurse two times a month for the purpose of exploring ways to develop a positive sense of self.
- Encourage the patient to express feelings associated with perceived self-limitations.
- Assist patient to explore strengths and limitations.
- Identify nonverbal and verbal expression of feelings of which the patient is not aware; support strengths and the ability to act for him- or herself. *Beliefs about oneself and associated feelings can be explained and altered to promote adaptive change and growth.*
- Encourage involvement in goal setting and verbalization by the patient of his or her responsibility for working toward goals; focus on "here-and-now" circumstances of the patient's situations; have reasonable expectations for progress. *Consistent, supportive feedback from the nurse assists the patient to feel less anxious and more trusting.*

Expected Outcome: The patient will engage in role-playing by the fourth outpatient session to test new interaction behaviors and will demonstrate self-confidence by using new social skills in other relationships by the eighth outpatient session.
- Promote use of new interaction skills with nurse during outpatient sessions.
- ▲ Assess the patient's patterns of behavior and communication themes that indicate the patient's readiness to change; seek mutual understanding with the patient about deficits in social skills; create a teaching plan with the patient for social skill development. *The patient's growth potential increases with the development of social skills.*
- ▲ Role-play social interactions with the patient to promote and reinforce skill development. Include other nurses or outpatients in the role-play. *Role-playing provides an experiential learning situation through which the patient gains understanding of his or her situation. Self-confidence and competence develop over time, based on the support and feedback gained from others in a role-playing learning situation.*
- Support the patient's growth, and encourage the use of skills in other social interactions. Have patient keep a journal of occasions when new skills were used.

Expected Outcome: The patient will develop a mutual working relationship with the nurse and will demonstrate understanding of how patterns of behavior facilitate or inhibit social interactions by the end of the outpatient sessions.
- View the patient as an adult capable of self-determination and self-responsibility.
- Support the patient's decision-making ability, and identify alternatives and options not considered by the patient.
- Express the beliefs and hope that the patient is capable of change, and assist the patient to understand the dynamics of dependent, independent, and interdependent behaviors in relationships. *Understanding a patient's strengths as well as limitations assists the nurse in supporting the patient's actions that build strength while addressing patterns of limitation. The nurse's response must consistently convey respectful feedback and a belief in the patient's capacity for self-determination.*

■ = nursing intervention; ▲ = collaborative intervention.

EVALUATION

Evaluation is ongoing throughout the therapeutic process. It is a process shared by the nurse and the patient. Ideally the patient participates in the goal-setting process and can therefore help evaluate outcomes. In the evaluation process, the nurse and the patient refer to goals and expected outcomes established earlier. Patient progress is discussed and goals are revised based on the mutual agreement of nurse and patient. Evaluation sessions are held regularly.

Specific outcomes can be evaluated by observing patterns of patient behavior and by patient self-reports. The patient develops a capacity to monitor anxiety and to take actions to promote effective social interaction. Interpersonal relationships are developed based on trust and mutuality. The patient's sense of self strengthens and permits satisfying and enjoyable relationships. Self-awareness promotes a realistic appreciation of one's strengths and limitations, one's capacity to define goals and to make decisions, and sufficient objectivity to evaluate one's behavior in social interactions. The patient is better able to enter into relationships with others through an increase in self-confidence and sense of autonomy.

If outcomes are not achieved, the nurse must reassess the patient situation to determine what is inhibiting progress. Often supervision of the nurse by a colleague or a clinical nurse specialist is sufficient to reassess and analyze the clinical situation and to determine appropriate nursing interventions that are congruent with the patient's needs. Interdisciplinary planning conferences contribute toward the development of a working nursing care plan.

◼ CASE STUDY WITH PLAN OF CARE

Ms. Wendy T. is a 23-year-old single woman, who arrived at a community mental health center stating she was distracted and unable to concentrate and was having difficulty making decisions. Ms. T. described herself as "alone and lonely." She stated that she was unable to make friends and that she felt a lack of confidence in her ability to maintain relationships. She said, "When I meet people, I feel uncomfortable and awkward. I am unable to talk to other people. I feel inadequate, so I try to leave." In her work situation, Ms. T. reported that she was having difficulty making decisions. She recently passed up a job promotion because "I could not decide what to do." Ms. T. described herself as quiet and shy since childhood. She lived with her family and only recently moved away from her family home for employment in the city. She stated that she did not feel prepared for life away from her family. She believed her loneliness interfered with her ability to make decisions. Ms. T. appeared shy and nonassertive in the initial interview and did not present herself with a sense of self-confidence. Her social discomfort was evident, as were her negative messages about herself. She requested assistance with her problem.

VIII

◼ PLAN OF CARE FOR MS. WENDY T.
Nursing Diagnosis: Impaired Social Interaction Related to Negative Self-Feelings and Perceived Incompetence in Relationships

---

Expected Outcome: Ms. T. will meet regularly with the nurse in a therapeutic one-to-one relationship.
- Establish a contract providing guidelines for one-to-one sessions, including the time, frequency, and place for sessions.
- Build a trusting relationship by communicating with Ms. T. that she is a person of worth and capable of growth and change.
- Construct a family tree to assess and understand Ms. T.'s position in her family relationships and the associated emotional responses to such relationships.
- Assess and appreciate family and cultural background, mores, norms, and values.

◼ = nursing intervention; ▲ = collaborative intervention.

Continued

■ **PLAN OF CARE FOR MS. WENDY T. — CONT'D**

Expected Outcome: Ms. T. will develop self-understanding by describing her perceptions of social interactions, including her feelings, behaviors, and thoughts.
- Use an empathic approach to help Ms. T. identify her feelings. Observe and comment on verbal and nonverbal expressions of behavior in a supportive and respectful manner.
- Encourage Ms. T. to identify her feelings as they occur in discussion with the nurse, to accept and understand her feelings, and to talk her feelings through with the nurse.
- In a supportive manner, point out ways that she avoids expression of her feelings.
- State hunches and conclusions about what Ms. T. is experiencing. Ask Ms. T. for feedback about this analysis.

Expected Outcome: Ms. T. will explore meaning of behavior and assess self-strengths, self-limitations, and deficits in social interactions.
- Assess Ms. T.'s strengths, limitations, and patterns of behavior. Listen for behavioral themes expressed.
- Support strengths. As Ms. T. demonstrates readiness, share perceptions of her behavior with her, and respond with empathy.
- Assist Ms. T. in understanding the meaning of her behavior. Share knowledge and experiences to enhance her understanding.

Expected Outcome: Ms. T. will evaluate how to develop effective social skills and how to set realistic goals to achieve desired change in behavior.
- Encourage goal setting in realistic and achievable steps.
- Support self-evaluation by affirming realistic goal setting or by kind confrontation of erroneous thinking.

Expected Outcome: Ms. T. will develop a realistic plan to achieve goals and will demonstrate willingness to take action.
- Support self-care activity, and assist Ms. T. in evaluating changes in behavior that will promote effective relationships with others. Stress that Ms. T. has a mutual relationship with the nurse.
- Devise plan to teach social interaction skills, and role-play in practice sessions.
- Encourage use of effective social skills in other relationships. Refer to young adult groups; support Ms. T.'s efforts to build social networks.

VIII

■■ **CRITICAL THINKING EXERCISES**

1. The therapeutic nurse-patient relationship is unique and offers a patient a corrective learning experience that can enhance behavioral functioning. What components in the therapeutic relationship with Ms. T. foster a corrective learning experience for her?

2. How important is it to assess patient strengths while providing nursing interventions for identified patient health deficits? How are Ms. T.'s strengths factored into the nursing assessment, expected outcomes, and interventions?

3. How do the concepts of mutuality and interdependence relate to the therapeutic nurse-patient relationship? Think of a patient with whom you are currently providing nursing care. Consider writing nursing outcomes that mutually include the patient as a partner in achieving health outcomes.

REFERENCES

1. American Psychiatric Association: *Diagnostic and statistical manual of mental disorders,* ed 4, Washington, D.C., 1994, The Association.
2. Burns DP: Focusing on ego strengths, *Arch Psychiatr Nurs* 5:202–208, 1991.
3. Dobson DJG and others: Effects of social skill training and social milieu treatment on symptoms of schizophrenia, *Psychiatr Serv* 46:376–380, 1995.

4. Forchuk C: Uniqueness within the nurse-client relationship, *Arch Psychiatr Nurs* 1:34–39, 1995.

5. Jahoda M: *Current concepts of positive mental health,* New York, 1958, Basic Books.

6. Kim MJ, McFarland GK, and McLane AM: *Pocket guide to nursing diagnoses,* ed 6, St. Louis, 1995, Mosby–Year Book.

7. Leininger M: Leininger's theory of nursing: cultural care, diversity, and universality, *Nurs Sci Quart* 4:152–160, 1988.

8. Montano CB: Recognition and treatment of depression in a primary care setting, *J Clin Psychiatry* 55(12):18–34, 1994.

9. Murray R and others: Components of an effective transitional residential program for homeless mentally ill clients, *Arch Psychiatr Nurs* 9:152–157, 1995.

10. North American Nursing Diagnosis Association: *NANDA nursing diagnoses: definitions and classification, 1995–1996,* Philadelphia, 1994, The Association.

11. Stuart GW and Sundeen SD: *Principles and practice of psychiatric nursing,* ed 5, St. Louis, 1995, Mosby–Year Book.

VIII

Social Isolation

▶

Social Isolation *is aloneness experienced by an individual that is imposed by others and that the individual views as a negative or threatening state.*[7]

OVERVIEW

Lack of contact with other people results in Social Isolation. Although individuals diagnosed by the nurse as socially isolated believe that their involvement with other people is limited by factors outside of their own control, in fact, many times they consciously or unconsciously isolate themselves. It is important for the nurse to determine the etiology of the isolation. Determination of the causes of the aloneness and the perception that the isolation makes the individual vulnerable to untoward consequences will dictate nursing interventions.

A person who experiences Social Isolation is often unable to make contact with others, although he or she may need or desire it. Psychological, physiological, or sociocultural factors can cause this isolation.[9] Isolation is subjective and may or may not be based in reality, but it exists whenever the person says it does and perceives it as imposed by others.[5] Because Social Isolation is subjective, the diagnosis must be validated by the individual. In other words, the nurse might suspect isolation, but until the individual acknowledges it, the diagnosis cannot be confirmed.

Social Isolation inherently includes aloneness, loneliness, deprivation, and unhappiness. It may involve the loss of social roles, social support, and environmental contact that the individual considers valuable, stimulating, and fulfilling.

Many factors may precipitate actual or perceived Social Isolation. One of the most common causes of Social Isolation is loss. The loss may be obvious, such as the death of a family member or a friend, or it may be more subjective, such as a move from familiar surroundings or the loss of functional abilities. Loss may also be perceptual—the person feels or thinks that he or she has limited chances for social interaction. An example of this is a depressed patient who says, "Old friends don't include me anymore," when in fact the friends are acting the same, but the individual perceives them as withdrawn. Loss, perceived or real, may trigger Social Isolation. Other factors that influence aloneness may have a physical or emotional basis. For instance, people who experience a loss of hearing may avoid others because communication is difficult and, many times, unrewarding; or people who are psychiatrically impaired, such as some schizophrenic patients, may view contact with others as dangerous or threatening. Environmental factors may also cause Social Isolation. Some examples of environmental origins are imprisonment or hospitalization in an isolation unit for communicable diseases.

One theory about the underlying causes of Social Isolation has been proposed by Gofman.[4] Gofman suggests that certain people or groups of people are stigmatized by society because of discernible defects that cause anxiety in the majority of the population. He speculates that individuals who are perceived as "different" are rejected, thus becoming socially isolated. Examples of this are a person who is crippled and must wear braces or a person with an indwelling tracheal tube that causes him or her to hiss when talking. People often withdraw from these individuals because they do not know how to respond; therefore the afflicted person becomes socially isolated. Stigmatization also occurs when a person has a dreaded disease, which causes discomfort in the community because of the population's perceptions about the communicability of the disease. Thus the diseased person is ostracized. A specific example of this is a patient with tuberculosis or acquired immunodeficiency syndrome (AIDS).

Other psychosocial causes of isolation are alienation, low self-esteem, and generalized coping difficulties. Alienation and low self-esteem are so interwoven that it is almost impossible to discern which is the cause and which the effect. However, both cause Social Isolation when a person feels that he or she does not belong because he or she is "unworthy" and "apart." These people feel shunned and see themselves as "outsiders." Therefore, because they feel and become alienated, other people treat them that way. For instance, this can occur when immigrants have language problems and are without support systems. Feelings of alienation may relate to ineffective efforts to gain attention or support.[6] An example of this are people who persist in addressing problems with methods that don't work, such as trying to get family members to visit by elaborating on minor physical problems and insisting that these problems are major, even though the son or daughter has told the parent that aches and pains are "normal."

Patients with personality disorders or chronic mental impairments are at greater risk for Social Isolation than those without such illnesses. Patterns of Social Isolation may also be predictive of mental disorders and suicide.

Family mobility may be a precursor to Social Isolation. For example, when an elderly couple moves to a warmer climate and finds the social climate cool and unresponsive, they may feel that they do not fit in and may tend to blame others. Consequently, they may not reach out to others, thereby suffering further isolation. Social Isolation is a major concern for elders and may be a precursor to loneliness.[3]

Families other than the elderly may also move. Although some of the family members may not become socially isolated, others will. For instance, the father may have new work associates, and the children may make new friends at school. But the mother who stays at home with preschool children in a neighborhood where all the other women work may experience unhappiness because she perceives her social world as very limited. The mother might need much more support from the family members than they need from her; this can result in her family resenting her clinging to them. The mother might then feel rejection and develop tension headaches. In addition to physical symptoms, Social Isolation may also result in low self-concept, disruption of one's support network, alterations in family process, or deterioration of social skills.

Changing community standards of involvement, which encourage people to be suspicious of others and "not to get involved" further promote Social Isolation. Community standards influence social interaction just as social interaction may influence community standards.[1]

ASSESSMENT

Assessment and diagnosis of Social Isolation depend on objective and subjective data. Feelings of loneliness and isolation need to be validated with the patient. Careful assessment of the social history is indicated when barriers or limitations are identified that inhibit relationships with others. Physiological, psychological, and sociocultural factors may influence the person's ability to develop and maintain relationships with others.

Subjective assessment of Social Isolation would include expressions of feelings of loneliness, the desire for more human contact, a loss of significant others, barriers to social contact, changes in living arrangements, and the adequacy of support systems.[2] Objective assessment may focus on physical limitations, disabilities, and environmental issues. Because individuals vary in their responses to isolation and aloneness, definitive objective indicators to this diagnosis are difficult to identify; therefore subjective patient responses are critical in making this diagnosis.[8]

The nurse must listen carefully to subjective cues. Does that patient feel lonely? Has the patient recently moved? Is there a lack of knowledge about available resources? Is there a sensory impairment?

When does the patient feel the most alone? Do physical barriers prevent the person from participating in desired activities? Does the patient feel rejected? What kind of relationships are desired?

Assessment of objective data includes observations of the patient who experiences difficulties in seeking help, initiating conversations, or responding to others. Self-report questionnaires may provide data about the patient's perception of his or her social skills; a social skills checklist may help identify behavioral patterns. Other data that might lead to consideration of a diagnosis of Social Isolation include physiological parameters such as changes in eating or sleeping habits.

Social Isolation may occur across the life span, with a rapid or an insidious onset. A young child who has been severely disfigured as a result of a burn injury may experience isolation almost overnight. An elderly male may experience isolation more gradually as his health weakens and his social network of family and friends diminishes. Social Isolation may be experienced in a variety of settings for a variety of reasons. Therefore the nurse must be aware of vulnerable populations at risk for Social Isolation, including the elderly, the physically compromised, the psychologically impaired, and those experiencing relocation stress or cultural shock.

It is well documented that social support provided through social networks influences health and well-being.[9] Social networks, such as families, friends, social groups, and communities, can facilitate or inhibit efforts for health protection and promotion. The nurse is able to assist people in assessing the strengths and limitations of the existing social support systems and subsequently aid them in modifying or developing a social support system. Supportive social networks can help decrease feelings of isolation.

■ Defining Characteristics

The presence of the following defining characteristics indicates that the patient may be experiencing Social Isolation:

- Evidence of physical or mental handicap or altered state of wellness

- Inappropriate or immature interests and activities for developmental stage and age
- Exhibits unacceptable behavior
- Sad or dull affect
- Hostility in behavior and voice
- Expresses feelings of aloneness imposed by others
- Expressions of inadequacy or lack of purpose in life
- Absence of supportive significant others (e.g., family, friends, or social group)
- Withdrawal and inability or refusal to communicate
- No eye contact
- Seeks to be alone
- Verbalization of feelings of aloneness and rejection imposed by others
- Expressions of being "different" and unable to meet expectations of others
- Insecure in social situations

■ Related Factors

The following related factors are associated with Social Isolation:

- Alteration in health
- Sensory deficits
- Impaired mobility
- Delay in accomplishing developmental tasks
- Alteration in physical appearance
- Body image disturbance
- Inadequate or loss of personal resources
- Chemical dependence
- Immature interests
- Alteration in mental status
- Unacceptable social behavior
- Impaired communication
- Inability to engage in satisfying personal relationships
- Divorce
- Homosexuality
- Poverty

DIAGNOSIS

■ Differential Nursing Diagnosis

There are three nursing diagnoses that are closely related to, and may be difficult to discriminate from, Social Isolation. These diagnoses are Impaired Social Interaction, Ineffective Individual Coping, and Risk for Loneliness. Like Social Isolation, a decrease in interactions or difficulty in relationships and societal participation may be characteristic of these diagnoses. These diagnoses may mimic Social Isolation, and, in fact, may be secondary to Social Isolation. The crucial differentiating factor is that Social Isolation is perceived as imposed by other and is not seen as originating in oneself.

■ Medical and Psychiatric Diagnoses

The category of psychiatric diagnosis that may appear to confound the diagnosis of Social Isolation would be thinking disorders that have paranoid ideation, such as paranoia or paranoid schizophrenia. Generally, in both of these conditions other psychopathology, such as delusions of persecution or ideas of reference, will allow the nurse to discern the difference.

OUTCOME IDENTIFICATION, PLANNING, AND IMPLEMENTATION

Outcomes for the socially isolated person are generally directed toward assisting the patient in identifying the causative factors of the isolation, decreasing or limiting the barriers to social contact, promoting social interaction and self-worth, improving meaningful relationships, and using community resources to limit isolation.

In planning care for those who are socially isolated, the nurse implements similar interventions and outcomes regardless of the cause of the Social Isolation. The focus is on helping the individual identify the reasons for the isolation and ways to alleviate it. This may include assisting the patient in identifying available social networks or in developing the skills needed to maintain relationships. For instance, these skills may include improving communication or meeting new people. The goal is to have increased opportunities for and to achieve success in interpersonal involvements. It is necessary to explore the causes of Social Isolation directly and openly. The nurse must convey an accepting attitude that will increase the individual's sense of self-worth. The nurse should assist in identifying acceptable social behaviors; positive reinforcement of these behaviors can enhance self-esteem and encourage repetition of those behaviors.

For some individuals, enhancement of social skills may be helpful. Others may feel embarrassed about their appearance and therefore anxious about social situations. A social skills training program would help improve social skills and decrease anxiety in social situations. Instruction and modeling of such skills can be helpful in achieving behavioral changes.

Research indicates that a variety of interventions are effective in decreasing Social Isolation in elders, including behavior modification techniques, mutual aid groups, therapeutic groups, and multipurpose senior centers. Nursing interventions that promote confidence and sharing will decrease loneliness and isolation.

In planning care, the nurse and the patient must consider the factors contributing to the isolation as well as discrepancies between the individual's perceptions and reality. The patient diagnosed with Social Isolation may lack objectivity, self-confidence, and self-worth. Nursing interventions that focus on providing a supportive and consistent environment help people gain confidence.[9] Open communication with honest feedback is an important strategy. Exploration of perceptions may assist the patient in gaining an understanding about his or her feelings and responses in social situations. Strengths and weaknesses should be identified; progress toward goals should be noted and encouraged. Involving patients in setting goals and planning care increases their sense of control and decreases isolation.

Encouraging participation in appropriate diversional activities will enhance the patient's interaction with others. The type of activity and frequency of participation will depend on the patient's health status and interests. Involvement with others is the first step in developing meaningful relationships. Realistic goals need to be planned with the patient, recognizing that success may not be achieved immediately.

VIII

A knowledge of community resources is essential for socially isolated individuals who experience physical barriers to social contact.[3] Although the socially isolated patient should be supported to maintain his or her independence, assistance is sometimes warranted. Assessment of the patient's present social network may indicate the need for more support in a particular area. For example, assistance may be needed with grocery shopping, transportation to medical appointments, or help with child care. Enhancing the patient's social network may limit feelings of isolation and helplessness and increase feelings of confidence and independence. The encouragement of self-care activities and the promotion of functional independence fosters independent actions and decreases helplessness and isolation.

◢ NURSING CARE GUIDELINES
Nursing Diagnosis: Social Isolation

Expected Outcome: The patient will acknowledge Social Isolation and identify its causes by the end of the first visit.
- Engage in active listening.
- Ask the patient about his or her perception of being socially isolated.
- Restate the patient's perceptions about the reason(s) he or she is socially isolated.
- Assist the patient in validating the causes of the Social Isolation he or she is experiencing.
  Exploration of the patient's perceptions assists him or her in understanding feelings about and responses to social situations.

Expected Outcome: The patient will verbalize a willingness to seek to end his or her Social Isolation.
- Assess the patient's motivation to alleviate Social Isolation.
- Assist the patient in making correlations between personal behavior and alleviation of Social Isolation.
- Discuss with the patient barriers to becoming socially active and the means to overcome these barriers.
  The patient's willingness to end feelings of Social Isolation is critical to making successful attempts to establish social relationships.

Expected Outcome: The patient will formulate a plan to become more involved with others by the second visit.
- Discuss with the patient possible opportunities to reach out to others.
- Support the patient's identification of short-term goals.
- Promote a realistic course of action.
- Encourage some risk taking.
- ▲ Suggest possible resources and actions.
- Encourage the patient to develop a realistic time frame for the achievement of long- and short-term goals.
- Support the patient's progress by giving positive feedback.
  Involving patients in setting goals increases their sense of control and decreases isolation.

Expected Outcome: The patient will become involved in activities with others by the end of the third visit.
- Give positive reinforcement for attempts patient makes to become more socially involved with others.
- Assist the patient to examine those behaviors that have contributed to success and those that have hindered success.
- Encourage the patient to continue involvement in social activities.
- Discuss with the patient ways to avoid relapse into Social Isolation.
  Reinforcement of positive behavior promotes independence and decreases feelings of helplessness.

■ = nursing intervention; ▲ = collaborative intervention.

EVALUATION

For the nursing diagnosis Social Isolation, expected outcomes are achieved when the individual can (1) identify causes and contributing factors of the isolation, (2) employ strategies for increasing meaningful relationships, (3) reduce barriers to social contact, (4) participate in selected social activities, (5) express increased confidence in social skills, (6) express increased self-worth, and (7) identify community resources that will assist in decreasing feelings of isolation. If the outcomes are not achieved, reevaluation and modification of goals and interventions may be indicated. Alternative strategies should be implemented if defining characteristics continue to be present. Referrals to other health care team members and community agencies may be indicated. Follow-up care is necessary for continued support of the individual and accomplishment of the desired outcomes.

▪ CASE STUDY WITH PLAN OF CARE

Mr. Justin Y., a 60-year-old man, lives alone in an apartment complex for senior citizens. Although Mr. Y. is functionally independent and capable of performing activities of daily living, he has gradually withdrawn from activities outside of his home. Before the death of his wife a year ago, Mr. Y. was actively involved in many of the daily apartment complex activities, enjoyed a large circle of friends, and frequently volunteered to help other residents in the building when the need arose. During the past year, however, Mr. Y. has discontinued all volunteer activities, no longer eats in the main dining room with other residents, and has very limited contact with friends. A community health nurse who is also the health consultant to the apartment complex made a home visit to Mr. Y. after a request from the apartment house manager. Mr. Y. was receptive to the home visit and eager to talk with the nurse.

During the assessment, Mr. Y. explained that since the death of his wife he had lost all interest in outside activities. He no longer enjoyed being with other residents because he felt as if he were a burden to them. He stated that his vision was getting poor and that his arthritis was getting painful and slowed him down. He felt that he was no longer able to help his friends and that he was probably a disappointment to them. Assessment data revealed that Mr. Y. had neglected to keep his medical appointments during the past year, had been taking his prescribed daily medications sporadically, and had poor nutritional intake for the past several months. It was determined that Mr. Y. was unable to engage in satisfying personal relationships secondary to the loss of his wife and his physical condition.

▪ PLAN OF CARE FOR MR. JUSTIN Y.
Nursing Diagnosis: Social Isolation Related to Inability to Engage in Satisfying Personal Relationships

---

Expected Outcome: Mr. Y. will develop satisfying social relationships as evidenced by (1) identification of his own behaviors that limit social activity, (2) identifying social activities in which he would be willing to participate, and (3) gradually increasing activities requiring social interaction.

- Encourage Mr. Y. to express his feelings about his Social Isolation.
- Assist Mr. Y. to examine the relationship between his feelings and his present lack of contact with others.
- Identify with Mr. Y. those things he can change and those things outside of his power to change.
- Stress the importance of maintaining health-related activities, such as adequate nutritional intake, keeping medical appointments, and taking medications as prescribed.
- Assist Mr. Y. in identifying opportunities for interaction and in setting goals for himself.

▪ = nursing intervention; ▲ = collaborative intervention.

Continued

▶ PLAN OF CARE FOR MR. JUSTIN Y. — CONT'D

- Encourage Mr. Y. to set up a weekly plan to eat in the residents' dining hall five times, take part in at least two group activities, initiate visits to two friends in the building, and to accept friend's offers to transport him to medical appointments.
- Encourage Mr. Y. to keep a record of his social interactions.
- Provide Mr. Y. with positive reinforcement.
- Assist Mr. Y. with referrals if needed, including those in the complex where he lives and others in the community.
- Allow Mr. Y. to progress at his own rate; review Mr. Y.'s progress and revise goals as needed.

■ CRITICAL THINKING EXERCISES

1. In what ways might Mr. Y.'s physical limitations influence his Social Isolation?
2. If the nurse visiting Mr. Y. found herself becoming impatient with Mr. Y.'s lack of progress, what should the nurse do?
3. How might the nurse respond if Mr. Y. said, "It seems I have two options to make my existence better. Either I can drink whiskey all day, or I can consider suicide"?

REFERENCES

1. Bandura A: *Social learning theory,* Englewood Cliffs, New Jersey, 1977, Prentice-Hall.
2. Bennett R, editor: *Aging, isolation, and resocialization,* New York, 1980, Van Nostrand Reinhold.
3. Clark MH: *Nursing in the community,* Norwalk, Connecticut, 1995, Appleton & Lange.
4. Gofman E: *Stigma,* Englewood Cliffs, New Jersey, 1963, Prentice-Hall.
5. Krause N.: Negative interaction and satisfaction with social support among other adults, *J Gerontol* 50B:59–73, 1995.
6. Moneyham L and Scott C: Anticipatory coping in the elderly, *J Geront Nurse* 21(7):23–27, 1995.
7. North American Nursing Diagnosis Association: *NANDA nursing diagnoses: definitions and classification,* 1995–1996, Philadelphia, 1994, The Association.
8. Pender NJ: *Health promotion in nursing practice,* ed 3, Norwalk, Connecticut, 1996, Appleton & Lange.
9. Sutherland D and Murphy E: Social support among elderly in two community programs, *J Geront Nurse* 21(2):31–34, 1995.

Risk for Violence: Self-Directed or Directed at Others

Risk for Violence: Self-Directed or Directed at Others *is a state in which an individual experiences aggressive behaviors that can be physically or verbally harmful to oneself, to others, or to an object.*[18]

OVERVIEW

Violence exists within a complex sociocultural matrix. Society determines what it does or does not consider to be an appropriate aggressive or violent response to a perceived threat. Therefore society accepts the use of some aggressive or violent behaviors, such as a soldier killing the enemy. However, society proscribes the same type of behavior in other situations (e.g., killing a civilian). The sanctions for the proscribed behavior may be violent also, but they are accepted by the society as necessary restraints against forms of violence that threaten the community. Thus society recognizes that appropriate levels of aggression and violence are needed or humankind would have difficulty surviving: such behavior enables an individual or group to defend against a perceived threat.

Currently our culture is experiencing what has been termed an "epidemic of violence."[24] This perception led the Centers for Disease Control and Prevention to place a top priority on violence prevention. So violence is now perceived as a public health issue because of its high mortality rate for young people, its staggering financial cost to society, and its ability to be prevented.[24] This epidemic affects the health care community directly, requiring an assessment of the Risk for Violence by the nurse.

If the individual enters the health care system as a result of inappropriate aggressive or violent responses, other health care problems usually exist and compound the Risk for Violence. Without an assessment of the Risk for Violence, appropriate interventions to mitigate the deleterious outcomes of violent behavior will not be instituted.

Although no comprehensive theory explains violence, research and applicable analyses have identified certain conditions that, if present, indicate a higher probability for violence. First, young males are more prone to violence than any other maturational group. Other risk groups include those who have a recent history for violence or involvement in the legal system, those who have recently been laid off,[2] women with abusive or violent partners,[9] and those with a condition of a schizoaffective disorder, psychosis, paranoid symptoms, or substance abuse.[11,13,16,18]

ASSESSMENT

Violent behavior exists sporadically and usually for brief periods of time. A patient entering the health care system needs at least a cursory assessment of Risk for Violence. The initial assessment can be quickly accomplished by determining whether any of the following risk factors are present. First, any young male is more prone to violence than any other maturational group. Additional information for an initial assessment can include fairly straightforward questions asked by the nurse. For example, questions related to whether the patient has recently harmed him- or herself or others or damaged property provides a recent historical propensity for engaging in violent behavior. The question "Do you have any current criminal charges pending, or have you been convicted of criminal charges?" will address the patient's involvement in the legal system. A nurse asking if the patient has encountered any crises or major problems lately will help identify a significant negative effect on the individual's perception of self and self-esteem. Negative crises or problems could include being laid off, the development of a serious or chronic illness, a perceived threat to oneself, being abused or physically hurt by someone (a victim), or overexposure to violent life experiences or TV. Also, drugs and violence are often associated, so asking "What recreational drugs do you use?" may elicit a pattern of drug use indicative of a Risk for Violence.

Despite the best assessment available at this time, the prediction of violence remains problematical. A current study found that clinicians predicted violence in psychiatric patients with an accuracy greater than chance—60%. However, that still leaves a large margin for error. The study also noted that clinicians had great difficulty predicting violence by women and may be missing cues indicating which women have a propensity for becoming violent.[15]

Although many risk factors for violence exist, the event itself has three phases: preassault, assault, and postassault.[17] To prevent the violent episode from progressing through the phases, the appropriate assessment of the preassault phase allows immediate interventions that will abort or diffuse the probability, severity, and/or duration of the incipient violence.

■ Risk Factors

The presence of the following behaviors, conditions, or circumstances renders the patient more vulnerable to Risk for Violence[2-4, 6-10, 12, 19-23]:

- Gender and age (young male)
- Medical conditions

- Brain tumor or brain damage
- Temporal lobe epilepsy
- Nutritional deficiencies
- Low neuroleptic blood level and medication noncompliance
- Body language
  - Rigid or taut body
  - Clenched teeth or fists
  - Very rapid, shallow breathing
  - Increased pacing
  - Increased excitement or agitation
  - Irritability
  - Defiance
  - Argumentative
  - Hostile or threatening verbalizations
- Psychiatric disorders
  - Dementias
  - Psychoactive substance–induced disorder
  - Command hallucinations
  - Paranoid schizophrenia
  - Mood disorders
  - Anxiety disorders
  - Personality disorders
  - Confusion or panic
- Posttraumatic stress disorder
- Experiences of violence within the family or community
- Fear of self or others
- Dependency on family member as primary caregiver
- Recent aggressive behavior and arrests
- Suicidal or homicidal behavior
- Temper tantrums
- Belief that behavior is not under personal control
- Hopelessness
- Vulnerable self-esteem
- Lack of self-control or poor impulse control
- Antisocial behavior
- Bullying others
- Intense interpersonal bonding
- Abusive behaviors
- Boasting about previous violent episodes
- Feeling that one's honor has been violated
- Increasing anxiety levels
- Belief that violence is justified
- Religious frenzy or trances

DIAGNOSIS

▪ Differential Nursing Diagnosis

Three nursing diagnoses have a possibility for violence because they can involve identified risk factors for violence and indicate the need to assess the potential Risk for Violence as a separate nursing diagnosis. Ineffective Individual Coping indicates the need for such a diagnosis if one of the ineffective behaviors includes behavior destructive to oneself or others. Impaired Social Interaction in some of the more disturbed situations that involve severe anxiety or altered thought processes could precipitate violent behaviors because the patient would not use alternative coping mechanisms. Altered Thought Processes includes delusions and command hallucinations, which can lead to violent behaviors. Therefore, if these diagnoses do include risk factors for violence, a separate diagnosis for the violence should be made. Although these diagnoses may involve a Risk for Violence, the risk factors of an individual being a young male with a recent history for violence have the greatest risk of any of the identified risk factors.

▪ Medical and Psychiatric Diagnoses

Alcohol and cocaine intoxication can include risk factors for violence as a result of impaired cognition, hallucinations, delusions, or mood alterations. In some instances, violence also may be used by substance abusers to acquire the resources to support their indulgence in recreational drugs. A borderline personality disorder may need a diagnosis of Risk for Violence if the patient's impulsivity, unstable emotions, or intense feelings have a history of resulting in violence because the offender exercises little control over his or her behaviors. The diagnosis of paranoid schizophrenia may or may not need a diagnosis of Risk for Violence, depending on the content of the delusions and hallucinations: persecutory content can lead to suicidal behaviors and grandiosity with anger can lead to violence against others. As with the nursing diagnosis, patients with these medical and psychiatric diagnoses may not be at risk for violent behaviors, depending whether or not the risk factors associated with violence are also pre-

sent. If such risk factors are present, then a separate diagnosis of Risk for Violence is needed.

OUTCOME IDENTIFICATION, PLANNING, AND IMPLEMENTATION

Violent episodes consist of three phases: preassault, assault, and postassault.[17] The episode can be aborted or altered during any of the three phases.

The probability of violence increases with the presence of certain risk factors, particularly if the individual is a young male and has a recent history of violence, a personality disorder, or uses recreational drugs. Individuals with brain damage or who experience psychotic states may react with violence for no apparent reason. Their provocation arises from an internal stimulus, such as confusion, delusions, hallucinations, or misperception. In many instances, medication helps prevent the assault phase. Observe for adverse reactions to the drugs, and make certain that the patient takes the medication as prescribed. Administer prn medications as needed. If prn medications are needed frequently, evaluate the patient's need for a medication change. It is common for patients to think that they do not need medication and therefore to be noncompliant about taking it, so provide patient education on the need for taking such medication. Patient education on reality testing, the need for taking medication, questioning the evidence that patients use to justify violent acts, and helping patients examine options and alternatives to using violence can help reduce violence. Because the perceived need to use violence may be reflective of the patients' cultural milieu, which requires violence for safety, alternative behaviors need to be taught within a paradigm consistent with their cultural milieu. Multiple interventions broadly grouped as environmental manipulations and approaches to the patient have to be adapted to the specific needs of a given patient. Such interventions include the reduction of stimuli by lowering lights, decreasing noise levels, requesting that people speak softly, improving poor air qual-

VIII

ity, reducing excessive heat and humidity, and providing quiet areas where individuals can go to regain control of themselves. Other interventions include suggesting that the patient take a shower, coaching the patient to take slow and deep breaths if breathing rapidly and shallowly, permitting or encouraging the patient to engage in an acceptable physical activity, such as playing sports, using a punching bag, or walking. It is also important to avoid getting into a power struggle with a patient about who is "the boss" or demanding that a patient alter nonthreatening behavior to achieve social propriety. A nonthreatening, nonconfrontational approach allows the patient to feel less threatened. The nurse's and the patient's perceptions of a given event are frequently noncongruent, particularly with psychiatric patients. These patients may explain a violent episode as just playing, wanting to stop objectionable behavior by the victim, or complaining of verbal abuse.[5,13]

Assault Phase

If the assault phase occurs, obtain physical control of the patient as a first priority. After staff gain physical control of the patient, that patient may be placed in restraints or seclusion to decrease the potential for further violence and injury. Explain to the patient in a calm, soothing voice what is being done and the reason for it. Although the patient may not appear to be responding to what is being said, it does influence the individual's perception of the event.

When a patient is in restraints or seclusion, the nurse needs to provide that patient with the means to maintain adequate hydration, nutrition, and personal hygiene. If medication is given during this period, it is usually given intramuscularly to have a rapid effect.

Postassault Phase

This phase involves the evaluation of the assault or violent episode and the responses of those who participated in or witnessed the event. This process enables the staff to determine what interventions were or were not effective in preventing the violent episodes of a given patient.

Determine whether the violent behavior was general and nondirected or goal-directed. If the patient incidently injured someone or disrupted the environment, the violent behavior was general and nondirected. Patients with this type of behavior may have an underlying medical problem, acute delirium, or panic behavior. Treatment and control of the underlying problem usually will enable the patient to control the violent behavior. Depending on the problem, the patient can be taught to recognize and to avoid situations or stimuli that will trigger the problem causing the violent behavior.

In goal-directed behavior, the patient chooses a target, for reasons that may or may not make sense to another individual. Patients who use this type of violence often have mental illness, feel threatened, or are trying to stop another person's perceived behavior.* Determine the patient's perceptions of the event. It is not unusual for the patient to feel that the staff overreacted or were punishing him or her. The patient may also believe that he or she was still in control of personal behavior and should not have been given medication or restrained or secluded. Without clarification of these perceptions, the patient may feel justified regarding the expressed behavior and continue to express hostility. With clarification, the patient may decide to eschew the use of violence to solve problems and try to learn other behavioral responses.

A variety of educational and psychotherapeutic interventions can assist patients in changing their perception of the need for violence. Educational interventions can decrease patients' stress, vulnerability, and hypersensitivity by teaching them skills to improve their interpersonal functioning. These interventions include but are not limited to job-seeking skills, skills for independent living, skills for the use of time, social and interpersonal skills, and the need to comply with a treatment regimen. Psychotherapeutic interventions assist patients to improve behavioral control by increasing anxiety tolerance, developing their ability to postpone gratification, improving impulse control, develop-

---

*References 2, 5–6, 8–9, 14, 16, 22.

ing realistic expectations, accepting responsibility for their actions, becoming self-reliant, acquiring a sense of autonomy and individuality, and con-structively verbalizing feelings. If working with a cross-cultural patient, use translators if available, and identify the cultural significance of the various nursing procedures and potential therapeutic modalities being considered as interventions. Then develop appropriate modifications of treat-ment and expected treatment outcomes. Not con-sidering the patients' sociocultural background can lead to feelings of rejection and alienation and develop vulnerable self-esteem. These are risk fac-tors for violence.

The staff also needs to evaluate their feelings and activities. Without assigning blame or preju-dice, a realistic assessment of how they might have

handled the situation differently can help the staff respond more effectively in the future. These ses-sions also help identify staff training needs in man-aging the aggressive or violent patient.

It is generally recognized that all staff need training if they are manage the aggressive, violent patient effectively. Identified areas of training include but are not limited to risk factors associ-ated with Risk for Violence, nonjudgmental com-munication skills, techniques for defusing a violent situation, principles of psychological assessment and interventions, cultural bases for violence, legal and ethical issues, and techniques for increasing staff teamwork. Even the federal Occupational Safety and Health Administration has started investigating institutions that expose their employ-ees to unreasonable risks of violence by patients.[1]

◢ NURSING CARE GUIDELINES
Nursing Diagnosis: Risk for Violence: Self-Directed or Directed at Others

Expected Outcome: The patient will rapidly defuse impending violent behavior as evidence by verbaliza-tion of feelings and behavior, indicating that the staff or the patient is able to control the situation; decreas-ing the need to use violence to solve problems; and using socially appropriate activities to express anger, verbalizing changes in cognitive values that indicate a decreasing need to use violence to solve problems.

- Evaluate patient for presence of risk factors, particularly for body language, active antisocial behavior, intoxication with alcohol or drugs, paranoid schizophrenia, and a history of recent violence *because these behaviors frequently occur before an immediate assault phase.*
- Use medication as needed before patient becomes violent *because medication will frequently assist the patient to control his or her behavior without resorting to violence.*
- Structure the environment to reduce stimuli by any means available; allow the patient to set the interac-tion distance; listen to what the patient actually says, and/or interrupt a treatment session or interview *because these allow the patient to reduce anxiety and fear, which increases the probability of the patient regaining control of his or her behavior.*
- ▲ Provide physical activities *to help the patient redirect the focus from a perceived threat to an appropri-ate and socially acceptable way of expressing feelings.*
- Verify that the patient takes medication as prescribed, and teach the necessity of taking these medica-tions as prescribed. *Low medication serum levels are implicated in relapses of psychiatric patients.*
- Avoid a tone of voice that suggests nagging, pessimism, indifference, or hostility. Also avoid direct con-frontation and responding to abusive language with abusive language *because patients respond to these staff behaviors defensively—sometimes violently—because they are perceived as a personal threat.*
- Determine patient's perception regarding the need for violence and the cultural or community parame-ters for violence *because this directly relates to whether or not this patient believes that the use of vio-lence is appropriate.*

■ = nursing intervention; ▲ = collaborative intervention.   *Continued*

VIII

◢ Nursing Care Guidelines — cont'd

▲ Provide those aspects of cognitive therapy (e.g., questioning evidence used, examining options and alternatives, and rehearsing more effective coping skills) that have been helpful for managing assaultive behavior *because they will help the patient decrease the use of violence as a coping strategy.*

Expected Outcome: The patient will incur no personal injuries and inflict no injuries to others if a violent episode occurs while in the health care system.

▪ Use trained and adequate staff to control the patient physically when necessary. *Trained and adequate staff decrease the frequency and severity of injuries to staff and patients.*

▲ Restrain, seclude, and medicate the patient as ordered. *This will help the patient regain control of acceptable behavior faster and will prevent the probability of patient or staff injuries.*

▪ Explain to the patient what is being done and why. *Patients frequently perceive the situation as less serious than the staff does.* This provides a reality check for the patient.

▲ Monitor closely for adverse reactions to the medication or the situation. *This will help prevent additional injury to the patient.*

▪ Assist patient to maintain adequate hydration, nutrition, and personal hygiene. *This allows the patient to maintain basic physical health while unable to provide the necessities for him- or herself.*

Expected Outcome: The patient will experience a decreased risk of violence as evidenced by fewer, less intense, and shorter violent episodes, with a decreased probability of injury; increased ability to sort out the feelings and thoughts related to violent episodes; increased ability to identify Risk for Violence and to initiate activities to defuse or control that potential.

▲ For general, nondirected violence, treat the underlying condition (e.g., toxic conditions) and avoid situations that trigger violent episodes. *The situation or condition reduces the individual's ability to inhibit violent behaviors, so avoidance of the situation or condition allows the individual to control the violent behavior.*

▲ For goal-directed violence, determine the patient's perception of the need for violence, implement appropriate educational and psychotherapeutic treatments to defuse or control the Risk for Violence, hold community and staff postassault sessions, train the staff to work as a team in the management of the aggressive, assaultive patient. *Education and training of the patient provide a context wherein the patient can change cognitive perceptions of the need for violence within a safe environment. The education and training of the staff improve the assessment of impending violence and decrease the probability of staff and patient injuries during violent episodes.*

EVALUATION

Preassault Phase

To evaluate the preassault phase, consider the interventions effective if violent behaviors are aborted or defused quickly, while the patient is in the care of the health care system. Any interventions initiated by the staff that indicate to the patient that the staff will control violent situations and will keep the environment safe enhance the probability of the patient defusing or aborting violent behavior. Sometimes patients will verbally or behaviorally demonstrate a decreased need to solve problems with violence. These behaviors indicate the effectiveness of the preassault interventions.

Assault Phase

To evaluate the assault phase, interventions are effective if physical injury and/or property damage is prevented or limited. If violence is not contained, serious injury, death, or major destruction of property will occur. A measure of effective interventions includes a decrease in the probable intensity and duration of the violent episodes. Patients with severe psychoses or toxic drug reactions can remain violent for several days or can exhibit several violent episodes. These patient may require intensive treatment and ongoing evaluation to bring the behavior under control. Another evaluation parameter involves the perceptions of the patient and the staff. If the patient perceives the interventions as beneficial and not punitive and if the staff perceives their interventions as therapeutic, then those interventions are effective. If patients and staff perceive the interventions as punitive, the patients will resort to violence when the opportunity presents itself and feel justified in doing it.

Postassault Phase

During this phase, the effectiveness of previous interventions is determined, and the identification

of appropriate interventions for continued treatment and prevention of further violence is specified. This process becomes the foundation for the successful treatment of violence and will function adequately only if it is done by the treatment team. The outcome has been achieved if patients exhibit an overall decrease in the frequency, duration, or intensity of violent episodes. Another positive outcome of this phase is an overall decrease in patient and staff injuries. One of the more rewarding outcomes occurs when a patient identifies and then initiates activities to defuse or control a situation that could lead to violence. Interventions also will be successful if the underlying risk factors are addressed, treated, and brought under control.

◤ CASE STUDY WITH PLAN OF CARE

Mr. Jonas J., a 21-year-old male with a diagnosis of paranoid schizophrenia, was admitted to a psychiatric unit because of an unprovoked assault on a family guest and because of increasing interpersonal problems. On admission, he said that he was just trying to make the guest stop lying about him. He denied having any hallucinations or delusions, but when he was alone he was observed by the nursing staff to move his lips as if talking to himself. At other times he was observed smiling to himself and nodding his head as if he were responding to some sort of internal stimuli. Mr. J. paced the halls continuously, with downcast eyes. When he attended unit activities, he maintained a distance of at least 6 to 8 feet between himself and other persons and would not participate, even when gently encouraged to do so. His appearance, behavior, conversation, cognition, and mood were in keeping with the diagnosis of paranoid schizophrenia. Mr. J. played basketball in high school and liked to talk about how aggressively he had played and how much he now missed playing the sport. Since

graduating from high school he has not developed any strong friendships and tends to prefer solitary pursuits, such as physical fitness, except for occasional get-togethers to play basketball. After finishing high school, he worked as an automobile mechanic until being fired 2 weeks ago. His parents stated that he was fired because of insubordination and numerous customer complaints about his hostility. However, Mr. J. stated that he was fired because his supervisor did not like him and had figured out a way to get rid of him. After his firing, Mr. J. stayed in his room listening to music and making no efforts to seek employment because he thought his previous employer would make certain he could not get another job. About 2 months ago, he broke up with his girlfriend "because she wanted to be better than I was." He made no attempt to find another girlfriend and ceased participating in family activities. His parents thought he was angry, but he denied having any strong feelings about his exgirlfriend or his family.

◤ PLAN OF CARE FOR MR. JONAS J.
Nursing Diagnosis: Risk for Violence: Directed at Others Related to an Alteration in Cognition Associated with a Diagnosis of Paranoid Schizophrenia

Expected Outcome: Mr. J. will abstain from violent behavior against others as evidenced by taking his medication as prescribed; refraining from acting on violent impulses while in the health care system; recognizing signs and symptoms indicative of impending violence and informing staff of this; identifying and

---

■ = nursing intervention; ▲ = collaborative intervention.　　　　　　　　　*Continued*

▶ PLAN OF CARE FOR MR. JONAS J.— CONT'D

verbalizing reasons for his violent behavior; participating in prescribed activities; and testing the reality of his perceptions with staff.

- ▲ Medicate as prescribed and give prn medication if symptoms increase.
- ▪ Monitor for increased pacing, clenched teeth or fists, or other signs of impending violence.
- ▪ Approach him in a nonconfrontational, nonthreatening manner.
- ▪ Teach the risks and benefits of taking medication.
- ▪ Teach appropriate ways to express his feelings of aggression and violence. Make provisions for him to use some of these methods on the unit.
- ▪ Assign one-to-one nurse to work on control of his suspiciousness and violent behavior.
- ▪ Assign him to nursing support and therapy groups.
- ▪ Interrupt interactions with Mr. J. if he needs to gain control of himself.
- ▲ Encourage Mr. J. to participate in prescribed therapies; set limits on aggressive and assaultive behavior during sessions; test his perceptions of reality while teaching him how others perceive him; and encourage him to use socially acceptable means of expressing violence.

▦ CRITICAL THINKING EXERCISES

1. What risk factors exist to indicate that Mr. Jonas J. would receive a nursing diagnosis of Risk for Violence: Directed at Others?
2. If Mr. Jonas J. were restrained or secluded for a violent episode, what criteria would you use to discontinue the treatment?
3. When evaluating the effectiveness of the nursing treatment plan, what changes would you make in the plan if Mr. Jonas J. had been secluded once and had verbally abused staff and other patients several times during the past week?

VIII

REFERENCES

1. Appelbaum PS and Dimiere RJ: Protecting staff from assaults by patients: OSHA steps in, *Psych Services* 46:333–334, 338, 1995.
2. Catalano R and others: Using ECA survey data to examine the effect of job layoffs on violent behavior, *Hosp Comm Psychiatry* 44:874–879, 1993.
3. Centerwall BS: Television and violence, *JAMA* 26a7:3059–3063, 1992.
4. Colenda CC and Hamer RM: Antecedents and interventions for aggressive behavior of patients at a geropsychiatric state hospital, *Hosp Comm Psychiatry* 42:287–292, 1991.
5. Crowner M and others: Psychiatric patients' explanations for assaults, *Psych Services* 46:614–615, 1995.
6. Durant RH, Pendergrast RA, and Cadenhead C: Exposure to violence and victimization and fighting behavior by urban black adolescents, *J Adol Health* 15:311–318, 1994.
7. Estroff SE and others: The influence of social networks and social support on violence by persons with serious mental illness, *Hosp Comm Psychiatry* 45:669–679, 1994.
8. Garza-Trevino ES: Neurobiological factors in aggressive behavior, *Hosp Comm Psychiatry* 45:690–699, 1994.
9. Grant CA: Women who kill: the impact of abuse, *Iss Ment Health Nurs* 16:315–326, 1995.
10. Grossberg GT and Manepalli J: The older patient with psychotic symptoms, *Psych Services* 46:55–59, 1995.
11. Grossman LS and others: State psychiatric hospital patients with past arrests for violent crimes, *Psych Services* 46:790–795, 1995.
12. Junginger J: Command hallucinations and the prediction of dangerousness, *Psych Services* 46:911–914, 1995.
13. Lanza ML: Origins of aggression, *J Psychosoc Nurs Ment Health Serv* 21:11–19, 1983.
14. Lanza ML and Kayne HL: Patient assault: a comparison of patient and staff perceptions, *Iss Ment Health Nurs* 16:129–141, 1995.
15. Lidz CW, Mulvey EP, and Gardner W: The accuracy of predictions of violence to others, *JAMA* 269:1007–1011, 1993.
16. Mulvey EP: Assessing the evidence of a link between mental illness and violence, *Hosp Comm Psychiatry* 45:663–668, 1994.
17. Rada RT: The violent patient: rapid assessment and management, *Psychosomatics* 22:101, 1981.
18. Roper JM and Anderson NLR: The interactional dynamics of violence, part I, *Arch Psychiatr Nurs* 5:209–215, 1991.

19. Saltzman LE and others: Weapon involvement and injury outcomes in family and intimate assaults, *JAMA* 267:3043–3047, 1992.

20. Straznickas KA, McNiel DE, and Binder RL: Violence toward family caregivers by mentally ill relatives, *Hosp Comm Psychiatry* 44:385–387, 1993.

21. Torrey EF: Violent behaviors by individuals with serious mental illness, *Hosp Comm Psychiatry* 45:653–662, 1994.

22. Valois RF and others: Correlates of aggressive and violent behaviors among public high school adolescents, *Soc Adol Med* 16:26–34, 1995.

23. Volvavka J and others: Characteristics of state hospital patients arrested for offenses committed during hospitalization, *Psych Services* 46:796–800, 1995.

24. White JH: Violence: a public health epidemic, *Health Prog* Jan-Feb:18–21, 1994.

VIII

Rape-Trauma Syndrome

▶ ──

Rape-Trauma Syndrome: Compound Reaction

▶ ──

Rape-Trauma Syndrome: Silent Reaction

▶ ──

IX

Rape-Trauma Syndrome. *Rape is a forced, violent sexual penetration against the victim's will and consent. The trauma syndrome that develops from this attack or attempted attack includes an acute phase of disorganization of the victim's lifestyle and a long-term process of reorganization of lifestyle.*

Rape-Trauma Syndrome: Compound Reaction *is an acute stress reaction to rape or attempted rape, experienced along with other major stressors, which include the reactivation of symptoms of a previous condition.*[13]

Rape-Trauma Syndrome: Silent Reaction *is a complex stress reaction to a rape in which an individual is unable to describe or discuss the rape.*[13]

OVERVIEW

Rape is an act of aggression and sexual violence. The purpose of rapists is to torment, control, humiliate, and violate the victim. The victims are not chosen based on physical appearance or attractiveness but on vulnerability. Infants, children, men, women, the elderly, and physically and mentally disabled persons are all potential victims. The physical, psychological, and emotional sequelae of rape are enormous and are further compounded by the reluctance of the victims to report the crime to law enforcement or even to their health care providers. This reluctance to report stems from

the persistent belief that the victims are somehow responsible for the sexual assault. Societal myths about rape are that victims dress in a way that invites assault, that victims put themselves into situations in which they deserve assault, or that rape only happens to certain kinds of people. This shifts responsibility for the crime from the perpetrators and places it on the victims. The victims subsequently suffer from guilt, shame, embarrassment, and the lack of a supportive network.

During the 1970s, victims' rights were furthered by a grass-roots movement initiated by feminists. The first crime victim assistance program in the United States was founded in Berkeley in 1972,[4] and it was a "rape crisis center." Work was done by volunteers, many of whom had been sexually victimized, and there was a loose consensus of services to be provided. In 1974, Burgess and Holmstrom published their research on Rape-Trauma Syndrome, thus providing a credible basis for intervention. The health care and mental health communities became aware of the sequelae of sexual victimization. In 1975, Congress established the National Center for the Prevention and Control of Rape, which developed programs, conducted research, and provided information to victims of rape.

Many agencies that started as "rape crisis centers" in the 1970s now have changed to "sexual assault centers" to reflect more accurately their emphasis on healing interventions and advocacy for survivors of all forms of predatory sexual acts. The definition of sexual assault is "a form of aggression and violence in which sex is the weapon."[22] Sexual abuse is the abuse of power by one individual over another as in sexual harrassment and child molestation. Rape represents sexual assault and sexual abuse in its most extreme form and is defined as "forced, violent sexual penetration against the victim's will and without the victim's consent."[11] In 1985, Burgess and Holmstrom provided a clinical definition of rape trauma as "the stress response pattern of the victim following forced, nonconsenting sexual activity."[4] Since the identification of Rape-Trauma Syndrome, rape trials frequently include expert testimony describing the symptoms and their significance. On appeal, admissibility of expert testimony on Rape-Trauma Syndrome has been addressed by the Supreme Courts of Colorado and Washington and the New York Court of Appeals.[9] In two of the three courts, Rape-Trauma Syndrome evidence was ruled scientifically reliable.

Burgess and Holmstrom have demonstrated that Rape-Trauma Syndrome meets the four criteria for posttraumatic stress disorder.[4] The primary criterion is that the stressor must be of significant magnitude to evoke distinguishable symptoms in almost everyone. In rape, the perpetrators use sexuality to express anger and power and to degrade and humiliate the victims.

The second criterion is intrusive imagery, in which the survivors have sudden recollections of the attacks. When confronted by circumstances similar to the rape, there may be the sudden fear that the event is recurring. Some victims have nightmares that contain elements of the rape. Research has shown that 93.3% of rape victims experienced one or more symptoms of intrusion and 72.8% experienced two or more symptoms of intrusive imagery.[24]

Numbing, the third major diagnostic criterion, is characterized by loss of interest in activities, detachment from others, and restricted affect.[8] The findings of one study, with a sample of prostitutes in the Netherlands[27] who had been subjected to sexual violence, demonstrated that there was a positive relationship between the severity of victimization and the frequency of dissociation and denial, which were labeled as numbing.

The fourth criterion consists of a combination of two of the following: hypervigilance, disturbance in sleep pattern, guilt, impairment of memory or concentration, avoidance of activities that arouse recollection, or increased symptoms that result from the event.[4] A study of sexual assault victims at a mean of 8 years years after the assault showed that three quarters of them asserted that sexual assault continued to affect their sexual relationships.[21] Fear and mistrust, decreased pleasure, flashbacks to the assault during sexual intimacy, decreased frequency of intercourse, obligatory sex, anger, avoidance, and emotional detachment were reported by survivors of rape.

Koss, Koss, and Woodruff[17] compared sexual assault victims with nonvictims and found that victims perceived themselves to be less healthy, reported more physical complaints and symptoms of emotional distress, and engaged in more injurious health behaviors than nonvictims. The number of visits to health care providers and outpatient medical costs were significantly increased for female sexual assault victims when compared to victims of crime resulting in injury with no threat of rape. A significant number of increased physician visits persisted over the 2-year length of the study. All body systems, with the exception of the skin and the eyes, were reported by sexual assault victims to have greater symptoms, and gynecological symptoms were the most frequent. Somatic symptoms reported by victims included pounding heartbeat, tension headaches, nausea, back pain, skin disorders, allergies, menstrual symptoms, and sudden weight change.[14] Physical symptoms decreased during the year following the sexual assault; however, psychological symptoms, including anxiety, fear, and depression, did not decrease.

Children—both male and female—are especially vulnerable to sexual molestation and rape. Adults who have been sexually molested in childhood report significantly more depression, obesity,

IX

and morbid obesity and experience more physician visits than adults not molested in childhood.[7] Adults who were childhood victims had increased incidence of irritable bowel syndrome, chronic constipation, asthma, headaches, insomnia, sexual dysfunction, overeating, and drug abuse. Psychologically, victims of child sexual abuse suffered depression, guilt, low self-esteem, relationship difficulties, suicidal thoughts, and memory lapses.[12] They rarely told caregivers about their history of sexual abuse.

Other researchers have described additional sequelae related to child sexual molestation. Almost one half of the women sexually abused as girls experience revictimization in adulthood, including rape, prostitution, and physical and emotional abuse.[28] They also have higher rates of unintended and aborted pregnancies. Up to 42% of homeless women were sexually abused as children.[1]

Men are at less risk than women for sexual assault. Incidence of male-male rape is unknown. A study of sexually assaulted homosexual men in a gay community showed that 27.6% had been sexually assaulted.[10] In addition, a study of medical school students found that gay students were two to three times more likely to report having sex against their will than heterosexual colleagues. Studies of incarcerated males revealed an estimated rape rate of 0.5% to 3.0%, and findings inferred that sexual aggression was for the purpose of asserting power.[19] There have been more incidents of multiple assailants and physical injury in male-male rape. However, men and women who are victims of sexual assault have an equally increased risk of developing major depression, drug dependence, phobias, panic disorders, and obsessive-compulsive disorders, whereas men are more likely to abuse alcohol.[5] Female-female rape appears to occur infrequently, but reliable data do not exist.

The use of rape as a deliberate tactic in war has been reported.[16,26] Rape was identified as a war crime by the United Nations Commission on Human Rights in 1993. A 10-day investigation by the United Nations concluded that 11,900 rapes occurred in the former Yugoslavia. The rapes were thought to be part of an "ethnic cleansing" with the expressed intent to impregnate. Other goals of rape include the destruction of family and societal bonds, the demoralization of the enemy, and the forced movement of women out of occupied areas. Japanese soldiers during World War II abducted between 100,000 and 200,000 Asian women for sexual slavery. Other large-scale reports of sexual victimization during war have occurred in Bangladesh (estimated between 250,000 and 400,000 rapes in 1971), in a village in Uganda (70% of the women were raped by soldiers in 1981), among the Vietnamese boat people in 1985, and under the Pol Pot reign in Cambodia.

Sexual torture victims treated by the Amnesty International Danish Medical Group and the International Rehabilitation and Research Center for Torture Victims demonstrated an overall incidence of sexual torture of 61% (80% of the victims were women and 56% were men).[20] Forty percent of sexually tortured victims subsequently developed sexual difficulties, which included lack of libido, lack of orgasm, loathing of sexual activity, and reliving torture during intercourse.

There are almost no scientific studies of rape prevalence or consequences in the nonindustrialized world.[16] There are some data to suggest that rape is a risk factor for suicide and murder in victim-blaming societies and that rates of pregnancy resulting from rape have cultural differences. The rate of sexually transmitted diseases also varies widely by country and community.

Rape-Trauma Syndrome: Compound Reaction shares the same criteria as Rape-Trauma Syndrome but in addition has reactivated symptoms of a previous condition, such as physical or psychiatric illness or drug or alcohol abuse. The trauma of sexual assault decreases over time for victims without previous mental health or substance abuse problems, whereas victims with those problems are at risk for greater severity and length of trauma.[25]

Rape-Trauma Syndrome: Silent Reaction occurs when victims have been raped but have not revealed the rape to anyone. In a study of 107 Ugandan women who had been raped by soldiers, only one half of the victims told anyone about the rape 7 years after the incident. However, they continued to acknowledge persistent problems related to the rape.[26]

ASSESSMENT

Rape-Trauma Syndrome

It has been estimated that more than 27% of all American women will be victims of attempted or completed rape in their lifetimes. Of those, only 12% report the assault to law enforcement. In the acute aftermath of rape, the role of nurses in intervention is to evaluate the extent of injury, collect forensic evidence, and address victims' concerns about pregnancy and sexually transmitted diseases. In planning for discharge, patients' social and personal resources need to be assessed.

Victims of sexual assault are excessive consumers of health care, and there is a need for nurses in the primary practice to recognize patterns that represent Rape-Trauma Syndrome.[14] One tool is a good sexual history as part of initial data gathering. The history should include the age of first intercourse and whether or not it was voluntary. A history investigating abuse is indicated for all patients who somatize or who overuse services. Situations that may trigger feelings related to a previous sexual assault are a pelvic or prenatal examination. Victims of child sexual abuse may demonstrate feelings of fear and helplessness when anticipating parenthood.

■ Defining Characteristics

The presence of the following defining characteristics indicates that the patient may be experiencing Rape-Trauma Syndrome:

Acute phase (from 1 to 6 weeks)
- Somatic symptoms, including pounding heartbeat, headaches, back pain, allergies, nausea, and skin disorders
- Muscle tension, soreness, and bruising
- Genitourinary symptoms: menstrual irregularities, pelvic pain, or vaginal discharge
- Sexually transmitted disease

- Recurrent gastrointestinal symptoms; irritable bowel syndrome, constipation, cramping, and change in appetite
- Sexual dysfunction
- Sleep pattern disturbance and fatigue
- Fear of violence and death
- Hypervigilance, low startle threshold
- Flashbacks of the rape
- Anger, anxiety, rage, revenge, and hysteria
- Numbing, memory lapse, and feelings of disengagement
- Powerlessness, helplessness, and hopelessness
- Shame, guilt, embarrassment, humiliation, and self-blame
- Fear of crowds or fear of being alone

Long-term phase
- Chronic genitourinary symptoms
- Chronic sexual dysfunction
- Unintended pregnancies
- Significant change in weight or an eating disorder (most notably bulimia)
- Persistent flashbacks, repetitive nightmares, fears, phobias, and anxieties
- Inability to trust and relationship instability
- Suicidal thoughts, depression, and low self-esteem
- Multiple victimizations
- Frequent presentations to health care providers
- Change in job, residence, and phone number
- Change in relationship to family (support seeking or isolation)

■ Related Factors

The following related factors are associated with Rape-Trauma Syndrome:

- Victim's age, gender, and sexual orientation
- Spouse or family blame the victim
- Inadequate support systems
- Cultural value of virginity or purity

Rape-Trauma Syndrome: Compound Reaction

■ Defining Characteristics

The presence of the following defining characteristics indicates that the patient may be ex-

IX

periencing Rape-Trauma Syndrome: Compound Reaction:

- All the defining characteristics listed for Rape-Trauma Syndrome
- Reactivation of previous drug or alcohol abuse
- Reactivation of previous physical or psychiatric illness

■ Related Factors

The following related factors are associated with Rape-Trauma Syndrome: Compound Reaction:

- Previous history of drug or alcohol abuse
- History of medical disorder that is chronic or in remission
- History of mental illness
- Male gender (vulnerability to substance abuse)
- Rape-Trauma Syndrome: Silent Reaction
- Unresolved grieving
- Multiple recent significant life changes

Rape-Trauma Syndrome: Silent Reaction

■ Defining Characteristics

The presence of the following defining characteristics indicates that the patient may be experiencing Rape-Trauma Syndrome: Silent Reaction:

- All the defining characteristics listed for Rape-Trauma Syndrome
- The unwillingness or inability to verbalize the experience of rape
- Abrupt changes in relationships or sexual behavior

■ Related Factors

The following related factors are associated with Rape-Trauma Syndrome: Silent Reaction:
- Intense guilt or shame
- Self-blame
- Denial
- Fear of retaliation from perpetrator
- Use of drugs or alcohol before the rape
- Fear of not being believed or validated by family or system

- Young age
- Spousal rape, same-sex rape, date rape
- Lack of support
- Children who have been bribed

DIAGNOSIS

■ Differential Nursing Diagnosis

Rape-Trauma Syndrome: Compound Reaction is differentiated from Rape-Trauma Syndrome by the reactivation of a prior physical or mental illness or prior drug or alcohol abuse. Previously well-controlled asthma or rheumatoid arthritis that are exacerbated after a rape are examples of Rape-Trauma Syndrome: Compound Reaction. Rape-Trauma Syndrome: Silent Reaction is characterized by the victims' inability or unwillingness to disclose the event. The Rape-Trauma Syndrome diagnoses are in the category of Post-Trauma Response and are different only because they are specific to victims of rape. Other traumatic events, such as war, disaster, near-death, torture, or accident, are categorized under the more general diagnosis of Post-Trauma Response. Rape victims may have subsequent Sexual Dysfunction as a result of Rape-Trauma Syndrome. The nursing diagnosis Sexual Dysfunction can be derived from a variety of etiologies, such as illness, medication side effects, or lack of a desirable partner. Anxiety, which is also a specific nursing diagnosis, can be a symptom of Rape-Trauma Syndrome. The source of anxiety in Rape-Trauma Syndrome is attributable to the rape and is generally characterized by hypervigilance and fearfulness.

■ Medical and Psychiatric Diagnoses

Postassault rape patients are more likely to interact with members of the health care community than the mental health community.[14] In a study with a sample of almost 1000 women, 63% of whom were African-American, the most common postassault symptom was tension headache, reported by more than one half of the subjects. Abdominal pain or nausea was reported by 44% of the subjects at 2 weeks after the assault and persisted for 21% 1 year later. Other presenting symptoms at 2 weeks included back pain, allergies, palpitations, and menstrual symptoms, all experienced by at least one quarter of the victims. Use of medical services remained elevated for rape victims even after symptoms were no longer significantly elevated. Among adolescents, the diagnoses of pregnancy and bulimia have been associated with prior sexual abuse. Possible psychiatric diagnoses relating to the effect of rape on sexual function include decreased desire dysfunction and decreased arousal dysfunction.[21] Sexual assault also predicted the onset of major depressive episodes, phobias, panic disorders, and obsessive-compulsive disorders.[5] Victims who have been assaulted in childhood are more likely to develop a psychiatric diagnosis than adult victims.

OUTCOME IDENTIFICATION, PLANNING, AND IMPLEMENTATION

Although the incidence and sequelae of rape are well documented, there is virtually no data on the effectiveness of nursing interventions. It is useful to conceptualize planning in terms of acute and long-term care. Acute intervention usually occurs in the emergency department, whereas long-term planning might occur in a primary care practice, a prenatal clinic, a birth control clinic, a drug rehabilitation program, or a mental health facility. Given the prevalence of sexual assault, familiarity with resources is critical for nurses who are willing to ask the client about sexual issues in any setting. It is important for patients and nurses to realize that healing is a process, not an event, and that the process will be different for each victim.

Rape-Trauma Syndrome

A desired outcome in the acute setting is that patients will retain optimum physical well-being following sexual assault. Male victims and prostitutes are the victims most likely to sustain serious injuries. Nursing interventions include prompt physical assessment and attention to all injuries. If elected by the patient, the importance of complying with care regimens, such as morning-after therapy for prevention of pregnancy and antibiotic therapy for prevention of sexually transmitted diseases, should be stressed. Complications and side effects should be discussed. Follow-up care for injuries or other concerns should be carefully explained. Written instructions are helpful for patients who may be overwhelmed by the surrounding events.

If desired, patients shall have all forensic evidence maintained and preserved in the event that they wish to pursue litigation. Nurses are responsible for explanations about the forensic examination and the implications of performing or not performing certain procedures. Nurses must be familiar with the protocol of the facility to ensure that proper procedures are followed regarding the collection and chain of evidence.

Another goal is that patients will feel safe and supported. From the time of triage, patients should be identified as high priority and not be left alone. Unconditional positive regard, reassurance that whatever each patient did was the best decision that could be made at the time, and empathetic listening constitute emotional support. Referral to sexual assault centers, victim advocate services, legal advocates, therapeutic agencies, and self-help groups may enhance physical, emotional, and spiritual healing.

An acute and long-term goal is that patients will be able to identify a positive social support network. Nurses should explain the importance of obtaining support and should assist patients to identify family or friends who can be caring and nonjudgmental. If possible, providing resources for support persons is valuable. Many sexual assault centers offer services to significant people in the patient's life, as well as a telephone crisis line that is available around the clock.

Long-term goals include patients' developing effective coping strategies to reinforce positive feelings of self-esteem and control. Assisting patients to identify behaviors that help to prevent revictimization is essential. Providing opportunities for

IX

decision making in regard to sexual relationships and contraception enhance a sense of control. Insights about the expected symptoms of Rape-Trauma Syndrome and the expectation that symptoms will improve is empowering for the victims.

In patients who show multiple presenting somatic symptoms or persistent psychological symptoms, a long-term goal is the cessation of these symptoms. They can persist for months or years, and they can lead to increased anxiety and fear that there is a devastating physical illness that is not being treated. Offering reassurance is an impor-

tant nursing intervention. Equally important is a thorough evaluation and treatment of symptoms to avoid misdiagnosis.

A major long-term goal is that patients will resume (or obtain) a satisfying lifestyle. For some victims, nursing intervention will lead to an increase in personal satisfaction. They may emerge from the traumatic event with increased self-esteem. The healing process leads to self-knowledge and a sense of purpose that can come from prevailing in adversity.

◢ NURSING CARE GUIDELINES
Nursing Diagnosis: Rape-Trauma Syndrome

Expected Outcome: The patient will retain optimum physical well-being following sexual assault. (For minor physical injuries, healing will usually occur in 1 to 2 weeks. For severe injuries, reconstruction and healing may take months or years.)

▲ Provide prompt physical assessment, treatment of injuries, and referral for medical treatment as needed. *Victims seek health care for reassurance of their physical condition.*[3]

▪ Inform patient regarding risks of sexually transmitted diseases and pregnancy, options available for treatment, and risks of treatment. *Education about options empowers the patient.*

▲ Provide precise written information regarding necessary follow-up for injuries, sexually transmitted disease testing and treatment, or possible pregnancy. *Nurses foster behaviors that promote self-care.*

Expected Outcome: The patient will have forensic evidence maintained and preserved for prosecution if desired. (This shall be accomplished as soon as possible after the rape and within 72 hours.)

▪ Explain the forensic examination and its purpose. *The patient may or may not want to pursue prosecution.*

▲ Perform forensic collection of evidence, adhering to protocols and chain of evidence. *Proper documentation and handling of evidence results in the ability of the prosecuting attorney to support the case against the assailant.*

▲ Notify law enforcement or Child or Adult Protective Services if desired by the patient or required by statute. *In some cases, criminal prosecution gives the patient a sense of empowerment. Nurses are mandatory reporters of abuse of children or the elderly.*

Expected Outcome: The patient will feel safe and supported in the acute care setting.

▪ Triage the patient as second in priority only to life-threatening emergencies. *Decrease the discomfort of the hospital experience by providing optimum, patient-centered care; enhance the timely preservation of evidence.*[2]

▲ Have a supportive person of the patient's choosing be present—either a nurse, victim advocate, social worker, or significant other. *Patients have identified the presence of a caring individual in the examination room as extremely helpful.*[18]

▪ = nursing intervention; ▲ = collaborative intervention.

- ▪ Provide reassurance, unconditional positive regard, and empathetic listening. *This creates security and trust, and establishes a base for development of a therapeutic alliance.*
- ▲ Refer patient to community resources, such as sexual assault centers, qualified therapists, self-help groups, telephone crisis lines, women's shelters, advocacy services, and legal services. *There is substantial efficacy of a group approach to treatment and a documented efficacy of specific psychotherapeutic approaches.*[15]

Expected Outcome: The patient will be able to identify a positive social support network before termination of the initial nurse contact.

- ▪ Explain the importance of emotional support from significant others during the healing process. *Emotional support results in decreased appearance of depression, anxiety, and fear.*[23]
- ▪ Assist patients to identify trusted friends and family. *Confiding in one or two friends results in less somatic complaints and feeling healthier.*[14]
- ▲ Identify community resources for use by the support persons. *Empowering patients' support networks enhances their ability to cope and the support people to provide help.*

Expected Outcome: The patient will develop effective coping strategies within 6 months to 1 year after the traumatic event.

- ▪ Provide education regarding the short- and long-term effects of rape or attempted rape and the process of healing. *It is important that patients know their reactions are normal and that they can recover.*[18]
- ▪ Assist the patient to identify behaviors that will minimize revictimization. *Patients may have behavior patterns that increase their vulnerability.*
- ▪ Assist patients in decision making regarding sexual relationships and birth control. *Help patients to establish areas of control.*

Expected Outcome: The patient will be free of somatic and psychological symptoms within 1 year of the traumatic event.

- ▪ Assist each patient to identify support people in whom they can confide. *Confiding in another person results in less somatic complaints and feeling healthier.*[14]
- ▲ Refer to specialist for persistent or debilitating psychological or somatic symptoms. *Early identification and treatment of disease may prevent long-term sequelae.*

Expected Outcome: The patient will resume (or obtain) a satisfying lifestyle within 1 year of the traumatic event.

- ▲ Identify expressions of depression, guilt, anxiety, fear, and anger; help to explore those feelings, and refer patient to counseling if indicated. *During a crisis, the patient is more open and accessible to intervention that will promote effective coping strategies.*[18]

IX

Rape-Trauma Syndrome: Compound Reaction

The stress of the traumatic event may exacerbate a chronic disease or make the victim vulnerable to reliance on alcohol or drugs. Assessment for specific symptoms of physical or psychiatric disease on a regular basis and early treatment or referral are essential to preventing complications or regression in healing.

Rape-Trauma Syndrome: Silent Reaction

The process of disclosure of sexual abuse or sexual assault is complex. For adults, the fear of invasive examinations and embarrassing interviews may inhibit disclosure. The failure to recognize that rape has occurred, as perhaps in spousal rape or date rape, may result in confusion and silence. The fear of retribution, such as physical violence from the perpetrator, or the fear of being without resources as a result of reporting spousal rape, may result in Rape-Trauma Syndrome: Silent Reaction. Children are often threatened or bribed into silence. When listening to a disclosure, the nurse should not display shock, dismay, or pity. For all victims of child sexual abuse, evaluation by a therapist who is skilled in treating young people is essential.

◀ NURSING CARE GUIDELINES

Nursing Diagnosis: Rape-Trauma Syndrome: Compound Reaction

Use applicable interventions from Rape-Trauma Syndrome in addition to the following:

Expected Outcome: The patient will achieve optimum well-being in regard to chronic or exacerbated physical condition. (The length of time for resolution is a function of the natural history of the disease and each patient's ability for resilience.)
- Perform a history and a physical examination that includes symptoms specific for the disease process. *Early detection of and intervention to ameliorate the disease may reduce symptoms and enhance the outcome.*
- ▲ Make arrangements for early referral to and collaboration with primary care provider. *This creates a multidisciplinary support network early in the disease process to promote healing.*

Expected Outcome: The patient will achieve optimum well-being in regard to chronic or exacerbated psychiatric conditions. (The length of time for resolution is a function of the natural history of the disease and the patient's ability for resilience.)
- Perform an assessment that includes symptoms specific to the psychiatric diagnosis. *Early detection and intervention may reduce symptoms and enhance the outcome.*
- ▲ Make arrangements for an early referral to and collaboration with a mental health professional. *This creates a multidisciplinary support network early in the disease process to promote healing.*

Expected Outcome: The patient will be free from alcohol and drugs. (Sobriety is measured 1 day at a time.)
- Maintain an open agenda with patients that regularly revisits drug and alcohol abuse. *Open and unconditional positive regard allows patient's to confide sensitive information.*
- ▲ Make arrangements for early referral to community resources for substance abuse. *This creates a multidisciplinary support network early in the disease process to promote healing.*

■ = nursing intervention; ▲ = collaborative intervention.

◀ NURSING CARE GUIDELINES

Nursing Diagnosis: Rape-Trauma Syndrome: Silent Reaction

Use applicable interventions from Rape-Trauma Syndrome in addition to the following:

Expected Outcome: The patient is able to disclose victimization and resultant feelings without pressure or coercion, taking as long as necessary.
- Provide an atmosphere in which there is unconditional positive regard. *This enables security and trust to develop and provides an opportunity for disclosure.*
- ▲ Refer patient to therapist skilled in sexual assault issues. *The silent reaction frequently involves complex issues, including child sexual abuse, that are best addressed by an expert.*

■ = nursing intervention; ▲ = collaborative intervention.

EVALUATION

Interventions that are initiated by emergency department nurses often have follow-up with professionals who are not nurses. It is nursing interventions in the emergency room that can have a critical positive effect on the necessary healing for sexual assault victims. Obtaining positive support for victims significantly decreases reports of physical symptoms at 1 year after the assault.[14] Nurses who are able to observe progress over time may be present in primary care, prenatal care, or psychiatric care settings. The Rape Trauma Symptom Rating Scale devised by Peter Divasto[6] can be useful for assessment or for charting progress over time (see Table 9).

Rape-Trauma Syndrome

Evaluation of optimal physical well-being can be accomplished by asking patients if all their physical needs were met as completely as possible in the emergency department. A review of the records can indicate needs identified and addressed by the emergency room personnel and the patient's responses. Evaluation of the appropriateness of forensic specimens can be tracked through chain-of-evidence records.

Feeling safe and supported is based on the patient's subjective recall and can be ascertained throughout the examination procedure, making modifications for patient comfort. The identification of a positive support person should be done before the patient leaves the acute care setting. If there is no available support person in a patient's social network, the need is identified immediately and arrangements for an advocate, counselor, or social worker are anticipated.

The development of effective coping strategies is a long-term goal. Depending on the maturity and resources of each patient, developing such strategies may take only a few weeks to as long as several years. Effective coping strategies will be demonstrated by patients meeting necessary obligations, such as keeping health care appointments or court hearings. The effective and appropriate utilization of resources, including professional, social, community, and financial resources, as well as the successful resolution of problems are indications of effective coping skills.

A satisfying lifestyle is a subjective value. Victims of chronic child sexual abuse by a close caregiver may require several years and often intense therapy to reach a level of satisfactory functioning, whereas rape victims who have healthy coping skills may find qualities in themselves that allow for spiritual growth through this painful experience. A useful tool for this evaluation is the Rape Trauma Symptom Rating Scale (see Table 9).

Rape-Trauma Syndrome: Compound Reaction

Within the context of psychiatric and physical diagnoses, maintenance of remission is the successful achievement of the goal. Constant vigilance for signs and symptoms of exacerbation is necessary with immediate therapeutic intervention or referral to prevent complications. As other issues contained in Rape-Trauma Syndrome are addressed and resolved, exacerbation of chronic diseases is less likely to occur as a result of rape trauma.

Rape-Trauma Syndrome: Silent Reaction

Successful resolution of somatic and psychological symptoms, along with the sense of a satisfying life, is a successful outcome for these patients. Tracking progress with the Rape Trauma Symptom Rating Scale may be helpful for evaluation. Victims of child sexual assault frequently have Rape-Trauma Syndrome: Silent Reaction. These patients have deep-seated issues about their self-esteem, trust, boundaries, body image, and relationships with members of the opposite sex. Healing frequently requires intensive therapy.

IX

TABLE 9 Rape Trauma Symptom Rating Scale

	5	4	3	2	1
Sleep disorder	No sleep; awake all night most nights; sleep-deprived state	Severe; 1–3 hours sleep per night; early morning awakening; nightmares	Moderate; difficulty falling asleep; nightmares	Mild; episodic nightmares; broken sleep	Sleeping well
Appetite	Hardly eating at all; prodded by others to eat	Severe; no appetite; eating out of habit	Moderate change; eating less food less frequently	Very little change; not quite as much food intake as before	No noticeable change
Phobias	Succumbed to fear; will not leave home, answer telephone, or talk with nonfamily	Severe; fears dominate life; seeking help; anxiety is immobilizing	Moderate suspicion; some fears expressed; change in lifestyle moderate	Mild suspicion; little change in lifestyle habits	Calm and relaxed
Motor behavior	Uprooting of life (job and home); no activities	Job or home change; reduction in activities; lack of interest, self-control	Restlessness and dissatisfaction with indecisiveness; reduction in activities	Mild restlessness; expressed desire to make changes in work or home life	Calm and relaxed
Relations	Denial of or from SOP(s)*; broken relationship with family, partner, friend	Severe tension, anxiety; relationship(s) disintegrating	Relationship(s) showing stress, nonsupportive, weakened	Relationship(s) intact, strained but supportive	SOP(s)* supportive, understanding, and patient
Self-blame	Overcome with shame; feels cannot forgive self	Severe guilt; blames self, feels dirty, cheap	Moderate guilt; feels responsible	Mild guilt; feels it can be overcome	Free from guilt; accepts event
Self-esteem	Feels worthless or hates self; completely unsatisfied with self	Disgusted with self	Disappointed with self; feels badly about self	Occasionally doubts self-worth	Feels good about self
Somatic reactions	Compounded symptoms directly related to the assault, plus reactivation of symptoms connected to a previous condition (e.g., heavy drinking, drug use)	Severe symptoms; distressing symptoms described, lifestyle disrupted	Moderate symptoms; ability to function but some disturbance of lifestyle	Mild symptoms; minor discomfort reported; ability to talk about discomfort and feeling of control over symptoms	No symptoms; none reported; symptoms denied when asked about a specific area

*SOP = significant other person(s).
Reprinted with permission from DiVasto P: *J Psychosoc Nurs* 23(2):34, 1985.

CASE STUDY WITH PLAN OF CARE

Mrs. R. May is a 66-year-old divorced woman who lives alone. She was raped in her home when she answered the door to an unknown man, who also took her cash, credit cards, jewelry, and keys. The man had said that his car had broken down and that he needed to use a phone, and Mrs. May was lured into a false sense of security. It was daylight and she lived in a safe neighborhood. Immediately after the assault, Mrs. May had the feeling that it wasn't real. She felt extremely ashamed and embarrassed, and she blamed herself for the sexual assault. Mrs. May decided not to tell anyone about the assault and robbery and focused her attention on changing her locks and replacing her credit cards. Gradually, over the next several days, Mrs. May began to experience anxiety and hypervigilance. Every time there was a knock on the door, she felt panic and relived parts of the assault. Her lack of appetite, nausea, stomach discomfort, and sleeplessness finally caused her to make an appointment with her care provider. She did not disclose the rape to anyone at the health care center. The symptoms did not resolve, and an adequate diagnosis could not be reached during the next several months and repeated office visits. During this time, Stacie, the office nurse, noted that Mrs. May appeared to be withdrawn and depressed, did not mention her family, and seemed nervous about examination procedures. In exploring those symptoms together, Mrs. May began to cry. She confided the rape to Stacie. She apologized for allowing the rape to occur by "being so stupid" and for being "so much trouble." Stacie diagnosed Mrs. May as having Rape-Trauma Syndrome: Silent Reaction related to self-blame and intense guilt and shame.

PLAN OF CARE FOR MRS. R. MAY
Nursing Diagnosis: Rape-Trauma Syndrome: Silent Reaction Related to Self-Blame and Intense Guilt and Shame

Expected Outcome: Mrs. May is able to disclose many aspects of the assault and her feelings as a result of the assault.
- Provide unconditional positive regard and acknowledge Mrs. May's feelings.
- Support decisions made as being the best possible under the circumstances.

Expected Outcome: Mrs. May will be able to identify a positive social support network.
- Encourage Mrs. May to contact the woman pastor in her church.
- Discuss daughter's possible reactions to Mrs. May's rape and her potential as support person.
▲ Assist Mrs. May in contacting sexual assault center to obtain advocate and information.
- Explain the importance of support.
▲ Refer her to counseling.

Expected Outcome: Mrs. May will be free of somatic and psychological symptoms.
- Explain Rape-Trauma Syndrome and provide reassurance that Mrs. May's symptoms are normal and that healing will occur.
▲ Work with primary care provider to evaluate specific symptoms and provide appropriate relief.
▲ Refer Mrs. May to counseling.

Expected Outcome: The patient will develop effective coping strategies.
- Assist in identifying actions that will make Mrs. may safer in her home and in public.

Expected Outcome: Mrs. May will resume a satisfying lifestyle.
▲ Refer Mrs. May to counseling.
- Reassure Mrs. May that her feelings are normal and will improve with time and appropriate interventions (i.e., therapy and support).

■ = nursing intervention; ▲ = collaborative intervention.

■ CRITICAL THINKING EXERCISES

1. How were Mrs. May's reactions to the sexual assault consistent with symptoms of Rape-Trauma Syndrome?
2. What qualities exhibited by Stacie, the nurse, enabled the process of identifying Rape-Trauma Syndrome?
3. What might be a reasonable period of time to expect to meet the patient outcome expectations successfully?

REFERENCES

1. Browne A: Family violence and homelessness: the relevance of trauma histories in the lives of homeless women, *Am J Orthopsychiatry* 63(3):370–384, 1993.
2. Burgess AW and Holmstrom LL: The rape victim in the emergency ward, *Am J Nurs* 73(10):1740–1745, 1973.
3. Burgess AW and Holmstrom LL: Crisis and counseling requests of rape victims, *Nurs Res* 23(3):196–202, 1974.
4. Burgess AW and Holmstrom LL: Rape trauma syndrome and post traumatic stress response. In AW Burgess, editor: *Rape and sexual assault,* New York, 1985, Garland Publishing.
5. Burnam MA and others: Sexual assault and mental disorders in a community population, *J Consult Clin Psychol* 56(6):843–850, 1988.
6. Divasto P: Measuring the aftermath of rape, *J Psychosoc Nurs* 85(2):33–35, 1985.
7. Felitti VJ: Long-term medical consequences of incest, rape and molestation, *South Med J* 84(3):328–331, 1991.
8. Foa EB, Riggs DS, and Gershuny A: Arousal, numbing, and intrusion: symptom structure of PTSD following assault, *Am J Psychiatry* 152(1):116–120, 1995.
9. Frazier AF and Borgida E: Rape trauma syndrome: a review of case law and psychological research, *Law Human Behav* 16(3):293–311, 1992.
10. Hickman FCI and others: Gay men as victims of nonconsensual sex, *Arch Sex Behav* 23(3):281–295, 1994.
11. Holmstrom LL and Burgess AW: Assessing trauma in the rape victim, *Am J Nurs* 75(8):1288–1292, 1975.
12. Hulme PA and Grove SK: Symptoms of female survivors of child sexual abuse, *Iss Ment Health Nurs* 15:519–532, 1994.
13. Kim MJ, McFarland GK, and McLane AM: *Pocket guide to nursing diagnosis,* ed 3, St. Louis, 1989, The CV Mosby Co.
14. Kimerling R and Calhoun KS: Somatic symptoms, social support, and treatment seeking among sexual assault victims, *J Consult Clin Psychol* 62(2):333–340, 1994.
15. Koss MP: Rape: scope, impact, interventions and public policy responses, *Am Psychologist* 48(10):1062–1069, 1993.
16. Koss MP, Heise L, and Russo NF: The global health burden of rape, *Psychol Women Quart* 18(4):509–537, 1994.
17. Koss MP, Koss PG, and Woodruff WJ: Deleterious effects of criminal victimization on women's health and medical utilization, *Arch Int Med* 151:342–348, 1991.
18. Ledray LE and Arndt S: Sexual assault victim: a new model for nursing care, *J Psychosoc Nurs* 32(2):7–12, 1994.
19. Lipscomb GH and others: Male victims of sexual assault, *JAMA* 267(22):3064–3066, 1992.
20. Lunde I and Ortmann J: Prevalence and sequelae of sexual torture, *Lancet* 336:289–291, 1990.
21. Mackey TF and others: Comparative effects of sexual assault on sexual functioning of child sexual abuse survivors and others, *Iss Ment Health Nurs* 12(1):89–112, 1991.
22. Minden P: The victim care service: a program for victims of sexual assault, *Arch Psychiatr Nurs* 3(1):41–46, 1989.
23. Moss M, Frank E, and Anderson A: The effects of marital status and partner support on rape trauma, *Am J Orthopsychiatry* 60(3):379–391, 1990.
24. Norris FH: Epidemiology of trauma: frequency and impact of different potentially traumatic events on different demographic groups, *J Consult Clin Psychol* 60(3):409–418, 1992.
25. Ruch LO and others: Repeated sexual victimization and trauma change during the acute phase of the sexual assault trauma syndrome, *Women Health* 17(1):1–19, 1991.
26. Swiss S and Giller JE: Rape as a crime of war: a medical perspective, *JAMA* 270(5):612–615, 1993.
27. Vanwesenbeeck I and others: Professional risk taking, levels of victimization, and well-being in female prostitutes in the Netherlands, *Arch Sex Behav* 24(5):503–515, 1995.
28. Wyatt GE, Guthrie D, and Notgrass CM: Differential effects of women's child sexual abuse and subsequent sexual revictimization, *J Consult Clin Psychol* 60(2):167–173, 1992.

Sexual Dysfunction

▶

Altered Sexuality Patterns

▶

Sexual Dysfunction *is the state in which problems with sexual function exist.*

Altered Sexuality Patterns *is the state in which an individual or the individual's partner expresses concern regarding the individual's sexuality.*

OVERVIEW

The term *human sexuality* refers to a part of human life that begins at birth and ends at death. It is intrinsic to our very existence and encompasses biological, psychological, and sociocultural aspects. Sexuality includes all aspects of people that involve being male or female, and it is a dynamic entity that changes over the life span. It is a basic human characteristic and cannot be separated from life events or from health. In every human life, there will be adaptations in the way sexuality is expressed. Adaptations will occur as people grow and change over time, as they interact with different sexual partners, and as they deal with physical and physiological alterations, such as acute or chronic illnesses, injury, disability, or changes related to childbearing.[10,15]

The problems of Sexual Dysfunction may be related to physical illness or psychological influences that cause a limitation in sexual desire and activity and subsequent difficulties in sexual performance, which is viewed as unsatisfying, unrewarding, or inadequate. Physical illness may influence one's sexuality in a systemic way, or it may interfere with neural, vascular, or hormonal components of the sexual response. Psychological influences may be traced to lack of knowledge about sexuality or sexual technique, guilt, anxiety, fear, relationship issues, or a history of sexual abuse.[9,16]

The diagnosis Altered Sexuality Patterns is multidimensional. Concerns regarding sexuality can be present at any point along the continuum from wellness to illness and may occur in conjunction with or independent of Sexual Dysfunction.

The diagnoses Sexual Dysfunction and Altered Sexuality Patterns are separate and distinct. However, the central theme of sexuality provides a similar basis for these diagnoses. Some overlapping of content is inevitable, especially in the areas of definition and assessment and, to an even greater degree, interventions, patient outcomes, and evaluation. This chapter will address both diagnoses, discuss their shared content as well as pointing out the uniqueness of each individual diagnosis.

The terms *gender identity* and *sex role* can be defined as one's internal sense of being male or female or the way we disclose ourselves to others as men or women. It is the conviction that one feels a part of the male or the female sex group. This concept of gender identity is thought to be developed through experience and implicit instruction.

The change in sexual performance that occurs in Sexual Dysfunction is that sex is viewed as unsatisfying, unrewarding, or inadequate. This loss or impairment may be devastating to the person for whom their ability to express sexuality is highly valued. The person who has experienced a biophysical crisis, such as surgical disfigurement or sexual assault, may also undergo a psychosocial crisis as well because that person may have to deal with a change in relationship, an altered body image, or a change in lifestyle. Sterilization, infertility, or a hysterectomy may affect a person's sense of worth as a sexual being. A person's inability to perform sexually can also create a crisis.

Sexual Dysfunction might be compared with sexual difficulties in that the latter results in occasional interference with sexual function, discomfort in the sexual relationship, and disinterest in sexual activity. whereas the former results in disruption of sexual function and severely strains the sexual relationship or sexual self-image. Sexual Dysfunction can usually be divided into three categories: disorders of sexual desire, disorders of arousal, and disorders of orgasm. Sex therapy is the most effective to treat Sexual Dysfunction.[1,2]

Altered Sexuality Patterns covers a wide range of defining characteristics and risk factors. A person's adaptation to these occurrences depends on the type of alteration, the meaning of the change to the patient, the patient's coping ability, and the response of his or her significant other. Each of these factors will influence the extent to which the alteration affects the patient's sexual satisfaction.

Persons may seek values clarification in hopes of relieving guilt or concerns about their sexuality. Teenagers and often adults exhibit a knowledge deficit regarding information or skills related to sexuality. Other problems perceived by patients might include a disinterest in sexual activity, inability to please or to be pleased by a partner, and problems in the timing of sexual activities.[5,12]

ASSESSMENT

Appropriate treatment of the patient relies on an accurate assessment. The majority of assessment data will come from the medical history and the sexual history. The nurse should have adequate background knowledge of sexual anatomy and physiology and should have participated in values clarification exercises to assure a level of comfort and competence. The subjective information

obtained by the sexual history is the most helpful in identifying a diagnosis and formulating a care plan. It is essential in this situation that the nurse be aware of his or her own feelings and values regarding sexuality. A nurse who communicates disapproval or is otherwise judgmental may interfere with the entire process of helping the patient. The approaches to obtaining the sexual history are varied and may be adapted according to the type of problem, the skills of the interviewer, and the expressed needs of the patient. It will help to define the patient's expectations and behavior patterns and to identify misconceptions, areas of difficulty, and the need for teaching and counseling.

The process of obtaining the sexual history may be therapeutic in itself. During the interview, the nurse gives permission to the patient to talk freely and openly about sexual concerns and answers some questions, which may provide information to the patient. The nurse may be able to confirm that the patient's concerns are acceptable. The privacy issues related to these diagnoses require special attention to the nurse's interview technique.

Suggesting answers or asking questions in a way that assumes or acknowledges the possibility that the patient has engaged in a particular activity makes it easier for the patient to discuss matters about which he or she might feel guilty or embarrassed. An example of this might be, "Many men have had some homosexual experience in their lifetimes. Have you had any concerns about this activity, Dave?" It is important to use language in a way to facilitate, not inhibit, communication. The use of appropriate terminology can convey professionalism and knowledge. It is important however, to differentiate euphemisms from colloquial language that the patient uses and to adapt to it because correcting the patient may inhibit communication. Positive feedback used effectively lets the patient know that the nurse has heard the information and accepts the patient as a person. The use of positive feedback need not indicate that all behaviors are condoned.

Several different approaches can be used in eliciting the sexual history. Assist the patient in relating information in chronological order. For patients with a diagnosis of Altered Sexuality Patterns, a brief sexual history may be sufficient. Inquire about the patient's current sexual role (e.g., husband) and how the patient feels about himself or herself as a sexual being, and then address concerns directly related to sexual function.

If Sexual Dysfunction is present, a more detailed history of the sexual problem is indicated. This would encompass a description of the problem as perceived by the patient, the patient's ideas about causes of the problem, and what the patient expects from treatment. Additionally, data should be collected and reviewed from the patient's physical findings, medical diagnoses, and mental status. It may also be appropriate to include the patient's sexual partner in the assessment process.

Sexual Dysfunction

Sexual Dysfunction is a common problem affecting most individuals at some point in their lives. Heterosexual and homosexual couples experience dysfunctions with similar causes and defining characteristics. There are differences between men and women in the defining characteristics of Sexual Dysfunction. The cause of this inhibited desire varies widely. Many medications taken by men and women have a negative effect on sexual desire. Also included in this category of related factors are drug and alcohol abuse. A wide range of psychological factors can have a profound effect on the libido; these may include stress (personal stress or stress in the relationship), depressions, anger, performance anxiety, or fear of pain associated with intercourse.

A major defining characteristic in men is impotence, more appropriately referred to as *erectile dysfunction*. The degree to which a man might experience this problem varies widely. Primary erectile dysfunctions arise from physical or emotional problems of sexual development; these are characterized by a man's not being able to achieve or maintain an erection long enough to have intercourse. Secondary erectile dysfunction occurs in a man who has previously functioned successfully. This inability to achieve a satisfactory erection is frequently a source of depression, frustration, and humiliation for the man. The commonly used term *impotence* implies both physical and emotional

failure. Subsequently, this depression and low self-esteem can also be causes of erectile dysfunction, and therefore it may become unclear which problem came first. Causes of erectile dysfunction may at times be unclear, but it is usually possible to differentiate between psychological and organic origins. Consideration of several issues helps identify causative factors: whether there is a complete inability to obtain an erection or the inability to maintain an erection; whether the dysfunction is present at all times or is episodic; whether the onset of the dysfunction is associated with significant life events; and whether the man's sexual desire (libido) is intact. Some of the many organic and psychogenic factors appear in the list of related factors.[2,11,15]

Another common Sexual Dysfunction in men is premature ejaculation. Individual experiences vary, and there is no precise definition, but it is generally accepted to be a loss of control over ejaculation. This may occur before entry or after a few thrusts. (This dysfunction occurs in nearly all men at one time or another, particularly when there has been no sexual activity for a long period of time.) As with erectile problems, increased anxiety about the problem reoccurring during subsequent sexual encounters can be a factor, with premature ejaculation becoming chronic.

One of the more common dysfunctions in women, in addition to inhibited sexual desire, discussed above, is orgasmic dysfunction. Women may be anorgasmic because of multiple factors. Inexperience, lack of information, insufficient stimulation, poor communication with the partner, and patterns established at an early age that interfere with sexual enjoyment are common causes. As with men, high expectations causing "performance anxiety" may lead to increased difficulty in becoming orgasmic.

Dyspareunia occurs in women and is characterized by painful penetration that may occur at any time during intercourse. The description of the pain or discomfort varies, as does its location (from external to vaginal or abdominal), but it is sufficient to create a dysfunctional sexual experience. The cause of dyspareunia is most often organic. One common cause is vaginal dryness or lack of lubrication, which may be the result of inadequate stimu-

IX

lation or hormonal factors, such as decreased estrogen. Other related factors include irritation related to vaginal infections, discomfort from certain contraceptive methods (such as foams, diaphragms, or condoms), or deep pelvic pain from the movement of certain uterine ligaments or from pelvic diseases, such as endometriosis, gonorrhea, or cervicitis. Dyspareunia may infrequently result from complex psychological problems usually associated with fear or anxiety.[7]

■ Defining Characteristics

The presence of the following defining characteristics indicates that the patient may be experiencing Sexual Dysfunction:

- Erectile dysfunction (male)
- Premature ejaculation (male)
- Retarded ejaculation (male)
- Orgasmic dysfunction (female)
- Dyspareunia (female)
- Vaginismus (female)
- Inhibited sexual desire (male and female)
- Alteration in achieving sexual satisfaction (male and female)
- Inability to achieved desired satisfaction (male and female)

■ Related Factors

The following related factors are associated with Sexual Dysfunction:

- Medical or surgical conditions: diabetes, neurological problems, urological problems, diseases causing central thalamic dysfunction, trauma to spinal cord, trauma to genital area
- Alcohol or drug abuse
- Use of prescription medications
- Decreased physiological drive (with aging)
- Lack of vaginal lubrication due to inadequate stimulation or decreased estrogen
- Vaginal infections
- Vaginal irritation
- Deep pelvic pain associated with movement of uterine ligaments, endometriosis, gonorrhea, or cervicitis
- Stress in general
- Stress in relationship

- Depression
- Anger
- Guilt
- Performance anxiety
- Fear of pain associated with intercourse
- Patterns established early in life that interfere with sexual enjoyment
- Poor communication with partner
- Lack of information
- Inexperience
- Immaturity (e.g., adolescence)

Altered Sexuality Patterns

The diagnosis Altered Sexuality Patterns encompasses all conditions or situations in which an individual expresses concern regarding his or her sexuality or in which there is a change in sexual behavior or activities. This diagnosis always occurs when Sexual Dysfunction is present but may also occur independently. There is wide variation in the degree to which a person can be affected and in the manifestations of the altered pattern(s).

Factors related to the diagnosis Altered Sexuality Patterns can be grouped into two categories—those of psychosocial or environmental origin and those relating to a lack of knowledge about appropriate responses to health-related transitions, changes in body function or structure, illness, or a prescribed medical treatment. Psychosocial or environmental factors may include lack of privacy, lack or absence of a significant other, poor communication with the sexual partner, conflicts with sexual orientation or variant preferences, or ineffective or absent role models. Health-related transitions that necessitate an adaptation may be normal life events, such as pregnancy and childbirth or menopause. Although these may be "normal" life events, a lack of knowledge may make it difficult to achieve a satisfactory adaptation, resulting in concern about sexual issues.

The presence of a developmental, physical, or mental disability can raise concerns regarding sexual behavior. This can be a lifelong issue, as when a disability exists from birth, or it can emerge at any stage of life, after an injury or disability occurs. Of course, these concerns may be present whether or not the disability or injury directly involves the sexual or reproductive organs. When there is a disability, one must deal with sexual concerns caused by physical problems that impose limits on movement and sensation, concerns that arise from lack of information, and concerns that arise from limits imposed by society.

Certain medical conditions can, by virtue of their physiological consequences to all body systems, cause one to experience Altered Sexuality Patterns. The disease process and the treatment have the potential of disrupting sexual patterns because of physiological changes or tissue injury. Body image changes are viewed as incompatible with maintaining a sexual relationship. Various therapies and drug treatments may also interfere with the ability to function sexually. Illness-related anxiety causes a decrease in the sex drive and sexual response, as does depression or grief. Illness may also cause physical separation from one's sexual partner.[14,16]

Cardiovascular disease, like many other chronic illnesses, has the ability to affect patterns of sexuality as well as most other facets of daily living. Patients who experience a myocardial infarction frequently express concern about their sexuality. Resumption of sexual activity after a coronary episode is influenced significantly by the presence of cardiovascular symptoms and fears of sudden death.[4,8]

In a long-term illness, such as chronic renal disease, psychosocial issues, including changes in sexual patterns, become critical concerns. Progressive deterioration occurs that affects all body systems. This deterioration, plus anxiety and a change in body image, cause sexual desire and functioning to diminish. Frequently there is a decrease in sex drive or performance related to uremia, which causes lethargy, listlessness, and peripheral neuropathy.

Research studies indicate that diabetic men have a higher incidence of Sexual Dysfunction than nondiabetic men. However, it should not be assumed that all of the sexual concerns reported in diabetes are organic. Such factors as use of certain medications, alcohol abuse, or poor control of the diabetes may create changes in sexual patterns. Diabetic men may experience erectile dysfunc-

tion, which is thought to be neurological in origin. Women report sexual problems and concerns related to first-stage arousal and vaginal lubrication that are sometimes additionally complicated by the presence of vaginitis.[6,13,17,20]

The physical consequences of sexually transmitted disease (e.g., vaginitis, cervicitis, lower abdominal pain, skin or mucous membrane lesions, or acquired immunodeficiency syndrome) interfere with sexual functioning. Prescribed treatments may also alter patterns of sexuality in that they may necessitate abstinence for a period of time. Emotional factors, such as feelings of guilt, shame, or stigma, also cause changes in previously established patterns of sexual expression.[16]

■ Defining Characteristics

The presence of the following defining characteristics indicates that the patient may be experiencing Altered Sexuality Patterns:

- Change in sexual behaviors or activities
- Verbal expression of concern regarding sexual behavior or activities

■ Related Factors

The following related factors are associated with Altered Sexuality Patterns:

- Medical conditions (e.g., diabetes, cardiac disease, renal disease, cancer, or sexually transmitted disease, such as acquired immunodeficiency syndrome)
- Trauma (e.g., sexual assault)
- Disability (e.g., developmental, physical, mental, or emotional)
- Childbearing (e.g., infertility, pregnancy, childbirth, postpartum period, lactation, contraception, and abortion)
- Knowledge deficit or skill deficit related to alternative responses to health-related transitions, altered body functions or structure, illness, or medical treatment
- Ineffective or absent role models
- Conflicts with sexual orientation or variant preferences
- Poor communication with partner
- Impaired relationship with significant other

- Lack or absence of significant other
- Lack of privacy

DIAGNOSIS

■ Differential Nursing Diagnosis

In these two diagnoses, perhaps more than most others, there is almost always a component of physical and psychological causes as well as symptoms. Frequently one symptom will be more apparent to the observer (the nurse) than the other. For example, Sexual Dysfunction and Altered Sexuality Patterns may appear as anxiety, depression, or ineffective family coping, as in instances when the sexual problem becomes a relationship problem. A thorough and accurate sexual history is the key tool to differentiate these diagnoses and plan appropriate interventions. The sexual history will also aid in distinguishing between a sexual alteration and a medical condition, such as a urological or gynecological problem.

■ Medical and Psychiatric Diagnoses

There are many medical and psychiatric diagnoses that are closely related to the nursing diagnoses Sexual Dysfunction and Altered Sexuality Patterns. In fact, it may be the nursing team members who first identify concerns of a sexual nature in patients with disease processes such as diabetes, cardiac disease, and neurological disorders. More apparent are sexually transmitted disease. The primary practitioner should include the sexual history assessment tool as part of the diagnostic process. Depression and anxiety are too often underdiagnosed and therefore go untreated. The sexual problems associated with these diagnoses are frequently seen as contributing factors to the depression or anxiety and are not recognized as possible symptoms of the underlying psychiatric illness.

OUTCOME IDENTIFICATION, PLANNING, AND IMPLEMENTATION

There are many types of nursing roles within the area of sexual health. Depending on the educational background and the skills of the nurse, there are opportunities to provide for the sexual health care needs of patients in multiple settings and situations. Patients may range from individuals to groups to communities and in home-, hospital-, or community-based settings.

The sexual health assessment initiates the process of helping the patient with his or her potential or actual expressed need. Patients with Sexual Dysfunction and Altered Sexuality Patterns may not directly seek help for their sexual problems. They may instead divulge their concerns during the sexuality portion of a more general health assessment.

There are many roles at different levels that enable nurses to assist patients with problems of sexual health. One of the most frequent interventions is education, or providing information. After the assessment process is complete, and based on the patient's needs, the nurse may intervene with appropriate information. Many patients benefit from basic knowledge of anatomy, physiology, and the sexual response cycle. The childbearing experience offers many opportunities for teaching women about their bodies and the changes that they experience during pregnancy, labor and delivery, and lactation. This is also an excellent time to get women to talk about how they feel about their bodies and to give them information regarding expressions of sexuality during this time. Teenagers need teaching and anticipatory guidance with regard to healthy sexuality, reproduction, contraception choices, and sexually transmitted disease. Certain prescription drugs are known to cause sexual changes in many people. Teaching should be done to ensure that these patients will be aware of these potential side effects and how they may affect their lives.

Another major role for nurses is counseling patients in regard to their sexuality. Counseling is the process of creating an atmosphere where the patient can feel comfortable and can express his or her thoughts and feelings openly. With the help of the nurse-counselor the patient can clarify the sexual problem and, one hopes, change the situation to reach a greater level of satisfaction. Sexual counseling may be for an individual or for a couple. Persons with Sexual Dysfunction and Altered Sexuality Patterns benefit from counseling in many situations. An example is a patient recovering from a myocardial infarction who becomes fearful of having intercourse. Discussing the situation with the nurse-counselor and acting on suggestions offered over a period of time, the patient would gradually decrease his or her anxieties and relax so that he or she could enjoy sexual intimacy while observing for the warning signs of cardiac stress.

Validating that the patient and the patient's sexual behavior are "normal" is an important role that the nurse can play. This may seem obvious, but many people wonder if their activities (e.g., masturbation or oral-genital sex) or even their fantasies are "perverted" or "dirty," and when a patient is able to open up to a health professional, it may be that the patient is merely seeking validation of what is acceptable. In allowing this and in ensuring the privacy and confidentiality that was displayed during the assessment process, the nurse becomes a patient advocate. It is the responsibility of the nurse to encourage patients to participate in decision making regarding their treatment plans and to support these decisions. By exhibiting a nonjudgmental and professional attitude, the nurse maintain the patient's dignity.

Nurses, as members of the health care team, may act as a referral source for patients with sexual problems. Referrals may include support or self-help groups, educational resources, or other professionals.

Occasionally nurses seek additional educational and clinical preparation and become sex therapists. These professionals offer intensive specialized therapy to patients with Sexual Dysfunction or Altered Sexuality Patterns.

◢ NURSING CARE GUIDELINES
Nursing Diagnosis: Sexual Dysfunction

Expected Outcome: The patient will seek and obtain appropriate medical or nursing intervention.
- Complete sexual history assessment.
- Make appropriate referrals for patients exhibiting any actual or potential condition that requires medical intervention.
- Assess and monitor the patient's and partner's level of knowledge and understanding of his or her dysfunction(s).

Expected Outcome: The patient will have increased knowledge and understanding of factors related to dysfunction(s) experienced.
- Provide the patient (and partner, when appropriate) with accurate information to increase the level of awareness.

Expected Outcome: The patient will exhibit behavior change that will result in more satisfying sexual function.
- Provide the patient with a safe, nonjudgmental atmosphere.
- Offer the patient (the couple) the opportunity for clarification of feelings concerning sexuality.
- Offer specific suggestions, when appropriate, for alteration in sexual activities that might result in elimination or reduction of dysfunction.

Expected Outcome: The patient will maintain a sense of personal dignity, and the patient's concerns regarding his or her sexuality will be alleviated.
- Provide the patient (the couple) with privacy and maintain confidentiality.
- Involve the patient (the couple) in decisions about plan of care.
- Validate the patient's feelings of normalcy.

■ = nursing intervention; ▲ = collaborative intervention.

IX

◢ NURSING CARE GUIDELINES
Nursing Diagnosis: Altered Sexuality Patterns

Expected Outcome: The patient (or couple) will seek and obtain appropriate counseling and intervention.
- Complete sexual history assessment.
- Make appropriate referrals for patients exhibiting any actual or potential condition that requires medical intervention.
- Assess and monitor the patient's and the partner's level of knowledge and understanding of his or her alteration in sexuality.

Expected Outcome: The patient will have increased knowledge and understanding of factors related to his or her Altered Sexuality Patterns.
- Provide the patient (and partner, when appropriate) with accurate information to increase the level of awareness.

Expected Outcome: The patient will exhibit behavior changes that will result in more satisfying sexual patterns of expressing sexuality.
- Provide the patient with a safe, nonjudgmental atmosphere.
- Offer the patient (or couple) opportunities for clarification of feelings concerning sexuality.
- Offer specific suggestions, when appropriate, for alteration in sexual activities that might result in greater satisfaction for patient or couple.

Expected Outcome: The patient will maintain a sense of personal dignity, and the patient's concerns regarding his or her sexuality will be alleviated.
- Provide the patient (or couple) with privacy and maintain confidentiality.
- Involve the patient (or couple) in decisions about plan of care.
- Validate the patient's feelings of normalcy.

■ = nursing intervention; ▲ = collaborative intervention.

EVALUATION

The effectiveness of the specified nursing interventions will depend on the patient's ability and willingness to accept the guidance and information provided. The time required to achieve the identified outcomes depends on the contributing or related factors and will vary for each patient. An ongoing assessment of the patient's progress will assist in evaluating the patient's response to a particular intervention (e.g., the provision of general information on sexual function) and provide data to guide the implementation of other interventions (e.g., specific suggestions for altering sexual activities).

◢ CASE STUDY WITH PLAN OF CARE

Mr. Theodore G. has recently been diagnosed with prostate cancer. Ted is a 57-year-old black male who has been married to Linda G. for 32 years. Ted owned a profitable dry cleaning business, which he sold last year. Ted and Linda had extensive plans to travel around the United States now that their son, Ted, Jr., had finished college and law school. All of this seemed to become insignificant when faced with the fact that Ted would be undergoing a radical prostatectomy followed by external-beam radiation therapy. During his preoperative admission testing, Linda G. had an opportunity to talk with Sara B., the urological clinical nurse specialist. Linda voiced her concerns about the future of Ted's sexual capabilities. They have always had a very fulfilling romantic relationship, and it has been a source of masculine validation and satisfaction for Ted. She worries about the psychological implications that impotence (erectile dysfunction) will have on Ted. Sarah set up a time to talk with Ted and Linda together about this issue, and she developed the following plan of care.

► PLAN OF CARE FOR MR. TED G.
Nursing Diagnosis: Sexual Dysfunction Related to Treatment for Prostate Cancer

Expected Outcome: Mr. and Mrs. G. will understand factors related to Sexual Dysfunction following treatment for prostate cancer by the time of the first postoperative visit.
- Conduct a thorough sexual assessment of Mr. G. individually and of Mr. and Mrs. G. as a couple.
- Provide the couple with accurate information regarding actual and potential sequelae of prostate cancer and the type of treatment Mr. G. will receive.

Expected Outcome: Mr. and Mrs. G. will understand options for sexual restoration following treatment for cancer before the end of the radiation therapy program.
- Provide Mr. and Mrs. G. with information and resources related to postoperative restorative options, such as penile prosthetic devices.

Expected Outcome: Mr. and Mrs. G. will achieve a high level of intimacy and sexual satisfaction through a successful sex therapy program within 6 months following the end of treatment for prostate cancer.
- Refer the couple to a counselor or therapist who can assist them in working through their feelings and frustrations related to this problem.
- Counsel the couple about exploring ways of achieving sexual intimacy through means other than intercourse.

■ = nursing intervention; ▲ = collaborative intervention.

► CASE STUDY WITH PLAN OF CARE

Judy F., age 47, is an attorney for a large corporation and works 50 to 60 hours per week. She has been married to Rob M. for 18 years, and they have a 10-year-old son. In spite of her busy work schedule, Judy plans her time to attend school and sports events that are important to her son, and she and Rob continue to have a romantic relationship, making time for private evenings several times a month. Judy has always had a very regular menstrual cycle and successfully planned her pregnancy for the time when her career was well established. She exercises regularly, eats a healthy vegetarian diet, and does not smoke or drink alcohol. Over the past 6 months, Judy has noticed her periods becoming irregular and sometimes heavier or lighter than she is used to. More recently, she has been experiencing night sweats and at times, even when she is very aroused, experiences vaginal dryness, which has interfered with the couple's lovemaking. She has consulted her gynecological nurse practitioner.

► PLAN OF CARE FOR MS. JUDY F.
Nursing Diagnosis: Altered Sexuality Patterns Related to Menopause

Expected Outcome: Judy will understand what menopause is and what it means, and she will explore her feelings related to this phase of her life within a mutually agreed upon time frame, related to counseling sessions.
- Provide Judy with literature and information on menopause.
- Refer her to a counselor who can help her deal with this unexpected (by her) new phase in her life.

Expected Outcome: Judy will make informed choices related to options, such as estrogen replacement therapy, within the next 6 months or as her symptoms progress.
- Provide Judy with information on treatment options, including hormone therapy, and the pros and cons of each option.

■ = nursing intervention; ▲ = collaborative intervention.   *Continued*

▛ PLAN OF CARE FOR MS. JUDY F. — CONT'D

Expected Outcome: Judy and Rob will explore ways of dealing with factors such as vaginal dryness, night sweats, and other physical symptoms that interfere with their intimacy.
- Conduct a physical examination to determine other causes for vaginal dryness.
- If none, provide information on options such as artificial lubricants, and suggest ways other than actual intercourse to achieve sexual intimacy.

▦ CRITICAL THINKING EXERCISES

1. Identify important factors and approaches in obtaining a sexual history. What factors or approaches would be used in the sexual assessment of Mr. and Mrs. G.?
2. Compare and contrast Sexual Dysfunction in men and women.
3. What information sources and content on menopause might be helpful to Judy F.?

REFERENCES

1. Ackerman MD: Consultation with clinical urology: expanded roles for health psychologists, *Health Psychologist* 4(1):3–4, 1992.
2. Ackerman MD, Montague DK, and Morganstern S: Impotence: help for erectile dysfunction, *Patient Care* 28(5):22–25, 29–30, 332, 1994.
3. American Cancer Society: *Cancer facts and figures,* Atlanta, 1993, The Society.
4. Beach EK and others: The spouse: a factor in recovery after acute myocardial infarction, *Heart Lung* 21(1):30–38, 1992.
5. Chambas K: Sexual concerns of adolescents with cancer, *J Pediatr Oncol Nurs* 8(4):165–172, 1991.
6. Frank D and Lang A: Disturbances in sexual role performace of chronic alcoholics: an analysis using Roy's adaptation model, *Iss Ment Health Nurs* 11:243, 1990.
7. Glatt A and others: The prevalence of dyspareunia, *Obstet Gynecol* 75:433, 1990.
8. Hamilton GA and Seidman RN: A comparison of the recovery period for women and men after an acute myocardial infarction, *Heart Lung* 22(4):308–315, 1993.
9. Kim M, McFarland G, and McLane A: *Pocket guide to nursing diagnoses,* ed 6, St. Louis, 1995, Mosby–Year Book.
10. LeMone P: Human sexuality in adults with insulin-dependent diabetes mellitus, *Image: J Nurs Scholarship* 25(2):101–105, 1993.
11. Morganstern B and Abrahams A: *The prostate sourcebook: managing problems with man's most troubled gland,* Los Angeles, 1993, Lowell House.
12. Plumbo MA: Clinical intervention framework for a sexual complaint of the perimenopause, *J Nurse-Midwif* 39(3):157–160, 1994.
13. Slob AK and others: Sexuality and psychophysiological functioning in women with diabetes mellitus, *J Sex Mar Ther* 16:59–69, 1994.
14. Taylor P: Beating the taboo . . . stoma and sexual difficulty, *Nurs Times* 90(13):51–53, 1994.
15. Waxman ES: Sexual dysfunction following treatment for prostate cancer: nursing assessment and interventions, *Oncol Nurs Forum* 20(10):1567–1571, 1993.
16. Wood N: *Human sexuality in health and illness,* ed 3, St. Louis, 1984, The CV Mosby Co.
17. Young EW, Koch PB, and Bailey C: Research comparing the dyadic adjustment and sexual functioning concerns of diabetic and nondiabetic women, *Health Care Women Int* 10:377–394, 1989.

IX

COPING—STRESS-TOLERANCE PATTERN

Impaired Adjustment

▶

Impaired Adjustment *is the state in which an individual is unable to modify his or her lifestyle or behavior in a manner consistent with a change in health status.*[6]

OVERVIEW

The nursing diagnosis Impaired Adjustment is seen in all clinical areas of nursing. It is important to note that this diagnosis is classified by NANDA under "Choosing" in the Taxonomy of Nursing Diagnoses.[6] The nurse should recognize that Impaired Adjustment does not occur because the patient cannot adjust or because the patient does not perceive a change in health status that results in a limitation. Rather, the individual "chooses" not to acknowledge the modifications necessary to deal with the limitations accompanying the health condition. Ignoring the consequences of the disability denotes a refusal to accept a change in health status, limiting to various degrees the activities of daily living and lifestyle. Therefore the individual behaves inconsistently with ability.

People with health limitations have always been a segment of the population in all societies. Disability transcends age, sex, race, and socioeconomic status. Folk tales and classical literary works contain many characters who are lame, blind, or frail. Western medical and nursing literature lists an abundance of conditions, illnesses, and diseases that result in impairment. *Disability* can be defined as an impairment that interferes with a person's ability to engage successfully in activities of daily living, such as walking, dressing, hearing, or seeing. Because people live longer

and because more infants with low birth weight survive, there is an increased chance of developing a disability.[7]

Although much of nursing involves healing the patient, another important aspect is assisting the patient in adjustment to limitations. Therefore rehabilitation is a vital component of nursing action. Unfortunately, adjustment to a change in health status sometimes does not occur. After evaluation, if the nurse decides that rehabilitation has not been successful, one possible explanation is that the patient's adjustment is impaired. To understand Impaired Adjustment, the nurse might refer to several theories that relate to this diagnosis. The main concepts to be considered are change, motivation, self-esteem, and locus of control, as well as the role of social support.

Change inherently causes some type of adjustment. Change is everywhere, and all human beings are exposed to its many forms during various times in life. People die and others are born; some get sick and some get well. But sometimes people do not get well. When individuals fail to regain their previous level of health, adjustments to the new level are necessary. In other words, the person must change. Essential to change is that the patient must acknowledge the problem and the need for change to overcome the problem. Many factors are involved in change. When seeking to identify the barriers that inhibit successful change, the nurse should attempt to discover problem areas that may be hindering a patient's adjustment (e.g., problems in trust, lack of family or group support, and goals that are unrealistic or incongruent with those of health care providers).

Lack of motivation can influence a person's reluctance to change. The relationship between change and motivation is frequently stressed by theorists and clinicians. Maslow, whose work focused on the motivational aspects of human behavior, theorized that an individual's activity or inactivity resulted from a personal hierarchy of needs.[4] If a need is not satisfied, then a person attempts to change that which blocks the fulfillment of the need. An example of this is the impairment of the need for self-actualization because of an illness that prevents independent function. In this situation, the individual will attempt to meet the need in other ways, such as minimizing the illness or overcompensating in other aspects of functioning. Frequently, highly motivated individuals treat disabilities with impatience, frustration, and sometimes depression. Moneyham and Scall note that the illness is frequently perceived as blocking fulfillment in various spheres of life, and many patients are concerned about the loss of control of their lives and the threat to their ability to live normally.[5] Many times the actual change does not upset the person, but the perceived limitation does. Weinstein, when describing the behaviors resulting from the patient's distress over limitations, includes (1) ignoring symptoms, (2) not taking prescribed medications, and (3) hoping that symptoms would just disappear without treatment.[8] All of these behaviors hinder successful adjustment. Like most dynamics of human behavior, motivation can be conscious and unconscious.

Conscious and unconscious aspects also influence a person's self-esteem, which is involved in Impaired Adjustment. Esteem is one of Maslow's broad categories of needs. Therefore, when real or perceived assaults occur that lower self-esteem, such as a condition that limits the person, the individual attempts to control that which inhibits the resolution of the need. In other words, self-esteem influences adjustment. Self-esteem has been defined and explained by many theories. Psychoanalytical, interpersonal, transactional, and existential schools of thought all provide concepts and ideas about the development of an individual's view of him- or herself. The nurse must recognize that self-esteem is highly complex component of

human beings and may influence attitudes toward recovery.

Locus of control is another complex concept related to an individual's adjustment to limitations. This theory also stresses perception as more important than real or actual consequences. In locus-of-control theory, the individual attributes his or her own performance and life situation to factors from within or factors outside of the self. Therefore, if people have an internal locus of control, they believe that they themselves are in control. If they have an external locus of control, they think and feel that outside forces, such as other people, are mainly responsible for what happens to them. Generally people have some but not complete control in coping with disabilities.[5]

Social support, especially from the family, influences success in adjustment. Bull and Jervis acknowledge that family, including a family's strength and effectiveness in coping, affects how people adjust to limiting conditions.[2] A family can provide a stable and loving atmosphere where individuals can accept health status changes and move toward independence. On the other hand, the family atmosphere can be such that illnesses and limitations are threatening because the family itself is unstable.

The reasons some people choose to adjust to the limitations accompanying a change in health status and others choose not to adjust remains a complex and not especially well-defined phenomenon. In summary, factors such as motivation, perception of threat to self-esteem, locus of control, and support systems all affect whether or not an individual adjusts. As with beauty, loss is in the eye of the beholder, and perceived loss can be more critical than actual loss. An understanding of the concepts relevant to Impaired Adjustment assists the nurse in understanding these patients, but caring for a person with a nursing diagnosis of Impaired Adjustment remains a challenge.

ASSESSMENT

Impaired Adjustment can be seen in all clinical nursing areas. It can occur in patients with heart and lung diseases, orthopedic conditions, complications of infectious illnesses, birth defects, diabetes, and chronic mental illnesses. These are just a few of a long list of conditions that may interfere with activities of daily living. Although most patients with a nursing diagnosis of Impaired Adjustment display physical limitations, the defining characteristics and related factors primarily focus on patients' psychological states.[6] Therefore the nursing actions focus on psychological factors, with consideration of selected social aspects.

Before assessing the patient, the nurse must assess his or her own feelings because these patients may resist interventions, causing the nurse to feel angry, frustrated, and helpless. In a clinical study, Carveth found that patients who were perceived to be difficult by nurses received lower quality care.[3] These patients may contend that they "know better" than the health care personnel and then exhibit behavior that negates or belies their knowledge. For example, a nurse works for more than an hour with a diabetic patient regarding diet, and the patient then says, "I know that diabetics should limit the amount of fat and refined sugar in their diets, but I'll probably be able to have a lot if I just figure out how to do it." The nurse feels as though the patient has not listened to a word during the patient education sessions. These patients often say, "Yes, but . . . ," which indicates that they understand what has been said but choose not to apply it to themselves. For instance, many patients with heart problems still smoke, although they are aware of the adverse affects of smoking.

In assessing a person for the diagnosis Impaired Adjustment, the nurse should be aware of factors related to change, motivation, self-esteem, and locus of control. Of special importance are the patient's verbalization of nonacceptance of health status change and the lack of involvement in solving problems or setting goals. The nurse can identify both of these areas through keen observation, careful questioning, and astute listening. For instance, a nurse observes nonverbal indications that a patient with arthritis might be having difficulty accepting a change in health status. In this case, the nurse could begin a conversation with a comment such as, "I noticed that you didn't seem to agree with your doctor when she was talking about your needing to exercise more. I'm wondering why." To assess the patient's ability to solve problems or set goals, the nurse might ask, "What do you see as the problems caused by your arthritis?" followed by "And how do you see these problems being handled?" Another method of obtaining this information would be to inquire about the patient's long- and short-term plans and goals regarding the specific limitations.

The latter strategy also addresses the lack of future-oriented thinking. To discover whether the person is suffering from an extended period of shock, disbelief, or anger regarding the limitation, the nurse should ask questions such as, "How do you feel about your condition?" or "How do you think these limitations will affect your future?" A lack of movement toward independence can be determined through questions about perceived limitations and strengths as well as a careful observation of the performance of activities of daily living.

For a thorough assessment, follow-up questions should be asked of the patient and family. Other staff members' evaluations of the patient can validate the nurse's hunches and conclusions. Feedback from the patient, family, and other staff members is important in processing the data the nurse has gathered.

■ Defining Characteristics

The presence of the following defining characteristics indicates that the patient may be experiencing Impaired Adjustment:

- Verbalization of nonacceptance of health status change
- Extended period of shock, disbelief, or anger regarding limitations
- Nonexistent or unsuccessful involvement in problem solving or goal setting
- Lack of progress toward independence
- Lack of future-oriented thinking

■ Related Factors

The following related factors are associated with Impaired Adjustment:

- Disability requiring changes in lifestyle

- Sensory overload
- Altered focus of control
- Incomplete grieving
- Impaired cognition
- Lack of motivation
- Low self-esteem
- Inadequate support systems

DIAGNOSIS

■ Differential Nursing Diagnosis

The diagnosis Impaired Adjustment can be difficult to discern from several other nursing diagnoses (e.g., Ineffective Individual Coping and Ineffective Management of Therapeutic Regimen: Individual). If, however, the clinician returns to the major defining characteristics of Impaired Adjustment (i.e., verbalization of nonacceptance of a change of health status and an inability to be involved in problem solving), then it becomes easier to determine the diagnosis. To make the diagnosis Impaired Adjustment, the nurse must hear the person say or imply that he or she does not accept the changes in health status and must observe the patient's unwillingness to be involved in problem solving.

■ Medical and Psychiatric Diagnoses

There are two broad categories of conditions that may confound identification of the diagnosis Impaired Adjustment. One category consists of physical illness with a sequelae of nonimprovement or limited improvement after treatment. Conditions falling into this category include progressive degenerative problems, such as arthritis and chronic pulmonary obstruction. The other category of conditions relates to the mental or behavioral status of the patient (e.g., affective disorders such as bipolar conditions and substance abuse, including alcoholism). To differentiate, the nurse must be an active team member communicating with physicians, social workers, and physical therapists to discern the underlying reason for the patient's verbalization of nonacceptance of the change in health status and the inability to participate in problem solving.

OUTCOME IDENTIFICATION, PLANNING, AND IMPLEMENTATION

Patient outcomes are specifically related to the defining characteristics of Impaired Adjustment. The long-term goal should focus on modification of the patient's lifestyle to coincide with the change in health status. To reach this goal, specific outcomes must be achieved.

The first outcome relates to the patient's developing an awareness of the change in health status and the demands that the change will place on his or her former lifestyle.[5] This outcome can be achieved by the nurse providing patients with opportunities to discuss the change in health status, the limitations resulting from the health status change, and the identification of those factors that have led to nonacceptance of the changes. Ongoing discussion between the patient and the nurse would reveal whether the outcome has been achieved or not.

The second outcome requires the patient to take an active role in identifying short-term goals that must be achieved to adapt his or her lifestyle to the change in health status.[1] This outcome can be addressed by the patient's identification of ways to take an active role in goal setting. This would include seeking ways to remedy those factors that have led to nonacceptance of mutual goal planning. The success of this outcome is measured by the patient listing specific short-term goals. Long-term evidence of success related to this outcome would be a patient-initiated approach to problem-solving activities.

The third outcome involves the patient's use of new strategies for coping with the change and for implementing a new lifestyle.[7] This outcome can be achieved by using problem-solving strategies. These strategies are addressed in more detail in the Nursing Care Guidelines. Evidence of success can be gleaned from conversations with the family and other health care team members that relate to identification and implementation of coping strategies that support adjustment to the change in lifestyle.

The nurse must bear in mind that the general nursing plan of care for persons with Impaired Adjustment focuses on the specific assessment findings. Theory provides the rationale for all stages of the nursing process. The use of information on change, motivation, self-esteem, locus of control, and support systems should direct nursing plans and interventions.

The care plan must be individualized for each patient through consideration of the effect that specific related factors have on the patient's physiological and psychosocial responses to the situation. The way in which a disability affects one's lifestyle and ability to cope will differ for each patient. For example, two patients who have arthritis may have severe functional limitations in using their hands and fingers. One of these patients may be an electrician who does fine, intricate work with his hands; the other may be an author who has always used a computer but now must dictate her work and have someone else transcribe it. The first patient's functional disability may threaten his livelihood, and he might seek a new career. The same functional disability creates difficulties and some expense for the second patient, but she can continue to pursue her career. Both of these patients will experience changes in their lifestyles in varying degrees; their usual coping mechanisms may or may not be effective in dealing with the challenges confronting each of them; and the support systems available in the past and the present may or may not be adequate.

Nursing intervention also should be individualized. Some patients might do well with a direct approach, whereas others might need a more indirect and subtle approach.

◢ **NURSING CARE GUIDELINES**

Nursing Diagnosis: Impaired Adjustment

Expected Outcome: The patient will verbalize awareness of changes in health status and their effects on lifestyle by the second home visit.
- Encourage the patient to describe his or her perceived changes in health and his or her feelings about the changes, especially regarding limitations. *Talking about perceptions and feelings can help the patient deal with the reality of the situation.*

Expected Outcome: The patient will take an active role in identifying realistic goals and the means to achieve these goals by the third home visit.
- Support the patient in attempts at goal formulation and problem solving.
- Focus on possible ways the patient can exhibit more independence and less dependence.
- ▲ Assist the patient in identifying others (e.g., family, significant others, and other health care providers) available to offer assistance.
- With the patient, evaluate on a regular basis the progress made in achieving set goals.
- Praise the patient's progress and work with him or her to overcome persistent interference in achieving set goals.
- With the patient, revise the goals as necessary; identify additional short-term goals that will support the patient in achieving long-term goals.
  Supporting the patient throughout the problem-solving process contributes to successful achievement of both short- and long-term goals.

Expected Outcome: The patient will use strategies that will assist him or her in coping with limitations and losses by the fourth home visit.
- Assist the patient in developing a sense of self-confidence by focusing on his or her strengths, abilities, and past achievements.
- Guide the patient in the identification of various coping strategies that he or she can use.

■ = nursing intervention; ▲ = collaborative intervention.

Continued

◢ NURSING CARE GUIDELINES — CONT'D

- Support the patient in the identification of ways in which he or she can schedule activities that allow for optimal participation.
- Assist the patient in initiating activities from which he or she can gain satisfaction.
- Encourage the patient to accept the assistance of family, significant others, and other health care providers as needed.
  Guiding the patient as he or she initiates strategies and engages in activities provides opportunities for immediate feedback and, if necessary, allows for a revision of the plan to assure success.

EVALUATION

In caring for patients with a nursing diagnosis of Impaired Adjustment, one would assume that the long-term goal is that the patient becomes better adjusted to the limitations arising from the changes in his or her health status. *Better* is a subjective word, but it does not connote movement toward a goal, which, for patients diagnosed with Impaired Adjustment, is to experience less impairment and more adjustment. The family's reaction must also be considered. Success may be measured by positive actions or fewer negative behaviors. The nurse must decide ahead of time the measures of success specific to each patient. Thus the patient outcomes and nursing interventions will be tailored to each patient.

▶ CASE STUDY WITH PLAN OF CARE

Mrs. Beverly R. is a 61-year-old home health patient who has had a stroke that has primarily affected her balance and walking. While in the hospital she fell several times getting out of bed to go to the bathroom. The hospital staff, including her primary nurse and physician, made several requests that she not get out of bed without a staff member present, but each time she laughed and said, "Well, you won't be around to help me next week, so I'm just practicing on my own. Soon I'll be as good as new." The hospital staff thought that her goal of being as "good as new" was unrealistic, yet they did not want to discourage her enthusiasm and her optimism about recovering. Although Mrs. R. had not injured herself, the staff expressed concern that she did not seem aware of her limitations, even though the dangers of overreaching her ability were explained to her. Mrs. R. was discharged to her home. According to the discharge notes, she had made excellent physical progress. She will begin attending physical therapy sessions as an outpatient at the end of the week. During the first home visit, the day after Mrs. R.'s discharge, the nurse noted that Mrs. R. was pleasant and cooperative but had not accepted her health limitations and how they affect her usual activities. Mrs. R.'s two daughters were present during the visit; they expressed concern that they cannot be available to her 24 hours a day because of their responsibilities for their own children.

▶ PLAN OF CARE FOR MRS. BEVERLY R.
Nursing Diagnosis: Impaired Adjustment Related to Mrs. R.'s Disability that Requires Changes in Her Lifestyle and Activities

Expected Outcome: Mrs. R. will verbalize her strengths and limitations and identify appropriate support systems to aid in her rehabilitation by the end of the first home visit.
- With Mrs. R. and her daughters, discuss her strengths and limitations as they relate to her disability and usual activities.

■ = nursing intervention; ▲ = collaborative intervention.

- Explore with Mrs. R. the limitations that she may have difficulty accepting and the reasons for such difficulty.
- Engage Mrs. R. in a discussion about things that she can and cannot control; have Mrs. R. make a list of these things.
▲ Discuss available support services, and provide Mrs. R. and her daughters information on services she might use (e.g., daily homemaking services or a home health aide two or three times a week to assist Mrs. R. with bathing).
- Discuss with Mrs. R. and her daughters possible schedules for the daughters to visit, and offer assistance in transporting Mrs. R. to physical therapy sessions and other activities Mrs. R. would like to participate in.
- Arrange with Mrs.. R. a mutually acceptable time for visits once a week over the next month.

Expected Outcome: Mrs. R. will take an active role in identifying personal goals and the means to achieve these goals by the second home visit.
- Explore realistic expectations with Mrs. R., her daughters, and the home health aide.
- With Mrs. R., list specific long- and short-term goals with appropriate means to achieve the identified goals.
- Have Mrs. R. identify target dates for achieving these goals.

Expected Outcome: Mrs. R. will focus on her strengths to overcome feelings of frustration and distress over things she cannot control by the second home visit.
- Discuss with Mrs. R. those things she is able to accomplish, with or without assistance.
- Encourage her to become involved in activities she can engage in with limited assistance (e.g., knitting, reading, and maintaining phone contact with friends).

Expected Outcome: Mrs. R. will continue to attempt independent activity with appropriate assistance from staff and family.
▲ Coordinate activities with the home health aide and the family.
- Assess Mrs. R.'s progress in relation to the goals she has established at each home visit.
- Encourage Mrs. R. to revise short-term goals as needed to support realistic achievement of the long-term goals.
▲ Positively reinforce Mrs. R.'s appropriate use of assistance.

■ CRITICAL THINKING EXERCISES

1. Explore your own feelings about people who refuse to take part in their own health planning.
2. What advice would you give Mrs. R. if one morning her home health aide did not appear?
3. How would you support Mrs. R.'s daughters, who express frustration that she tries to do too much?
4. Why must all nursing interventions be documented on the home health record?

REFERENCES

1. Blair C: Combining behavior management and mutual goal setting to reduce physical dependency in nursing home residents, *Nurs Res* 44:160–165, 1995.
2. Bull MJ and Jervis LL: Hospitalized elders: the difficulties families encounter, *J Geront Nurs* 21(6):19–23, 1995.
3. Carveth JA: Perceived patient deviance and avoidance by nurses, *Nurs Res* 44:173–178, 1995.
4. Clark MJ: *Nursing in the community,* Norwalk, Connecticut, 1992, Appleton & Lange.
5. Moneyham L and Scall C: Anticipatory coping in the elderly, *J Geront Nurs* 21(7):23–28, 1995.
6. North American Nursing Diagnosis Association: *NANDA nursing diagnoses: definitions and classification, 1995–1996,* Philadelphia, 1994, The Association.
7. Smith CM and Maurer FA: *Community health nursing: theory and practice,* Philadelphia, 1995, WB Saunders Co.
8. Weinstein A: *Asthma: the complete guide to self-management of asthma and allergies for patients and their families,* New York, 1987, McGraw-Hill.

X

Ineffective Community Coping

▶

Potential for Enhanced Community Coping

▶

Ineffective Community Coping *is a pattern of community activities for adaptation and problem solving that is unsatisfactory for meeting the demands or needs of the community.*

Potential for Enhanced Community Coping *is a pattern of community activities for adaptation and problem solving that is satisfactory for meeting the demands or needs of the community but can be improved for management of current and future problems and stressors.*

OVERVIEW

Even though the concept of community health diagnosis has been discussed for more than 20 years,* specific diagnostic labels had not been articulated before NANDA accepted these diagnoses in 1994. Diagnostic labels for communities are needed so that communities and providers will have systematic and consistent ways of communicating interpretations of community responses to health problems and life processes. Incorporation of these and other community diagnoses in the NANDA Taxonomy enhances knowledge development of community responses. For example, community health nurses in one state (n = 190) had low levels of confidence in caring for ethnically diverse communities, including types of social supports,

use of family and kin supports, and use of social resources.[5] If schools of nursing and community health agencies include community diagnoses in curricula, it will draw attention to gaps in knowledge such as these and will support knowledge development about community phenomena. Coping is an accepted diagnostic concept for individuals and families, making it an appropriate choice for inclusion of community diagnosis in the NANDA Taxonomy.

Generally, the term *community* has referred to (1) designated geographic areas (e.g., political districts or towns), (2) specific locations with an environmental problem, such as hazardous waste contamination, and (3) special interest groups or aggregates. Jakob proposed, however, that the word *community* be reserved only for geographic areas in which people have a sense of belonging to the community, and the word *population* be used for special interest groups or populations (e.g., persons with HIV).[18] Because of the complexity of community systems and the ambiguity of the term *community,* an operational definition can be developed by asking the questions who, what, why, where, when, and how.[36] Neufeld and Harrison suggest that the "who" of the community be included in the diagnostic label.[31]

The usual ways of community coping are described by Anderson and McFarlane as the "normal line of defense," an application of Betty Neuman's model for nursing.[2] Maglacas, chief scientist for nursing of the World Health Organi-

---

*References 1, 3, 10, 14, 17, 29, 30, 34, 35.

zation, explained nursing's role in the goal of health for all as focused on two key dimensions, health stability and health potential.[26] *Health potential* refers to the capacity to cope with environmental or psychosocial demands or stresses. Community competence, an ability to solve problems effectively, was described as a major indicator of community health.[11]

The diagnosis Ineffective Community Coping was included in a validation study of four other new diagnoses.[22] Concerns were expressed by nurse experts in the study that this should be a wellness diagnosis as well as a problem diagnosis. The diagnosis Potential for Enhanced Community Coping was developed by Lunney in response to these concerns.

In Lunney's validation study, 44 of 59 nurses who provided data had more than 4 years' experience working with communities as well as families and individuals, making them eligible to validate this diagnosis. The 44 nurses were from 17 states in the United States, and 1 was from Canada. Respondents had a range of 4 to 40 years of experience in community health nursing (M = 19.4 years). For 23% (n = 11), the highest degree held was a bachelor's degree, whereas 49% (n = 21) had master's degrees and 28% (n = 12) had doctoral degrees. The mean age of the sample was 47 years (n = 41) with a range of 29 to 66.

Methods described by Fehring were used for analysis of data.[7] Subjects rated each defining characteristic on a scale of one (almost never present) to five (almost always present). The defining characteristics were presented in alphabetical order to minimize the effect of order on the ratings. A space was provided for respondents to list additional defining characteristics. The weighted means of these responses were computed to differentiate defining characteristics as major, minor, and low relevance.

The overall diagnostic content validity score for Ineffective Community Coping was .69, indicating adequate validity of the diagnosis and defining characteristics. None of the defining characteristics were identified as major because the weighted means were under .80 (see Table 10), but two defining characteristics approached this level with means of .77. The weighted means of the defining characteristics were all above .50, indicating that until clinical validation studies are done these should be considered as minor cues for the diagnosis.

Of the 44 experts, 36 agreed with the diagnostic label and 8 disagreed. Thirty-five experts agreed with the definition and 9 disagreed. Twenty experts (45%) rated the diagnosis as frequently useful or almost always useful. The remaining ratings were sometimes useful (n = 11), seldom useful (n = 10), and not useful (n = 3). A report of this study was submitted to NANDA in 1991, and the two diagnoses were accepted and staged at level 1.4 in 1994.

Despite support for this diagnostic label, however, the issue was raised in this study and through personal communication with a few nurses that concepts such as "coping" may not be appropriate for communities and populations because the underlying meaning pertains to individuals, not groups. Other labels besides coping were considered (e.g., Ineffective Problem Solving), but these other concepts, too, were developed specifically for individuals. Lunney proposed that labels used for individuals are acceptable until labels developed specifically for communities are available.[22] This issue would make an excellent topic for a consensus conference of community health nursing experts.

The treatment of coping at a community level is likely to be more economical, as well as more successful in achieving positive outcomes, than the diagnosis and treatment of each individual in a community that demonstrates problems with coping. Stressors are experienced by geographic communities (e.g., internal or external wars[6]) and aggregates within communities (e.g., women who have been raped by their husbands).[5] Nurses who are able to obtain the larger view, through community and aggregate assessment, are able to diagnose community health status, including coping, thus having accurate diagnoses to guide the devel-

TABLE 10   Weighted Means of Defining Characteristics for Ineffective Coping, *n* = 44

Defining Characteristic	Weighted Mean
Deficits in communication methods	.77
Deficits in community participation	.77
Stressors perceived as excessive	.72
Community does not meet its own expectations	.68
Excessive community conflicts	.68
High illness rates	.68
Expressed difficulty in meeting demands for change	.64
Expressed vulnerability	.56

opment of health programs. Nurses have great potential to facilitate the health of communities (e.g., the Healthy Cities Project in Indianapolis).[9] Various nursing theories can be used to guide assessment and interventions.[16,17,25] A focus on communities and populations is consistent with the principles of primary health care as advocated by the World Health Organization.[38]

ASSESSMENT

To determine community diagnoses, a community assessment needs to be conducted and analyzed.° Community assessment is best conducted in partnership with community members.[2,21] Many different frameworks were suggested in the past for community assessment, the most frequent being the epidemiological model.[8] But since the epidemiological model is mainly focused on the distribution and determinants of disease, the Functional Health Patterns provide a more holistic framework for nurses to assess community health.[13,20]

Assessment parameters for the diagnosis of community coping are (1) number and types of stressors (e.g., crime rate, problems with illegal drugs, inadequate housing, and absent landlords); (2) the usual coping strategies of the community (e.g., apathy, assertiveness and problem solving, or

mixed behaviors); (3) specific community responses to stress (e.g., sense of unity and purpose, denial, powerlessness, hopelessness); (4) information that is available for problem solving (e.g., political, economic, health, recreation, and religious); and (5) available support systems (e.g., churches, health agencies, crisis intervention centers, senior citizen centers, peers, volunteers, and government agencies).[13,20,21] Graduate and undergraduate nursing students at Hunter-Bellevue School of Nursing demonstrated that use of the parameters enabled them to interpret the status of community coping with community members. The nursing process with community as client is based on a professional-community partnership.[2]

The diagnostic process applies to the diagnosis of communities, as it does to individuals and families.[13,19] Particular care should be taken that ethical standards are applied as nurses mentally consider the diagnosis Ineffective Community Coping because this label may be used to "blame the victim." When the existence of community stress is an issue of societal neglect in meeting the needs of a community (e.g., state laws that allow men to rape their wives) the effectiveness of community or population coping should not be the focus of nursing care.

Ineffective Community Coping

There were no major defining characteristics for Ineffective Community Coping identified in the validation study.[22] The minor defining characteris-

---

° References 1, 2, 13, 15, 17, 21, 33.

tic, community does not meet its own expectations, is a cue that the community is not solving problems in a way that is satisfactory to its members. A key to the diagnosis of Ineffective Coping is comparison of community indicators with the community's own goals and wishes. The nursing diagnosis of Ineffective Coping is made with members of the community so that the applied standards and goals are those of the community, not those of the nurse.

Communication and the development of good relationships within communities are considered important characteristics of healthy communities.[11] The establishment of a collective base for community action is dependent on relationships, communication, and participation. The three defining characteristics, deficits in community participation, deficits in communication methods, and excessive communication conflicts, indicate that members of the community are not working together to solve community problems and to manage community stressors.

Subjective evaluations of community problems from key members of the community are necessary for making community diagnoses.[2,24] Three types of subjective data that should be sought by nurses in making this diagnosis are the defining characteristics (1) expressed difficulty in meeting demands for change, (2) expressed vulnerability, and (3) stressors perceived as excessive. These data indicate that community strategies may be inadequate to meet the demands of problem solving and adaptation.

Studies have shown that high illness rates are an indication of stress and ineffective coping for individuals and families. Logically, high illness rates are also an indication of stress and ineffective coping in a community.

■ Defining Characteristics
The presence of the following defining characteristics indicates that the community may be experiencing Ineffective Community Coping:

- Community does not meet its own expectations
- Deficits in community participation

- Deficits in communication methods
- Excessive community conflicts
- Expressed difficulty in meeting demands for change
- Expressed vulnerability
- Stressors perceived as excessive
- High illness rates

■ Related Factors
The following related factors are associated with Ineffective Community Coping:

- Deficits in social support
- Inadequate resources for problem solving
- Powerlessness

Potential for Enhanced Community Coping

This wellness diagnosis was not validated before its submission to NANDA, but it has been used by Lunney and others. The use of the wellness diagnosis indicates that there are risk factors for Ineffective Community Coping but that a problem does not actually exist. Risk factors can be minimized through interventions for health promotion and health protection.

The defining characteristics of this diagnosis are the problem-solving and stress management behaviors of the community. The diagnosis is applied when these behaviors are evident, but there are one or more areas of concern, such as excessive stressors (current or predicted), that require interventions for health promotion or health protection.

A major defining characteristic is deficits in one or a few strategies for coping with problems or stressors at the present time or predicted for the future. Indications of community coping are active planning by the community for predicted stressors; active problem solving by the community when faced with issues; agreement that the community is responsible for stress management; positive communication among community members; positive communication between this community or population and the larger community; programs available for recreation and relaxation; and resources sufficient for managing stressors.

X

■ Defining Characteristics

The presence of the following defining characteristics indicates that the community may be experiencing Potential for Enhanced Community Coping:

Major

- Deficits in one or a few of the characteristics that indicate effective coping (see minor characteristics)

Minor

- Active planning by community for predicted stressors
- Active problem solving by community when faced with issues
- Agreement that the community is responsible for stress management
- Positive communication among community members
- Positive communication between the community or population and the larger community
- Programs available for recreation and relaxation
- Resources sufficient for managing stressors

■ Related Factors

There is no need for consideration of related factors with the diagnosis Potential for Enhanced Community Coping.

DIAGNOSIS

■ Differential Nursing Diagnosis

Because there is only one other community-level diagnosis approved by NANDA, there is no overlap of related diagnoses. Nurses are cautioned, however, not to use this diagnosis when the number and types of stressors are overwhelming to a community and coping is not the issue. In many instances, community coping should not be the focus of nurses; the focus should be the relief of stressors from political and societal forces.

■ Medical and Psychiatric Diagnoses

Because communities do not have medical and psychiatric diagnoses, this section does not apply.

OUTCOME IDENTIFICATION, PLANNING, AND IMPLEMENTATION

Assessment and interventions for community health are generally collaborative with a broad range of community workers (e.g., public health specialists, physicians, social workers, and community members). Interventions can be initiated and carried out by nurses with community members, but because interventions are often conducted by a community team, the interventions below are designated as collaborative.

Communities and populations need to have a sense of power to solve problems and adapt to change.[26,27] Interventions for the outcome, the community or population will express the power to solve problems, will help the community or population to feel a sense of worth, clarify values, organize for optimum use of community energy, set realistic and achievable goals, and recognize community strengths.

Social support was identified as a contributing factor to coping in numerous studies.[27] The community may not demonstrate support of its own members, especially if members of the community experience stigma.[12] People who are undervalued by others in society are at risk of deficits in social support. An outcome for a community or population experiencing deficits in social support is that the community or population will obtain additional social supports.

External factors in the environment that contribute to the stress levels of communities are also amenable to nursing interventions. The foci in these cases are the public health or societal problems (e.g., lack of jobs or housing, prejudicial policies, and lack of governmental planning for health promotion and health protection). Working to influence health policy, and advocating for communities are interventions that support community coping by focusing on environmental factors.

■ NURSING CARE GUIDELINES

Nursing Diagnosis: Ineffective Community Coping

Expected Outcome: The community or population will express a sense of power to solve problems.
- ▲ Help the community or population develop coping strategies that promote group pride. *A sense of positive worth is a resource for power and coping.*[27]
- ▲ Share knowledge pertaining to community problems and issues with the community or population. *Knowledge is necessary for power and coping.*
- ▲ Develop leadership programs, and support leaders who have a sense of community problems. *Community leaders are needed for problem solving. Leadership within a community or population supports goal attainment.*
- ▲ Assist the community or population to negotiate other systems. *Resources from other communities, political forces, and private enterprises can be obtained through negotiation.*
- ▲ Assist the community or population with goal setting. *Clearly defined goals enable communities or populations to identify effective strategies for meeting goals.*
- ▲ Work with the community or population to increase awareness of oppressed group behavior that is not helpful for coping. *Theories of stigma and oppressed group behavior indicate that stigmatized and oppressed groups may not value each other and may use ineffective strategies, such as demeaning each other and internal conflict.*
- ▲ Plan with members of the community or population to obtain stronger financial bases. *Monetary support for programs is a resource for power and problem solving.*
- ▲ Sensitize key members of the community or population to symptoms of ineffective coping (e.g., attacking and blaming each other, recurring conflicts, and nonparticipation in problem solving). *Ineffective coping strategies are often habitual and unnoticed. Awareness may promote positive change.*

Expected Outcome: The community will obtain additional social supports.
- ▲ Offer support. *To some degree, the support of health providers substitutes for other supports.*
- ▲ Provide information to the community or population about the relationship of social support and coping. *Knowledge of the importance of support will enable the community to make decisions about obtaining additional support.*
- ▲ Role model support behaviors. *Role modeling may help the community or population to learn new ways of interacting and supporting one another.*
- ▲ Assist the community or population to identify and mobilize supports. *There may be supports in place that the community or population was not using or did not recognize.*
- ▲ Sensitize others to the needs of the population. *Other groups may have been unaware of this community or population's need for support or the advantages of supporting this community or population.*

■ = nursing intervention; ▲ = collaborative intervention.

■ NURSING CARE GUIDELINES

Nursing Diagnosis: Potential for Enhanced Community Coping

Expected Outcome: The community or population will improve problem-solving activities.
- ▲ Identify key leaders in the community. *Collaboration with key leaders is necessary to establish a partnership.*
- ▲ Encourage valuing of the community or population. *Positive attitudes toward the community or population are essential for enhanced coping.*
- ▲ Share community assessment data on risk factors pertaining to coping with key persons (e.g., politicians and the media).

■ = nursing intervention; ▲ = collaborative intervention.   *Continued*

X

▪ **NURSING CARE GUIDELINES — CONT'D**

> ▲ Assist community groups to work toward reducing risk factors. *Commitment of the community or population to reduce risk factors will enhance coping.*
> ▲ Facilitate rational thinking by members of the community or population. *Rational decision making is associated with effective coping.*

EVALUATION

Evaluation is conducted with members of the community or population. Health providers and community members look for positive coping behaviors, such as the establishment of committees and groups for problem solving and the identification and effective use of resources for coping. Data for evaluation can be found in local newspapers and other media sources, at community board meetings, and at meetings of large community groups, such as at churches and schools.

▪ **CASE STUDY WITH PLAN OF CARE**

The geographic community of X was a culturally homogeneous neighborhood in a large city of the Northeast. One day, a teenager from the neighborhood was accused of stealing items from a grocery store that was owned by a family from a different culture than persons in the neighborhood. The shopkeeper called the police to arrest the boy. The teenage friends of the boy who were nearby created a major incident by trying to prevent the police from arresting the boy. The focus of their anger was the man who owned the store. The teenagers claimed that the store owner was prejudiced against persons of their culture and that he lied about the boy to the police. The police made the arrest without anyone getting hurt, but soon after this community members gathered near the store to express their anger at the store owner. Angry demonstrations occurred regularly over the next few weeks, and anger escalated to rage. The store owner was afraid for his safety.

A community health nurse who lived in the neighborhood and worked for a local home health agency was concerned that the anger being expressed by the community reflected general problems, such as high unemployment and poverty, rather than a problem with the owner of the grocery store. The coping behaviors of groups in the community seemed to be less effective than needed for the situation. The nurse attended a community board meeting to express her perception of the current problem, to obtain support from community leaders to address the real issues, and to facilitate improved problem solving regarding this issue.

▪ **PLAN OF CARE FOR COMMUNITY X**
Community Diagnosis: Potential for Enhanced Community Coping

Expected Outcome: Community X will develop an accurate description of the problem.
- ▪ Provide community members with data to support the need to develop an accurate description of the problem so that problem solving will be effective.
- ▪ Explain the theory that increased rage leads to violence and that additional problems will occur if community anger leads to violence.
- ▪ Suggest the establishment of a community task force to address the problem, including teenagers who are leaders in the demonstrations.
- ▪ Obtain support from the home health agency to work with the community in assessment, diagnosis, and planning for improved coping.

▪ = nursing intervention; ▲ = collaborative intervention.

- Obtain financial support from local businesses to conduct a thorough community assessment for identification of underlying problems that lead to irrational anger.

Expected Outcome: Community X will participate in problem solving.
- Provide leadership in task force activities, explain the relationship of present concerns to the health of the community.
- Attend community board meetings and meetings of other groups to speak in favor of rational problem solving.
- Write letters to newspapers and draw media attention to positive coping strategies.
- Suggest long-range problem solving for substantive problems, such as unemployment and poverty.

■ CRITICAL THINKING EXERCISES

1. What are six possible explanations other than the actual diagnosis for community X that could have been considered during the diagnostic reasoning process?

2. What are two common assumptions that should be challenged in situations like that of community X?

3. What are three types of specialized knowledge needed to implement the nursing interventions for community X?

REFERENCES

1. American Nurses' Association: *Standards of community health nursing* (revised), Washington, D.C., 1986, The Association.
2. Anderson ET and McFarlane JM: *Community as partner: theory and practice in nursing,* ed 2, Philadelphia, 1996, JB Lippincott Co.
3. Anderson ET, McFarlane JM, and Helton A: Community as client: a model for nursing practice, *Nurs Outlook* 34:220–224, 1986.
4. Bernal H and Froman R: The confidence of community health nurses in caring for ethnically diverse populations, *Nurs Res* 19:201–203, 1987.
5. Campbell JC and Alford P: The dark consequences of marital rape, *Am J Nurs* 89:946–949, 1989.
6. Coler M: Axial representation of community mental health nursing diagnosis of a country at war: El Salvador, *Nurs Diagnosis* 4:63–69, 1993.
7. Fehring R: Methods to validate nursing diagnoses, *Heart Lung* 16:625–629, 1987.
8. Finnegan L and Ervin N: An epidemiological approach to community assessment, *Pub Health Nurs* 6:147–151, 1989.
9. Flynn B, Rider M, and Ray D: Healthy cities: the Indiana model of community development in public health, *Health Ed Quart* 18:331–347, 1991.
10. Freeman RB: Community health diagnosis, *Community health nursing practice*, Philadelphia, 1970, WB Saunders Co.
11. Goeppinger J, Lassiter PG, and Wilcox B: Community health is community competence, *Nurs Outlook* 30:464–467, 1982.
12. Goffman E: *Stigma: notes on management of spoiled identity*, Englewood Cliffs, New Jersey, 1963, Prentice-Hall.
13. Gordon M: *Nursing diagnosis: process and application,* ed 3, St. Louis, 1994, Mosby–Year Book.
14. Hamilton P: Community nursing diagnosis, *Adv Nurs Sci* 5(3):21–36, 1983.
15. Hanchett E: *Community health assessment: a conceptual tool,* New York, 1979, John Wiley & Sons.
16. Hanchett E: *Nursing frameworks and community as client: bridging the gap,* Norwalk, Connecticut, 1988, Appleton & Lange.
17. Higgs ZR and Gustafson DL: *Community as client: assessment and diagnosis,* Philadelphia, 1985, FA Davis.
18. Jakob DF: Nursing diagnosis case study: community system as client. In ME Hurley, editor: *Classification of nursing diagnoses: proceedings of the Sixth Conference,* St. Louis, 1986, The CV Mosby Co.
19. Kneeshaw MF and Lunney M: Nursing diagnoses: not for individuals only, *Geriatr Nurs* 10:246–247, 1989.
20. Kriegler NF and Harton MK: Community health assessment tool: a patterns approach to data collection and diagnosis, *J Comm Health Nurs* 9:229–234, 1992.
21. Lunney M: A framework to analyze a taxonomy of nursing diagnosis. In Kim MJ, McFarland GK, and McLane AM, editors: *Classification of nursing diagnoses: proceedings of the Fifth National Conference,* St. Louis, 1984, The CV Mosby Co.
22. Lunney M: *Proposed new nursing diagnosis, Ineffective Coping: Community,* submitted to the North American Nursing Diagnosis Association, 1991.

X

23. Lunney M: Nursing diagnosis of community as client, *Proceedings of the 1991 Spring Institute, Association of Community Health Nursing Educators,* Chicago, 1992, The Association.

24. Lunney M and others: *Community diagnosis: analysis and synthesis of the literature,* paper presented at the Spring Institute, Association of Community Health Nursing Educators, San Antonio, Texas, 1994.

25. Lunney M and others: Community diagnosis: to be or not to be? *Proceedings of the 1993 Spring Institute, Association of Community Health Nursing Educators,* Chicago, 1994, The Association.

26. Maglacas AM: Health for all: nursing's role, *Nurs Outlook* 36:66–71, 1988.

27. May R: *Power and innocence: a search for the sources of violence,* New York, 1972, WW Norton.

28. Miller JF: *Coping with chronic illness: overcoming powerlessness,* Philadelphia, 1993, FA Davis.

29. Mueke MA: Community health diagnosis in nursing, *Pub Health Nurs* 1:23–35, 1984.

30. Nettle C and others: Community nursing diagnosis, *J Comm Health Nurs* 6:135–145, 1989.

31. Neufeld A and Harrison MJ: The development of nursing diagnoses for aggregates and groups, *Pub Health Nurs* 7:251–255, 1990.

32. Porter EJ: The nursing diagnosis of population groups. In McLane AM, editor: *Classification of nursing diagnoses: proceedings of the Seventh Conference,* St. Louis, 1987, The CV Mosby Co.

33. Public Health Nursing Directors of Washington: *Public health nursing functions with core public health functions,* Olympia, Washington, 1993, Washington State Department of Health.

34. Rodgers S: Community as client—a multivariate model for analysis of community and aggregate health risk, *Pub Health Nurs* 1:210–222, 1984.

35. Schultz P: When client means more than one: extending the foundational concept of person, *Adv Nurs Sci* 10:71–86, 1987.

36. Shamansky S and Pesznecker B: A community is . . . , *Nurs Outlook* 29:182–185, 1981.

37. Sills GM and Goeppinger J: The community as a field of inquiry in nursing. In Werley HH and Fitzpatrick JJ, editors: *Annual review of nursing research,* vol 3, New York, 1985, Springer.

38. World Health Organization: *Primary health care,* Geneva, 1978, The Organization.

X

Defensive Coping

▶ ──

Defensive Coping *is the state in which an individual repeatedly projects false positive self-evaluation based on a self-protective pattern that defends against underlying perceived threats to positive self-regard.*[73]

OVERVIEW

The process of coping has received attention from a variety of disciplines. Observations regarding how individuals cope with the events in their lives have underscored how differently they may respond even in the same situation. Whereas some may cope effectively, others experience distress and difficulty.

When an individual experiences a real or imagined event, he or she responds to regain a sense of equilibrium or well-being.[2,49] The event could be writing an examination, planning a visit to the dentist, or being diagnosed with cancer. The event creates demands for a person and evokes a set of response strategies. The strategies are feelings (emotions), thoughts (cognitions), and behaviors (actions) elicited to maintain or regain a sense of balance or well-being. If the person's usual responses to an event do not achieve the desired balance, distress and anxiety occur; in other words, if the demands of the event exceed the resources of the individual, he or she becomes uncomfortable. Other response strategies will be needed to cope with the emerging discomfort and anxiety. Coping with life events is an ongoing, dynamic process that occurs similarly in life-threatening events and "daily hassles." In this chapter, *coping* is defined as "the ways in which individuals manipulate their environment in service of themselves or

the ways in which they manipulate themselves to better fit the environment."[13] Thus coping refer to any attempts to ward off, to reduce, or to assimilate an existing or expected demand (or stressor) by intrapsychic effort (cognition- or emotion-related) or by action (field-related).

According to Lazarus and Folkman,[49] coping strategies serve two fundamental purposes. These include (1) managing or altering the problem (event) causing the distress and (2) regulating the emotional response to the problem. The first category is problem-focused coping, and the second is emotion-focused coping. Relatively little is known about why an individual chooses a particular strategy or combination of strategies in a given situation.[24,71] However, we do know that individuals may select the same strategies for a variety of situations and yet select different strategies for the same situation at different times.[41,62]

An explanation for the variation in individual responses has emerged from work in cognitive appraisal. *Cognitive appraisal* is the process in which an individual categorizes an event and its various aspects and judges its effect on his or her well-being.[49] It is largely evaluative, is focused on meaning, and occurs constantly during an individual's waking hours. When confronted with an event, the individual engages in primary appraisal and judges the event as irrelevant, benign, positive, or stressful by asking the question "Am I in trouble or will I benefit, now or in the future?" Secondary appraisal involves answering the question "What can be done about this situation?" and assessing the coping options against the demands of the event. These appraisals may be at a conscious or an unconscious level and are conducted

X

through the individual's existing knowledge, experiences, self-concept, needs, attitudes, and life goals. The individual will judge the situation using his or her own unique frame of reference (cognitive map) and personal ideas about what is important.

This interaction between determining what is at stake and whether coping resources are sufficient for the event will shape the degree of stress and the emotional reaction that the individual feels. The stress does not arise from the event itself but from the interaction between the person and the environment.[49] Individual variation results from the unique nature of cognitive appraisal.

A person's selection of a coping strategy is based on his or her appraisals. In general, emotional-focused strategies are selected when the appraisal concludes that nothing can change a harmful or threatening environment. Certain coping strategies serve to protect the individual or act as buffers against the emotional distress.[48] The problem-solving forms of coping are chosen when conditions are considered amenable to change or to challenge. As we learn more about the coping process, we realize that individuals use a wide variety of strategies. The key to understanding any particular individual's responses lies in understanding his or her cognitive appraisal and exploring its specific dimensions. To judge the effectiveness of specific coping strategies or responses requires a clear understanding of the purpose they serve for the individual. Those purposes are derived from the meaning that the person assigns to a particular event through his or her cognitive appraisal.

Meaning may be assigned to an event through an assessment of its perceived harm, threat, or challenge to an individual's sense of self and the occurrences that will maintain the individual's personal integrity.[25] Meaning is integrally linked to identity, providing the basis of continuity between the past and present frames of reference for interpreting the potential consequences of events. The sense of self (self-system) is the image or picture of oneself as distinct and different from other people.[8,77] It consists of one's conceptions of who one is at a particular point in one's life course. It includes the notions of self-concept and self-esteem. Self-con-

cept incorporates the perception of what one is like (self-identity), one's worth as a person (self-evaluation), and one's aspirations for growth and accomplishment (self-ideal). This repertoire of beliefs about one's nature is in part an organization of the interpersonal motives and attitudes that an individual considers centrally important.[23] Self-esteem refers to the feelings associated with the self-evaluation or judgment of one's worth and may emerge from comparisons between what one is like and what one aspires to be.

All individuals presumably have a global self-concept with an associated global self-esteem. This basic level of self-esteem is learned during childhood through the appraisals of significant others, may be relatively stable throughout one's lifetime,[16] and is evidenced in behaviors across a wide variety of situations. Basic self-esteem contains physical, social, personal, family, school, peer, and behavioral aspects. Individuals with relatively high self-esteem are better students, are less depressed, display better physical health, and enjoy better social relationships than those with lower self-esteem.[32] The functional level of self-esteem may change daily as one judges one's performance in a variety of situations, such as school, work, family, peer relationships, and physical well-being. It arises from the ongoing evaluation of interactions with other people and events, the person's notions about what is important, and discrepancies between a person's ideal self and the perceived self in specific situations. Functional self-esteem may vary throughout an individual's lifetime as he or she undertakes different tasks and roles, such as marrying or parenting.[66] It can exceed or fall below basic self-esteem. Severe, acute, or chronic stress, such as that occurring with acute or chronic illness or the sudden loss of a person or object, may alter functional self-esteem.[4,19,27,64]

A person's perception of events tends to reinforce his or her self-concept and self-esteem.[16] Self-esteem in adults is influenced by perceived levels of success in employment and interpersonal and parenting roles. Adults may perceive a discrepancy between how they are performing and how they expect to perform and therefore experience lowered self-esteem. The resulting behavior may reflect passivity, helplessness, powerlessness, decreased decision making, and despondency. Of particular interest is the concept of defensive self-esteem. Coopersmith[17] describes individuals with marked differences between their reported self-view and their behavior. Specifically, these individuals reported high self-evaluations in reaction to low underlying self-evaluations resulting from poor performance and low status. Reporting high self-esteem based on denial or avoidance of negative personal information has been described as "role-faking"[60] to meet perceived demands in a situation. It is a self-protective maneuver that defends against a perceived gap between the ideal self and the real self.[35,38,67]

An event appraised as harmful or threatening to the self-concept will evoke coping strategies to protect what is important to the individual (self-esteem) and defend against a painful experience. Psychoanalytic theory has provided descriptions of mechanisms that defend the self-concept against dangerous or unpleasant feelings. These defense mechanisms incorporate distorted interpretations of reality, including a distorted self-concept, repression, projection, fantasy, displacement, and sublimation. The literature describing the coping strategies that individuals use during life events provides clear evidence that defensive strategies are indeed used. These mechanisms include daydreaming; the use of alcohol or drugs; sleeping; ignoring; joking about, or denying the situation; blaming oneself or others; just focusing on the day; and getting away by oneself.[7,53,69,76]

Ego-oriented psychological models describe a hierarchy of coping and defense mechanisms, implying that some processes are automatically superior to others.[30,57,74] The implication is that a person has coped with the situation and met the demands successfully or that a person has defended and coped ineffectively or inadequately.[51] According to Lazarus and Folkman,[49] this hierarchial assumption should be abandoned, and the coping process and the coping outcome should be considered independently. The effectiveness of coping and defending must be considered for each person individually. Both can work well or poorly in particular persons, contexts, and occasions. "No one strategy is considered inherently better than another. The goodness (efficacy or appropriateness) of a strategy is determined only by its effect in a given encounter and its effects over the long term."[49]

Studies of crisis situations have emphasized the primary importance of maintaining self-esteem to manage the situation.* An individual's sense of self can be disrupted by a physical injury or a traumatic event. The resulting need to consider different images of oneself can threaten self-esteem. Defense mechanisms may be used to avoid or defend against emotional pain, resulting in a retreat from full awareness of what is happening. These defenses may conserve energy by reducing the amount of emotional coping and by providing a buffer that allows time to collect oneself and to mobilize problem-focused strategies. In some instances, this can mean holding a distorted view of the personal image and abilities for a period of time. Particularly in unexpected events, seeking relief through avoidance and disavowal—redefining a situation or the self view—can serve to obliterate the threatening reality of the situation, maintain self-esteem, and allow time for other coping responses to emerge. Also, the distress an individual feels often influences processes of thinking and perceiving.[39] In times of crisis, individuals can have trouble defining who they are and the skills they possess; they may have difficulty making decisions or solving problems. The resulting confusion and anxiety additionally threaten the already vulnerable self-esteem and can cause ineffective coping.[12,45,75]

Defense mechanisms may be helpful in protecting the self from overwhelming unpleasant feelings, particularly on a short-term basis.[5,15,31,68] However, defense mechanisms do close the cognitive field to further input, and they do not allow further cognitive appraisal as new information becomes available that could reduce the threat.

---

*References 1, 5, 18, 33, 35, 68.

The use of these mechanisms is inappropriate when the emotional response (1) prevents seeking and cooperating with treatment for illness, (2) interferes with everyday functioning, (3) evokes behavior that causes more pain and distress than the event itself, or (4) evokes responses that appear as conventional psychiatric symptoms. However, it is important to recognize that not all events are amenable to resolution through problem solving. Many irremediable events, such as natural disasters, disease, aging, and losses, can demand the use of defensive strategies to manage emotions and maintain self-esteem and a positive outlook in the face of overwhelming loss and harm.

Life events such as illness, bereavement, divorce, job loss, or aging can cause people to use defense mechanisms when the sense of self is threatened. When an individual is uncertain about his or her ability to cope with a particular event or to enact a specific role, he or she may develop self-doubt and fear of failure and humiliation. As a defense against failure and low self-esteem, the behavior pattern defensive coping may emerge.

ASSESSMENT

The set of observations previously outlined has contributed to the development of the nursing diagnosis Defensive Coping. The main characteristic of an individual who has this behavior is a tendency to present the self more favorably in response to perceived failure. This may be manifested as a denial of obvious problems or weaknesses and as grandiosity. The individual has a high need for social approval, yet is uncomfortable with intimacy and self-disclosure and is unable to acknowledge personal failures openly. Blame is projected onto someone or something else, and expressions of self-competency are unrealistic or exaggerated. There is difficulty perceiving reality. In some instances, the person may have a superior attitude toward others and ridicule or laugh hostilely at them. Difficulty in establishing and maintaining relationships is evident. In therapeutic environments, lack of participation in therapy, lack of follow-through, and self-neglect have been reported. This concept of defending one's self-

esteem is validated in a study by Norris and Kunes-Connell[60] in which 15 of 27 subjects with low self-esteem displayed characteristics such as those previously described.

Whether an event is appraised as threatening to one's self-esteem depends on the environment and the person. Regardless of whether the event is real, anticipated, or imagined, or whether the appraisal is realistic or unrealistic, the coping behaviors are based on the perceptions of the individual. Events that occur suddenly or that are unpredictable, uncontrollable, or ambiguous present a greater sense of threat. If the event impinges on ideas or goals that are important to the individual, the threat will be heightened. The individual's level of knowledge, skills, and coping abilities will influence feelings of threat. An appraisal of harm or threat occurs when an individual believes or feels that his or her coping resources are insufficient to meet the demands of a particular situation. If a similar situation has happened in the past, the previous experience will provide the frame of reference regarding the individual's ability to manage it. Evidence now leads us to believe that an individual's social support (sense of being cared for) has an influence on feelings of distress.[3,7,11] The capability to overcome uncertainty, to maintain motivation, to cope, and to maintain an emotional balance are also considered important personal factors.[14] In general, ego strength and increased self-esteem reduce vulnerability to stress.[49]

A loss or change in significant roles and appraisals that create unrealistic self-expectations may lead to self-esteem disturbance. *Self-esteem disturbance* is defined as "negative feelings or conception of self including social self or self capabilities."[60] According to Coopersmith,[17] self-appraisals are based on (1) the ability to influence personally significant others (power), (2) the sense of being accepted and valued as worthwhile (significance), (3) the ability to meet performance demands successfully in terms of personal goals (competence), and (4) behaving according to one's moral and ethical beliefs and values (virtue). Situations perceived as harmful or threatening to these dimensions may lead to low self-esteem. The resulting behavior to cope with low self-esteem depends on an individual's coping response style and availability of resources. Generally individuals will resort to coping strategies they have used in the past.

Almost any medical condition has the potential for being perceived as threatening. Not only may the condition be life threatening, but the illness and treatment also may threaten the person's role in the family, ability to work, or potential for achieving desired goals. The psychosocial effect of illness is vividly described in professional and popular literature.° The loss of a breast may alter a woman's sense of femininity; the loss of a limb may require an occupational change; and the death of a spouse forces a person to view him- or herself as single. Whether the loss or threat is observable or evident, the self-esteem disturbance can be similar. A woman who has had a hysterectomy may feel a threat to her self-esteem, as does a woman who has suffered burns to her hands and face. The words of sociologist Arthur Frank, speaking from a personal perspective, underscore the transforming experience that can accompany illness. Illness "leaves no aspect of life untouched . . . your relationships, your work, your sense of who you are and who you might become, your sense of what life is and ought to be—these all change, and the change is terrifying."[28]

How a person copes with a particular acute illness or a permanent disability depends on how the aspects of the event affect the individual and the unique meaning he or she assigns to these aspects. The type of illness; the location, rate of onset, and progression of symptoms; the degree of reversibility; and the functional impairment all have personal meaning for an individual.[43,52] Individuals who perceive their illness as a weakness or a failing may attempt to escape by denying it. Illness perceived as an enemy may also evoke coping strategies that defend against attack and danger. Low self-esteem with defensive behaviors has been described by battered women in a women's shelter, alcohol and drug abusers in treatment, hospitalized psychiatric patients, and patients with chronic physical illness.[60]

Assessment needs to occur on two dimensions. First, the nurse needs to assess the interaction between the person and the environment (the event) and the effectiveness of the coping strategies. Are the strategies accomplishing the individual's desires without undue harm to oneself or to others? Second, the context surrounding self-esteem must be established to understand the behavioral observations and to ensure that appropriate intervention strategies are initiated.

The immense complexity and variation in human response has to some degree hampered efforts to measure coping in a standardized manner. Much ambiguity and confusion exists in the field because of inconsistencies in the defining terminology and the boundaries for the concept.[43] A controversial issue in the measurement of coping is the use of specific criteria to define success. Coping success is defined differently by various people.

Much of the work in measuring coping has focused on the process of coping. This approach has resulted in a list of individual specific strategies for a particular situation[26,41,62] or a description of how individuals manage current problem situations.[37] Measurement of the outcomes of coping has included describing how a particular event has changed aspects of life functioning[21,54] or using surrogate measures of emotional distress.[6,56] This last approach is based on the assumption that noncoping will cause measurable emotional distress. Inherent in all measures of coping is the question of what constitutes "normal." What is normal when one confronts death, accidents, or life-threatening illnesses?

The standardized measurement of ego strength and psychological defense mechanisms has been methodologically problematical[72]; the validation of existing tools has also been doubtful. Perhaps the best known defense scale is the Defense Mechanisms Inventory (DMI).[33] It was designed to identify defenses used in dealing with conflict and was based on the assumption that the major function of defenses is to resolve conflicts between the perceptions of the individual and his or her internalized values. Gutmann[34] developed an ego styles instrument (TAT) that measures three styles of coping with the environment: (1) active, (2) pas-

X

°References 3, 10, 22, 44, 61, 64, 65, 70, 78–80.

sive, and (3) magical. The last approach is characterized by gross interpretations and distortions of stimuli that reflect misperceptions of the environment and ego regression.

The formal measurement of self-esteem has also suffered from methodological difficulties, including ambiguities and inconsistencies in defining the concept and a wide range of theoretical perspectives.[8] A major issue concerns the appropriateness of using the ratings of the individual and an objective person. The defining characteristics for Self-Esteem Disturbance include objective observations and subjective statements from the person, thus suggesting that both types of measures are necessary. Other issues focus on the global nature of measurement devices, the stability of self-esteem, the human need to provide socially desirable information about oneself, and the need for approval. Lawson and McGrath[47] developed the Social Self-Esteem Inventory in an attempt to overcome these shortcomings. This instrument was used in the Norris study cited earlier and has a high level of reliability ($r = 0.88$). Preliminary work with this instrument supports the idea that self-esteem can be differentiated into basic self-esteem, functional self-esteem, and defensive self-esteem. Reviews of self-esteem measures are available by Gilberts[32] and Breytspraak.[8]

Data collected for clinical assessment will depend in large measure on the context of the situation and the time constraints. Ultimately the goal of assessment is to determine whether the individual's resources correlate with the demands of the event and whether the desirable goals are met. Important areas for data collection are as follows:

1. The nature of the situation (the event)
   - Determine the specific event at issue
   - Assess the event for unexpectedness, predictability, controllability, and duration
   - Assess the potential for harm or threat (especially to functional self-esteem)
2. The individual
   - Appearance: briefly note sex, apparent age, ease of deportment, overt signs of distress, composure
   - Perception of the event: ask the individual to explain in his or her own words the perception of and the (assigned) meaning to the event, including harm or threat to self-esteem
   - Coping resources and goals: ask the individual to describe the ability to manage this type of situation; what he or she would consider important objectives (goals)
   - Self-concept: ask the individual to describe his or her sense of self, including self-worth, personal competence, and achievement of ideals or aspirations
   - Past coping: ask the individual to describe how successful coping has been in the past
3. The context of the situation
   - Determine the individual's past experiences with similar events
   - Determine available social support (supportive or tangible)
   - Assess the individual's ability to deal with uncertainty, motivation to cope, usual coping patterns, and knowledge and abilities
   - Identify other concurrent events and concerns
   - Identify any discrepancy between the ideal self and the perceived self in the current situation
4. Coping strategies and outcome
   - Identify the emotional, behavioral, and cognitive responses to the event and the purpose they serve for the individual, such as solving problems or controlling emotions
   - Assess the extent to which the desired outcomes are achieved
   - Identify the individual's skills, communication patterns, and interactions with others

A key aspect of this assessment is understanding the individual's cognitive appraisal of the situation and the purpose served by his or her specific coping strategies. The environment must be supportive and nonjudgmental for the individual to reveal this information.

■ Defining Characteristics

The presence of the following defining characteristics indicates that the patient may be experiencing Defensive Coping[9]:

- Denial of obvious weaknesses or problems

- Projection of blame or responsibility
- Rationalization of failures
- Hypersensitivity to slight criticism (defensiveness)
- Projection of heightened sense of capabilities (grandiosity)
- Superior attitude toward others
- Hostile laughter or ridicule of others
- Difficulty in establishing and maintaining relationships
- Difficulty in testing the reality of perceptions
- Lack of follow-through or participation in treatment or therapy

■ Related Factors

The following related factors are associated with Defensive Coping:

- Appraisal of the event by family members or significant others
- Concurrent events (demands) in the family or social system
- Family dynamics and functioning
- Coping resources in the family or social system (informational, tangible, and financial)

DIAGNOSIS

■ Differential Nursing Diagnosis

Several nursing diagnoses are closely related to Defensive Coping. There could be difficulty discriminating one from another. These diagnoses include Body Image Disturbance, Self-Esteem Disturbance, and Altered Role Performance. Each of these diagnoses identifies specific disruptions for individuals evidenced by subsequent emotional distress. Negative perceptions of oneself and one's capabilities are prominent. Defensive Coping would emerge as a response to these disruptions and contain a falsely positive appraisal of oneself and one's capabilities. Other nursing diagnoses that could be related to the diagnosis of Defensive Coping are Ineffective Individual Coping and Impaired Adjustment. Each of these diagnoses reflects an ineffective pattern of adjustment or managing change in which the individual acknowledges difficulties. Defensive Coping be-

havior works to protect the individual against perceived threats and maintains a closed perceptual set. To some degree the individual does not openly acknowledge the threat.

■ Medical and Psychiatric Diagnoses

Defensive Coping could be observed with a wide range of medical diagnoses. Acute and chronic illnesses have the potential to threaten one's self-concept. Surgery, trauma, and treatments have the potential to alter body image and body function. Illnesses that require a change in lifestyle (e.g., myocardial infarction, arthritis, AIDS, and chronic lung disease) may also be associated with Defensive Coping. Defensive Coping could also be observed with a range of psychiatric disorders, including anorexia, bulimia, impulse control disorder, and substance abuse. Unresolved grief may also be associated with Defensive Coping.

OUTCOME IDENTIFICATION, PLANNING, AND IMPLEMENTATION

The expected outcome of the nursing interventions for the patient exhibiting Defensive Coping is that the person will regain a sense of balance or well-being. In particular, a patient will feel a reduction in distress and a movement toward a desired goal without undue cost. Johnson and Lauver[42] suggest that successful coping can be measured by the patient's emotional comfort and ability to resolve problems and to resume usual activity.

A major issue in evaluating coping is the lack of criteria to judge the success of the patient's coping behavior. Coping success is different for various patients and is based in part on personal opinion and preferences. The efficacy (appropriateness) of the coping strategies must be evaluated for the patient concerned in the specific situation. For one patient it may be very important to use denial and avoidance, whereas for another the same strategy creates additional difficulties.[55] The coping outcome must be assessed within the context of the interaction between the event and the patient.

The nature of the nursing interventions depends on the assessment of the interaction between the event and the patient and the specific expected outcomes identified by the patient and the nurse. The nursing response will be directed toward preventing further loss of self-esteem or confronting and working with the patient to change behaviors consistent with patient readiness.

Whether defensive self-esteem is used to defend against basic low self-esteem or functional low self-esteem will also make a difference in the interventions. Functional self-esteem is expected to be more amenable to alteration. Enhancing an adult's self-esteem involves as a first step exploring the discrepancies with the patient's self-concept.[19] In particular, these discrepancies often exist between the patient's expectations of him- or herself and his or her perception of current abilities. Second, it is necessary to identify and to change the thoughts that cause negative feelings and low self-esteem. These thoughts include minimizing accomplishments, overgeneralizing, and magnifying negatives. Involvement in decision making and problem solving, particularly in areas that affect their lifestyles, can enhance self-esteem in older adults.[60] Self-esteem can be enhanced for adults through (1) promoting security by defining clear expectations and setting well-defined limits, (2) providing a positive identity through acceptance and recognition, (3) communicating a sense of belonging through strong family ties and encouraging group and social concern, and (4) providing purpose by encouraging realistic goal setting and conveying faith in the patient's ability to achieve.[19]

Fundamentally nursing interventions must be based on a clear idea why the patient exhibits the behaviors he or she does. Once the patient is understood, interventions can be generally directed toward reducing the sense of harm or stress and increasing the patient's confidence in his or her coping resources.[12] The nurse needs to observe and assess carefully and to engage in active listening and supporting. Initially, when the individual perceives an overwhelming threat, he or she will strive to protect the self-concept (image and integrity). Nursing behavior needs to focus on preserving the patient's integrity and at the same time

to deal with the behavior the patient has selected (e.g., denial, bragging, and joking). The nurse must seek to reduce the stressful aspects of a situation and to correct any misperception gently.

When a patient's defensive behavioral choices result from different stages of adapting, and when in time the patient moves away from the original closed cognitive stance, the nurse must pace him- or herself with the patient's progress, helping the patient adapt to the situation.[40] This process involves exploring realistic interpretations of the event—why it is threatening, what is required to meet the demands of the situation, and what abilities the patient possesses. In turn, the nurse may need to help the patient acquire new knowledge and skills and to provide support and guidance to aid the patient in maintaining a reasonable emotional balance during the transition period. Specific approaches to assist with functional self-esteem disturbances include designing clearly defined, mutually agreeable goals; identifying specific strategies to accomplish the goals; establishing realistic time frames for achieving the goals; and facilitating the patient's recognition of and challenge of distortions in thinking, especially about his or her ideal self and perceived self in the situation. Other health professionals and community agencies may need to be consulted and the patient's relationships with significant others maintained or strengthened.

If a patient continues to need particular defenses for managing distress, the nurse must think very carefully about more appropriate interventions. In certain instances, interventions aimed at helping the patient "face the truth" could leave a previously "defended" person defenseless and perhaps do more harm than good. In addition, it has been suggested that "well-defended" individuals are not susceptible to intervention. The most appropriate approach is one of support and patience. This can create a dilemma for health professionals when they believe that the defensive stance retards the patient's ability to deal with real threats that are amenable to resolution. The nurse must be aware of the necessity to discriminate between his or her needs and those of the patient.

◢ NURSING CARE GUIDELINES
Nursing Diagnosis: Defensive Coping

Expected Outcome: The patient will not suffer further insult to self-esteem.
- Support the patient's personhood, uniqueness, and right to be involved in decision making.
- Seek to understand the patient's perspective of the situation and what is stressful or threatening to him or her and to the sense of self. *Enhancing an individual's sense of self-esteem involves as a first step exploring the discrepancies within his or her self-concept.*
- Gently clarify misconceptions.
- When possible, reduce stressful aspects of the event.
- Encourage maintenance of social networks, including support from family, neighbors, and clergy.
- If necessary, assist the patient to become aware of behaviors that are harmful to others, such as ridiculing them.

Expected Outcome: The patient will express a realistic appraisal of the event, its demands, and the coping resources available.
- Assist the patient to explore the nature and characteristics of the event, its demands, and the coping resources required and to identify the discrepancies between the ideal and perceived roles in the situation. *Pace intervention to the patient's readiness for assistance because a period of denial may be present.*

Expected Outcome: The patient will become comfortable with ideal and perceived roles and develop competency to manage the situation.
- Assist the patient to identify desired goals.

Expected Outcome: The patient will verbalize a sense of personal integrity and of movement toward desired goals.
- Set realistic and concrete goals with the patient.
- Identify specific strategies for achieving goals.
- Set realistic time frames for reaching goals.
- Review capabilities and learning from past experiences.
- Explore patterns of thinking (especially negative thoughts).
- Teach necessary knowledge and skills.
- Acknowledge progress toward desired goals.
- Encourage the patient to maintain social networks.
- Encourage the expression of fears and concerns.
  Pacing interventions with the patient's progress helps the patient adapt to the situation.

■ = nursing intervention; ▲ = collaborative intervention.

EVALUATION

The nurse uses observation of and interaction with the patient to evaluate the effectiveness of the nursing interventions. The desired effect must be defined in the context of the particular situation and the desired outcome identified by the patient. The nurse must be able to separate his or her own idea of effective outcomes from the patient's. Each patient will define coping success differently, and different strategies may be selected for achieving desired goals.

The efficacy of any strategy must be determined on the basis of its success in achieving the desired outcome for the patient, and any interventions must be evaluated accordingly.

☞ CASE STUDY WITH PLAN OF CARE

Mr. Edward S. is a 35-year-old male who is married and has two children. He teaches physical education at the local high school. He was admitted to the coronary care unit with a diagnosis of acute myocardial infarction 4 days ago and was transferred today to the general nursing unit. Mr. S. had no history of heart disease and up until admission ran 10 miles daily. He prides himself on having the "physical conditioning of a 20-year-old." Mr. S. has had little hospital exposure, with the exception of the death of his 70-year-old father from heart disease 5 years ago and the birth of his children. During the first few days on the general unit, Mr. S. made frequent trips to the stairwell. When the nursing staff questioned him about these trips, Mr. S. retorted, "Surely, as a health professional, you know that muscles have to be used to be maintained. I've been in bed long enough! It's been 4 days already. A man in my shape needs to be exercising. I have been going up and down the stairs to keep my muscles in shape. After all, I'm the coach, and we have a big game next week. I need to be able to keep up with the boys or we won't win the game. What business is it of yours, anyway?" The next day Mr. S. discussed his athletic abilities and his intent to return to the playing field. He ridicules those around him who are not in good physical shape, including the hospital staff. One nurse reports that Mr. S. attributes his hospitalization to that "idiot medical student in emergency who can't tell the difference between chest pain and a cardiac arrest!"

☞ PLAN OF CARE FOR MR. EDWARD S.

Nursing Diagnosis: Defensive Coping Related to Myocardial Infarction and Threat to Self-Esteem

---

Expected Outcome: Mr. Edward S. will not experience further insult to his sense of self.
- Encourage Mr. S. to describe the events surrounding his hospitalization and his appraisal and perceptions of the situation.

Expected Outcome: Mr. S. will demonstrate no increase in climbing the stairs.
- Encourage Mr. S. to describe his perception of his roles at work and what he believes is required to perform these roles.

Expected Outcome: Mr. S. will discuss his perceptions with the nurses.
- Determine whether there are role inconsistencies between Mr. S.'s ideal self and his perceived self secondary to his hospitalization.
- Assess Mr. S.'s knowledge of cardiac status, exercise, and myocardial infarction.
- Correct any misconceptions Mr. S. may hold about cardiac physiology and disease.
- Reduce stressful aspects, such as noise, when possible.
- Acknowledge Mr. S.'s abilities, achievements, and right to make informed decisions regarding his care.
- Assist Mr. S. to appraise his situation realistically.
- Provide information regarding disease.
- Assist Mr. S. to define concrete goals for exercise.

■ = nursing intervention; ▲ = collaborative intervention.

■ CRITICAL THINKING EXERCISES

1. How would you describe the coping process?
2. What assessment parameters need to be present to establish a nursing diagnosis of Defensive Coping?
3. What assessment data would lead the nurse to select a supportive approach?

REFERENCES

1. Adams JF and Lindermann E: Coping with long-term disability. In Coelho GV, Hamburg DA, and Adams JE, editors: *Coping and adaptation*, New York, 1974, Basic Books.
2. Antonovsky A: *Health, stress and coping*, San Francisco, 1981, Jossey-Bass Publishers.
3. Balder L and DeNour AK: Couple's reactions and adjustments to mastectomy, *Int J Psychiatry Med* 14(3):265–270, 1984.
4. Barnard D: Healing the damaged self, *Perspect Biol Med* 33(4):535–546, 1990.
5. Bean G and others: Coping mechanisms of cancer patients: a study of 33 patients receiving chemotherapy, *CA* 30:257–259, 1980.
6. Beck AT and others: Inventory for measuring depression, *Arch Gen Psychiatry* 4:561–569, 1961.
8. Breytspraak LM and George LK: Self-concept and self-esteem. In Mangen DJ and Peterson WA, editors: *Research instruments in social gerontology: clinical and social psychology*, vol 1, Minneapolis, 1981, University of Minnesota Press.
9. Carroll-Johnson RM: *Classification of nursing diagnoses: proceedings of the Eighth Conference*, Philadelphia, 1989, JB Lippincott Co.
10. Cassileth BR and others: Psychological analysis of cancer patients and their next of kin. *Cancer* 55:72–76, 1985.
11. Cassileth BR and others: Psychological status in chronic illness, *N Eng J Med* 311:506–511, 1985.
12. Clark S: Nursing diagnosis: ineffective coping. I. A theoretical framework. II. Planning care, *Heart Lung* 16(6):670–674, 1984.
13. Cobb S: Social support as a moderator of life stress, *Psychosom Med* 35:375–389, 1973.
14. Coelho GV, Hamburg DA, and Adams JE: *Coping and adaptation*, New York, 1974, Basic Books.
15. Cohen F and Lazarus RS: Active coping processes, coping dispositions and recovery from surgery, *Psychosom Med* 35:375–389, 1973.
16. Colenda C and Dougherty LM: Positive ego and coping functions in chronic pain and depressed patient, *J Geriatr Psychiatry Neurol* 3(1):48–52, 1990.
17. Coopersmith S: *Antecedents of self-esteem*, San Francisco, 1967, Freeman, Cooper.
18. Cornwell C and Schmitt M: Perceived health status, self-esteem and body image in women with rheumatoid arthritis or systemic lupus erythematosus, *Res Nurs Health* 13:99–107, 1990.
19. Crouch MA and Straub V: Enhancement of self-esteem in adults, *Family Community Health* 6:65–78, 1983.
20. Curbow B and others: Self-concept and cancer in adults, *Soc Sci Med* 31(2):115–128, 1990.
21. Derogatis LR: *Scoring and procedures manual for PAIS*, Baltimore, 1976, Clinical Psychometric Research.
22. Draup K: Psychosocial aspects of coronary heart disease, *West J Nurs Res* 4(3):257–271, 1982.
23. Epstein S: Anxiety, arousal and the self-concept. In Sarason GI and Seilberger CD, editors: *Stress and anxiety*, Washington, D.C., 1976, Hemisphere Publishing.
24. Feifel H, Strack S, and Nagy VT: Coping strategies and associated features of medically ill patients, *Psychosom Med* 49:616–625, 1987.
25. Fife B: The conceptualization of meaning in illness, *Soc Sci Med* 38(2):309–316, 1994.
26. Folkman S and Lazarus RS: An analysis of coping in a middle-aged community sample, *J Health Soc Behav* 21:219–239, 1980.
27. Foltz AT: The influence of cancer on self-concept and quality of life, *Semin Oncol Nurs* 3(4):303–312, 1987.
28. Frank A: *At the will of the body*, Boston, 1991, Houghton Aldine.
29. Friedenbergs I and others: Assessment and treatment of psychosocial problems of the cancer patient: a case study, *Cancer Nurs* 3:111–119, 1981.
30. Freud A: *The ego and the mechanisms of defense*, New York, 1946, International Universities Press.
31. George JM and others: The effect of psychological factors of physical trauma on recovery from oral surgery, *J Behav Med* 3:291–310, 1980.
32. Gilberts R: The evaluation of self-esteem, *Family Community Health* 6:29–49, 1983.
33. Gleser G and Ihilevich D: An objective instrument for measuring defense mechanisms, *J Consult Clin Psychol* 33(1):51–60, 1969.
34. Gutmann DL: An exploration of ego configuration in middle and later life. In Neugarten and others, editors: *Personality in middle and later life*, New York, 1964, Atherton Press.
35. Heidrich SM, Forsthoff CA, and Ward SE: Psychological adjustment in adults with cancer: the self as mediator, *Health Psychol* 13(4):346–353, 1994.
36. Heidrich SM and Ward SE: The role of the self in adjustment to cancer in elderly women, *Oncol Nurs Forum* 19(10):1491–1496, 1992.
37. Heim E and others: Coping with breast cancer over time and situation, *J Psychosom Res* 37(5):523–542, 1993.
38. Higgins ET: Self-discrepancy: a theory relating to self and affect, *Psychol Rev* 94:319–340, 1987.
39. Hoff LA: *People in crisis: understanding and helping*, Toronto, 1978, Addison-Wesley.

X

40. Hymovich DP and Hagopian GA: *Chronic illness in children and adults: a psychosocial approach,* Philadelphia, 1992, WB Saunders Co.

41. Ilfield FW: Coping styles in Chicago adults: description, *Human Stress* 6:2–10, 1980.

42. Johnson JE and Lauver DR: Alternative explanations of coping with stressful experience associated with physical illness, *Adv Nurs Sci* 11(2):39–52, 1989.

43. Kahana E, Faischild T, and Hakana B: Adaptation. In Mangen DJ and Peterson WA, editors: *Research instruments and social gerontology, vol I, clinical and social gerontology,* Minneapolis, 1981, University of Minnesota Press.

44. Kiely WF: Coping with severe illness, *Adv Psychosom Med* 8:105–118, 1981.

45. Lamb MA and Sheldon TA: The sexual adaptation of women treated for endometrial cancer, *Cancer Pract* 2(2):103–113, 1994.

46. Lampic C and others: Coping, psychosocial well-being and anxiety in cancer patients at follow-up visits, *Acta Oncologica* 33(8):887–894, 1994.

47. Lawson M and McGrath S: The social self-esteem inventory, *Ed Psychol Measure* 39:109–125, 1978.

48. Lazarus RS: *Emotion and adaptation,* New York, 1991, Oxford University Press.

49. Lazarus RS and Folkman S: *Stress, appraisal and coping,* New York, 1984, Springer Publishing.

50. Lewis F: Patient response to illness and hospitalization, *Radiography* 52(602):91–93, 1986.

51. Lindstrom TC: Defence mechanisms and some notes on their relevance for the caring profession, *Scand J Caring Sci* 3(3):99–104, 1989.

52. Lipowski ZJ: Psychosocial aspects of disease, *Ann Int Med* 71(6):1197–1206, 1969.

53. Mages NL and Mendelsohn GA: Effects of cancer on patients' lives: a peronological approach. In Stone GC, Cohen F, and Adler NE, editors: *Health psychology,* San Francisco, 1979, Jossey-Bass Publishers.

54. Marrow GR and others: Development of brief measures of psychosocial adjustment to medical illness applied to cancer patients, *Gen Hosp Psychiatry* 3:79–88, 1981.

55. McHugh P and others: The efficacy of audiotapes in promoting psychological well-being in cancer patients: a randomized controlled trial, *Brit J Cancer* 71(2):388–392, 1995.

56. McNair PM, Loor M, and Drappelman L: *POMS manual,* San Diego, 1971, Education and Industrial Testing Services.

57. Menniger K: Regulatory devices of the ego under major stress, *Int J Psychoanal* 35:412–420, 1954.

58. Moos RH and Tsu VD: The crisis of physical illness: an overview. In Moos R, editor: *Coping with physical illness,* New York, 1977, Plenum Publishing.

59. Neugarten B, Havinghurst R, and Tobin S: The measurement of life satisfaction, *J Gerontol* 16:134–143, 1961.

60. Norris J and Kunes-Connell M: Self-esteem, *Nurs Clin North Am* 20(4):745–761, 1985.

61. Northhouse L: The impact of cancer on the family: an overview, *Int J Psychiatry Med* 14(3):215–242, 1984.

62. Pearlin LI and Schoolar C: The structure of coping, *J Health Soc Behav* 19:2–21, 1978.

63. Pearlman RA and Uhlmann RF: Quality of life in chronic disease: perceptions of elderly patients, *J Gerontol* 43(2):25–30, 1988.

64. Platzer H: Body image—helping patients to cope with changes, *Intensive Care Nurs* 3(3):125–132, 1987.

65. Rawlinson E: Quality of life after treatment for laryngeal cancer: the patient's perspective, *Can J Radiog Radiother Nucl Med* 14(4):125–127, 1983.

66. Reasoner RW: Self-esteem through the life span, *Family Community Health* 6:11–18, 1983.

67. Rosenberg M: *Conceiving the self,* Malabar, Florida, 1986, Robert E Krieges.

68. Rosensteil A and Roth S: Relationships between cognitive activity and adjustment in four spinal-cord-injured individuals: longitudinal investigation, *J Human Stress* 35–43, March 1981.

69. Ruberman W and others: Psychosocial influences on mortality after myocardial infarction, *N Eng J Med* 311(9):552–559, 1984.

70. Schain WS and others: Mastectomy versus conservative surgery and radiation therapy, *Cancer* 73(4):1221–1228, 1994.

71. Shapiro DE and others: Cluster analysis of the medical coping modes questionnaire: evidence for coping with cancer styles?, *J Psychosom Res* 38(2):151–159, 1994.

72. Swan GE and others: The rationality/emotional defensiveness scale—II. Convergent and discriminant correlational dialysis in males and females with and without cancer, *J Psychosom Res* 36(4):349–359, 1992.

73. Turkat D: Defensiveness in self-esteem research, *Psychol Rec* 28:129–135, 1978.

74. Valliant GE: *Adaptation to life,* Boston, 1977, Little, Brown.

75. Vincent KG: The validation of a nursing diagnosis, *Nurs Clin North Am* 20(4):631–664, 1985.

76. Viney LL and Westbrook MT: Coping with chronic illness: strategy preferences, changes in preferences and associated emotional reactions, *J Chronic Dis* 37(6):489–502, 1984.

77. Weiner CL and Dodd MF: Coping amid uncertainty: an illness trajectory perspective, *Scholarly Inquiry Nurs Prac* 7(1):17–31, 1993.

78. Weisman AD: *Coping with cancer,* New York, 1979, McGraw-Hill Book Co.

79. Wellisch D and others: Evaluation of psychosocial problems of the homebound cancer patient, *Psychosom Med* 45:11–21, 1983.

80. Williams GH: Quality of life and its impact on hypertensive patients, *Am J Med* 82(1):48–105, 1987.

Family Coping: Potential for Growth

▶

Ineffective Family Coping: Disabling

▶

Ineffective Family Coping: Compromised

▶

Family Coping: Potential for Growth *is the effective managing of the patient's adaptive tasks by family members or a designated support person while exhibiting a desire and readiness for enhanced personal or family growth and health.*[9]

Ineffective Family Coping: Disabling *is the incapacitating behavior by family members or a designated support person to address effectively essential tasks required for adaptation to the health challenge.*[9]

Ineffective Family Coping: Compromised *is insufficient, ineffective, or compromised support, comfort, assistance, or encouragement by family members or a designated support person who may be needed by the patient to perform adaptive tasks related to his or her health challenge.*[9]

OVERVIEW

Family coping is best understood within a family context.[6, 8, 11, 12] For example, a young father reported, "Our 11-year-old son had a rare blood disease, unresponsive to chemotherapy. By exploring our family coping behaviors, new health-promoting family behaviors were developed at an important time in our family's life cycle. I believe that we coped well, learning to raise both our family and our children."

Coping is a process of adapting to an ever-changing environment, including new or recurring health challenges.[6, 11] Coping strategies are often divided into two categories: (1) problem-focused actions, such as providing care, transportation, or shopping, and (2) emotion-focused actions, such as affirmation, denial, or support. Depending on the situation, coping may be at an individual, family, or community level.[6, 11] When coping strategies are used at an individual level within a family, knowledge and responses are limited. However, when a family can have a conversation about each other's perceptions and their perceptions as a family as they relate to the health challenge, each member gains additional knowledge of other family members' perceptions as well as the family unit's perceptions of the experience. For example, families who do not have meaningful conversations about a presenting health challenge often have a number of individual reactions and a greater risk of increasing family chaos. If a family provides opportunities to strengthen the family unit by nurturing family relationships, offering flexibility or new roles and expanding strong social networks, effective family coping is experienced.[2, 8, 11]

Family coping is challenged by increasingly variable, complex family structures.[8, 11, 12] Some families gather by self-initiation to provide support, but the families are not the family structures that are recognized legally. Other family structures include nuclear families, blended families, extended families, adoptive families, single-parent families, foster families, and step-families. These families can also be subcategorized to include legitimate, revitalized, reassembled, and combination families. Currently a broad definition of *family* is needed to encompass the diversity of family forms in contemporary society.[11] Because the family may vary depending on the health challenge, for purposes of this discussion *family* is defined as "who the family says it is."[10,11]

Families can vary tremendously in how they do their work or how they cope with stressful events, including health challenges.[1–4,13,14] Rolland's integrative treatment model illustrates the impact of sudden, moderate-to-severe, and chronic illness on families.[11] Sudden health events, such as a ruptured cerebral aneurysm, moderate-to-severe events causing sudden incapacitation, such as a spinal cord tumor, or rapid relapse events, such as reocclusion of a coronary artery, require families to reorganize quickly and efficiently to respond to the health event. Chronic illness, such as renal failure, Alzheimer's disease, or AIDS, requires long-term caregiving and can often jeopardize family health physically and psychosocially.

Diagnoses related to family coping are guided by the Family Systems Theory, in which the matrix of identity is the family.[6,8,11] This theory offers a conceptual framework that focuses on the family and total family unit perceptions; the complexity of interacting family variables, such as typology, vulnerability, subsystem boundaries, transactional patterns, life cycle stages, and coping; and family health and competence, rather than family pathology. Family responses to transitions and hardships are viewed as a natural, predictable aspect of family life.

Family coping is evolutionary, multifaceted, and shaped over time. Family coping responses are learned skills.[1,3,13,14] During stressful events, families learn to cope; these coping skills become intrafamilial strengths, which are then used to protect the family during future transition and change. Some families are limited in the number

and types of family coping responses. Examples of effective family coping responses include mutual respect for the individuality of family members, effective communication of thoughts and feelings, and health-promoting behaviors during the health challenge. Manipulation, denial, anger, and avoidance are examples of ineffective family coping behaviors. Any family that has experienced serious health challenges understands that effective coping can best occur within a supportive environment that is individual, family-focused, and collaborative over the care continuum. Family coping involves *familying,* a chosen point of view of how the family will lead its life and will give meaning to all that happens in its life.[2]

ASSESSMENT

Family coping is assessed during a family health-illness cycle, health promotion and risk-reduction programs, or consultation related to family-specific requests. Several approaches are identified in the literature.[2,6,8,11,12] The nurse assesses individuals and the whole family system related to the presenting health challenge through a structured family interview process and informal family contacts. In complex family situations, an interdisciplinary interview process may be selected, using the expertise of the nurse, the social worker, and the family therapist.

During a family assessment it is important to determine (1) how the health challenge affects individual members as well as the total family, (2) whether the health challenge is in phase or out of phase in the family life stage, and (3) the unique meaning the family assigns to the health challenge.[11] For example, a single, 35-year-old mother of two teenagers who has an acute myocardial infarction may be also facing parent-adolescent value issues. This out-of-phase illness may exhaust coping strategies and may explain increased family anxiety. This family will demonstrate much different family coping mechanisms than a family at another family life stage.

In assessing family coping skills or strategies, it is important to know how families view their roles, their problem-solving actions, and the work they need to do. For example, some families view their role as direct care providers, whereas other families see their role as care managers. Families who cultivate many healthy coping strategies are better prepared. Those families with dysfunctional family behaviors experience more stress and have limited coping skills.

Factors influencing family coping are dynamic, interactive, and multifaceted. The most common are culture, ethnicity, and spirituality. Cultural influences include intragenerational relationships among family members; family values, rules, and rituals; family relationships; and family interactions with the external environment.[7] Examples are numerous. Americans focus on an intact nuclear family. Black families include kin and community. Italians tend to disregard the nuclear family concept and view their family as a three- or four-generational family. In African-American families the family members hold a rich, extensive network of shared responsibility, such as taking turns in phoning, visiting, or running errands in caring for older adults.[11] In Native American families it is important to be present with a member during birthing, illness, and death. Cultural sensitivity directs appropriate family outcomes in assessing family coping. Family rules, according to Satir, are shaped by culture and ethnicity, such as rules for withholding anger, overresponsibility, and lack of affection. She suggests that there are no bad families but that there are bad rules.[12] Some families who hold rigid beliefs about personal responsibility and control may cope effectively during the early stages of a health challenge but may progress to ineffective coping as the health challenge becomes prolonged.

Spirituality influences a family's coping response. A family's spiritual dimension is not restricted to religious beliefs and practices but includes family faith belief systems, formal or informal.[2,9,11] Families who perceive spirituality as a meaningful resource often engage in the discipline of quiet prayer or religious practices. These family actions are perceived as helpful in strengthening family coping during a family health challenge.

There are numerous family coping assessment tools available for use.[5,6,11] Some clinicians prefer to begin with a generic tool that will guide direction for various additive assessment tools. The family genogram is a useful tool in illustrating a family tree of significant multigenerational patterns and interactions of important family events horizontally across family members and vertically through the generations. This process focuses a family on sharing its history and on identifying family influences and coping patterns over time. Assessing family members' degree of exposure to health challenges and beliefs about coping through generations is important. For example, some families may cope well with crisis and loss but are unable to cope effectively with chronic illness, possibly because it has not been a lived family experience or is considered a family stigma. Other families may have limited coping skills and repeat dysfunctional patterns of denial, lack of preparation, and flight from terminal illness.[8] A family history of effective coping with moderate-to-severe constant stressors is a good predictor of how a family will adjust to health challenges that demand continuous caregiving activities.[11]

Assessing family coping along a care continuum is especially important for families adapting to chronic health challenges of a family member. Rolland's model supports assessing illness type, time phase, and family functioning.[11] Selected parameters include the following:

- The family belief system related to the health challenge
- The meaning of the health challenge for the family
- The impact of the health challenge on individuals and on family development
- Multigenerational family coping strategies with previous health challenges, loss, and crisis
- The family's planning for medical crises
- The family's capacity to handle home-based, medical caregiving
- The family's health- or illness-oriented communication, role exchanges, and extrafamilial support, including the use of community resources

X

Family Coping: Potential for Growth

Families experiencing effective coping may desire opportunities for growth. These may include a verbalized desire for a healthier lifestyle, exploring family myths, or expanding social networks.

■ Defining Characteristics

The presence of the following defining characteristics indicates that the family may be experiencing Family Coping: Potential for Growth:

- Family member(s) describes event or crisis as an opportunity for self-growth in values, priorities, goals, or relationships
- Family member(s) evidences movement toward health-promoting and enriching lifestyle consistent with maturational processes and treatment modalities and generally chooses experiences that optimize wellness
- Family member(s) expresses interest in individual contact or in a group that has experienced a similar situation

■ Related Factors

The following related factors are associated with Family Coping: Potential for Growth:

- Adaptive tasks effectively addressed to support goals of self-actualization to emerge
- Optimal level of family adjustment to previous family stress event(s)
- Appropriate social support and resources available

Ineffective Family Coping: Disabling

When ineffective family coping is disabling, some degree of family dysfunction exists. This may be sudden or chronic. For example, a family can exhibit a closed family system in which family members must be cautious about what they say and with whom they communicate. There can be a family myth that all family members are to think and feel the same way. If additional family stress events occur, family stress increases, and the family becomes more disabled in its coping behaviors. As the family becomes more disabled, isola-

tion from friends, community, and church begins to increase. In turn, the family becomes more alone, more neglectful of relationships, less competent in interacting with extrafamilial support systems, and unhealthy in family dynamics.

Successful coping as perceived by the family does not necessarily mean effective coping. For example, when a family uses withdrawal to face a health challenge, such as verbal, physical, sexual, or chemical abuse by family members, family anxiety may be decreased. This may be perceived by the family as successful coping; however, the situation continues as a pattern, so in reality there is ineffective family coping, which becomes disabling. The family may not always perceive itself to be immobilized or incapacitated but is clearly unable to adapt therapeutically to the health challenge.

■ Defining Characteristics

The presence of the following defining characteristics indicates that the family may be experiencing Ineffective Family Coping: Disabling:

- Verbalization of inability to cope
- Neglectful care of the patient related to basic human needs or health interventions
- Distortion of the health problem, including denial and prolonged overconcern
- Intolerance as expressed by agitation, depression, or hostility
- Abandonment
- Actions or decisions that are detrimental to the economic or psychosocial well-being of the patient
- Fostering of patient's development of learned helplessness or inactive dependence

■ Related Factors

The following related factors are associated with Ineffective Family Coping: Disabling:

- Long-term unexpressed feelings of guilt, anxiety, hostility, or despair of family member(s)
- Highly ambivalent family relationships
- Chronic pattern of defensiveness and resistance to treatment related to underlying anxiety of family member(s)

X

- Rigidity in function and roles among family members
- Highly ambivalent family relationships
- Depletion of family's supportive capacity

Ineffective Family Coping: Compromised

When family functioning is perceived as compromised, there is distress and limited energy for health promotion within the family. This can be temporary or long-term. Compromised family coping exists when behaviors are insufficient, ineffective, or accommodated. When family coping is consistently marked by a pattern of compromise, family growth is generally minimal or absent.[6,11]

Nurses are in a unique position to observe when a family's effective coping skills have begun to change.[2,11] Examples include reported feelings of powerlessness, the inability to share feelings or utilize support resources, and the resignation of individual or family preferences to accommodate a family member during a crisis or health challenge. When family behaviors are insufficient, there is usually an inadequate response, which may be verbalized as family inadequacy. This is often associated with a knowledge deficit related to family coping skills, family management of the situational stress, or family tasks during family life cycle transitions.[8,11] When family behaviors are ineffective, there are unsatisfactory outcomes that are generally related to a multiplicity of factors, such as mistiming, inappropriate or unhealthy coping skills, inadequate knowledge base, underutilization of extrafamilial resources, and underfunctioning by selected family members. When Ineffective Family Coping is associated with accommodation, generally some family members feel that their preferences have been overridden by other family members, which can result in feelings of powerlessness, guilt, or distress.

■ Defining Characteristics

The presence of the following defining characteristics indicates that the family may be experiencing Ineffective Family Coping: Compromised:

Subjective

- The patient expresses a concern about response of family to the health challenge
- Family expresses fear, guilt, or anxiety regarding the presenting health or situational challenge
- Family member(s) describes a knowledge deficit associated with coping skills or effective support behaviors

Objective

- Assistive or supportive family behaviors resulting in unsatisfactory outcomes
- Limited or absent personal family communication during a time of need
- Overprotective or underprotective family behaviors

■ Related Factors

The following related factors are associated with Ineffective Family Coping: Compromised:

- Inadequate or incorrect information or understanding by family member(s)
- Temporary preoccupation by family member(s) that results in ineffective actions
- Temporary family disorganization and alteration in family roles
- Concurrent situational or developmental family crises
- Chronicity of health challenge that exhausts the family's supportive capacity
- Family history of limited or ineffective coping strategies
- Altered family dynamics that result in temporarily unhealthy behaviors
- Lack of mutual support among family members

DIAGNOSIS

■ Differential Nursing Diagnosis

Family Coping: Potential for Growth is a wellness-oriented nursing diagnosis. This diagnosis may be related to a family's desire to improve family nutrition and relational communication and to expand play activities. In these situations, a clinical judgment is made about a family in transition from a specific level of wellness to a higher

X

level of wellness. Ineffective Family Coping: Disabling refers to an immobilized family who cannot therapeutically adapt to the health challenge. The disabling behavior may be related to family resistance to treatment, chronicity of the health challenge, or depletion of the family's support systems. Ineffective Family Coping: Compromised, temporary or long-term, is usually marked by insufficient, ineffective, or accommodated family behaviors. The individual or family system and how a family does its work in responding to a health challenge differentiates the cluster of family coping diagnoses from other nursing diagnoses. The diagnosis Ineffective Community Coping focuses on a community-level diagnosis. Individual Coping: Ineffective is an example of a patient diagnosis. Altered Family Processes is an example of a family-level diagnosis that focuses on alterations in family function and dynamics that may be related to a situational crisis, an economic crisis, or a history of ineffective coping strategies.

■ Medical and Psychiatric Diagnoses

Family coping nursing diagnoses focus on human responses to health. They are interrelated to selected medical and psychiatric diagnoses and require collaboration in assessment, interventions, care planning, and evaluation. Two examples are offered. The nursing diagnosis Ineffective Family Coping: Disabling can be related to eating disorders, explosive disorder, or avoidance disorder. The nursing diagnosis Ineffective Family Coping: Compromised can be related to phase-of-life problems, adjustment disorder, or avoidance disorder.

OUTCOME IDENTIFICATION, PLANNING, AND IMPLEMENTATION

The critical expected family outcome related to the cluster of family coping nursing diagnoses is effective family coping with a sense of family well-being. Success in achieving this outcome will be determined over time by recognizing the family relationship system and patterns as well as family mastery in improving the quality of relationships. Nursing interventions are purposeful and include

consistent, planned reevaluation. In preparing to meet with a family, the nurse must exercise control to have a safe environment and must focus on building a therapeutic relationship. As the family story unfolds, active listening is important. Family members must be encouraged to share perceptions and feelings that are relevant to the situation. Following an initial assessment, appropriate interventions are offered and explained. Then a family agreement is reached to try these interventions. During the family session, the nurse assists the family to gain insights and to reassess ways that the family receives new insights. In closing the session, the nurse assists the family in choosing a course of action and determines if the situation has been reframed since the opening of the family session. Future family sessions are scheduled as appropriate.

Nursing interventions can be categorized into five major areas: (1) assessing the individual or family system's cognitive appraisal and behavioral skills; (2) strengthening family competence; (3) facilitating family education; (4) enhancing family caring and emotional responsiveness over the care continuum; and (5) expanding extrafamilial resource opportunities to enhance family growth when appropriate.

How a family does its work or adapts to the sudden or chronic health challenge is a critical indicator of effective or ineffective family coping.[1-4, 13, 14] The underlying issue is generally about power—*family power*. Healthy family power nourishes the spirit of family life. When there is a misuse of family power, it takes many forms and disguises, such as hostility, blame, control, avoidance, rejection, forgetting, and neglect. Often, working through family power issues is difficult because of fear: fear of things that could happen and fear of things that require action (e.g., "I fear that my family cannot handle this illness"); fear of failure, rejection, or loss (e.g., "I fear that my family will fail"); and fear of life experiences (e.g., "I fear that my family will not be able to handle this"). Assessing individual and family coping strengths and gaining mutual agreement on desired family outcomes directs nursing or interdisciplinary interventions.

Family Coping: Potential for Growth

Outcomes identified for this nursing diagnosis focus on enhancing family health-promoting behaviors, such as learning new strategies to improve the quality of family relationships, health, nutrition, or play. The nurse provides the family with techniques to improve family relationships, such as the discipline of quiet story telling or intimacy exercises. It is also important to identify family enrichment opportunities, such as healthy food selections, family enhancement programs, and cultural events and to suggest cultivation of family leisure through activities such as hiking and reading.

Ineffective Family Coping: Disabling

Outcomes related to this nursing diagnosis focus on family identification of their predominant family relational behaviors, such as avoidance, forgetting, or neglect; improved, effective family expression of feelings among members and with others; and a demonstrated family attitude to learn new lifestyle coping patterns. Identification of outcomes will be family-specific related to the disabling behaviors exhibited. When family behavior is addictive, such as gambling, substance abuse, or alcoholism, nursing interventions focus on a referral to a family counselor or a program that specializes in addiction interventions. Over the care continuum, the nurse can continue to explore the family's perceptions in overcoming the disabling family behavior by asking the family about new insights, available options, and the next steps to take. At some point the nurse can explore family fears related to relapse and can assist the family to identify family strengths to cope effectively.

Ineffective Family Coping: Compromised

Outcomes related to this diagnosis focus on recognizing family relationship patterns, acknowledging the effect of family communication on individual members and others, and learning new strategies to improve family decision making. Nursing interventions initially focus on family awareness exercises related to family perceptions, coping strategies, types of family decision making, and extrafamilial resources available. Additional interventions are determined by family awareness and preferences. For example, when a family uses accommodation as their type of family decision making, some family member's choices are devalued. The nurse can explore with the family the types of family decision making, including the strengths and limitations of each. In turn, family decision making options can be purposefully chosen with potential for increasingly effective, health-promoting family coping behaviors.

X

◢ **NURSING CARE GUIDELINES**

Nursing Diagnosis: Family Coping: Potential for Growth

Expected Outcome: Family members will engage in health-promoting behaviors, such as healthy nutrition, regular exercise, nurturing extrafamilial relationships, and expression of hope, as identified by the family and within the family's established timeline.
- Establish a healthy relationship with the family *to enhance the nurse's effectiveness in therapeutic family interventions.*
- Assist the family to identify meaningful health-promoting behaviors *to strengthen family competence and health.*
- ▲ Facilitate appropriate resources as needed (e.g., support groups, respite care, nutrition counselor, sleep evaluation clinic, or spiritual director).

Expected Outcome: Family members will express positive feelings related to family growth within 3 months.
- Assist the family in using effective communication skills (e.g., "I feel . . . ," "I perceive . . . ," "I prefer . . . "),

---

■ = nursing intervention; ▲ = collaborative intervention.   *Continued*

■ **NURSING CARE GUIDELINES — CONT'D**

active listening to one another, and honest, direct communication *to enhance a sense of nurturance and support.*

- Facilitate experiences in which the family can be supportive of one another *to promote a trusting family relationship.*
▲ Assist family in expressing perceptions related to family growth *to reinforce family strengths.*

■ **NURSING CARE GUIDELINES**
Nursing Diagnosis: Ineffective Family Coping: Disabling

Expected Outcome: The family will control or terminate abusive coping behaviors and use effective coping skills prioritized according to need within 6 weeks.
- Respect each family member's individual responses (e.g., withdrawal, resistance, anger, blame, or verbal assault); intervene appropriately with practice sessions, goal setting, and supportive caring *to develop healthy family coping skills.*
- Determine the family unit composition, family dynamic, range of family coping behaviors, and the effect of the presenting health challenge on the family system *to support family competence (not failure).*
▲ Assist family to appraise the presenting health challenge and the degree of effectiveness of family coping *to promote the maintenance of family control and self-esteem.*
▲ Assess readiness of the family to adapt alternative ways of responding to the presenting health challenge *to support family competence (not failure).*

Expected Outcome: The family will utilize family and human services to preserve the family's supportive capacity within 2 weeks.
- Provide information about appropriate and available external family resources *to assist the family in understanding that professional assistance is viewed as normal (not pathological) and that through such experiences most families work to strengthen family competence.*
- Provide a climate for family decision making *to promote the maintenance of family control and competence.*
▲ Assist the family in locating and using resources *to assist the family's supportive capacity.*
▲ Monitor family perceptions about their resources and their experiences in accessing and using resources, facilitating changes as needed *to preserve the supportive capacity of family members over time.*

■ = nursing intervention; ▲ = collaborative intervention.

■ **NURSING CARE GUIDELINES**
Nursing Diagnosis: Ineffective Family Coping: Compromised

Expected Outcome: The family will appropriately express feelings and accurately appraise the presenting health challenge within 1 month.
- Establish weekly family conferences.
- Determine the family unit composition, family dynamic, range of family coping behaviors, and the effect of presenting health challenge on the family system *to support family competence (not failure).*
- Assist family members to verbalize distress from their own perspective and from a family perspective *to expand the family's cognitive appraisal skills.*

■ = nursing intervention; ▲ = collaborative intervention.

X

- Establish a healthy relationship with family *to enhance the nurse's effectiveness in therapeutic family intervention.*
- Assist family to appraise the presenting health challenge and the degree of effectiveness of family coping *to promote the maintenance of family control and self-esteem.*

Expected Outcome: Family members will verbalize educational needs and expectations for individuals and for the family by the fourth family conference.

- Present an overview of potential family educational areas, such as relational communication skills, coping skills, attention-focusing skills, and problem-solving skills *to expand the family's knowledge base and coping strategies.*
- ▲ Assist family to prioritize needs to strengthen family competence.
- ▲ Develop a teaching plan for these needs, including a family assessment of outcomes *to promote family growth through the experience of being a family within an educational climate.*

Expected Outcome: The family will utilize extrafamilial resources to preserve family strengths on a temporary basis, beginning in 2 weeks.

- Provide an overview of appropriate and available extrafamilial resources *to expand the family's knowledge base and coping strategies.*
- Provide a climate for family decision making regarding the type of extrafamilial resources preferred *to promote the maintenance of family control and competence.*
- ▲ Monitor family perceptions regarding access to resources and their experience in utilizing extrafamilial resources *to preserve the supportive capacity of family members over time.*

Expected Outcome: Family members will express positive feelings related to family strengths and growth within 3 months.

- Assist family in using effective communication skills, active listening to one another, or honest, clear communication, such as "I cope by . . . ," "When this happens, I feel . . . ," and "I prefer . . ." *to promote family competence and health.*
- Facilitate experiences in which family members can practice being supportive and relational to one another (e.g., role playing, script acting, and modeling) *to promote family growth within an educational climate.*
- Assist family in expressing feelings from an individual and family perspective (e.g., "I feel that I am . . ." and "I feel that my family is angry, withdrawing") *to strengthen family coping skills by practice and refinement.*

Expected Outcome: Family members will verbalize satisfaction with the continuity of family care and their competence in developing effective behaviors within 6 months.

- Provide regular family conferences for supportive and informational sharing *to enhance the continuity of family competence and caring.*
- Provide opportunities for the family to share feelings about the quality and continuity of family care; refine nursing interventions as appropriate *to affirm healthy family coping behavior changes.*
- ▲ Affirm family competence in healthy coping behaviors with honest appraisals and through personal affirmation *to revitalize family integrity and competence.*

EVALUATION

Evaluation related to family coping is based on the achievement of family outcomes. Refinement of nursing interventions may be required, not because the interventions were inappropriate but because family dynamics are in constant change, because new or emergent data contributes to new priorities, and because referrals to other professionals may be indicated. The evaluation process requires consistent, ongoing evaluation with participation by the family and health professionals. Of importance is continuity provided by the same nurse(s) across the care continuum so that family competence can be strengthened and family growth affirmed.

X

Family Coping: Potential for Growth

Family reporting will provide the nurse and the family with the most definitive evaluation of achievement of expected family outcomes related to this nursing diagnosis. Growth areas can include increased family discoveries, nurturing, caring, and connection; respect for individual family members' needs; mutual trust; commitment to and shared responsibility for the family; flexibility of family roles; and a sense of play and humor. One question for a family might be, "As a family what is important at this time to enjoy family health?"

Ineffective Family Coping: Disabling

The measures to evaluate success in family coping will be formative (i.e., family member perceptions) and cumulative (i.e., family changes over time). Initially there would be family acknowledgment of distress with the health challenge. Over time healthy family coping skills would be evidenced by open, honest family expressions and a reported decrease in family distress. Family idealization of professional resources and learning opportunities would be perceived as generally helpful. Finally, the family would demonstrate and verbalize healthy family energy in meeting the presenting health challenge, with a healthy balance between individual and family commitments. A question for this family might be, "Do you have any new insights related to your family's coping with fear related to a relapse of unhealthy family behaviors?"

Ineffective Family Coping: Compromised

Successful family outcomes related to this nursing diagnosis are achieved when the family (1) demonstrates and communicates a decrease in family distress; (2) demonstrates a deeper commitment to the individual or family system and shared responsibility; (3) uses appropriate external familial resources; and (4) perceives and communicates family growth toward effective family coping. A question for this family might be, "How do you perceive your family communication among yourselves and with other families?"

Case Study with Plan of Care

David A., a 39-year-old, married farmer with two children, is in his third week of recovery from triple-vessel, myocardial revascularization. His wife, Abby, is an attentive mother and homemaker. Their daughter, Jane, is 14 years old, a tenth-grade honor student, and a star athlete. Their son, Joe, is a happy, energetic, well-adjusted 6-year-old. After a cardiac rehabilitation class one evening, Mr. A. expresses interest to his wife in working on stress management and healthy food choices. The next morning Mrs. A. places a call to the cardiac rehabilitation nurse, Diane, for a family appointment. Diane makes a diagnosis of Effective Family Coping: Potential for Growth. The following care plan was initiated.

X

Plan of Care for the David A. Family

Nursing Diagnosis: Effective Family Coping: Potential for Growth Related to Health-Promoting Behaviors in Prevention Health Checks, Nutrition, and Stress Management

Expected Outcome: The David A. family will improve health-promoting behaviors in the areas of health prevention checks, improved nutrition choices, and stress management within 4 weeks.

- ▪ Establish a healthy relationship with family.
- ▲ Facilitate cardiac health risk appraisal screening within 2 weeks for family members.
- ▲ Facilitate family nutritional counseling through Healthy Choice hospital program.
- ▲ Help family access books and videotapes on stress management.

▪ = nursing intervention; ▲ = collaborative intervention.

Expected Outcome: The David A. family members will know their status related to modifiable cardiac risk factors, will consistently make healthy nutritional choices, and will communicate their feelings and perceptions regularly.

- Provide information update on cardiac risk factors and nutrition as needed.
- Assist family in using effective communication skills (e.g., "I feel . . . ," "I perceive . . . ," "I prefer . . . "), active listening to one another, and honest, direct communication.
- ▲ Assist family in expressing perceptions related to family growth.

Expected Outcome: The David A. family will identify various stress management techniques and their perceptions regarding their usefulness to them as an individual or family system by the third family conference.

- Provide an opportunity of appropriate and available stress management resources.
- ▲ Facilitate practice session related to the various stress management modalities (e.g., stress identification, exercise, guided imagery, and music therapy).
- Assist family in using effective communication skills, active listening to one another, or honest, clear communication, such as "I cope by . . . ," "When this happens, I feel . . . ," and "I prefer . . . ."
- ▲ Assist family members to express feelings related to family strengths and growth over time; evaluate in 3 months.

■■ CRITICAL THINKING EXERCISES

1. How could the A. family's well-being be compromised if Mr. A. were to become permanently disabled?

2. How might caregivers lend support to families to live well during uncertainties of health challenges and the threatened loss of a family member?

3. Have you reflected on your own multigenerational and family history as related to coping, your health beliefs, and your current life cycle stage? What have you discovered? What implications can your own family history have on the way you approach your practice?

4. Families coping with chronic health challenges often need to deal with multiple systems and professionals. Because these systems are often disengaged from one another, how can you best assist families to cope with processes and systems that are unfamiliar?

REFERENCES

1. Bull MJ, Maruyama G, and Luo D: Testing a model for posthospital transition of family caregivers for elderly persons, *Nurs Res* 44(3):132–138, 1995.

2. Dossey BM and others: *Holistic nursing,* Gaithersburg, Maryland, 1995, Aspen Publishers.

3. Fink SV: The influence of family resources and family demands on the strains and well-being of caregiving families, *Nurs Res* 44(3):139–146, 1995.

4. Langner SR: Finding meaning in caring for elderly relatives: loss and personal growth, *Holist Nurs Pract* 9(3):75–84, 1995.

5. Loos F and others: Circular question: a family interviewing strategy, *DCCN* 90(1):46–53, 1990.

6. McCubbin H and Thompson A, editors: *Family assessment inventories for research and practice,* Madison, Wisconsin, 1987, University of Wisconsin, Madison.

7. McGoldrick M, Pearce J, and Giordano J, editors: *Ethnicity and family therapy,* New York, 1982, The Guilford Press.

8. Minuchin S: *Families and family therapy,* Cambridge, Massachusetts, 1974, Harvard University Press.

9. North American Nursing Diagnosis Association: *NANDA nursing diagnoses: definitions and classification, 1995–1996,* Philadelphia, 1994, The Association.

10. Robinson CA: Beyond dichotomies in the nursing of persons and families, *Image* 27(2):116–120, 1995.

11. Rolland JS: *Families, illness & disability: an integrative treatment model,* New York, 1994, Basic Books.

12. Satir V: *Cojoint family therapy: your many faces,* Palo Alto, California, 1967, Science and Behavior Books.

13. Schaefer KM: Women living in paradox: loss and discovery in chronic illness, *Holist Nurs Pract* 9(3):63–74, 1995.

14. Snelling J: The effects of chronic pain on the family unit, *J Adv Nurs* 19(3):543–551, 1994.

X

Ineffective Individual Coping

Ineffective Individual Coping *is impairment of adaptive behaviors and problem-solving abilities of a person in meeting life's demands and roles.*[7]

OVERVIEW

Coping is a process by which a person manages the ever-changing environment. From a beginning awareness that a condition exists, to dealing with the emotions generated by it, to a specific, deliberate action on it, to considering the effects of the action on a life goal, the range of the process is great. For the individual at a given time, the behaviors noted are often the best that he or she can do given a particular genetic, developmental, biological, and situational context. Effective coping implies adaptation to the environment, successful accomplishment of the tasks associated with growth and development, and management of problems. Some aspects of the environment and events in the life cycle are more critical or problematic to an individual and are labeled stressful. A person with an acute health crisis, such as a broken leg or a chronic disease, or someone undergoing treatment for a particular condition, is experiencing stress. Changes in lifestyle, in one's role in the family or work situation, or in one's body can be perceived as stressful. If a person is coping effectively with a stressful event, then the adjustment or recovery is enhanced.

Disease and maladaptation, even death, are believed to be long-term consequences of stress and are related to Ineffective Individual Coping. A decrease in psychological well-being and social functioning is experienced. More immediate effects or outcomes are noted in changes in affect, in the quality of interpersonal encounters, and in physiological response.[3,4,6,9]

Lazarus and others describe a model that focuses on the regulation of the emotions and management of the person-environment transaction. "Coping refers to the person's cognitive and behavioral efforts to manage (reduce, minimize, master, or tolerate) the internal and external demands of the person-environment transaction that is appraised as taxing or exceeding the person's resources."[3,11] Two appraisals precede coping: (1) a primary appraisal considers the effects on oneself and one's goals, values, and commitments. The person asks him- or herself about the possibilities of being perceived as incompetent, being endangered of one's life or health or those of another or of losing the love of an important person; and (2) a secondary appraisal identifies the actions possible; that is, what can be changed; what cannot be changed but must be accepted; what can improve chances for a positive outcome; and what actions need to be delayed or postponed. During these appraisals one arrives at conclusions regarding the threat to oneself, the meaning of the event, its predictability, and the degree of control possible.

Coping strategies or modes can be divided into two major groupings: problem-focused strategies and emotion-focused strategies. Problem-focused strategies are actions to identify or change the effects of the event, stress, or illness or cognitive activities generated by the event, stress, or illness. Emotion-focused strategies are actions to change or control feelings and emotional states generated by the events, stress, or illness.

The Ways of Coping Checklist (WOC and WOCR)[10] is an inventory of adult coping strategies in eight categories: problem-focused coping, wishful thinking, distancing, emphasizing the problem, self-blame, tension reduction, self-isolation, and seeking social supports. Other studies[1,2,4,5,10-17] have identified strategies such as increasing activity; making self statements; praying, hoping, and relying on religious or philosophical beliefs; ignoring pain, diverting attention, and denial; and preoccupation with objects of meaning.

Leventhal and Nerenz[10] have also conceptualized coping as part of a self-regulating system. The first stage of their model is the preattentive stage and appraisal process in which perceptual representation and interpretation occur. The stimulus first enters the perceptual system through the sense organs, where it is registered, and a perceptual representation is generated. The sense organs then relay the input to the central nervous system. Emotions affect the process by intensifying body sensations. By further processing, aspects of the stimulus event stimulate the recall and perception memories, which again may activate other memories. The relationships among memory structure, the input, and one's attending to the information determine when the information reaches conscious awareness. Emotional memory structures are more powerful and demand greater attention. The schemata of past experiences assists in interpreting the event—in other words, mental images about what was felt, seen, heard, and smelled, what the symptom was called, how long it lasted, its cause, and its prognosis. The interpretation of the stimulus occurs as it is given labels, causal relationships, time structures, and consequences. Leventhal and Nerenz stress the importance of distinguishing between the types of memory for determining the effect on the coping process. Perceptual memory—memory of the visual, auditory, and tactile sensations of an event—is associated with automatic responding. Therefore interpretation of an event using more of the emotional schemata leads to automatic responding. Abstract and conceptual memory is related to more conscious, volitional responding.

The response or coping stage follows the complex appraisal process. The representations of the

events, stress, or illness and the interrelated factors direct the plan and actions. For example, the meaning of the label *diabetic* to the patient will give the patient ideas of where to go for help, and in what medication and diet regimen the patient may be asked to participate. Fears, anxiety, or other emotions aroused by the thought of AIDS will promote behaviors to regulate or cope with these emotions. The amount of time believed to be necessary to make a plan of action or to carry it out will influence the coping actions taken. The patient's ability to postpone satisfaction or to endure will also influence the timing.

Health problems are particularly demanding of emotional coping resources. The threat to the self is great. The dependence on others for assistance of all types increases. The feelings generated may overwhelm abilities to do what is necessary: problem solving is delayed. Lifestyle changes may be easy while in a hospital, but not at work or in the home. If treatment is extended for months or habits or daily routines altered for years, the time dimension will affect the plan and the action.

The patient tends to repeat actions found useful in the past. Medications used the last time are thought to work this time. Fear may cause the patient to postpone a needed visit to a clinic. Beliefs, values, and goals also influence the strategies used or planned. The nurse deals differently with the cocaine habit of an unemployed, homeless man than with the cocaine habit of a college student studying to become a chemist.

Perceptions of the self as able to identify problems, make plans, and act greatly affect the patient's use of available resources. In other words, self-esteem is important. Being able to visualize oneself as thin, or not smoking, or free from pain is also useful. One's knowledge and skill base affects coping. Observing others who are successfully handling the event, stress, or illness further enhances development. The opportunity to practice or try it out for oneself is reinforcing.

The last stage of Leventhal and Nerenz's model is the monitoring stage, which involves the appraisal process again. The patient evaluates the change in distress, the coping responses, and the objective effect on the illness or the event. The appraisal is related to several factors. First, the setting of reasonable goals is important. When goals are set too high, are unrealistic and very abstract, are extremely concrete and minute, or when they demand an unreasonable time sequence, the patient may conclude that he or she cannot make a difference and thus effect change. Second, the feedback system is important in the appraisal process. The model has two basic types of feedback: emotional and objective. Leventhal and Nerenz proposed that the key sign of disruption of problem-solving behavior is awareness of affect. As the problem-solving behavior becomes less effective in coping with the stresses, the person focuses less on acquiring and processing information and more on emotional responses. Emotional expressions are pleas for assistance or social support. Reevaluation is signaled by intense emotions.

Finally, the recurring appraisal or interpretation of the event, stress, or illness and the coping are dynamic. Change does occur; transitions are made. Perhaps most important, one perceives things differently, feels more sure of oneself, plans for oneself, takes pleasure in the actions taken, sees the progress made, and knows his or her desires.

ASSESSMENT

The nurse assesses information regarding the patient's experience with the event, stress, or illness, the actions being taken to deal with the consequences of the event, stress, or illness, and the outcomes desired.[1,4,7,9,10-14] Important considerations include the effects of age, sex, specific illness, procedure(s), treatment(s), and socioeconomic status. Of extreme importance are the effects of the support system, including the nurse and other members of the health care team, in making an event less threatening or a situation more tolerable or understandable, in meeting basic needs for food, safety, and caring, and in validating the fears and emotion being experienced. Specifically, the nurse should address the following parameters: the complex situation being experienced; coping style; the coping style demanded by a particular event, stress, or illness or the family,

community, or culture; the degree of anxiety; the effects of time on the event, stress, or illness; the opportunity for control over important outcomes; the timing of coping strategies; any information or teaching gaps; and the effects of stress on the 11 Functional Health Patterns.

■ Defining Characteristics

The presence of the following defining characteristics indicates that the patient may be experiencing Ineffective Individual Coping:

Physiological
- Stress-related illness (e.g., diabetes or hypertension)
- Stress-related symptoms (e.g., back pain, frequent colds)
- Drug abuse or dependence
- Accident-prone behavior

Psychological
- Engaging in lifestyles with risk to health
- Increased anxiety
- Unhappiness or dissatisfaction
- Lack of future orientation and hopelessness
- Pessimism
- Focus on oneself
- Use of defensive patterns (e.g., denial, dissociation, hypervigilance, and projection)

Social
- Nonproductive lifestyle
- Lack of functioning in usual social roles
- Nonperformance of activities of daily living
- Inappropriate behavior in social situations
- Lack of concern for and detachment from usual social supports

■ Related Factors

The following related factors are associated with Ineffective Individual Coping:

Physiological
- Memory loss
- Sensory or perceptual impairment
- Nervous system impairment
- Disease process
- Previous psychiatric treatment
- Complications

Psychological

- Impaired self-efficacy or self-concept
- Powerlessness
- Lack of hardiness
- Lowered self-competency
- Personality disorder
- Conflict arising from incompatible motives or goals
- Inaccurate appraisal of stress, event, or illness
  - Inability to recognize source of threat
  - Inability to redefine or interpret threat correctly
  - Inability to find meaning for the event
  - Inability to identify the skills, knowledge, and abilities one has to cope with the threat
  - Lack of clear, realistic goals or outcomes
  - Unresolved memories of past threats or negative experiences
- Inaccurate response repertoire
  - Difficulty in expressing feelings, especially anger, guilt, and fear
  - Use of behavior destructive to oneself or others
  - Inability to seek out or to learn new skills and knowledge needed
  - Inability to deal with tangible consequences of stress, event, or illness
  - Increasing emotional responsiveness or lack of objective responsiveness
  - Defensive avoidance of dealing with threatening situations
  - Lack of palliative skills
- Inappropriate deployment of coping resources
- Inability to develop alternative goals, plans, actions, and rewards
- Lack of ability to transfer knowledge and skills to actual resolution of problem
- Giving up hope and spiritual values
- Social withdrawal
- Difficulty in using problem-solving skills and decision-making skills
- Lack of assertiveness behaviors
- Impaired communication skills
- Concerns or fears about initiating action
- Lack of an appropriate coping response because there is no cognitive cue to action
- Lack of supportive social network

- Overuse or underuse of certain responses
- Life cycle or stage of development

Social

- Stress, event, or illness
- Loss of loved one
- Threat to life
- Threat to security or lack of employment
- Pain
- Multiple repetitive stressors over time
- Lack of supportive social network

Situation or context

- Lack of resources
- Social or cultural instability
- Lack of available treatment
- Exhaustion of available treatment

Spiritual

- Giving up hope and spiritual values

DIAGNOSIS

■ Differential Nursing Diagnosis

The diagnosis Ineffective Individual Coping is a very broad category that encompasses the whole process of coping.[7] Consequently, there are nursing diagnoses that focus on just a part or an aspect of the process. It is useful as a beginning diagnosis; then, as more and more data is gathered about a patient, the nurse can be more specific in the diagnosis. For example, the diagnosis Fear or Anxiety may be more appropriate because the patient may be dealing with this aspect of the process and may only acknowledge these feeling states and claim no desire to look at the whole. He or she may be overwhelmed by a particular situation and only be willing to deal with information about a disease or disorder; the diagnosis Knowledge Deficit would be more appropriate than Ineffective Individual Coping. Nursing diagnoses need to be "patient friendly" or understood at least partially by the patient and provide the nurse a focus for planning interventions.

Some nurses prefer focusing on a part of the coping process instead of the whole. Nursing diagnoses such as Caregiver Role Strain, Grieving, Pain, Post-Trauma Response, Rape-Trauma Syn-

X

drome, and Relocation Stress Syndrome already identify the event, stress, or illness as one of the first steps of the process of coping. The nursing diagnoses Ineffective Denial, Defensive Coping, Social Isolation, and Health-Seeking Behaviors (Specify) identify the method a patient is using in handling the event, stress, or illness.

At this point, there is no definitive research to assist the nurse in the selection of one diagnosis over another. However, the data needs to support the diagnosis; the patient needs to acknowledge the diagnosis as an aspect of the problem that he or she and the nurse are working together on; and the nurse needs to conceptualize the diagnosis as useful in his or her practice.

■ Medical and Psychiatric Diagnoses

The major illnesses, especially chronic illnesses and diseases associated with impending death, are commonly related to increased stress, and therefore the nurse may frequently find the diagnosis

Ineffective Individual Coping useful. A few examples are cancer, stroke, heart disease, or surgery, accidents, suicide attempts, major depression, and schizophrenia.

OUTCOME IDENTIFICATION, PLANNING, AND IMPLEMENTATION

The expected outcomes for the nursing diagnosis Ineffective Individual Coping were selected to describe the steps in the coping process.[9,10] First is appraising the events; then, using the facts to redefine the event, stress, or illness. The patient will appropriately express his or her feelings as necessary and identify them as related to the event, stress, or illness. Then the patient will experience decreasing emotional responsiveness and increasing objectivity and problem-solving ability. Finally, the patient will be able to deal with and evaluate the event, stress, or illness.

◢ NURSING CARE GUIDELINES
Nursing Diagnosis Ineffective Individual Coping°

Expected Outcome: The patient will accurately appraise the event, stress, or illness.
- Assist patient to determine the what, who, why, where, when, and how of the event, stress, or illness. *If the stimulus and related actions of the patient remain out of conscious awareness, the opportunities to take effective action are decreased. Discussion with another person makes the event, stress, or illness more real—less a dream or fantasy—and decreases the need for less mature defense mechanisms.*
- Seek time sequences, beliefs about what should or should not be, and roles of important people involved. *Further clarification of the event, stress, or illness and associated beliefs and expectations of others reduces patient fear and anxiety and increases patient knowledge.*
- Identify areas that cannot be recalled or described. *Areas that are not available to the conscious mind may require further exploration with a therapist.*
- Give empathetic responses to expressions of feelings *because this assists the patient to accept his or her feeling state and enhances the nurse-patient relationship.*

Expected Outcome: The patient will use new facts or knowledge to redefine the threat, stress, or illness.
- Provide preparatory information to changes, treatment, tests, and so on because *facts have the potential of reducing the threat and increasing the patient's ability to cope effectively.*
- Describe the sound, smell, taste, feel, and appearance of the treatment. *Impacting as many of the five senses as possible increases the learning curve.*

■ = nursing intervention; ▲ = collaborative intervention.
°References 1, 2, 4, 5, 8, 10, 12, 16, 17.

- Explain the causes of the sensation *that provide the facts for the patient to use when he or she is coping with new or strange, often painful, sensations.*
- Give information about how long the pain, procedure, or treatment will last *because, if the time is known the discomfort may be more tolerable and may offer the patient hope of an end.*

Expected Outcome: The patient will express feelings appropriately and identify them as related to the event, stress, or illness.
- Assist in identifying feelings with names that are acceptable and understandable to the patient *because a named state is less fearful and less threatening than one that is unnamed.*
- Validate the feelings expressed because *this increases the patient's sense of being understood and valued.*
- Encourage description of feelings *because they become less overwhelming when expressed.*
- Ask questions and make comments that relate the feelings being experienced to the event, stress, or illness *that makes them more attached to a specific situation and less generalized or attached to other situations, events, or people.*

Expected Outcome: The patient will have decreased emotional responsiveness.
- Give feedback about the behavior and feeling states observed and expressed *to assist patient in becoming aware of his or her feeling states. Fear, anger, helplessness, and feelings of rejection overwhelm objective rational processes.*
- Use distraction, distancing, relaxation, instruction, listening, and directing activity *as ways to offer relief from intense emotions.*
- Teach relaxation techniques, distraction, removing self from the situation via mind or body, taking time, seeking help, and so on *to increase the patient's coping skills. Management of one's emotional response needs to be achieved before problem solving can proceed.*
- Provide the opportunity for practice and use in real situations *because this increases the possibility of future use and enhances learning.*

Expected Outcome: The patient will have increased objectivity and the ability to solve problems, make decisions, and communicate needs.
- Teach problem-solving, decision-making, and communication skills *because the patient needs to take action to learn coping skills for regulating emotions and maintaining self-control and for problem solving.*
- Provide opportunity for practice and use in real situations *because this increases the possibility of use by the patient in his or her real life.*

Expected Outcome: The patient will evaluate the strategies used to deal with the event, stress, or illness.
- Explore past situations in which effective coping behaviors were demonstrated. *Recalling a past experience with similar circumstances assists the patient in believing in his or her capacity to deal with the threat, stress, or illness.*
- Provide feedback and instruct patient on how to obtain it from others. *Feedback provides data to help in evaluation of one's actions.*
- Teach conceptual model for understanding coping and stress. *Having a conceptual model or framework to look at a disease process or coping process or one's own reactions helps an individual evaluate his or her actions.*

EVALUATION

Using the expected outcomes as goals, the nurse and the patient together can arrive at a consensus of achievement. To what extent have the defining characteristics been reduced or modified? Probably the most important aspect of the evaluation is the new question raised, the challenge to an old idea held by nurse and patient, or the action avoided—in other words, a discovery of a new goal.

▶ CASE STUDY WITH PLAN OF CARE

Mr. John R., a 29-year-old, separated black male, walked into the HMO stating he had a severe sore throat, could not eat, had not worked for a day, and was feeling "awful." He wanted to see the doctor and get a prescription for an antibiotic. The medical record revealed two episodes within the last 9 months of complaints of a sore throat, culture of organism, and antibiotic treatment. The separation from his wife was a year ago. He had not had a physical in 2 years. During the assessment interview, the nurse gathered the following information. Mr. John R., appeared tired, presented his problem in short, terse statements, was irritable about the clinic's slowness, and expressed a need to get back to work. Within the past 3 weeks he had been required to work overtime because of deadline penalties, and his boss said that the patient's promotion, due in 2 months, depended on his performance now. The patient said that in general things were fine. His wife apparently was happy without him, and he was too busy to care or to think about that relationship now. He made one remark about his boss. "What do you do with a nervous boss?" He described his diet as fast food "taken on the run." He obtains about 6 hours of sleep per night and awakes one or two times near morning. He has infrequent contact with his family, who live in the area.

▶ PLAN OF CARE FOR MR. JOHN R.

Nursing Diagnosis: Ineffective Individual Coping Related to Increased Stress at Work and Limited Coping Strategies

Expected Outcome: Mr. John R. will report increased information on, and consequences to self, of stressors experienced.
- Give Mr. R. stress management pamphlet and encourage him to read it.
- Raise questions, encourage data gathering, and promote an attitude of openness to new information.

Expected Outcome: Mr. John R. will report change in diet, sleep pattern, and ability to set work limits.
- Monitor diet and sleep patterns.
- Note sections of above pamphlet on techniques for stress management and request that Mr. R. try one during the week and report when he calls back after antibiotic treatment.

Expected Outcome: Mr. John R. will describe one or two ways to handle nervous boss and deal with self.
- Set time to discuss idea of how to handle nervous boss when he calls in after antibiotic treatment.

■ = nursing intervention; ▲ = collaborative intervention.

X

▦ CRITICAL THINKING EXERCISES

1. If Mr. John R. does not wish to discuss his "nervous boss," nor has he read stress management material, what stage of the coping process does this indicate? What would one intervention be?
2. What signs or symptoms would indicate a referral for stress counseling? Marital counseling?
3. How would the nurse document an ongoing concern about Mr. John R.'s ability to cope?

REFERENCES

1. Benjamin LS: Good defenses make good neighbors. In Conte HR and Putchik R, editors: *Ego defenses: theory and measurement,* New York, 1995, John Wiley & Sons.
2. Davis TMA and others: Undergoing cardiac catheterization: the effects of informational preparation and coping style on patient anxiety during the procedure, *Heart Lung* 23(1): 140–150, 1994.
3. Folkman S and others: Dynamics of a stressful encounter: cognitive appraisal, coping and encounter outcomes, *J Pers Soc Psychol* 50(5):992–1003, 1986.
4. Folkman S, Chesney MA, and Christopher-Richards A: Stress and coping in caregiving partners of men with AIDS, *Psychiatr Clin North Am* 17(1):35–53, 1994.

5. Good M: Relaxation techniques for surgical patients, *AJN* 95(5):39–43, 1995.

6. Holahan CJ and Moos RH: Life stresses and mental health: advances in conceptualizing stress resistance. In Avison WR and Gotlib IH, editors: *Stresses and mental health: contemporary issues and prospects for the future,* New York, 1994, Plenum Press.

7. Kim MJ, McFarland GK, and McLane AM: *Pocket guide to nursing diagnoses,* ed 6, St. Louis, 1995, Mosby–Year Book.

8. Kumasaka LMKB and Dungan JM: Nursing strategy for initial emotional response to cancer diagnosis, *Cancer Nurs* 16(4):296–303, 1993.

9. Lazarus RS and Folkman S: *Stress, appraisal and coping,* New York, 1984, Springer Publishing.

10. Leventhal H and Nerenz DR: A model for stress research with some applications for control of stress disorder. In Meichenbaum D and Jarenko ME, editors: *Stress reduction and prevention,* New York, 1983, Plenum Press.

11. Meichenbaum D and Fitzpatrick D: Constructivist narrative perspective on stress and coping: stress inoculation applications. In Golberger L and Breznitz S, editors: *Hand-book of stress: theoretical and clinical aspects,* ed 2, New York, 1993, Free Press.

12. Mishel MH and Sorenson DS: Revision of the Ways of Coping Checklist for a clinical population, *West J Nurs Res* 15(1):59–76, 1993.

13. Palmer S and Dryden W: *Counseling for stress problems,* London, 1995, Sage Publications.

14. Ryan-Wenger NM and Copland SG: Coping strategies used by black school-age children from low-income families, *J Pediatr Nurs* 9(1):33–40, 1994.

15. Sharrer VW and Ryan-Wenger MN: A longitudinal study of age and gender differences of stressors and coping strategies in school-aged children, *J Pediatr Health Care* 9:123–130, 1995.

16. Snow DL and Kline ML: Preventive interventions in the workplace to reduce negative psychiatric consequences of work and family stress. In Mazure CM, editor: *Does stress cause psychiatric illness,* Washington, D.C., 1995, American Psychiatric Press.

17. Solomon Z: *Coping with war-induced stress,* New York, 1995, Plenum Press.

X

Ineffective Denial

▶

Ineffective Denial *is a state in which an individual unconsciously disowns unpleasant or painful reality to the detriment of health to reduce anxiety or fear.*

OVERVIEW

Denial is the negation of unpleasant reality. The term can be used in everyday language as simply saying "no." From a mental health perspective, denial is generally viewed as a more specific unconscious process used to protect the individual from the anxiety of accepting reality.[3,8,18] Conscious denial would be the same as lying. Herein lies the crux of the difficulty in nursing interventions related to denial. Ideally nurses use a process of mutually identified concerns to work on with patients. However, by definition a patient cannot agree that denial is an issue. Therefore the determination that denial is an ineffective rather than an effective coping strategy requires careful observation and assessment.

There are several frameworks for understanding denial. Common understandings of denial include the classic psychoanalytical view of denial as a defense mechanism, the cognitive view of denial as a cognitive strategy, and the stress adaptation view of denial as a healthy coping strategy. The earliest view of denial was to understand it as a defense mechanism. Freud[14] developed this perspective in the context of his analytical theory in 1923. The purpose of all defense mechanisms is to alter perceived reality so that it is more comfortable.[31] Other defense mechanisms include such processes as repression, suppression, and projection. Viewed from this perspective, denial is seen as relatively fixed, and the individual could be overwhelmed with anxiety if the denial were successfully challenged.

Dorpat[8] describes the process of denial as developing through the following phases: (1) preconscious appraisal of a threat, (2) painful affects and defensive actions, (3) cognitive arrest, and (4) screen behavior. For example, a person may be given information about a potentially life-threatening diagnosis. This information would be the threat. The person receives the information about the diagnosis but is not yet conscious of having heard it. The person feels uncomfortable and avoids accepting the information as personally relevant. During cognitive arrest the person may seem to "freeze up" and simply not hear what is said. The screen behavior involves an explanation for the uncomfortable feelings or explains away what was heard. In this example, the person may say (and believe), "I'm sure there has been a mix-up on the test results."

Another framework used to understand denial is cognitive dissonance.[9] Cognitive dissonance results when conflicting messages are received, or information is received that is incongruent with one's personal beliefs. The conflicting information creates anxiety. One method of reducing this anxiety is to deny the conflictual message.[11]

Using the same example of a person receiving a potentially life-threatening diagnosis, the message that one is dying may be inconsistent with one's self-view as a healthy person. From a cognitive dissonance perspective, one could reject the first message and deny the seriousness of the illness or even its very existence. Another option would be to alter the self-view to that of an unhealthy

X

person. The other alternative would be to add a third belief or message to explain the perceived discrepancy, such as "Healthy people also die" or "Dying is a normal part of living and can coexist with health." Westwell and Forchuk[32] describe using a "back door" approach rather than directly confronting denial. The back door involves assessing which messages are in conflict and addressing a less threatening aspect of the conflict.

Denial has also been described as a normal coping strategy. For example, Kubler-Ross[16] identified denial as a normal, early response to grief. Lazarus and Folkman also view denial as a potentially helpful coping strategy. They identify two means to cope with stress: problem-focused and emotion-focused strategies. Denial is seen as an example of an emotion-focused strategy in that it does not change the reality of the stressful situation but how the individual feels about the situation. Because some situations cannot be changed (e.g., impending death), emotion-focused strategies are needed to cope. From this perspective the denial would only be seen as ineffective if it prevented some adaptive response.

There have been a number of studies that support the view of denial as a healthy coping strategy by finding improved health outcomes among individuals using denial in the early phase of illness.[10, 20, 28] For example, patients with myocardial infarction using denial were found to have less pain[4] and be more likely to survive hospitalization.[15] Fewer studies have explored the longer-term implications of using denial. One example is Dean and Surtees's study.[7] In this study women with breast cancer who used denial in the initial months had less recurrence 6 to 8 years later than women using any other coping mechanism.

Regardless of the framework used to understand denial, a commonality is that denial serves a protective function. Nurses must not assume that denial is maladaptive, and they must be cautious about intervening to change denial. It can be difficult to determine whether or not denial is ineffective as a coping strategy. The nurse must first ascertain that denial exists and then determine whether the use of denial is creating more prob-

lems for the person than the potential absence of denial. Nurses must be sensitive to the issues the patient is grappling with, must understand the patient's need for denial, and must pace all interventions accordingly.[32] Frequently the best intervention is no intervention.

ASSESSMENT

The main characteristic of denial is the protection from fear or anxiety it gives an individual faced with a threatening situation by allowing disavowal of the reality of the situation. *Anxiety* is a diffuse apprehension that is vague in nature and associated with feelings of uncertainty and helplessness,[23] and *fear* is the feeling of dread associated with an identifiable source. The appraisal of situations as stressful or threatening arises from the meaning persons give to experiences. Precipitating stressors are usually either threats to physical integrity or threats to the self-system. Threat appraisals can range from minimal, in which little stress is experienced, to extreme, characterized by intense emotions, such as fear.[19] Denial closes the mind to whatever could be threatening. Denial in the context of illness is considered ineffective when the person fails to engage in appropriate problem-focused coping, such as seeking medical attention or adhering to a treatment regimen. However, as discussed above, denial may be protective or adaptive. To make the diagnosis of Ineffective Denial, the nurse must first determine whether the patient is denying and, if so, determine whether the denial is maladaptive.

Denial may arise in any threatening situation. However, the patient must have appraised the issue as a threat for denial to occur. Assessment of denial requires the nurse's appraisal and understanding of the patient's patterns of coping. To understand how the person is coping, the nurse must observe the patient in many types of encounters and in different situations. Denial is an unconscious process. Therefore nurses must observe behavior that may indicate that denial is present. Westwell and Forchuk[32] identified ten points to consider when assessing for denial. The nurse

X

must first recognize that denial may be operating when a person does not acknowledge the obvious; for example, when a patient does not acknowledge the relationship between his or her condition and lifestyle. During assessment the patient's knowledge about and understanding of the illness, event, or situation sheds light on whether or not Ineffective Denial is present. For example, denial may be present if the patient ignores, minimizes, or disputes the reality of the illness, event, or situation. A patient with a myocardial infarction who does not follow the prescribed treatment and acts as if nothing has changed may be using denial as a means of coping with the threat to personal integrity.

It may take several interviews to assess Ineffective Denial. A key aspect of the assessment is to understand the meaning assigned to the event by the person and the purpose served by the denial. Ultimately the goal of assessment is to determine if the person's coping patterns fit the demands of the event or situation. To assess the patient's perception and the meaning assigned to the situation, ask how much is being experienced and how much harm or threat he or she feels in the situation. Ask the patient to describe his or her ability to manage the situation and what he or she sees as important goals. Assess the person's ability to deal with uncertainty, as well as his or her motivation, knowledge, abilities, and usual coping patterns. The nurse should consider what the person gains from using denial as a coping strategy.

Often behavior that may be initially viewed as denial on closer examination is not denial.[6,30] For example, noncompliance does not necessarily mean denial. The nurse needs first to understand the patient's perspective, and on further examination the patient may have a good reason not to comply with a particular treatment plan or may perhaps lack important information. Lazarus[18] points out that people cannot deny something about which they have not been informed. Some behavior labeled as denial may actually be inadequate communication.[6,30]

Denial is indicated when persons faced with a threatening situation state that they are not fearful. Hackett, Cassem, and Wishnie[15] identified three levels of denial in patients hospitalized in a coronary care unit. Major deniers consistently denied fear. A total of 40% of the patients were major deniers. Fifty-two percent of the sample were partial deniers and initially denied fear but later acknowledged some fear. The remaining 8% were minimal deniers, who readily admitted fear.

During assessment, the nurse must be careful not to conclude that a patient is denying based solely on the fact that he or she does not wish to talk about the illness. For example, some patients may know very well that they have cancer but prefer not to talk about it.[17] Individuals who do not acknowledge having cancer are not denying the diagnosis if they were never told of it or were not cognitively able to understand what was told to them.

The fact that a patient delays seeking treatment does not necessarily indicate denial. Safer and colleagues[29] interviewed 93 patients seeking medical treatment and found that those who delayed coming for treatment had not denied their symptoms. They had thought a great deal about their symptoms and the negative consequences of being ill. Although they were aware of their symptoms, they did not take any action. They displayed inappropriate coping, but not because of denial.

Nurses must be aware of their own responses to denial.[32] Knowing their own feelings, nurses can prevent themselves from acting on them inappropriately. Nurses unaware of their feelings may also blame the patient for their discomfort. Nurses may respond to their uncomfortable feelings by confronting the patient with "reality," ignoring the patient's use of denial and thereby creating a distance between themselves and the patient. Using confrontation is a common error nurses make when facing a person in denial. The nurse may believe that pointing out reality will resolve the patient's oversight. However, confrontation often increases the patient's anxiety and therefore the need for denial. Instead, nurses need to accept the protective function of denial. Patients use denial to avoid the intolerable feeling generated by conflicting thoughts, feelings, and attitudes. Nurses should respect the patient's need for this protection. At the same time, while assessing for denial, it is important not to reinforce the denial. In a caring nurse-patient relationship, nurses can agree with parts of the patient's statements that are true without accepting or confronting the parts they believe are not true.[12]

A key point in the assessment of denial is determining whether or not denial is creating a problem for the patient. Although denial cannot be directly confirmed, the effect or influence of denial may be observed.[12] An example of denial is a patient who is abusing alcohol and/or other substances but is unwilling to acknowledge that a problem exists. Wing and Hammer-Higgins[33] found several determinants of denial in alcoholics. Persons needing external motivation for seeking treatment are in denial. For example, a family member, the court, or a health care professional may have coerced a patient into treatment, and yet the patient may still deny that he or she has a problem. Individuals with alcoholism often use denial by refusing to acknowledge connections between life problems and drinking. They blame others for personal problems and for initiating treatment; minimize the extent or the effects of drinking; rationalize that drinking is necessary for coping, stress reduction, or social interaction; and express anger at staff, accusing them of incompetence.[33] Thus denial in alcohol abuse stems from a failure to recognize the salience of the negative effects of alcohol use and a failure to recognize that there is a current inability to cope with this difficulty.[25]

Assessment of denial must also focus on uncovering the underlying thoughts, feelings, and issues. Because denial serves a protective function, identifying the specific thoughts or emotions in conflict may illuminate the dynamics of the denial. In this way the nurse may hypothesize what feelings and issues the denial is protecting the person from experiencing. The nurse shares what he or she has hypothesized may be the underlying issues and feelings with the patient to facilitate the patient's ability to work through the conflict. Instead of confrontation, the nurse uses open-ended questions and active listening and explores the patient's values and beliefs about his or her experiences, perceptions, and expressions of the situation. As values and beliefs are discussed, the meaning of the conflicts may become apparent for the nurse and the patient. This is a very different process than approaching a patient with a fixed hypothesis about the thoughts and feelings underlying the denial and then attempting to gather data to prove them.[32]

■ Defining Characteristics

The presence of the following characteristics indicates that the patient may be experiencing denial:

- Presence of a perceived threat
- Lack of perception of the personal relevance of the symptoms or threat
- Partial or inconsistent expression of fear and anxiety when in a threatening situation
- Minimizes or fails to recognize symptoms
- Inability to admit the effect of the illness on life pattern
- Allowing others to decide that treatment is needed

The presence of the following characteristics in combination with any of the characteristics above indicates that the patient may be experiencing Ineffective Denial:

- Required self-care action not being carried out
- Delays seeking or refusing medical attention to the detriment of health
- Health outcomes are not met because of the use of denial

■ Related Factors

The following related factors are associated with Ineffective Denial:

- Inability to tolerate the consequences of a chronic and/or terminal illness or any other threatening situation
- Fear of death
- Fear of pain
- Fear of separation
- Fear of the loss of autonomy
- Feelings of increased stress or anxiety
- Feelings of inadequacy, low self-esteem, guilt, loneliness, or despair
- Feelings of omnipotence
- Negative feelings associated with stigma or stereotype of an illness

X

- The context of the situation in which denial is occurring (e.g, drug use, alcohol use, smoking, obesity)

DIAGNOSIS

■ Differential Nursing Diagnosis

The nurse must be careful not to confuse Noncompliance, Ineffective Individual Coping, Knowledge Deficit, and Defensive Coping with Ineffective Denial. The nursing diagnosis Noncompliance describes a person desiring to follow a therapeutic regime who is prevented from doing so by factors such as a lack of understanding, inadequate finances, and instructions that are too complex. The person using Ineffective Denial may not even recognize that he or she has a particular illness, so there is no reason even to desire to follow a particular treatment plan. Knowledge Deficit can be distinguished from Ineffective Denial because a person cannot deny what they don't know.[18] Ineffective Individual Coping describes a wide range of impairment of adaptive behaviors and problem-solving abilities preventing a person from meeting life's demands and role. Ineffective Denial, however, describes a very particular coping strategy. Furthermore, the main characteristic of denial is a disavowal of fear or anxiety when faced with a threatening situation, which is not a feature of Ineffective Individual Coping. Defensive Coping is also closely related to Ineffective Denial. Denial may be present as a feature of Defensive Coping. However, the diagnosis Defensive Coping is to be used when projection of blame, rationalization of failures, and hypersensitivity to slight criticism are also present.

■ Medical and Psychiatric Diagnoses

Ineffective Denial can be a human response to any major threatening or serious illness. Most commonly, patients diagnosed with cancer, AIDS, or with a myocardial infarction may initially use denial. Considerable research has shown that denial is adaptive in the acute phase of illness.[4, 10, 20, 21, 24] Some research has even suggested that long-term denial is adaptive,[7, 10, 28, 29] whereas other research indicates that it constitutes maladaptive coping.[21] However, if the denial interferes with the person's potential to achieve optimum health, quality of life, or sense of well-being, Ineffective Denial may be an appropriate diagnosis. There is a large body of literature addressing the maladaptive use of denial in patients diagnosed with psychoactive substance use disorders* and overcoming the denial is the first step to the successful treatment of any substance abuse disorder.[22, 27]

OUTCOME IDENTIFICATION, PLANNING, AND IMPLEMENTATION

When planning care for persons diagnosed with Ineffective Denial, interventions are directed toward facilitating the patient's ability to gain insight into their denial and the detrimental effects of the denial on their health. If the denial is not detrimental to their health, the denial may be adaptive, and no interventions are required. The nurse should not use confrontation but instead should use a caring, nonjudgmental approach in exploring the nature of the denial by discussing the beliefs, values, and perceptions of the patient concerning the threatening situation. When the patient gains insight and understanding into the relationship of the denial on health, the patient will be able to use more appropriate defense mechanisms in coping with the threatening situation.

Another outcome for patients experiencing Ineffective Denial is acceptance of the reality of the situation by no longer using denial. Providing information and creating a supportive environment empowers patients to use more appropriate coping behaviors and health-seeking behavior.

---

*References 1, 2, 5, 13, 25, 26, 33.

◢ **NURSING CARE GUIDELINES**
Nursing Diagnosis: Ineffective Denial

Expected Outcome: The patient will gain insight into the detrimental relationship of their denial on their health as evidenced by statements demonstrating an understanding of the threatening situation.
- Assess the nature of the threat. *Assessing the nature of the threat uncovers its presence and meaning and whether or not denial is a deterrent to health and well-being.*
- Consider no intervention if the denial is not a deterrent to the patient's health and well-being. *Adaptive denial temporarily protects the patient from psychological harm.*
- Do not use confrontation. *Confrontation increases anxiety and the need for denial.*
- Discuss with the patient his or her values, beliefs, and perceptions of the threatening situation. *As values and beliefs are discussed, insight into the denial conflicts may be gained.*

Expected Outcome: The patient accepts the reality of the threatening situation as evidenced by health-seeking behavior.
- Provide information to correct any misperceptions the patient may have. *Factual information presented in a caring, nonjudgmental way may help the patient focus on his or her behaviors and gain an understanding of the relationship between behaviors and health.*
- Provide a supportive environment. *A supportive environment allows the patient to feel free and safe to ask questions and gain a deeper understanding of the nature of their denial.*

■ = nursing intervention; ▲ = collaborative intervention.

EVALUATION

To evaluate nursing interventions related to Ineffective Denial the nurse assesses whether or not the patient has moved toward acceptance or continues to use Ineffective Denial as a means to deal with the threatening situation. Denial may be effective when there are no detriments to health. The denial is ineffective if the denial persists and the patient's health continues to be adversely affected. Interventions for Ineffective Denial are successful when there is an absence of defining characteristics and the patient has accepted and understands the negative impact of denial on health. Instead, the patient uses health-seeking behavior and alternate coping strategies in dealing with the threat.

X

▶ **CASE STUDY WITH PLAN OF CARE**

A nurse practitioner is giving a job-related physical examination to Mr. James C. in a primary health care clinic. The examination was precipitated by concerns of lost time at work. Lab work indicated that his liver enzymes were at an elevated level, although no gross abnormalities were noted. During the health history, Mr. C. admitted to drinking about 10 beers each evening but stated that he does not have any problems with alcohol. He stated that he does not understand why his employer requested he get a physical examination because "I don't have any problems . . . everyone gets sick occasionally." The nurse expressed concern about the pattern of alcohol use, the pattern of work absence, and the elevated level of liver enzymes and is now considering referral for a drug assessment program to determine if drug counseling is required. Upon hearing this suggestion, Mr. C. became angry and stated, "There is no way I'm an alcoholic . . . I will never go anywhere that assesses drinking problems. I would rather quit my job first." Rather than confront the denial directly, the nurse asked the patient, "What is an alcoholic?" Mr. C. replied, "Someone who drinks every day, loses control, and no longer can work." The nurse stated, "I can see why you say you are not an alcoholic. You still have a job, you feel you have control,

Continued

▶ CASE STUDY WITH PLAN OF CARE — CONT'D

and some days you do not drink. There are many different definitions of alcoholism, and I really don't know if you fit any of them. That is why I am suggesting an assessment. The definition that I use is that when one's physical or mental health is detrimentally affected, including one's job or family, or if any legal problems arise from the use of alcohol, further assessment is needed. You have problems with your liver that may be associated with your use of alcohol, and it seems that your work may be affected by your drinking."

▶ PLAN OF CARE FOR MR. JAMES C.

Nursing Diagnosis: Ineffective Denial Related to the Use of Alcohol and Stigma of Being Labeled an Alcoholic

Expected Outcome: Mr. C. will seek further exploration of an alcohol problem.
- Assess the impact of the denial.
- Assess nature of threat in accepting difficulty with alcohol.
- Be aware of own responses to the denial by not responding to the anger.
- Convey an attitude of acceptance of the patient.
- Do not use confrontation.

Expected Outcome: Mr. C. will have a more realistic understanding of what it means to have alcoholism.
- Review definition of alcohol dependence and categories of symptoms.
- Discuss Mr. C.'s current life situation and the impact of alcohol use.
- Discuss with Mr. C. his values and beliefs that illuminate his negative view of alcoholism and his personal inability to accept problems related to alcohol use.
- Provide information about further alcohol assessment programs when Mr. C. requests it.
- Provide a supportive environment that allows Mr. C. to feel safe to ask questions.

■ = nursing intervention; ▲ = collaborative intervention.

■ CRITICAL THINKING EXERCISES

1. What is the impact of the denial on the patient's health?
2. What statements and behaviors reflect the patient's denial?
3. From the patient's perspective, what purpose does denial serve?
4. What are the patient's perceptions, values, and beliefs concerning the threatening situation?
5. What alternative coping mechanisms and health-seeking behaviors are evident when the patient is no longer using Ineffective Denial to deal with the threatening situation?

REFERENCES

1. Allan CA: Acknowledging alcohol problems: the use of the Visual Analogue Scale to measure denial, *J Nerv Ment Diseases* 179:620–625, 1991.
2. Amodeo M and Liftik J: Working through denial in alcoholism, *J Contemp Human Serv* 73:131–135, 1990.
3. Bereznitz S: The seven kinds of denial. In Breznitz S, editor: *The denial of stress,* New York, 1983, International Universities Press.
4. Billing E and others: Denial, anxiety, and depression following myocardial infarction, *Psychosomatics* 21:639–645, 1980.
5. Bishop DR: Clinical aspects of denial in chemical dependency, *Individ Psychol* 42:199–209, 1991.
6. Cousins N: Denial: are sharper definitions needed?, *JAMA* 248:210–212, 1982.
7. Dean C and Surtees PG: Do psychological factors predict survival in breast cancer?, *J Psychosom Res* 33:561–569, 1989.
8. Dorpat TL: The cognitive arrest hypothesis of denial, *Int J Psychoanal* 64:47–58, 1983.
9. Festinger L: *A theory of cognitive dissonance,* Evanston, Illinois, 1957, Row, Peterson and Company.
10. Folks DG and others: Denial: predictor of outcome following coronary bypass surgery, *Int J Psychiatry Med* 18:57–66, 1988.
11. Forchuk C: Cognitive dissonance: denial, self-concepts and the alcoholic stereotype, *Nurs Papers* 16:57–69, 1984.

12. Forchuk C and Westwell J: Denial, *J Psychosoc Nurs* 25(6): 9–13, 1987.

13. Frances R, Franklin J, and Borg L: Psychodynamics. In Galanter M and Kleber H: *Textbook of substance abuse treatment*, Washington, D.C., 1994, American Psychiatric Press.

14. Freud S: *The standard edition of the complete psychological works of Sigmund Freud (1923–1935): the ego and the id and other works*, vol 19, London, 1961, The Hogarth Press and Institute of Psychoanalysis.

15. Hackett TP, Cassem NH, and Wishnie HA: The coronary care unit: an appraisal of its psychological hazards, *N Eng J Med* 279:1370, 1968.

16. Kubler-Ross E: *On death and dying*, New York, 1969, Macmillan.

17. Lazarus RS: Stress and coping as factors in health and illness. In Cohen J, Cullen JW, and Martin LR, editors: *Psychosocial aspects of cancer*, New York, 1982, Raven Press.

18. Lazarus RS: The costs and benefits of denial. In Bereznitz S, editor: *The denial of stress*, New York, 1983, International Universities Press.

19. Lazarus RS and Folkman S: *Stress, appraisal and coping*, New York, 1984, Springer Publishing.

20. Leiker TJ: The role of the addiction nurse specialist in a general hospital setting, *Nurs Clin North Am* 24(1):137–149, 1989.

21. Levenson JL and others: Denial predicts favorable outcome in unstable angina pectoris, *Psychosom Med* 46:25–32, 1984.

22. Levine J and others: The role of denial in recovery from coronary heart disease, *Psychosom Med* 49:109–117, 1987.

23. Mai FM: Graft and donor denial in heart transplant recipients, *Am J Psychiatry* 143:1159–1161, 1986.

24. May R: *The meaning of anxiety*, New York, 1977, Pocket Books.

25. McMahon J and Jones BT: The change process in alcoholics: client motivation and denial in the treatment of alcoholism within the context of contemporary nursing, *J Adv Nurs* 17:173–186, 1992.

26. Metzger L: *From denial to recovery: counseling problem drinkers, alcoholics, and their families*, San Francisco, 1988, Jossey-Bass.

27. Miller H: Addiction in a coworker: getting past the denial, *Am J Nurs* 90:73–75, 1990.

28. Prince R, Frasure-Smith N, and Rolicz-Woloszyk E: Life stress, denial and outcome in ischemic heart disease patients, *J Psychosom Res* 26:23–31, 1982.

29. Safer MA and others: Determinants of three stages of delay in seeking care at a medical clinic, *Med Care* 17:11–29, 1979.

30. Shelp EE and Perl M: Denial in clinical medicine: a reexamination of the concept and its significance, *Arch Intern Med* 145:697–699, 1985.

31. Vaillant GE: Theoretical hierarchy of adaptive ego mechanisms, *Arch Gen Psychiatry* 24:107–118, 1971.

32. Westwell J and Forchuk C: Denial: buffer and barrier, *Canadian Nurse* 85(9):16–18, 1989.

33. Wing DM and Hammer-Higgins P: Determinants of denial: a study of alcoholics, *J Psychosoc Nurs* 33:13–17, 1993.

X

Post-Trauma Response

Post-Trauma Response *is the intense, sustained emotional response of an individual to a traumatic experience or a natural or man-made disaster.*

OVERVIEW

Post-Trauma Response is characterized by a range of emotional responses from fear and anger to flashbacks and psychic numbing. Post-Trauma Response (PTR) affects those who participated in war-related combat; those who are victims of rape, childhood physical and/or sexual abuse, and kidnapping; those who survived automobile accidents and natural or man-made disasters; and those whose emotional or physical survival or that of a loved one is threatened.

PTR can have an acute or a long-term phase or both. In the acute phase, the patient may experience shock and disbelief followed by intense fear and anxiety. Some individuals appear calm and controlled during this phase, giving the impression of coping well. However, it may be difficult for some victims to express their feelings or acknowledge the extent of the trauma to themselves and others. For example, some rape victims may be discouraged from expressing their feelings because of cultural or religious beliefs. In the acute phase, the PTR patient will express feelings of terror, shock, disbelief, embarrassment, and anger.

In the long-term phase, which begins within a few days to several months after the traumatic event, the patient may have flashbacks (revisualizations of the traumatic scene that seem real), intrusive thoughts, and nightmares in which the event is reenacted. Victims may be preoccupied with the traumatic event and may have difficulty concentrating on work or other matters of daily living. Some continue to deny the trauma and will develop emotional numbing, which may lead to total amnesia about the event.[5] Others feel depressed and hopeless.[1,4,5,6]

The long-term effects of trauma from childhood physical or sexual abuse can have a significant impact on the personality and interpersonal relationships of the adult survivor. The individual may develop chronic feelings of low self-esteem and suicidal feelings accompanied by suicidal acts, and he or she may become a substance abuser or physically abusive in adult relationships.[10] Dissociation, a psychological defense mechanism by which the individual separates emotionally from a traumatized body, may persist into adulthood, resulting in sexual dysfunction or, in its extreme form, multiple personality disorder.[1,9]

Recent films about the Vietnam War have portrayed the consequences of PTR. Veterans have been depicted as having flashbacks of being shot or watching their friends die in battle. The sights, sounds, and smells of the battlefield remain vivid in their memories for years. For some, the war has never ended because of the daily intrusion of flashbacks and nightmares into their cognitive and emotional lives. The veterans of World War II and the Vietnam War, as well as civilian victims of war and political oppression, have also been studied and have been found to be suffering varying degrees of PTR.[5,7,8]

In contrast, some victims of PTR remain in denial about the event. Although it serves an important role in healthy coping, denial can render

X

the individual emotionally numb, disinterested, and withdrawn from life. Unfortunately these victims often "slip though the cracks" of the support systems designed to help them adjust to the traumatic experience. When family and friends try to reach out, the sufferer who is denying may react with hostility and rejection, further widening the gap and aggravating maladaptive responses.

Those who survive disasters in which others died or were seriously injured may suffer the long-term consequences of PTR. They may feel guilty for being spared when others died, ashamed that they did not do enough to save others, and helpless.

Alcohol and drug abuse may result when the victim of PTR tries to cope with the impact of the trauma. In an attempt to avoid or to numb themselves to anxiety, depression, and shame, victims may drink or use other drugs. However, substance abuse aggravates the symptoms of PTR, and the patient becomes increasingly alienated from pretrauma relationships and commitments.

Impaired interpersonal relationships occur in the long-term phase. The individual may withdraw from friends and family. He or she may feel increasingly limited in interactions with people, self-conscious, and distrustful of others.

ASSESSMENT

Most healthy, emotionally stable people experience some degree of shock, anxiety, and ongoing fear after an event such as automobile accident or a criminal assault. A victim failing to express some anxiety or fear after a traumatic episode should be regarded as unusual by the nurse. However, depending on the role played by the victim of the disaster, the reaction may be difficult to assess.

For instance, the driver of a car who survives an automobile accident in which others were seriously injured or killed may be unable to express the conflicting, confusing feelings of the threat to his or her own life and sense of responsibility for the passengers. The driver may have assisted the others immediately after the accident, exposing him- or herself to the gruesome sight of physical trauma and to the sounds of pain and suffering. The driver may have suffered personal injury that he or she may not have noticed until the police and rescue squads arrived to assist the wounded. The driver may feel shock and disbelief, fear, guilt, and shame but may not express any personal concern, only concern for the passengers. This person may develop flashbacks, nightmares, and intrusive thoughts in the aftermath of the accident. The nurse needs to be aware of the potential for a delayed response in this type of scenario.

Victims of trauma who suffered "invisible" damage (e.g., childhood sexual abuse or emotional abuse) and those who suffered physical abuse that was not reported or investigated exhibit PTR symptoms that are often confused with other psychiatric disorders. It is not uncommon for an adult survivor of childhood abuse to seek treatment for anxiety and depression and to be incorrectly given a diagnosis of personality disorder or anxiety disorder. It is essential that a thorough history be taken, including questions about child abuse, to diagnose and treat all trauma victims accurately.[3,9]

The nurse must consider many factors regarding the patient with PTR. What was the nature of the trauma? Was the patient alone or with others? Was there loss of life or physical trauma to others or to a loved one? Did the patient experience loss of personal property, livelihood, or social status? These questions can yield important information about the likelihood of a mild or severe emotional response by the patient.

It is unusual for a person to fail to express some degree of anxiety and depression in the aftermath of trauma. However, not all victims of trauma experience the serious and unremitting reactions associated with PTR. What makes one person more likely than another to develop PTR?

Research suggests that individuals who have a high exposure to stressful events throughout the life cycle are at greater risk for PTR not only because of the adverse impact of experiencing repeated stress but because of the increased likelihood of exposure to trauma.[12] Therefore factors such as unstable family relations and socioeconomic disadvantage correlate positively with higher exposure to trauma and the development of PTR.[3,8,16] Maturity of coping mechanisms, support systems, and cultural and religious beliefs about expressing emotions are other factors that contribute to PTR. Children are at risk for PTR not only because of their innocence but because they may observe the severe effects of the traumatic event on their parents or other adults to whom they naturally look for care, comfort, and reassurance.[2,11]

When children are the victims of a disaster, the nurse must consider the child's developmental stage and the impact on the child's continuing emotional development. Twenty-five survivors of the Chowchilla school bus kidnapping in 1976 were the subjects of a 4-year follow-up study.[14] The children who experienced the most severe reactions to this trauma were assessed as having had prior vulnerabilities, such as family dysfunction and social isolation. The study also identified important differences in the ways children respond to trauma. They are more likely to exhibit pessimism about the future, superstitiousness, distorted or incorrect memories about the trauma, thought suppression, post-traumatic play and reenactment, and fear of dying young.

The nurse is most likely to encounter the victim of trauma in (1) the acute care setting shortly after the event, (2) in the community mental health center several days, weeks, or months after the event, or (3) in the rehabilitation setting years after the traumatic experience. Depending on the setting, the nurse will be assessing for phase-specific symptoms of PTR.

In the acute care setting, the nurse must first observe the patient's physical status and attend to his or her immediate needs for help. The nurse can assess the emotional response simultaneously. Is the patient crying? Can the patient be comforted? Does the patient react with fear and suspiciousness to the ministrations of the nurse and other caregivers? If the patient is unconscious, the nurse should speak with family members or friends who arrive with the patient. Are they able to discuss the incident and their concerns about their loved one?

How do they seem to be coping with the initial shock, fear, and anxiety? Are they expressing emotions appropriate to the circumstances, or are they minimizing, trivializing, or joking about the event? These observations can provide valuable data about the patient's coping in the immediate hours after the trauma.

In the community mental health setting, the nurse will interview the self-referred patient or the one referred by a doctor, a friend, an employer, or a family member. The source of the referral is important because it frequently indicates the willingness of the victim to discuss the traumatic event. A self-referred patient is more likely to acknowledge his or her problems and may be more motivated to accept help developing effective coping strategies. The patient who seeks treatment on the recommendation of another person may not be as aware of post-traumatic difficulties and may not accept professional help. Patients who seek help under duress or to appease others may reluctantly acknowledge their suffering because of their fear of losing control of their emotional stability. The nurse must respect the patient's need for emotional distance while offering support in whatever ways are accepted.

The nurse in the rehabilitation setting is likely to encounter patients—perhaps war veterans— who display chronic dysfunction associated with PTR.[7] The patient may have been coping maladaptively for years through drug or alcohol abuse, social isolation, and, possibly, sociopathic behavior. The sufferer may not have made the transition from the military setting or the combat zone to civilian life. The patient may be depressed and display the cognitive impairments associated with PTR: flashbacks, intrusive thoughts, poor reality testing, and poor concentration. The nurse in the rehabilitation setting will be assessing for physiological, psychological, interpersonal, and occupational functioning.

Nursing assessment of the PTR patient is an ongoing, dynamic process, regardless of the setting in which the patient presents. Each PTR victim will have a unique set of circumstances that will require specific, caring nursing assessment.

The assessment guide in the box on page 846 provides a focus for assessing the patient.

■ Defining Characteristics

The presence of the following defining characteristics indicates that the patient may be experiencing Post-Trauma Response:

- Flashbacks of the traumatic event triggered by visual, auditory, and olfactory stimuli
- Nightmares
- Intrusive thoughts
- Impaired concentration, memory, and cognition
- Emotional numbing, including amnesia and confusion about the event
- Denial of the effect of the trauma
- Avoidance of situations or persons that remind the victim of traumatic event
- Excessive fearfulness, worrying, and obsessiveness over recurrence of traumatic event
- Guilt
- Dissociation
- Impaired interpersonal relationships; social withdrawal
- Abusive relationships
- Impaired occupational or academic functioning; withdrawal from activities and commitments
- Alcohol and drug abuse
- Helplessness and hopelessness; suicidal thoughts and behaviors
- Common characteristics in children and adolescents: post-traumatic play and reenactment; impaired time orientation for traumatic event; limited view of the future; fear of dying young; superstitiousness; pretrauma family dysfunction

■ Related Factors

The following related factors are associated with Post-Trauma Response:

- War-related combat exposure
- Disasters such as floods, fires, and earthquakes
- Domestic violence or exposure to gang or community criminal activity
- Rape
- Assault
- Childhood physical and/or sexual abuse
- Torture
- Kidnapping
- Catastrophic illness
- Accidents
- Preexisting emotional disorders
- Previous experience of trauma
- Limited community supports

DIAGNOSIS

■ Differential Nursing Diagnosis

Patients suffering from PTR may present with features similar to the following nursing diagnoses: Sleep Pattern Disturbance, Sensory/Perceptual Alterations, Altered Thought Processes, Ineffective Individual Coping, and Impaired Adjustment. Whereas the patient with PTR will present with some similar complaints, he or she will also have experienced a recent or past traumatic experience from which the most severe of the complaints can be dated. The neurobiological response will appear more dramatically in Post-Trauma Response than in the other diagnoses, and the patient will likely be more fearful and anxious when exposed to the possibility of reexperiencing the traumatic event or to similar circumstances.[5,15]

■ Psychiatric Diagnoses

Related psychiatric diagnoses include anxiety disorders (e.g., panic or phobias), dissociative disorders, adjustment disorders, major depressive disorder, substance-related disorders, and personality disorders (especially borderline, avoidant, and obsessive-compulsive). These diagnoses coexist in some individuals with PTR and may have been present before the patient experienced the severe traumatic event. The patient must be treated concurrently for any of the above diagnoses and PTR and may be best managed by professionals with expertise in dual diagnoses, such as Substance Abuse and PTR. Psychotherapy and psychopharmacology approaches for PTR should treat the patient's mood, anxiety, and personality disorders as well.

X

ASSESSMENT GUIDE FOR TRAUMA

PHYSIOLOGICAL IMPAIRMENT ASSOCIATED WITH THE TRAUMA
- Nature of the injury; long-term disability
- Patient's response to medical regimen
- Prostheses or devices used to compensate for impairment
- Involvement in rehabilitation program
- Actual or potential effect of injuries on body image and self-esteem
- Neurobiological changes related to fight-or-flight response

EMOTIONAL FUNCTIONING
- Ability to express feelings associated with the traumatic event
- Evidence of prolonged denial
- Receptivity of patient to caregivers and significant others
- Use of drugs or alcohol to cope with feelings
- Hyperarousal and exaggerated startle responses[11]
- Degree of anxiety, despair, depression, and helplessness
- Suicidal thoughts and actions
- Adaptive and maladaptive coping patterns
- Significant history related to previous exposure to traumatic experiences
- Preexisting mental health disorder

COGNITIVE FUNCTIONING
- Presence of flashbacks, intrusive thoughts, and nightmares
- Inability to concentrate on work, academic, or recreational activities
- Obsessive thoughts and discussion about the trauma
- Impaired judgment

INTERPERSONAL RELATIONSHIPS
- Quality of interpersonal relationships before the traumatic event
- Significant others with whom patient maintains regular contact
- Receptivity of patient to efforts of significant others
- Evidence of alienation from pretrauma relationships
- Communication skills

PROFESSIONAL AND COMMUNITY SUPPORTS
- Supportive responses from patient's work or professional colleagues, organizations, church groups, and school
- Community supports available to the patient (e.g., victim's support group, rape crisis center, Veteran's Administration)
- Patient's receptivity to use of community supports

OUTCOME IDENTIFICATION, PLANNING, AND IMPLEMENTATION

The nursing plan of care for the patient experiencing Post-Trauma Response should focus primarily on providing him or her with emotional support and assisting in the integration of the traumatic experience into the victim's life to achieve specified outcomes.

The first outcome addresses the patient's feelings as being appropriate to the effect of the trauma on his or her life. Initially the patient may not be receptive to expressing feelings about and reactions to the trauma. The nurse must respect the patient's need to avoid or deny feelings. Denial is an expected and healthy coping mechanism in the initial phases of recovery. Denial can help the patient do what is necessary to regain strength and a positive self-image.[6] The nurse can be available when the patient is ready to talk, most likely when recovering from injuries or when the threat of the disaster occurring again has passed. Healthy denial may give way to outbursts of anger, anxiety, and depression. A consistent, supportive response from the nurse is necessary to help the patient sort through confusing and overwhelming feelings.

The second outcome focuses on the patient experiencing increasingly longer periods free of impaired concentration. The patient will need assistance in performing cognitive functions and concentrating on tasks because of the occurrence of intrusive thoughts and flashbacks. The nurse's presence and acceptance of the patient's experience will help him or her learn techniques to improve concentration and encourage a return to work or academic responsibilities.

The patient's maintenance of old interpersonal relationships and development of new ones is the focus of the third outcome. Family and friends will benefit from the nurse's explanations of the patient's difficulties. The patient may need to reexamine some relationships that may be self-defeating or abusive. Survivors of childhood physical and sexual abuse often seek out such abusive relationships in an effort to master and control the outcome of similar experiences. The patient needs to evaluate the positive and negative aspects of these relationships, discarding some and resuming others with those who will accept and support him or her through recovery. New and healthy relationships may be fostered by the patient's involvement in support groups and through new, constructive social contacts.

The fourth outcome relates to abstinence from drug and alcohol use. Patients who have difficulty expressing their emotions about the trauma often turn to drugs or alcohol to induce psychological numbing. Appropriate psychopharmacological agents are available to assist the patient cope with the anxiety, depression, and impaired concentration that result from traumatic experience. Verbalization of feelings, relaxation techniques, and support groups often fill the void for the patient.[13,15]

The patient's integration of the traumatic experience into his or her self-perception is addressed in the fifth outcome. A long-term task for the patient is the integration of the traumatic experience into a realistic perspective. Some patients feel their lives are ruined by the trauma and feel hopeless about overcoming the deleterious effects. The nurse must understand and explore these attitudes, while encouraging the patient to consider prior skills, qualities, and supports that may be employed in the aftermath of the trauma. Renewal of spiritual ties may assist the patient to feel unity with other victims, from whom emotional strength can be garnered and to whom the patient may be a source of hope. Acceptance is the final stage of the grieving process; the nurse must help the patient understand that this is a slow but necessary stage to complete.

Finally, the nurse must be aware of how he or she is affected emotionally by the patient with PTR. The intense nature of the patient's reactions and need for support may be draining. The nurse may feel revulsion on seeing the patient's injuries or hearing a description of the experience. Some nurses identify with the patient and begin to fear being traumatized themselves. It is important that the nurse maintain an open, nonjudgmental attitude with the patient. Equally important is validation of the patient's feelings of fear, depression, rage, and dread. It will benefit the nurse to share these feelings with colleagues, to be aware of the need for intermittent breaks from work with patients with PTR, and to be aware of fears based on personal, painful life experiences. Attending to personal emotional needs will enable the nurse to continue the important supportive and rehabilitative work with the patient.

X

◢ **NURSING CARE GUIDELINES**
Nursing Diagnosis: Post-Trauma Response

Expected Outcome: The patient will express feelings appropriate to the effect of the trauma on his or her life within a few days to 2 weeks in the acute stage and within 1 to 2 months in the long-term stage.
- Allow the patient to focus on the recovery of physical health while medical status is compromised.
- Introduce discussion of the emotional effect of the trauma when the patient seems ready.
- Explain to patient and family that as physical recovery progresses, more extreme emotional responses may occur.
- Assist the patient to deal with altered physical status.
- Help the patient verbalize feelings of loss, inadequacy, low self-esteem, and distorted body image.
  In the early stages of the nurse-patient relationship, it is essential to let the patient lead the way and establish the pace. Allowing the patient to focus on concrete goals, such as recovery from physical injury, will increase his or her ability to talk about the traumatic experience.

Expected Outcome: The patient will experience increasingly longer periods free of impaired concentration within 2 weeks to a month in the acute stage and within 2 to 4 months in the chronic stage.
- Encourage the patient to talk about the traumatic event and how it interferes with current life goals.
- Accept patient's fears associated with thoughts and revisualizations; provide an understanding response that acknowledges how real the thoughts seem to the patient.
- ▲ Teach relaxation techniques—progressive relaxation, deep breathing, and imagery. *Providing the patient with alternative ways of coping and expressing oneself will allow him or her to sort through the maze of feelings, thoughts, memories, and reactions that have resulted from the trauma.*
- Expose the patient to other calming activities—listening to music, drinking warm milk before bedtime, and taking walks.
- Encourage structured time during the day and involvement in meaningful activities. *Structure and realistic goal attainment can minimize opportunities to dwell on the confusing aspects of the trauma, and they provide the patient with a break from intrusive thoughts.*

Expected Outcome: The patient will maintain old interpersonal relationships and develop new ones within several weeks to 1 year after the trauma.
- Arrange family meetings while the patient is hospitalized to discuss how they can support and assist the patient.
- Discuss with family and significant others the meaning of the patient's withdrawal.
- Empathize with the family's plan while encouraging family members to maintain involvement with patient. *The patient's family and significant others are key to recovery. They can assist the nurse in helping the patient reestablish pretrauma involvements and in arranging the necessary adaptations to allow the patient to continue life or to develop new pursuits and interests.*

Expected Outcome: The patient will abstain from alcohol and drug use throughout the course of therapy and for 2 years following the traumatic event.
- ▲ Refer for psychopharmacological evaluation and treatment.
- ▲ Refer for individual or group psychotherapy.
- ▲ Refer to Alcoholics Anonymous or Narcotics Anonymous.
- Encourage family support and involvement in Al-Anon or other survivor support groups.
- Maintain drug-free environment except for prescribed, therapeutic medications.
- Discourage association with individuals or groups actively using illicit drugs.
- Encourage the patient to discuss uncomfortable feelings that drug use may have repressed.
- ▲ Encourage the patient to become involved in activities and occupational rehabilitation and to make the necessary adaptations in participation because of injuries or other limitations resulting from the trauma.

■ = nursing intervention; ▲ = collaborative intervention.

- Discuss and teach alternatives to substance abuse that may provide a more satisfying state of well-being (e.g., religious affiliation, physical exercise, yoga, and meditation).
Substance abuse resulting from a traumatic experience or as a premorbid condition in the PTR patient may aggravate many symptoms, such as depression, poor concentration, and difficulty functioning and performing pretrauma activities and responsibilities. Research indicates that many patients benefit from psychopharmacological treatment, particularly the serotonin reuptake inhibitors (SRI) classification of antidepressants. Providing the patient with alternative forms of self-soothing helps him or her regain confidence in his or her ability to cope with the painful memories and fears associated with the traumatic experience.

Expected Outcome: The patient will integrate the traumatic experience into his or her self-perception and entire life experience within several months to 2 years of treatment.
- Encourage the patient to discuss the traumatic experience in the context of his or her whole self and life course.
- Discourage the patient from using feelings about trauma to avoid responsibility for oneself and one's life goals.
- ▲ Contact community resources (e.g., Survivors of Trauma, Victims' Assistance, and Veterans' Administration), and encourage the patient to utilize them.
- Encourage the patient to share the experience with others and to offer support to other victims of trauma. *Traumatic experiences can reshape the person's sense of self to the extent that it may define him or her for the rest of his or her life. For a child, a traumatic experience may be the defining one of his or her life. Yet life goes on, and the individual's life history predates the traumatic event. Being able to draw from past experiences and strengths will assist the patient in placing the traumatic event into an appropriate perspective from which he or she can learn to face challenges in the future and regain a more positive and accurate sense of self.*

EVALUATION

Evaluation of the patient with PTR is based on his or her subjective report of improvement in emotional, social, physical, and cognitive functioning. The nurse will also make objective observations of the patient's response to psychotherapy, support groups, and, if relevant, to psychotropic medication. Collaboration among the nurse, the patient, significant others, and other caregivers will yield the most information about the patient's progress.

In general the nurse will evaluate the following desired behaviors:

- Response to medical regimen; resolution of physiological injuries
- Emotional coping; management of anxiety and adaptation to altered body image
- Cognitive abilities
- Abstinence from drug and alcohol use
- Interpersonal relationships
- Integration of trauma into the patient's life experience and self-image

Recovery from a traumatic experience is a long-term process that will occur over several years and possibly for the patient's entire life. Having suffered PTR once may make an individual vulnerable to reexperiencing the adverse effects of trauma in the future or even to being more sensitive to predictable, albeit stressful, life events, such as the death of a loved one, changes in job status, and physical illness.[3] Those patients who show little or no progress toward the alleviation of the most severe symptoms should be referred for long-term psychotherapy, and ongoing psychopharmacological treatment. Some patients may benefit from an assisted-living environment to support them through the difficult process of reintegration into the community, the job market, and the pretrauma social and family milieu.

X

CASE STUDY WITH PLAN OF CARE

Ms. Ruth C. referred herself to the community mental health center 5 months after an automobile accident in which the car she was driving was hit head-on by a car driven by a drunk driver. Ms. C., a 25-year-old white law student, sustained a broken leg and clavicle and cuts to her upper body, including her face. She was hospitalized for 2 weeks after the accident, then spent 1 month with her mother in her hometown. When she returned to her law classes, she had difficulty concentrating on her studies, was afraid of driving an automobile, and felt depressed and tearful whenever she thought of or talked about the accident. She felt embarrassed by the temporary scars that were visible on her face and hands, and she felt uncomfortable when anyone asked about them. She had been refusing offers to socialize with her friends and would end telephone conversations with her family abruptly. She stated, "I don't understand why I'm so upset. Why can't I concentrate at school? Why am I so fearful? I should feel lucky to be alive, but I'm so angry." Ms. C. had no significant medical illnesses or injuries before the accident. When she was in her freshman year of college, her father died from a heart attack. She spent all of her semester breaks at home helping her mother adapt to the loss of her husband and assisting her two younger siblings. Ms. C. felt that she had been helpful to her family during this crisis but had not taken time to consider how she was coping with the sudden death of her father to whom she never felt emotionally close. She had passed up several opportunities to work and study during summer vacations so she could be available to her family.

Ms. C. had no preexisting mental health or emotional disorder. She states that her family has been supportive of her through her ordeal but that it is not characteristic of them to talk to each other about their feelings. She has two close female friends with whom she is more comfortable expressing her feelings. She had been dating a fellow law student about 1 month before the accident but has not returned his phone calls since she resumed classes. Ms. C. belongs to a Lutheran church near the law school and attends services regularly. She had been involved in an ethical discussion group at the church before the accident. A victims-of-trauma support group meets monthly through the community mental health center.

PLAN OF CARE FOR MS. RUTH C.
Nursing Diagnosis: Post-Trauma Response Related to Automobile Accident

Expected Outcome: Ms. C. will benefit from short-term, focused psychotherapy (10 to 15 sessions) to assist her in exploring the myriad emotional reactions she has had to the automobile accident, her injuries, and the immediate and long-term effects on her life.
- Establish a trusting, supportive relationship with Ms. C. through twice-weekly sessions for 3 to 4 weeks.
- Convey an attitude of acceptance for the range of feelings she expresses.
- Encourage Ms. C. to continue to talk with her two friends about the accident and to voice her feelings about injuries and ongoing treatment she must withstand.
▲ Refer Ms. C. to the victims support group offered through the community mental health center.

Expected Outcome: Ms. C. will accept altered body image related to injuries within 6 months to 1 year.
- Encourage Ms. C. to continue medical treatments and other self-care activities appropriate to her stage of recovery.
- Encourage Ms. C. to express feelings about facial scars, and explore ways to increase comfort with her appearance.

Expected Outcome: Ms. C. will accept support offered by friends and family within 2 to 3 weeks of initiation of treatment.
- Encourage Ms. C. to meet with friends for a few hours each week in nonthreatening social situations.
- Explore concerns about contact with family; encourage Ms. C. to write letters if phone calls are awkward.
- Support her attendance at church services and church activities.

■ = nursing intervention; ▲ = collaborative intervention.

Expected Outcome: Cognitive functioning will return to pretrauma level within 2 to 3 months.
- Assist Ms. C. to set up a realistic study schedule that will not tax her physically and emotionally.
- Discuss options that may decrease stress while she continues to recover from trauma, such as reducing academic credit load and requesting extensions on papers, assignments, and examinations.
- Teach relaxation exercises; encourage Ms. C. to revive herself with calming activities (e.g., listening to music and meditation).

Expected Outcome: Ms. C. will integrate the effect of the accident into her total life experience through ongoing self-evaluation of adaptation to the traumatic experience.
- Encourage Ms. C. to review her previous life history and evaluate the permanent versus temporary changes in life goals, skills, and accomplishments.
- Encourage Ms. C. to attend a victims-of-trauma support group and offer herself as a source of hope and positive coping to others.
- Discuss stages of grieving process with Ms. C., and encourage her to understand the importance of dealing with the tasks of each stage to resolve the acute and long-term effects of the trauma on her life.

■ CRITICAL THINKING EXERCISES

1. How does the case of Ms. C. illustrate the point that the traumatic event itself is the most significant factor in the development of Post-Trauma Response?
2. Describe some related factors that may have contributed to the onset of Post-Trauma Response in Ms. C.
3. Is Ms. C. at risk for Post-Trauma Response in the future? Why?
4. What strengths does Ms. C. bring to the experience of trauma that may be mobilized to assist her during recovery?

REFERENCES

1. American Psychological Association: *Diagnostic and statistical manual of mental disorders,* ed 4, Washington, D.C., 1994, The Association.
2. Armsworth M and Holaday M: The effects of psychological trauma on children and adolescents, *J Counsel Dev* 72(1): 49–52, 1993.
3. Breslau N, Davis G, and Andreski P: Risk factors for PTSD-related traumatic event: a prospective analysis, *Am J Psychiatry* 154:4, 1995.
4. Burgess A and Holstrom L: Rape trauma syndrome, *Am J Psychiatry* 131:981, 1974.
5. Foa E, Riggs D, and Gershuny B: Arousal, numbing, and intrusion: symptoms structure of PTSD following assault, *Am J Psychiatry* 152:1, 1995.
6. Horowitz M: *Stress-response syndromes,* New York, 1976, Jason Aronson.
7. Kulka R and others: *Trauma and the Vietnam war generation,* New York, 1990, Brunner/Mazel.
8. Lee K and others: A 50-year prospective study of the psychological sequelae of World War II combat, *Am J Psychiatry* 152:4, 1995.
9. McCann L and Pearlman L: *Psychological trauma and the adult survivor,* New York, 1990, Brunner/Mazel.
10. North American Nursing Diagnosis Association: *NANDA nursing diagnoses: definitions and classification, 1995–1996,* Philadelphia, 1994, The Association.
11. Schwartz E and Perry B: The post-traumatic response in children and adolescents, *Psych Clin North Am* 17:2, 1994.
12. Southwick S and others: Psychobiologic research in post-traumatic stress disorder, *Psych Clin North Am* 17:2, 1994.
13. Sutherland S and Davidson J: Pharmacotherapy for post-traumatic stress disorder, *Psych Clin North Am* 17:2, 1994.
14. Terr L: Chowchilla revisited: the effects of psychic trauma four years after a school bus kidnapping, *Am J Psychiatry* 140:1543, 1983.
15. Vander Kolk B and others: Fluoxetine in post-traumatic stress disorder, *J Clin Psych* 55(12): 517–522, 1994.
16. Weisman G: Adolescent PTSD and developmental consequences of crack dealing, *Am J Orthopsychiatry* 63:553, 1993.

X

VALUE-BELIEF PATTERN

Spiritual Distress

▶ ─────────────────────────────

Potential for Enhanced Spiritual Well-Being

▶ ─────────────────────────────

Spiritual Distress *is a disruption in the life principle that pervades a person's entire being and that integrates and transcends one's biological and psychological nature.*

Potential for Spiritual Well-Being *is the process of an individual's developing or unfolding of mystery through harmonious interconnectedness that springs from inner strength.*[17]

OVERVIEW

The construct of holism and holistic care has been accepted by nurses for many years. Nursing views the person as a balance of mind, body, and spirit. Each dimension affects and is affected by the other. Spirituality is a resource that assumes various degrees of prominence throughout life. Furthermore, holistic nursing is supported by an inherent spirituality on the part of the patient and the nurse. The need for spiritual care as a part of holism has been well documented in the literature. Nursing, with this tradition of caring for the whole person, needs then to reexamine periodically its "care of the soul" if it is to remain faithful to the philosophy of holistic nursing. Limiting spiritual care to the identification of patients' religious affiliation, however, denies the patient truly holistic care.

Confusion exists regarding the meaning of the words *spirituality* and *religion*. This ambiguity is not limited just to the nursing literature. In addition, nursing has experienced difficulty differentiating the spiritual nature of individuals from the religious aspects of an individual's life. Until recently, *religion* and *spirituality* were frequently used interchangeably and synonymously. Used in this manner, they could be seen as specific ritual practices or beliefs related to one's relationship with God, a higher being, or an organized religion, or they could be viewed as a unifying force or framework for values, codes, and relationships that provide an individual with meaning and purpose. Emblen[10] conducted an exhaustive study of the use of these two terms in the nursing literature for the last 30 years, from which she formulated definitions. *Religion* refers to faith, beliefs, and practices that nurture a relationship with a superior being or power. *Spirituality* alluded to a dynamic principle, or an aspect of the person that related to God or gods, other persons, or aspects of personal believing or material nature. It may be more precise to think of religion and spirituality in this manner. In this way all persons, including atheists and agnostics, have a spiritual dimension that must be addressed.

Burnard[5] has argued for the spiritual exigencies of atheists and agnostics. He defined their spiritual needs in terms of a search for meaning. *Spiritual distress* may be described as the failure to invest life with meaning and can be a very painful situation for the patient. Meaning may be found within the context of a set of religious beliefs, or, alternatively, meaning may be found through adherence to a particular ideological viewpoint: philosophical, psychological, sociological, or political.

XI

Others take the view that there is no meaning to life except that which they as individuals invest in it. Proponents of "New Age" religion have a belief in the "Universe" or the collective unconscious. They see themselves as cocreators of a new humanity. "New Agers," as they are sometimes called, put much emphasis on dreams and on ancient rituals and cults from the past. They celebrate the seasons, wanting to be in tune with the rhythm of the earth and the energy of the sun. They reenact and update the rituals of passage of human life from birth through adulthood and marriage to death.[8]

Brennan[3] defines *spirituality* as an essential, intrinsic, and intangible quality or state of being that may be conscious or unconscious. It is a continuous behavior or process throughout life that allows one to relate with God, a higher being, or others, to find meaning and purpose in life, and to act with courage and serenity when facing the crises of life.

The concept of spirituality and of Spiritual Distress, according to Heliker,[11] is hard to grasp in that the definition is dependent on the perspective of the conceiver, thereby limiting its generality. The roots of one's spirituality are culture-bound and pertain not only to oneself but to the many. Furthermore, spirituality ought to be perceived as a process or a journey, in which change and flexibility are inherent.

Religious beliefs are an integral part of some cultures and may influence the way in which a patient seeks and cooperates with health care regimens. Nursing must broaden its perspective regarding spirituality and widen its knowledge base of transcultural philosophy and spirituality. Global perspectives must be incorporated into any discussion of spirituality. Oriental teaching emphasizes enlightenment and liberation from the demands and illusions of the sensorial, time-bound world. Western teachings stress bonding with the natural world and commitment to exploring the mysterious element of time. Philosophical and theological perspectives must be considered. A patient with a sin consciousness may require a much different approach than one whose belief system includes an individual capacity for the divine. Pain, suffering, and disease, as well as

health, take on different meanings. One's spiritual dimension may bring fear and isolation from others or promote community and compassion. Dualistic philosophical views of the world, separation of body and soul, produce a one-sided spirituality that may prevent a sense of holism. Tradition, symbolism, and ritual must be recognized as a part of spirituality but not all of it.

Although nursing espouses holistic care, the application of spirituality in the clinical arena is often less than adequate. In this era of personal and familial disintegration, patients may depend on nurses to assist them in finding wholeness and meaning. The nurse may be the one health care professional who has continuous, intimate access to patients. Some patients are particularly in need of quality spiritual care.

As has been noted, the spiritual needs of persons include a search for meaning, a sense of hope, forgiveness, and love. Van Heukelen[23] describes the spiritual needs of children as including love, relatedness, forgiveness, meaning, and purpose. Their spiritual beliefs are often influenced by their parents, significant others, teachers, and friends. Moral and cognitive development will also affect the level of their spirituality.

According to Bearon and Koenig,[1] older persons commonly connect their religious beliefs with those about health and illness. The nurse must assess these beliefs appropriately to facilitate the person's understanding his or her illness in the context of his or her religion. Those who face the reality of death need to experience a sense of meaning for their lives as lived, as well as acquiescence for what has not been.[12]

The spiritual dimension has been identified as a means for the elderly to cope. Nelson[16] reports that elderly persons with high self-esteem are more intrinsically oriented to religion and less depressed. In her review of studies of depression and aging, she also reported that religion was used to help the elderly adjust to the adversities associated with growing old in this society. It is especially important in the dying process.

During critical illness, patients may be confronted with fundamental questions about their

XI

value system and sources of inner support. Several studies have been reported concerning the importance of spirituality to those patients with terminal illness. Patients with cancer often report an increased sense of spirituality, a rise in existential concerns, and a use of religion as a coping strategy.[13,15] Spiritual well-being was studied in patients with AIDS.[6] Participants who were higher in spiritual well-being tended to be more hopeful. Spiritual well-being was also inversely related to levels of anxiety in adults diagnosed with cancer.

The relationships between health, locus of control, and helpfulness of prayer as a direct coping mechanism before having cardiac surgery were studied by Saudia and others.[21] Ninety-six percent of respondents indicated that prayer was used as a coping mechanism, with 70% giving it the highest rating.

Spiritual care was defined by Johnston Taylor, Armenta, and Highfield[14] as health-promoting attendance to responses to stress that affect the spiritual perspective of an individual or group. They noted that spiritual care may be influenced by narrow views of spirituality, fear of incompetence, uncertainty regarding personal spiritual and religious beliefs and values, and discomfort with the conditions that frequently bring spiritual needs to the surface. Some nurses believe that spiritual care is not within the domain of nursing. Lack of time and a focus on physical problems also may interfere with the provision of spiritual care.

Nurses are sometimes reluctant to discuss spirituality because they take seriously their responsibility not to discuss or impart their own philosophy or religious view to patients, who may already be vulnerable, confused, or in a crisis and who may have difficulty with abstraction and reality. Although reluctance to discuss spiritual concerns with patients is not the same as denial of spiritual needs, the results are often the same.

Nurses who are able to venture beyond themselves can best share the spiritual needs of others or at least recognize the spiritual dimension. The ability to diagnosis Spiritual Distress becomes a skill most professionals will find threatening and frustrating. To journey with a patient in this dimen-

sion, one must first recognize one's own spiritual journey and be willing to share the process.

ASSESSMENT

To understand and to identify the spiritual manifestation of crises caused by illness, suffering, and death in patients, nurses must have knowledge about the spirit of a person and what are valid cues to Spiritual Distress. A list of defining characteristics has been compiled by NANDA. Inclusion of the spiritual assessment in the nursing history conveys its importance as an influence and as a coping strategy. When patients are prompted to reflect on their spiritual values and how they have coped in the past, they may recognize how their spiritual resources have provided them with meaning.

Duff[9] notes that the nurse decides whether or not to assist the patient who is experiencing Spiritual Distress or Potential for Enhanced Spiritual Well-Being at two critical points. The first is when the nurse decides whether to include or disregard the verbal and nonverbal cues the patient gives. The second critical point is when the nurse decides whether to implement actions based on the nursing diagnosis. The nurse must decide whether or not to hear the spiritual needs of the patient. For a nurse ascribing to the concept of holism, the decision to address spirituality is a simple one.

DiMeo[7] suggests three steps to assessing patients regarding their spiritual needs. First, ask if they wish to see a chaplain or their clergyperson. In addition, question them as to any specific religious practices that are important to them. These first nonintrusive inquiries can set the stage for more in-depth sharing. Second, be alert for any indications of Spiritual Distress. If a patient questions the meaning of life or the purpose of suffering or illness, take time to listen and note their concerns. Third, be aware of the common religious tenets of the population in which one serves.

To perform a proper assessment, it is important first to be familiar with the codes and practices of traditional religious denominations as well as more modern associations (e.g., New Age religions) that address the spiritual nature of persons. Although it may be impossible to know everything about all groups, it is important that one have at least a working knowledge of the beliefs of the major population of patients one serves. The beliefs of certain groups may conflict with certain medical regimens (e.g., the refusal of blood and blood components by Jehovah's Witnesses). In addition, certain groups may deviate slightly from the majority view or position within a particular region. Suggested guidelines for nursing assessment and interventions are heavily laden with emphasis upon religiosity—religious articles and religious practices. Although the narrowness of this vision may be recognized, these assessment guides can be very useful with most patients.

The initial assessment of a patient should include questions that might lead to the need for a more in-depth spiritual assessment. There are several tools available in the nursing literature that may assist the nurse to evaluate fully the spiritual aspects of the patient. O'Brien[18] developed a spiritual assessment guide to investigate a patient's spiritual beliefs and practices. The areas in which a patient is assessed are general spiritual beliefs, personal spiritual beliefs, identification with institutionalized religion, spiritual or religious support systems and rituals, and Spiritual Distress or deficit. The Spiritual and Religious Concerns Questionnaire was developed by Silber and Reilly[22] to measure hospitalized adolescents' spiritual and religious concerns and needs objectively. Paloutzian and Ellison[19] developed a Spiritual Well-Being Scale that measures a person's religious and existential well-being. This scale is particularly helpful with the elderly and the terminally ill.

Many nurses seek cues in the patient's environment: a rosary, a bible or prayerbook, a religious medallion. Verbal cues include a mention of a procedure at variance with a patient's religious beliefs or a confession as to why the suffering should be occurring. Behavioral clues might be the rejection of certain foods or praying at certain times.

Weatherall and Creason[24] in a validation study of the nursing diagnosis Spiritual Distress found that the cues males presented were different from those presented by females in their study. Cues presented by men were related to relationships with others. They expressed feelings of hopelessness, cried, and chose not to participate in usual religious practices. Women, on the other hand, had a tendency to question the meaning of suffering, verbalized a concern about their relationship with God, and expressed inner conflicts about their beliefs.

In the patient with no specific religious beliefs or affiliations, the nurse must be alert for comments that indicate meaning or lack of meaning in the patient's life. Questions such as "How has your illness affected the way you view life?" or "What does this illness mean for you and for your life?" may elicit this information. Patients are often willing to talk to nurses about how their illness has affected their feelings about God or faith and to receive assistance to identify a purpose for what has transpired.

As part of an assessment of Spiritual Distress, a nurse may become aware of guilt and unfinished business with others that need to be addressed to decrease feelings of anxiety and distress. The nurse should recognize that anger may indicate the need for forgiveness. Nurses may ask open-ended questions to elicit more information, always aware that a patient may or may not choose to discuss the matter.

The nurse's own assessment skills, the use of spiritual assessment guides, and an awareness of spiritual needs will assist the nurse in making the diagnosis Spiritual Distress or identifying Potential for Enhanced Spiritual Well-Being. The following specific defining characteristics and related factors have been suggested by NANDA[17] and the literature.

Spiritual Distress

■ Defining Characteristics

The presence of the following defining characteristics indicates that the patient may be experiencing Spiritual Distress:

- Expresses concern or questions the meaning of life and existence, of suffering, death, and/or belief systems

- Anger toward God, supreme being, or others
- Regards illness as a punishment
- Expresses feelings of guilt and engages in self-blame
- Verbalizes inner conflict about beliefs and relations with deity
- Unable to participate in usual religious practices
- Seeks spiritual assistance
- Questions moral or ethical implications of therapeutic regimen
- Gallows humor
- Displacement of anger toward religious representatives
- Description of nightmares or sleep disturbances
- Alterations in behavior and mood evidenced by anger, crying, withdrawal, preoccupation, anxiety, hostility, apathy, and so forth

■ Related Factors

The following related factors are associated with Spiritual Distress:

- Illness or threat to well-being
- Loss of meaningful roles
- Separation from religious, family, or cultural ties
- Challenges belief and value system (e.g., due to moral or ethical implications of therapy or due to intense suffering)

Potential for Enhanced Spiritual Well-Being

■ Defining Characteristics

The presence of the following defining characteristics indicates that the patient may be experiencing Potential for Enhanced Spiritual Well-Being:

- Unfolding mystery: one's experiences about life's purpose and meaning, mystery, uncertainty, and struggles
- Harmonious interconnectedness
- Inner strengths: a sense of awareness, self-consciousness, sacred source, unifying force, inner core, and transcendence
- Relatedness, connectedness, harmony with oneself, others, God or a higher power, and the environment

■ Related Factors

The related factors that may be associated with Spiritual Distress may also be present with Potential for Enhanced Spiritual Well-Being.

DIAGNOSIS

■ Differential Nursing Diagnosis

A caution must be noted about possible confusion between the spiritual and the psychological. Psychological and spiritual assessment are readily interchanged. Boutell and Bozett[2] found that most nurses assessed patients for fears, feelings of hope, and sources of strength and considered these psychological or emotional issues rather than spiritual. Less frequently assessed were integration, love of God, meaning in suffering, and transcendence. This finding was also reported by Piles.[20] She noted that the spiritual dimension had been subsumed as a subcategory of psychosocial nursing and was minimally addressed.

Nursing diagnoses that might be confused with Spiritual Distress are Anxiety, Fear, Grieving, and Hopelessness. The common thread running through these nursing diagnoses is the psychological or emotional component. It might be argued that the presence of any or all of these nursing diagnoses may be related to the state of Spiritual Distress.

To discern which diagnosis is most accurate, the nurse must obtain a careful nursing history and assessment. Listening to the patient's verbal cues and behavioral cues is paramount. The recognition of the defining characteristics thus plays an integral part in this process. Many of the related factors will be similar. The major cues to the diagnosis of Spiritual Distress or Potential for Enhanced Spiritual Well-Being revolve around the issues of the belief system, relationship to God or a higher power, and the search for ultimate meaning.

■ Medical and Psychiatric Diagnoses

Serious illness can challenge a person's spirituality—his or her beliefs, values, and sense of meaning. It can also rouse feelings of anger, frustration, hopelessness, fear, and guilt. Any illness that threatens life in any way, is debilitating, or causes prolonged pain and suffering may be related to Spiritual Distress and Potential for Enhanced Spiritual Well-Being. Some pathophysiological conditions (e.g., cancer and heart disease) can cause an individual to come face to face with his or her mortality and the meaning of life and death. Certain treatments (e.g., abortions, amputations, sterilization surgeries, blood transfusions, and contraceptive medications, to name but a few) can generate cognitive dissonance or conflict between the spiritual values, belief systems, and physical needs.

Spiritual Distress may also be a nursing diagnosis related to some mental health disorders, such as the affective disorders (i.e., depression, anxiety and adjustment disorders, and substance abuse disorders). Expressions of hopelessness, helplessness, anger, guilt, and the need for forgiveness and healing found in these disorders may be related intrinsically to the nursing diagnosis Spiritual Distress.

OUTCOME IDENTIFICATION, PLANNING, AND IMPLEMENTATION

Establishing expected outcomes is the next step in caring for the patient with Spiritual Distress. Expected outcomes will determine the plan of action. Outcomes dealing with the spiritual nature must be developed with the patient if they are to be meaningful. Whenever possible, they should be measurable. However, because spirituality is a process, it may be very difficult to establish a time frame. In some cases the ability to discuss spiritual concerns with a nurse, a significant other, or a spiritual confidant will result in immediate relief of Spiritual Distress. In many cases, however, a significant amount of time for integration will be necessary. Although NANDA has determined that Spiritual Distress and Potential for Enhanced Spiritual Well-Being are distinct nursing diagnoses, in reality the goal of a nursing care plan addressing Spiritual Distress is to assist the patient in achieving spiritual well-being. Therefore the ultimate outcomes should be the same for both diagnoses.

In many cases, the process toward spiritual well-being will only begin during the nurse-patient interaction. In some settings (e.g., hospice, home health, or nursing home) and in some cases (e.g., terminal illness) the nurse will have the opportunity to see the patient through to the conclusion of life.

Nursing interventions for patients with Spiritual Distress may be classified into nine general areas: presence, active listening, spiritual counseling, values clarification, reminiscence therapy, crisis intervention, truth telling, relaxation therapy, and music therapy.[2] All of these interventions depend on the ability of the nurse to develop a close nurse-patient relationship built on trust, openness, and mutual respect. Presence is paramount to all of these interventions and is indeed the first and foremost intervention. In many cases, presence alone will be enough to assist a patient toward spiritual well-being.

◀ **NURSING CARE GUIDELINES**
Nursing Diagnosis: Spiritual Distress

Expected Outcome: The patient will experience a greater sense of purpose, meaning, and hope in living with an illness.
- Be available to listen to the patient's concerns and feelings. *Listening is an intervention by which the nurse establishes a relationship with the patient. It means entering the frame of reference of the patient, and it allows the patient to verbalize his or her concerns.*
- Provide time just to be present with the patient. *Presence forms the basis of all nursing interventions and demonstrates a willingness on the part of the nurse to be there for the patient.*

■ = nursing intervention; ▲ = collaborative intervention.
Continued

■ NURSING CARE GUIDELINES — CONT'D

- Question the patient about past beliefs and spiritual experiences to assist him or her in putting this event into a wider perspective. *Focusing on past strengths enables the patient to assess and accept his or her abilities to face crises with strength and courage.*
- Pray with the patient if appropriate. *Many patients have acknowledged that prayer is used as a coping mechanism, allows them to seek divine intervention, and thus provides them with a sense of peace, hope, and strength.*
- ▲ Contact usual spiritual counselor or clergyperson if one exists. *Relationships that have been established with spiritual counselors and clergypersons can be a source of strength for a person facing a crisis of life.*

Expected Outcome: The patient will express decreased feelings of guilt and will experience a sense of forgiveness.
- Using reminiscence therapy, encourage the patient to express past hurts and guilt.
- Assist the patient to "heal memories." *The use of reminiscence therapy allows a patient to review his or her life and identify those persons or areas of his or her life where forgiveness is necessary. It also allows an opportunity to deal with feelings of anger, guilt, or other emotions that have been repressed.*
- If appropriate, tell the patient that God loves and accepts people as they are. *This is a tenet of most religions, based on the Judeo-Christian tradition.*
- ▲ If the patient so desires, contact the respective clergyperson for a reconciliation service. *Specific religious denominations provide their members with a formal mechanism by which forgiveness may be sought.*

Expected Outcome: The patient will verbally express anger and will discuss his or her feelings with another person.
- Assist patient to recognize and express feelings of anger.
- Reassure the patient that feelings of anger are normal and acceptable.
- Assist patient to seek ways of resolving feelings of anger. *Clarification and naming of feelings and emotions allow the patient to deal with them realistically. Once brought into the open, the feelings can then be dealt with in a constructive fashion.*
- ▲ If necessary, make appropriate referrals to clergypersons, social workers, and psychologists. *Deep-seated or long-repressed feelings often need specialized assistance that an individual nurse may feel unable to handle. Patients belonging to certain Christian sects may feel the need to seek reconciliation through sacramental or counseling sessions with their specific clergy.*

Expected Outcome: The patient will accept him- or herself.
- Provide time and presence for patient to verbalize concerns.
- Be an advocate for the patient's needs. *Patients who have a poor sense of self or who have placed their needs after others will often require the nurse to help them identify their own needs and be reassured that their needs are just as important as others.*
- Use therapeutic touch to comfort the patient. *Therapeutic touch is a means for the nurse to convey to patients that they are worthwhile and that the nurse is accepting and present for them.*

Expected Outcome: The patient will have a sense of belonging, even though he or she is separated from religious practices.
- Inform the patient of available religious resources within the institution.
- Maintain diet within religious practice as long as it is not detrimental to health.
- Allow patient to continue to wear religious objects or clothing whenever possible.
- Make necessary arrangements for important religious rituals (e.g., anointing of the sick).
- Encourage visits from clergy and church members. *Continued contact with familiar rites and rituals will lessen the pain of separation that the patient might be experiencing and provide a sense of continued participation.*

■ = nursing intervention; ▲ = collaborative intervention.   *Continued*

Expected Outcome: The patient will have a clearer understanding and perception of personal beliefs and values.
- Use values clarification.
- Provide accurate information concerning procedures and treatments.
- Support patient in making an individual, informed decision.
- ▲ Refer the patient to other disciplines as necessary. *Clarifying the values and belief system can be a therapeutic intervention. The patient can be assisted to find peace, hope, and meaning in his or her individual choices.*

Expected Outcome: The patient will establish meaningful relationships with him- or herself, God, and others.
- Encourage the patient to take responsibility for his or her own life.
- Encourage the patient to make positive choices. *Making personal choices and taking responsibility will help to alleviate cognitive dissonance if it exists. It will also assist the patient in accepting him- or herself as a mature individual who has some control over his or her life.*
- ▲ Encourage contact with clergy and other significant others.

Expected Outcome: The patient will develop inner peace through a decrease in somatic complaints and emotional distress.
- Instruct the patient in relaxation techniques, music therapy, and centering prayer. *Relaxation techniques, music therapy, and other methods have been documented in the literature as means to decrease somatic complaints through the release of endorphins.*

◀ **NURSING CARE GUIDELINES**
Nursing Diagnosis: Potential for Enhanced Spiritual Well-Being

Expected Outcome: The patient will maintain previous relationships with his or her God or higher being.
- Provide quiet time for prayer, meditation, visit from clergy, and so on. *The health care environment often affects the ability of the patient to practice familiar and meaningful religious practices. The nurse as patient advocate can provide the quiet time necessary for prayer and meditation.*
- Allow the patient an opportunity to verbalize his or her feelings about this life event and its relationship to the spiritual self. *Persons with a well-developed sense of spirituality and a relationship with a supreme being will want to make the necessary connections between the life event and this relationship.*

Expected Outcome: The patient will continue spiritual practices not detrimental to health.
- Provide access whenever possible to religious services or programs.
- Encourage patient to continue to practice rituals that are not in conflict with medical regimen. *Continued contact with familiar rites and rituals will lessen the pain of separation that the patient may be experiencing and will provide a sense of continued participation.*

Expected Outcome: The patient will express continued spiritual harmony and wholeness.
- ▲ Provide opportunity for patient to pray with others or have members of his or her own religious group present.

■ = nursing intervention; ▲ = collaborative intervention.

XI

EVALUATION

In actuality the achievement of spiritual health and well-being is a lifelong process. Evaluation of Spiritual Distress or Potential for Enhanced Spiritual Well-Being consists of examining with the patient each outcome behavior suggested in the Nursing Guidelines for an improvement, a change for the better, or maintenance of usual healthy spiritual practices. Only the patient will be able to discern and report if the expected outcome has been met.

Spiritual Distress

The absence of or decrease in the defining characteristics of Spiritual Distress indicates that spiritual needs are being fulfilled. Outcome criteria will include expressing some or all of the following: a sense of purpose, meaning, inner peace, and hope; an acceptance of oneself and the ability to live with one's illness if necessary; a decrease in feelings of guilt, if they have been expressed, or a reconciliation with a particular person if appropriate; a sense of God's love and forgiveness; the absence of or less cognitive dissonance as related to certain health practices and religious beliefs and values; and continued support of meaningful religious practices.

Potential for Enhanced Spiritual Well-Being

Outcome criteria that should be evaluated for the patient with Potential for Enhanced Spiritual Well-Being will include maintenance of a previous state of spiritual well-being or, in some cases, a more enhanced state of well-being due to a deeper relationship with God or a higher power because of the new life event. Spiritual practices not detrimental to the health care regimen will be continued. The patient will express a deeper sense of wholeness and peace of mind.

▥ CASE STUDY WITH PLAN OF CARE

Mrs. Jane B., a 48-year-old computer executive, became tearful and emotional after being advised that a mass in her abdomen would require surgery and probably a permanent colostomy, followed by a course of chemotherapy. She apologized for her tears, stating that she must not let her family see her upset. After expressing her apprehension about why she should be faced with this illness, Jane spoke about her isolation from God. Although she had been raised in a fairly religious family that attended church regularly, she had stopped doing so over the years. She continued to cry and expressed fear of "not having the strength to make it through the coming ordeal." She then commented that she felt her "sins are coming back to haunt me." She verbalized her anger at God for allowing this to happen to her. When asked if she wished to see a clergyperson, she stated that there would be no point to it because God could never forgive her because she had failed to practice her faith. She questioned her nurse, "What is the point of it all?"

▥ PLAN OF CARE FOR MRS. JANE B.
Nursing Diagnosis: Spiritual Distress Related to an Illness and Threat to Well-Being, a Loss of Meaning, Sense of Guilt, and Separation from Previous Religious Ties

---

Expected Outcome: Mrs. B. will experience a greater sense of purpose, meaning, and hope in living with her illness.
- Be available to listen to Mrs. B.'s feelings and experiences.
- Encourage Mrs. B. to verbalize her fears and concerns.
- Encourage Mrs. B. to reminisce about her past experiences, about what her life has meant to her, and how she has coped in the past.

■ = nursing intervention; ▲ = collaborative intervention.

Expected Outcome: Mrs. B. will express her feelings of anger and discuss her feelings with another person.
- Assist Mrs. B. to recognize and express her feelings of anger.
- Reassure Mrs. B. that feelings of anger are normal and acceptable at this time.
- Assist Mrs. B. in identifying how she might resolve her feelings of anger.

Expected Outcome: Mrs. B. will express decreased feelings of guilt and experience a feeling of forgiveness.
- Assist Mrs. B. in clarifying her feelings of guilt.
- Reassure Mrs. B. that God is a forgiving God and that He accepts people as they are.

Expected Outcome: Mrs. B. will establish a meaningful relationship with God.
- Encourage Mrs. B. to explore and discuss her relationship with God.
- Make appropriate referral to chaplain or clergyperson if Mrs. B. desires this.

■ CRITICAL THINKING EXERCISES

1. How might you assist Mrs. B. in identifying her abilities to deal with the upcoming surgery, colostomy, and chemotherapy?
2. Mrs. B. feels that she must hide her feelings from her family. How might you use values clarification to explore these feelings with her?
3. What strategies could you use to respond to Mrs. B.'s feelings that God could never forgive her?
4. What response would you give to Mrs. B. when she asks, "What is the point of it all?"

REFERENCES

1. Bearon L and Koenig H: Religious cognitions and use of prayer in health and illness, *Gerontologist* 30(2):249–253, 1990.
2. Boutell K and Bozett F: Nurses' assessment of patients' spirituality: continuing education implications, *J Contin Ed Nurs* 26(4):155–160, 1990.
3. Brennan R: Concept analysis: spirituality, Unpublished manuscript, 1991.
4. Bulechek GM and McCloskey JC: *Nursing interventions: treatments for nursing diagnoses,* Philadelphia, 1985, WB Saunders Co.
5. Burnard P: Spiritual distress and the nursing response: theoretical considerations and counseling skills, *J Adv Nurs* 12:377–382, 1987.
6. Carson V and others: Hope and essential well-being: essentials for living with AIDS, *Perspect Psychiatr Care* 26(2):28–34, 1990.
7. DiMeo E: Rx for spiritual distress, *RN* 54(3):22–24, 1991.
8. Dominic, PA: Accompanying New-Age people, *Review for Religious* 54(3):339–352, 1995.
9. Duff V: Spiritual distress: deciding to care, *J Christian Nurs* 11(1):29–31, 1994.
10. Emblen J: Religion and spirituality according to current use in nursing literature, *J Prof Nurs* 8:41–47, 1992.
11. Heliker D: Reevaluation of a nursing diagnosis: spiritual distress, *Nurs Forum* 27(4):15–20, 1992.
12. Hungelmann J and others: Spiritual well-being in older adults: harmonious interconnectedness, *J Religion Health* 24(2):147–153, 1985.
13. Johnson SC and Spilka B: Coping with breast cancer: the roles of clergy and faith, *J Religion Health* 30:21–33, 1992.
14. Johnston Taylor E, Armenta M, and Highfield M: Spiritual care practices of oncology nurses, *Oncol Nurs Forum* 22(1):31–39, 1995.
15. Mickley JR, Soeken K, and Belcher A: Spiritual well-being, religiousness, and hope among women with breast cancer, *Image* 24:267–272, 1992.
16. Nelson PB: Intrinsic/extrinsic religious orientation of the elderly: relationship to depression and self-esteem, *J Geront Nurs* 16(2):29–37, 1990.
17. North American Nursing Diagnosis Association: *NANDA nursing diagnoses: definitions and classification, 1995–1996,* Philadelphia, 1994, The Association.
18. O'Brien ME: The need for spiritual integrity. In Yura H and Walsh MB, editors: *Human needs and the nursing process,* Norwalk, Connecticut, 1982, Appleton-Century-Crofts.
19. Paloutzian RF and Ellison CW: Loneliness, spiritual well-being, and quality of life. In Peplau L and Perlman D, editors: *Loneliness: a source book of current theory, research, and therapy,* New York, 1982, John Wiley & Sons.
20. Piles C: Providing spiritual care, *Nurse Educator* 15(1):36–41, 1990.

XI

21. Saudia TL and others: Health locus of control and helpfulness prayer, *Heart Lung: J Crit Care* 20(1):60–65, 1991.

22. Silber TJ and Reilly M: Spiritual and religious concerns of the hospitalized adolescent, *Adolescence* 20(77):217–224, 1985.

23. Van Heukelen J: Assessing the spiritual needs of children and their families. In Shelley JA, editor: *The spiritual needs of children,* Downers Grove, Illinois, 1982, Intervarsity Press.

24. Weatherall J and Creason NS: Validation of the nursing diagnosis, spiritual distress. In McLane AM, editor: *Classification of nursing diagnosis: proceedings of the Seventh Conference,* St. Louis, 1986, The CV Mosby Co.

XI

NANDA-Approved Nursing Diagnoses

▶

This list represents the NANDA-approved nursing diagnoses for clinical use and testing (1994).

Pattern 1: Exchanging

1.1.2.1	Altered Nutrition: More Than Body Requirements
1.1.2.2	Altered Nutrition: Less Than Body Requirements
1.1.2.3	Altered Nutrition: Risk for More Than Body Requirements
°1.2.1.1	Risk for Infection
°1.2.2.1	Risk for Altered Body Temperature
1.2.2.2	Hypothermia
1.2.2.3	Hyperthermia
1.2.2.4	Ineffective Thermoregulation
1.2.3.1	Dysreflexia
1.3.1.1	Constipation
1.3.1.1.1	Perceived Constipation
1.3.1.1.2	Colonic Constipation
1.3.1.2	Diarrhea
1.3.1.3	Bowel Incontinence
1.3.2	Altered Urinary Elimination
1.3.2.1.1	Stress Incontinence
1.3.2.1.2	Reflex Incontinence
1.3.2.1.3	Urge Incontinence
1.3.2.1.4	Functional Incontinence
1.3.2.1.5	Total Incontinence
1.3.2.2	Urinary Retention
1.4.1.1	Altered (Specify Type) Tissue Perfusion (Renal, Cerebral, Cardiopulmonary, Gastrointestinal, Peripheral)
1.4.1.2.1	Fluid Volume Excess
1.4.1.2.2.1	Fluid Volume Deficit
°1.4.1.2.2.2	Risk for Fluid Volume Deficit
1.4.2.1	Decreased Cardiac Output
1.5.1.1	Impaired Gas Exchange
1.5.1.2	Ineffective Airway Clearance
1.5.1.3	Ineffective Breathing Pattern
1.5.1.3.1	Inability to Sustain Spontaneous Ventilation
1.5.1.3.2	Dysfunctional Ventilatory Weaning Response (DVWR)
°1.6.1	Risk for Injury
1.6.1.1	Risk for Suffocation
°1.6.1.2	Risk for Poisoning
°1.6.1.3	Risk for Trauma
°1.6.1.4	Risk for Aspiration
°1.6.1.5	Risk for Disuse Syndrome
1.6.2	Altered Protection
1.6.2.1	Impaired Tissue Integrity
1.6.2.1.1	Altered Oral Mucous Membrane
1.6.2.1.2.1	Impaired Skin Integrity
°1.6.2.1.2.2	Risk for Impaired Skin Integrity
†1.7.1	Decreased Adaptive Capacity: Intracranial
†1.8	Energy Field Disturbance

Pattern 2: Communicating

2.1.1.1	Impaired Verbal Communication

Pattern 3: Relating

3.1.1	Impaired Social Interaction
3.1.2	Social Isolation
†3.1.3	Risk for Loneliness
3.2.1	Altered Role Performance
3.2.1.1.1	Altered Parenting
°3.2.1.1.2	Risk for Altered Parenting
†3.2.1.1.2.1	Risk for Altered Parent/Infant/Child Attachment
3.2.1.2.1	Sexual Dysfunction
3.2.2	Altered Family Processes
3.2.2.1	Caregiver Role Strain
°3.2.2.2	Risk for Caregiver Role Strain
†3.2.2.3.1	Altered Family Processes: Alcoholism

°Diagnoses with modified label terminology in 1994. This change was recommended by the NANDA Taxonomy Committee and adopted to remain consistent with the ICD.
†New diagnoses added in 1994 classified at level 1.4 using new critieria for staging (see reference later in this book).
From North American Nursing Diagnosis Association: *NANDA nursing diagnoses: definitions and classification, 1995–1996,* Philadelphia, 1994, The Association.

3.2.3.1	Parental Role Conflict
3.3	Altered Sexuality Patterns

Pattern 4: Valuing

4.1.1	Spiritual Distress (Distress of the Human Spirit)
†4.2	Potential for Enchanced Spiritual Well-Being

Pattern 5: Choosing

5.1.1.1	Ineffective Individual Coping
5.1.1.1.1	Impaired Adjustment
5.1.1.1.2	Defensive Coping
5.1.1.1.3	Ineffective Denial
5.1.2.1.1	Ineffective Family Coping: Disabling
5.1.2.1.2	Ineffective Family Coping: Compromised
5.1.2.2	Family Coping: Potential for Growth
†5.1.3.1	Potential for Enhanced Community Coping
†5.1.3.2	Ineffective Community Coping
5.2.1	Ineffective Management of Therapeutic Regimen (Individuals)
5.2.1.1	Noncompliance (Specify)
†5.2.2	Ineffective Management of Therapeutic Regimen: Families
5.2.3	Ineffective Mangement of Therapeutic Regimen: Community
†5.2.4	Effective Management of Therapeutic Regimen: Individual
5.3.1.1	Decisional Conflict (Specify)
5.4	Health-Seeking Behaviors (Specify)

Pattern 6: Moving

6.1.1.1	Impaired Physical Mobility
°6.1.1.1.1	Risk for Peripheral Neurovascular Dysfunction
†6.1.1.1.2	Risk for Perioperative Positioning Injury
6.1.1.2	Activity Intolerance
6.1.1.2.1	Fatigue
°6.1.1.3	Risk for Activity Intolerance
6.2.1	Sleep Pattern Disturbance
6.3.1.1	Diversional Activity Deficit
6.4.1.1	Impaired Home Maintenance Management
6.4.2	Altered Health Maintenance
6.5.1	Feeding Self-Care Deficit
6.5.1.1	Impaired Swallowing
6.5.1.2	Ineffective Breastfeeding

6.5.1.2.1	Interrupted Breastfeeding
6.5.1.3	Effective Breastfeeding
6.5.1.4	Ineffective Infant Feeding Pattern
6.5.2	Bathing/Hygiene Self-Care Deficit
6.5.3	Dressing/Grooming Self-Care Deficit
6.5.4	Toileting Self-Care Deficit
6.6	Altered Growth and Development
6.7	Relocation Stress Syndrome
†6.8.1	Risk for Disorganized Infant Behavior
†6.8.2	Disorganized Infant Behavior
†6.8.3	Potential for Enhanced Organized Infant Behavior

Pattern 7: Perceiving

7.1.1	Body Image Disturbance
7.1.2	Self-Esteem Disturbance
7.1.2.1	Chronic Low Self-Esteem
7.1.2.2	Situational Low Self-Esteem
7.1.3	Personal Identity Disturbance
7.2	Sensory/Perceptual Alterations (Specify) (Visual, Auditory, Kinesthetic, Gustatory, Tactile, Olfactory)
7.2.1.1	Unilateral Neglect
7.3.1	Hopelessness
7.3.2	Powerlessness

Pattern 8: Knowing

8.1.1	Knowledge Deficit (Specify)
†8.2.1	Impaired Environmental Interpretation Syndrome
†8.2.2	Acute Confusion
†8.2.3	Chronic Confusion
8.3	Altered Thought Processes
†8.3.1	Impaired Memory

Pattern 9: Feeling

9.1.1	Pain
9.1.1.1	Chronic Pain
9.2.1.1	Dysfunctional Grieving
9.2.1.2	Anticipatory Grieving
°9.2.2	Risk for Violence: Self-Directed or Directed at Others
°9.2.2.1	Risk for Self-Mutilation
9.2.3	Post-Trauma Response
9.2.3.1	Rape-Trauma Syndrome
9.2.3.1.1	Rape-Trauma Syndrome: Compound Reaction
9.2.3.1.2	Rape-Trauma Syndrome: Silent Reaction
9.3.1	Anxiety
9.3.2	Fear

NANDA-Approved Nursing Diagnoses Categorized by Functional Health Patterns

Health-Perception—Health-Management Pattern

Health-Seeking Behaviors (Specify)
Altered Health Maintenance
Ineffective Management of Therapeutic Regimen
Effective Management of Therapeutic Regimen
Ineffective Management of Therapeutic Regimen: Families
Ineffective Management of Therapeutic Regimen: Community
Noncompliance (Specify)
Risk for Infection
Risk for Injury
Risk for Trauma
Risk for Perioperative Positioning Injury
Risk for Poisoning
Risk for Suffocation
Altered Protection
Energy Field Disturbance

Nutritional-Metabolic Pattern

Altered Nutrition: More Than Body Requirements
Altered Nutrition: Risk for More than Body Requirements
Altered Nutrition: Less Than Body Requirements
Ineffective Breastfeeding
Interrupted Breastfeeding
Effective Breastfeeding
Ineffective Infant Feeding Pattern
Impaired Swallowing
Risk for Aspiration
Altered Oral Mucous Membranes

Adapted from Gordon M: *Manual of nursing diagnosis, 1997–1998,* St. Louis, 1997, Mosby.

Fluid Volume Deficit
Risk for Fluid Volume Deficit
Fluid Volume Excess
Risk for Impaired Skin Integrity
Impaired Skin Integrity
Impaired Tissue Integrity
Risk for Altered Body Temperature
Ineffective Thermoregulation
Hyperthermia
Hypothermia

Elimination Pattern

Colonic Constipation
Perceived Constipation
Constipation
Diarrhea
Bowel Incontinence
Altered Urinary Elimination
Functional Incontinence
Reflex Incontinence
Stress Incontinence
Urge Incontinence
Total Incontinence
Urinary Retention

Activity-Exercise Pattern

Activity Intolerance
Risk for Activity Intolerance
Fatigue
Impaired Physical Mobility
Risk for Disuse Syndrome
Bathing/Hygiene Self-Care Deficit
Dressing/Grooming Self-Care Deficit
Feeding Self-Care Deficit
Toileting Self-Care Deficit
Diversional Activity Deficit
Impaired Home Maintenance Management

Dysfunctional Ventilatory Weaning Response
Inability to Sustain Spontaneous Ventilation
Ineffective Airway Clearance
Ineffective Breathing Pattern
Impaired Gas Exchange
Decreased Cardiac Output
Altered Tissue Perfusion (Specify Type)
Dysreflexia
Disorganized Infant Behavior
Risk for Disorganized Infant Behavior
Potential for Enhanced Organized Infant Behavior
Risk for Peripheral Neurovascular Dysfunction
Altered Growth and Development

Sleep-Rest Pattern

Sleep Pattern Disburbance

Cognitive-Perceptual Pattern

Pain
Chronic Pain
Sensory/Perceptual Alterations (Specify)
Unilateral Neglect
Knowledge Deficit (Specify)
Altered Thought Processes
Acute Confusion
Chronic Confusion
Impaired Environmental Interpretation Syndrome
Impaired Memory
Decisional Conflict (Specify)
Decreased Adaptive Capacity: Intracranial

Self-Perception—Self-Concept Pattern

Fear
Anxiety
Risk for Loneliness
Hopelessness
Powerlessness
Self-Esteem Disturbance
Chronic Low Self-Esteem
Situational Low Self-Esteem
Body Image Disturbance
Risk for Self-Mutilation
Personal Identity Disturbance

Role-Relationship Pattern

Anticipatory Grieving
Dysfunctional Grieving
Altered Role Performance
Social Isolation or Social Rejection
Social Isolation
Impaired Social Interaction
Relocation Stress Syndrome
Altered Family Processes
Altered Family Processes: Alcoholism
Altered Parenting
Risk for Altered Parenting
Parental Role Conflict
Risk for Altered Parent/Infant/Child Attachment
Caregiver Role Strain
Risk for Caregiver Role Strain
Impaired Verbal Communication
Risk for Violence: Self-Directed or Directed at Others

Sexuality-Reproductive Pattern

Altered Sexuality Patterns
Sexual Dysfunction
Rape-Trauma Syndrome
Rape-Trauma Syndrome: Compound Reaction
Rape-Trauma Syndrome: Silent Reaction

Coping—Stress-Tolerance Pattern

Ineffective Individual Coping
Defensive Coping
Ineffective Denial
Impaired Adjustment
Post-Trauma Response
Family Coping: Potential for Growth
Ineffective Family Coping: Compromised
Ineffective Family Coping: Disabling
Ineffective Community Coping
Potential for Enhanced Community Coping

Value-Belief Pattern

Spiritual Distress (Distress of Human Spirit)
Potential for Enhanced Spiritual Well-Being

Home Health Care Classification (HHCC) System*

Overview

The Home Health Care Classification (HHCC) System is a unique system designed to document nursing care through its standardized nomenclature. The nomenclature was developed by Saba and others [4,5] from empirical data as part of a national research study.[6] The HHCC nomenclature is designed to record and track the clinical care process for an entire episode of care of patients in the home and ambulatory care settings.

This nomenclature consists of the Home Health Care Classification: Nursing Diagnoses and the Home Health Care Classification: Nursing Interventions.[3] They are structured according to 20 nursing care components and used to index, code, and classify the six steps of the nursing process.[1]

The HHCC nomenclature is presented in Tables C-1, C-2, and C-3. Table C-1 consists of the 20 HHCC nursing components used to assess the patient. A nursing component is a cluster of elements that represent a functional, physiological, psychological, health behavior pattern.

Table C-2 consists of 145 HHCC nursing diagnoses (50 two-digit major categories and 95 three-digit subcategories). A nursing diagnosis is a clinical judgment,

based on the assessment of the patient, that forms the basis for the selection of the nursing interventions needed to achieve the desired outcome.[2]

Table C-2 is preceded by the coding structure and three modifiers (1 = improved, 2 = stabilized, or 3 = deteriorated), which are used to provide the outcome goal for each diagnosis. These three modifiers are also used to document and measure the actual outcome as compared to the expected outcome.

Table C-3 consists of the 160 HHCC nursing interventions (60 two-digit major categories and 100 three-digit subcategories). A nursing intervention is a single treatment or service performed to achieve an outcome for a specific diagnosis.

Table C-3 is preceded by the coding structure and four modifiers (1 = assess/monitor, 2 = care/perform, 3 = teach/instruct, and/or 4 = manage/coordinate), which are used to identify the type of nursing intervention action. The four modifiers expand the data dictionary fourfold, resulting in 640 HHCC nursing interventions.

The HHCC nursing disgnoses and HHCC nursing interventions are structured according to the 20 care components and coded according to ICD-10.[7] The HHCC System nomenclature is used for computer-based patient records (CPR). It is also used to identify a nursing minimum data set and to track the nursing care process across time, different settings, and geographic locations.

*By Virginia K. Saba, EdD, RN, FAAN, FACMI, Georgetown University School of Nursing.

TABLE C-1 Home Health Care Classification—20 Nursing Components: Alphabetic Index with Codes

A	Activity Component	H	Medication Component	O	Self-Care Component
B	Bowel Elimination Component	I	Metabolic Component	P	Self-Concept Component
C	Cardiac Component	J	Nutritional Component	Q	Sensory Component
D	Cognitive Component	K	Physical Regulation Component	R	Skin Integrity Component
E	Coping Component	L	Respiratory Component	S	Tissue Perfusion Component
F	Fluid Volume Component	M	Role Relationship Component	T	Urinary Elimination Component
G	Health Behavior Component	N	Safety Component		

Home Health Care Classification (HHCC): Nursing Diagnoses with Expected Outcomes/Goals and Coding Structure

The coding structure for the Home Health Care Classification of nursing diagnoses (see Table C-2) is described below. The structure is used when coding home health nursing diagnoses, including an expected outcome/goal. The coding structure consists of five alphanumeric characters: the first character is a letter of the alphabet representing the home health care component; the second and third characters are numbers representing the major home health care nursing diagnoses; a fourth character is blank or a decimal digit representing a diagnostic subcategory; and the fifth character is a modifier in the form of a decimal digit (1, 2, or 3) representing the expected outcome/goal.

Coding Structure

- Home health care component (first character): Letter of the alphabet from A to T
- Nursing diagnosis, major category (second and third characters): 01 to 50
- Nursing diagnosis, subcategory (fourth character): decimal digit from 1 to 9
- Discharge status/goal (fifth character): 1 to 3 (1 = improved, 2 = stabilized, 3 = deteriorated; use only one)

TABLE C-2 Home Health Care Classification of Nursing Diagnoses and Coding Scheme: 50 Major Categories and 95 Subcategories[1]

A ACTIVITY COMPONENT	08.2 Knowledge Deficit of Dietary Regimen
01 Activity Alteration	08.3 Knowledge Deficit of Disease Process
01.1 Activity Intolerance	08.4 Knowledge Deficit of Fluid Volume
01.2 Activity Intolerance Risk	08.5 Knowledge Deficit of Medication Regimen
01.3 Diversional Activity Deficit	08.6 Knowledge Deficit of Safety Precautions
01.4 Fatigue	08.7 Knowledge Deficit of Therapeutic Regimen
01.5 Physical Mobility Impairment	09 Thought Processes Alteration
01.6 Sleep Pattern Disturbance	
02 Musculoskeletal Alteration	**E COPING COMPONENT**
	10 Dying Process
B BOWEL ELIMINATION COMPONENT	11 Family Coping Impairment
03 Bowel Elimination Alteration	11.1 Compromised Family Coping
03.1 Bowel Incontinence	11.2 Disabled Family Coping
03.2 Colonic Constipation	12 Individual Coping Impairment
03.3 Diarrhea	12.1 Adjustment Impairment
03.4 Fecal Impaction	12.2 Decisional Conflict
03.5 Perceived Constipation	12.3 Defensive Coping
03.6 Unspecified Constipation	12.4 Denial
04 Gastrointestinal Alteration	13 Post-Trauma Response
	13.1 Rape-Trauma Syndrome
C CARDIAC COMPONENT	14 Spiritual State Alteration
05 Cardiac Output Alteration	14.1 Spiritual Distress
06 Cardiovascular Alteration	
06.1 Blood Pressure Alteration	**F FLUID VOLUME COMPONENT**
	15 Fluid Volume Alteration
D COGNITIVE COMPONENT	15.1 Fluid Volume Deficit
07 Cerebral Alteration	15.2 Fluid Volume Deficit Risk
08 Knowledge Deficit	15.3 Fluid Volume Excess
08.1 Knowledge Deficit of Diagnostic Test	15.4 Fluid Volume Excess Risk

[1]Adapted from North American Nursing Diagnosis Association: *Taxonomy 1: revised,* St. Louis, 1990, The Association.

G HEALTH BEHAVIOR COMPONENT

16   Growth and Development Alteration

17   Health Maintenance Alteration

18   Health-Seeking Behavior Alteration

19   Home Maintenance Alteration

20   Noncompliance
     20.1   Noncompliance of Diagnostic Test
     20.2   Noncompliance of Dietary Regimen
     20.3   Noncompliance of Fluid Volume
     20.4   Noncompliance of Medication Regimen
     20.5   Noncompliance of Safety Precautions
     20.6   Noncompliance of Therapeutic Regimen

H MEDICATION COMPONENT

21   Medication Risk
     21.1   Polypharmacy

I METABOLIC COMPONENT

22   Endocrine Alteration

23   Immunological Alteration
     23.1   Protection Alteration

J NUTRITIONAL COMPONENT

24   Nutrition Alteration
     24.1   Body Nutrition Deficit
     24.2   Body Nutrition Deficit Risk
     24.3   Body Nutrition Excess
     24.4   Body Nutrition Excess Risk

K PHYSICAL REGULATION COMPONENT

25   Physical Regulation Alteration
     25.1   Dysreflexia
     25.2   Hyperthermia
     25.3   Hypothermia
     25.4   Thermoregulation Impairment
     25.5   Infection Risk
     25.6   Infection, Unspecified

L RESPIRATORY COMPONENT

26   Respiration Alteration
     26.1   Airway Clearance Impairment
     26.2   Breathing Pattern Impairment
     26.3   Gas Exchange Impairment

M ROLE RELATIONSHIP COMPONENT

27   Role Performance Alteration
     27.1   Parental Role Conflict
     27.2   Parenting Alteration
     27.3   Sexual Dysfunction

28   Communication Impairment
     28.1   Verbal Impairment

29   Family Processes Alteration

30   Grieving
     30.1   Anticipatory Grieving
     30.2   Dysfunctional Grieving

31   Sexuality Patterns Alteration

32   Socialization Alteration
     32.1   Social Interaction Alteration
     32.2   Social Isolation

N SAFETY COMPONENT

33   Injury Risk
     33.1   Aspiration Risk
     33.2   Disuse Syndrome
     33.3   Poisoning Risk
     33.4   Suffocation Risk
     33.5   Trauma Risk

34   Violence Risk

O SELF-CARE COMPONENT

35   Bathing/Hygiene Deficit

36   Dressing/Grooming Deficit

37   Feeding Deficit
     37.1   Breastfeeding Impairment
     37.2   Swallowing Impairment

38   Self-Care Deficit
     38.1   Activities of Daily Living (ADLs) Alteration
     38.2   Instrumental Activities of Daily Living (IADLs) Alteration

39   Toileting Deficit

P SELF-CONCEPT COMPONENT

40   Anxiety

41   Fear

42   Meaningfulness Alteration
     42.1   Hopelessness
     42.2   Powerlessness

43   Self-Concept Alteration
     43.1   Body Image Disturbance
     43.2   Personal Identity Disturbance
     43.3   Chronic Low Self-Esteem Disturbance
     43.4   Situational Self-Esteem Disturbance

Q SENSORY COMPONENT

44   Sensory/Perceptual Alteration
     44.1   Auditory Alteration
     44.2   Gustatory Alteration
     44.3   Kinesthetic Alteration
     44.4   Olfactory Alteration
     44.5   Tactile Alteration
     44.6   Unilateral Neglect
     44.7   Visual Alteration

Continued

TABLE C-2 Home Health Care Classification of Nursing Diagnoses and Coding Scheme: 50 Major Categories and 95 Subcategories—cont'd

45	Comfort Alteration	**S**	**TISSUE PERFUSION COMPONENT**
	45.1 Acute Pain	48	Tissue Perfusion Alteration
	45.2 Chronic Pain		
	45.3 Unspecified Pain	**T**	**URINARY ELIMINATION COMPONENT**
		49	Urinary Elimination Component
R	**SKIN INTEGRITY COMPONENT**		49.1 Functional Urinary Incontinence
46	Skin Integrity Alteration		49.2 Reflex Urinary Incontinence
	46.1 Oral Mucous Membrane Impairment		49.3 Stress Urinary Incontinence
	46.2 Skin Integrity Impairment		49.4 Total Urinary Incontinence
	46.3 Skin Integrity Impairment Risk		49.5 Urge Urinary Incontinence
	46.4 Skin Incision		49.6 Urinary Retention
47	Peripheral Alteration	50	Renal Alteration

Home Health Care Classification (HHCC): Nursing Interventions with Type of Intervention Action and Coding Structure

The coding structure for the Home Health Care Classification of nursing interventions (see Table C-3) is described below. The structure is used when coding home health nursing interventions, including type of intervention action. The coding structure consists of five alphanumeric characters: the first character is a letter of the alphabet representing the home health care component; the second and third characters are numbers representing the major home health nursing interventions;

the fourth character is blank or a decimal digit representing an intervention subcategory; and the fifth character is a modifier in the form of a decimal digit (1, 2, 3, or 4) representing the type of intervention action.

Coding Structure

- Home health care component (first character): Letter of the alphabet from A to T
- Nursing intervention, major category (second and third characters): 01 to 50
- Nursing intervention, subcategory (fourth character): decimal digit from 1 to 9
- Type of intervention action (fifth character): 1 to 4 (1 = assess, 2 = care, 3 = teach, 4 = manage; use only one)

TABLE C-3 Home Health Care Classification of Nursing and Interventions and Coding Scheme: 60 Major Categories and 100 Subcategories

A	**ACTIVITY COMPONENT**		05.1 Range of Motion
01	Activity Care		05.2 Rehabilitation Exercises
	01.1 Cardiac Rehabilitation		
	01.2 Energy Conservation	**B**	**BOWEL ELIMINATION COMPONENT**
02	Fracture Care	06	Bowel Care
	02.1 Cast Care		06.1 Bowel Training
	02.2 Immobilizer Care		06.2 Disimpaction
03	Mobility Therapy		06.3 Enema
	03.1 Ambulation Therapy	07	Ostomy Care
	03.2 Assistive Device Therapy		07.1 Ostomy Irrigation
	03.3 Transfer Care		
04	Sleep Pattern Control	**C**	**CARDIAC COMPONENT**
05	Rehabilitation Care	08	Cardiac Care
		09	Pacemaker Care

D   COGNITIVE COMPONENT
10   Behavior Care
11   Reality Orientation

E   COPING COMPONENT
12   Counseling Service
    12.1   Coping Support
    12.2   Stress Control
13   Emotional Support
    13.1   Spiritual Comfort
14   Terminal Care
    14.1   Bereavement Support
    14.2   Dying/Death Measures
    14.3   Funeral Arrangements

F   FLUID VOLUME COMPONENT
15   Fluid Therapy
    15.1   Hydration Status
    15.2   Intake/Output
16   Infusion Care
    16.1   Intravenous Care
    16.2   Venous Catheter Care

G   HEALTH BEHAVIOR COMPONENT
17   Community Special Programs
    17.1   Adult Day Center
    17.2   Hospice
    17.3   Meals-on-Wheels
    17.4   Other Community Special Program
18   Compliance Care
    18.1   Compliance with Diet
    18.2   Compliance with Fluid Volume
    18.3   Compliance with Medical Regime
    18.4   Compliance with Medication Regime
    18.5   Compliance with Safety Precautions
    18.6   Compiance with Therapeutic Regime
19   Nursing Contact
    19.1   Bill of Rights
    19.2   Nursing Care Coordination
    19.3   Nursing Status Report
20   Physician Contact
    20.1   Medical Regime Orders
    20.2   Physician Status Report
21   Professional/Ancillary Services
    21.1   Home Health Aide Service
    21.2   Medical Social Worker Service
    21.3   Nurse Specialist Service
    21.4   Occupational Therapist Service
    21.5   Physical Therapist Service
    21.6   Speech Therapist Service
    21.7   Other Ancillary Service
    21.8   Other Professional Service

H   MEDICATION COMPONENT
22   Chemotherapy Care
23   Injection Administration
    23.1   Insulin Injection
    23.2   Vitamin B_{12} Injection
24   Medication Administration
    24.1   Medication Actions
    24.2   Medication Prefill Preparation
    24.3   Medication Side Effects
25   Radiation Therapy Care

I   METABOLIC COMPONENT
26   Allergic Reaction Care
27   Diabetic Care

J   NUTRITIONAL COMPONENT
28   Gastrostomy/Nasogastric Tube Care
    28.1   Gastrostomy/Nasogastric Tube Insertion
    28.2   Gastrostomy/Nasogastric Tube Irrigation
29   Nutrition Care
    29.1   Enteral/Parenteral Feeding
    29.2   Feeding Technique
    29.3   Regular Diet
    29.4   Special Diet

K   PHYSICAL REGULATION COMPONENT
30   Infection Control
    30.1   Universal Precautions
31   Physical Health Care
    31.1   Health History
    31.2   Health Promotion
    31.3   Physical Examination
    31.4   Physical Measurements
32   Specimen Analysis
    32.1   Blood Specimen Analysis
    32.2   Stool Specimen Analysis
    32.3   Urine Specimen Analysis
    32.4   Other Specimen Analysis
33   Vital Signs
    33.1   Blood Pressure
    33.2   Temperature
    33.3   Pulse
    33.4   Respiration
34   Weight Control

L   RESPIRATORY COMPONENT
35   Oxygen Therapy Care
36   Respiratory Care
    36.1   Breathing Exercises

Continued

TABLE C-3   Home Health Care Classification of Nursing and Interventions and Coding Scheme: 60 Major Categories and 100 Subcategories—cont'd

36.2   Chest Physiotherapy
36.3   Inhalation Therapy
36.4   Ventilator Care
37   Tracheostomy Care

M   ROLE RELATIONSHIP COMPONENT
38   Communication Care
39   Psychosocial Analysis
    39.1   Home Situation Analysis
    39.2   Interpersonal Dynamics Analysis

N   SAFETY COMPONENT
40   Abuse Control
41   Emergency Care
42   Safety Precautions
    42.1   Environmental Safety
    42.2   Equipment Safety
    42.3   Individual Safety

O   SELF-CARE COMPONENT
43   Personal Care
    43.1   Activities of Daily Living (ADLs)
    43.2   Instrumental Activities of Daily Living (IADLs)
44   Bedbound Care
    44.1   Positioning Therapy

P   SELF-CONCEPT COMPONENT
45   Mental Health Care
    45.1   Mental Health History
    45.2   Mental Health Promotion
    45.3   Mental Health Screening
    45.4   Mental Health Treatment
46   Violence Control

Q   SENSORY COMPONENT
47   Pain Control

48   Comfort Care
49   Ear Care
    49.1   Hearing Aid Care
    49.2   Wax Removal
50   Eye Care
    50.1   Cataract Care

R   SKIN INTEGRITY COMPONENT
51   Decubitus Care
    51.1   Decubitus Stage 1
    51.2   Decubitus Stage 2
    51.3   Decubitus Stage 3
    51.4   Decubitus Stage 4
52   Edema Control
53   Mouth Care
    53.1   Denture Care
54   Skin Care
    54.1   Skin Breakdown Control
55   Wound Care
    55.1   Drainage Tube Care
    55.2   Dressing Change
    55.3   Incision Care

S   TISSUE PERFUSION COMPONENT
56   Foot Care
57   Perineal Care

T   URINARY ELIMINATION COMPONENT
58   Bladder Care
    58.1   Bladder Instillation
    58.2   Bladder Training
59   Dialysis Care
60   Urinary Catheter Care
    60.1   Urinary Catheter Insertion
    60.2   Urinary Catheter Irrigation

REFERENCES

1. American Nurses Association: *Standards of clinical nursing practice,* Washington, D.C., 1991, The Association.
2. North American Nursing Diagnosis Association: *Taxonomy I: revised,* St. Louis, 1990, The Association.
3. Saba VK: *Home health care classification (HHCC) of nursing diagnoses and interventions,* revised ed, Washington, D.C., 1994, The Author.
4. Saba VK: The classification of home health care nursing diagnoses and interventions, *Caring* 10(3):50–57, 1992.
5. Saba VK: Home health care classification, *Caring* 10(5):58–60, 1992.
6. Saba VK and Zuckerman AE: A new home health care classification method, *Caring* 10(10):27–34, 1992.
7. World Health Organization: *International statistical classification of diseases and related health problems: tenth revision,* Geneva, Switzerland, 1992, The Organization.

Nursing-Sensitive Outcomes Classification (NOC)

Abuse Cessation Evidence that the victim is no longer abused.

Abuse Protection Protection of self or dependent others from abuse.

Abuse Recovery: Emotional Healing of psychological injuries due to abuse.

Abuse Recovery: Financial Regaining monetary and legal control or benefits following financial exploitation.

Abuse Recovery: Physical Healing of physical injuries due to abuse.

Abuse Recovery: Sexual Healing following sexual abuse or exploitation.

Abusive Behavior Self-Control Management of own behaviors to avoid abuse and neglect of dependents or significant others.

Acceptance: Health Status Reconciliation to health circumstances.

Adherence Behavior Self-initiated action taken to promote wellness, recovery, and rehabilitation.

Aggression Control Ability to restrain assaultive, combative, or destructive behavior toward others.

Ambulation: Walking Ability to walk from place to place.

Ambulation: Wheelchair Ability to move from place to place in a wheelchair.

Anxiety Control Ability to eliminate or reduce feelings of apprehension and tension from an unidentifiable source.

Balance Ability to maintain body equilibrium.

Blood Transfusion Reaction Control Extent to which complications of blood transfusions are minimized.

Body Image Positive perception of own appearance and body functions.

Body Positioning: Self-Initiated Ability to change own body positions.

Bowel Continence Control of passage of stool from the bowel.

Bowel Elimination Ability of the gastrointestinal tract to form and evacuate stool effectively.

Breastfeeding Establishment: Infant Proper attachment of an infant to and sucking from the mother's breast for nourishment during the first 2 to 3 weeks.

Breastfeeding Establishment: Maternal Maternal establishment of proper attachment of an infant to and sucking from the breast for nourishment during the first 2 to 3 weeks.

Breastfeeding Maintenance Continued nourishment of an infant through breastfeeding.

Breastfeeding Weaning Process leading to the eventual discontinuation of breastfeeding.

Cardiac Pump Effectiveness Extent to which blood is ejected from the left ventricle per minute to support systemic perfusion pressure.

Caregiver Adaptation to Patient Institutionalization Family caregiver adaption of role when the care recipient is transferred outside the home.

Caregiver Emotional Health Feelings, attitudes, and emotions of a family care provider while caring for a member or significant other in the home.

Caregiver Lifestyle Disruption Disturbances in the lifestyle of a family member due to caregiving.

Caregiver-Patient Relationship Positive interactions and connections between the caregiver and care recipient.

Caregiver Performance: Direct Care Provision by family care provider of appropriate personal and health care for a family member or significant other.

Caregiver Performance: Indirect Care Arrangement and oversight of appropriate care for a family member or significant other over an extended period of time.

These outcomes were developed by the Iowa Outcomes Project (1996) with funding from Sigma Theta Tau International and the National Center of Nursing Research (NIH 1R01NR03437-01, M. Johnson and M. Maas, Co-Pis). Copyright © Nursing-Sensitive Outcomes Classification, 1996.

Caregiver Physical Health Physical well-being of a family care provider while caring for a family member or significant other over an extended period of time.

Caregiver Stressors The extent of biopsychosocial pressure on a family care provider caring for a family member or significant other over an extended period of time.

Caregiver Well-Being Primary care provider's satisfaction with health and life circumstances.

Caregiving Endurance Potential Factors that promote family care provider continuance over an extended period of time.

Child Adaptation to Hospitalization Child's adaptive response to hospitalization.

Circulation Status Extent to which blood flows unobstructed, unidirectionally, and at an appropriate pressure through large vessels of the systemic and pulmonary circuits.

Cognitive Ability Ability to identify person, place, and time.

Comfort Level Feelings of physical and psychological ease.

Communication Ability to receive, interpret, and express spoken, written, and nonverbal messages.

Communication: Expressive Ability Ability to express and interpret verbal and/or nonverbal messages.

Communication: Receptive Ability Ability to express and interpret verbal and/or nonverbal messages.

Compliance Behavior Actions taken on the basis of professional advice to promote wellness, recovery, and rehabilitation.

Concentration Ability to focus on a specific stimulus.

Coping Actions to manage stressors that tax an individual's resources.

Decision Making Ability to choose between two or more alternatives.

Dignified Dying Maintaining personal control and comfort with the approaching end of life.

Distorted Thought Control Ability to self-restrain disruption in perception, thought processes, and thought content.

Electrolyte and Acid Base Balance Balance of the electrolytes and nonelectrolytes in the intracellular and extracellular compartments of the body.

Endurance Extent that energy enables a person's activity.

Energy Conservation Extent of active management of energy to initiate and sustain activity.

Fluid Balance Balance of water in the intracellular and extracellular compartments of the body.

Grief Resolution Adjustment to actual or impending loss.

Growth A normal increase in body size and weight.

Health Belief: Perceived Ability to Perform Personal conviction that one can carry out a given health behavior.

Health Belief: Perceived Control Personal conviction that one can influence a health outcome.

Health Belief: Perceived Resources Personal conviction that one has adequate means to carry out a health behavior.

Health Belief: Perceived Threat Personal conviction that a health problem is serious and has potential negative consequences for lifestyle.

Health Beliefs Personal convictions that influence health behaviors.

Health Orientation Personal view of health and health behaviors as priorities.

Health-Promoting Behavior Actions to sustain or increase wellness.

Health-Seeking Behavior Actions to promote optimum wellness, recovery, and rehabilitation.

Hope Presence of internal state of optimism that is personally satisfying and life-supporting.

Hydration Amount of water in the intracellular and extracellular compartments of the body.

Identity Ability to distinguish between self and nonself and to characterize one's essence.

Immobility Consequences: Physiological Compromise in physiological functioning due to impaired physical mobility.

Immobility Consequences: Psycho-Cognitive Extent of compromise in psycho-cognitive functioning due to impaired physical mobility.

Immune Hypersensitivity Control Extent to which inappropriate immune responses are suppressed.

Immune Status Adequacy of natural and acquired appropriately targeted resistance to internal and external antigens.

Impulse Control Ability to self-restrain compulsive or impulsive behaviors.

Infection Status Presence and extent of infection.

Information Processing Ability to acquire, organize, and use information.

Joint Movement: Active Range of motion of joints with self-initiated movement.

Joint Movement: Passive Range of motion of joints with assisted movement.

Knowledge: Breastfeeding Extent of understanding conveyed about lactation and nourishment of infant throught breastfeeding.

Knowledge: Diet Extent of understanding and skills conveyed about diet.

Knowledge: Disease Process Extent of understanding conveyed about a specific disease process.

Knowledge: Energy Conservation Extent of understanding and skills conveyed about energy conservation techniques.

Knowledge: Health Behaviors Extent of understanding conveyed about the promotion and protection of health.

Knowledge: Health Resources Extent of understanding conveyed about health care resources.

Knowledge: Infection Control Extent of understanding conveyed about prevention and control of infection.

Knowledge: Medication Extent of understanding conveyed about the safe use of medication.

Knowledge: Personal Safety Extent of understanding conveyed about preventing unintentional injuries.

Knowledge: Prescribed Activity Extent of understanding and skills conveyed about prescribed activity and exercise.

Knowledge: Substance Use Control Extent of understanding conveyed about managing substance use safely.

Knowledge: Treatment Regimen Extent of understanding and skills conveyed about a specific treatment regimen.

Leisure Participation Use of restful or relaxing activities as needed to promote well-being.

Loneliness The extent of emotional, social, or existential isolation response.

Memory Ability to retrieve cognitively and to report previously stored information.

Mobility Level Ability to move purposefully.

Mood Equilibrium Appropriate adjustment of prevailing emotional tone in response to circumstances.

Muscle Function Adequacy of muscle contraction needed for movement.

Neglect Cessation Evidence that substandard care is corrected.

Neurological Status Extent to which the peripheral and central nervous systems receive, process, and respond to internal and external stimuli.

Neurological Status: Autonomic Extent to which the autonomic nervous system coordinates visceral function.

Neurological Status: Central Motor Control Extent to which skeletal muscle activity (body movement) is coordinated by the central nervous system.

Neurological Status: Consciousness Extent to which an individual arouses, orients, and attends to the environment.

Neurological Status: Cranial Sensory Motor Function Extent to which spinal nerves convey sensory and motor information.

Normal Physical Aging Physical changes that commonly occur with adult aging.

Nutritional Status Extent to which nutrients are available to meet metabolic needs.

Nutritional Status: Biochemical Measures Body fluid components and chemical indices of nutritional status.

Nutritional Status: Body Mass Congruence of body weight, muscle, and fat to height, frame, and gender.

Nutritional Status: Energy Extent to which nutrients provide cellular energy.

Nutritional Status: Food and Fluid Intake Amount of food and fluid taken into the body over a 24-hour period.

Nutritional Status: Nutrient Intake Adequacy of nutrients taken into the body.

Oral Health Condition of the mouth, teeth, gums, and tongue.

Pain Control Behaviors Personal actions to control pain.

Pain: Disruptive Effects Observed or reported disruptive effects of pain on emotions and behavior.

Pain Level Amount of reported or demonstrated pain.

Parent-Infant Attachment Demonstration of an enduring affectionate bond between a parent and infant.

Parenting Provision of an environment that promotes optimum growth and development of dependent children.

Parenting: Social Safety Parental actions to avoid social relationships that might cause harm or injury.

Participation: Health Care Decisions Personal involvement in selecting and evaluating health care options.

Physical Maturation: Female Normal physical changes in the female that occur with the transition from childhood to adulthood.

Physical Maturation: Male Normal physical changes in the male that occur with the transition from childhood to adulthood.

Play Participation Use of activities as needed for enjoyment, entertainment, and development by children.

Psychosocial Adjustment: Life Change Psychosocial adaptation of an individual to a life change.

Quality of Life An individual's expressed satisfaction with current life circumstances.

Respiratory Status: Gas Exchange Alveolar exchange of CO_2 or O_2 to maintain arterial blood gas concentrations.

Respiratory Status: Ventilation Movement of air in and out of the lungs.

Rest Extent and pattern of diminished activity for mental and physical rejuvenation.

Risk Control Actions to eliminate or reduce actual, personal, and modifiable health threats.

Risk Control: Alcohol Use Actions to eliminate or reduce alcohol use that poses a threat to health.

Risk Control: Drug Use Actions to eliminate or reduce drug use that poses a threat to health.

Risk Control: Immunization Actions to obtain immunity from a preventable communicable disease.

Risk Control: Sexually Transmitted Disease (STD) Actions to eliminate or reduce behaviors associated with sexually transmitted disease.

Risk Control: Tobacco Use Actions to eliminate or reduce tobacco use.

Risk Control: Unintended Pregnancy Actions to reduce the possibility of unintended pregnancy.

Risk Detection Actions taken to identify personal health threats.

Role Performance Congruence of an individual's role behavior with role expectations.

Safety Behavior: Fall Prevention Individual or caregiver actions to minimize factors that might result in falls.

Safety Behavior: Home Physical Environment Individual or caregiver actions to minimize environmental factors that might cause physical harm or injury in the home.

Safety Behavior: Personal Individual or caregiver efforts to control behaviors that might cause physical injury.

Safety Status: Falls Occurrence Number of falls in the past week.

Safety Status: Physical Injury Severity of injuries from accidents and trauma.

Self-Care: Activities of Daily Living (ADLs) Ability to perform the most basic physical tasks and personal care activities.

Self-Care: Bathing Ability to cleanse own body.

Self-Care: Dressing Ability to dress self.

Self-Care: Eating Ability to prepare and ingest food.

Self-Care: Grooming Ability to maintain kempt appearance.

Self-Care: Hygiene Ability to maintain own hygiene.

Self-Care: Instrumental Activities of Daily Living (IADLs) Ability to perform activities needed to function in the home or community.

Self-Care: Nonparenteral Medication Ability to administer oral and topical medications to meet therapeutic goals.

Self-Care: Oral Hygiene Ability to care for own mouth and teeth.

Self-Care: Parenteral Medication Ability to administer parenteral medications to meet therapeutic goals.

Self-Care: Toileting Ability to toilet self.

Self-Esteem Personal judgment of self-worth.

Self-Mutilation Restraint Ability to refrain from intentional self-inflicted (nonlethal) injury.

Sleep Extent and pattern of sleep for mental and physical rejuvenation.

Social Interaction Skills An individual's use of effective interaction behaviors.

Social Involvement Frequency of an individual's social interactions with persons, groups, or organizations.

Social Support Perceived availability and actual provision of reliable assistance from other persons.

Spiritual Well-Being Personal expressions of connectedness with self, others, higher power, all life, nature, and the universe that transcend and empower the self.

Substance Addiction Consequences Compromise in health status and social functioning due to substance addiction.

Suicide Self-Restraint Ability to refrain from gestures and attempts at killing self.

Symptom Control Behavior Personal actions to minimize perceived adverse changes in physical and emotional functioning.

Symptom Severity Extent of perceived adverse changes in physical and emotional functioning.

Thermoregulation Balance among heat production, heat gain, and heat loss.

Thermoregulation: Neonate Balance among heat production, heat gain, and heat loss during the neonatal period.

Tissue Integrity: Skin and Mucous Membranes Structural intactness and normal physiological function of skin and mucous membranes.

Tissue Perfusion: Abdominal Organs Extent to which blood flows through the small vessels of the abdominal viscera and maintains organ function.

Tissue Perfusion: Cardiac Extent to which blood flows through the coronary vasculature and maintains heart function.

Tissue Perfusion: Cerebral Extent to which blood flows through the cerebral vasculature and maintains brain function.

Tissue Perfusion: Peripheral Extent to which blood flows through the small vessels of the extremities and maintains tissue function.

Tissue Perfusion: Pulmonary Extent to which blood flows through the pulmonary vasculature and maintains arterial blood gas concentrations.

Transfer Performance Ability to change body locations.

Treatment Behavior: Illness or Injury Personal actions to palliate or eliminate pathology.

Urinary Continence Control of the elimination of urine.

Urinary Elimination Ability of the urinary system to filter wastes, conserve solutes, and to collect and discharge urine in a healthy pattern.

Vital Signs Status Temperature, pulse, respiration, and blood pressure within expected range for the individual.

Well-Being An individual's expressed satisfaction with health status.

Will to Live Desire, determination, and effort to survive.

Wound Healing: Primary Intention The extent to which cells and tissues have regenerated following intentional closure.

Wound Healing: Secondary Intention The extent to which cells and tissues in an open wound have regenerated.

Nursing Interventions Classification (NIC): Intervention Labels and Codes

6400 Abuse Protection
°6402 Abuse Protection: Child
°6404 Abuse Protection: Elder
1910 Acid-Base Management
1911 Acid-Base Management: Metabolic Acidosis
1912 Acid-Base Management: Metabolic Alkalosis
1913 Acid-Base Management: Respiratory Acidosis
1914 Acid-Base Management: Respiratory Alkalosis
1920 Acid-Base Monitoring
4920 Active Listening
4310 Activity Therapy
°1320 Acupressure
7310 Admission Care
3120 Airway Insertion and Stabilization
3140 Airway Management
3160 Airway Suctioning
6410 Allergy Management
°6700 Amnioinfusion
3420 Amputation Care
2210 Analgesic Administration
°2214 Analgesic Administration: Intraspinal
2840 Anesthesia Administration
4640 Anger Control Assistance
4320 Animal-Assisted Therapy
5210 Anticipatory Guidance
5820 Anxiety Reduction
6420 Area Restriction
4330 Art Therapy
3180 Artificial Airway Management
3200 Aspiration Precautions
4340 Assertiveness Training
6710 Attachment Promotion

5840 Autogenic Training
°2860 Autotransfusion
1610 Bathing
0740 Bed Rest Care
°7610 Bedside Laboratory Testing
4350 Behavior Management
°4352 Behavior Management: Overactivity/Inattention
°4354 Behavior Management: Self-Harm
°4356 Behavior Management: Sexual
4360 Behavior Modification
°4362 Behavior Modification: Social Skills
4680 Bibliotherapy
5860 Biofeedback
6720 Birthing
°0550 Bladder Irrigation
4010 Bleeding Precautions
4020 Bleeding Reduction
°4021 Bleeding Reduction: Antepartum Uterus
4022 Bleeding Reduction: Gastrointestinal
4024 Bleeding Reduction: Nasal
°4026 Bleeding Reduction: Postpartum Uterus
4028 Bleeding Reduction: Wound
4030 Blood Products Administration
5220 Body Image Enhancement
0140 Body Mechanics Promotion
1052 Bottle Feeding
0410 Bowel Incontinence Care
°0412 Bowel Incontinence Care: Encopresis
0420 Bowel Irrigation
0430 Bowel Management
0440 Bowel Training
°1054 Breastfeeding Assistance
5880 Calming Technique
4040 Cardiac Care
4044 Cardiac Care: Acute
4046 Cardiac Care: Rehabilitative
4050 Cardiac Precautions

°Interventions new to the second edition.
Developed from McCloskey JC and Bulechek GM, editors:
Nursing Interventions Classification (NIC), ed 2, St. Louis,
1996, Mosby–Year Book.

7040 Caregiver Support
0762 Cast Care: Maintenance
0764 Cast Care: Wet
2540 Cerebral Edema Management
°2550 Cerebral Perfusion Promotion
6750 Cesarean Section Care
2240 Chemotherapy Management
3230 Chest Physiotherapy
6760 Childbirth Preparation
4060 Circulatory Care
°4064 Circulatory Care: Mechanical Assist Device
4070 Circulatory Precautions
6140 Code Management
4700 Cognitive Restructuring
4720 Cognitive Stimulation
4974 Communication Enhancement: Hearing Deficit
°4976 Communication Enhancement: Speech Deficit
4978 Communication Enhancement: Visual Deficit
°5000 Complex Relationship Building
°2260 Conscious Sedation
0450 Constipation/Impaction Management
1620 Contact Lens Care
°7620 Controlled Substance Checking
5230 Coping Enhancement
3250 Cough Enhancement
5240 Counseling
6160 Crisis Intervention
°7640 Critical Path Development
7330 Culture Brokerage
1340 Cutaneous Stimulation
5250 Decision-Making Support
°7650 Delegation
6440 Delirium Management
°6450 Delusion Management
°6460 Dementia Management
°7050 Developmental Enhancement
0460 Diarrhea Management
1020 Diet Staging
7370 Discharge Planning
5900 Distraction
°7920 Documentation
1630 Dressing
5260 Dying Care
2560 Dysreflexia Management
4090 Dysrhythmia Management
1640 Ear Care
1030 Eating Disorders Management
2000 Electrolyte Management
2001 Electrolyte Management: Hypercalcemia
2002 Electrolyte Management: Hyperkalemia

2003 Electrolyte Management: Hypermagnesemia
2004 Electrolyte Management: Hypernatremia
2005 Electrolyte Management: Hyperphosphatemia
2006 Electrolyte Management: Hypocalcemia
2007 Electrolyte Management: Hypokalemia
2008 Electrolyte Management: Hypomagnesemia
2009 Electrolyte Management: Hyponatremia
2010 Electrolyte Management: Hypophosphatemia
2020 Electrolyte Monitoring
°6771 Electronic Fetal Monitoring: Antepartum
°6772 Electronic Fetal Monitoring: Intrapartum
°6470 Elopement Precautions
4104 Embolus Care: Peripheral
4106 Embolus Care: Pulmonary
4110 Embolus Precautions
6200 Emergency Care
°7660 Emergency Cart Check
5270 Emotional Support
°3270 Endotracheal Extubation
0180 Energy Management
1056 Enteral Tube Feeding
6480 Environmental Management
6481 Environmental Management: Attachment
    process
6482 Environmental Management: Comfort
°6484 Environmental Management: Community
6486 Environmental Management: Safety
6487 Environmental Management: Violence Preven-
    tion
°6489 Environmental Management: Worker Safety
°7680 Examination Assistance
0200 Exercise Promotion
°0202 Exercise Promotion: Stretching
0221 Exercise Therapy, Ambulation
0222 Exercise Therapy: Balance
0224 Exercise Therapy: Joint Mobility
0226 Exercise Therapy: Muscle Control
1650 Eye Care
7690 Fat Prevention
7100 Family Integrity Promotion
7104 Family Integrity Promotion: Childbearing Family
7110 Family Involvement
7120 Family Mobilization
6784 Family Planning: Contraception
6786 Family Planning: Infertility
6788 Family Planning: Unplanned Pregnancy
7130 Family Process Maintenance
7140 Family Support
7150 Family Therapy
1050 Feeding

°7160 Fertility Preservation
3740 Fever Treatment
°6500 Fire-Setting Precautions
6240 First Aid
0470 Flatulence Reduction
4120 Fluid Management
4130 Fluid Monitoring
4140 Fluid Resuscitation
2080 Fluid Electrolyte Management
1660 Foot Care
1080 Gastrointestinal Intubation
5242 Genetic Counseling
5290 Grief Work Facilitation
°5294 Grief Work Facilitation: Perinatal Death
5300 Guilt Work Facilitation
1670 Hair Care
6510 Hallucination Management
°7960 Health Care Information Exchange
°5510 Health Education
°7970 Health Policy Monitoring
6520 Health Screening
7400 Health System Guidance
3780 Heat Exposure Treatment
1380 Heat/Cold Application
2100 Hemodialysis Therapy
4150 Hemodynamic Regulation
4160 Hemorrhage Control
°6800 High-Risk Pregnancy Care
7180 Home Maintenance Assistance
5310 Hope Instillation
5320 Humor
2120 Hyperglycemia Management
4170 Hypervolemia Management
5920 Hypnosis
2130 Hypoglylcemia Management
3800 Hypothermia Treatment
4180 Hypovolemia Management
6530 Immunization/Vaccination Administration
°4370 Impulse Control Training
°7980 Incident Reporting
3440 Incision Site Care
6820 Infant Care
6540 Infection Control
°6545 Infection Control: Intraoperative
6550 Infection Protection
°7410 Insurance Authorization
2590 Intracranial Pressure (ICP) Monitoring
6830 Intrapartal Care
°6834 Intrapartal Care: High-Risk Delivery
4190 Intravenous (IV) Insertion
4200 Intravenous (IV) Therapy

4210 Invasive Hemodynamic Monitoring
°6840 Kangaroo Care
°6850 Labor Induction
°6860 Labor Suppression
°7690 Laboratory Data Interpretation
°5244 Lactation Counseling
6870 Lactation Suppression
°6560 Laser Precautions
°6570 Latex Precautions
5520 Learning Facilitation
5540 Learning Readiness Enhancement
°3460 Leech Therapy
4380 Limit Setting
°3840 Malignant Hyperthermia Precautions
3300 Mechanical Ventilation
3310 Mechanical Ventilatory Weaning
2300 Medication Administration
2301 Medication Administration: Enteral
2302 Medication Administration: Interpleural
°2303 Medication Administration: Intraosseous
2304 Medication Administration: Oral
2305 Medication Administration: Parenteral
2306 Medication Administration: Topical
°2307 Medication Administration: Ventricular Reservoir
2380 Medication Management
°2390 Medication Prescribing
5960 Meditation
4760 Memory Training
4390 Milieu Therapy
°5330 Mood Management
°8020 Multidisciplinary Care Conference
4400 Music Therapy
4410 Mutual Goal Setting
1680 Nail Care
2620 Neurological Monitoring
6880 Newborn Care
6890 Newborn Monitoring
6900 Nonnutritive Sucking
°7200 Normalization Promotion
1100 Nutrition Management
1120 Nutrition Therapy
5246 Nutritional Counseling
1160 Nutritional Monitoring
1710 Oral Health Maintenance
1720 Oral Health Promotion
1730 Oral Health Restoration
°8060 Order Transcription
°6260 Organ Procurement
0480 Ostomy Care
3320 Oxygen Therapy
1400 Pain Management

5562 Parent Education: Adolescent
5564 Parent Education: Childbearing Family
5566 Parent Education: Childrearing Family
°7440 Pass Facilitation
4420 Patient Contracting
2400 Patient Controlled Analgesia (PCA) Assistance
7460 Patient Rights Protection
°7700 Peer Review
°0560 Pelvic Floor Exercise
1750 Perineal Care
2660 Peripheral Sensation Management
4220 Peripherally Inserted Central (PIC) Catheter Care
2150 Peritoneal Dialysis Therapy
°4232 Phlebotomy: Arterial Blood Sample
°4234 Phlebotomy: Blood Unit Acquisition
°4238 Phlebotomy: Venous Blood Sample
°6924 Phototherapy: Neonate
6580 Physical Restraint
°7710 Physician Support
4430 Play Therapy
°6590 Pneumatic Tourniquet Precautions
0840 Positioning
°0842 Positioning: Intraoperative
0844 Positioning: Neurologic
0846 Positioning: Wheelchair
°2870 Postanesthesia Care
1770 Postmortem Care
6930 Postpartal Care
°7722 Preceptor: Employee
°7726 Preceptor: Student
°5247 Preconception Counseling
6950 Pregnancy Termination Care
6960 Prenatal Care
°2880 Preoperative Coordination
5580 Preparatory Sensory Information
5340 Presence
3500 Pressure Management
3520 Pressure Ulcer Care
3540 Pressure Ulcer Prevention
°7760 Product Evaluation
1460 Progressive Muscle Relaxation
1780 Prosthesis Care
°7800 Quality Monitoring
6600 Radiation Therapy Management
6300 Rape-Trauma Treatment
4820 Reality Orientation
5360 Recreation Therapy
°0490 Rectal Prolapse Management
8100 Referral
4860 Reminiscence Therapy

°7886 Reproductive Technology Management
°8120 Research Data Collection
3350 Respiratory Monitoring
7260 Respite Care
6320 Resuscitation
°6972 Resuscitation: Fetus
°6974 Resuscitation: Neonate
6610 Risk Identification
6612 Risk Identification: Childbearing Family
5370 Role Enhancement
6630 Seclusion
5380 Security Enhancement
2680 Seizure Management
2690 Seizure Precautions
5390 Self-Awareness Enhancement
1800 Self-Care Assistance
1801 Self-Care Assistance: Bathing/Hygiene
1802 Self-Care Assistance: Dressing/Grooming
1803 Self-Care Assistance: Feeding
1804 Self-Care Assistance: Toileting
5400 Self-Esteem Enhancement
4470 Self-Modification Assistance
4480 Self-Responsibility Facilitation
5248 Sexual Counseling
°8140 Shift Report
4250 Shock Management
4254 Shock Management: Cardiac
4256 Shock Management: Vasogenic
4258 Shock Management: Volume
4260 Shock Prevention
7280 Sibling Support
6000 Simple Guided Imagery
1480 Simple Massage
6040 Simple Relaxation Therapy
3584 Skin Care: Topical Treatments
3590 Skin Surveillance
1850 Sleep Enhancement
4490 Smoking Cessation Assistance
5100 Socialization Enhancement
7820 Specimen Management
5420 Spiritual Support
0910 Splinting
°7830 Staff Supervision
2720 Subarachnoid Hemorrhage Precautions
4500 Substance Use Prevention
4510 Substance Use Treatment
4512 Substance Use Treatment: Alcohol Withdrawal
4514 Substance Use Treatment: Drug Withdrawal
4516 Substance Use Treatment: Overdose
6340 Suicide Prevention
°7840 Supply Management

5430 Support Group
5440 Support System Enhancement
°2900 Surgical Assistance
°2920 Surgical Precautions
2930 Surgical Preparation
6650 Surveillance
°6656 Surveillance: Late Pregnancy
6654 Surveillance, Safety
7500 Sustenance Support
3620 Suturing
1860 Swallowing Therapy
5602 Teaching: Disease Process
5604 Teaching: Group
5606 Teaching: Individual
5608 Teaching: Infant Care
5610 Teaching: Preoperative
5612 Teaching: Prescribed Activity/Exercise
5614 Teaching: Prescribed Diet
5616 Teaching: Prescribed Medication
5618 Teaching: Procedure/Treatment
5620 Teaching: Psychomotor Skill
5622 Teaching: Safe Sex
°5624 Teaching: Sexuality
7880 Technology Management
°8180 Telephone Consultation
3900 Temperature Regulation
°2902 Temperature Regulation: Intraoperative
5465 Therapeutic Touch
5450 Therapy Group
1200 Total Parenteral Nutrition (TPN)
5460 Touch
0940 Traction/Immobilization Care

1540 Transcutaneous Electrical Nerve Stimulation (TENS)
0960 Transport
6360 Triage
5470 Truth Telling
1870 Tube Care
1872 Tube Care: Chest
1874 Tube Care: Gastrointestinal
°1875 Tube Care: Umbilical Line
1876 Tube Care: Urinary
1878 Tube Care: Ventriculostomy/Lumbar Drain
°6982 Ultrasonography: Limited Obstetric
°2760 Unilateral Neglect Management
°0570 Urinary Bladder Training
0580 Urinary Catheterization
0582 Urinary Catheterization: Intermittent
0590 Urinary Elimination Management
°0600 Urinary Habit Training
0610 Urinary Incontinence Care
°0612 Urinary Incontinence Care: Enuresis
0620 Urinary Retention Care
5480 Values Clarification
°2440 Venous Access Devices (VAD) Maintenance
3390 Ventilation Assistance
7560 Visitation Facilitation
6680 Vital Signs Monitoring
1240 Weight Gain Assistance
1260 Weight Management
1280 Weight Reduction Assistance
3660 Wound Care
3662 Wound Care: Closed Drainage
3680 Wound Irrigation

Assessment Guide for Adult Patient

General Information

Name   Address/Phone
Age
Allergies

Pattern Assessment

Assess not only complaints, limitations, and problems but also what is being done to alleviate the problem or problems, as well as positive health practices and current and previous coping skills and strengths.

Health-Perception—Health-Management Pattern

- Perception of own health state? Chief complaint?
- Previous illness or surgery?
- Past and current health-seeking behaviors?
- Resources for health maintenance?
- Current treatments? On any prescription medications?
- Adherence to therapeutic recommendations?
- Presence of risk factors for injury? Infection?
- Prevention practices?
- Health promotion practices?

Nutritional-Metabolic Pattern

- Appetite?
- Weight loss or gain?
- Nutritional status? Diet? Special diet?
- Fluid intake?
- Drug and alcohol consumption?
- Ability to swallow?
- Breastfeeding (if applicable)?
- Skin, tissue, or mucous membrane integrity (including oral cavity)?

By Gertrude K. McFarland, DNSc, RN, FAAN.

- Dentures?
- Body temperature?

Elimination Pattern

- Bowel elimination? Bowel habits?
- Urinary elimination habits and patterns?
- Urinary incontinence?

Activity-Exercise Pattern

- Physical mobility?
- Range of motion?
- Fatigue level?
- Self-care ability?
- Growth and development (in relation to age group norms)?
- Recreation and leisure activities?
- Home maintenance?
- Respirations?
- Shortness of breath?
- Coughing?
- Cyanosis?
- Breath sounds?
- Pulse (rate? rhythm? peripheral pulses?)
- Blood pressure?
- Edema?
- Extremities (cold? cyanosis?)
- Changes in mental status?

Sleep-Rest Pattern

- Sleep habits? Feel rested?
- Rest habits?
- Problem?
- Methods to promote sleep and relaxation?

Cognitive-Perceptual Pattern

- Level of consciousness?
- Speech? Pupils? Eyes?
- Ability to see, feel, taste, touch, and smell?

- Special aids?
- Pain? Discomfort? How are these managed?
- Hallucinations? Delusions?
- Awareness of both sides of body?
- Health care self-management knowledge?
- Mental status?
- Memory?
- Judgment?
- Ability to concentrate?
- Decision-making ability?
- Education?

Self-Perception—Self-Concept Pattern

- Any perceived threat or danger?
- Apprehension? Tension?
- Restlessness?
- Mood change? Depressed? Anxious?
- Ability to mobilize energy on own behalf? Passivity?
- Perceived control over situations?
- Perception and feelings about self? Self-worth?
- Body image? Personal identity?
- Risk factors for self-mutilation?

Role-Relationship Pattern

- Significant loss? Grieving?
- Ability to perform roles? Occupation? Employment?
- Marital status?
- Interpersonal interactions?
- Significant others? Social support network? Any interpersonal difficulties? Any caregiver difficulties?
- Family structure and system? Any difficulties?
- Attitude of family and significant others toward illness?
- Parenting practices and problems?
- Communication skills?
- Risk factors for self-harm?
- Risk factors for other-directed physical injury (if relevant)?

Sexuality-Reproductive Pattern

- Sexuality patterns? Satisfaction? Dysfunctions?
- Contraceptives (use or problems)?
- Menstrual history?
- History of sexual abuse?

Coping—Stress-Tolerance Pattern

- Current stressors? Life challenges?
- Recent major life changes? Recent relocation?
- Emotional state?
- Response and adjustment to trauma?
- Methods to deal with stressors?
- Degree and quality of family support available?
- Potential for family growth during stress?

Value-Belief Pattern

- Overall life beliefs and values?
- Religious affiliation and importance of religion?
- Religious practices? Which ones are desired while in hospital?
- Desire for chaplain visit?

Discharge Planning

- Projected date of discharge?
- Health care system resources?
- Community resources?
- Social network resources (family, friends, neighbors)?
- Assistance needed?
- Health care teaching needed?

REFERENCES

1. Gordon M: *Nursing diagnoses: process and application,* ed 3, St. Louis, 1994, Mosby–Year Book.
2. McFarland GK, Wasli E, and Gerety EK: *Nursing diagnoses and process in psychiatric mental health nursing,* Philadelphia,1992, JB Lippincott Co.

NANDA Diagnoses Received for Review and Developmental Staging

1.0 Received for development (consultation from DRC)
1.1 Label only
Alteration in Preservation/Quality of Life
Cardiac Rhythm, Potential for Alteration in (High Risk)
Cardiac Rhythm, Alteration in Dyspnea
High Risk for Impaired Skin Integrity: Pressure Ulcer
Impaired Alcohol Drinking Patterns (Dysfunctional)
Idiopathic Fecal Incontinence
Self-Care Deficit: Medication Administration
Spasticity
Urinary Filtration, Impaired

NANDA has accepted the following labels as a group for development from the ANA Psychiatric Mental Health Nursing Group:

Motor Behavior, Disorganized
Catatonia
Hyperactivity
Hypoactivity
Motor Behavior, Bizarre
Psychomotor Agitation
Psychomotor Retardation
Recreation, Age-Inappropriate
Recreation, Antisocial
Recreation, Bizarre
Restlessness
Self-Care, Potential for Alteration
Altered Eating:
    Binge-Purge Syndrome

From North American Nursing Diagnosis Association: *NANDA nursing diagnoses: definitions and classification, 1995–1996,* Philadelphia, 1994, The Association.

Nonnutritive Ingestion
Pica
Unusual Food Ingestion
Refusal to Eat
Rumination
Sleep/Arousal Patterns, Potential for Alteration
Altered Sleep/Arousal Pattern:
    Decreased Need for Sleep
    Hypersomnia
    Insomnia
    Nightmares/Terrors
    Somnolence
    Somnambulism
Decision Making, Potential for Alteration
Decision Making, Altered
Judgment, Potential for Alteration
Judgment, Altered
Knowledge, Potential for Alteration
Altered Knowledge Processes:
    Agnosia
    Intellectual Functioning, Altered
Learning, Potential for Alteration
Learning Processes, Altered
Memory, Potential for Alteration
Altered Memory:
    Amnesia
    Distorted Memory
    Long-Term Memory Loss
    Memory Deficit
    Memory Loss, Short-Term
Altered Thought Processes:
    Abstract Thinking, Altered
    Concentration, Altered
    Problem Solving, Altered
    Confusion Disorientation
    Delirium
    Delusions
    Ideas of Reference

Magical Thinking
Obsessions
Suspiciousness
Thought Insertion
Community Maintenance: Potential for Alteration
Altered Community Maintenance:
    Community Safety Hazards
    Community Sanitation Hazards
Environmental Integrity, Potential for Alteration
Environmental Integrity, Altered
Home Maintenance, Potential for Alteration
Altered Home Maintenance:
    Home Safety Hazards
    Home Sanitation Hazards
Feeling States, Potential for Alteration
Altered Feeling States:
    Anger
    Elation
    Envy
    Grief
    Guilt
    Sadness
    Shame
Affect Incongruous in Situation
Flat Affect
Feeling Processes: Potential for Alteration
Altered Feeling Processes:
    Lability
    Mood Swings
Abuse Response Patterns, Potential for Alteration
Communication Processes, Potential for Alteration
Nonverbal Communication, Altered
Altered Verbal Communications:
    Aphasia
    Bizarre Content
    Confabulation
    Ecolalia
    Incoherent
    Mute
    Neologisms
    Nonsense Word Salad
    Stuttering
Conduct/Impulse Processes, Potential for Alteration
Suicidal Ideation
Altered Conduct/Impulse Processes:
    Accident-Prone
    Aggressive Violent Behavior Toward Environment

Delinquency
Lying
Physical Aggression Toward Others
Physical Aggression Toward Self:
    Suicide Attempts
    Promiscuity
    Substance Abuse
    Truancy
    Vandalism
    Verbal Aggression Toward Others
Role Performance, Potential for Alteration
Parental Role Deficit
Play Role, Altered
Student Role, Altered
Work Role, Altered
Sexuality, Potential for Alteration
Sexual Behavior Leading to Intercourse, Altered
Sexual Conception Actions, Altered
Sexual Development, Altered
Sexual Intercourse, Altered
Sexual Relationships, Altered
Variation of Sexual Expressions, Altered
Social Interaction, Potential for Alteration
Altered Social Interaction:
    Bizarre Behaviors
    Compulsive Behaviors
    Disorganized Social Behaviors
    Social Intrusiveness
    Social Isolation? Withdrawal (Note: Social Isolation occurs on prior NANDA lists; this is included here for sake of clarity. It may represent indications for review and/or revision of the present nursing diagnosis.)
    Unpredictable Behaviors
Attention: Potential for Alteration
Altered Attention:
    Hyperalertness
    Inattention
    Selective Attention
Altered Comfort Pattern:
    Discomfort
    Distress
Self-Concept, Potential for Alteration
Sexual Identity, Altered
Gender Identity, Altered
Self-Concept, Undeveloped
Sensory Perceptions, Potential for Alteration
Auditory Hallucinations
Gustatory Hallucinations

Kinesthetic Hallucinations
Olfactory Hallucinations
Tactile Hallucinations
Visual Hallucinations
Illusions
Circulation, Potential for Alteration
Elimination, Potential for Alteration
Encopresis
Skin Elimination, Altered
Endocrine/Metabolic Processes: Potential for
   Alteration
Hormone Regulation, Altered
Premenstrual Stress Syndrome, Altered
Gastrointestinal Processes: Potential for Alteration
Absorption, Altered
Digestion, Altered
Musculoskeletal Processes: Potential for Alteration
Coordination, Altered
Equilibrium, Altered
Mobility, Altered
Motor Planning, Altered
Muscle Strength, Altered
Posture, Altered
Range of Motion, Altered
Reflex Patterns, Altered
Muscle Twitching
Equilibrium, Altered
Neuro/Sensory Processes: Potential for Alteration
Level of Consciousness, Altered
Auditory Sensory Acuity, Altered
Gustatory Sensory Acuity, Altered
Olfactory Sensory Acuity, Altered
Tactile Sensory Acuity, Altered
Visual Sensory Acuity, Altered
Seizures
Anorexia
Oxygenation: Potential for Alteration
Physical Regulation Processes: Potential for Alter-
   ation
Altered Immune Response
Meaningfulness: Potential for Alteration
Helplessness
Loneliness
Spirituality, Potential for Alteration
Spritual Despair
Values, Potential for Alteration
Altered Values:
   Conflict with Social Order
   Inability to Internalize Values

Unclear Values
1.2   Label and Definition Only
Activity Level, Excessive
Decisional Conflict, Family: Required
Feeding Drive, Impaired
Terminal Illness Reponse
1.3   Label and Defining Characteristics or Risk Fac-
      tors Only
1.4   Label, Definition, and Defining Characteristics or
      Risk Factors Present
Acute Confusion
Altered Family Processes: Alcoholism
Chronic Confusion
Decreased Adaptive Capacity: Intracranial
Disorganized Behavior: Infant
Effective Management of Therapeutic Regimen:
   Individual
Energy Field Disturbance
High Risk for Positioning Perioperative Injury
Impaired Environmental Interpretation Syndrome
Ineffective Coping: Community
Ineffective Management of Therapeutic Regimen:
   Communities
Ineffective Management of Therapeutic Regimen:
   Families
Loneliness, High Risk for
Memory, Impaired
Potential for Enhanced Organized Infant Behavior
Potential for Enhanced Coping: Communities
Risk for Altered Parent/Infant/Child Attachment
Risk for Disorganized Behavior: Infant
Spiritual Well-Being, Potential for Enhanced
2.0   Accepted for Clinical Development:
      Authentication/Substantiation
2.1   Label, Definition, Defining Characteristics, or
      Risk Factors and Literature
         Review Present
2.2   Case Study
2.3   Clinical Studies
3.0   Clinically Supported: Validation and Testing
3.1   °
3.2   °
3.3   °
4.0   Revision: Refinement
4.1   °
4.2   °
4.3   °

_____

°Criteria under development.

Index

▶

A

Abdominal angina, 435
Abdominal muscles
  in diaphragmatic breathing, 317
  exercises to strengthen bladder support, 280
Abdominal surgery, postoperative complications of, 423
Abdominal X-ray exam, 253
Abdominoperineal resection, 273
Acceptance, in grieving process, 680
Accessory muscles of respiration, 311–312, 427
Accidents; *see* Injury
Acculturation stress, 720, 722
Acetaminophen, antidiuretic hormone levels altered by, 179
Achondroplasia, growth and development in, 363
Acidosis, 424
Acquired immunodeficiency syndrome; *see* AIDS
Activities of daily living; *see also* Self-Care
  aging effects on, 409
  assessment of functional ADL status, 410–411
  cognitive impairment and, 480–485, 497–501
  complications of immobility/inactivity and, 336
  definition of, 409
  developmentally disabled and, 370
  energy for
    conservation regimens to improve, 358
    insufficient to complete, 296–297, 299–300
  factors influencing individual's approach to, 409
  limitations on
    incidence of, 409
    psychological effects of sudden, 296–297
  motor skills basic to, 411
  related to Unilateral Neglect, 543–550
Activity
  definition of, 296
  lack of leisure; *see* Diversional Activity Deficit
Activity Intolerance, 296–306
  assessment of, 297–300
    related factors in, 300
    usual lifestyle patterns, 297–298
  case study of, 304–305
  causes of, 296–297
  defining characteristics of, 299–300
  differential nursing diagnosis of, 300
  evaluation in, 304
  functional limitations leading to, 299–300
  medical/psychiatric diagnoses related to, 300
  nursing care guidelines for, 302–303

Activity Intolerance—cont'd
  outcomes expected for, 300–304
  overview of, 296–297
  planning and implementation in, 300–304
  related to Constipation, 254
  related to Risk for Disuse Syndrome, 300
  related to Sleep Pattern Disturbance, 457
  related to Stress Incontinence, 275
  sedentary lifestyle contributing to, 299
  situational limitations leading to, 299–300
  structural limitations leading to, 299–300
  versus Fatigue, 357
Activity Intolerance, Risk for
  assessment of, 297–298
  differential nursing diagnosis of, 300
  evaluation in, 304
  medical/psychiatric diagnoses related to, 300
  planning and implementation in, 300–301
  related to Risk for Disuse Syndrome, 334
Activity-Exercise Pattern
  assessment in, 15
  guidelines for assessing usual, 297–298
  human need for, 296
  nursing diagnoses in
    Activity Intolerance, 296–306
    Altered Growth and Development, 361–374
    Altered Tissue Perfusion, 421–440
    Decreased Cardiac Output, 322–331
    Disorganized Infant Behavior, 385–394
    Diversional Activity Deficit, 341–348
    Dysfunctional Ventilatory Weaning Response, 441–452
    Dysreflexia, 349–354
    Fatigue, 355–360
    Impaired Gas Exchange, 307–321
    Impaired Home Maintenance Management, 375–384
    Impaired Physical Mobility, 395–399
    Inability to Sustain Spontaneous Ventilation, 441–452
    Ineffective Airway Clearance, 307–321
    Ineffective Breathing Pattern, 307–321
    Potential for Enhanced Organized Infant Behavior, 385–394
    Risk for Activity Intolerance, 296–306
    Risk for Disorganized Infant Behavior, 385–394
    Risk for Disuse Syndrome, 332–340
    Risk for Peripheral Neurovascular Dysfunction, 400–407
    Self-Care Deficit, 408–420
  psychological effects of sudden limits on, 296

Brain injury
  causing Unilateral Neglect, 543–550
  in children, 464
  impaired swallowing in, 231
  increased intracranial pressure in, 463–470
Brazelton Neonatal Behavioral Assessment Scale, 365
Breast milk
  advantages of, 154, 160
  colostrum, 159, 160
  composition of, 150, 156, 160
  digestion of, 150
  expression of, 150, 155, 156, 159, 162
  foremilk, 156
  hind, 150, 156
  HIV and, 152
  immunological advantages of, 151, 159, 160
  iron content of, 160
  mature milk, 160
  medications and, 168–169
  neonatal jaundice and, 151, 169–170
  production of, 155, 156
  pumping; *see* Breast milk pumping
  storing of, 167, 173, 174–175
  substitutes for, 156
  supply of, 156, 171, 174
  transitional milk, 159–160
  types of, 159
Breast milk pumping
  breast shields and, 154
  during maternal illness, 164, 169
  techniques for, 171–174
Breastfeeding
  advantages of, 154, 160
  assessment tools for, 152
  breast cancer and, 152, 153, 162
  decision to, 160
  effective; *see* Breastfeeding, Effective
  engorgement, 170, 171, 172
  frequency of, 150, 155, 156
  ineffective; *see* Breastfeeding, Ineffective
  infections and, 168
  interruption of; *see* Breastfeeding, Interrupted
  jaundice and, 151, 169–170
  maternal medications and, 151, 168–169
  medical conditions interfering with, 152, 153, 161
  neonatal conditions that may interrupt, 169
  nutritional needs of infant, 160
  nutritional needs of mother, 163, 164
  prior experiences with, 151–152, 161
  psychological attachment and, 160
  reasons for discontinuing, 149
  supplemental feedings and, 152, 155, 156
  switch feeding, 154, 155, 156
  techniques recommended for, 154, 156, 163, 164
  weaning, 160
Breastfeeding, Effective, 159–166
  assessment of, 161–162
  case study of, 164–165
  defining characteristics of, 161–162
  differential nursing diagnosis of, 162

Breastfeeding, Effective—cont'd
  evaluation in, 164–165
  medical/psychiatric diagnoses related to, 162
  nursing care guidelines for, 163
  overview of, 159–161
  planning and implementation in, 162–164
  related factors in, 162
  versus Ineffective Breastfeeding, 162
Breastfeeding, Ineffective, 149–158
  assessment of, 149–153
  case study of, 157
  defining characteristics of, 153
  differential nursing diagnosis of, 153
  evaluation in, 156
  medical/psychiatric diagnoses related to, 153
  nursing care guidelines for, 155
  outcomes expected for, 153–156
  overview of, 149
  planning and implementation in, 153–156
  related factors in, 153
  versus Ineffective Infant Feeding Pattern, 153, 193
Breastfeeding, Interrupted, 167–177
  assessment of, 167–170
  case study of (related to prematurity), 175–176
  conditions that may lead to, 167–170
  defining characteristics of, 170
  differential nursing diagnosis of, 170–171
  evaluation in, 175
  medical/psychiatric diagnoses related to, 171
  nursing care guidelines for, 172–174
  overview of, 167
  planning and implementation in, 171–176
  reasons for, 151
  related factors in, 170
  versus Ineffective Breastfeeding, 170–171
  versus Ineffective Infant Feeding Pattern, 171
Breasts
  biopsy, breastfeeding and, 168
  cancer of, breastfeeding and, 152, 153, 162
  changes in with pregnancy, 161
  fibrocystic disease of, 161
  mastitis, 151, 161
  surgery, breastfeeding and, 151, 168
Breath sounds, 309, 315, 325
  in impaired tissue perfusion, 424, 425, 426
Breathing
  control center for, 308, 425
  diaphragmatic, 317
  paradoxical, 311
  postoperative abnormalities in, positioning injury and, 68
  respiratory alternans pattern of, 427
  retraining, 316–317
  work of, 309, 441–443
Breathing Pattern, Ineffective, 307–321
  assessment of, 310–312
  in asthma patient, 311
  causes of, 310–311
  in COPD patient, 311–312
  defining characteristics of, 312